THE ROUTLEDGE HANDBOOK OF PALEOPATHOLOGY

The Routledge Handbook of Paleopathology provides readers with an overview of the study of ancient disease.

The volume begins by exploring current methods and techniques employed by paleopathologists as means to highlight the range of data that can be generated, the types of questions that can be methodologically addressed, our current limitations, and goals for the future. Building on these foundations, the volume introduces a range of diseases and conditions that have been noted in the fossil, archaeological, and historical record, offering readers a foundational understanding of pathological conditions, along with their potential etiologies. Importantly, an evolutionary and highly contextualized assessment of diseases and conditions will be presented in order to demonstrate the need for adopting anthropological, biological, and clinical approaches when exploring the past and interpreting the modern world. The volume concludes with the contextualization of paleopathological research. Chapters highlight ways in which analyses of health and disease in skeletal and mummified remains reflect political and social constructs of the past and present. Health and disease are tackled within evolutionary perspectives across deep time and generationally, and the nuanced interplay between disease and behavior is explored.

The volume will be indispensable for archaeologists, bioarchaeologists, and historians, and those in medical fields, as it reflects current scholarship within paleopathology and the field's impact on our understanding of health and disease in the past, the present, and implications for our future.

Anne L. Grauer, PhD, is a Professor in the Department of Anthropology at Loyola University Chicago, USA.

THE ROUTLEDGE HANDBOOK OF PALEOPATHOLOGY

Edited by Anne L. Grauer

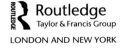

LONDON AND NEW YORK

cover image: © Getty Images

First published 2023
by Routledge
4 Park Square, Milton Park, Abingdon, Oxon OX14 4RN

and by Routledge
605 Third Avenue, New York, NY 10158

Routledge is an imprint of the Taylor & Francis Group, an informa business

© 2023 selection and editorial matter, Anne L. Grauer; individual chapters, the contributors

The right of Anne L. Grauer to be identified as the author of the editorial material, and of the authors for their individual chapters, has been asserted in accordance with sections 77 and 78 of the Copyright, Designs and Patents Act 1988.

All rights reserved. No part of this book may be reprinted or reproduced or utilised in any form or by any electronic, mechanical, or other means, now known or hereafter invented, including photocopying and recording, or in any information storage or retrieval system, without permission in writing from the publishers.

Trademark notice: Product or corporate names may be trademarks or registered trademarks, and are used only for identification and explanation without intent to infringe.

British Library Cataloguing-in-Publication Data
A catalogue record for this book is available from the British Library

ISBN: 978-0-367-64067-5 (hbk)
ISBN: 978-0-367-67358-1 (pbk)
ISBN: 978-1-003-13099-4 (ebk)

DOI: 10.4324/9781003130994

Typeset in Bembo
by codeMantra

To my family for their love, support, and good humor.
And to all the makers of gin.

CONTENTS

List of Figures   *xi*
List of Boxes and Tables   *xiii*
List of Contributors   *xv*
Foreword   *xxx*
Acknowledgments   *xxxvi*

1. Introduction   1
   Anne L. Grauer

PART I
Applications, Methods, and Techniques in Paleopathology   **17**

2. The Macroscopic Study of Human Skeletal Paleopathology   19
   Simon Mays

3. Differential Diagnosis and Rigor in Paleopathology   43
   Jo Appleby

4. Epidemiology and Mathematical Modeling   64
   Samantha L. Yaussy

5. Paleohistopathology: History, Technical Aspects, and Diagnostic Challenges   82
   Sandra Assis and Hans H. de Boer

6. Paleoradiology   105
   Chiara Villa and Marie Louise Jørkov

7	Isotopes in Paleopathology *Chris Stantis and Ellen J. Kendall*	118
8	Genetics and Genomics *Susanna Sabin and Anne C. Stone*	136
9	Parasitology and Paleopathology *Aida R. Barbera, Morgana Camacho and Karl Reinhard*	158
10	Historical Sources, Historiography, and Paleopathology *Piers D. Mitchell*	180
11	Osteobiography and Case Studies *Alexis T. Boutin*	192
12	Mummified Remains *Ken Nystrom, Dario Piombino-Mascali, Jane E. Buikstra and Lucía Watson Jiménez*	210

PART II
Investigating Diseases and Conditions of the Past — 229

13	"Sticks and Stones May Break My Bones": Traumatic Injuries in Paleopathology *Jennifer F. Byrnes and Katherine Gaddis*	231
14	Developmental Conditions in Paleopathology *Anne R. Titelbaum, Scott E. Burnett and D. Troy Case*	250
15	Tumors and Neoplastic Diseases: Assessing Antiquity and Pondering Prevalence *Casey L. Kirkpatrick*	271
16	Treponemal Infection *Brenda J. Baker*	292
17	Here and Now, There and Then: Two Mycobacterial Diseases Still with Us Today *Charlotte A. Roberts, Kelly E. Blevins, Kori Lea Filipek and Aryel Pacheco Miranda*	306
18	Paleopathology of Infectious Diseases *Olivier Dutour*	324

19	Metabolic and Endocrine Diseases *Megan B. Brickley and Brianne Morgan*	338
20	Dental Disease *Jaime Ullinger and Tisa Loewen*	360

PART III
Theoretical Approaches and New Directions — 379

21	Ethical Considerations for Paleopathology *Carlina de la Cova*	381
22	Synthesizing Stress in Paleopathological Perspective: Theory, Method, Application *Daniel H. Temple and Haagen D. Klaus*	397
23	Theoretical Approaches to the Paleopathology of Infants, Children, and Adolescents: Structural Violence as a Holistic Interpretive Tool in Paleopathology *Siân E. Halcrow and Gwen Robbins Schug*	417
24	Issues of Gender, Identity, and Agency in Paleopathology *Pamela K. Stone and Adam Netzer Zimmer*	435
25	Disability and Care in the Bioarchaeological Record: Meeting the Challenges of Being Human *Lorna Tilley*	457
26	Defining the Margins, Embodying the Consequences *Madeleine Mant and Lauren September Poeta*	482
27	Interpreting Trauma and Social Violence from Skeletal Remains *Debra L. Martin, Aurora Marcela Pérez-Flórez, Claira Ralston and Ryan P. Harrod*	502
28	The Developmental Origins of Health and Disease: Implications for Paleopathology *Rebecca Gowland and Jennifer L. Caldwell*	520
29	Disease in the Fossil Record *Florian Witzmann and Patrick Asbach*	541
30	Zooarchaeology and the Paleopathological Record *László Bartosiewicz and Khashaiar Mansouri*	557

31	Plagues and Pandemics *Sharon N. DeWitte, Ziyu R. Wang and Saige Kelmelis*	576
32	Public Perceptions of Paleopathology and the Future of Outreach *Kristina Killgrove and Jane E. Buikstra*	593
33	Big Pictures in 21st-Century Paleopathology: Interdisciplinarity and Transdisciplinarity *Jane E. Buikstra, Elizabeth W. Uhl and Amanda Wissler*	625

Index   *637*

FIGURES

2.1	Numbers of publications in the bibliometric study mainly or solely directed at paleopathology using macroscopy as the sole means of studying skeletal lesions versus those that supplement macroscopy with medical imaging alone, microscopy alone or both medical imaging and microscopy.	22
2.2	Macroscopic appearance of taphonomic damage versus lytic in vivo lesions in various states of remodeling.	28
3.1	Mentions of differential diagnosis in the American Journal of Physical Anthropology (AJPA), *International Journal of Osteoarchaeology* (IJO), and *International Journal of Paleopathology* (IJPP) from the 1960s to 2020.	44
4.1	The multistate model of morbidity and mortality described by Usher (2000) and further applied by DeWitte and Wood (2008).	72
6.1	Healed malaligned fracture of a right tibia (a) photograph; (b) radiograph; (c) coronal CT scan.	109
6.2	Mandible with pronounced destruction due to treponemal disease (syphilis): (a) photograph; (b) radiograph; (c) axial CT scan; (d) coronal CT scan.	110
6.3	A right humerus showing sign of osteoarthritis on the head: (a) photograph; (b) lateral X-ray; (c) coronal CT scan; (d) axial CT scan; (e) sagittal CT scan.	111
6.4	A right femur showing signs of osteomyelitis at the distal end due to a fracture: (a) photograph frontal view; (b) photograph posterior view; (c) X-ray; (d–f) coronal CT scans.	111
7.1	Carbon ($\delta^{13}C$) and nitrogen ($\delta^{15}N$) stable isotope incremental dentine collagen data for an adolescent with tuberculosis, showing the onset of wasting from around seven years of age.	125
8.1	Decision tree for incorporating an ancient DNA component into a project.	143
9.1	The Pathoecology Lab at the School of Natural Resources.	160
13.1	Illustrations of fracture types. (A) Transverse fracture; (B) Spiral fracture; (C) Comminuted fracture; (D) Impacted fracture; (E) Greenstick fracture; and (F) Oblique fracture.	235

Figures

13.2	Illustration of fracture healing process. (a) Hematoma formation; (b) Soft callus formation; (c) Hard callus formation; (d) Remodeling of hard callus.	239
14.1	Osteogenesis imperfecta in a 20th c. young adult female.	253
14.2	Anomalies of the foot.	257
14.3	Developmental anomalies of the axial skeleton.	258
18.1	Comparison of age distribution of acute osteomyelitis at the end of the 19th century (Lannelongue, 1879) and at the mid-20th century (Trueta, 1959).	330
18.2	Paleopathological cases of chronic osteomyelitis: (a) Right tibia, showing the involucrum and the cloacal opening; (b) Diaphysis of femur displaying bifocal osteomyelitis; (c) Complete sclerosis of the medullar canal characteristic of Garré's sclerosing osteomyelitis.	332
18.3	Three paleopathological examples of joint fusion due to infectious arthritis: (a) left ulna; (b) right humerus, radius, and ulna fused at elbow joint; (c) left femur fused to os coxae.	334
19.1	Generic bone with varying cortical thicknesses illustrating basic principles underlying lesion formation occurring in the four basic biological mechanisms that results in porotic lesions.	348
19.2	Porotic lesions of the orbit Individual SMB217 (1.3 years), St. Martin's UK	350
19.3	Systemic evaluation and interpretation of porotic lesions.	353
20.1	Illustration of (a) dental caries, (b) dental calculus, (c) periapical lesions, and (d) AMTL.	362
20.2	Illustration of abfraction.	367
20.3	Illustration of irritation of dentinal tubules that can lead to dental sensitivity and dental hypersensitivity.	367
22.1	Commonly used phenotypic alterations associated with stress experience in paleopathology.	398
22.2	Scurvy is an increasingly scrutinized indicator of preadult biological stress in paleopathology. A chronic insufficiency of vitamin C leads to production of subperiosteal hemorrhages and osseous responses to inflammation in multiple anatomic sites.	403
22.3	Enamel surface and perikymata spacing profile of a right mandibular second incisor for individual 194 from the Takasago site, Hokkaido, Japan.	405
22.4	Enamel cross-striations each representing approximately one day of growth.	405
25.1	Examples of BoC application – Man Bac Burial 9 and the Nasca Boy.	467
29.1	Examples of pathological lesions in the fossil record.	545
29.2	Fossil evidence of Paget's Disease of Bone.	551
30.1	Parodontal disease in sheep. 1: Neolithic Endrőd 23B, Hungary; 2: Neolithic Tell Karanovo, Bulgaria; 3: Chalcolithic Horum Höyük, Anatolia/Turkey; 4: Chalcolithic Polyanitsa, Bulgaria.	562
30.2	The distribution of pathological lesions by body region in domestic animals.	564
30.3	Healed fracture of a horse left third metacarpal showing slight dislocation and shortening (Early Iron Age Stična, Slovenia).	567
30.4	The number of bilateral zoonoses shared by humans and various animals as a function of the time since domestication.	568

BOXES AND TABLES

Boxes

8.1	Glossary of Terms	136
8.2	Ethical Checkpoint: Data Management	140
8.3	Ethical Checkpoint: Initiating a Genomics Project	142
8.4	Ethical Checkpoint: Data Mining	146
16.1	Current Issues in the Paleopathological Diagnosis of Treponemal Disease	294

Tables

2.1	Numbers of publications (2011–2019) devoted specifically to paleopathology that are reliant upon macroscopy alone, split by focus on different classes of pathology	22
2.2	A dual process model of paleopathological diagnosis	25
2.3	Some kappa values reported for recording of macroscopic lesions in paleopathology	34
3.1	Approaches to diagnosis in paleopathology	46
3.2	Sources of information for generating and refining differential diagnosis	50
3.3	Updated modified Istanbul Terminological Protocol and suggested abbreviations for use in tables of diagnostic criteria	53
3.4	Factors potentially affecting lesion severity, morphology, and distribution in the skeleton	54
3.5	Criteria for indicating certainty in overall diagnosis alongside suggested abbreviations	57
3.6	Factors affecting disease likelihood	57
4.1	Maximum likelihood estimates of k_2 with nominal standard error (SE) and likelihood ratio tests of the hypothesis that $k_2 = 1$ (i.e., no selectivity), in the study of Black Death mortality applying the multistate model produced by Usher (2000)	74
5.1	The hierarchical organization of bone	89

9.1	Selected helminths of humans and their archaeological recovery potential	168
13.1	Summary of characteristics of fracture mechanisms and fracture timing	237
14.1	Terms used in the paleopathological literature to describe variations of skeletal morphology	250
15.1	Types of neoplastic diseases that can affect the skeleton	274
18.1	Physiopathogeny of common specific and non-specific infection observed in skeletal paleopathology	327
18.2	Comparison of percentage skeletal distribution of hematogenous osteomyelitis on two clinical series observed in 1879 and in 2010	330
19.1	Typical sites for hemorrhagic lesions in scurvy	340
19.2	Key lesions of impaired mineralization: Rickets and Osteomalacia	342
19.3	Lesions in anemia	344
24.1	Common biological characteristics used in defining a bimorphic model of sex in humans	437
25.1	'Constants of care'	464
25.2	The four stages of the bioarchaeology of care	466
25.3	Summaries of selected bioarchaeology of care case studies	468
30.1	Frequencies of periodontal disease among caprines in 36 zooarchaeological assemblages from Europe and Southwest Asia Incidence is significantly ($p=0.000$) higher in assemblages from Europe	563
32.1	Most engaging peer-reviewed articles in the *International Journal of Paleopathology* (as of 27 December 2021) and their category codes	595
32.2	Paleopathology press releases in *Science Daily* from January–December 2021	597
32.3	Characteristics of paleopathology articles in *Forbes* (2015–2020)	601
32.4	Pearson correlation of word frequency with popularity of *Forbes* articles	612
32.5	Frame matrix for *Forbes* articles related to violence	614

CONTRIBUTORS

Jo Appleby, PhD, is currently an Associate Professor in the School of Archaeology and Ancient History at the University of Leicester, UK. Her research interests include human ageing, the archaeology and anthropology of cremation, the association between mortuary practices and taphonomy, and the British and European Bronze Age.

Patrick Asbach, MD, is currently a Professor of Radiology at the Charité – Universitätsmedizin Berlin, Germany. His medical clinical area of expertise is musculoskeletal and abdominal magnetic resonance imaging. His research interests include paleopathology with focus on disease of the spine. His clinical research emphasis is imaging of the extracellular matrix in liver diseases. He serves as Editor of the *European Journal of Radiology*. His publications include books on urogenital and rectal cancer imaging and numerous journal articles and book chapters.

Sandra Assis, PhD, is a Researcher at the CRIA – Centre for Research in Anthropology (FCSH, NOVA University, Lisbon), Portugal. She holds a Master's degree in Human Evolution and a PhD in Biological Anthropology from the University of Coimbra, Portugal. Her research interests include the study and diagnosis of infectious diseases and trauma, with particular emphasis on the application of histological methods. She is the author of numerous research papers on the field of paleopathology. Key publications include articles in the *Journal of Anatomy*, the *American Journal of Physical Anthropology*, *Microscopy and Microanalysis*, *Pathobiology*, and the *International Journal of Paleopathology*.

Brenda J. Baker, PhD, is an Associate Professor of Anthropology and Curator of Nubian Collections in the Center for Bioarchaeological Research, School of Human Evolution and Social Change, at Arizona State University. She is also the Director of the ASU Bioarchaeology of Nubia Expedition (BONE). Her research integrates archaeology and biological anthropology to investigate the lifeways of past people, particularly in Cyprus, the Nile Valley, and the USA. Her interest in paleopathology and fascination with treponemal disease began as an undergraduate. She is founding co-editor-in-chief of *Bioarchaeology International* and has served as an Associate Editor for *International Journal of Paleopathology* and currently for the *Journal of Human Evolution*. Her publications include *The Osteology of Infants and Children*

(Texas A&M University Press) and two edited volume, *Migration and Disruptions: Toward a Unifying Theory of Ancient and Contemporary Migrations* and *Bioarchaeology of Native American Adaptation in the Spanish Borderlands* (both from University Press of Florida), as well as numerous journal articles and book chapters.

Aida R. Barbera is a PhD student at the CELAT research center and the Biomolecular Laboratory at Université Laval in Québec, Canada. Her research focuses on the relationship between foodways, sanitation, and parasitic infectious diseases in historic urban centers in Northeast North America using archaeoparasitological approaches. She is also interested in using bioarchaeology, as well as botanical and palynological techniques, to gain a better understanding of cultural changes, health, and human adaptations. She received her MSc in Osteoarchaeology at The University of Edinburgh, Scotland. Her publications include "Attempting to simplify methods in parasitology of archaeological sediments: An examination of taphonomic aspects" in the *Journal of Archaeological Sciences: Reports* (2020).

László Bartosiewicz, PhD, serves as a Professor Emeritus of the Osteoarchaeological Research Laboratory at Stockholm University, Sweden. His research has focused on animal-human relationships throughout human history, based on the study of animal remains from archaeological sites of various periods in Europe, Southwest Asia, and South America. He was elected president of the International Council for Archaeozoology between 2006–2010 and 2010–2014. In addition to numerous journal articles, he is author of the books *Animals in the Urban Landscape in the Wake of the Middle Ages* (Tempus Reparatum), and *Shuffling Nags, Lame Ducks: The Archaeology of Animal Disease* (Oxbow Books), and senior author of the monograph *Draught Cattle: Their Osteological Identification and History* (Koninklijk Museum voor Midden-Afrika) and co-editor of several volumes on the topic of archaeozoology.

Kelly E. Blevins, PhD, is currently a Postdoctoral Research Associate in the Department of Archaeology at Durham University, UK. She specializes in human paleopathology and bioarchaeological applications of ancient DNA (aDNA). Her research interests include genomic evolution and paleoepidemiology of mycobacterial pathogens that cause tuberculosis and leprosy, as inferred through the recovery and analysis of their ancient and modern genomes. Her publications include book chapters and journal articles on pathogen phylogenomics including ("Evolutionary history of Mycobacterium leprae in the Pacific Islands", *Philosophical Transactions of the Royal Society B*) and the value and ethics of aDNA in bioarchaeological research ("Paleogenómica y bioarqueología en México" – *Cuicuilco Revista de Ciencias Antropológicas*). Her research has been funded by a Fulbright-García Robles fellowship in Mexico City, Mexico and a National Science Foundation Doctoral Dissertation Research Improvement Grant.

Hans H. de Boer, MD, PhD, is a full-time forensic pathologist at the Victorian Institute of Forensic Medicine and faculty member of the Department of Forensic Science of Monash University, both in Melbourne, Australia. He publishes regularly on subjects within forensic pathology, forensic anthropology, disaster victim identification, and paleopathology. He currently sits on the advisory board of the *International Journal of Legal Medicine* and the advisory board of the Forensic Anthropology Society Europe (FASE). He is also the current chair of the Interpol DVI sub-working group for pathology and anthropology.

Alexis T. Boutin, PhD, is a Professor and Graduate Coordinator in the Department of Anthropology at Sonoma State University. Her research draws on human skeletal remains, archaeological contexts, and ancient texts from ancient Near Eastern, Gulf, and eastern Mediterranean cultures to explore embodied personhood in all of its intersectional iterations, especially through osteobiographical narratives. Her recent projects in California emphasize community collaboration and stakeholder-oriented interpretation and outreach. She is the co-founder and past co-chair (with Sabrina Agarwal) of the Bioarchaeology Interest Group of the Society for American Archaeology. She has co-edited two volumes: *Breathing New Life into the Evidence of Death: Contemporary Approaches to Bioarchaeology* (SAR Press) and *Remembering the Dead in the Ancient Near East: Recent Contributions from Bioarchaeology and Mortuary Archaeology* (University Press of Colorado) and published numerous book chapters and journal articles.

Megan B. Brickley, PhD, is currently a Professor and Tier 1 Canada Research Chair in the Bioarchaeology of Human Disease in the Department of Anthropology, McMaster University, Canada. Her primary research interests are use of paleopathology in bioarchaeology, and interdisciplinary research on past human health and disease. She has served as past-Chair of the British Association of Biological Anthropology and Osteoarchaeology, an Associate Editor of *American Journal of Physical Anthropology*, and the President of the Paleopathology Association. Her publications include two co-authored and six edited books and over 80 journal papers and book chapters.

Jane E. Buikstra, PhD, is a Regents' Professor in the School of Human Evolution and Social Change at Arizona State University (USA), where she was the Inaugural Director of the Center for Bioarchaeological Research. She received MA and PhD degrees from the University of Chicago and holds an Honorary Doctor of Science degree from Durham University (UK). She is a member of the National Academy of Sciences, the American Academy of Arts and Sciences, a Fellow of the American Association for the Advancement of Science, a Fellow of the American Association of Forensic Sciences (AAFS), and a Diplomate of the American Board of Forensic Sciences. She was the Inaugural Editor of the *International Journal of Paleopathology* and is the President of the Center for American Archeology. She has received numerous awards including the Charles R. Darwin Lifetime Achievement Award (AAPA), the Fryxell Award for Interdisciplinary Science (Society for American Archaeology), the T. Dale Stewart Award (AAFS), the Pomerance Award for Scientific Contributions to Archaeology (Archaeological Institute of America), The Lloyd Cotsen Prize for Lifetime Achievement in World Archaeology. She has authored over 200 articles and 25 books.

Scott E. Burnett, PhD, is a Professor of Anthropology at Eckerd College. His primary research interests include the use of developmental variation in the skeleton to better understand human biology, evolution, and lifeways. His work also extends to dental anthropology, including studies on dental wear, methodological biases, and intentional dental modification. He has served as President of the Dental Anthropology Association and as Chair of the Comparative Cultures Collegium at Eckerd College. His published works include the co-edited volume, *A World View of Bioculturally Modified Teeth* (University Press of Florida) and more than two dozen book chapters and articles.

Jennifer F. Byrnes, PhD, D-ABFA, is currently an Assistant Professor in the Department of Anthropology at the University of Nevada, Las Vegas. Within the field of bioarchaeology, she is interested in questions focusing on disability and impairment in past human groups, particularly within historical institutional contexts. Her work has focused on injuries resulting from trauma and/or pathology that leave interpretable bony changes. Her research in the realm of forensic anthropology focuses on personal identification, such as radiographic comparison, as well as demographic trends within forensic anthropology casework. Her publications include the edited volume *Bioarchaeology of Disability and Impairment* (Springer Press), *The Marginalized in Death: A Forensic Anthropology of Intersectional Identity in the Modern Era*, articles in the *Journal of Forensic Sciences*, as well as multiple book chapters.

Jennifer L. Caldwell, PhD, MPH, is currently an Assistant Professor of Population Health and Health Equity at Pennington Biomedical Research Center at Louisiana State University. Her research interests include exploring genetic variation in Legacy African Americans using biocultural anthropology as a basis for exploration, and creating effective methods of community engagement in diverse populations. Her current research involves developing better communication techniques between cardiogenomic health providers and patient populations in order to improve patient understanding of their genetic risk of sudden cardiac death. Her most recent publication is "Evolutionary perspectives on African North American genetic diversity: Origins and prospects for future investigations". In addition to her genetic research, she develops community engagement, diversity, equity, and inclusion paradigms for research and practice.

Morgana Camacho, PhD, is a biologist with parasitology diagnosis experience. Her research has focused on the impact of biodegradation and experimental water percolation on Ascaris lumbricoides eggs survival in stratigraphically intact sediment cores collected from Sernambetiba shell mounds (sambaqui). She has also demonstrated that 30 years of negative paleoparasitological results in these types of archaeological sites is due to taphonomic processes associated with intense bioactivity. She has conducted research and published on the paleoepidemiology, pathoecology, and taphonomy of Ancestral Pueblo sites based on the archaeoparasitological analyses, where she documented pinworm infection through time and demonstrated that ancient data can be used to understand epidemiological data. She has published in journals including *Archaeological and Anthropological Sciences*, *Acta Tropica*, and the *Korean Journal of Parasitology*.

D. Troy Case, PhD, is a Professor of Anthropology and Head of the Department of Sociology and Anthropology at NC State University in Raleigh. His research interests include metric and morphological variation of the limbs, sex and stature estimation methods in a forensic anthropological context, and mortuary analysis among the Ohio Hopewell and, most recently, among Iron Age burials from Thailand. He has served as an Associate Editor for the journal *Bioarchaeology International* and is currently a member of its Advisory Board. Publications include a co-authored book, *The Scioto Hopewell and Their Neighbors: Bioarchaeological Documentation and Cultural Understanding*, an edited volume entitled *Gathering Hopewell: Society, Ritual, and Ritual Interaction*, as well as many journal articles and book chapters.

Carlina de la Cova, PhD, is currently an Associate Professor of Anthropology at the University of South Carolina, Columbia. Her research interests include examining the biological impact of inequality, marginalization, institutionalization, and the Great Migration amongst 20th Americans. de la Cova's current work focuses on the relationship between social race, class, and the social origins of anatomical collections and the social stigma of dissection in 19th- and early 20th-century America. She has published numerous articles and book chapters humanizing individuals in anatomical collections. In addition to her academic work, de la Cova is a member of the prestigious Sherlock Holmes literary society, the Baker Street Irregulars, and is a deputy corner in Richland County, South Carolina.

Sharon N. DeWitte, PhD, is currently a Distinguished Professor of Anthropology at the University of South Carolina. She is a biological anthropologist who specializes in paleodemography and paleoepidemiology. She is particularly interested in infectious diseases and famine conditions in the past, and focuses on determining how factors such as sex, gender, social status, developmental stress, nutritional status, and geographic origin affected risks of mortality during such crises. For over 15 years, her research has primarily focused on trends in health and demography before, during, and after the 14th-century outbreak of bubonic plague, the "Black Death", in England. She is also interested in expanding the tools available to bioarchaeologists to examine health in the past in ways that put them in dialogue with human biologists studying living people. She has served on the editorial boards of the *American Journal of Physical Anthropology*, *Evolutionary Anthropology*, and *PLOS One*. She co-edited The *Bioarchaeology of Urbanization: The Biological, Demographic, and Social Consequences of Living in Cities* (Springer); other publications include articles in the *American Journal of Human Biology, American Journal of Physical Anthropology, Annals of Human Biology, International Journal of Paleopathology, Journal of Archaeological Science,* and *Proceedings of the National Academy of Sciences*.

Olivier Dutour, MD, PhD, is currently a Professor and Chair in Biological Anthropology, Paleopathology, and Paleoepidemiology at the Ecole Pratique des Hautes Etudes, Université PSL (Paris Sciences & Lettres) Paris and Researcher at the PACEA Research Unit (CNRS-Université de Bordeaux, Ministère de la Culture). His research interest includes reconstructing the health conditions of past populations, with a focus on infectious diseases. He has served as Director-at-Large of the Paleopathology Association, President of the Groupe des Paléopathologistes de Langue Française, and member of the Editorial Board of the *International Journal of Osteoarchaeology*. His publications include numerous articles and book chapters, two books: *La Paléopathologie* (CTHS Press), *Hommes Fossiles du Sahara* (CNRS Press), and seven co-edited volumes, among them: *Origins of Syphilis in Europe* (CAV, Errance); *Tuberculosis, Past and Present* (Golden Book-TB Foundation); and *Plague, from Epidemics to Societies* (Firenze University Press).

Kori Lea Filipek, PhD, is currently an Associate Professor in Biomedical and Forensic Science at the University of Derby in the UK. Her publications include numerous journal articles and book chapters, and her research interests include paleopathology, multi-isotopic and trace element analyses in paleopathology, social identity and inequalities, disability, care and treatment in the past, and forensic archaeology and anthropology. She is an advocate for historically underrepresented groups in archaeology and currently serves as the secretary for the BABAO's Equality, Diversity, and Inclusion committee, and is a member of the Black Trowel Collective. She is a Fellow of the Higher Education Academy and is passionate about teaching and public outreach, working with the British Council, the Sutton Trust, Skype a Scientist!, the London Science Museum, the Manchester Science Festival, and the North East Raising Aspiration Partnership. She also serves as the Program Coordinator for Transylvania Bioarchaeology and is a Co-director for the Jucu de Sus Necropolis Project.

Katherine Gaddis, MA, is currently a doctoral student in the Department of Anthropology at the University of Nevada, Las Vegas. Her current research interests involve exploring biocultural theories of ageing as they relate to the interpretation of health and disease across the lifespan. Her recent work has focused on the application of interdisciplinary methods to the assessment of traumatic injuries and pathological conditions observed in the skeletal remains of a late-medieval Prussian population. Her publications include an article in the *International Journal of Osteoarchaeology*.

Rebecca Gowland, PhD, is currently a Professor in the Department of Archaeology, Durham University, and Deputy Executive Dean for People and Culture in the Faculty of Social Sciences and Health. Her research interests include social theory, infant and non-adult bioarchaeology, maternity, the life course, and social inequality. She also collaborates with international NGOs on forensic humanitarian casework and training. In her faculty role she seeks to address intersectional inequities in higher education, including gender, race, LGBTQ+, and disability. Her publications include three edited volumes and one co-authored book; *Social Archaeology of Funerary Remains* (Oxbow); *Care in the Past: Archaeological and Interdisciplinary Perspectives* (Oxbow); *The Mother Infant Nexus in Anthropology* (Springer); *Human Identity and Identification* (Cambridge); and numerous articles and book chapters.

Anne L. Grauer, PhD, is a Professor in the Department of Anthropology at Loyola University Chicago. Her research interests include exploring the effects of inequity on health and disease in 19th-century urban centers in the USA. She has served as the President of the Paleopathology Association and the American Association of Biological Anthropologists, and is the Editor-in-Chief of the *International Journal of Paleopathology*. She is a fellow of the American Academy for the Advancement of Science and was awarded the Gabriel W. Lasker Award for Distinguished Service by the American Association of Physical (Biological) Anthropologists. Her publications include four edited volumes: *Bodies of Evidence* (John Wiley & Sons); *Sex and Gender in Paleopathological Perspective* (Cambridge University Press); *Companion to Paleopathology* (John Wiley & Sons); *Biological Anthropology of the Human Skeleton* (co-edited) (Wiley/Blackwell), and numerous journal articles and book chapters.

Siân E. Halcrow, PhD, is a Professor and leader of the Biological Anthropology Research Group in the Department of Anatomy at the University of Otago in New Zealand. Her research focuses on the examination of the agricultural transition in prehistory with a focus on infant and child bioarchaeology. Dr. Halcrow also has a research interest in the ethics of bioarchaeological practice. She has published extensively, with more than 110 papers and chapters, including a co-edited volume *The Mother-Infant Nexus in Anthropology: Small Beginnings, Significant Outcomes* (Springer), and is the co-Editor-in-Chief of *Bioarchaeology International* and an academic editor at *PLOS ONE*. Siân is the proud mother to two wonderful children.

Ryan P. Harrod, PhD, is the Dean of Academic Affairs/Chief Academic Officer, Garrett College and an Affiliate Professor of Anthropology in the Department of Anthropology, University of Alaska Anchorage. His area of specialization is bioarchaeology with a focus on ancient and historic human remains. The majority of his work has focused on the ways that violence was used as a strategy for social control necessary in marginal environments with shrinking resources in the region prior to European contact. The significance of this research is that it further develops an understanding of bioarchaeological research on social inequality and climate change as it is reflected in the presence of non-lethal trauma, activity-related changes to the skeleton, and pathological conditions. Ryan Harrod has co-authored and co-edited several books including *The Bioarchaeology of Climate Change and Violence* (co-authored with Debra Martin) Springer (2014), *Bioarchaeology: An Integrated Approach to Working* *with Human Remains* (co-authored with Debra Martin and Ventura Perez) Springer (2013), *The Bioarchaeology of Violence* (co-edited with Debra Martin and Ventura Perez) University Press of Florida (2012).

Lucía Watson Jiménez, PhD, earned her degree in Anthropology from Archeology at Wroclaw University (Poland). Her research is focused on understanding the ways of life and death of the Central Andes past societies from the bioarchaeological perspective. She is a culture advisor, university professor, member of the HORUS team, and co-director of Dr. Andrew Nelson's bioarchaeological project "Mummies as microcosms". Her recent publication is "Los fardos de Ancón-Perú (800d.C-1532d.C) Una perspectiva bioarqueológica de los cambios sociales en la Costa Central del Perú (BAR); Camino al Titicaca. Tramo La Raya-Desaguadero" (https://qhapaqnan.cultura.pe/publicaciones/camino-al-titicaca-tramo-la-raya-desaguadero). Most of her articles and contributions focus on Andean bioarchaeology from the Central Coast of Peru.

Marie Louise Jørkov, PhD, is currently an Associate Professor in Biological and Forensic Anthropology and Manager of the Anthropological Collection in the Department of Forensic Medicine at the University of Copenhagen. Her research interests include the study of health and disease in 18th- and 19th-century urban centers in Denmark and explores the link between paleodiet and paleopathology. She has used several imaging techniques such as CT, digital X-ray, and photogrammetry as diagnostic tools and documentation in paleopathology.

Saige Kelmelis, PhD, is currently an Assistant Professor in the Department of Anthropology and Sociology at the University of South Dakota. Her areas of specialty include bioarchaeology, paleodemography, and paleoepidemiology. Her research interests include exploring the effects of urbanization, industrialization, emerging diseases, and climate change on human demography and health in past populations. She has served as a program committee member of the American Association of Biological Anthropologists. Her publications include a chapter in *The Bioarchaeology of Urbanization* edited volume and journal articles in *American Journal of Physical Anthropology, Anthropologischer Anzeiger, Earth-Science Reviews,* and *Journal of Archaeological Science: Reports.*

Ellen J. Kendall, PhD, is a Wellcome Trust Early Career Research Fellow at Durham University (UK), with research interests in early life diet and health, archaeological theory and lifecourse approaches, interactions between social identity and disease, the paleopathology of malaria, and isotopic paleopathology. Her current project focuses on the role of historical climate change in modifying the balance of benefit and risk for past human health in wetlands. She is also the Treasurer for the Society for the Study of Childhood in the Past (SSCIP). She recently co-edited her first book with Routledge, *The Family in Past Perspective: An Interdisciplinary Exploration of Familial Relationships through Time.*

Kristina Killgrove, PhD, is an Affiliated Researcher at UNC Chapel Hill and the Ronin Institute. Her research interests include understanding the life histories of ancient Romans through analysis of their skeletal remains. A self-trained science communicator, she has published in *Forbes, Mental Floss, Science Uncovered,* and *Smithsonian Magazine,* and earned awards for her outreach from the Society for American Archaeology and the American Anthropological Association. Her current projects involve bioarchaeological work at the sites of

Oplontis and Gabii in Italy, and she has published peer-reviewed work on dietary isotopes, mobility and migration, and paleopathology in historic Europe.

Casey L. Kirkpatrick, PhD, is a Postdoctoral Researcher at the Max Planck Institute for Evolutionary Anthropology, an Adjunct Research Professor in the Department of Anthropology at the University of Western Ontario, and the Head of Osteology on the BYU Egypt Excavation Project. Her research interests include paleo-oncology, paleopathology, archaeogenetics, and dental anthropology. She is also a co-founder and former Executive Director of the Paleo-oncology Research Organization (PRO), which is devoted to the study of cancers and other neoplastic diseases in ancient remains and maintains the Cancer Research in Ancient Bodies (CRAB) database. Along with her PRO colleagues, she designed and guest edited a special issue for the *International Journal of Paleopathology* (IJPP), entitled "Paleo-oncology: Taking Stock and Moving Forward". She has also co-authored a number of publications including Kirkpatrick, C., Campbell, R. & Hunt, K. (2018), "Paleo-oncology: Taking stock and moving forward" IJPP, 21: 3–11.; Ragsdale, B., Kirkpatrick, C. & Campbell, R. (2018) "Morphological analysis of dry bone specimens: General principles and differential diagnosis" IJPP, 21: 27–40; and Hunt, K., Roberts, C. & Kirkpatrick, C. (2018) "Taking Stock: A systematic review of archaeological evidence of cancers in human and early hominin remains" IJPP, 21: 12–26.

Haagen D. Klaus, PhD, is an Associate Professor of Anthropology at George Mason University. His research spans skeletal physiology, ancient health, stress, and infectious disease, mortuary practices, violence, method and theory in bioarchaeology, and the archaeology of the pre-Hispanic and Colonial Central Andes. Since 2002, he has directed the Lambayeque Valley Biohistory Project in Peru. He has co-edited and co-authored volumes such as *Diet, Nutrition, and Foodways on the North Coast of Peru: Bioarchaeological Perspectives on Adaptive Transitions* (Springer), *Bones of Complexity: Bioarchaeological Case Studies of Social Organization and Skeletal Biology* (University Press of Florida), and *Ritual Violence in the Ancient Andes: Reconstructing Sacrifice on the North Coast of Peru* (University of Texas), along with publications in the *American Journal of BIological Anthropology, Latin American Antiquity, American Journal of Human Biology,* and *International Journal of Paleopathology*. He currently serves as an editoral board member of the American Journal of Biological Anthropology.

Tisa Loewen received her MA in Anthropology from New York University in 2018. She is currently a PhD candidate at Arizona State University in the School of Human Evolution and Social Change and recipient of the National Science Foundation Doctoral Dissertation Research Award. As a bioarchaeologist, her research focuses on population change, human variation, admixture, and the embodied in-between experiences of past and modern people. Specifically, she utilizes dental traits to understand population genetics in the Iron Age and Roman Adriatic. Her expertise also includes analyses utilizing fragmentary and commingled human remains and her service entails prioritizing NAGPRA, collections ethics, mentorship, and support of underrepresented minorities in biological anthropology and archaeology.

Madeleine Mant, PhD, is an Assistant Professor in Anthropology of Health at the University of Toronto Mississauga. Her research integrates bioarchaeology, medical history, and medical anthropology to investigate the health experiences of people through time, with a focus upon trauma and infectious disease. She is a co-editor of *Routledge's Advances in the*

History of Bioethics and has co-edited three volumes: *The History and Bioethics of Medical Education: "You've Got to Be Carefully Taught"* (Routledge); *Bioarchaeology of Marginalized People* (Elsevier Academic Press); and *Beyond the Bones: Engaging with Disparate Datasets* (Elsevier Academic Press) in addition to paleopathological and medical historical journal articles.

Khashaiar Mansouri, DVM, is a former graduate and now intern at the Bovine Reference Laboratory, Razi Vaccine and Serum Research Institute (Agricultural Research, Education and Extension Organization) in Karaj, Iran. His current research focuses on the *Mycobacterium tuberculosis* complex (MTC).

Debra L. Martin, PhD, is a Distinguished Professor of Anthropology at the University of Nevada, Las Vegas and is an expert in human osteology and bioarchaeology. She conducts research in the areas of nonlethal violence and inequality, gender differences and paleopathology, and the bioarchaeology of human experience with a focus on groups living in risky and challenging desert environments. She is the Editor for *American Antiquity* and is the Series Editor for *Bioarchaeology and Social Theory*, Springer. Her recent publications include co-editing *Bioarchaeology of Violence* (UPF) and *Bioarchaeological and Forensic Perspectives on Violence* (Cambridge), *Massacres* (UPF) as well as co-authoring *Bioarchaeology of Climate Change and Violence* (Springer). Recently she authored "Masculinity and Violence in Small Scale Societies" in *Current Anthropology*. She is the Director of the NSF-funded Belen Bioarchaeology Project examining the morbidity and mortality profiles of formerly enslaved New Mexicans (circa 1850).

Simon Mays, PhD, is currently the Senior Human Skeletal Biologist for Historic England, an organization that, inter alia, provides advice to the UK government on archaeological matters in England. He also holds visiting positions in archaeology at the Universities of Southampton and Edinburgh. He is currently an Associate Editor for the *International Journal of Paleopathology*. He has more than 250 academic publications which, as well as focusing on paleopathology, range across areas including ancient biomolecules, ethics and human remains, and medieval folk beliefs. He has recently collaborated with Megan Brickley and Rachel Ives on the production of a second edition of *The Bioarchaeology of Metabolic Bone Disease* (2020), and his book, *The Archaeology of Human Bones*, has now (2021) passed into a third edition.

Aryel Pacheco Miranda, PhD, earned an MA in Forensic Anthropology and Bioarchaeology, and is a PhD candidate at Durham University. He is an Assistant Professor in the Department of Anthropology at the Universidad de Chile, a member of the Sociedad Chilena de Antropología Biológica (SOCHIAB), and the representative of SOCHIAB on the Consejo de Monumentos Nacionales (Chile). His research interests are focused on Andean bioarchaeology, mainly in paleopathology, paleodiet, and mobility of Pre-Columbian communities who inhabited the North of Chile (Atacama Desert). Since 2003, he has excavated, analyzed, and/or supervised the analyses of more than 1,500 human remains in Chile and Perú. His publications include book chapters, "Bioarchaeology in Chile: What it is, where we are, and where we want to go" (2018); "Violence in Northern Chile during the Late Intermediate Period (1000–1450 CE) revisited utilising three archaeological indicators" (2016); and journal articles on diet, mobility, violence, artificial cranial modification, and paleopathologies.

Piers D. Mitchell, MD, works part of the week in the Department of Archaeology at the University of Cambridge, and the remainder as a hospital doctor in the NHS. His research interests focus upon archaeological and textual evidence for disease in past populations, and he is the Director of the Cambridge Ancient Parasites Laboratory. He has served as President of the British Association for Biological Anthropology and Osteoarchaeology, and also of the Paleopathology Association. He is Editor-in-Chief of the Cambridge University Press Book Series *Cambridge Texts in Human Bioarchaeology and Osteoarchaeology.*

Brianne Morgan, MSc, is currently a PhD candidate in the Department of Anthropology at McMaster University, Ontario, Canada. Her PhD research involves investigating skeletal manifestations of scurvy and anemia co-occurrence and examining the implications of these conditions for 19th-century communities in Quebec, Canada. Her other research interests include digital skeletal imaging methods and skeletal trauma analysis. She has published journal articles in both the *American Journal of Physical Anthropology* and the *International Journal of Paleopathology.*

Ken Nystrom, PhD, is a Professor in the Department of Anthropology at the State University of New York at New Paltz (USA). He received his BA from the University of Minnesota-Duluth (1997), and MS (1999) and PhD (2005) from the University of New Mexico. Nystrom's research has covered a wide range of topics including the reconstruction of mortuary behavior, trepanation and trauma, dental health, sex-specific post-manumission migration patterns, long bone cross-sectional geometry, post-marital residence patterns, and the impact of conquest on regional-level genetic homogeneity. Most recently, his focus has been on how bioarchaeology can speak to social inequality in the past and its connection to the present.

Aurora Marcela Pérez-Flórez has a degree in Biology and a Master's degree in Physical Anthropology. She is currently a doctoral student in Physical Anthropology at the Escuela Nacional de Antropología e Historia (ENAH) in Mexico, finishing a doctoral thesis entitled: Bioarchaeology of Violence in Monte Albán. Her main areas of interest are the analysis of bone trauma and violence in ancient and modern populations. She has been trained in Colombia, Mexico, and in the USA. She has participated in national and international congresses and has publications on the analysis of bone trauma. Her recent publication is "The Inhabitants of Monte Albán: A Bioarchaeological Approach" in *The Routledge Handbook of Mesoamerican Bioarchaeology*. In 2019, she was invited as an affiliate instructor to work with Dr. Ryan Harrod in the Department of Anthropology at the University of Alaska at Anchorage. Currently, she works as a forensic advisor for the project "Strengthening the Rule of Law in Mexico" at the Deutsche Gesellschaft für Internationale Zusammenarbeit (GIZ) GmbH, program funded by the German Federal Foreign Office (AA), and is a Professor of Forensic Anthropology at the Escuela Nacional de Antropología e Historia.

Dario Piombino-Mascali, PhD, is a biological anthropologist specialized in mummy studies. He acts as a research professor at the Institute of Biomedical Sciences at Vilnius University and is an honorary inspector of the Department of Cultural Heritage and Sicilian Identity. He has lectured in different organizations, such as the Universities of Messina, Cranfield, Tartu, and Catania, and is the current scientific curator of the Capuchin Catacombs at Palermo. A National Geographic explorer, he was often featured in different local and international media and has published numerous articles in both medical and archaeological journals.

Lauren September Poeta, BA, is an Anishinaabe (Wiikwemkoong Unceded Territory) and British MA candidate in the Department of Anthropology at Western University in London, Ontario. She is a Project Associate in the Office of Indigenous Initiatives at Western University. Her MA research interests include non-destructive methods in bioarchaeology and how diverse lived experiences are translated to mortuary identity. For her thesis, she is investigating variability in the funerary treatment of non-adults and the expression of their social and physiological age categories in the Pre-Columbian funerary record of Peru. She is currently serving as the Student Representative for the Canadian Association of Biological Anthropology /l'Association Canadienne d'Anthropologie Biologique.

Claira Ralston, MS, is a PhD candidate in the Department of Anthropology at the University of Nevada, Las Vegas. Her research addresses issues of identity, inequity, health and disease, marginalization, settler colonialism, and creeping genocide in the North American Southwest. Her dissertation research explores how social institutions shaped gendered inequities in experiences of disease and trauma among the pre-contact occupants of Turkey Creek Pueblo (AZ W:9:123/AZ W:10:78), an early aggregated pueblo in the Point of Pines region of east-central Arizona (AD 1225–1286). She is a part time instructor of anatomy at the Kirk Kerkorian School of Medicine and formerly served as a part time investigative assistant for the Clark County Office of the Coroner-Medical Examiner (2017–2020). In this position she participated in mass-fatality identification and recovery efforts, including those relating to the Route 91 Harvest Festival shooting in Las Vegas (2017) and the Butte County California Camp Fire (2018). She is the Site Supervisor for the NSF-funded Historic Belen Bioarchaeology Project, which is a collaborative, community-engaged project examining the physiological consequences of Spanish colonial programs of marginalization, domination, and assimilation within a community of freed Indigenous indentured servants and slaves known as Genízaros.

Karl Reinhard, PhD, is a Fulbright Scholar and Professor. He has conducted parasitological research since 1981 and his MS and PhD research focused on this topic. That research defined the roles of diet, agriculture, and urbanization on the emergence and control of infection. It elucidated the epidemiology of select species and defined a quantitatively rigorous science. Parallel to parasitological work, he conducts paleonutrition study of Southwestern cultures. He collected dietary observations from Southwestern USA and northern Mexico sites. These data reveal 11,000 years of dietary development. With this database, he explores the relation of diet to the evolution of non-insulin-dependent diabetes mellitus. Since 2017, he expanded nutrition research into gut microbiome applications.

Gwen Robbins Schug, PhD, is a Professor in the Department of Biology at the University of North Carolina Greensboro. Her research is focused on how history, society, and culture guide human responses to crisis and adaptive challenges. She is primarily interested in the role of social inequality in shaping health experiences and resilience in the face of climate and environmental changes. She is also interested in the ethics of human skeletal collections, their origins, curation, and use in teaching and research. She has worked in India and has recently begun projects in Oman and Italy. She is the editor of *The Routledge Handbook of the Bioarchaeology of Climate and Environmental Change* (2020) and *A Companion to South Asia in the Past* (2016), author of the book, *Bioarchaeology and Climate Change* (2011) and more than 40 articles and book chapters. She is the co-Editor-in-Chief of *Bioarchaeology International* and an academic editor at *PLOS ONE*. She is a mother to four children, three dogs, two cats, and welcomed her first grandchild in 2022.

Contributors

Charlotte A. Roberts, PhD, is a bioarchaeologist and Emeritus Professor (since 2020) in the Department of Archaeology, Durham University, England. Her research lies in the study and contextual interpretation of our ancestors' health and well-being, and specifically the origin and evolution of infectious diseases. Elected to the British Academy as a Fellow in 2014 in recognition of excellence in bioarchaeological research, she has presented her research at conferences across the globe, supervised over 30 PhD students, and been involved in public engagement activities all her academic life (talks, exhibitions, production of resources). She has published over 200 book chapters and journal papers, authored/co-authored five books (e.g., *Leprosy. Past and Present; The Bioarchaeology of Tuberculosis: A Global Perspective on a Re-Emerging Disease; Health and Disease in Britain: From Prehistory to the Present Day; Human Remains in Archaeology: A Handbook* and *The Archaeology of Disease*, both the latter having been translated into Chinese), and been involved with four co-edited books (e.g., *Palaeopathology and Evolutionary Medicine: an integrated approach; The Backbone of Europe: Health, Diet, Work and Violence over Two Millennia; A Global History of Paleopathology: Pioneers and Prospects; The Past and Present of Leprosy*).

Susanna Sabin, PhD, is currently a public health scientist. Her research interests include methods development for pathogen genomics, microbial population genomics, and metagenomics. She has completed postdoctoral work at Arizona State University's Center for Evolution and Medicine with Dr. Anne C. Stone and Dr. Jeffrey Jensen and completed her doctoral research at the Max Planck Institute for the Science of Human History in the Department of Archaeogenetics. Her publications include work on molecular dating of the *Mycobacterium tuberculosis* complex, a metagenomic study of ancient cesspit sediments, and metagenomic examinations of human dental calculus.

Chris Stantis, PhD, has been a postdoctoral researcher at three different institutions over the course of this book's creation. Starting the draft at Bournemouth University in the United Kingdom, editing from the Department of Anthropology at the Smithsonian National Museum of Natural History, and seeing the final publication while at the University of Utah, she is, to be honest, very tired. At the time of publication, she serves as Treasurer for the Paleopathology Association and Communications Officer for the IsoArcH Association. She hasn't gotten the hang of writing about herself in third person, but she likes writing about isotopes. She especially enjoys using isotopic data to place past humans in their local environment, both physical and social.

Anne C. Stone, PhD, is Regents' Professor in the School of Human Evolution and Social Change at the Arizona State University. At ASU, she is a member of the Center for Bioarchaeological Research, the Center for Evolution & Medicine, and the Institute of Human Origins. Stone was elected fellow of the American Association for the Advancement of Science (AAAS) (2011) and of the National Academy of Sciences, USA (2016). She currently serves on the scientific executive committee of The Leakey Foundation, the advisory board for the Center of Excellence for Australian Biodiversity and Heritage, and as an Associate Editor for *Philosophical Transactions of the Royal Society*. Stone's research focuses on the analysis of ancient and modern genetic data to investigate population history and adaptation in humans, other animals, and pathogens. She is particularly interested in the evolutionary history of *Mycobacterium tuberculosis* and *M. leprae* (which cause tuberculosis and leprosy, respectively) and their biogeography in relation to human migrations and interactions.

Pamela K. Stone, PhD, is currently a Visiting Associate Professor in the Department of Sociology and Anthropology at Mount Holyoke College. Her research interests include bioarchaeological and biocultural dialogues of health, gender, race, and identity. She has served as a member on the Executive Board of the American Anthropological Association. She was also a member and chair of two executive committees for the American Anthropological Association, Committee on Ethics and the Committee on the Status of Women in Anthropology, as well as treasurer for the Association of Feminist Anthropologists. Her publications include one co-authored book *Bodies and Lives in Victorian England: Sex, Science, and the Affliction of Being Female* (Routledge Press/with L.S. Sanders), two edited books, *Bioarchaeological Analyses and Bodies: New Ways of Knowing Anatomical and Skeletal Collections* (Springer Press), and *Childbirth Across Cultures Ideas and Practices of Pregnancy, Childbirth and the Postpartum* (Springer Press/co-editor H. Selin), and numerous journal articles and book chapters.

Daniel H. Temple, PhD, is currently an Associate Professor and Chair in the Department of Sociology and Anthropology at George Mason University. His research explores stress and life history using incremental microstructures of enamel, estimations of adult body size, and skeletal growth. He uses long bone biomechanics, dental indicators of diet, and mortuary practices to understand resilience and adaptability in hunter-gatherer communities. He has worked with ancestral remains from Japan, Siberia, Florida, Alaska, and the American Southwest. This work has resulted in more than 40 peer-reviewed articles and book chapters in journals such as the *American Journal of Physical Anthropology, PLOS One, International Journal of Osteoarchaeology, American Journal of Human Biology,* and *American Antiquity.* He has also published one edited volume *Hunter-Gatherer Adaptation and Resilience: A Bioarchaeological Perspective* (Cambridge University Press) and acts as an Associate Editor for the *American Journal of Physical Anthropology.*

Lorna Tilley, PhD, works as an Independent Researcher and gained her PhD from the Australian National University in 2013. She came to archaeology late, from a background which included health outcomes assessment and public health policy; this experience informed development of the Bioarchaeology of Care approach. Her publications include *Theory and Practice in the Bioarchaeology of Care* (2015) and, with Alecia Schrenk, the edited volume *New Developments in the Bioarchaeology of Care: Further Case Studies and Expanded Theory* (2017). Together with Tony Cameron, she developed the Index of Care, the online tool designed to assist in bioarchaeology of care analysis. She has authored journal articles and book chapters on aspects of disability and health-related care in the past, and with Ken Nystrom served as guest editor for a special section on Mummy Studies and the Bioarchaeology of Care in the *International Journal of Paleopathology* (2019).

Anne R. Titelbaum, PhD, is an Assistant Professor in the Department of Basic Medical Sciences at the University of Arizona College of Medicine-Phoenix, where she teaches Clinical Anatomy to medical, allied health, and anthropology graduate students. Her research interests include developmental variation, traumatic injury, and musculoskeletal stress. Her primary area of investigation is Andean South America, with a focus on prehistoric populations from northern coastal and highland Peru. She has served as the Treasurer of the Paleopathology Association and is currently an Associate Editor for the *International Journal of Paleopathology.* Her publications include discussions of archaeological developmental anomalies such as brachydactyly, Madelung's deformity and possible Léri-Weill dyschondrosteosis, os odontoideum, block vertebrae, and radioulnar synostosis.

Contributors

Elizabeth W. Uhl, DVM, PhD, DACVP, is a veterinary pathologist with diagnostic expertise in musculoskeletal pathology. She is currently a Professor in the Department of Pathology, College of Veterinary Medicine at The University of Georgia and was recognized as an AAVMCC/APTR One Health Scholar. Her research is varied and includes characterization of a rat model of virus-induced asthma, FIV pathogenesis, Cryptosporidium infections in mammals and reptiles, miRNA expression in canine lymphoma, and codon usage in morbilliviruses. Her current research interests include animal paleopathology, the evolutionary origins and historical impacts of human and animal diseases, and the comparative pathomechanics of degenerative joint disease. Her most recent publications include a chapter on pathogens infecting both humans and animals in *Palaeopathology and Evolutionary Medicine* (Oxford University Press), an interdisciplinary investigation of the origins of canine distemper, a review of the pathology of vitamin D deficiency in domesticated animals, functional analysis of the equine navicular apparatus, and the development of a whole-body 3D equine skeletal model for functional postural analysis of equine degenerative joint disease.

Jaime Ullinger, PhD, is currently a Professor in the Department of Sociology and Anthropology at Quinnipiac University. Her research interests include bioarchaeological reconstructions of health, disease, and biological relatedness in the Bronze Ages of Southwest Asia and Eastern Europe. She is currently a co-director of the Bioanthropology Research Institute at Quinnipiac University (BRIQ) and serves as an Associate Editor for *Dental Anthropology*.

Chiara Villa, PhD, is currently an Associate Professor of Forensic Anthropology and Forensic Imaging in the Department of Forensic Medicine at the University of Copenhagen. Her field of expertise is the human skeleton, both in forensic and archaeological context. In particular, she investigates how bone changes with age, diseases, and traumas crossing scales and merging evidence from the microscopic scale to 3D whole-body. She has used several 3D imaging techniques, like CT, photogrammetry, surface scanner, 3D printing in her research. She is also involved in many multidisciplinary projects, e.g., mummy studies and projects in cultural heritage, veterinary science, and paleontology.

Ziyu R. Wang, PhD, is currently a Research Scientist in the Department of Genome Sciences at the University of Washington. She is a biological anthropologist who trained to specialize in ancient pathogen genomics and infectious disease dynamics. She is especially interested in studying the effects of pathogens' genomic variation on their protein functions and how these effects contribute to the dynamics of infectious disease, such as virulence factors and disease transmission. Her current research focuses on developing cutting edge tools in bioengineering and functional genomics to address questions to better understand the impact of genome variations on human health and disease. She has been a National Science Foundation Fellow and a member of American Association of Physical Anthropologists.

Amanda Wissler, PhD, is an NSF Postdoctoral Research Fellow with the University of South Carolina. She is a biological anthropologist specializing in bioarchaeology, paleopathology, and paleoepidemiology. Her research interests include examining the social, cultural, and biological forces that shape health and survival during major epidemiological events such as the 1918 influenza pandemic and how to leverage past anthropological knowledge to inform current-day public health initiatives. She is a Research fellow at the Cleveland Museum of Natural History Physical Anthropology Laboratory examining the long-term impacts of the 1918 flu on population health and demography and at the Centre for Advanced Study at the Norwegian Academy of Science and Letters with the Centre for Pandemics and Society studying the impact of the 1918 flu pandemic on Indigenous peoples of Alaska. Her work has been published in *Bioarchaeology International, American Journal of Biological Anthropology*, and *the Scandinavian Journal of Public Health*.

Florian Witzmann, PhD, is a paleontologist and currently curator for fossil fishes and amphibians at the Museum of Natural History Berlin and an Associate Professor (Privatdozent) at the Humboldt University Berlin, Germany. His research interests include the fish-to-tetrapod transition and paleopathology of fossil vertebrates, especially Paleozoic and Mesozoic amphibians and reptiles. The focus of his paleopathological research lies on vertebral pathologies and congenital abnormalities. He is one of the chief editors of *Fossil Record* and edited the mini-series: "Palaeopathology – a fresh look at ancient diseases in the fossil record" in the *Journal of Zoology*. His publications include numerous journal articles and book chapters.

Samantha L. Yaussy, PhD, is currently a Temporary Assistant Professor in the Department of Sociology and Anthropology at Utah State University. Her research interests include exploring how factors such as socioeconomic status, developmental stress, biological sex, and age intersected to affect frailty and risks of mortality in the past. Dr. Yaussy's work examines the bioarchaeological evidence for the developmental origins of health and disease hypothesis and demonstrates the potential for intersectional perspectives to inform our understanding of life and death in the past. Her previous research on intersectionality, frailty, and mortality in England was funded by the National Science Foundation (2017), and her current research project on intersectionality in 16th- and 17th-century Hungary has been awarded a Cobb Professional Development Grant (2021) by the American Association of Biological Anthropologists. In recognition of her research accomplishments, Dr. Yaussy was awarded the University of South Carolina Breakthrough Graduate Scholar Award (2019) and the Rhude M. Patterson Trustee Fellowship (2017). Her recent publications include "Intersectionality and the interpretation of past pandemics" *Bioarchaeology International*, 2022, and "The intersections of industrialization: Variation in skeletal indicators of frailty by age, sex, and socioeconomic status in 18th- and 19th-century England" *American Journal of Physical Anthropology*, 2019.

Adam Netzer Zimmer is a PhD candidate in the Department of Anthropology at the University of Massachusetts Amherst, also working in collaboration with the Faculty of Social Sciences at the University of Iceland. Their dissertation research focuses on the rise of race-based anatomical science in 19th- and early 20th-century Iceland and the US and is also interested in queer and feminist perspectives in bioarchaeology and forensic anthropology, particularly focusing on the history of science. Their work has been supported by a Fulbright-National Science Foundation Arctic Research Grant, an NSF Graduate Research Fellowship, the Armelagos-Swedlund Biocultural Anthropology Dissertation Award, and a Leifur Eiríksson Foundation Fellowship. Previously, he was the Laboratory Manager for the UMass Taphonomic Research Facility and is currently the co-primary director of the Rivulus Dominarum Transylvanian Bioarchaeology project in Baia Mare, Romania.

FOREWORD

Like everything in life, the modes of generating knowledge are always changing and reconfiguring themselves. It is good news to have a *Handbook of Paleopathology* that accounts for that vitality. This handbook proposes topics that bridge the gap between the past and our current problems as a society. Social inequality, individual and structural violence, resilience at different levels, mobility, carefulness, vulnerable groups, non-adults, gender roles, and ethical issues are some of them. Promoting creative configurations in our professional practices and encouraging the search for alternative relationships is part of the current challenges. In relation to the ethical aspects of our practice, there is a long way to go. We, together with other social actors, need to learn and promote experiences of honest controversies. Faced with the variety of conflicts that we are experiencing in different parts of the world, building spaces of trust may be a good alternative. Finally, there are many ways of reading or rereading a book, necessitating encounters at all levels (multi-inter and transdisciplinary). Thus, from our different experiences and formative paths, the themes of this new *Handbook of Paleopathology* invite us to think and rethink about our perspectives and relationships. As Marcel Proust proposes, the act of discovery does not consist only in going out to look for new lands, but in learning to see the old land with new eyes.

Dr. Ricardo A. Guichón
CONICET, Laboratorio de Ecología Evolutiva Humana (LEEH), EUEQ, FACSO,
Universidad Nacional del Centro de la Provincia de Buenos Aires, Quequén, Argentina

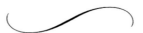

Agreeing to write a foreword for a book of this nature and significance is both an honor and a tremendous charge. It is indeed an honor to be picked among a thousand other fellow researchers to be part of this great edited volume. However, this also brings a great responsibility, as one is tasked with introducing world renowned and highly acclaimed researchers who need no introduction. The editor and contributors deserve a congratulatory note for having brought this project to fruition. Every few years a project of this magnitude is commissioned focusing on various areas within paleopathology. Contributors emphasize methodologies, analytical technics, and interpretations. Despite this, there remains gaps in the literature that collates the broader aspects of paleopathology. These gaps are addressed by Grauer and contributors in this book.

As noted by some contributors, the problem of compartmentalizing knowledge and publishing on specific topics in limited publication outlets serves as a challenge and a stumbling block for the growth of the discipline. This book addresses this issue by paying attention to the evolution of paleopathology and how its sub-specialties have developed and evolved into robust key routes for the better understanding of past human morbidity and mortality. Some of the relatively "new" areas of research include paleo-oncology, paleontological paleopathology, and parasitology. These sub-specialties testify to the need for multidisciplinary and transdisciplinary approaches in paleopathological studies.

As can be expected, human remains in the form of fossils, mummies, skeletons, and teeth form the core source of information for paleopathological research and are essential subjects of observation in this book. It is particularly interesting to see how single or populations of human remains, past and present, are used to assess ancient diseases (for instance, when exploring paleoepidemiology, pandemics, and plagues), whether they are linked to infectious disease, metabolic disorders, stress, endocrine disease, developmental conditions, dental diseases, or neoplastic diseases. In addition to studies based on human remains, contributions using secondary sources such as coprolites, historical records, microbial species, parasites, and faunal remains clearly play an important role in paleopathology. Thus, the book solidifies the need for researchers and students to look beyond human remains in their pursuit of knowledge of the origins and evolution of diseases.

Focusing on the development of methods and techniques of investigation is also essential to paleopathology. Analytical approaches covered in this volume cover microscopy, macroscopy, histology, medical imaging in its various forms, stable isotope analysis, and genetic and genomic analysis (of humans, parasites, and microbes). Moreover, new standards are offered on how best to use analytical approaches, including differential diagnosis, to recognize diseases at the individual and community levels. The call for inclusion of broad-based theoretical frameworks, such as social theory including gender, identity, disability, and agency in paleopathology, is also noteworthy, as these approaches are new and vital components to the interpretation of morbidity and mortality. It is often said that in order to develop a solution to a problem, we first have to understand the source of the problem. In this book, many chapters tackle ancient, historical, and present-day social inequities that lead to marginalization, structural violence, and social violence, and bring to light how they have negatively impacted the health and wellness of past populations. In addition, discussions of disability and care for others in the past are tackled. Despite the limitations associated with paleopathology and the well-known osteological paradox, these contributions provide a framework that can be used for the development and advancement of strategies for healthcare providers and policy developers today.

In conclusion, a common thread throughout the chapters is the detailed presentation of the origins and history of methods, techniques, our understanding of particular diseases, and theoretical approaches, alongside discussion of interpretations, analytical approaches, and the potential for growth and improvement. The quality of these presentations demonstrates a deep knowledge and understanding by all authors. This offers a great service to current and future students seeking a deep-time perspective of the field of paleopathology and to researchers interested in the development, evolution, and potential of the field. Moreover, the accessible language used throughout the volume, alongside details and theoretical foundations, renders the volume truly accessible for readers in many disciplines and interested members of the public. In all, this volume contributes greatly to our understanding of health and disease in the past and the role that paleopathology can play in shedding light on current and future socioeconomic issues that impact disease globally. This renders paleopathology a discipline that contributes substantially to new knowledge-based socio-economic strategic goals of many individuals, civil and other groups, as well as national governments around the world.

Dr. Morongwa Nancy Mosothwane
Associate Professor, Faculty of Humanities: History
University of Botswana, Gabarone, Botswana

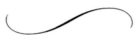

Tracking the traces of diseases suffered by ancient people requires navigating through uncertainly and ambiguity caused by evidence lost due to the passage of time. However, paleopathology, the study of ancient human diseases, has made remarkable progress over the past decades. Application of novel techniques and analytical tools enabled us to gain new insight into human diseases of the past. Paleopathology is now emerging from a practice of conjecture into the realm of robust inquiry based on scientific evidence.

Researchers living in areas of the world privy to a wealth of scientific information are fortunate. They can easily access and share knowledge, allowing them to move the field of paleopathology forward. However, in many regions of the world, paleopathological inquiry is limited by the lack of communication and knowledge, and Asia is not an exception. There are still only vague assumptions about the environments in which ancient Asian populations lived and how conditions affected their health and disease status. In Asia today, well-written and edited books can serve as beacons for those who hope to conduct rigorous research in paleopathology.

In this regard, I am happy that Dr. Grauer, my esteemed colleague who has authored several books and articles that I owe much of my research, is releasing a new book on paleopathology. Based on the composition of the chapters, the *Routledge Handbook of Paleopathology* covers important subjects that researchers encounter in their fieldwork. The authors who have contributed chapters are excellent and highly respected in their respective fields. I have no doubt that Dr. Grauer's new book will shine bright where it is desperately needed: the countries of Asia, once the cradle of ancient civilizations.

Dr. Dong Hoon Shin
Professor and Chair, Bioanthropology and Paleopathology Lab, Department of Anatomy/Institute of Forensic Science, Seoul National University College of Medicine, Seoul, South Korea

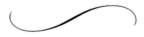

Foreword

A View from South America

The first two decades of the 21st century have witnessed remarkable progress in paleopathology across the globe. Books on a variety of topics have emerged, illustrating new approaches to research on human remains. This volume represents a significant step forward in updating our ever-growing discipline, reflecting a period of exciting developments.

In South America, as in many other regions of the world, paleopathology has advanced in new and intriguing ways (Guillén, 2012; Rojas-Sepúlveda & Rivera-Sandoval, 2019; Suby & Luna, 2019). The pioneering studies of many colleagues, mostly since the 1980s and 1990s, have stimulated a new 21st-century forum for research communication; the Paleopathology Association Meeting in South America (PAMinSA) held its first meeting in 2003. In part due to these meetings, increasing numbers of new researchers and students from South America have markedly advanced the discipline. Most of the studies have been based on archaeological remains from past hunter-gatherers and complex societies who inhabited the subcontinent until recent times, a richness and diversity that is found in few other regions of the world.

This high-quality South American scholarship has resulted in increasing numbers of paleopathological and bioarchaeological papers published in prestigious English language journals, including studies of infectious diseases (e.g., Costa-Junqueira et al., 2009; Arriaza et al., 2010; Ramos Van Raap & Scabuzzo, 2021), trauma and violence (e.g., Gordon, 2015), degenerative joint diseases and pattern activities (e.g., Rojas-Sepúlveda et al., 2008), oral diseases (e.g., Bernal & Luna, 2011; Fabra & Gonzalez, 2015), and many other subjects. Valuable results are also published in Spanish, with abstracts in English, many available on a free website that compiles many of the highly ranked scientific journals from Hispano-America (i.e. http//scielo.org). Hence, all paleopathologists can easily become acquainted with this high-quality global resource and use it to anchor their studies.

Considerable South American research includes the newest methodological approaches in paleopathology, such as imaging techniques and biogenomics, reviewed here in Chapters 6 and 8, respectively. Likewise, theoretical discussions are underway, several treated here, including rigor in differential diagnosis and degrees of certainty (Chapter 2), health and stress concepts (Chapter 22), the bioarchaeology of care model (Chapter 25), and the bioarchaeology of gender (Chapter 24), among others. Studies of South American mummies (Chapter 11), specifically from the Andean region, have also made unparalleled contributions to cultural and pathological knowledge of past populations (Lombardi & Arriaza, 2020). Moreover, several countries of South America are pioneering in forensic anthropology. Numerous new developments in forensics are produced, including new methods for age and sex estimation, in both adults and non-adults (Luna et al., 2017; Rabelo Maciel et al., 2021). The FASE (Forensic Anthropology in Europe; http://forensicanthropology.eu/osteological-collections/#page-content) website reports ten documented skeletal collections from Argentina (4), Brazil (3), Chile (1), and Colombia (2), (e.g., Isaza & Monsalve Vargas, 2012; Salceda et al., 2012; Sanabria Medina, 2016), which will be helpful in advancing our knowledge and evolution of past diseases in the region.

To balance the great challenges posed by the Sars-Cov-2 pandemic, the internet has facilitated new and more frequent interactions between colleagues around the world. Online conferences are continuously available, and scholars from South America have joined numerous meetings and webinars, unavailable previously. These ways of "being in touch" offer opportunities not only to incorporate new techniques, methods, and theoretical approaches, but also to share South American paleopathological data. These contacts are facilitated, not only with other regions around the globe but also among South American researchers. As an example, the first Webinar of Biological Anthropology arranged by scholars from Perú, Colombia, Uruguay, Argentina, Brazil, and Chile took place in 2020, as well as other regional conferences and online meetings.

Bioarchaeology and paleopathology are constantly expanding in South America. The many published results advance global knowledge and techniques. Our regional challenges include (as always) funding issues and institutional support. South American paleopathologists are well advised to become more connected with the rest of the world, and to include our results in international meetings, conferences, and journals, if we want to be part of a more complex, collaborative, and very exciting discipline. I am confident that this new book will stimulate further interest in paleopathology by South American scholars.

Dr. Jorge Suby
Researcher at the National Council for Science and Technology (CONICET-Argentina).
Bioarchaeological Research Group. Department of Archaeology, Faculty of Social Sciences,
University of the Center of Buenos Aires Province, Argentina

References

Arriaza, B. T., Amarasiriwardena, D., Cornejo, L., Standen, V, Byrne, S., Bartkus, L. & Bandak, B. (2010). Exploring chronic arsenic poisoning in pre-Columbian Chilean mummies. *Journal of Archaeological Science* 37(6):1274–1278. https://doi.org/10.1016/j.jas.200.12.030.

Bernal, V. & Luna, L. (2011). The development of dental research in Argentinean biological anthropology: current state and future perspectives. *Homo. Journal of Comparative Human Biology* 62:315–327. https://doi.org/10.1016 /j.jchb.2011.08.004.

Costa-Junqueira, M. A., Matheson, C., Iachetta, L., Llagostera, A. & Appenzeller, O. (2009). Ancient leishmaniasis in a highland desert of Northern Chile. *PloS ONE* 4(9):1–7.

Fabra, M., González, C. V. (2015). Diet and oral health of populations that inhabited Central Argentina (Córdoba Province) during late Holocene. *International Journal of Osteoarchaeology* 25(2):160–175. https://doi.org/10.1002/oa.2272.

Gordón, F. (2015). Bioarchaeological patterns of violence in North Patagonia (Argentina) during the late Holocene: implications for the study of population dynamics. *International Journal of Osteoarchaeology* 25(5):625–636. https://doi.org/10.1002 /oa.2325.

Guillén, S. A. (2012). History of paleopathology in Peru and Northern Chile: from head hunting to head counting. In Buikstra, J. E. & Robert, C. A. (Eds.), *The Global History of Paleopathology: Pioneers and Prospects*, pp. 312–329. New York: Oxford University Press. https://doi.org /10.1093/acprof:osobl/9780195389807.003.0039.

Isaza, J., Monsalve Vargas, T. (2012). Características biológicas de la colección osteológica de referencia de las Universitdad de Antioquia; Informe preliminar. *Boletin de Antropologia*, 25.

Lombardi, G., Arriaza, B. (2020). South American mummies. In Shin, D. H. & Bianucci, R. (Eds.), *The Handbook of Mummy Studies*. Singapore: Springer. https://doi.org/10.1007/978-981-15-1614-6_25-1.

Luna, L. H., Aranda, C. M., Santos, A. L. (2017). New method for sex prediction using the human non-adult auricular surface of the ilium in the Collection of Identified Skeletons of the University of Coimbra. *International Journal of Osteoarchaeology* 27(5):898–911.

Rabelo Maciel, D., Fidalgo, D., Costa, C., Wesolowski, V., Michel Crosato, E. & Haye Biazevic, M. G. (2021). Estimation of age at death based on the analysis of third molar mineralization in individuals from Brazilian archaeological populations. *Bulletin of the International Association for Paleodontology* 15(2):58–65.

Ramos van Raap, M. A. & Scabuzzo, C. (2021). Infectious diseases in North Eastern Argentina: treponematosis and its connection with population concentration. *International Journal of Osteoarchaeology* 31(2):293–302. DOI:10.1002/oa.2951.

Rojas-Sepúlveda. C. & Rivera-Sandoval, J. (2019). Paleopathology in Northwestern South America (Venezuela, Colombia, Ecuador, and Peru). In Ubelaker, D. & Colantonio, S. (Eds.), *Biological Anthropology in Latin America*, pp. 217–238. Smithsonian Contributions to Anthropology number 51. Washington, DC: Smithsonian Institution Scholar Press.

Rojas-Sepúlveda, R., Ardagna, Y. & Dutour, O. (2008). Paleoepidemiology of vertebral degenerative disease in a Pre-Columbian Muisca series from Colombia. *American Journal of Physical Anthropology* 135(4):416–430.

Salceda. S. A., Desántolo, B., García Mancuso, R., Plischuk, M. & Inda, A. M. (2012). The 'Prof. Dr. Rómulo Lambre' Collection: an Argentinian sample of modern skeletons. *HOMO – Journal of Comparative Human Biology* 63:275–281.

Sanabria Medina, C. (2016). *Patología y Antropología Forense de la Muerte: – La Investigación cientifico-judicial de la muerte y la tortura, desde las fossa clandestinas, hasta la audiencia pública*. Bogotá, Colombia: Forensic Publisher LLD.

Suby, J. A. & Luna, L. H. (2019). Paleopathology in Southern South America. Recent advances and future challenges. In Ubelaker, D. & Colantonio, S. (Eds.), *Biological Anthropology in Latin America*, pp 311–324. Smithsonian Contributions to Anthropology number 51. Washington, DC: Smithsonian Institution Scholar Press.

ACKNOWLEDGMENTS

I don't have the words to adequately thank the extraordinary scholars who generously agreed to contribute to this volume. We began this endeavor weeks before the horrors of the COVID pandemic were fully realized and knew nothing of the isolation, fear, hardship, and heartbreak that lay ahead. Your candor, generosity, and perseverance on personal and professional levels were astonishing and deeply appreciated. Many thanks are also owed to all the chapter reviewers, as you beautifully modeled how comments and critique can be insightful, respectful, encouraging, and compassionate. Thanks, too, to the great team at Routledge (Taylor and Francis) Books: Manas Roy, Editorial Assistant and Gabrielė Gaižutytė, Senior Production Editor; and at codemantra, Gayathree Sekar, Project Manager. Special thanks go to Taylor Emery and Alexis Martinez for helping with the time-sucking task of creating an index.

1
INTRODUCTION

Anne L. Grauer

The field of paleopathology, like many scientific disciplines, has changed profoundly over the past decades. Technological advances, new theoretical approaches, and the inclusion of diverse voices in the creation of and discourse surrounding data collection and analysis have influenced all aspects of our understanding of health and disease in the past. These strides have also contributed to the increasing complexity of our field; a complexity that necessitates multidisciplinary collaboration between medical, biological, and social scientists, as well as humanists, to address significant questions in a contextually rich manner. The interpretation of disease now extends beyond the recognition of its presence in the past to include deep archaeological and social contexts within which human and animal pathology is rooted, sophisticated means to detect the presence and evolution of pathogens and host responses, and ways in which our research informs the future. It also includes existential reflection on social and political privilege, past and present. Subsequently, we have moved beyond a limiting definition of "violence" from direct trauma to recognizing and confronting social violence—the deeply embedded structural inequities that have privileged a few and inexcusably harmed others. In parallel, efforts to decolonize academic fields, including paleopathology, are being organized, as evidenced in this volume.

What's in a Name? Everything.

By nature of its name, research within the field of paleopathology (*paleo* = ancient, *pathology* = the study of disease) ought to be straightforward. It is not. In fact, the very definitions of the terms *paleo* and *pathology* have changed since the inception of the discipline and reflect its contributors and their intellectual environments. The definitions also influence the questions we ask, the data we collect, and our understanding of the past (Buikstra, 2010; Grauer, 2012). For instance, some of the earliest exploration into ancient disease reported on pathological conditions in fossil remains in non-human taxa recovered from mountainous and cavernous regions of Europe (see, for instance, Esper, 1774; Goldfuss, 1810; and Schmerling, 1835). Later, 19th-century and early 20th-century physicians and anatomists, such as Sir Marc Armand Ruffer (1859–1917), Frederic Wood Jones (1879–1954), and Grafton Elliot Smith (1871–1937), centered their attention on diagnosing disease in Egyptian mummified remains, in part influenced by French occupation of the country in the 18th century and

British occupation in the 19th and early 20th centuries, and the public's growing romanticized colonialist construction of the cultural past. The foci of North American scholars rested on living and deceased Native Americans (see for instance Hrdlicka (1908) and Hooton's analysis of skeletal remains of Pecos Pueblo individuals (1930)), as they were seen to represent present-day vestiges of "primitive" and "savage" past human life, had sacred burial grounds that were legally unprotected from archaeological excavation and looting, and held little to no political power to advocate for themselves or their ancestors.

Throughout the 20th century, the *paleo* aspect of the field of paleopathology continued to center on the analysis of human remains of individuals or groups accessible to researchers with resources to travel and undertake scientific research, access to education, and the socio-political authority to disinter and dislocate human remains. The timescale of inquiry (i.e., millennia or centuries), therefore, was less of an impetus for exploration than the "fortuitous" access to mummified and/or skeletonized human remains. Recognizing these biases is essential, as the extraordinary number of analyses completed on North and South American, British and European, and North African human remains is not a gauge of the importance of these populations in human history, but rather reflects axes of power during centuries of colonization. Hence, *paleo* for many of these decades has been defined through a decidedly Western lens that centers on distinctions between prehistory/history, precolonial/colonial, preindustrial/industrial, and views time as linear and progressive. Lost and/or overlooked are insights into cyclical aspects of health and disease, traditional knowledge impacting illness and treatment, and experiences of peoples over the vast geographical areas of Asia and much of the African continent.

Definitions of the term *pathology* have also changed over time. Throughout much of the 19th and up to the late 20th century, a decidedly biomedical model was adopted to explain the presence of disease. That is, the human body could be expected to function "normally" unless affected by singular causal agents such as pathogenic invasion or malfunctioning organs. Paleopathological investigations sought to identify changes to the human skeleton or in mummified remains linked to specific known diseases (see Chapter 12 on mummified remains, this volume). Midway through the 20th century, however, paradigmatic changes took place that increased both the scope and complexity of the concept of disease (Mason, 1975, and see Chapter 22 on the concept of stress, this volume). Selye (1957, 1973), for instance, revealed that measurable biomolecular changes took place in the body provoked by environmental conditions such as cold temperatures or excessive and prolonged exercise. These changes reduced an individual's tolerance to other injuries or pathogens and, when prolonged, eventually led to death. He labeled this pathophysiological response the General Adaptation Syndrome (GAS). Concomitantly, other researchers such as Audy (1971) and Dever (1976) argued that simplistic disease models ignored deleterious physiological and psychological stress factors that contributed to or caused disease, and that failure to recognize the impact of adverse social and environmental conditions impeded health practice and policy.

Changing Models of Disease

The changing models of disease influenced paleopathological research (Grauer, 2018). First, they led researchers to appreciate the scientific value of lesions devoid of a specific etiology. Macroscopically recognizable skeletal changes, such as diffuse periosteal reaction linked to the body's generalized response to inflammation or infection, or dental conditions such as enamel hypoplasia, linked to childhood dental development disruption, provided essential information about responses to stressors within individuals or populations, regardless of whether the stress could be identified. Goodman et al. (1984), Huss-Ashmore et al. (1982), and Lewis and Roberts (1997), for instance, use these "multiple stress indicators" or "non-specific stress indicators" to explore the roles that infection, nutrition, subsistence changes, and social environment play in human health and disease in the past. Even lesions associated with single-origin etiologies were re-evaluated in light of the recognizably complex interplay between hosts and stressors. Identifying the presence of tuberculosis and/or leprosy in the past, for instance, sheds light on far more than the antiquity of the disease or host contact and response to pathogens; their presence is deeply intertwined with human social interactions, the interface between humans and animals, availability of and access to resources, and host immune competence (Roberts & Buikstra, 2008; Roberts, 2020, and see Chapters 17 on mycobacterial infections, and 18 on infectious disease, this volume). Importantly, new models of health and disease appreciate that environmental factors, human biology, and culture, working in consort, can exacerbate and/or ameliorate states of stress or disease (Goodman & Armelagos, 1989; Temple & Goodman, 2014).

The Roots of Paleopathology

Under the Influence of Medicine

The field of paleopathology has global roots, albeit nurtured and amplified in some areas of the world and less well known, if not squelched, in others. The European and North American origins of the discipline have been outlined well by Moodie (1923), Jarcho (1966), Brothwell and Sandison (1967), Angel (1981), and Buikstra and Cook (1980), and more recently by Buikstra (2010) and Grauer (2018). These chronicles elucidate trends within paleopathology that, for the most part, follow the field's inextricable links to Western intellectual traditions, contemporary paradigms, and social and political power (see Chapter 10 on historical sources of knowledge, this volume). For instance, as mentioned previously, the earliest forays into paleopathology were conducted by 19th-century and early 20th-century European medically trained anatomists and physicians who sought to identify diseases of the past and catalogue their antiquity. Sir Marc Armand Ruffer (1859–1917), in particular, whose work linked known clinical manifestations of disease to identifiable lesions on Egyptian mummified and skeletal remains, earned him the moniker "Pioneer of Paleopathology" (Sandison, 1967). In following decades, clinical knowledge, supported by clear descriptions and increasingly sophisticated imaging technology, provided foundations for rigorous diagnoses. Anderson (1969, 1982) and Møller-Christensen (1961, 1965), for instance, offered refined diagnostic criteria for recognizing leprosy in human remains based on their extensive clinical and archaeological knowledge, while Hackett (1976) and Rogers and Waldron (1995) closely examined skeletal manifestations of treponematosis and joint disease, respectively. However, contributions to our understanding of disease in the past were also made by medically trained doctors such as Karl von Baer (1860) from Estonia and Yoshikiyo Koganei (1894, 1934) and Kiyono and Hoshijima (1922) from Japan, whose names rarely show up in publications.

The Roles of Physical Anthropology and Archaeology

Paleopathology was also influenced by other fields. The late 18th- and early 19th-century intent of physical anthropology to examine human populations and to classify them into types or groups led Ernest Hooton (1887–1954) to include a population-based study of noted pathological conditions within his typological analysis of Native American skeletal remains from Pecos Pueblo, New Mexico (Hooton, 1930). He linked pathological conditions to the group's diet, the presence of infectious disease, and the changing environment. Similarly, Aleš Hrdlička (1869–1943) adopted a population approach in his published report on pathological conditions witnessed on the skeletons of "Ancient Peruvians" whose remains were collected from excavations or left behind as "debris" from looters (Hrdlička, 1914).

Archaeology also influenced paleopathological research. The early emphasis on cataloguing and reporting excavated materials to preserve the past was criticized mid-century, and a "New Archeology" was introduced positing that quantitative scientific investigation of mortuary remains offered insight into social dimensions of the past (see Willey & Phillips, 1958; Binford & Binford, 1968; Saxe, 1970; Binford, 1971). These researchers argued that social responses to environmental change were predictable and that aspects of social interactions, such as "social status", could be readily identified in the archaeological record. The subsequent critiques of "New Archeology", posed by Hodder (1982), Shanks and Tilley, (1982), and Earle and Pruecel (1987), to name a few, countered that human behavior was far from predictable and universally absolute. They asserted that most archaeological interpretation was "deterministic" and "positivist", with little to no objective "truth" at its core. These paradigmatic approaches influenced the rise of a bioarchaeological approach toward interpreting human skeletal remains (Buikstra, 1977). As Armelagos and Van Gerven (2003) and Buikstra and Beck (2006) clearly articulate, understanding the presence and evolution of human disease requires researchers to carefully place skeletal analysis deeply within archaeological contexts. Recognizing skeletal changes does not *ipso facto* provide a definitive diagnosis nor does it offer insight into host/pathogen relationships, the multifactorial aspects of human health and disease, or human adaptation. Rather, the complex ecological, climatic, and social conditions within which the individual(s) lived must be explored. So began a rift between paleopathological practice in Europe and the United States, whereby European practitioners with medical backgrounds honed their skills in diagnosis of single cases, while their American counterparts with anthropological training explored the presence and social aspects of disease within populations (Roberts, 2006; Mays, 2010).

Legacies of Colonialism, Privilege, and Racism

Essential to confront, and inescapable to ignore, is the fact that the roots of paleopathology worldwide are entangled within centuries of colonialism, scientific racism, and social inequity. Early European physicians, for instance, exercised their colonial social and political privilege by collecting the mummified and skeletal remains of ancient Egyptians in the name of scientific inquiry. Even the first "Paleopathology Club", which met in 1973 and later became the Paleopathology Association, an international scientific organization, began as a gathering to unwrap the mummified remains of an individual from 7th to 8th century BC Egypt. Throughout Europe and the United States, vast collections of skeletal remains were amassed by physicians and anthropologists, alike, to assist with teaching, serve as bases for research, and/or simply kept as curiosities. Roberts and Mays (2011) report that over 80,000 human remains are currently curated in UK institutions alone, while in the US, well over 100,000 human remains disinterred from Native American sites are held in federally funded institutions, with over 57,000 repatriated under the Native American Graves Protection and Repatriation Act (Buikstra, 2019). These figures do not include the vast number of remains that make up medical/anatomical collections such as the Robert J. Terry, the Hamann-Todd, and the W. Montague Cobb collections in the US, or the identified human osteology collections in Portugal (Ferriera, et al., 2021), Brazil (Cunha et al., 2018), and Italy (Carrara et al., 2018). And, importantly, the tally ignores the estimated peak of 60,000 skeletons per year exported from India and sold over a 150-year period to universities, hospitals, schools, and the general public until the ban in 1985 (Agarwal, 2022).

As astonishing as these numbers are, the key issue is not the quantity of human remains in collections worldwide; it is whose bodies were relegated to become "specimens". It is well known that 19th-century medical doctors and students in the US, needing practice in anatomy, pathology, and surgery, met their needs by hiring grave robbers to disinter the recently buried (often African American decedents) and acquired bodies of individuals who had died in institutions without family members to collect and bury them (Nystrom, 2011, 2017; Watkins, 2018). Soppol (2002) argues that it wasn't uncommon for those of greater economic means to feel it was the poor's duty to offer themselves to the professionalization of physicians as restitution for their dependence on taxpayers. In the UK and Europe, extensive excavation of human remains over the past century has yielded thousands of skeletons available for paleopathological investigation, but excavations rarely take place in cemeteries with elaborately marked graves or alongside churches with affluent parishioners. Hence, it is clear that the human remains we use to understand disease in the past reflect centuries of power and privilege at the expense of the poor, marginalized, and disenfranchised; individuals without political power and who never gave consent (Rankin-Hill, 2016; Blakey, 2020a; de la Cova, 2020). The same has been argued for skeletal remains in identified human skeletal collections (collections where the name and information about the individual has been retained) and for unidentified anatomical collections amassed through commercial means (Muller et al., 2017, and see Chapter 21 on ethical considerations, this volume). In these circumstances, laws may have been followed and care taken in the curation of each individual; but while it might be legal (now or in the past) to excavate or buy and sell human bodies and body parts, the remains of the wealthy, politically powerful, and socially connected are *not* the ones whose bodies are exhumed or curated in collections without consent (Alfonso & Powell, 2006; Williams & Ross, 2021). These are the legacies of our discipline. These are our roots. Recognizing the vestiges of power and privilege is the first step in moving forward to decolonize our field.

Branching Out

Toward Improvement of Standardization and Rigor

Paleopathology has moved forward in many directions since its inception (Grauer, 2023). For one, considerable focus has been placed on standardizing data collection. Jarcho's (1966) concern that paleopathology suffered from unsystematic data collection and weak methodological work has been met with efforts in the US (see Rose et al., 1991; Buikstra & Ublaker, 1994; Harris and Rose, 1995; and *Osteoware* developed by researchers at the Smithsonian National Museum of Natural History, https://naturalhistory.si.edu/research/anthropology/programs/repatriation-office/osteoware). In Britain, Brickley and McKinley (2004), Roberts and McConnell (2004) and Mitchell and Brickley, (2018) provide guidance in recording skeletal changes that are clear, systematic, reproducible, and comparable. These efforts have contributed to the use of coherent terminology that reduces misinterpretation: for instance, the use of the medical term "erosion" is not suitable for paleopathology since it could ambiguously refer to both antemortem and taphonomic processes. In 1992, the Paleopathology

Association compiled of list of terms to encourage clear communication between researchers (see Buikstra, 2016). More recently, Manchester et al. (2016) have produced an extensive document defining hundreds of suitable terms organized into categories such as functional and systemic anatomy, physiology, pathology, radiology, and taphonomy. Terms are predicated upon an understanding of biological and taphonomic processes, not merely physical description, allowing this massive guide to enhance effective communication within and beyond the field of paleopathology.

Rigor in diagnosis has also received considerable attention. Compendia specifically designed to assist with disease diagnosis in dry bone specimens, such as Steinbock (1976), Ortner and Putschar (1981), Aufderheide and Rodriquez Martin (1998), Ortner (2012), and most recently Buikstra (2019), emphasize pathophysiological bases for disease processes in bone and place pathological conditions into archaeological contexts. The need for scientific rigor has also been tackled by Appleby et al. (2015), Klaus (2015), Buikstra et al. (2017), Lawler (2017), Mays (2020), (and see Chapters 2, on data collection and protocols, 3 on rigor and differential diagnosis, and 16 on treponemal infections, this volume), to name a few. They warn of the dangers of spurious diagnoses without differential diagnosis (clearly outlining other possible diagnoses and why these are less reasonable options) and address the importance of utilizing modern clinical data to inform conclusions. Continued work to ensure that paleopathological diagnoses and interpretations are based on sound evidence will strengthen our field immeasurably (Zuckerman et al., 2016).

Technological Advancement

In many scientific fields, technology has played an important role in advancing knowledge. The field of paleopathology is no exception. Sophisticated imaging techniques have allowed us to view pathological changes without destruction to bone and other tissues (Öhrström et al., 2010; Miccichè et al., 2018; Morrone et al., 2021; and see Chapter 6 on imaging techniques, this volume). Microscopy, contributing to the growth of paleohistopathological study of tissues, has advanced appreciably in spite of the considerable challenges posed by the effects of tissue damage over time and the need to limit destruction of valuable mummified and skeletal remains (see Chapter 5 on histology, this volume). Biomolecular applications to paleopathology, including stable isotope and genetic analyses, have also contributed profoundly to our field. Assessing the isotopic signatures of human and animal tissues offers insight into local ecologies, patterns of migration, and diet—all factors contributing to disease past and present (Scorrano, 2018; Toyne & Turner, 2020; and see Chapters 7 on stable isotopes and 20 on dental disease, this volume). Analyses of biomolecules such as DNA (aDNA) of bacteria and proteins (proteomics) move us substantially closer to understanding the presence, evolution, and human response to pathogens (Orlando et al., 2021; and see Chapter 8 on genetics, this volume). In spite of the methodological, computational, and ethical obstacles faced in biomolecular analyses, of which there are many, genetic, genomic, and proteomic studies have captured the presence of pathogenic bacteria, such as *Mycobacterium* (associated with tuberculosis and leprosy) and *Yersinia* (associated with the plague) and viruses such as *Variola* (associated with smallpox) (Mühlemann et al., 2020), to name a few.

The Importance of Social Theory

Technological advancement, however, is not a paleopathological a panacea—it does not answer all questions or, as the public may think, render obsolete other avenues of inquiry.

Introduction

Acknowledging the complexity of disease has also contributed to our field. Gone are simplistic notions that disease is characterized by interactions between a pathogen and a host (or, for that matter, that detecting pathogenic DNA informs us about *disease*). The creation of biocultural models mapping the interplay between varied dimensions of human life alongside human biology, and bioarchaeological models that adapted these models to explore the past, disclose the many variables that contribute to and/or mitigate human disease (Zuckerman & Martin, 2016). Current research has investigated the effects of comorbidity in the past, as numerous conditions provoke or are intricately linked to other conditions. Researchers such as Meyer (2016), for instance, warn against precise diagnoses of specific vitamin-related deficiencies in light of the ways that nutritional deficiency and metabolic disease can elicit similar osteological responses (or none at all) and the fact that these two conditions are often found together in human populations. Similarly, van Schaik (2018), Lockau and Atkinson (2018), and Brickley et al. (2020; and see Chapter 19 on metabolic and endocrine diseases, this volume) directly confront the limitations, complexities, and promise of evaluating the effects of comorbidity in the archaeological record. Alongside the concept of comorbidity, the theory of syndemics (synergistic epidemics) posits that the presence of two or more disease clusters within a population exacerbates the effects of conditions and intensifies disease burden. Researchers exploring paleosyndemics, such as Sattenspiel and Herring (2010), Robbins Schug and Halcrow (2022), and Larsen and Crespo (2022), offer new ways to interpret co-occurring diseases such as leprosy and plague epidemics in medieval Europe, or the relationship between mal- or undernutrition and infectious disease, or socio-economic oppression and chronic disease.

The complexity of the human disease experience has also been tackled head on by intricately weaving social theory into the discourse surrounding health and disease in the past; an approach often referred to as social bioarchaeology (Agarwal & Glencross, 2011, and see the series *Bioarcheology and Social Theory*, D. Martin, Series Editor, Springer). Here, humans are seen as active participants in all dimensions of their lives, throughout their life course, and not simply passive reactors to the world around them. The approach requires deep introspection on the part of researchers and reflexive thought on the limitations produced by the personal lens through which we see the world (Watkins, 2020). Although the ways in which social theories are now used to inform our understanding of past diseases are too vast to discuss in this short space, a few examples provide insight into the promise of these applications.

Through the lens of feminism and queer theory, for instance, scholars such as Geller (2008, 2009), Hollimon (2011), and Stone and Zimmer (Chapter 24 on issues of gender and agency, this volume) have explored how definitions (and thus preconceived notions) of sex and/or gender have led to distorted conclusions about variation in disease presence and susceptibility. Differences in pathological conditions noted between individuals deemed "female" or "male" do not verify the presence of division of labor, nor does the *a priori* assertion that division of labor was present uniformly lead to differences in disease experiences, especially when the estimation of "biological sex" is problematic (Klales, 2020) and evidence of disease rarely, if ever, are limited to a single group (e.g., Standen et al., 1997). Disability theories, too, inform paleopathology (see Chapter 25 on disability and impairment, this volume). As an example, the medical model of disability views physical change as a functional impairment. Paleopathologists noting morphological changes in bone often conclude that an individual's ability to 'function normally" was impacted, that the individual was productively limited, and was, in fact, *dis*abled. However, adopting the modern stigma-laden label of "disabled" for individuals in the past does the field of paleopathology a gross disservice. It obscures the potential to understand the nuanced ways that individuals and groups treated human variation in the past, which, in fact, may be far different than now (Marstellar et al., 2011; Tilley & Oxenham, 2011). Adopting a social, rather than medical model of disability, which views the concept of "disabled" as a social construct that varies between individuals, families, and communities (Oliver, 2013, and see Chapter 14 on congenital and developmental disorders, this volume), and is centered deeply in identity, has far greater potential to shed light on the presence and effects of disease on lives of individuals in the past (see Chapters 11 on osteobiographies and case studies, and 15 on tumors and neoplasm, this volume). Lastly, theories of violence, which often center on interpersonal aggression and the male predilection for the behavior (Pinker, 2012), have been replaced in paleopathology with a far less reductionist view that recognizes the cultural complexity and ranges of behavior (Martin & Harrod, 2015; Mosothwane, 2017; Tung, 2021), the varying participants (Redfern, 2006, Redfern & Roberts, 2019), and the insidious ways that social and economic power can lead to structural violence (Mant et al., 2021, and see Chapters 13 on trauma, 23 on infants and children, 26 on social marginalization, and 27 interpreting violence, this volume). In all, adoption of social theory into paleopathology has brought us far from our roots of hunting for the oldest or most severe case of a disease and has allowed us to hypothesize about causes, effects, transmission, and evolution of disease over time and space (see Chapters 20 on dental disease, 28 on evolutionary approaches, and 29 disease in the fossil record, this volume).

Looking Back and Moving Forward

Looking back as a way to move forward is a uniquely paleopathological approach that provides powerful perspectives on disease past, present, and future. Buikstra and Roberts (2012), for instance, in their volume *The Global History of Paleopathology: Pioneers and Prospects*, aggregate the perspectives of over 90 authors worldwide who provide biographies of key figures in the field, snapshots of work conducted across the globe, and future developments. The varied voices reflect both the roots and future of the discipline, with much work being conducted in the past and present by European, UK, and North American-trained scholars, but with a sensitivity to the imperative of broadening the scope and amplifying diverse voices. The edited volume *New Directions in Biocultural Anthropology* (Zuckerman & Martin, 2016) centers attention on the powerful biocultural model that informs us not only about health, disease, and diet, past and present, but also about identity, especially aligned with race, politics, violence, and inequity. Indeed, perspectives adapted from paleopathology contribute to our understanding of current issues and future outcomes. In Buikstra's (2019) edited volume, for instance, authors tackle essential contemporary issues, including the public's misinformed view of violence in the past and subsequent 'modern' attitudes (see Redfern & Fibiger, 2019, and Chapter 32 on paleopathology in the public eye, this volume), the continued trope that genetic data supports "races" as biological and absolute categories that explain differences in disease experience (see Stojanowski, 2019), the stance that gender is binary and sexuality heteronormative (see Geller, 2019), and that 'family' or 'kin' is singularly defined by biological relationship (see Johnson, 2019), to name a few.

In fact, paleopathologists have a great deal to say about our future. The biological and social effects of climate change can be viewed through an paleopathological lens. Nerlich and Lösch (2009), as well as Robbins Schug (2021) and Robbins Schug et al. (in press), offer many examples of groups that dealt with the consequences of and adapted to environmental change. There are myriad lessons to be learned as we navigate through climatic changes today. Similarly, epidemics are not new in human (or animal) populations (see Chapters 4 on epidemiology, and 31 on plagues and pandemics, this volume). Knowledge of their presence throughout history allows for modern predictions and offers insight into how disease spread can be mitigated (e.g., Fangerau, 2010; DeWitte, 2016; Galassi et al., 2020). Emerging and re-emerging diseases can also be evaluated with assistance from paleopathology. Barrett et al. (1998) and Roberts and Buikstra (2008) recognized that pathogens in the past, as well as now, rely on complex ecosystems that often center more on human behavior than human biology (and see Chapter 17 on mycobacterial infections, this volume). Altering the environment, human migration, maintaining close social connections, and effects of oppression and inequity can allow infrequent host/pathogen interactions to amplify and travel quickly. The complexity of human/animal interactions is equally essential to note, as the long evolutionary history of human and animal contact, along with modern human/animal associations, has influenced the paths of zoonotic infection (Bendry et al., 2019; Uhl et al., 2019; Bendry & Fournié, 2020; Littleton et al., 2022, and see Chapters 9 on parasitology, and 30 on faunal analyses, this volume). The ONE Health approach, or as Buikstra et al. suggest—taking a ONE Paleopathology approach (see Chapter 33 on the future in paleopathology, this volume), which advocates adopting an evolutionary perspective of disease that incorporates the complex interactions between the environment, all non-human organisms, and humans—has the potential to profoundly contribute to our understanding disease in the past, the present, and in the future.

Confronting and Deconstructing the Legacies of Colonialism and Racism

The undeniably colonial and racist roots of medicine and physical anthropology, and thus paleopathology, are essential legacies to confront if paleopathology is to truly move forward (Walker, 2000; Lambert, 2012). Arguably, these efforts are not new; they have simply been ignored or worse, forcibly marginalized (Blakey, 2020a, 2020b). The New York African Burial Ground Project, which formally began in 1991 (Blakey & Rankin-Hill, 2004, GSA, 2009), serves as an exemplar for inter- and transdisciplinary research, as well as for publically engaged bioarchaeology. The project modeled ways in which researchers from many disciplines and with varying approaches and voices could develop innovative and unified strategies to understand the lived experiences of enslaved Africans living in 17th and 18th-century New York City. The project also modeled how community engagement could positively influence paleopathological inquiry. Input from invested community members, more broadly defined than biologically related descendants, was actively sought prior to the commencement of scientific analysis. Questions posed by community members about their own past and the lives of those interred in the burial ground were as critical to explore as the often limited questions posed by most paleopathologists. For instance, rather than seeking to record the types of diseases present in the population, community members sought to understand ways in which individuals and the community adapted to and overcame extreme oppression. They sought to find a holistic understanding of the past, predicated by resilience and power (La Roche & Blakey, 1997). Projects such as the recent excavation and analysis of the colonial-era burials at Belen, New Mexico build on these foundations (Ralston, et al., 2022).

Efforts to confront issues of race, racism, and colonialism within bioarchaeology and paleopathology continue (see Chapter 21 on ethical considerations, this volume). Critical race theory and black feminist pedagogy, in particular, have cast a bright light on long-standing vestiges of colonialism and consequential inequities. Scholars such as Watkins (2020), Williams (2021), de la Cova (2020), Lans (2019, 2021), and Muller (2020) make clear how skeletal and anatomical collections used by bioarchaeologists and paleopathologists to create baseline data from which inference about the past can be made is deeply problematic. Individuals whose bodies make up most collections had neither the power nor option to consent. The social violence suffered in the past resonates to the present with the repeated use of their bodies within a system of privilege. However, it is essential to move beyond the recognition of historical and modern power dynamics toward praxis. How might we decolonize the collections and begin reparation? Candid and difficult conversations within paleopathological and bioarchaeological communities, supported by professional organizations such as the Paleopathology Association and the American Association of Biological Anthropologists, hopefully provide initial steps toward remediation. We have far to go.

The "Handbook of Paleopathology"

The intent of this volume is to provide readers with a snapshot of the field of paleopathology and fuel for discussion. The three parts tackle essential aspects of the discipline: methods and techniques that we use to understand the past; specific diseases and conditions frequently explored in skeletal and mummified remains; and theoretical approaches that profoundly influence our interpretations and conclusions. Although this organization appears intuitive, upon reading the chapters, it is evident that the rubrics are not discrete. Chapters centered on methods and techniques offer readers fundamental details alongside applications of their approach. Authors focusing on diseases and conditions dive into foundations upon which diagnoses are made and how diagnosis leads to interpretations and conclusions. Weaving this all together are authors who introduce ways in which biological and social theories place health and disease into greater context. In fact, the authors exemplify the holistic nature of our field. Human biology, health, and disease cannot be understood devoid of human culture, behavior, and the broader environment, and conversely, human culture, behavior, and the broader environment cannot be evaluated without considering the roles that human biology, health, and disease play, regardless of place or time.

An equally important aspect of this volume is the focus on deeply rooted biases and ethical concerns. Scientific inquiry is steeped in structural violence; the effects of which reverberate through many chapters in this volume. Chronicling the discipline's history and drawing attention to the pervasive roles of power and privilege in the production (and exaltation) of scientific knowledge does not remedy the perpetuation of inequity; it only exposes it. Contributors to this volume embody many identities and offer varied voices to begin the decolonization of our discipline. They encourage reflection and reflexivity. Understanding disease in the past requires recognition of the whole person and their complex environments. Our field is best served when multidisciplinary teams converge to address significant questions in a humanistic and contextually enriched manner. This is the future of paleopathology.

References

Agarwal, S. (2022). The legacy and disposability of brown bodies: the bioethics of skeletal anatomy collections from India. *American Journal of Biological Anthropology* 177(S73):2.

Agarwal, S. C. & Glencross, B. A. (2011). *Social Bioarchaeology*. Chichester: Wiley-Blackwell.

Alfonso, M. P. & Powell, J. (2006). Ethics of flesh and bone, or ethics in the practice of paleopathology, osteology, and bioarchaeology. In Cassman, V., Odegaard, N. & Powell, J. (Eds.), *Human Remains: Guide for Museums and Academic Institutions*, pp 5–20. Lanham, MD: AltaMira Press.

Anderson, J. G. (1969). *Studies in the Medieval Diagnosis of Leprosy in Denmark: An Osteological, Historical and Clinical Study*. Copenhagen: Costers Bogtrykkeri.

Anderson, J. G. (1982). The osteo-archaeological diagnosis of leprosy. In Haneveld, G. & Perizonius, W. (Eds.), *Proceedings of the Fourth European Meeting of the Paleopathology Association, Middelburg-Antwerpen*, pp. 221–226. Utrecht: BV Eleinkwijk.

Angel, J. L. (1981). History and development of paleopathology. *American Journal of Physical Anthropology* 56: 509–515.

Appleby, J., Thomas, R. & Buikstra, J. (2015). Increasing confidence in paleopathological diagnosis: application of the Istanbul terminological framework. *International Journal of Paleopathology* 8:19–21. https://doi.org/10.1016/j.ijpp.2014.07.003

Armelagos, G. J. & Van Gerven, D. P. (2003). A century of skeletal biology and paleopathology: contrasts, contradictions, and conflicts. *American Anthropologist* 105(1):51–62.

Audy, J.R. (1971). Measurement and diagnosis of health. In Shepard, P. (Ed.), *Environ/Mental: Essays on the Planet as a Home*, pp. 140–162. Boston, MA; Houghton, MI: Mifflin.

Aufderheide, A. C. & Rodríguez-Martin, C. (1998). *The Cambridge Encyclopedia of Human Paleopathology*. Cambridge: Cambridge University Press.

Baer, K. (1860). Die makrokephalen im boden der krym und österreichs, verglichen mit der bildungs-abweichung welche blumenbach macrocephalus genannt hat. *Memmories de l' Academy Imperial des Sciences de St. Petersburg* VII Serie. T. II. N6.

Barrett, R., Kuzawa, C., McDade, T. & Armelagos, G. (1998). Emerging and re-emerging infectious diseases: the third epidemiological transition. *Annual Review of Anthropology* 27:247–271.

Bendrey, R., Cassidy, J. P., Fournié, G., Merrett, D., Oakes, R. & Taylor, G. M. (2019). Approaching ancient disease from a One Health Perspective: interdisciplinary review for the investigation of zoonotic brucellosis. *International Journal of Osteoarchaeology* 30(1):99–108.

Bendrey, R. & Fournié, G. (2020). Zoonotic brucellosis from the long view: can the past contribute to the present? *Infection Control & Hospital Epidemiology* 42(4):505–506.

Binford, L. (1971). Mortuary Practices: their study and their potential. In Brown, J. A. (Ed.), *Approaches to the Social Dimensions of Mortuary Practices*, pp. 6–29. Washington, DC: Society for American Archaeology.

Binford, S. R. & Binford, L. (1968). *New Perspectives in Archaeology*. Chicago: Aldine Press.

Blakey, M. L. (2020a). Archaeology under the blinding light of race. *Current Anthropology* 61: 184–197.

Blakey, M. L. (2020b). Understanding racism in physical (biological) anthropology. *American Journal of Biological Anthropology* 175(2):316–325.

Blakey, M. & Rankin-Hill, L. (2004). *New York African Burial Ground: Skeletal Biology Report*. Department of Sociology and Anthropology, Washington, DC: Howard University.

Blakey, M. & Rankin-Hill, L. (2009). The skeletal biology of the New York African Burial Ground, Part I. In the US General Services Association, *The New York African Burial Ground: Unearthing the African Presence in Colonial New York, Volume 1*. Washington, DC: Howard University Press.

Brickley, M., Ives, R. & Mays, S. (2020). *The Bioarchaeology of Metabolic Bone Disease*. London: Academic Press.

Brickley, M. & McKinley, J. I. (2004). *Guidelines to the Standards for Recording Human Skeletal Remains*. IFA Paper No. 7. Southampton: BABAO and the Institute of Field Archaeologists.

Brothwell, D. & Sandison, A. T. (1967). Editorial prolegomenon: the present and future. In Brothwell, D. & Sandison, A.T. (Eds.), *Disease in Antiquity: A Survey of the Diseases, Injuries and Surgery of Early Populations*, pp. xi–xiv. Springfield, IL: Charles C. Thomas.

Buikstra J. E. (1977). Biocultural dimensions of archaeological study: a regional perspective. In Blakely, R.L. (Ed.), *Biocultural Adaptation in Prehistoric America*, pp. 67–84. Southern Anthropological Society Proceedings, No. 11. Athens, GA: University of Georgia Press.

Buikstra, J. E. (2010). Paleopathology: a contemporary perspective. In Larsen, C.S. (Ed.), *Companion to Biological Anthropology*, pp. 395–411. Chichester: Wiley–Blackwell.

Buikstra, J. E. (2016). Nomenclature in paleopathology. Accessed May 2022 at: https://paleopathology-association.wildapricot.org/resources/Documents/PPA%20Monographs/Nomenclature%20in%20Paleopathology.pdf.

Buikstra, J. E. (2019a). Knowing your audience: reactions to the human body, dead and undead. In Buikstra, J. E. (Ed.), *Bioarchaeologists Speak Out: Deep Time Perspectives on Contemporary Issues*, pp. 19–58. Cham, Switzerland: Springer.

Buikstra, J. E. (2019b). *Ortner's Identification of Pathological Conditions in Human Skeletal Remains*, 3rd Edition. London: Academic Press.

Buikstra, J. E. (2019c). *Bioarchaeologists Speak Out: Deep Time Perspectives on Contemporary Issues*. Cham: Springer.

Buikstra, J. E. & Beck, L. (2006). *Bioarchaeology: The Contextual Analysis of Human Remains*. San Diego, CA: Elsevier Inc.

Buikstra, J. E. & Cook, D. C. (1980). Palaeopathology: an American account. *Annual Reviews in Anthropology* 9:433–470.

Buikstra, J. E., Cook, D. C. & Bolhofner, K. L. (2017). Introduction: scientific rigor in paleopathology. *International Journal of Paleopathology* 19:80–87.

Buikstra, J. E. & Roberts, C. A. (2012). *The Global History of Paleopathology: Pioneers and Prospects*. Oxford: Oxford University Press.

Buikstra, J. E. & Ubelaker, D. H. (1994). *Standards for Data Collection from Human Skeletal Remains: Proceedings of a Seminar at The Field Museum of Natural History Organized by Jonathan Haas*. Research Series No. 44. Fayetteville: Arkansas Archaeological Survey.

Carrara, N., Scaggion, C. & Holland, E. (2018). The Tedeschi collection: a collection of documented and undocumented human skeletal remains at the museum of anthropology, Padua University (Italy). *American Journal of Physical Anthropology* 166(4):930–933.

Cunha, E., Lopez-Capp, T. T., Inojosa, R., Marques, S. R., Moraes, L. O. C., Liberti, E., … & Soriano, E. (2018). The Brazilian identified human osteological collections. *Forensic Science International* 289:449.e1–449.e6.

de la Cova, C. (2020). Making silenced voices speak: restoring neglected and ignored identities in anatomical collections. In Cheverko, C., Prince-Buitenhuys, J. & Hubbe, M. (Eds.), *Theoretical Approaches in Bioarchaeology*, pp. 150–169. New York: Routledge.

Dever, G. E. A. (1976). An epidemiological model for health policy analysis. *Social Indicators Research* 2(4): 453–466.

DeWitte, S. (2016). Archaeological evidence of epidemics can inform future epidemics. *Annual Review of Anthropology* 34:63–77.

Earle, T. K. & Preucel, R. W. (1987). Processual archaeology and the radical critique. *Current Anthropology* 28(4):501–538.

Esper, J. F. (1774). *Ausführliche Nachricht von Neuentdeckten Zoolithen Unbekannter Vierfüsiger Thiere, und Denen sie Enthaltenden, so Wie Verschiedenen Andern Denkwürdigen Grüften der Obergebürgischen Lande des Marggrafthums Bayreuth*. Nürnberg: Georg Wolfgang Knorr.

Fangerau, H. (2010). Paleopathology and the history of medicine: the example of influenza pandemics. *Der Urologe A* 49(11):1406–1410. DOI: 10.1007/s00120-010-2435-0

Ferreira, M. T., Coelho, C., Makhoul, C., Navega, D., Gonçalves, D., Cunha, E. & Curate, F. (2021). New data about the 21st century identified skeletal collection (University of Coimbra, Portugal). *International Journal of Legal Medicine* 135(3):1087–1094.

Galassi, F., Ingaliso, L. & Varotto, E. (2020). The Covid-19 pandemic as a communication responsibility and opportunity for paleopathology. *Paleopathology Newsletter* 91:13.

Geller, P. L. (2008). Conceiving sex: fomenting a feminist bioarchaeology. *Journal of Social Archaeology* 8(1):113–138.

Geller, P. L. (2009). Identity and difference: complicating gender in archaeology. *Annual Review of Anthropology* 38:65–81.

Geller, P. L. (2019). The fallacy of the transgender skeleton. In Buikstra, J. E. (Ed.), *Bioarchaeologists Speak Out: Deep Time Perspectives on Contemporary Issues*, pp. 231–242. Cham: Springer.

Goldfuss, G. A. (1810). *Die Umgebungen von Muggendorf. Ein Taschenbuch für Freunde der Natur und Alterthumskunde. Fränkische Schweiz*. Erlangen: Verlag Johann Jakob Palm.

Goodman, A. H. & Armelagos, G. J. (1989). Infant and childhood morbidity and mortality risks in archaeological populations. *World Archaeology* 21(2):225–243.

Goodman, A. H., Martin, D. L., Armelagos, G. J. & Clark, G. (1984). Indications of stress from bone and teeth. In Cohen, M. N. & Armelagos, G. J. (Eds.), *Paleopathology at the Origins of Agriculture*, pp. 13–44. New York: Academic Press.

Grauer, A. L. (2012). Introduction: the scope of paleopathology. In Grauer, A. L. (Ed.), *Companion to Paleopathology*, pp. 1–14. Chichester: Wiley-Blackwell.

Grauer, A. L. (2018). A century of paleopathology. *American Journal of Physical Anthropology* 165:904–914.

Grauer, A. L. (2023). Paleopathology. In Pollard, A. M., Armitage, R. A. & Makarewicz, C. (Eds.), *Handbook of Archaeological Sciences, Second Edition*, pp. 19–32. London: Wiley.

GSA (2009). *The New York African Burial Ground: Unearthing the African Presence in Colonial New York*. Washington DC: Howard University Press. https://www.gsa.gov/about-us/regions/welcome-to-the-northeast-caribbean-region-2/about-region-2/african-burial-ground/introduction-to-african-burial-ground-final-reports

Hackett, C. (1976). *Diagnostic Criteria of Syphilis, Yaws and Treponarid (Treponematoses) and of Some Other Diseases in Dry Bone: For Use in Osteo-Archaeology*. Berlin: Springer-Verlag.

Harris, R. & Rose, J. C. (1995). *Standardized Osteological Database (Computer Software)*. Fayetteville: Center for Advanced Spatial Technology, University of Arkansas.

Hodder, I. (1982). *Symbolic and Structural Archaeology*. Cambridge: Cambridge University Press.

Hollimon, S. E. (2011). Sex and gender in bioarchaeological research. In Agarwal, S. C. & Glencross, B. A. (Eds.), *Social Bioarchaeology*, pp. 312–332. Chichester: Wiley-Blackwell.

Hooton, E. A. (1930). *The Indians of Pecos Pueblo: A Study of their Skeletal Remains*. New Haven, CT: Yale University Press

Hrdlicka, A. (1908). *Physiological and Medical Observations Among the Indians of Southwestern United States and Northern Mexico*. Smithsonian Institution Bureau of American Ethnology Bulletin 34. Washington: Government Printing Office.

Hrdlička, A. (1914). *Anthropological Work in Peru in 1913, with Notes on the Pathology of the Ancient Peruvians*. Smithsonian Miscellaneous Collections Volume 21(number 18). Washington, DC: Smithsonian Institution.

Huss-Ashmore, R., Goodman, A. H. & Armelagos, G. J. (1982). Nutritional inference from paleopathology. *Advances in Archaeological Method and Theory* 5:395–474.

Jarcho, S. (1966). The development and present condition of human palaeopathology in the United States. In Jarcho, S. (Ed.), *Human Palaeopathology*, pp. 3–30. New Haven, CT: Yale University Press.

Johnson, K. (2019). Opening up the family tree: promoting more diverse and inclusive studies of family, kinship, and relatedness. In Buikstra, J. E. (Ed.), *Bioarchaeologists Speak Out: Deep Time Perspectives on Contemporary Issues*, pp. 201–230. Cham: Springer.

Kiyono, K. & Hoshijima, H. (1922). Paleopathology—particularly on the bone diseases of the ancient and indigenous Japanese. *Japanese Journal of Microbiology* 16:1–16.

Klales, A. (2020). *Sex Estimation of the Human Skeleton: History, Methods, and Emerging Techniques*. London: Academic Press.

Klaus, H. (2015). Paleopathological rigor and differential diagnosis: case studies involving terminology, description, and diagnostic frameworks for scurvy in skeletal remains. *International Journal of Paleopathology* 19:96–110.

Koganei, Y. (1894). *Beiträge zur physischen Anthropologie der Aino I. Untersuchungen am Skelet*. Mittheilungen aus der Medicinischen Facultät der Keiserlich-Japanischen Universität; II Band.

Koganei, Y. (1934). A study on the statistics of dental caries. *Journal of the Anthropological Society of Nippon* 49:331–353.

Lambert, P. (2012). Ethics and issues in the use of human skeletal remains in paleopathology. In Grauer, A. L. (Ed.), Companion to Paleopathology, pp. 17–33. New York: Wiley-Blackwell.

Lans, A. (2019). Black feminist science. *Anthropology News*. Accessed March 18, 2019 at: https://doi.org/10.1111/AN.1118

Lans, A. (2021). Decolonize this collection: integrating black feminism and art to re-examine human skeletal remains in museums. *Feminist Anthropology* 2:130–142.

La Roche, C. & Blakey, M. (1997). Seizing intellectual power: the dialogue at the New York African Burial ground. *Historical Archaeology* 31(3):84–106.

Larsen, C. S. & Crespo, F. (2022). Paleosyndemics: a bioarchaeological and biosocial approach to study infectious diseases in the past. *Centaurus* 64(1). DOI: 10.1484/J.CNT.5.130031

Lawler, D. F. (2017). Differential diagnosis in archaeology. *International Journal of Paleopathology* 19:119–123.

Lewis, M. E. & Roberts, C. A. (1997). Growing pains: the interpretation of stress indicators. *International Journal of Osteoarchaeology* 7:581–586.

Littleton, J., Karstens, S. & Busse, M. (2022). Human-animal interactions and infectious disease: a view for bioarchaeology. *Bioarchaeology International* 6(1–2):133–148.

Lockau, L. & Atkinson, S. (2018). Vitamin D's role in health and disease: how does the present inform our understanding of the past? *International Journal of Paleopathology* 23:6–14.

Mant, M., de la Cova, C. & Brickley, M. B. (2021). Intersectionality and trauma analysis in bioarchaeology. *American Journal of Physical Anthropology* 174(4): 583–594. https://doi.org/10.1002/ajpa.24226

Manchester, K., Ogden, A. & Storm, R. (2016) Nomenclature in palaeopathology. *Paleopathology Newsletter* 175.

Marsteller, S. J., Torres-Rouff, C. & Knüdson J. (2011). Pre-Columbian Andean sickness ideology and the social experience of leishmaniasis: a contextualized analysis of bioarchaeological and paleoathological data from San Pedro de Atacama, Chile. *International Journal of Paleopathology* 1: 24–34.

Martin, D. L. & Harrod, R. P. (2015). Bioarchaeological contributions to the study of violence. *American Journal of Physical Anthropology* 156(S59):116–145.

Mason, J. W. (1975). A historical overview of the stress field. *Journal of Human Stress* 1(1): 6–12, 1(2):22–36.

Mays, S. A. (2010). Human osteoarchaeology in the UK 2001–2007: a bibliometric perspective. *International Journal of Osteoarchaeology* 20:192–204.

Mays, S. A. (2020). A dual process model for paleopathology. *International Journal of Paleopathology* 31:89–96.

Meyer, A. (2016). Assessment of diet and recognition of nutritional deficiencies in paleopathological studies: A review. *Clinical Anatomy* 29(7):862–869

Miccichè, R., Carotenuto, G. & Sìneo, L. (2018). The utility of 3D medical imaging techniques for obtaining a reliable differential diagnosis of metastatic cancer in an iron age skull. *International Journal of Paleopathology* 21:41–46.

Mitchell, P. & Brickley, M. (2018). *Updated Guidelines to the Standards for Recording Human Remains*. Chartered Institute for Archaeologists. British Association for Biological Anthropology and Osteoarchaeology. https://www.babao.org.uk/assets/Uploads-to-Web/14-Updated-Guidelines-to-the-Standards-for-Recording-Human-Remains-digital.pdf

Møller-Christensen, V. (1961). *Bone Changes in Leprosy*. Copenhagen: Munksgaard.

Møller-Christensen, V. (1965). New knowledge of leprosy through palaeopathology. *International Journal of Leprosy* 33:603–610.

Moodie, R. L. (1923). *Paleopathology: An Introduction to the Study of Ancient Evidences of Disease*. Urbana: University of Illinois Press.

Morrone, A., Pagi, H., Tõrv, M. & Oras, E. (2021). Application of reflectance transformation imaging (RTI) to surface bone changes in paleopathology. *Anthropologischer Anzeiger; Bericht Uber die Biologisch-anthropologische Literatur* 78(4):295–315.

Mosothwane, M. (2017). The Osteological composition of the alleged victims of the xhosa cattle-killing saga from Edward street cemetery, King William's town, South Africa. *Journal of Conflict Archaeology* 12:163–176.

Mühlemann, B., Vinner, L., Margaryan, A., Wilhelmson, H., Castro, C., de la, F., Allentoft, M. E., ... & Sikora, M. (2020). Diverse variola virus (smallpox) strains were widespread in northern Europe in the viking age. *Science* 369(6502). https://doi.org/10.1126/science.aaw8977

Muller, J. L. (2020). Reflecting on a more inclusive historical bioarchaeology. *Historical Archaeology* 54:202–211.

Muller, J. L., Pearlstein, K. E. & de la Cova, C. (2017). Dissection and documented skeletal collections: embodiments of legalized inequality. In Nystrom, K. (Ed.), *The Bioarchaeology of Dissection and Autopsy in the United States*, pp.185–201. Cham, Switzerland: Springer.

Nerlich, A. G. & Lösch, S. (2009). Paleopathology of human tuberculosis and the potential role of climate. *Interdisciplinary Perspectives on Infectious Diseases* 2009: 437187. https://doi.org/10.1155/2009/437187

Nystrom, K. (2011). Postmortem examinations and the embodiment of inequality in 19th century United States. *International Journal of Paleopathology* 1(3–4), 164–172.

Nystrom, K. (2017). *The Bioarchaeology of Dissection and Autopsy in the United States*. Cham, Switzerland: Springer.

Öhrström, L., Bitzer, A., Walther, M. & Rühli, F. (2010). Technical note: terahertz imaging of ancient mummies and bone. *American Journal of Physical Anthropology* 142(3):497–500.

Oliver, M. (2013). The social model of disability: thirty years on. *Disability & Society* 28(7):1024–1026.

Orlando, L., Allaby, R., Skoglund, P., Sarkissian, S. D., Stockhammer, P., Ávila-Arcos, M., ... & Warinner, C. (2021). Ancient DNA analysis. *Nature Reviews Methods Primers* 1(14). https://doi.org/10.1038/s43586-020-00011-0

Ortner, D. J. (2012). Differential diagnosis and issue in disease classification. In Grauer, A. L. (Ed.), *A Companion to Paleopathology,* pp. 250–267. Chicester: Wiley-Blackwell.

Ortner, D. J. & Putschar, W. G. J. (1981). *Identification of Pathological Conditions in Human Skeletal Remains*. Smithsonian Contributions to Anthropology, No. 28. Washington: Smithsonian Institution Press.

Pinker, S. (2012). *The Better Angels of Our Nature: Why Violence Has Declined*. United Kingdom: Penguin Publishing Group.

Ralston, C., Stone, P. & Martin, D. (2022). Colonized bodies and descendent voices: collaborative narratives and learning to decolonize the past through bioarchaeological work in Belen, New Mexico. *American Journal of Biological Anthropology* 177(S73):149.

Rankin-Hill, L. (2016). Identifying the First African Baptist Church: Searching for historically invisible people. In Zuckerman, M. K. & Martin, D. L. (Eds.), *New Directions in Biocultural Anthropology*, pp. 133–156. Hoboken: Wiley-Blackwell.

Redfern, R. (2006). A bioarchaeological analysis of violence in iron age females: a perspective from Dorset, England (fourth century BC to the first century AD). In Davis, O., Sharples, N. M. & Waddington, K. (Eds.), *Changing Perspectives on the First Millennium BC: Proceedings of the Iron Age Research Student Seminar*, pp.139–160. Barnsley: Oxbow.

Redfern, R. & Fibiger, L. (2019). Bioarchaeological evidence for prehistoric violence: use and misuse in the popular media. In Buikstra, J. E. (Ed.*), Bioarchaeologists Speak Out: Deep Time Perspectives on Contemporary Issues*, pp. 59–78. Cham: Springer.

Redfern, R. & Roberts, C. (2019). Trauma. In Buikstra, J. (Ed.), *Ortner's Identification of Pathological Conditions in Human Skeletal Remains* (3rd ed.), pp. 78–90. London: Academic Press.

Robbins Schug, G. R. (2021). *The Routledge Handbook of the Bioarchaeology of Climate and Environmental Change*. New York: Routledge.

Robbins Schug, G. R. & Halcrow, S. E. (2022) Building a bioarchaeology of pandemic, epidemic, and syndemic diseases: lessons for understanding COVID-19. *Bioarchaeology International* 6(1–2):1–22.

Robbins Schug, G. W., Buikstra, J., DeWitte, S., Baker, B., Berger, E., Buzon, M., … & Zakrzewski, S. (Submitted manuscript). *Perspective: Climate Change, Human Health, and Challenges to Resilience in the Holocene*. PNAS.

Roberts, C. A. (2006). A view from afar: bioarchaeology in Britain. In Buikstra, J. E. & Beck, L. (Eds.), *Bioarchaeology: The Contextual Analysis of Human Remains*, pp. 417–439. San Diego, CA: Elsevier Inc.

Roberts, C. A. (2020). *Leprosy Past and Present*. Gainesville: University of Florida Press.

Roberts, C. A. & Buikstra, J. E. (2008). *The Bioarchaeology of Tuberculosis: A Global View on a Reemerging Disease*. Gainesville: University of Florida Press.

Roberts, C. A. & Connell, B. (2004). Guidance on recording palaeopathology. In Brickley, M. & McKinley, J. I. (Eds.), *Guidelines to the Standards for Recording Human Skeletal Remains*, pp. 34–39. IFA Paper No. 7. Southampton: BABAO and the Institute of Field Archaeologists.

Roberts, C. A. & Mays, S. (2011). Study and restudy of curated skeletal collections in bioarchaeology: A perspective on the UK and the implications for future curation of human remains. *International Journal of Osteoarchaeology* 21(5):626–630.

Rogers, J. & Waldron, T. (1995). *A Field Guide to Joint Disease in Archaeology*. New York: John Wiley & Sons, Inc.

Rose, J. C., Anton, S., Aufderheide, A., Buikstra, J. & Eisenberg, L. et al. (1994). *Association Skeletal Database Committee Recommendations*. Detroit: Paleopathology Association

Sandison, A. T. (1967). Sir Marc Armand Ruffer (1859–1917): pioneer of palaeopathology. *Medical History* 11(2):150–156.

Sappol, M. (2002). *A Traffic of Dead Bodies: Anatomy and Embodied Social Identity in Nineteenth-Century America*. Princeton: Princeton University Press.

Sattenspiel, L. & Herring, A. (2010). Emerging themes in anthropology and epidemiology: geographic spread, evolving pathogens, and syndemics. In Larsen, C. (Ed.), *A Companion to Bioarchaeology*, pp. 167–178. New York: Wiley

Saxe, A. A. (1970). *Social Dimensions of Mortuary Practices*. Ph.D. Dissertation, University of Michigan.

Schmerling, M. (1835). Description des ossements fossiles à l'état pathologique provenant des cavernes de la province de liège. *Bulletin des la Société Géologique de France* 7: 51–61.

Scorrano, G. (2018). The stable isotope method in human paleopathology and nutritional stress analysis. *Anthropology and Archaeology Open Access* 1(5). https://doi.org/10.31031/AAOA.2018.01.000523

Selye, H. (1957). *The Stress of Life*. London: Longmans, Green and Co.

Selye, H. (1973). The evolution of the stress concept. *American Scientist* 61: 692–699.

Shanks, M. & Tilley, C. (1982). Ideology, symbolic power and ritual communication: A reinterpretation of neolithic mortuary practices. In Hodder, I. (Ed.), *Symbolic and Structural Archaeology*, pp. 129–154. Cambridge: Cambridge University Press.

Standen, V., Bernardo, G., Arriaza, T. & Santoro, C. M. (1997). External auditory exostosis in prehistoric Chilean populations: a test of the cold water hypothesis. *American Journal of Physical Anthropology* 103:119–129.

Steinbock, R. T. (1976). *Paleopathological Diagnosis and Interpretation*. Springfield, IL: Charles C. Thomas.

Stojanowski, C. (2019). Ancient migrations: Biodistance, genetics, and the persistence of typological thinking. In Buikstra, J. E. (Ed.), *Bioarchaeologists Speak Out: Deep Time Perspectives on Contemporary Issues,* pp. 181–200. Cham: Springer.

Temple, D. & Goodman, A. (2014). Bioarchaeology has a "health" problem: conceptualizing "stress" and "health" in bioarchaeological research. *American Journal of Physical Anthropology* 155:186–191.

Tilley, L. & Oxenham, M. F. (2011). Survival against the odds: modeling the social implications of care provision to seriously disabled individuals. *International Journal of Paleopathology* 1: 35–42.

Toyne, J. M. & Turner, B. L. (2020). Linking isotope analysis and paleopathology: an Andean perspective. *International Journal of Paleopathology* 29:117–127.

Tung, T. A. (2021). Making and marking maleness and valorizing violence: a bioarchaeological analysis of embodiment in the Andean Past. *Current Anthropology* 62(S23):S125–S144. https://doi.org/10.1086/712305.

Uhl, E. W., Kelderhouse, C., Buikstra, J., Blick, J. P., Bolon, B. & Hogan, R. J. (2019). New world origin of canine distemper: interdisciplinary insights. *International Journal of Paleopathology* 24:266–278.

van Schaik, K., Vinichenko, D. & Rühli, F. (2014). Health is not always written in bone: using a modern comorbidity index to assess disease load in paleopathology. *American Journal of Physical Anthropology* 154(2):215–221.

Walker, P. (2000). Bioarchaeological ethics: a historical perspective on the value of human remains. In Katzenberg, M. A. & Saunders, S. R. (Eds.), *Biological Anthropology of the Human Skeleton*, pp. 3–40. New York: Wiley-Liss.

Watkins, R. (2018). Anatomical collections as the anthropological other: some considerations. In Stone, P. (Ed.), *Bioarchaeological Analyses and Bodies: Bioarchaeology and Social Theory*, pp. 27–47. Cham, Switzerland: Springer.

Watkins, R. (2020). An alter(ed)native perspective on historical bioarchaeology. *Historical Archaeology* 54:17–33.

Willey, G. R. & Phillips, P. (1958). *Method and Theory in American Archaeology*. Chicago: University of Chicago Press.

Williams, S. E. & Ross, A. H. (2021). Ethical dilemmas in skeletal collection utilization: implications of the black lives matter movement on the anatomical and anthropological sciences. *Anatomical Record* 305:860–868.

Zuckerman, M., Harper, K. & Armelagos, G. (2016). Adapt or die: three case studies in which the failure to adopt advances from other fields has compromised paleopathology. *International Journal of Osteoarchaeology* 26:375–383.

Zuckerman, M. & Martin, D. (2016). *New Directions in Biocultural Anthropology*. New York: Wiley-Blackwell.

PART I

Applications, Methods, and Techniques in Paleopathology

2
THE MACROSCOPIC STUDY OF HUMAN SKELETAL PALEOPATHOLOGY

Simon Mays

About 15 years ago, a colleague and I submitted a proposal for an edited volume on paleopathology (Pinhasi & Mays, 2008). In our "Analytical Approaches" section of the book, we had been careful to propose chapters on the various methods used in the examination of skeletal lesions, such as histology, radiography and CT-imaging. The publisher elicited comments from reviewers on our proposal, one of whom asked why we did not include a chapter on the role of macroscopic (i.e., naked-eye) examination of remains. The truth was that we had simply overlooked the need for such a thing. As this is the one approach that is universally applied, and has formed the foundation of paleopathological investigation since the dawn of our discipline, this might seem a surprising omission. Our first response was, naturally, to ask the reviewer to contribute such a chapter to our book (which she kindly did – Grauer, 2008). We then pondered why we had neglected to commission one in the first place. It is worth briefly recapitulating what we felt were the main reasons for this oversight because, given the continued paucity of discussions explicitly devoted to the role of macroscopy in paleopathology, it seems likely that they persist today.

Compared with techniques for examining skeletal lesions such as microscopy or medical imaging, the notion that a paleopathologist identifies and records the lesions seen with the naked eye seems so commonplace and obvious that we may not think of it as a "technique" at all. Second, because a process uses the naked eye, it is easy to assume that it is uncomplicated: provided that recording and description of lesions is done carefully and precisely, and that proper terminology is used, one might assume that there is little more to say on the matter. Third, there may be a tendency in science to equate progress with technical innovations in methods. Such innovations occur very rapidly in imaging and microscopy. It may be easy to fall into a trap of associating increased prominence of such techniques with a more "up-to-date" discipline; conversely, a reliance mainly or entirely on observing with the naked eye may seem unsophisticated and redolent of the past. Of course, these lines of reasoning were, and are, profoundly mistaken. In this chapter, I will emphasize the centrality of macroscopic examination of skeletal abnormalities to paleopathology, and that other techniques, such as medical imaging and microscopy, whilst clearly important, should normally be considered as playing secondary, supporting roles.

The primacy of macroscopy has shaped the development of paleopathology, both in terms of method and theory. We have originated, and over the years refined, dry bone criteria for the diagnosis of a wide variety of skeletal disorders. Being able to observe directly bone alterations means that we can identify lesions more reliably and describe their surface morphology in much finer detail in skeletal paleopathology than is possible in biomedical disciplines that are reliant upon imaging techniques such as radiography or CT. Standard clinical CTs produce image stacks with resolutions of approximately 0.5 mm (Waltenburger et al., 2021), so CT scans of surface bone lesions customarily provide crude renditions of what we can see in much finer detail with the naked eye (e.g., Lopez et al., 2017: Figures 2 and 3 vs. Figure 6D). When it comes to visualizing bone density changes, an alteration of about 40% is needed before lesions become visible radiographically (Ortner, 1991). Studies have repeatedly shown that many lesions that are readily apparent macroscopically are invisible radiographically (Rogers et al., 1990; Biehler-Gomez et al., 2019; van Schaik et al., 2019). Although imaging and microscopy of lesions obviously have vital roles to play in allowing visualization of features that cannot be seen with the naked eye, either because they are too small or because they are partially or entirely hidden within the bone, this does serve to emphasize that it is our ability to assess bony alterations using macroscopy that is probably the key methodological strength of our discipline.

The basis of paleopathology in macroscopy has some important higher-level theoretical implications. Advances in a discipline take place not just through advances in techniques, but through advances in theoretical frameworks. I have argued elsewhere that, in paleopathology, we have been slow to consider the epistemological frameworks that underpin our work and within which the identification of disease takes place (Mays, 2018a). This is in contrast to cognate disciplines. For example, in clinical sciences, explicit theoretical models have been applied to deconstruct the cognitive processes involved in diagnosing disease. Producing accurate theoretical models in this way potentially helps us to understand biases and limitations in our work, and may help us to improve our procedures, including how we impart skillsets in pedagogic settings (Mays, 2020). However, in order to do this successfully, we need to acknowledge the central role of macroscopy in paleopathology and explicitly define and understand its specific role in diagnosis in our discipline.

An alternative to "diagnostic paleopathology" instead simply focuses on lesions, using their frequency and/or severity as a general index of physiological stress in the sense originally formalized by Selye (reviewed by Bush, 1991 and Temple & Goodman, 2014). In this contribution, I examine the role of macroscopy in both diagnostic and 'stress indicator' approaches to paleopathology. The chapter is divided into two main parts. The first is a bibliometric study. The aim of this is to investigate the extent to which paleopathology relies on macroscopic study of remains alone, versus that to which macroscopy is supplemented by the two other main methods of examining pathological lesions: medical imaging techniques (radiography, CT) and microscopy (principally light microscopy and scanning electron microscopy). The second part of the work focuses upon the role of macroscopy at a theoretical and methodological level.

Bibliometric Analysis

Methods

This part of the work draws principally upon a subset of a large database assembled for the purposes of evaluating publication trends in osteoarchaeology since 2011 (Mays, 2021). The part of the data used here consists of all publications in the database published in the period 2011–2019[1] devoted specifically (N=773) or substantially (N=49) to paleopathology (these latter are either osteobiographic studies of single or some few skeletons or else general descriptive studies of larger groups; they include analysis of other osteological data in addition to information on pathology) where macroscopy is used alone or else is supplemented by imaging and/or microscopy. For this analysis, macroscopy is defined as gross examination of remains with the naked eye, perhaps augmented with low power magnification (e.g., through a hand lens) and/or with basic measurements using hand-held instruments (e.g., callipers). The 822 papers analyzed were drawn from nine international peer-reviewed journals: *International Journal of Paleopathology, American Journal of Physical Anthropology, Bioarchaeology International, International Journal of Osteoarchaeology, Journal of Archaeological Science, Journal of Archaeological Science Reports, Anthropological Science, Anthropologischer Anzeiger* and *Homo Journal of Comparative Human Biology*. Publications were classified into case, population, or methodological studies. This follows previous practice (Mays, 1997a, 2010, 2019), but briefly, case studies are those where the prime aim is the study of one or some few skeletons on an individual-by-individual basis. I also include osteobiographical studies within this classification. Although the aims of osteobiography differ from those of the paleopathological case study, the paleopathology component of an osteobiography bears similarities with a case study (Hosek & Robb, 2019), so for the current purposes they are not distinguished. Population studies are those where the aim is to shed light on disease in one or more earlier populations. Methodological studies involve developing paleopathological methods. The papers specifically devoted to paleopathology were additionally classified, following previous practice (Mays, 1997a, 2010, 2019), according to the principal class of disease upon which they are focused (arthropathy, congenital/developmental, dental disease, general (where the focus is on more than one type of disease), infection, metabolic disease, neoplastic disease, non-specific stress, trauma).

Although the main purpose of this section is to give an overall picture of recent practice, several specific hypotheses are also investigated. Given the increased availability and rapid technical advances that have taken place in both imaging and microscopy (Conlogue et al., 2020; Portier et al., 2020; Welsh et al., 2020), the hypothesis is tested that reliance on macroscopy alone has declined over time. As well as examining trends in that respect during the period 2011–2019, in order to extend the time depth for this particular part of the analysis, entries relating to publications mainly or principally concerned with paleopathology in a previously assembled bibliometric database (Mays, 1997a) were also studied. These publications (N=113) appeared in the period 1991–1995. In that original bibliometric work (Mays, 1997a), data on whether macroscopy was augmented with imaging and/or microscopic study of skeletal lesions was not collected, so these data were added to that database specifically for this part of the study (all other bibliometric analyses presented here relate solely to the much larger 2011–2019 data set). With regard to the extent to which different types of study rely on macroscopy alone, it was secondly hypothesized that given the relative rapidity of macroscopic study compared with imaging and microscopy, population-level studies would more frequently rely on macroscopy alone. Imaging and microscopy are of more value in some classes of disease than for others, and macroscopic recording protocols are regularly employed for some conditions but not for others (Mays, 2012a): the third hypothesis was that there would be an interaction between the reliance on macroscopy alone and the type of disease that was the focus of the work. Publications cannot be considered independent data points as required by inferential statistical tests. Nevertheless, such tests are applied, but only as a general aid to testing these hypotheses and to identifying other patterning in the data. Because of the non-independence of data points, levels of statistical significance will not be as great as test statistics suggest.

Results

The majority (428/822=52%) of publications during the period 2011–2019 relied on macroscopy alone. Over the period 2011–2019 (Figure 2.1), there was no time trend (Kolmogorov-Smirnov, Z=0.67, p=0.76) in this respect. There was also no time trend over the longer term:

the proportion reliant on macroscopy alone among the 1991–1995 publications was similar (60/113 = 53%).

Of the 394 publications where macroscopy was supplemented by other methods, in 276 this consisted of imaging the remains, in 72 this consisted of applying microscopy and in 46 publications both of these approaches were applied. More population than case studies relied on macroscopy alone (248/330=75% vs. 132/375=35%; chi-square=112.8, p<0.00001). There was a significant interaction (chi-square=56.3, p<0.00001) between the frequency with which studies relied on macroscopy alone and the type of pathology that was the focus of the work. Studies focusing on multiple diseases, arthropathies, non-specific stress, dental disease and trauma tended to rely on macroscopy alone more frequently than studies focusing on the other types of conditions (Table 2.1).

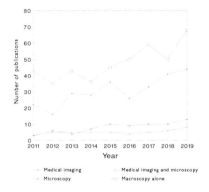

Figure 2.1 Numbers of publications in the bibliometric study mainly or solely directed at paleopathology using macroscopy as the sole means of studying skeletal lesions versus those that supplement macroscopy with medical imaging alone, microscopy alone or both medical imaging and microscopy. Data split by year of publication.

Table 2.1 Numbers of publications (2011–2019) devoted specifically to paleopathology that are reliant upon macroscopy alone, split by focus on different classes of pathology

	Disease class									
	General	Arthropathy	Non-specific stress	Dental	Trauma	Infection	Metabolic	Congenital	Neoplastic	Total
All publications										
Macroscopy alone	40 (66%)	37 (65%)	40 (62%)	65 (61%)	113 (57%)	44 (43%)	25 (38%)	23 (35%)	9 (18%)	396
Total	61	57	65	106	197	102	66	65	51	770
Population studies only										
Macroscopy alone	29 (91%)	17 (100%)	36 (82%)	58 (81%)	54 (71%)	17 (74%)	11 (41%)	–	–	222
Total	32	17	44	72	76	23	27			291

A small number of studies (N=3) do not fit into any of these categories and were omitted.
For population studies alone, figures for congenital and neoplastic disease are omitted because population studies focusing on these disease classes are few (three in each case).

Discussion

Of the three types of papers considered here, it is solely case studies where only a minority of publications are reliant upon macroscopy alone. The difference between case reports where only about one-third of publications rely on macroscopy alone, and population studies where this figure is approximately three-quarters, can be understood both in terms of differences in the specific nature of these two types of studies and in terms of the purpose of supplementing macroscopy with other means of study, which may differ somewhat between these two types of publication.

Case reports in paleopathology serve a number of purposes (Mays, 2012b). They may be used to shed light on the history of particular diseases or on medico-historical debates concerning the geographic spread or distribution of diseases in the past. They are widely used to present cases of conditions not well-described in more general works, and to present differential diagnosis, a procedure that is not usually covered in detail in laboratory manuals. Case reports, and most population studies, have a common need for accurate diagnosis. Augmentation of macroscopic observation with imaging/microscopy is used for that purpose in both types of study. However, given the aims of the case report, they are naturally more often directed at the less well-studied conditions that present more diagnostic difficulties, rather than at those that are readily identified by existing macroscopic standards. For example, among the papers directed at arthropathies, all the population studies in the bibliometric survey relied on macroscopy alone (Table 2.1). These were principally studies of osteoarthritis (e.g., Domett et al., 2017; Becker, 2019), for which there are standard diagnostic protocols based on macroscopic changes (e.g., Rogers & Waldron, 1995). Case reports in arthropathies less often rely on macroscopy alone (5/21=24%). A factor here is that these tend to concentrate on the rarer forms of arthritis – erosive arthropathies (e.g., Tesi et al., 2019) or other forms of joint disease (e.g., Manzon et al., 2017) – that require careful differential diagnosis for which the radiological appearance is often critical.

There are also differences between case studies and population studies in the way in which macroscopy is supplemented by other techniques. Although in each type of publication, imaging is more frequently applied than microscopy as a supplementary technique, this pattern is more marked in case reports than in population studies: among the former where macroscopy is supplemented by other methods 223/240=93% apply imaging compared with 55/74=74% of the latter, p=<0.001 by chi-square (diagnostic paleopathology only, i.e., excludes stress indicator studies). The purpose of supplementing macroscopy in case reports may be partly for purposes of describing the case rather than being strictly necessary for diagnostic purposes. Imaging, particularly CT imaging, is suited to this, as it enables morphology of lesions extending into the internal structure of bone to be shown more fully than is possible using photographic record of macroscopic alterations. Although these images may not have a decisive bearing on the diagnosis, it may help to give a reader a more detailed and thorough view of the pathological alterations present, which is likely to be helpful should they encounter similar cases. (An example of this is the CT scan in the study of dwarfism by Slon et al. (2013), which gives a usefully detailed view of cranial morphology that photography could not adequately capture.) There may also be other factors in the increased augmentation of macroscopy with imaging in case reports over population studies. Where case reports identify cases of disease from particularly early time periods, or cases that might challenge received wisdom in medico-historical debates, there may be a perceived need to demonstrate that the remains have been thoroughly evaluated in anticipation that the validity of a diagnosis might be questioned.

Although the case study clearly has a value in paleopathology, they are cited less often than other types of publications (Mays, 2012b). Quantitative, hypothesis-driven research is the hallmark of scientific endeavor, so commentators have argued that the capacity of the case report to advance the discipline is rather limited and that population studies have the potential to make a more substantial contribution (Armelagos & van Gerven, 2003; Roberts, 2006; Rühli et al., 2016). Three out of every four publications in the bibliometric survey in this, more important area of applied research, were dependent upon unaided macroscopy. This emphasizes the centrality of macroscopy in paleopathological endeavor. Application of macroscopic criteria for lesion recording and disease identification enables greater rapidity of data gathering. This facilitates study of large numbers of skeletons helping to enable sufficient statistical power to adequately test hypotheses. Application of macroscopy is also well suited to studies by researchers traveling between collections held in disparate locations. This sort of large-scale study is becoming increasingly common in some areas of the discipline to investigate eco-geographic distribution of disease in the past. Examples include the study of vitamin D deficiency in Europe (Mays et al., 2018; Veselka et al., 2021), dental disease in South America (Menéndez, 2016), and indicators of stress or "health" on a global scale (Steckel & Rose, 2002; Steckel et al., 2018).

The centrality of macroscopy is reflected in other types of publications as well. Laboratory manuals of paleopathology have long taken the form of atlases illustrating the skeletal changes wrought by various diseases. They have consistently included radiological images and histological slides alongside macroscopic images of diseased remains. In more recent texts, CT scans have become more numerous relative to plain film radiographs (although the latter still predominate), and in the realm of microscopy, we are starting to see more scanning electron micrographs rather than light microscope slides. What has not changed, however, is that the texts are dominated by macroscopic illustrations of dry bones (compare early texts such as Steinbock, 1976, Ortner & Putschar, 1985 with Lewis, 2018, Buikstra, 2019). This predominance of images of dry bones is likely to continue as existing macroscopic diagnostic criteria are refined and updated (for example, for various metabolic diseases – summarized in Brickley et al., 2020) and new ones continue to be developed, for diagnostic purposes (for example, for malaria – Smith-Guzman, 2015), or for facilitating accurate quantification of lesion prevalence (e.g., Davies-Barrett et al., 2019).

The ability of population studies to place a high reliance on macroscopy alone is facilitated by the development of dry bone diagnostic criteria for the more common specific diseases and for the identification of commonly used non-specific indicators of stress. The only exception to the pattern whereby population studies normally rely on macroscopy alone is for metabolic disease (Table 2.1). Here the low proportion of unaugmented macroscopy studies is largely due to works on osteoporosis. Osteoporosis produces no diagnostic gross lesions; radiological or microscopic study is essential to identify the loss of bone mass or microstructural integrity that characterize the condition (Beauchesne & Agarwal, 2014; Curate & Tavares, 2018). Studies of neoplastic and congenital disease also rarely use macroscopy unaided (Table 2.1). This may reflect the fact that these are rare conditions that are most usually described in case reports, and that in these classes of disease augmenting macroscopy with imaging in particular, aids diagnosis. For neoplasms, this helps in distinguishing among the various different types (Brothwell, 2008; Ragsdale et al., 2018), and for congenital conditions for fully describing changes in syndromic conditions and for distinguishing changes of congenital origin from those stemming from other causes (e.g., bony ankylosis due to infection/trauma) (e.g., Rivollat et al., 2014; Marchewka et al., 2017).

The Role of Macroscopy in the Diagnostic Process

Traditionally, in paleopathology, it has been said that the diagnostic process begins with a systematic recording of lesions, followed by differential diagnosis. However, it has recently been pointed out (Mays, 2020) that this is probably not an accurate representation of the way we actually work. Recording of lesions is not a passive process conducted by minds empty of diagnostic thoughts, but rather it is part of a more complex process of testing diagnostic hypotheses. The diagnostic process in paleopathology has been understood using a particular theoretical approach – a dual process model (DPM) (Mays, 2020). DPM is also a useful tool for helping us to understand the role of macroscopy in this process.

DPMs recognize that human cognition is a result of both Type 1 (intuitive) and Type 2 (analytical) thought processes. Type 1 processes are effortless recognition of objects or situations as of a type that have been encountered previously. In an osteological context, an example would be recognition of a bone as a femur or a humerus. Type 2 processes are slower, reflective and effortful. The application of specific procedural approaches in order to arrive at conclusions based on evidence, such as hypothesis testing in science, are Type 2 processes. DPMs have been useful in deconstructing the processes involved in clinical diagnosis. Like clinical diagnosis, paleopathological diagnosis results from a combination of Type 1 and Type 2 processes. Although the precise rubric followed in diagnosis will vary from cases to case (depending, *inter alia*, upon the nature and complexity of the condition (Mays, 2020)), a formal model, applicable in less routine cases, together with a worked example, is reproduced in Table 2.2.

In essence, the first step in diagnosis is the generation of a diagnostic hypothesis or hypotheses. These generally spring to mind, via Type 1, intuitive processes, upon initial, macroscopic examination of the skeleton. There is a close analogy with a physician who forms diagnostic hypotheses in the first stages of a clinical encounter with a patient. In the mind of an experienced clinician, diseases are represented as "illness scripts" – knowledge structures in memory relating to particular illnesses. They provide a link between observations made in a patient and particular diseases. Similarly, provisional diagnoses spring to mind for the paleopathologist upon initial macroscopic examination of the skeleton by the activation of "skeletal disease scripts", knowledge structures in memory relating macroscopic skeletal changes to particular diseases (Mays, 2020). In humans, visual pattern recognition is an especially rapid process. In clinical practice, the generation of diagnostic hypotheses occurs

Table 2.2 A dual process model of paleopathological diagnosis

Step	Principal DPM mode	Actions	Example
STEP 1	Type 1	Gestalt view of skeleton results in activation of skeletal disease scripts and hypothesized diagnosis or preferred diagnosis plus differentials	Adult female skeleton, ca. 75% complete. Lytic lesions on 6th and 7th thoracic vertebrae; periostitis 6th and 7th rib heads. Diagnostic hypothesis: tuberculosis
STEP 2	Type 2	Add (further) differential diagnoses using literature (e.g., from case studies of skeletons with the same diagnosis as the hypothesized diagnosis in this case, lab manuals)	Differential diagnoses (in perceived rank order of likelihood after tuberculosis): Brucellosis Mycoses Pyogenic osteomyelitis Metastatic cancer

(Continued)

Step	Principal DPM mode	Actions	Example
STEP 3	Type 2	Systematically record lesions in skeleton that are relevant to investigating the competing diagnoses. During this process further script activation may occur and further relevant lesions may be discovered. These may also occur if imaging/microscopic studies are conducted. Procedures during recording of lesions might include (i) Searching specifically for evidence that might undermine one's favored hypothesis (ii) Ignoring lesions that are not a feature of any of the differential diagnoses but indicate co-existing conditions	A further lesion, periosteal new bone on a fragment of the body of a scapula, was discovered. No new diagnostic hypotheses occurred. No imaging or microscopic studies were thought necessary (i) Bones were closely examined for the presence of endosteal fiber bone in trabecular elements; none was found. Had it been present, this would have countermanded the leading hypothesis (tuberculosis) and the other infectious disease differential diagnoses but would potentially have been consistent with metastatic cancer (Mays et al., 1996). (ii) Porotic hyperostosis of the orbital roofs was present. This was ignored for the current diagnostic purposes as it is not a feature of any of the differential diagnoses and has a very different pathophysiology (Brickley et al., 2020: 35–38).
STEP 4	Type 2	Conduct systematic differential diagnosis, drawing on both comparative and biological approaches (Mays, 2018a) as described in the literature (e.g., Klaus & Lynnerup, 2019)	Differential diagnosis suggested the most likely option was tuberculosis. This was subsequently supported by aDNA analysis which indicated the presence of *M. tuberculosis*.

This table reproduced from Mays, 2020: Table 1.

especially readily and rapidly in subdisciplines such as dermatology, where gross appearance of lesions is of particular importance diagnostically (Lowenstein et al., 2019). The primacy of macroscopy in paleopathology means that the activation of skeletal disease scripts occurs with similar facility and rapidity when skeletal remains are examined. Following the second step in Table 2.2, in which further diagnostic hypotheses are added using the literature, there then follows a third step of data gathering. It is at this stage that there is systematic macroscopic recording of lesions. The lesions to be recorded should be those relevant to testing the hypotheses generated in steps 1 and 2. Because skeletons often show alterations that are the result of more than one condition, simply listing all lesions unguided by any diagnostic hypotheses would result in an incoherent list of features that could not be meaningfully combined into a diagnostic framework. Explicitly tying the recording of lesions to testing diagnostic hypotheses prevents this (Mays, 2020). Again, this approach echoes that in clinical practice where the gathering of signs and symptoms from the patient is structured according the diagnostic hypotheses in the mind of the physician (Monteiro & Norman, 2013; Mamede & Schmidt, 2017). It is at this stage in the process that decisions will be made as to whether medical imaging and microscopy of lesions will be used to augment macroscopic observation.

It is clearly impossible to conduct imaging or microscopic studies of every skeleton in a collection, nor of every bone in every skeleton that is pathological. In a diagnostic context, these techniques need to be applied in a selective, purposive manner to help test diagnostic hypotheses. Knowledge of the diseases identified as possible diagnoses will indicate how likely it is that imaging and/or microscopy of lesions already identified macroscopically and/or other skeletal parts will be helpful for differential diagnosis. It is thus the results of macroscopy that determine if and how these supplementary methods will be applied. Three examples help to illustrate this. An adult male skeleton from Wharram Percy showed fine-grained subperiosteal deposits of new bone on multiple skeletal elements, together with fine cortical pitting (Mays et al., 1996). Macroscopic study of post-depositional breaks showed fiber bone deposition in some trabecular bone elements and in the medullary cavities of some long-bones. Among the hypothesized diagnoses was metastatic carcinoma. In metastatic cancer, metastases are most frequent in the axial skeleton and are rare in the distal parts of the appendicular skeleton (Lipton & Vigorita, 2015). Therefore, to help evaluate this diagnostic hypothesis, the skeletal remains were fully radiographed in order to provide an overall picture of the distribution of endosteal alterations. In another case from Wharram Percy, detailed in Table 2.2, metastatic cancer was considered as a differential diagnosis. It was noted that the presence of endosteal fiber bone would have argued in favor of that option, but this change was absent on macroscopic inspection at the numerous post-depositional breaks in the remains. This, together with the morphology of the vertebral and rib lesions, made it an unlikely diagnosis. So, macroscopy led to the judgment that radiography or other imaging was unnecessary. In some skeletons from a 19th-century hospital site in The Netherlands, macroscopic changes suggestive of osteomalacia were present, but firm diagnosis required microscopic study of a bone sample to verify defective mineralization at the microstructural level. In that instance (van der Merwe et al., 2018), the nature of the diagnosis hypothesized on the basis of macroscopy meant that the expected microstructural alterations would be systemic, so there was no need to sample from lesions. Any elements with high trabecular bone contents, such as ribs, would form good targets (van der Merwe et al., 2018).

The Macroscopic Identification of Pseudopathology

Taphonomic damage is ubiquitous in archaeological skeletal remains. Whether diagnostic or stress-indicator based, a preliminary step in any paleopathological analysis is to distinguish in vivo lesions from post-depositional damage. Fundamentally, the only way in which bone can respond to disease is by removal or formation of bone. Very occasionally, it may be questionable whether a deposit is bone or calcified soft tissue, or whether it is of post-depositional origin (e.g., Flohr et al., 2014; Cook & Patrick, 2014), but generally the problem is distinguishing holes or breaks in bone that represent disease or injury from taphonomic damage. In practice, making this distinction in skeletal remains almost always relies on macroscopy.

In distinguishing lytic lesions from taphonomic damage, it is the macroscopic morphology of the margins that is key. Taphonomic defects tend to have rather irregular, ragged edges. In vivo lesions usually, but not invariably, tend to be more regular in morphology and even if there is no visible new bone production, the margins are usually to a greater or lesser extent, remodeled. These effects are most pronounced in slow growing lesions and are least when bone destruction is rapid. Lesion margins comprised of cortical bone indicate very slow growing or quiescent lesions; well-remodeled trabecular bone may suggest a more

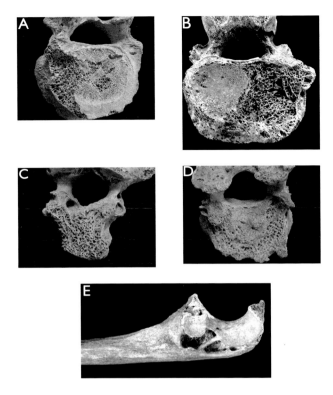

Figure 2.2 Macroscopic appearance of taphonomic damage versus lytic in vivo lesions in various states of remodeling. (a) Taphonomic defect in a vertebral body exposing ragged, unremodeled trabecular bone. (b–e) In vivo lytic lesions showing progressively greater degrees of remodeling. (b). Slight thickening of trabecular elements indicate that the cavity on the right side of the inferior surface of the vertebral body is of in vivo not taphonomic origin. (c) Trabecular elements on the surface of this vertebral body are thicker than in (b), indicating greater remodeling. (d) There is partial cortication of the surface on this vertebral body. (e) In this ulna, the margins of the lytic lesion in the proximal metaphysis are fully corticated. A likely explanation of the differing states of the bone surfaces in sequence (b–e) is that they lay at the margins of progressively slower expanding abscesses or other soft tissue lesions; alternatively each may have been an initially rapidly expanding soft tissue lesion which subsequently became quiescent and the different extents of remodeling arose due to differences in elapsed time between lesion quiescence and death permitting different degrees of consolidation of bony margins. Specimens in (b) – (e) each come from a burial where tuberculosis was diagnosed on the basis of the pictured lesions and from alterations elsewhere in the skeleton. (b) and (e) are from burials 0459 and 2127 from 11th century AD School Street, Ipswich, England (Mays, 1989), and (c) and (d) are from burial G438 (11th–12th century AD) from Wharram Percy (Mays, 2007).

rapidly expanding area of destruction, and minimally remodeled trabecular margins indicate a still more aggressive lesion (Figure 2.2).

It is usually rapidly progressing osteolytic lesions that initiated just prior to death, such as those that occur in malignant cancers that tend to present the most problems in recognition. Examples of such lesions exist in anatomical collections in individuals documented to have died of cancer. If similar lesions were found in archaeological remains, distinguishing them from post-depositional defects might be challenging, particularly if they were overlain with taphonomic damage (e.g., Klaus & Lynnerup, 2019: Figure 5.2). Occasionally, other types of lytic lesions may also resemble taphonomic damage. Soil erosion may sometimes produce defects with smooth edges that may imitate remodeled margins. There may be a close resemblance, for example, between cranial vault destruction due to treponemal disease and taphonomic damage (e.g., Rao et al., 1996: Figures 2–4; Lopez et al., 2017: Figures 2–4). Nevertheless, with a little experience, true lytic lesions tend to "jump out" at one from within the myriad taphonomic defects that characterize archaeological skeletal remains. Distinguishing true from pseudopathology by eye becomes largely an intuitive (Type 1 in DPM terms) process. Rarely is more detailed consideration of a lesion needed to determine this.

Perhaps reflecting the rapidity with which pseudopathology is eliminated by the experienced eye (and the fact that doubtful cases do not reach publication), most publications in paleopathology make no mention of this stage in the work, on the basis that it would be tedious and unnecessary in most cases to describe this step.[2] However, occasionally it is considered. Micarelli et al. (2019) discuss it as a preliminary stage in their cataloguing of lytic lesions in a skeleton that they eventually ascribe to mycotic infection. More often, those publications that do discuss pseudopathology consider it as a differential diagnosis, after they have described the alterations in the remains. Lieverse et al. (2014) and Klaus (2018) do this for remains showing lytic changes those authors concluded were due to metastatic cancer, as does Klaus (2017) for two skeletons with pitting he subsequently inferred was due to scurvy, and Lopez et al. (2017) for cranial defects in an individual who they felt had treponemal disease.

Although it may be convenient within the case study publication format to cover the topic of pseudopathology in the discussion of differential diagnosis, this is not indicative of how this stage of work slots into the diagnostic process in the laboratory. For one thing, whether a hole or other cavity in bone is a true lesion or not is generally something that is obvious from the start, rather than something that remains to be resolved once one has got to the differential diagnosis stage. Second, identifying true lesions from taphonomic damage is something that is carried out on a lesion-by-lesion basis, whereas differential diagnosis is something that considers the relevant skeletal changes as a whole.

Referring to the case example in Table 2.2, the identification of the vertebral lesions that are the prime alterations we wish to interpret, as true lesions rather than taphonomic damage was a Type 1 identification (in DPM terms) that occurred in Step 1 – in other words, there was instantaneous macroscopic recognition that they were not taphonomic. Exclusion of taphonomic origin thus occurred even prior to the activation of the skeletal disease script for tuberculosis. Confirmation that no further lytic lesions existed (i.e., that all remaining defects were post-depositional) occurred, again rapidly by Type 1 processes, as the skeleton was examined systematically in Step 3, so that by the time the formal differential diagnosis was instituted (Step 4) the question of pseudopathology had already been dealt with.

Macroscopy in Stress Indicator Paleopathology

In the bibliometric survey, the overwhelming majority of stress indicator studies focused on one or more of the following: porotic hyperostosis (PH, usually in the orbital roofs but sometimes also in the cranial vault), subperiosteal new bone deposits (PNB), or dental enamel hypoplasia (DEH). These occur frequently in many skeletal collections, facilitating statistical analyses. Stress indicators are generally studied using macroscopy alone (Table 2.1).

Because PNB and PH are surface alterations, macroscopy is well suited for their recognition in skeletal remains. For PH (and for porotic bony alterations in general), care needs to be taken in distinguishing normal from abnormal porosity. Careful evaluation of pore morphology, in some instances coupled with morphological comparison with normal individuals of similar ages, may be needed, especially in the young whose bones are often rather porous. In the very young, care is also needed in the identification of abnormal PNB, as layers of periosteal new bone formation may be normal findings in individuals in the first months of life (Brickley et al., 2020: 54–55), and apposition of bone in normal growth of infants and young children macroscopically resembles the woven bone deposited in response to disease (Lewis, 2018: 132). Many studies that use subperiosteal new bone as a stress indicator fail to specify how they deal with this problem. Others offer a range of solutions, for example, limiting study to adolescents and adults (Davies-Barrett et al., 2019), excluding perinates and infants (Rohnbogner & Lewis, 2017), including all ages from birth onwards but only considering lesions in the middle third of the diaphysis (Wheeler, 2012), or making case-by-case judgmental decisions in young individuals (Novak et al., 2017).

Although the state of remodeling of both lytic and proliferative lesions may vary considerably within a particular disease (e.g., Figure 2.2), it may nevertheless have diagnostic relevance, potentially helping to distinguish conditions that are characteristically rapidly progressing and aggressive, such as cancers, from those where lesions may be slower developing. Identification of bone lesions as active or inactive (remodeled) at death is potentially important, as it enables us to infer whether the disease that caused the lesion was present at the death of the individual (and, depending upon the condition, may be implicated in cause of death) or whether the lesion represents a relic of an earlier disease episode from which the individual recovered. This is beginning to assume increased prominence in some population studies of specific diseases – for example, vitamin D deficiency (e.g., Mays et al., 2006; Watts & Valme, 2018) – in order to investigate age profiles in disease occurrence. In stress indicator or other studies, where no close diagnosis is attempted, study of active versus healed lesions has been used to shed light on questions concerning the relative ability of different populations, or subsections of a single population, to survive and recover from episodes of disease (e.g., Mays, 1997b; DeWitte, 2014; Pinhasi et al., 2014).

Distinguishing active from inactive lesions in PNB or PH is reliant on their macroscopic appearance. For proliferative lesions, woven bone indicates bone actively depositing at time of death. Woven bone is readily distinguished macroscopically by its finely porous appearance. Lamellar bone indicates a lesion that was no longer depositing bone at time of death. Lamellar bone deposits are more coarsely pitted/striated, and pits have rounded, remodeled edges (Weston, 2008). The distinction between active and inactive PNB thus has a firm basis in pathophysiology. For PH, distinctions used by most authors can be traced back to a publication by Mensforth et al. (1978). Assuming, as was common at that time, that anemia was the cause of lesions, they associated pores with sharp margins with active lesions, whereas remodeled lesions were associated with loss of smaller pores, together with rounding of the margins of pores that remained. However, since that publication, there has been recognition that porosity of the orbital roofs and cranial vault may arise due to a variety of different causes. These include rickets and scurvy, where it occurs due to different pathophysiological mechanisms (Mays, 2018b; Brickley et al., 2020: 35–37). In vitamin D deficiency, it arises as a result of deficient mineralization of the growing bone surface, in scurvy as a result of deposition of porous new bone and/or vascular inflammatory response; versus diploic hyperplasia coupled with resorption of overlying cortical bone in anemia. The biological basis for imposition of a single standard for distinguishing active from healed porous lesions is therefore unclear and potentially problematic.

DEH and PH occur in specific areas of the skeleton, potentially speeding data capture as only those parts need to be examined for lesions. PNB, on the other hand, can potentially occur anywhere on the skeleton, but data capture can be streamlined if lesions are sought only in specific skeletal elements. For example, some workers have sought PNB solely on the tibia (e.g., DeWitte, 2014; Judd et al., 2018; Yaussy et al., 2019), with the rationale that this is a robust bone that survives regularly in ancient remains, and that in most populations it is the element that most frequently shows PNB (Larsen, 2015: 88). As well as increasing the efficiency of data capture, this strategy helps maintain sample size and enables clear criteria for entry of a skeleton into a study to be defined, aiding calculations of prevalence rates.

When macroscopy is augmented by other methods in stress indicator studies, this usually involves studies of DEH where microscopy is used to help evaluate defects. For DEH work, macroscopic recording has the familiar benefits of facilitating examination of large samples with the greater statistical power that this confers. However, microscopy offers a number of advantages. It is a more objective way of recording defects; it allows much smaller defects to be identified with confidence; it permits more accurate estimates of the timing of formation of DEH; it mitigates the biasing effects of differential visibility of defects in different parts of the tooth and in different teeth have on interpreting age-at-insult data; it also enables the duration of the event that produced the defect to be estimated (Hillson, 2014, 2019).

As regards DEH, macroscopy is suited to producing small amounts of data about larger numbers of individuals; microscopy provides larger amounts of data, but given its more time-consuming and sometimes destructive nature, perhaps from smaller numbers of skeletons. Selective application of microscopy to a subsample of cases, when limitations on resources, permissions for destructive analyses or other constraints apply, is one way of resolving this tension between approaches. For example, Temple et al. (2013) found that frequency of macroscopic DEH was greater among early hunter gatherers from Japan than among those from Alaska. Out of that study group of 113, they were able to conduct a microscopic analysis of teeth from 35 individuals, which showed that despite having an overall lower prevalence of macroscopic defects, the duration of the insults that produced defects was about 40 days in the Alaskans, twice as long as in the Japanese. Putting these results together they suggested that the Alaskans may have suffered from longer duration, seasonal nutritional problems with few fall-back options owing to the nature of their environment. The Japanese likely had a more diverse resource base so that even though food insecurities were frequent, the greater range of fall-back foods meant that seasonal and other food insecurities may have been relatively brief. Coupling the coarse-grained data from the macroscopic work with the finer grained information from the microscopic study enabled a more nuanced understanding of subsistence differences between these two groups of Pacific Rim hunter gatherers.

Presenting the Results of Macroscopic Observation: Description and Images

Careful description of lesion location and morphology, coupled with a good skeletal inventory, is essential in paleopathology (Grauer, 2008). A skeletal diagram showing the elements preserved, as well as those that are diseased is often a good way of conveying this information. In description, the proper use of terminology is key (e.g., Ortner & Putschar, 1985: 36; Ragsdale, 1992; Buikstra & Ubelaker, 1994; Lovell, 2000; Ortner, 2012; Buikstra, et al., 2017). Following long debate, best practice as regards descriptive terminology for macroscopic observations has recently been published by the Paleopathology Association (Manchester et al., 2017).

Although correct terminology in description is important, because of the visual nature of paleopathology, images rather than words are perhaps even more vital in presenting lesions. Traditional photography is well-suited to conveying the fine morphological detail that is so often pivotal to lesion interpretation. In laboratory manuals, images are important because they are key to the comparative approach to diagnosis in which morphology of alterations in known cases of disease are used to help identify disease from lesions in unknown archaeological skeletons (Mays, 2018a). Aspects of lesions other than the purely diagnostic, such as whether they are likely to be active or inactive at death, are also best conveyed using images. It would be impossible to prepare a laboratory manual in paleopathological diagnosis using text descriptions alone, nor to convey the appearance of active versus healed lesions; good photographic images are essential for these purposes.

In the primary literature, where case studies are described, new methods are demonstrated, and population studies are presented, photographic images of pathological lesions are ubiquitous in order to convey our findings and our methods to our readers. Study of images (radiographs and CT scans, but mainly photographs) of skeletal lesions is a chief means by which readers evaluate diagnoses offered in paleopathological publications, and they form the prime focus for debates over diagnosis conducted at conferences and other meetings. In methodological or population studies, good photographs should be presented, not only of "classic cases" of the disease(s) under study, but also (and probably more importantly) of less clear-cut examples, so that readers can understand how more ambiguous and diagnostically difficult cases were dealt with. In addition, if study of remodeled versus active lesions, or lesions of different grades of severity was germane to a work, photographs of *exempla* should be presented so readers can evaluate them. Adequate photographic documentation of studies is facilitated by the use of supplementary data sections of journals.

Despite the primacy of photographic images in our discipline, by comparison with the attention devoted to descriptive terminology, there is little prominence accorded to the methods needed to produce a good photographic record as part of the descriptive process. Making effective photographs of skeletal lesions is not always straightforward. Shadows cast into the interior of lytic lesions may make lighting them difficult. Subtle lesions, such as minor subperiosteal deposits of new bone, may be difficult to visualize and may require experimentation with orientation and lighting conditions. Given the centrality of photography in recording the macroscopic appearance of lesions, the importance of making appropriate choices concerning which lesions are to be photographed and which of these are to be selected for presentation in publications, and the difficulties that sometimes attend making satisfactory images, it is surprising that laboratory manuals do not devote significant space to it (but Smith (2013) has a short but useful section on photography for the beginning paleopathologist). This stands in contrast to clinical sciences, where there are practical handbooks devoted to medical photography (e.g., Pasquali, 2020).

How Reliable Is Macroscopic Lesion Identification? The Question of Observer Error

When quantitative data are used to test hypotheses, the extent to which variation in data reflects variation in the variable of interest rather than inconsistency on the part of the observer(s) is a crucial measure of data quality. In population-based studies in paleopathology, data regarding bony lesions comprise observations, recorded on a nominal or ordinal scale (e.g., presence/absence or by grades of severity), which directly or indirectly form the basis of analysis. However, studies rarely report measures of inter- or intra-observer error in lesion recording. By contrast, in osteometric studies in physical anthropology, reporting measures of observer error has been routine. This split in approaches between metric (i.e., ratio scale data) and nominal/ordinal variables even extends to particular papers. In cases where stress indicators are recorded both as ratio scale data (e.g., vertebral neural canal size, fluctuating asymmetry in osteometric dimensions) and as macroscopic presence of lesions, if there is any report of observer error, it is normally only the former that is assessed (e.g., Watts, 2015; Gawlikowska-Sroka et al., 2017; Hagg et al., 2017). It might be suggested that this reflects a widespread belief that macroscopic lesion recognition should be reliable for a competent practitioner. However, this seems an unlikely explanation. For example, the difficulties in repeatability for macroscopic recording of DEH (especially inter-observer error) have long been realized (e.g., Goodman & Rose, 1990; Hillson, 1992, 2014), but nevertheless few DEH studies report observer error. The lack of attention paid to observer error in recording of nominal or ordinal data in paleopathology stands in contrast to other fields. In social sciences, psychology and biomedical fields, theory and methods from the statistical reliability literature are routinely employed in order to assess the validity of a wide variety of subjectively recorded categorical data (Schrout, 1998; Wilde et al., 2013; O'Connor & Joffe, 2020).

A wide variety of indices can be used to quantify observer error in categorical data. They can be classified into those that are adjusted for chance agreement and those that are not. An example of the latter is simple percentage agreement (for example, percentage agreement between observers concerning presence/absence or grading of lesions). A caveat with that approach is that even if scoring was random, we would expect some concordance between observations merely by chance. There are a number of statistics that estimate agreement by chance using various methods, and then use that as a basis for calculating chance-adjusted indices of observer concordance.

In paleopathology, whether we should use chance-adjusted measures of agreement or not, and if so, which statistic is likely to be most suitable (each has its own statistical properties and, hence, its own strengths and weaknesses) are non-trivial (and, indeed, intriguing) questions and, in contrast with the situation in other disciplines, we have given them little explicit consideration. The answers to these questions are likely different in different research settings rather than being generic. An additional point to consider is that, although it is invariably the question they wish to address, no index will tell a researcher whether observer error is at a level that is acceptable for their particular study. That decision will always rest with the judgment of the researcher (O'Connor & Joffe, 2020).

In research involving categorical data, one particular chance-adjusted observer concordance measure, the kappa statistic, is widely used in diverse fields in social and biomedical sciences (Viera & Garrett, 2005; Zhao et al., 2012; Feng, 2014; Erdmann et al., 2015; O'Connor & Joffe, 2020). The original form (Cohen, 1960) has been extended to assess concordance between more than two observers, making it useful for assessing observer error within research teams. A weighted kappa may be applied to observer error in ordinal variables taking into account degree of disagreement (Fliess et al., 2003: 598–626) (i.e., so that a discrepancy between "slight" and "severe" grades of lesion expression would carry greater weight than between "slight" and "moderate"). Absolute values of kappa range from zero (no agreement) to one (+1 is compete agreement).

Because it allows for agreement by chance, kappa is lower than percentage agreement. Kappa tends to be lower for polytomous than dichotomous variables (Maclure & Willett, 1987). It also varies with prevalence, especially when this is very high or low – for example, for rare findings, a low kappa may not reflect low levels of percentage agreement (Viera & Garrett, 2005). Hence, for rare lesions its ability to reflect observer agreement accurately is compromised (Gwet, 2008). This sensitivity to prevalence also means that lesion prevalence in the test sample used to assess observer error should resemble that in the study group as a whole. Several rules of thumb have been proposed to help with the question of what constitutes an acceptable value (Landis & Koch, 1977; Altman, 1991; Schrout, 1998; Fleiss et al., 2003: 604; McHugh, 2012), but as might be expected given the above discussion, these are rather subjective and differ quite a bit between authors.

Because kappa (and other measures of concordance) each have their strengths and weaknesses, it may be best to use more than one measure when assessing observer error. One approach would be to use a combination of chance adjusted and non-chance adjusted measures – McHugh (2012), for example, recommends the use of kappa in conjunction with percentage agreement. Another review (Zhao et al., 2012) ranks different observer concordance indices according to how conservative they are and suggests that combinations from both the liberal and conservative ends of the spectrum be employed.

In paleopathology, results of any particular observer error test for some particular lesion will depend, *inter alia*, upon the recording methods used, the taphonomic condition of the assemblage, the conditions under which observations were taken, the experience of the observer(s) and, for kappa and many other measures, lesion prevalence or other factors that affect how the level of chance agreement is estimated (see Zhao et al., 2012 for a detailed discussion of this last). Observer error of any particular lesion is study-specific rather than generalizable. It seems reasonable therefore, to suggest that observer error should be quantified routinely in biocultural studies in paleopathology.

A few paleopathology studies have reported observer error in macroscopic lesion observation. Some report percentage agreement, for example, Danforth et al. (1993), Mays (1995) and Amoroso et al. (2014) for DEH, and Waldron and Rogers (1991) for osteoarthritis. However, more are beginning to use the kappa statistic, probably because it is the most popular measure in other disciplines, particularly biomedical studies, and (I suspect) because it is offered in widely used statistical software packages. Some recent studies where repeatability has been assessed using this measure are given in Table 2.3. Although the difficulties of determining what is an "acceptable" kappa value have already been alluded to, consensus is that those above about 0.8 are indicative of strong observer concordance. The high values for DEH, both compared with this figure, and with the other lesions listed in Table 2.3, seem quite surprising given the acknowledged difficulties in its macroscopic recording. However, the methodological differences between studies (e.g., in scoring procedures), and the multiple other factors that can affect kappa values (Zhao et al., 2012) make comparisons and interpretation difficult.

Table 2.3 Some kappa values reported for recording of macroscopic lesions in paleopathology

Lesion	N	Lesion frequency	Intra- or inter-observer	Scoring method	Kappa value	Reference
Linear dental enamel hypoplasias	50	–	Intra	0, 1, >1 lines	0.81	Guatelli-Steinberg (2003)
	72	–	Intra	0, 1, >1 lines	0.63	Temple (2007)
	12	–	Intra	0, 1–2, >2 lines	0.86	Amoroso et al. (2014)
	12	–	Intra	p/a	1.0	Amoroso et al. (2014)

Lesion	N	Lesion frequency	Intra- or inter-observer	Scoring method	Kappa value	Reference
	10?	–	Intra	p/a	>0.8[1]	Fabra & González (2015)
Dental caries	–	–	Intra	p/a	0.93	Wasterlain et al. (2009)
	180[2]	48/180	Intra	p/a; five point scale of observer confidence in lesion	0.62[3]	Liebe-Harkort et al. (2010)
	180[2]	48/180	Inter	p/a; five point scale of observer confidence in lesion	0.41[4]	Liebe-Harkort et al. (2010)
Lesions ascribed to osteoarthritis[5]	1560	–	Intra	p/a; three to four category ordinal scales	0.78[6]	Zampetti et al. (2016)
	520	–	Inter	p/a; three to four category ordinal scales	0.44[6]	Zampetti et al. (2016)
Periosteal new bone	?	–	Intra	Four category nominal scale	0.68	Biehle-Gomez et al. (2020)

Notes
For linear dental enamel hypoplasias, N refers to number of teeth; for dental caries, tooth surfaces; for lesions ascribed to osteoarthritis to number of articular surfaces. For scoring method, p/a denotes presence/absence.
[1]Kappa >0.8 also reported for presence/absence of 'abscess' in 320 teeth in 10 individuals.
[2]Tooth surfaces on 20 loose teeth.
[3]Mean results for four observers.
[4]Mean of comparisons among four observers.
[5]Eburnation, loss of joint morphology, marginal lipping, porosity, joint surface osteophytes.
[6]Median of figures for five indicators.

Conclusions

Macroscopy is a method universally applied to the study of lesions in skeletal paleopathology and has formed the foundation of study since the dawn of the discipline. The analysis of peer-reviewed publications used here indicates that the majority use macroscopic study of lesions as their sole method of analysis. The extent to which this is the case appears to have remained unchanged at least over the past decade and probably over the last 25 years, despite the great advances that have occurred during those periods in medical imaging and microscopy. Population studies are particularly reliant on unaided macroscopy. It is these, rather than case reports, that are the more widely cited and the more important and influential type of applied paleopathological research. The key position of macroscopic study of lesions within our discipline could hardly be clearer.

With regard to epistemological theory in diagnostic paleopathology, adequate recognition of the role and nature of visual assessment of lesions is vital for effective deconstruction, and hence the understanding, of the diagnostic process. This potentially helps us to improve our procedures, including how we impart diagnostic skills in a pedagogic setting, and in aiding our understanding of biases and limitations in our work. In diagnostic paleopathology, macroscopy provides the basis for diagnostic hypotheses, and it is the main means of recording lesions relevant to testing those hypotheses. The diagnostic hypotheses generated by macroscopy enable decision making as to whether imaging or microscopy of remains would be helpful and, if so, which techniques should be used and to which lesions/skeletal elements they should be applied. The central role of macroscopy in our work therefore persists regardless of whether we also apply other methods of examining lesions. Our ability to directly examine lesions with the naked eye is the key methodological strength in paleopathology; other observational methods are normally subservient to this.

With regard to presentation of results of macroscopy, an important step toward scientific rigor has been the widespread recognition of the need for precision in terminology for lesion description. However, in a science where inferences are primarily based on the visual appearance of lesions, the image, primarily the photographic image, is key to presenting our observations. Compared with the efforts at securing correct use of terminology, relatively little prominence has been given to discussing best practice in photography. Perhaps it is time we turned out attention toward 'paleopathological photography' and accorded it a status within our own discipline comparable to the prestige which medical photography appears to enjoy within the clinical sciences.

With regard to methodology, recording of macroscopic lesions that are to be used in quantitative studies (whether to enable diagnosis or to use as stress indicators) is essentially a process of imposing upon our observations categories that are useful to our research aims (e.g., lesion presence/absence; active versus inactive; grades of severity). Looking at the problem in this rather broad way allows us to draw parallels, both at the methodological and at a more general theoretical level, with other disciplines, often very different from our own, that use categorical data. One area where this may be useful is in the issue of observer error in categorical data. This is a problem that has been considered in a wide variety of disciplines, particularly in the social sciences, but has been rather under-discussed with reference to lesion recording in paleopathology. Reporting of observer error in lesion identification needs to be a standard practice in quantitative paleopathology. This has been recommended for some time (e.g., Buikstra & Ubelaker, 1994: 183–184; Mays, 1998: 157; Di Gangi & Moore, 2013), but it has simply failed to happen. In other disciplines (e.g., O'Connor & Joffe, 2020), authoring and reviewing criteria for publication of studies based on subjectively recorded categorical data in peer-reviewed journals include measures of observer error. Alterations in policy by editors in journals in paleopathology toward requiring measures of observer error in lesion recording might be a ready means of accomplishing this important step toward greater rigor in our own discipline. There needs concomitantly to be research into the strengths and weaknesses of different measures of observer concordance in the different types of studies undertaken, and the data sets customarily generated, in paleopathology. We cannot assume that concordance measures used by other disciplines (or those that happen to be included in readily available statistical software packages!) are necessarily suited to our own data. That would help give workers a framework for making appropriate choices of concordance statistics for their macroscopic observations of lesions as they plan their research projects.

Notes

1. The year 2019 was the last complete year for which data were available at time of writing.
2. I refer here to cases of disease. Distinguishing perimortal trauma from post-mortem breaks to bone is a different matter and one that elicits significant discussion due to its frequently difficult nature.

References

Altman, D. G. (1991). *Practical Statistics for Medical Research*. London: Chapman & Hall.

Amoroso, A., Garcia, S. J. & Cardoso, H. F. V. (2014). Age at death and linear enamel hypoplasias: testing the effects of childhood stress and adult socioeconomic circumstances on premature mortality. *American Journal of Human Biology* 26:461–468.

Armelagos G. J. & Van Gerven, D. P. (2003). A century of skeletal biology and paleopathology: contrasts, contradictions and conflicts. *American Anthropologist* 105:53–64.

Beauchesne, P. & Agarwal, S. C. (2014). Age-related cortical bone maintenance and loss in an imperial Roman population. *International Journal of Osteoarchaeology* 24:15–30.

Becker, S. K. (2019). Labor across an occupational and gendered taskscape: bones and bodies of the Tiwanaku state (A.D. 500–1100). *Bioarchaeology International* 3:118–141.

Biehler-Gomez, L., Tritella, S., Mertino, F., Campobasso, C. P., Franchi, A., Spairani, R., Sardanelli, F. & Cattaneo, C. (2019). The synergy between radiographic and macroscopic observation of skeletal lesions in dry bone. *International Journal of Legal Medicine* 133:1611–1628.

Biehler-Gomez, L., Indra, L., Martino, F., Campobasso, C. P. & Cattaneo, C. (2020). Observer error in bone disease description: a cautionary note. *International Journal of Osteoarchaeology* 30:607–615.

Brickley, M., Ives, R. & Mays, S. (2020). *The Bioarchaeology of Metabolic Bone Disease* (2nd edition). London: Elsevier.

Brothwell, D. (2008). Tumours and tumour-like processes. In Pinhasi, R. & Mays, S. (Eds.), *Advances in Human Paleopathology*, pp. 253–281. Chichester: Wiley.

Buikstra, J. E. (2019). *Ortner's Identification of Pathological Conditions in Human Skeletal Remains* (3rd edition). London: Academic Press.

Buikstra J. E. & Ubelaker, D. H. (1994). *Standards for Data Collection from Human Skeletal Remains*. Arkansas Archaeological Survey Research Series No. 44. Fayetteville: Arkansas Archaeological Survey.

Buikstra, J. E., Cook, D. C. & Bolhofer, K. L. (2017). Introduction: scientific rigor in paleopathology. *International Journal of Paleopathology* 19:80–87.

Bush, H. (1991). Concepts of health and stress. In Bush, H. & Zvelebil. M. (Eds.), *Health in Past Societies. Biocultural Interpretations of Human Skeletal Remains in Archaeological Contexts*. British Archaeological Reports International Series 567. Oxford: Tempus Reparatum.

Cohen, J. (1960). A coefficient of agreement for nominal scales. *Educational Psychological Measurement* 20:37–46.

Conlogue, G. J., Nelson, A. J. & Lurie, A. G. (2020). Computed tomography (CT), multidetector computed tomography (MDCT), micro-CT, and cone-beam computed tomography (CBCT). In Conlogue, G. J. & Beckett, R.G. (Eds.), *Advances in Paleoimaging: Applications in Paleoanthropology, Bioarchaeology, Forensics and Cultural Artifacts*, pp. 111–178. Boca Raton: CRC.

Cook, D. C. & Patrick, R. R. (2014). As the worm turns: an enigmatic calcified object as pseudopathology. *International Journal of Osteoarchaeology* 24:123–125.

Curate, F. & Tavares, A. (2018). Maternal mortality, marital status and bone mineral density in young women from the Coimbra identified skeletal collection. *Anthropologischer Anzeiger* 75:233–242.

Danforth, M. E., Herndon, K. S. & Propst, K. B. (1993). A preliminary study of patterns of replication in scoring linear enamel hypoplasias. *International Journal of Osteoarchaeology* 3:297–302.

Davies-Barrett, A. M., Antoine, D. & Roberts, C. A. (2019). Inflammatory periosteal reaction on ribs associated with lower respiratory tract disease: a method for recording prevalence from sites with differing preservation. *American Journal of Physical Anthropology* 168:530–542.

DeWitte, S. N. (2014). Differential survival among individuals with active and healed periosteal new bone formation. *International Journal of Paleopathology* 7:38–44.

Di Gangi, E. A. & Moore, M. K. (2013). Application of scientific method to skeletal biology. In Di Gangi, E. A. & Moore, M. K. (Eds.), *Research Methods in Human Skeletal Biology*, pp. 29–59. New York: Academic Press.

Domett, K., Evans, C., Chang, N., Tayles, N. & Newton, J. (2017). Interpreting osteoarthritis in bioarchaeology: highlighting the importance of a clinical approach through case studies from prehistoric Thailand. *Journal of Archaeological Science: Reports* 11:762–773.

Erdmann, T. P., De Mast, J. & Warrens, M. J. (2015). Some common errors of experimental design, interpretation and inference in agreement studies. *Statistical Methods in Medical Research* 24:920–935.

Fabra, M. & González, C.V. (2015). Diet and oral health of populations that inhabited central Argentina (Córdoba Province) during Late Holocene. *International Journal of Osteoarchaeology* 25:160–175.

Feng, G. C. (2014). Intercoder reliability indices: disuse, misuse and abuse. *Quality and Quantity* 48:1803–1815.

Fleiss, J. L., Levin, B. & Paik, M. C. (2003). *Statistical Methods for Rates and Proportions* (3rd edition). Chichester: Wiley.

Flohr, S., Kierdorf, U., Jankauskas, R., Püschel, B. & Schultz, M. (2014). Diagnosis of stapedial footplate fixation in archaeological human remains. *International Journal of Paleopathology* 6:10–19.

Gawlikowska-Sroka, A., Dabrowski, P., Szczurowski, J., Dzieciolowska-Baran, E. & Staniowski, T. (2017). Influence of physiological stress on presence of hypoplasia and fluctuating asymmetry in a medieval population from the village of Sypniewo. *International Journal of Paleopathology* 19:3–52.

Goodman, A. H. & Rose, J. C. (1990). Assessment of systemic physiological perturbations from dental enamel hypoplasias and associated histological structures. *Yearbook of Physical Anthropology* 33:59–110.

Grauer, A. L. (2008). Macroscopic analysis and data collection in paleopathology. In Pinhasi, R. & Mays, S. (Eds.), *Advances in Human Paleopathology*, pp. 57–76. Chichester: Wiley.

Guatelli-Steinberg, D. (2003). Macroscopic and microscopic analyses of linear enamel hypoplasia in plio-pleistocene South Africa hominins with respect to aspects of enamel development and morphology. *American Journal of Physical Anthropology* 120:309–322.

Gwet, K. L. (2008). Computing inter-rater reliability and its variance in the presence of high agreement. *British Journal of Mathematical and Statistical Psychology* 61:29–48.

Hagg, A. C., van der Merwe, A. E. & Steyn, M. (2017). Developmental instability and its relationship to mental health in two historic Dutch populations. *International Journal of Paleopathology* 17:42–51.

Hillson, S. (1992). Dental enamel growth, perikymata and hypoplasia in ancient tooth crowns. *Journal of the Royal Society of Medicine* 85:460–466.

Hillson, S. (2014). *Tooth Development in Human Evolution and Bioarchaeology*. Cambridge: Cambridge University Press.

Hillson, S. (2019). Dental pathology. In Katzenberg, M. A. & Grauer, A. L. (Eds.), *Biological Anthropology of the Human Skeleton* (3rd edition), pp. 295–333. Chichester: Wiley-Blackwell.

Hosek, L. & Robb, J. (2019). Osteobiography: a platform for archaeological research. *Bioarchaeology International* 3:1–15.

Judd, M. A., Walker, J. L., Miller, A.V., Razhev, D., Epimakhov, A.V. & Hanks, B. K. (2018). Life in the fast lane: settled pastoralism in the central Eurasian steppe during the middle bronze age. *American Journal of Human Biology* 30:e23129.

Klaus, H. (2017). Paleopathological rigor and differential diagnosis: case studies involving terminology, description and diagnostic frameworks for scurvy in skeletal remains. *International Journal of Paleopathology* 19:96–110.

Klaus, H. (2018). Possible prostate cancer in northern Peru: differential diagnosis, vascular anatomy, and molecular signalling in the paleopathology of metabolic bone disease. *International Journal of Paleopathology* 21:147–157.

Klaus, H. & Lynnerup, N. (2019). Abnormal bone: considerations for documentation, disease process identification and differential diagnosis. In Buikstra, J. E. (Ed.), *Ortner's Identification of Pathological Conditions in Human Skeletal Remains* (3rd edition), pp. 59–89. London: Academic Press.

Landis, J. R. & Koch, G. C. (1977). The measurement of observer agreement for categorical data. *Biometrics* 33:159–174.

Larsen, C. S. (2015). *Bioarchaeology. Interpreting Behavior From the Human Skeleton* (2nd edition). Cambridge: Cambridge University Press.

Lewis, M. (2018). *Paleopathology of Children: Identification of Pathological Conditions in the Human Skeletal Remains of Non-Adults*. London: Academic Press.

Liebe-Harkort, C., Ástvaldsdóttir, Á. & Tranaeus, S. (2010). Quantification of dental caries by osteologists and odontologists – a validity and reliability study. *International Journal of Osteoarchaeology* 20:525–539.

Lieverse, A. R., Temple, D. H. & Bazaliiskii, V. I. (2014). Paleopathological description and diagnosis of metastatic carcinoma in an Early Bronze Age (4588±34 Cal. BP) forager from the cis-Baikal region of eastern Siberia. *PloS ONE* 9(12):e113919.

Lipton, J. E. & Vigorita, V. J. (2015). Metastatic bone disease. In V. J. Vigorita (Ed.), *Orthopaedic Pathology* (3rd edition), pp. 1033–1080. Philadelphia: Wolters Kluwer.

Lopez, B., Lopez-Garcia, J. M., Costilla, S., Garcia-Vazquez, E., Dopico, E. & Pardiñas, A. F. (2017). Treponemal disease in the old world? Integrated palaeopathological assessment of a 9th–11th century skeleton from north-central Spain. *Anthropological Science* 125:101–114.

Lovell, N. C. (2000). Paleopathological description and diagnosis. In Katzenberg, M. A. & Saunders, S. R. (Eds.), *Biological Anthropology of the Human Skeleton* (1st edition), pp. 217–248. Chichester: Wiley-Liss.

Lowenstein, E. J., Sidlow, R. & Ko, C. J. (2019). Visual perception, cognition and error in dermatologic diagnosis: diagnosis and error. *Journal of the American Academy of Dermatology* 81(6):1237–1245.

Maclure, M. & Willett, W. C. (1987). Misinterpretation and misuse of the kappa statistic. *American Journal of Epidemiology* 126:161–169.

Mamede, S. & Schmidt, H. G. (2017). Reflection in medical diagnosis: a literature review. *Health Professions Education* 3:15–25.

Manchester, K., Ogden, A. & Storm R. (2017). Nomenclature in Palaeopathology. Palaeopathology Association. Accessed January 2021 at: https://paleopathology-association.wildapricot.org/resources/Documents/Nomenclature%20in%20Palaeopathology%20Web%20Document.pdf.

Manzon, V. S., Ferrante, Z., Giganti, M. & Gualdi-Russo, E. (2017). On the antiquity of Legge-Calvé-Perthes disease: skeletal evidence from early iron age Italy. *HOMO: Journal of Comparative Human Biology* 68:10–17.

Marchewka, J., Borowska-Strungińska, B., Czuczkiewicz, J. & Kliś, K. (2017). Cervical spine anomalies: children in one of the oldest churches in Poland. *International Journal of Osteoarchaeology* 27:926–934.

Mays, S. A. (1989). *The Anglo-Saxon Human Bone From School Street, Ipswich, Suffolk*. AML Report 115/89. Portsmouth: Historic England.

Mays, S. A. (1995). The relationship between Harris lines and other aspects of skeletal development in adults and juveniles. *Journal of Archaeological Science* 22:511–520.

Mays, S. A. (1997a). A perspective on human osteoarchaeology in Britain. *International Journal of Osteoarchaeology* 7:600–604.

Mays, S. A. (1997b). Life and death in a mediaeval village. In De Boe, G. & Verhaege, F. (Eds.), *Death & Burial in Mediaeval Europe. Papers of the 'Mediaeval Europe Brugge 1997' Conference*, Volume 2, pp. 121–125. Zellik: Instituut voor het Archeologisch Patrimonium.

Mays, S. A. (1998). *The Archaeology of Human Bones* (1st edition). London: Routledge.

Mays, S. A. (2007). The human remains. In Mays, S., Harding, C. & Heighway, C. (Eds.), *Wharram, A Study of Settlement on the Yorkshire Wolds. XI The Churchyard*, pp. 77–192; 337–397. York University Archaeological Publication 13. York: York University.

Mays, S. A. (2010). Human osteoarchaeology in the UK 2001–2007: a bibliometric perspective. *International Journal of Osteoarchaeology* 20:192–204.

Mays, S. A. (2012a). The relationship between palaeopathology and the clinical sciences. In Grauer, A. L. (Ed.), *A Companion to Paleopathology*, pp. 285–309. Oxford: Wiley-Blackwell.

Mays, S. A. (2012b). The impact of case reports relative to other types of publication in palaeopathology. *International Journal of Osteoarchaeology* 22:81–85.

Mays, S. A. (2018a). How should we diagnose disease in paleopathology? Some epistemological considerations. *International Journal of Paleopathology* 20:12–19.

Mays, S. A. (2018b). Micronutrient deficiency diseases. In Trevathan, W. (Ed.), *The International Encyclopaedia of Biological Anthropology*. Chichester: Wiley.

Mays, S. A. (2019). *Palaeopathology in South America and beyond: A Bibliometric Perspective*. Paper presented at the 2019 Palaeopathology Association Meeting in South America (PAMinSA), Brazil: Sao Paulo.

Mays, S. A. (2020). A dual process model for palaeopathological diagnosis. *International Journal of Paleopathology* 31:89–96.

Mays, S. A. (2021). A content analysis by bibliometry of the first ten years of the International Journal of Paleopathology. *International Journal of Paleopathology* 34:217–222.

Mays, S. A., Strouhal, E., Vyhnánek, L. & Němečková, A. (1996). A case of metastatic carcinoma of medieval date from Wharram Percy, UK. *Journal of Paleopathology* 8(1):33–42.

Mays, S. A., Brickley, M. B. & Ives, R. (2006). Skeletal manifestations of rickets in infants and young children in an historic population from England. *American Journal of Physical Anthropology* 129:362–374.

Mays, S. A., Prowse, T., George, M. & Brickley, M. (2018). Latitude, urbanisation, age and sex as risk factors for vitamin D deficiency disease in the Roman empire. *American Journal of Physical Anthropology* 167:484–496.

McHugh, M. L. (2012). Interrater reliability: the Kappa statistic. *Biochemia Medica* 22:276–282.

Menéndez, L. P. (2016). Spatial variation of dental caries in late Holocene samples of southern South America: a geostatistical study. *American Journal of Human Biology* 28:825–836.

Mensforth, R. P., Lovejoy, C. O., Lallo, J. W. & Armelagos, G. J. (1978). The role of constitutional factors, diet, and infectious disease in the etiology of porotic hyperostosis and periosteal reactions in prehistoric infants and children. *Medical Anthropology* 1(2):1–59.

Micarelli, I., Paine, R. R., Tafuri, M. A. & Manzi, G. (2019). A possible case of mycosis in a post-classic burial from La Selvicciola (Italy). *International Journal of Paleopathology* 24:25–33.

Monteiro, S. M. & Norman, G. (2013). Diagnostic reasoning: where we've been, where we're going. *Teaching and Learning in Medicine* 25(S1):S26–S32.

Novak, M., Howcroft, R. & Pinhasi, R. (2017). Child health in five early medieval Irish sites: a multidisciplinary approach. *International Journal of Osteoarchaeology* 27:398–408.

O'Connor, C. & Joffe, H. (2020). Intercoder reliability in qualitative research: debates and practical guidelines. *International Journal of Qualitative Methods* 19:1–13.

Ortner, D. J. (1991). Theoretical and methodological issues in paleopathology. In Ortner, D. J. & Aufderheide, A. C. (Eds.), *Human Paleopathology: Current Syntheses and Future Options*, pp. 5–11. Washington: Smithsonian Institution Press.

Ortner, D. J. (2012). Differential diagnosis and issues in disease classification. In Grauer, A. L. (Ed.), *A Companion to Paleopathology*, pp. 250–267. Oxford: Wiley-Blackwell.

Ortner, D. J. & Putschar, W. G. J. (1985). *Identification of Pathological Conditions in Human Skeletal Remains*. Washington: Smithsonian Institution.

Pasquali, P. (Ed.) (2020). *Photography in Clinical Medicine*. Cham: Springer.

Pinhasi, R. & Mays, S. (2008). *Advances in Human Paleopathology*. Chichester: Wiley.

Pinhasi, R., Timpson, A., Thomas, M. & Šlaus, M. (2014). Bone growth, limb proportions and non-specific stress in archaeological populations from Croatia. *Annals of Human Biology* 41:127–137.

Portier, H., Jaffré, C., Kewish, C. M., Chappard, C. & Pallu, S. (2020). New insights in osteocyte imaging by synchrotron radiation. *Journal of Spectral Imaging* 9:a3.

Rao, V.V., Vasulu, T. S. & Rector Babu, A. D. W. (1996). Possible paleopathological evidence of treponematosis from a megalithic site at Agripalle, India. *American Journal of Physical Anthropology* 100:49–55.

Ragsdale, B. D. (1992). Taskforce on terminology: provisional wordlist. *Paleopathology Newsletter* 78:7–8.

Ragsdale, B. D., Campbell, R. A. & Kirkpatrick, K. L. (2018). Neoplasm or not? general principles of morphologic analysis of dry bone specimens. *International Journal of Paleopathology* 21:27–40.

Rivollat, M., Castex, D., Haurat, L. & Tillier, A-M. (2014). Ancient Down syndrome: an osteological case from Saint-Jean-des-Vignes, northeastern France, from 5th–6th century AD. *International Journal of Paleopathology* 7:8–14.

Roberts, C. (2006). A view from afar: bioarchaeology in Britain. In Buikstra, J. & Beck, L. (Eds.), *Bioarchaeology: The Contextual Analysis of Human Remains*, pp. 417–439. New York: Elsevier.

Rogers, J. & Waldron, T. (1995). *A Field Guide to Joint Disease*. Chichester: Wiley.

Rogers, J., Watt, I. & Dieppe, P. (1990). Comparison of visual and radiographic detection of bony changes at the knee joint. *British Medical Journal* 300:367–368.

Rohnbogner, A. & Lewis, M. (2017). Poundbury Camp in context – a new perspective on the lives of children from urban and rural Roman England. *American Journal of Physical Anthropology* 162:208–228.

Rühli, F. J., Galassi, F. M. & Haeussler, M. (2016). Palaeopathology: current challenges and medical impact. *Clinical Anatomy* 29:816–822.

Schrout, P. E. (1998). Measurement reliability and agreement in psychiatry. *Statistical Methods in Medical Research* 7:301–317.

Slon, V., Nagar, Y., Kuperman, T. & Hershkovitz, I. (2013). A case of dwarfism from the Byzantine city of Rehovot-in-the-Negev, Israel. *International Journal of Osteoarchaeology* 23:573–589.

Smith, M. O. (2013). Paleopathology. In Di Gangi, E. A. & Moore, M. K. (Eds.), *Research Methods in Human Skeletal Biology*, pp. 181–217. New York: Academic Press.

Smith-Guzmán, N. E. (2015). The skeletal manifestations of malaria: an epidemiological approach using documented skeletal collections. *American Journal of Physical Anthropology* 158:624–635.

Steckel, R. H. & Rose, J. C. (Eds) (2002). *The Backbone of History: Health and Nutrition in the Western Hemisphere*. Cambridge: Cambridge University Press.

Steckel, R. H., Larsen, C. S., Roberts, C. A. & Baten, J. (Eds.) (2018). *The Backbone of Europe. Health, Diet, Work and Violence Over Two Millennia*. Cambridge: Cambridge University Press.

Steinbock, R.T. (1976). *Paleopathological Diagnosis and Interpretation*. Springfield: Charles C Thomas.

Temple, D. H. (2007). Dietary variation and stress among prehistoric Jomon foragers from Japan. *American Journal of Physical Anthropology* 133:1035–1046.

Temple, D. H. & Goodman, A. H. (2014). Bioarchaeology has a "health" problem: conceptualising "stress" and "health" in bioarchaeological research. *American Journal of Physical Anthropology* 155:186–191.

Temple, D. H., McGroarty, J. N., Guatelli-Steinberg, D., Nakatsukasa, M. & Matsumura, H. (2013). A comparative study of stress episode prevalence and duration among Jomon period foragers from Hokkaido. *American Journal of Physical Anthropology* 152:230–238.

Tesi, C., Giuffra, V., Fornaciari, G., Larentis, O., Motto, M. & Licata, M. (2019). A case of erosive polyarthropathy from medieval northern Italy (12th–13th centuries). *International Journal of Paleopathology* 25:20–29.

van der Merwe, A. E., Veselka, B., van Veen, H. A., van Rijn, R. R., Colman, K. L. & de Boer, H. H. (2018). Four possible cases of osteomalacia: the value of a multidisciplinary diagnostic approach. *International Journal of Paleopathology* 23:15–25.

van Schaik, K., Eisenberg, R., Bekvalac, J., Glazer, A. & Rühli, F. (2019). Evaluation of lesion burden in a bone-by-bone comparison of osteological and radiological methods of analysis. *International Journal of Paleopathology* 24:171–174.

Veselka, B., Brickley, M. B. & Waters-Rist, A. L. (2021). A joint medico-historical and paleopathological perspective on vitamin D deficiency prevalence in post-medieval Netherlands. *International Journal of Paleopathology* 32:41–49.

Viera, A. J. & Garrett, J. M. (2005). Understanding interobserver agreement: the kappa statistic. *Family Medicine* 37:60–363.

Waldron, T. & Rogers, J. (1991). Inter-observer variation in coding osteoarthritis in human skeletal remains. *International Journal of Osteoarchaeology* 1:49–56.

Waltenburger, L., Rebay-Salisbury, K. & Mitteroecker, P. (2021). Three-dimensional surface scanning methods in osteology: a topographical and geometric morphometric comparison. *American Journal of Physical Anthropology* 174:846–858.

Wasterlain, S. N., Hillson, S. & Cunha, E. (2009). Dental caries in a Portuguese identified skeletal sample from the late 19th and early 20th centuries. *American Journal of Physical Anthropology* 140:64–79.

Watts, R. (2015). The long-term impact of developmental stress. Evidence from later medieval and post-medieval London (AD1117–1853). *American Journal of Physical Anthropology* 158:569–580.

Watts, R. & Valme, S-R. (2018). Osteological evidence for juvenile vitamin D deficiency in a 19th century suburban population from Surrey, England. *International Journal of Paleopathology* 23:60–68.

Welsh, H., Nelson, A., van der Merwe, A., de Boer, H. & Brickley, M. (2020). An investigation of the use of micro-CT analysis of bone as a new diagnostic method for paleopathological cases of osteomalacia. *International Journal of Paleopathology* 31:23–33.

Weston, D. A. (2008). Investigating the specificity of periosteal reactions in pathology museum specimens. *American Journal of Physical Anthropology* 137:48–59.

Wheeler, S. M. (2012). Nutritional and disease stress of juveniles from the Dakhleh Oasis, Egypt. *International Journal of Osteoarchaeology* 22:219–234.

Wilde, D., Katz, D. L., Elmore, J. G., Wilde, D.M.G. & Lucan, S.C. (2013). *Jekel's Epidemiology, Biostatistics, Preventive Medicine and Public Health* (4th edition). Philadelphia: WB Saunders.

Yaussy, S. L. (2019). The intersections of industrialisation: variation in skeletal indicators of frailty by age, sex and socioeconomic status in 18th and 19th century England. *American Journal of Physical Anthropology* 170:116–130.

Zampetti, S., Mariotti, V., Radi, N. & Balcastro, M. G. (2016). Variation of skeletal degenerative joint disease features in an identified Italian modern skeletal collection. *American Journal of Physical Anthropology* 160:683–693.

Zhao, X., Liu, J. & Deng, K. (2012). Assumptions behind intercoder reliability indices. *Communication Yearbook* 36:419–480.

3
DIFFERENTIAL DIAGNOSIS AND RIGOR IN PALEOPATHOLOGY

Jo Appleby

It is no exaggeration to say that without rigorous and accurate differential diagnosis, there is no paleopathology. The process of identifying diseases with similar osteological features and then narrowing them down to those that can adequately explain the lesions observed on a skeleton is key to everything else that follows, whether that is estimation of past health and disease (e.g., Milner & Boldsen, 2017), understanding the development and spread of infectious disease (e.g., Zuckerman et al., 2016) or assessing the likely care requirements of sick individuals (e.g., Tilley, 2015, and see Chapter 25, this volume). Rigorous differential diagnosis in paleopathology is a complex process, and Buikstra et al. (Buikstra et al., 2017) have rightly noted that no practitioner will have every skill necessary to carry out all aspects of the process for every pathological condition. For commonly encountered pathological conditions, it will be possible for most bioarchaeologists to diagnose the condition. For rarer conditions, or more rarely encountered manifestations of common conditions, paleopathologists need to collaborate with others, whether they be other paleopathologists, bioarchaeologists, or specialists in cognate fields. There is every advantage in collaboration, and no shame in admitting personal defeat. Often, a precise diagnosis will not be possible even with every possible expert and diagnostic technique: under these circumstances it is always better to sacrifice precision than accuracy in diagnosis. In recording specific lesions, precision and accuracy are both required.

This chapter outlines the process of differential diagnosis and discusses key considerations to be taken into account in each step. It does not attempt to set out the differential diagnosis of specific diseases or pathologies: the reader is directed elsewhere in this volume for those. In addition to differential diagnosis itself, this chapter discusses the mental processes involved in differential diagnosis, alongside consideration of how differential diagnosis should be addressed in publication.

Differential diagnosis is a process that can be divided into a number of steps. While those steps are not necessarily sequential (Mays, 2020), it is worth setting out each step separately in order to explore what is required for each. Exactly how many steps are involved in differential diagnosis is partly a matter of semantics, but roughly, it involves:

1 Systematically observing skeletal lesions
2 Recording lesions precisely and accurately

DOI: 10.4324/9781003130994-4

3 Considering the full appropriate range of possible diagnoses
4 Accurately ruling out diagnoses that do not fit the lesions observed and assessing the likelihood of those that remain
5 Clearly communicating steps one through four in the site archive and publications

Interest in Differential Diagnosis

While the process of differential diagnosis has always been part of paleopathology, it has not always been at the forefront of scholarly attention. A quick search of the *American Journal of Physical (now Biological) Anthropology* reveals that no articles from the 1960s and only 15 in the 1970s mention differential diagnosis (Figure 3.1). Of course, this doesn't mean that differential diagnosis wasn't taking place: many paleopathologists at the time had backgrounds in clinical medicine and differential diagnosis would have been a key part of their medical training. What it does mean is that differential diagnosis wasn't being discussed, theorized, and/or argued about in the scholarly literature, and this has implications for its rigor.

Interest in differential diagnosis has increased every decade, with a tripling of articles between the 1970s and 1980s and again between the 1980s and 1990s (likely helped by the appearance of the *International Journal of Osteoarchaeology* in 1991). Only in the last ten years or so, though, has the discussion of differential diagnosis taken off, with a leap from 149 articles in the 2000s to 401 articles in the 2010s. Whether this jump was driven by the appearance of the *International Journal of Paleopathology*, or whether this journal reflects an increased desire to discuss the theoretical underpinnings of paleopathology (including differential diagnosis), is hard to tell, but researchers are now engaging ubiquitously with differential diagnosis in a way that was rare a few decades ago.

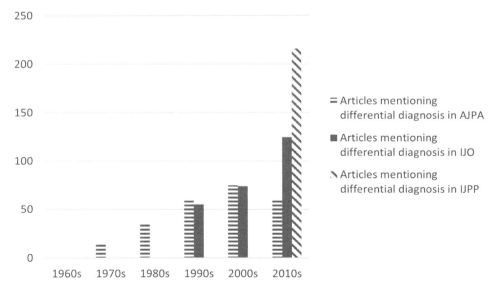

Figure 3.1 Mentions of differential diagnosis in the American Journal of Physical Anthropology (AJPA), *International Journal of Osteoarchaeology* (IJO), and *International Journal of Paleopathology* (IJPP) from the 1960s to 2020.

Epistemological Approaches to Differential Diagnosis

Mays (2018) has noted that there are two broad approaches to differential diagnosis: the comparative approach and the biological approach. Until recently, the comparative approach has dominated. The comparative approach uses a target sample/reference sample approach: that is, lesions noted in individuals within a reference sample with a clinically known disease are compared to lesions in an unknown archaeological individual. As Mays notes, when there is a lack of correspondence between the noted lesions and particular diseases, this can result in flawed results. Sources of information used in the comparative approach include pathology museum collections, anatomical collections, and clinical studies. Each of these has advantages for use in paleopathology (see Table 3.1) but also harbors significant disadvantages. The flaws inherent to specific sources of information are accompanied by a significant flaw that they have in common: the use of a comparative approach allows paleopathologists to identify disease in skeletonized remains without fully understanding the biological processes underlying the lesions observed. This may compromise the accuracy of differential diagnosis (as described by Klaus 2017 in relation to scurvy and anemia) and may also hamper our ability to improve the diagnostic criteria for specific diseases. Recently, many paleopathologists have made an argument for adopting the biological approach (e.g., Ortner, 2011, 2012; Ragsdale & Lehmer, 2012; Buikstra et al., 2017; Klaus, 2017; Brickley, 2018; Grauer, 2018; Mays, 2018; Klaus & Lynnerup, 2019) in which lesions are specifically considered in relation to the pathophysiology of disease. This approach has the advantage of avoiding some of the systematic biases associated with museum and anatomical collections, as well as allowing for the identification of lesions that are not represented in the clinical literature, but that are plausibly explained by a known disease process. Nevertheless, it is not entirely problem-free. The biological/pathophysiological approach allows paleopathologists to identify disease via discussion of disease mechanisms even when a lesion has not been identified in either museum collections or clinical practice, so long as the mechanism (and hence the lesion) is plausible. There is a degree of risk that this can lead to circular arguments of cause and effect. This potential has led to lengthy arguments in the paleopathological literature (see, for example, the two decades of discussion over the significance of porotic lesions of the sphenoid bone in diagnosing scurvy, e.g., Ortner & Ericksen, 1997; Melikian & Waldron, 2003; Brickley & Ives, 2006; Waldron, 2008; Stark, 2014; Klaus, 2017; Snoddy et al., 2018). As Klaus (2017:108) notes, the "necessary but potentially conflicting needs of conservatism and creativity in paleopathological problem solving" both need to be taken into account. I would add to this that a degree of pragmatism must accompany conservatism as well as creativity in paleopathological decision-making: such arguments underpin the ongoing need for research into the association between specific conditions and skeletal lesions.

The pathophysiological approach can help to decrease errors in both lesion recording and diagnosis. For example, much of the over-diagnosis of iron-deficiency anemia noted by Ortner (2012:251) could have been avoided had researchers been more familiar with the processes leading to lesion formation. Biehler-Gomez's et al. (2020) recent cautionary tale over inconsistencies in lesion recording between individuals was based on the creation of a check-list of pathological features. One wonders whether researchers might have been more accurate and consistent in their observations had they been focusing on the underlying pathological processes rather than on identifying the presence or absence of particular kinds of pathological alteration to bone.

Table 3.1 Approaches to diagnosis in paleopathology

Approach	Data from	Advantages	Disadvantages
Comparative approach	Pathology museum collections	– Show progression of disease in the absence of modern treatment – Dry bone preparations allow direct comparison with archaeological skeletons	– Rare expressions of disease are over-represented (and vice versa) – Documentation is variable (and may be absent) – Diagnostic methods are unknown – Presence of multiple conditions in a single individual is often not documented
Comparative approach	Anatomical skeletal collections	– Often show progression of disease in the absence of modern treatment (earlier anatomical collections only) – May have documented cause of death – Likely to show fuller range of disease expression than pathology museum collections including subtle expressions	– Non-fatal conditions may not be documented, leading to circular arguments about disease presence and expression – Diagnostic methods may be unknown.
Comparative approach	Modern imaging studies of living subjects	– Often include data from hundreds or thousands of subjects – Most indicate diagnostic criteria used	– Untreated advanced cases unlikely to be seen, limiting range of skeletal expression of lesions – Diseases that are rare in modern contexts may not be covered – Imaging may be limited to specific body parts, skewing understanding of lesion distribution – Some lesions are not visible on plain film radiographs – Some anatomical locations are hard to visualize on plain film radiographs.
Biological approach	Pathophysio-logical approach	– Feasible where no adequate dry bone or imaging data exists – Rooted in specific biological processes	Reliability of approach and competing hypotheses can be difficult to differentiate in the absence of clinical studies focusing on the bony lesions of relevance (N.B. this highlights the need for clinical researchers and paleopathologists to work together)

Source: Data from Mays, 2018.

Observing Skeletal Lesions: Normal vs. Abnormal Variation and the Importance of Taphonomy

Before a rigorous and accurate differential diagnosis can be carried out, all lesions of relevance need to be observed and abnormal bone securely differentiated from normal bone. Lynnerup and Klaus (2019:47) note that there are a limited range of abnormal bone phenotypes because skeletal changes are biologically and evolutionarily constrained. All pathological reactions involve abnormal bone formation, abnormal bone loss/absence, or a combination of the two. The first job of the paleopathologist is thus to identify abnormal bone through systematic investigation of all preserved skeletal elements and to exclude all instances of post-mortem change.

In order to identify abnormal bone created during a person's life, a paleopathologist must have an excellent understanding of normal skeletal variation and be able to recognize bone changes produced by post-mortem taphonomic processes. In both cases, there is no substitute for experience: understanding normal and abnormal bone requires familiarity with a wide range of skeletons of different ages, sexes, from different periods of time and geographic origin, and with different ecological and environmental conditions that contribute to post-mortem bone change. The identification of abnormal bone is thus a process that improves with experience. For instance, during training in paleopathology, students often struggle to differentiate normal porosity created by metaphyseal blood supply (often misclassified as pathological change), vascular impressions in bone (frequently mistaken for sharp-force trauma), and infant woven bone, which is often erroneously ascribed to infection/inflammation leading to periostosis.

Taphonomic damage creates an extra layer of complexity of the diagnostic process. Corron et al. (2017:2) recommend considering taphonomy as the first diagnostic possibility when undertaking paleopathological analysis and suggest using the term "taphognomonic" to refer to bone modifications specific to a particular taphonomic agent, action, or factor (2017:17). Experienced observers ought to be able to identify commonly encountered taphonomic changes. However, they can be difficult to recognize when moving between regions or periods or when working within contexts outside one's experience. For example, taphonomic processes can differ in temperate and tropical climates, and human bone recovered from caves will typically (but not always) have a much more complex taphonomic history than those recovered from graves.

Important to consider, however, is that taphonomic damage to bone does not rule out the presence of pathological changes to that bone. Hence, when both taphonomic damage and pathological conditions are present, it can be complicated to differentiate between the two. An important step in differential diagnosis is thus to indicate the degree of certainty that a bony change is related to a pathological, rather than taphonomic process. Description of taphonomic processes should be provided alongside the description of bony lesions, rather than separately, so that the two can be clearly understood by the reader, but with clear explanation of which bony changes are ante-mortem, peri-mortem, or post-mortem (Buikstra et al., 2017:84).

Taphonomic analysis has developed significantly in the last decades, driven partly by the increasing role of bioarchaeology in paleopathological analysis and by the increasing interest in forensic taphonomy. Both the actions and mechanisms of taphonomic processes are understood far better now than they were ten years ago. It is recommended that recent primary taphonomic literature be consulted alongside relevant textbooks (e.g., Schotsmans et al., 2017 and references therein), in order to accurately differentiate taphonomic processes from pathological ones. It is essential that paleopathologists understand the specific ways in which taphonomy affects bone structure, just as they need to understand the pathophysiology of the conditions they are diagnosing.

Fragmentation of skeletons and individual skeletal elements also complicates differential diagnosis: in a commingled skeletal assemblage, it may not be possible to identify which skeletal elements belong to which individual. Under these circumstances, the ability to undertake differential diagnosis may be limited. Approaches that allow dispersed skeletal elements to be reunited, such as pair matching, will often be impossible for pathological bone. For commingled assemblages, therefore, the best approach is usually to record lesions systematically by skeletal element. Because not all skeletal elements are present, it will often only be possible to classify diseases into broad categories (for example, see Assis et al., 2018) in commingled remains. Cremated bone offers another challenge due to extreme fragmentation, warping, and damage to bone surfaces. McKinley (1997:131) notes that, while it is often possible to identify lesions in cremated bone, it is frequently impossible to move from the recording of lesions to diagnosis of a specific pathological condition. Histological analysis can sometimes aid in the understanding of the pathophysiology of a specific lesion in cremated bone (see, for example, Nováček & Schultz, 2020), but because cremated bone is typically incomplete, a differential diagnosis may remain impossible.

In distinguishing abnormal from normal bone, demographic variation in response to disease must be considered. Lewis (2017: 8) notes that five key factors cause differences in the nature and frequency of disease expression in children compared to adults: rapid bone remodeling; bone plasticity; the presence of cartilaginous growth plates; the periosteum (which is looser, thicker, and more active); and the presence of large amounts of red bone marrow. Of particular importance is the fact that the presence of woven bone is normal in infants, but usually considered pathological in individuals over the age of two. Although age-related changes in bony response in adults are less frequently discussed, differences in bony responses in older adults should also be considered: factors such as differences in rates of bone turnover, reduced response to mechanical loading (Borgiani et al., 2019), and reduced bone mass compared to younger adults should be considered when identifying pathological bone, and especially in relation to taphonomic factors. Such considerations mean that the identification of abnormal bone needs to be tailored to the circumstances of the individual being analyzed, and this is also true of the later stages in the differential diagnosis process.

Recording the Skeletal Lesions Precisely, Accurately, and Consistently

Recording skeletal lesions must be thorough, accurate, consistent, and clearly communicated in order to allow accurate diagnosis and reduce inter-observer error. Mays (see Chapter 2, this volume) covers this in more detail, but the basic principles are covered here. Ortner (2012:250) notes that the names we apply to the abnormalities encountered in human paleopathology, and how we classify these abnormalities, often make a big difference between confusion and understanding. Indeed, a basic component of any scientific discipline is rigor in defining and using terms. Similarly, Klaus (2017:98) notes that terms used are not just a matter of communication, as precise use of terminology enables a fuller understanding of disease processes. Many paleopathologists have decried the use of the tautological term 'pathological lesion', but although irritating, it is unlikely to cause significant confusion. Terms used to describe anatomy, lesions, and their positioning, though, need to be recorded in a way that is precise and unambiguous since variation in recording the same skeletal lesion will lead to error both in diagnosis and interpretation. Anatomical and directional terminology should follow current international standards published in the *Terminologia anatomica* (FIPAT, 2019). It is worth noting that there have been a number of changes relating to skeletal anatomy in the *Terminologia anatomica* of 2019 in comparison to the previous version. Chmielewski and Domagala (2020) highlight many of these, alongside commonly misused anatomical terms. When discussing congenital anomalies, it may also be necessary to consult the *Terminologia Embryologica* (FIPAT, 2017). Specialist terminology for physical anthropology, to be published as the *Terminologia Anatomica Anthropologica*, is currently in development. Within paleopathology, lesion descriptions should use the terms defined in *Nomenclature in Paleopathology* (Manchester et al., 2016). While many paleopathologists follow these guidelines, a review of articles published in 2021 in the *International Journal of Paleopathology* indicates that non-standard terms are still being employed. It is also notable that *Nomenclature in Paleopathology* is very rarely cited in the materials and methods sections of paleopathology papers, making it difficult to establish how widely used it is (for example, it received no citations in articles published in the *International Journal of Paleopathology* between January and June 2021). Given the importance of standard terminology, it is recommended that *Nomenclature in Paleopathology* is not just used in practice, but is routinely cited in methods. When *Nomenclature in Paleopathology* definitions are insufficiently precise, authors must be clear on how terms are defined. It is also worth consulting Ragsdale (1992:8) on terms to be avoided in description of lesions.

Considering the Full Appropriate Range of Possible Diagnoses

Mays (2020:90) has noted that while there is an expanding literature on differential diagnosis, there is relatively little discussion of the processes to be followed in order to achieve a successful differential diagnosis. This is particularly important for the identification of plausible conditions that could form part of a diagnosis: how can a paleopathologist ensure that the full range of plausible diagnoses is considered while excluding those that are not realistic in a manner that is consistent and rigorous? In addition, how do we ensure that all plausible diagnoses are fully considered and that we do not concentrate our efforts on proving a favored diagnosis (Buikstra et al., 2017:80)? Lawler (2017:120) notes that it requires expertise, experience, and research effort, while Mays (2020) emphasizes that generating a potential list of conditions for differential diagnosis cannot be accomplished from an intellectual blank slate. Intuitive ideas about likely diagnoses will present themselves from the moment the skeleton is first observed, and there is no way for the researcher to avoid this. He therefore suggests that we should formally integrate this intuitive reasoning into the diagnostic process using approaches from cognitive science and script theory. In this model, "disease scripts" are activated when the researcher first observes a skeleton, suggesting potential diagnoses. These intuitive diagnoses will be dependent on the expertise and previous experiences of the observer. The initial data set is then expanded through a thorough literature search, which is used to generate potential alternative diagnoses. Systematic recording of lesions (including imaging or other diagnostic techniques) is then undertaken in order to evaluate the proposed possibilities, at which point it is possible that new potential diagnoses may present themselves. Only after these steps are completed can a systematic differential diagnosis be undertaken.

Mays (2020) and others (e.g., Buikstra et al., 2017) emphasize using a literature search to generate a list of possible conditions, but the sources used by paleopathologists, in reality, are much wider than this. Table 3.2 offers different sources of information and their advantages and disadvantages, emphasizing the value of a wide range of resources. During the earlier stages of data gathering, a maximal list of potential diagnoses and emphasis on identifying all potential causes of a lesion/lesions is essential. Using informal sources of data (such as asking a colleague's opinion) is therefore as valid as other approaches, as long as it is followed up by a thorough examination of the clinical literature and systematic exclusion of conditions that cannot explain all aspects of the lesions.

It is worth briefly considering what might be "plausible" for a given case. "Plausible" cases include all conditions expected to be part of the differential diagnosis by a well-informed researcher. Thus, even if it is possible for a paleopathologist to rule out a condition on the basis of casual observation, if that condition is a part of the differential diagnosis, the justification for exclusion must be as thoroughly documented as more likely diagnoses.

Table 3.2 Sources of information for generating and refining differential diagnosis. N.B. This list is indicative rather than definitive

Data source	Advantages	Disadvantages	Use for
Paleopathology atlases	– Give an overview of many conditions – May list differential diagnoses	– Do not always promote detailed understanding of biology of disease processes – Images offer limited view of disease expression (images frequently show severe disease expression)	Initial evaluation of diagnostic possibilities, alongside other sources
Condition-specific paleopathological literature	– Considers expression of disease in skeletonized archaeological remains – Biological processes typically (although not universally) well described and explained	– Danger of circular argument in the absence of clinically confirmed cases – Published cases may over-emphasize severe disease	Refining diagnostic possibilities
Paleopathologist colleagues (in person or via specialist groups such as the Paleopathological Association)	May have previous experience of similar disease presentations	– Potential for confirmation bias – Potential for misinterpretation of photographic information when consulted remotely (cf. Biehler-Gomez et al., 2020)	Initial evaluation of diagnostic possibilities, alongside other sources
Online paleopathological resources (e.g., Digitized Diseases)	Enables comparison with 3D models of well-described pathological specimens that would otherwise be inaccessible	– Resource may not be updated, so may not take changes in understanding of disease process into account – Limits to resolution of scanning	Initial evaluation of diagnostic possibilities, alongside other sources

Data source	Advantages	Disadvantages	Use for
Radiopaedia (online resource)	– Case studies may indicate typical and unusual expressions of disease – Explicitly targets areas of the world with poorer access to medical care so may include more examples of advanced cases of untreated disease than western medical texts	Limited to conditions visible on radiographs; variable peer review	Initial evaluation of diagnostic possibilities, alongside other sources
General orthopedic texts	Give an overview of relevant conditions and introductions to disease processes	– May be primarily radiographic – May not consider all bony lesions in archaeological skeletons – Expense of texts may mean scholars lack access to up-to-date edition	Initial evaluation of diagnostic possibilities, alongside other sources
Modern primary clinical literature	Diagnostic criteria fully set out and linked to biological processes of disease	Treatment of modern cases means full range of disease expression is unlikely to be seen in western examples (literature from areas without universal access to medical care may be helpful in this regard and should be sought out)	Refining diagnostic possibilities
Historical primary clinical literature	– Indicate disease progression in the absence of modern treatment – May devote more attention to lesion manifestations than modern sources, which tend to focus on treatment	– Historical (mis) understandings of anatomy, biology, and disease process may complicate interpretation – Disease classifications may change over time – Texts may be written (and illustrations prepared) by those who have never seen the condition – Biases in recording may relate to the recipient of the text (Mitchell, 2011)	Refining diagnostic possibilities (with careful attention to potential misinformation)

(Continued)

Data source	Advantages	Disadvantages	Use for
Medical specialists	Significant expertise in specific conditions of interest	– May lack familiarity with appearance of lesions in dry bone – May lack familiarity with appearance of untreated advanced disease – May lack familiarity with diseases that are uncommon in modern medical contexts N.B. Clinicians may need to be warned of the relative fragility of archaeological bone	– Refining diagnostic possibilities in dialogue with the paleopathologist – Especially useful for more unusual disease presentations.

Accurately Ruling Out Diagnoses That Do Not Fit Lesions Observed and Accurately Assessing the Likelihood of Those That Remain

Once a potential list of conditions has been compiled, the process of differential diagnosis depends upon the compatibility, sensitivity, and specificity of the lesions associated with a condition, alongside the significance of lesion distribution within the body. A lesion is a highly sensitive indicator for a disease if it is usually present when the disease is present, and it is a highly specific indicator of a disease if it is rarely associated with other conditions. In reality, sensitivity tends to increase as specificity decreases, and vice versa (Milner & Boldsen, 2017).

For each potential disease or condition posited by differential diagnosis, the first step is to generate an exhaustive list of the skeletal lesions associated with the condition and the concomitant pathophysiology. This is based on the relevant clinical and paleopathological literature and should not rely exclusively on general paleopathology textbooks, no matter how useful these are in providing an overview of pathological conditions that affect the skeleton. The next step is to consider whether each lesion observed on the skeletal remains is compatible with the lesions associated with the condition. Compatibility should be identified through identification of the pathophysiology of the lesion formation process and not through a process of "ribbon matching" (Ortner, 2011:6) with lesions in known cases of the disease. Additional analyses may need to be carried out at this stage to refine the diagnostic options. This may involve photography, radiology, computed tomography, histology, electron microscopy, mineralogy, bacteriological, parasitological, or genetic analyses (Lawler, 2017:122). Careful consideration of additional techniques involving destructive analysis is essential. Before any destructive approaches are used, both their diagnostic potential and ethical considerations must be thoroughly evaluated alongside consultation with interest groups and stakeholders.

Of course, just because a lesion is *compatible* with a disease, does not ensure that it is *diagnostic* of that disease. Table 3.3 offers an updated version of the modified Istanbul Terminological Protocol (Appleby et al., 2015) that can be used to associate the presence of a lesion with the likelihood of a disease diagnosis, alongside suggested abbreviations. Importantly, the updated modified Istanbul Terminological Protocol uses additional categories

Table 3.3 Updated modified Istanbul Terminological Protocol and suggested abbreviations for use in tables of diagnostic criteria

Lesion criteria	Definition	Abbreviation
Diagnostic of	Pathognomonic lesion, not associated with other conditions	+++
Typical of★	Usually associated with the condition	++
Highly consistent with★★	Lesion can be associated with the condition and there are few other possible causes	++
Consistent with	Can be associated with the condition	+
Pathophysiologically consistent with	Consistent with the pathophysiology of the condition, but previously unreported in the clinical literature	+/−
Not consistent with	Not consistent with the condition	−
Undefined	Currently undefined, but with possible lesion involvement	?

★"Typical of" denotes lesions that are relatively sensitive indicators of a condition.
★★"Highly consistent with" denotes lesions that are relatively specific indicators of a condition.
Source: Adapted from Appleby et al., 2015 and Klaus 2017, Table 3.3.

from Klaus (2017:Table 3). These make it possible to indicate that a lesion is compatible with the pathophysiology of a condition, even if the indicator has not been described in the clinical literature, and to recognize cases where the expression of a disease in the skeleton is incompletely understood. The term "typical of" is used to report lesions that are relatively sensitive indicators of a condition, while 'highly consistent with' is used to report lesions that are relatively specific indicators of a condition. When a lesion appears incompatible with the pathophysiology of a condition, it is important to consider whether that condition should be ruled out or whether it could be associated with a co-occurring disease process.

Differential diagnosis in paleopathology is not simply a matter of considering whether lesions associated with a condition are present. Consideration of whether and why lesions which might be expected to be associated with a particular disease (i.e., highly sensitive lesions) might be absent is equally important. On that basis, it is important to consider whether a condition would normally be associated with additional lesions, and if so, whether they are present, absent, or unobservable. Thorough recording should have identified obvious lesions earlier in the recording process, but it is possible that more subtle lesions may have been overlooked, especially if lesions are not macroscopically visible and are only apparent through the use of other techniques, such as radiography (Mays, 2020, Table 2). While absence of evidence is famously not evidence of absence, the absence of lesions that are sensitive indicators of a condition is a critical factor in the evaluation of diagnoses. In these cases, researchers should bear in mind the osteological paradox: the absence of lesions may indicate absence of disease but may also indicate that death took place before lesions developed. In addition, factors that affect lesion expression must be considered (Table 3.4).

Once a full consideration of a lesion or lesions has been completed, viable diagnostic options should become clear. Table 3.5 offers terms to express certainty in diagnosis and their definitions. When a condition is classified as "cannot be", it can be ruled out from the diagnoses. All remaining diagnostic options should be discussed based on their likelihood: a definitive diagnosis can be identified as "certain to be", while lesser degrees of certainty can be indicated with "highly likely to be", "could be", and "unlikely to be". The assessment of

Table 3.4 Factors potentially affecting lesion severity, morphology, and distribution in the skeleton

Factor	Explanation	Example
Age of onset	Changes in anatomy during growth affect bony response to disease. Immune response varies over the life course (Simon, et al., 2015). Lewis (2017) discusses disease expression in children in more detail	Marrow hyperplasia associated with anemia is present only in skeletal areas retaining red marrow, meaning that porosity of the orbit roof only develops in children
Sex	– Females tend to have stronger immune responses than males, which can affect both susceptibility to disease and disease severity (generally estrogens increase immune competence, whereas androgens reduce it) – Sex hormones affect bone remodeling (DeWitte, 2017) – Pregnancy uncouples bone formation and resorption (Black et al., 2000) and has complex effects on immune response (Mor & Cardenas, 2010)	Adult females worldwide tend to have worse oral health than males, with greater prevalence and severity of dental caries. Several underlying factors explain this: there is a correlation between estrogen levels and caries rates; saliva flow rate is lower in women than men; the antimicrobial function and buffering capacity of saliva are reduced in pregnancy; food cravings in pregnancy can increase intake of foods that create a cariogenic environment (Lukacs, 2017).
Nutritional status	– Nutritional inadequacy affects immune response – Specific nutritional deficiencies, as well as under- and overnutrition, can affect bone remodeling (Seibel, 2002) – Nutritional inadequacy may enhance the effects of deleterious alleles	Scurvy reduces osteoblastic activity, which may reduce the expression of pathological conditions involving bone formation (Schattmann et al., 2016)
Speed and effectiveness of treatment	– Quick and effective treatment may prevent a condition becoming chronic and thus prevent skeletal involvement, while slow but effective treatments may enable complete healing of lesions – Treatment that slows disease progression may enable survival for long enough for skeletal lesions to develop – Ineffective treatment may have no effect or may be associated with more severe disease	A study of documented South African skeletons showed that since the introduction of antibiotics, the prevalence of spinal lesions in tuberculosis has decreased, but overall levels of skeletal involvement have increased (Steyn & Buskes, 2016)

Factor	Explanation	Example
Whether lesions are active, healed, or recurrent	Healed lesions may be harder to distinguish from normal anatomical variation than active lesions and may become completely remodeled	Active rickets in children is easier to diagnose than healed rickets in adults, where deformity may have been corrected through growth and modeling (Brickley & Mays, 2019: 541)
Co-occurrence of different conditions	Effects of one condition on bone modeling and remodeling may inhibit or exaggerate the effects of another	Where rickets and scurvy co-occur, each affects the other: scurvy reduces osteoblastic activity, which inhibits the production of unmineralized osteoid, whereas rickets inhibits bone mineralization and therefore limits new bone formation and calcified matrix accumulation (Schattmann et al., 2016:64)
Genes (alleles) affecting disease expression	Presence or absence of multiple risk-associated alleles can increase or decrease expression of disease	Alleles affect the expression of some erosive arthropathies. For example, different alleles associated with psoriatic arthritis are associated with different phenotypic characteristics (FitzGerald et al., 2015)
Activity patterns	High activity levels might increase disease severity or might be protective against severe disease	Large cystic lesions in rheumatoid arthritis are most commonly associated with individuals who continue heavy physical activity (Castillo et al., 1965)
Bone former/bone loser status	Tendency to form or lose bone may affect the appearance of lesions	There is evidence for an inverse relationship between osteoarthritis and osteoporosis (Im & Kim, 2014)
In infectious disease:		
Adequacy of immune response	– A strong immune response may allow the patient to recover before the disease becomes chronic, reducing the likelihood and severity of skeletal lesions – Immune response may affect the expression of the disease	Leprosy infection can lead to no noticeable disease, mild disease (tuberculoid type), or more severe disease (lepromatous type), which is typically the type that affects the skeleton. The primary reason for the variability in expression of leprosy is the immune response (Ridley & Jopling, 1966; Roberts & Buikstra, 2019)
Virulence and other aspects of biology of causative agents	More virulent disease-causing organisms may cause death before skeletal lesions develop or slow recovery, allowing a condition to become chronic and skeletal lesions to develop	Early descriptions of syphilis suggest that it was considerably more virulent in the first few years after its introduction and then became less so (Knell, 2004)

(Continued)

Factor	Explanation	Example
Size of inoculum	The larger the inoculum, the more likely that clinical disease will develop and the more severe the infection is likely to be	Study of household contacts of tuberculosis patients has shown that household contacts with more intense exposure were more likely to develop disease than those with less intense exposure (Acuña-Villaorduña et al., 2018)
Portal of entry	Different parts of the body and anatomical structures respond differently to inoculation by a pathogen	*Streptococcus* causes septic sore throat and mastoiditis when entering through the mouth, erysipelas when entering through the skin and osteomyelitis and endocarditis when entering as a result of penetrating trauma (Ragsdale & Lehmer, 2012: 236).
Causative agent	The frequency with which an infectious disease spreads to bone in diseases that can affect the skeleton varies according to the behavior of the pathogen	In cases of disseminated Cryptococcosis, bone involvement is present around 10% of the time, whereas with disseminated coccidioidomycosis, bone involvement is present around 50% of the time (Ortner, 2003:326)
Evolution of causative agent	Host-pathogen evolution means that the severity and effects of disease on the skeleton are likely to change over time	Limited research currently exists on specific changes in bony response to pathogen evolution, although it is speculated that this may have occurred with many infectious diseases (for example, syphilis; Knell, 2004). Future aDNA research in tandem with paleopathological analysis may clarify changes in disease processes

Source: Adapted and expanded from Mays, 2018:16.

likelihood should be based on the analysis of lesions, but should also take into account external factors affecting the likelihood of a particular disease (Table 3.6). At this stage, as in earlier stages, it is essential that researchers share their decision-making process. Presenting how and why different diagnostic possibilities were weighted allows future paleopathologists to utilize the process in their own research. This is particularly important when lesions have been identified as pathophysiologically consistent or previously undefined for particular conditions/diseases. In many cases, precise diagnosis is unrealistic or impossible. In these instances, providing an association with a disease category will be more accurate than an attempt to over-refine the diagnosis (cf. Jacobi & Danforth, 2002; Ragsdale & Lehmer, 2012; Buikstra et al., 2017). There are a variety of ways to categorize pathological conditions. To avoid ambiguity and allow consistency, it is recommended that researchers use the VITAMIN (Vascular, Innervation/Mechanical, Trauma/repair, Anomaly, Metabolic, Inflammatory/Immune, Neoplastic) criteria of Ragsdale and Lehmer (Ragsdale & Lehmer, 2012), whenever possible. This classificatory system considers the behavior of bone at a cellular level, which makes it particularly suitable when diagnosis follows a pathophysiological approach.

Table 3.5 Criteria for indicating certainty in overall diagnosis alongside suggested abbreviations

Diagnostic certainty	Definition	Abbreviation
Certain to be	Pathognomonic lesion(s) is/are present	+++
Highly likely to be	No pathognomonic lesions are present, but lesions are typical of the condition or highly consistent with the condition	++
Could be	Either: Lesions present are compatible with the condition but non-specific Or: Lesions present are compatible with the condition, but additional lesions that would typically be expected with this condition are absent or unobservable	+
Unlikely to be	Either: Some lesions are incompatible with the condition, but they may represent a separate condition Or: Lesions present are very unusual for this condition	-/+
Cannot be	Either: All lesions present are incompatible with this condition Or: Some lesions present are incompatible with this condition and co-presence of this condition with another that could explain incompatible lesions is not plausible	-

Table 3.6 Factors affecting disease likelihood*

Factor	Explanation	Example
Age of onset	Certain conditions are limited to particular age groups or predominantly develop before or after specific ages	Multiple myeloma is predominantly a disease of the elderly (Turesson et al., 2010)
Sex	Certain conditions are only or predominantly present in specific sexes	Around 99% of cases of breast cancer are associated with women only 1% with men (Giordano, 2018)
Gender	Gendered patterns of behavior will affect disease risk and potentially severity because (i) gender is associated with particular occupations/tasks; (ii) gender is associated with different nutritional status and diet; (iii) gender may be associated with living conditions	The ratio of female:male leprosy patients varies according to a number of factors including whether women work outside the household (which increases exposure risk) and gendered differences in access to healthcare. In some countries, women wait significantly longer than men before seeking treatment (Le Grand, 1997)

(Continued)

Factor	Explanation	Example
Social status	Social status will affect disease risk and severity because (i) status is often associated with occupations/tasks; (ii) status may be associated with differential access to nutrition and diet; (iii) status may be associated with living conditions	People of lower socioeconomic status are at increased risk of TB in many societies worldwide due to crowded living conditions, poor nutrition, and poor access to medical treatment (e.g., Spence et al., 1993; Pelissari & Diaz-Quijano, 2017)
Ethnic group/population	The frequency of specific genes in interaction with environmental and behavioral factors will affect the likelihood of disease in different populations.	Gaucher's disease frequency is related to genetic mutations and is typically present in around 1/111,111 worldwide, but is present in approximately 1/855 Ashkenazi Jews (Burrow et al., 2011:60). In contrast, the causal factors underlying multiple myeloma are much more poorly understood, but there was a 2-3 times higher incidence of multiple myeloma amongst black American people in comparison with white American people between 1973 and 2005, and the age of onset was typically 4 years younger amongst black people than white people (Waxman et al., 2010). Research has so far failed to uncover genetic candidates that explain this difference (Padala et al., 2021)
Geographic location	This may affect the presence of disease-causing organisms, as well as environmental and nutritional risk factors for disease.	Coccidioidomycosis infection occurs only in the Western hemisphere in some southern states of the USA, Central, and South America due to the distribution of the pathogen *Coccidioides immitis* (Grauer & Roberts, 2019:442)
Time period/archaeological horizon	This may relate to whether a disease is present, as well as to how common it is. For infectious disease, this might include consideration of the period when a zoonosis made the transition to human populations and how effectively it spread. For non-infectious disease it might relate to patterns of human behavior (see below)	Malaria was absent in Mauritius until 1865. Anopheles mosquitoes were introduced into the country after the 1864 opening of a steamship line with Madagascar, whereas the Plasmodium parasite was probably already present in immigrant workers who arrived from India from 1834 onwards (Lambrechts et al., 2011). Only when both parasite and mosquito were present, did the disease spread widely.

Factor	Explanation	Example
Behavior/occupation	Risk factors for different diseases and conditions are associated with human activity.	In Britain, phosphorous necrosis ('phossy jaw') was caused by phosphorous poisoning in the matchstick industry during the industrial revolution (Roberts et al., 2016)

*This table deliberately includes social factors that must be assessed contextually, as well as biological factors such as age and sex. The likelihood of a condition being present is affected by complex inter-relationships between factors.

Source: Adapted and expanded from Ortner 2003, Chapter 3.

Clearly Communicating Steps in Archiving and Publication of Results

Although the focus of this chapter is on the process of differential diagnosis, how paleopathologists communicate that process is also critically important to discuss. Differential diagnosis is a process of understanding and to some extent resolving uncertainty. However, it is also a process of communicating that uncertainty. If we fail to do this, differential diagnosis becomes a "black box" process in the published literature, and readers are forced to rely blindly on trust rather than on evidence and the peer review process.

Within paleopathology, differential diagnosis is an expected process and ought to be a requisite component of every publication. Still, publications appear where differential diagnosis is absent, which is concerning since they tend to be those where non-specialists interact with paleopathological data. Although there are worthy exceptions, in site reports and non-specialist publications, it is common for diagnosed pathological conditions to be presented as fact without reference to the differential diagnosis process or the degree of certainty associated with the diagnosis. This is important because it generates a false sense of certainty in our data, which may not be warranted, and allows mistakes and inaccuracies to remain unidentified. Hence, the differential diagnosis process should be available to readers, even if as an appendix. When this is not possible, the differential diagnosis must be part of the site archive. This is particularly important as reburial of human remains renders future evaluation impossible. A paleopathological diagnosis should never have to be taken on trust.

Conclusion

Because bone is constrained in its response to disease, differential diagnosis in paleopathology will always be a complex and somewhat limited process. In many cases, the diagnostic options cannot be reduced to a single condition even with the most rigorous approach. The role of the paleopathologist is to ensure that skeletal lesions are recorded thoroughly and accurately, using standardized terminology and indicating uncertainties, alongside the strength of those uncertainties. Differential diagnosis should follow the pathophysiological approach, whereby diagnosis is based on the specific effects of a condition on bone rather than a process of asserting that one lesion simply looks like another published image (Ortner, 2011:6). While rigor in recording and diagnosis is essential to the success and future of paleopathology, so too is the communication of process. Attention to these details will assist specialists and non-specialists alike for centuries to come.

Acknowledgments

Sarah Inskip kindly read a draft of this paper. My sincere thanks to Anne Grauer for being possibly the most patient editor in the history of academic publishing after my writing plans were interrupted by the SARS-CoV-2 pandemic.

References

Acuña-Villaorduña, C., Jones-López, E. C., Fregona, G., Marques-Rodrigues, P., Gaeddert, M., Geadas, C., … & Dietze, R. (2018). Intensity of exposure to pulmonary tuberculosis determines risk of tuberculosis infection and disease. *European Respiratory Journal* 51:1701578. DOI:10.1183/13993003.01578–2017

Appleby, J., Thomas, R. & Buikstra, J. (2015). Increasing confidence in paleopathological diagnosis – Application of the Istanbul terminological framework. *International Journal of Paleopathology* 8:19–21. https://doi.org/10.1016/j.ijpp.2014.07.003

Assis, S., Henderson, C. Y., Casimiro, S. & Alves Cardoso, F. (2018). Is differential diagnosis attainable in disarticulated pathological bone remains? A case-study from a late 19th/early 20th century necropolis from Juncal (Porto de Mos, Portugal). *International Journal of Paleopathology* 20:26–37. DOI:10.1016/j.ijpp.2017.10.007

Biehler-Gomez, L., Indra, L., Martino, F., Campobasso, C. P. & Cattaneo, C. (2020). Observer error in bone disease description: a cautionary note. *International Journal of Osteoarchaeology* 30:607–615. https://doi.org/10.1002/oa.2885

Black, A. J., Topping, J., Durham, B., Farquharson, R. G. & Fraser, W. D. (2000). A detailed assessment of alterations in bone turnover, calcium homeostasis, and bone density in normal pregnancy. *Journal of Bone and Mineral Research* 15:557–563. https://doi.org/10.1359/jbmr.2000.15.3.557

Borgiani, E., Figge, C., Kruck, B., Willie, B. M., Duda, G. N. & Checa, S. (2019). Age-related changes in the mechanical regulation of bone healing are explained by altered cellular mechanoresponse. *Journal of Bone and Mineral Research* 34:1923–1937. https://doi.org/10.1002/jbmr.3801

Brickley, M. & Ives, R. (2006). Skeletal manifestations of infantile scurvy. *American Journal of Physical Anthropology* 129(2):163–172. https://doi.org/10.1002/ajpa.20265

Brickley, M. B. (2018). Cribra orbitalia and porotic hyperostosis: a biological approach to diagnosis. *American Journal of Physical Anthropology* 167:896–902. doi:https://doi.org/10.1002/ajpa.23701

Brickley, M. B. & Mays, S. (2019). Metabolic disease. In Buikstra, J. E. (Ed.), *Ortner's Identification of Pathological Conditions in Human Skeletal Remains* (third edition), pp. 531–566. London: Academic Press.

Buikstra, J. E., Cook, D. C. & Bolhofner, K. L. (2017). Introduction: scientific rigor in paleopathology. *International Journal of Paleopathology* 19:80–87. https://doi.org/10.1016/j.ijpp.2017.08.005

Burrow, T. A., Barnes, S. & Grabowski, G. A. (2011). Prevalence and management of Gaucher disease. *Pediatric Health, Medicine and Therapeutics* 2:59–73. https://doi.org/10.2147/PHMT.S12499

Castillo, B., El Sallab, R. & Scott, J. (1965). Physical activity, cystic erosions, and osteoporosis in rheumatoid arthritis. *Annals of the Rheumatic Diseases* 24:522–527. http://dx.doi.org.ezproxy4.lib.le.ac.uk/10.1136/ard.24.6.522

Chmielewski, P. P. & Domagała, Z. A. (2020). Terminologia anatomica and its practical usage: pitfalls and how to avoid them. *Folia Morphologica* 79:198–204. https://doi.org/10.5603/FM.a2019.0086

Corron, L., Huchet, J. B., Santos, F. & Dutour, O. (2017). Using classifications to identify pathological and taphonomic modifications on ancient bones: do "taphognomonic" criteria exist? *Bulletins et mémoires de la Société d'Anthropologie de Paris* 29(1):1–18. http://doi.org/10.1007/s13219-016-0176-3

DeWitte, S. N. (2017). Sex and frailty: patterns from catastrophic and attritional assemblages in medieval Europe. In Agarwal, S. C. & Wesp, J. K. (Eds.), *Exploring Sex and Gender in Bioarchaeology*, pp. 189–221. Albuquerque: University of New Mexico Press.

FIPAT, (2017). *Terminologia Embryologica*. Last accessed at: https://fipat.library.dal.ca/te2/

FIPAT, (2019). *Terminologia Anatomica*. Last accessed at: https://fipat.library.dal.ca/ta2/

FitzGerald, O., Haroon, M., Giles, J. T. & Winchester, R. (2015). Concepts of pathogenesis in psoriatic arthritis: genotype determines clinical phenotype. *Arthritis Research & Therapy* 17:115. https://doi.org/10.1186/s13075-015-0640-3

Giordano, S. H. (2018). Breast cancer in men. *New England Journal of Medicine* 378:2311–2320. https://doi.org/10.1056/NEJMra1707939

Grauer, A. L. (2018). A century of paleopathology. *American Journal of Physical Anthropology* 165:904–914. https://doi.org/10.1002/ajpa.23366

Grauer, A. L. & Roberts, C. A. (2019). Fungal, viral, multicelled parasitic, and protozoan infections. In Buikstra. J. E. (Ed.), *Ortner's Identification of Pathological Conditions in Human Skeletal Remains* (third edition), pp. 441–478. London: Academic Press.

Im, G.-I. & Kim, M.-K. (2014). The relationship between osteoarthritis and osteoporosis. *Journal of Bone and Mineral Metabolism* 32:101–109. https://doi.org/10.1007/s00774-013-0531-0

Jacobi, K. P. & Danforth, M. E. (2002). Analysis of interobserver scoring patterns in porotic hyperostosis and cribra orbitalia. *International Journal of Osteoarchaeology* 12:248–258. https://doi.org/10.1002/oa.619

Klaus, H. D. (2017). Paleopathological rigor and differential diagnosis: case studies involving terminology, description, and diagnostic frameworks for scurvy in skeletal remains. *International Journal of Paleopathology* 19:96–110. DOI:10.1016/j.ijpp.2015.10.002

Klaus, H. D. & Lynnerup, N. (2019). Abnormal bone: considerations for documentation, disease process identification, and differential diagnosis. In Buikstra, J. E. (Ed.), *Ortner's Identification of Pathological Conditions in Human Skeletal Remains* (third edition), pp. 59–89. London: Academic Press.

Knell, R. J. (2004). Syphilis in renaissance Europe: Rapid evolution of an introduced sexually transmitted disease? *Proceedings. Biological sciences* 271(Suppl 4):S174–S176. https://doi.org/10.1098/rsbl.2003.0131

Lambrechts, L., Cohuet, A. & Robert, V. (2011). Encyclopedia of biological invasions. In Daniel, S. & Marcel, R. (Eds.), *Malaria Vectors*, pp. 442–445. Berkeley: University of California Press.

Lawler, D. F. (2017). Differential diagnosis in archaeology. *International Journal of Paleopathology* 19:119–123. https://doi.org/10.1016/j.ijpp.2016.05.001

Le Grand, A. (1997). Women and leprosy: A review. *Leprosy Review* 68(3):203–211. doi:http://doi.org/10.5935/0305-7518.19970028

Lewis, M. (2017). *Paleopathology of Children: Identification of Pathological Conditions in the Human Skeletal Remains of Non-Adults*. London: Academic Press.

Lukacs, J. R. (2017). Bioarchaeology of oral health: sex and gender differences in disease. In Agarwal, S. C. & Wesp, J. K. (Eds.), *Exploring Sex and Gender in Bioarchaeology*, pp. 263–290. Albuquerque: University of New Mexico Press.

Lynnerup, N. & Klaus, H. D. (2019). Fundamentals of human bone and dental biology: structure, function, and development. In Buikstra, J. E. (Ed.), *Ortner's Identification of Pathological Conditions in Human Skeletal Remains* (third edition), pp. 35-48. London: Academic Press.

Manchester, K., Ogden, A. & Storm, R. (2016). Nomenclature in palaeopathology. *Paleopathology Association Newsletter*. Last accessed at: https://paleopathology-association.wildapricot.org/Nomenclature-in-Paleopathology

Mays, S. A. (2018). How should we diagnose disease in palaeopathology? Some epistemological considerations. *International Journal of Paleopathology* 20:12–19. https://doi.org/10.1016/j.ijpp.2017.10.006

Mays, S. A. (2020). A dual process model for paleopathological diagnosis. *International Journal of Paleopathology* 31:89–96. https://doi.org/10.1016/j.ijpp.2020.10.001

McKinley, J. I. (1997). Bronze age 'barrows' and funerary rites and rituals of cremation. *Proceedings of the Prehistoric Society* 63:129–145.

Melikian, M. & Waldron, T. (2003). An examination of skulls from two British sites for possible evidence of scurvy. *International Journal of Osteoarchaeology* 13(4):207–212. https://doi.org/10.1002/oa.674

Milner, G. R. & Boldsen, J. L. (2017). Life not death: epidemiology from skeletons. *International Journal of Paleopathology* 17:26–39. 10.1016/j.ijpp.2017.03.007

Mitchell, P. D. (2011). Retrospective diagnosis and the use of historical texts for investigating disease in the past. *International Journal of Paleopathology* 1:81–88. https://doi.org/10.1016/j.ijpp.2011.04.002

Mor, G. & Cardenas, I. (2010). Review article: the immune system in pregnancy: a unique complexity. *American Journal of Reproductive Immunology* 63:425–433. https://doi.org/10.1111/j.1600-0897.2010.00836.x

Nováček, J. & Schultz, M. (2020). Palaeopathological investigations of cremated human remains – Methodological and comparative study on the example of traces of pathological conditions in the skull. *Anthropologischer Anzeiger; Bericht Uber die Biologisch-Anthropologische Literatur* 78:59–81. https://doi.org/10.1127/anthranz/2020/1259

Ortner, D. J. (2003). Background data in paleopathology. In Ortner, D. J. (Ed.), *Identification of Pathological Conditions in Human Skeletal Remains* (second edition), pp. 37–44. Amsterdam: Academic Press.

Ortner, D. J. (2011). Human skeletal paleopathology. *International Journal of Paleopathology* 1(1):4–11. https://doi.org/10.1016/j.ijpp.2011.01.002

Ortner, D. J. (2012). Differential diagnosis and issues in disease classification. In Grauer, A. L. (Ed.), *A Companion to Paleopathology*, pp. 250–267. Chichester: Blackwell.

Ortner, D. J. & Ericksen, M. F. (1997). Bone changes in the human skull probably resulting from scurvy in infancy and childhood. *International Journal of Osteoarchaeology* 7:212–220.

Padala, S. A., Barsouk, A., Barsouk, A., Rawla, P., Vakiti, A., Kolhe, R., Kota, V. & Ajebo, G. H. (2021). Epidemiology, staging, and management of multiple myeloma. *Medical Sciences* 9(1):3. Last accessed at: https://www.mdpi.com/2076-3271/9/1/3

Pelissari, D. M. & Diaz-Quijano, F. A. (2017). Household crowding as a potential mediator of socio-economic determinants of tuberculosis incidence in Brazil. *PLOS ONE* 12(4):e0176116. https://doi.org/10.1371/journal.pone.0176116

Ragsdale, B. D. (1992). Task force on terminology: provisional word list. *Paleopathology Association Newsletter* 78:7–8.

Ragsdale, B. D. & Lehmer, L. M. (2012). A knowledge of bone at the cellular (histological) level is essential to paleopathology. In Grauer, A. L. (Ed.), *A Companion to Paleopathology*, pp. 225–249. Chichester: Blackwell.

Ridley, D. & Jopling, W. (1966). Classification of leprosy according to immunity. *International Journal of Leprosy and other Mycobacterial Diseases* 34:255–273.

Roberts, C. A. & Buikstra, J. E. (2019). Bacterial infections. In Buikstra, J. E. (Ed.), *Ortner's Identification of Pathological Conditions in Human Skeletal Remains* (third edition), pp. 321–439. London: Academic Press.

Roberts, C. A., Caffell, A., Filipek-Ogden, K. L., Gowland, R. & Jakob, T. (2016). 'Til poison phosphorous brought them death': a potentially occupationally-related disease in a post-medieval skeleton from north-east England. *International Journal of Paleopathology* 13:39–48. https://doi.org/10.1016/j.ijpp.2015.12.001

Schattmann, A., Bertrand, B., Vatteoni, S. & Brickley, M. (2016). Approaches to co-occurrence: scurvy and rickets in infants and young children of 16–18th century Douai, France. *International Journal of Paleopathology* 12:63–75. https://doi.org/10.1016/j.ijpp.2015.12.002

Schotsmans, E. M. J., Márquez-Grant, N. & Forbes, S. L. (2017). *Taphonomy of Human Remains: Forensic Analysis of the Dead and the Depositional Environment*. New York, United Kingdom: John Wiley & Sons, Incorporated.

Seibel, M. J. (2002). Nutrition and molecular markers of bone remodelling. *Current Opinion in Clinical Nutrition & Metabolic Care* 5(5):525–531. https://doi.org/doi:10.1097/00075197-200209000-00011

Simon, A. K., Hollander, G. A. & McMichael, A. (2015). Evolution of the immune system in humans from infancy to old age. *Proceedings of the Royal Society B: Biological Sciences* 282(1821):20143085. doi:https://doi.org/doi:10.1098/rspb.2014.3085

Snoddy, A. M. E., Buckley, H. R., Elliott, G. E., Standen, V. G., Arriaza, B. T. & Halcrow, S. E. (2018). Macroscopic features of scurvy in human skeletal remains: a literature synthesis and diagnostic guide. *American Journal of Physical Anthropology* 167:876–895. 10.1002/ajpa.23699

Spence, D. P., Hotchkiss, J., Williams, C. S. & Davies, P. D. (1993). Tuberculosis and poverty. *British Medical Journal* 307(6907):759–761. https://doi.org/10.1136/bmj.307.6907.759

Stark, R. J. (2014). A proposed framework for the study of paleopathological cases of subadult scurvy. *International Journal of Paleopathology* 5:18–26. https://doi.org/10.1016/j.ijpp.2014.01.005

Steyn, M. & Buskes, J. (2016). Skeletal manifestations of tuberculosis in modern human remains. *Clinical Anatomy* 29:854–861. https://doi.org/10.1002/ca.22688

Tilley, L. (2015). *Theory and Practice in the Bioarchaeology of Care*. Cham, Switzerland: Springer.

Turesson, I., Velez, R., Kristinsson, S. Y. & Landgren, O. (2010). Patterns of multiple myeloma during the past 5 decades: stable incidence rates for all age groups in the population but rapidly changing age distribution in the clinic. *Mayo Clinic Proceedings* 85:225+. https://doi-org.ezproxy4.lib.le.ac.uk/10.4065/mcp.2009.0426

Waldron, T. (2008). *Palaeopathology*. Cambridge: Cambridge University Press.

Waxman, A. J., Mink, P. J., Devesa, S. S., Anderson, W. F., Weiss, B. M., Kristinsson, S. Y., McGlynn, K. A. & Landgren, O. (2010). Racial disparities in incidence and outcome in multiple myeloma: a population-based study. *Blood* 116:5501–5506. https://doi.org/10.1182/blood-2010-07-298760

Zuckerman, M. K., Harper, K. N. & Armelagos, G. J. (2016). Adapt or die: three case studies in which the failure to adopt advances from other fields has compromised paleopathology. *International Journal of Osteoarchaeology* 26:375–383. https://doi.org/10.1002/oa.2426

4
EPIDEMIOLOGY AND MATHEMATICAL MODELING

Samantha L. Yaussy

Introduction

Epidemiology is broadly defined as "the study of the distribution and determinants of health-related states or events in specified populations, and the application of this study to the control of health problems" (Porta, 2016: 95). Given this focus on controlling and curtailing contemporary health problems, modern epidemiology pays relatively little attention to the distribution and determinants of diseases and pathological conditions in past populations. Rather, population-level analyses of health and disease in the distant past are often considered to be adjacent to or subsumed under the discipline of paleopathology, which studies pathological conditions found in ancient human remains. As such, the relatively young field of paleoepidemiology encompasses an interdisciplinary approach to the study of disease determinants, patterns of disease susceptibility and risks of mortality, and health outcomes associated with disease in past human populations (Cohen & Crane-Kramer, 2003; Souza et al., 2003; Dutour, 2008).

Despite its close relationship with paleopathology, the objectives and analytical methods employed by paleoepidemiology are distinct and reflect the focus of the field on population-level patterns and processes. For instance, whereas paleopathology has historically examined the remains of one individual or a small number of individuals for the presence of highly distinctive skeletal lesions that can be attributed to a specific disease (i.e., differential diagnosis), paleoepidemiology has, from the outset, been concerned with associating the existence of skeletal lesions with the occurrence of specific diseases or conditions and, by extension, the risk of death those diseases or conditions posed to particular groups of people in the past. Likewise, the methodologies, theoretical approaches, and research pursuits of modern epidemiological studies and those of paleoepidemiological studies overlap to a degree, but the two fields remain distinct. Modern epidemiology and paleoepidemiology have a shared interest in patterns of morbidity and mortality within populations or population subsets, as well as the effects of social and biological variables on survivorship and health. However, the clinical trials, cohort studies, and case-control studies familiar to modern epidemiologists are largely inaccessible to paleoepidemiologists, who operate within the constraints imposed by the archaeological record, which includes a shortage of soft tissue and other contextual information, presumably silent subjects, and biased skeletal samples. Under these circumstances, the characterization of health conditions in past communities requires the development of new techniques and models or the modification of existing methods to overcome the shortcomings of the data that are available.

History of Paleoepidemiology

In anthropology, the first indication of interest in examining the epidemiological aspects of past societies through their skeletal remains was a study of the Pecos Indians conducted by Earnest Hooton (1930). Widely lauded as the foundation for modern skeletal biology, Hooton's research was also the first to incorporate paleoepidemiological measures into its analyses and interpretations, including basic statistics on mortality and skeletal lesion frequencies (Buikstra & Cook, 1980; Armelagos & Van Gerven, 2003). It would be more than a decade before another anthropologist would explore patterns of health at the population level. Lawrence Angel, a student of Hooton, investigated temporal changes in the frequencies of pathological conditions like arthritis and porotic hyperostosis (a lesion typically found on the cranium and often associated with the presence of anemia) in his studies of skeletal samples from Greece, Cyprus, and Anatolia and connected his findings to changing ecological and cultural factors (Angel, 1946, 1966, 1969). In the 1950s, a handful of other anthropologists, including Marcus Goldstein (1953, 1957) and James Roney Jr. (1959), would publish studies of skeletal lesion frequencies and their relationships to biological and cultural factors of interest, such as age, sex, and time period. Though few and far between, early paleoepidemiological studies of how host and environmental factors influenced patterns of health and disease at the population level contrasted starkly with the descriptive approaches to paleopathology that were popular at the time, which identified and described lesions in a single individual or skeletal element with little or no reference to the larger population from which the deceased came.

Paleoepidemiological investigations would make a further leap forward in the 1970s and 1980s, when paleopathologists became more interested in observing changes in the health of populations over time to better understand human life in the past (Washburn, 1953). Particularly, researchers at this time would exhibit a greater appreciation for the relationship between pathological conditions and the cultural and environmental contexts of these transitional periods. For example, several studies at this time would associate skeletal lesion frequencies with the changing cultural and environmental landscape during the transition from the hunting and gathering to the agricultural mode of subsistence (e.g., Lallo et al., 1977; Lallo et al., 1978; Goodman et al., 1980, 1984; Cohen & Armelagos, 1984; Cohen, 1989). Skeletal indicators or lesions indicative of pathological conditions—such as dental enamel hypoplasia, cribra orbitalia, ante-mortem tooth loss, dental caries, skeletal lesions associated with infection, degenerative joint disease, and trauma—were used to assess health in pre-agricultural and agricultural populations from numerous global contexts. In brief, the studies would conclude that skeletal indicators of health and disease increased in frequency throughout the transition to agriculture, and negative health outcomes were likely exacerbated by increased population density, increased sedentism, and the extension and intensification of group interactions (e.g., long-distance trade). Perhaps the most substantial contribution of this era in paleopathology was the establishment of a general approach to paleoepidemiology in which researchers collect skeletal data from two or more comparable sites or samples, compile skeletal indicator or lesion frequencies, and compare these frequencies across space (e.g., sites within a regional exchange network), time periods (e.g., across the transition from hunting and gathering to an agricultural subsistence economy), or cultural categories of interest (e.g., high vs. low status) (DeWitte & Stojanowski, 2015).

Within the past three decades (1990–2020), paleoepidemiological researchers have continued to generate scholarship following the basic approach that was established in the 1970s and 1980s and have produced studies that extend and problematize the earlier examination of the health consequences related to the transition to agriculture (Steckel & Rose, 2002; Douglas, 2006; Bocquet-Appel & Bar-Yosef, 2008; Bocquet-Appel et al., 2008; Lambert, 2009; Pinhasi & Stock, 2011; Cohen & Crane-Kramer, 2012; Harper & Armelagos, 2013), examine the consequences of European colonization in terms of population-level health experiences in Native American populations (Thomas, 1990a, 1990b, 1990c; Ubelaker, 1992; Verano & Ubelaker, 1992; Baker & Kealhofer, 1996; Larsen et al., 2001; Jones & DeWitte, 2012), and investigate the health consequences of urbanization and industrialization (Lewis, 2002; Lewis & Gowland, 2007; Zuckerman, 2014; Kelmelis & Pedersen, 2019; Betsinger & DeWitte, 2020).

The Osteological Paradox

In addition to a sustained interest in the disease experiences of populations in a variety of contexts, scholars during the past three decades have sought to remedy the deficiencies of earlier paleoepidemiological studies and address the limitations imposed by skeletal samples from archaeological contexts. Of particular interest to paleoepidemiological studies that use skeletal indicator frequencies to examine population-level trends in health over time are the conceptual and methodological challenges presented in a paper titled "The Osteological Paradox: Problems of Inferring Prehistoric Health from Skeletal Samples" (Wood et al., 1992b). Previous reviews of the Osteological Paradox, the challenges it poses to paleopathology and paleoepidemiology, and the reactions of the bioarchaeological community to its publication have been printed elsewhere (Wright & Yoder, 2003; Siek, 2013; DeWitte & Stojanowski, 2015) and need not be recapitulated in this chapter. However, in recent years, paleoepidemiological and paleopathological researchers have grappled with and attempted to address the issues of hidden heterogeneity in frailty and selective mortality and therefore deserve mention here, especially given that the methodological approaches used by such studies have expanded the statistical and mathematical models employed by bioarchaeologists in their study of health and disease in the past.

Hidden Heterogeneity in Frailty

Hidden heterogeneity in frailty refers to the fact that individuals in a population differ in their susceptibility to different diseases and other stressors, which, by extension, generates variation in risks of death among members of the population that is often unobservable (Wood et al., 1992b). This issue stems from the nature of bioarchaeological and paleopathological work in that scholars are attempting to reconstruct the lived experiences and health conditions of past populations using skeletal samples, which are inherently biased. One source of bias in skeletal samples is due to the fact that, in living populations, individuals vary in terms of their risks of dying at a given age, meaning that all populations exhibit heterogeneous frailty (Vaupel et al., 1979). There are many sources of variation in frailty, including biological differences (e.g., differences in immune responses due to genetic or hormonal factors), variation in exposure to disease vectors (e.g., differences in risk-taking behaviors among population subgroups), variation in environmental factors, and nutritional variation (DeWitte & Stojanowski, 2015), and not all of these sources of differential frailty will be visible or accessible in a skeletal sample. As a result, when bioarchaeological studies examine patterns of health and disease at the population (or aggregate) level, individual or subgroup variation in the age-standardized relative risk of death (i.e., heterogeneous frailty) may be obfuscated or "hidden" (Wood et al., 1992b).

Selective Mortality

Selective mortality is the concept that heterogeneity in frailty influences risk of death and thus the composition of the skeletal samples being studied by bioarchaeologists (Vaupel & Yashin, 1985; Wood et al., 1992b). In brief, selective mortality generates bias because individuals in a population who are the frailest are more likely to die (or be "selected" for mortality) compared to their less-frail peers, meaning that skeletal samples are biased collections composed of individuals who exhibited the highest frailty for their given age group. As a result, the use of skeletal indicator frequencies to directly estimate the prevalence of a particular disease or diseases in the once-living population is a flawed exercise, because skeletal lesions—if they are caused by conditions that increased the risks of death—will inevitably overestimate the prevalence of the condition in the living population of interest (Wood et al., 1992b).

Differentiating 'Good Health' From 'Poor Health'

A further challenge to bioarchaeological studies is the potential for skeletal indicators of physiological stress to simultaneously indicate relatively good and relatively poor health in individuals from the same skeletal sample. Traditionally, paleopathological studies assumed that skeletal indicators could serve as direct measures of health, meaning that an individual with skeletal lesions was in relatively poor health and an individual without skeletal lesions was relatively healthy. However, this assumption overlooks the fact that many of the skeletal indicators observed in paleopathological studies (e.g., periosteal new bone formation) take weeks or months to manifest in the skeleton in response to trauma, disease, or other physiological insults. Consequently, individuals who do not exhibit a particular skeletal indicator of stress may have been frailer than their peers who survived bouts of malnutrition, traumatic injuries, or infections for a sufficient period of time for the skeletal indicators to form (Ortner, 1991; Wood et al., 1992b). In other words, the absence of a particular skeletal indicator may indicate relatively poor health, and the presence of that skeletal indicator may indicate relatively good health.

Despite these challenges to paleopathological and paleoepidemiological research, recognition of the problems posed by heterogeneous frailty and selective mortality has prompted some scholars to explicitly examine how skeletal indicators and factors such as sex or socioeconomic status that may coincide with underlying frailty affect patterns of mortality or survival at the population level (e.g., Usher, 2000; Boldsen, 2005a, 2005b, 2007; DeWitte & Wood, 2008; Kreger, 2010; Wilson, 2010; Redfern & DeWitte, 2011a; DeWitte & Hughes-Morey, 2012; DeWitte et al., 2016; Hughes-Morey, 2016; Yaussy & DeWitte, 2019; Yaussy, 2019; McFadden & Oxenham, 2020). Some of the analytical methodologies employed by these studies are explored below as examples of statistical techniques and mathematical models that may be of use to future paleoepidemiological studies of the lives and health experiences of past populations.

Current Approaches

Current approaches to paleoepidemiology rely heavily on mathematical models and statistical analyses to better characterize the disease experiences of past populations. Survival analysis, hazard models, multistate models, regression, and hierarchical log-linear analyses have all been proposed in recent years as ways of reaching beyond the simple lesion frequencies that were foundational to the field nearly a century ago to more accurately understand health and disease conditions in past communities. Additional topics of great interest and importance to the discipline (such as sensitivity, specificity, prevalence, relative risk, and odds ratios) have been covered elsewhere (Boldsen & Milner, 2012; Klaus, 2013; Milner & Boldsen, 2017) and will not be repeated here. Rather, the approaches discussed below include mathematical models and statistical analyses that are being incorporated into paleoepidemiological research and show promise in terms of overcoming the challenges of the Osteological Paradox to better understand the lived experiences of populations in the past.

Kaplan-Meier Survival Analysis

Kaplan-Meier survival analysis has been one of the most widely used statistical approaches in both modern epidemiological and paleoepidemiological studies. Kaplan-Meier survival analysis is a nonparametric method that was developed to estimate the probability of survival past a given time point, also known as a survival function (Kaplan & Meier, 1958). In modern epidemiological studies, the Kaplan-Meier method is often used to examine variation in the time to an event of interest, such as disease-specific survival times. In these analyses, researchers collect data on the time that has elapsed until the event of interest for each study participant, the status of the participant at the end of the study (i.e., event occurrence or censored), and the study group that the participant was in. Censorship is particularly important in modern epidemiological studies, as it describes a situation in which the time-to-event (or survival time) cannot be determined for a particular study participant, perhaps because the participant dropped out of the study, could not be reached for follow-up, or survived beyond the end of the study period (Rich et al., 2010). For modern epidemiological studies, censoring can generate serious issues in terms of the traditional ways that data may be described (such as average survival time), and the Kaplan-Meier method overcomes this issue by incorporating censored cases into the analysis (Singer et al., 2003). Therefore, the Kaplan-Meier method estimates the probability of surviving (or not experiencing the event of interest) past a particular time point, while also taking into consideration the existence of censored cases. In paleopathological studies, censoring is typically not an issue, given that the "study participants" (i.e., the individuals in the skeletal sample) have all reached the event of interest (i.e., death) and can be included in the study if the relevant areas of the skeleton are complete enough to estimate age at death.

The survival function (or survival curve) produced by the Kaplan-Meier method consists of a series of horizontal steps (which represent survival duration) connected by vertical lines (which represent the change in cumulative survival probability between different points in time). In studies comparing the survivorship of two groups, the Kaplan-Meier survival curve serves as an effective visual aid to depict the difference in survival between the two groups. In brief, a sizeable gap between the survival functions for each group indicates a difference in survivorship. However, additional tests are necessary to determine if the survival distributions were equal (i.e., if the difference in survivorship visible in the survival curves is statistically significant). The most common statistic for comparing the survival functions of two groups is the Mantel-Cox log-rank test (Bland & Altman, 2004), although the Breslow and Tarone-Ware tests are also available in common statistical software packages like SPSS. The log-rank test investigates the null hypothesis that there is no difference in the survival distributions of the two groups being examined.

Kaplan-Meier Survival Analysis in Paleopathological Studies

In paleopathological and bioarchaeological studies, Kaplan-Meier survival analysis has been used to study survivorship in individuals with specific diseases like tuberculosis (Blondiaux et al., 2015) and leprosy (Boldsen, 2005b, 2008; Boldsen et al., 2013; Torino et al., 2015), but it has also been used to study survival in particular contexts of interest to paleopathologists, including studies of urban and rural differences in survivorship (Redfern et al., 2016; Walter & DeWitte, 2017), pre- and post-epidemic changes in survivorship (DeWitte, 2014b, 2014c, 2015), and the survival advantages or disadvantages associated with certain skeletal lesions or pathological conditions (DeWitte, 2014a; Yaussy & DeWitte, 2019). A recent example of a bioarchaeological study using Kaplan-Meier survival analysis to examine the difference in survivorship associated with a particular skeletal lesion is a study by McFadden and Oxenham (2020), which examined the relationship between survival time and cribra orbitalia, a lesion often associated with the presence of anemia and/or vitamin deficiencies, in samples including and excluding subadults. Importantly, the study represents a growing interest in using paleoepidemiological approaches to study the challenges of the Osteological Paradox, including the potential for a skeletal lesion to differentially represent resilience or frailty in different samples or contexts. McFadden and Oxenham apply Kaplan-Meier survival analysis to age at death data extracted from the Global History of Health Project, including 33 European skeletal samples and 19 American skeletal samples. The authors find that, in a majority of cases, the relationship between cribra orbitalia presence and survivorship changed based on whether subadults were included in the analyses. For instance, in 28 out of 33 of the European samples, survivorship was lower for individuals with cribra orbitalia lesions when subadults and adults were included in the analysis. However, when subadults were excluded from the analysis, only 12 out of 33 of the European samples exhibited reduced survivorship among individuals with cribra orbitalia lesions, and the remaining 16 European samples exhibited a nonsignificant relationship between cribra orbitalia presence and survivorship. McFadden and Oxenham conclude that the association between cribra orbitalia and survival is most apparent in subadult individuals, and cribra orbitalia is indicative of physiological stress and thus is associated with an increased risk of death in subadults. In contrast, the presence of cribra orbitalia among adults may be associated with frailty or resilience in different populations or contexts and depends heavily on etiology and environmental variables.

Hazard Models

In recent years, paleoepidemiological studies have also found hazard models—fully parametric models of the age pattern of mortality—to be appropriate for comparisons of the age at death distributions of multiple separate skeletal samples (Wood et al., 1992a; Wood et al., 2002). Hazard models of mortality are considered to be an alternative to model life tables, such as those developed by Coale and Demeny (1983) and Weiss (1973). In earlier studies of human variation in mortality patterns, model life tables were vital in that they provided an age pattern of mortality with the limited information typical of bioarchaeological data. However, the glaring disadvantage of model life tables is that age patterns of mortality vary from population to population, meaning that the results are only accurate if the selected table corresponds closely to the population being studied (Gage, 1988; Wood et al., 2002). In an effort to improve studies of variation in mortality patterns in human populations, a number of mathematical models describing mortality across the lifespan have been developed and applied in paleopathological and bioarchaeological studies (Gage, 1989; Wood et al., 1992b). The primary benefit of these parametric models of mortality is that they can smooth and correct variation in age-specific mortality that is produced by small sample sizes, which are a common problem in paleopatholgical studies (Gage, 1988; Wood et al., 2002).

The Gompertz, Gompertz-Makeham, and Siler Models of Mortality in Paleopathology

Though a number of parametric models of mortality have been developed over the years, the most commonly employed hazard models in paleopathological and bioarchaeological studies have been the Gompertz, Gompertz-Makeham, and Siler models of mortality. The Gompertz-Makeham model (Makeham, 1860) is a modification of the earlier Gompertz model of mortality (Gompertz, 1825), which describes the acceleration in mortality that occurs across the adult portion of the lifespan. The original Gompertz model includes a single component (i.e., the aging or senescent component of mortality) consisting of two parameters that describe the overall level of adult mortality (α) and the increasing risk of death associated with advancing age (β). Thus, the Gompertz mortality function for a given age (a) is:

$$h(a) = \alpha e^{\beta a}$$

The modification proposed by Makeham (1860) involved the addition of a second component that captures age-independent mortality in adulthood (α_1), such as that produced by car crashes, lightning strikes, infectious diseases, and other causes of death that are unrelated to senescence. Therefore, the Gompertz-Makeham mortality function for a given age (a) is:

$$h(a) = \alpha_1 + \alpha_2 e^{\beta a}$$

The Gompertz and Gompertz-Makeham models fit human mortality curves between the ages of 30 and 85, which can be described as relatively low mortality at young adult ages, followed by increasing risk of death with age (Gage, 1989; Finch, 1994). As a result, the two models of mortality are used frequently in paleopathological and bioarchaeological studies to assess variability in adult mortality and in many cases include a covariate acting upon the parameters of the given hazard model to examine variation in risk of death associated with other variables of interest, such as burial type or sex (e.g., DeWitte, 2010; Redfern & DeWitte, 2011a, 2011b; DeWitte, 2014c; Wilson, 2014; DeWitte, 2015; Yaussy, DeWitte, & Redfern, 2016; DeWitte & Yaussy, 2020). For example, a study by DeWitte (2009) examined the effect of sex on risk of death in a skeletal sample associated with the Black Death (*c.* 1347–1351) in London and two comparative nonepidemic samples from Denmark. The results indicated that the estimated value of the parameter representing the effect of the sex covariate did not significantly differ from zero, suggesting that the Black Death was not selective with respect to sex among adults. As the study by DeWitte (2009) demonstrates, the Gompertz and Gompertz-Makeham hazard models are one way to examine variation in mortality patterns across populations and contexts and investigate how additional variables affect those patterns of mortality among adults.

Another parametric model of mortality, the Siler competing hazards model, further expands the scope of the Gompertz and Gompertz-Makeham models to include the earliest ages of the human lifespan (i.e., subadults). Originally developed for animal populations (Siler, 1979), the Siler model has been tested on human populations and found to fit human mortality data as well as or better than other models (Gage & Dyke, 1986; Gage, 1988; Gage & Mode, 1993). The Siler model adds a third component to the Gompertz-Makeham model described above, and this component represents the rapid decline in risk of death during the earliest years of life. As a result, the Siler mortality function for a given age (*a*) is:

$$h(a) = \alpha_1 e^{-\beta_1 a} + \alpha_2 + \alpha_3 e^{\beta_2 a}$$

The three components of the Siler model correspond to the independent yet competing causes of death operating throughout an individual's life: the immature or juvenile component (i.e., risk of death is high at birth and declines rapidly with age), the age-independent component (i.e., risk of death that is unrelated to age), and the senescent component (i.e., risk of death is low at younger ages and increases with adult age). As a result, the Siler model allows for the estimation of the typical curve of human mortality across the entire lifespan, in which mortality is high at birth, declines during childhood, then increases again in adolescence or adulthood (Gage, 1988). Like the Gompertz and Gompertz-Makeham models, the Siler model can be applied to relatively small sample sizes—making it ideal for bioarchaeological studies of variation in mortality across populations—and it smooths random variation in age-specific mortality without imposing a particular age pattern on the data (Gage, 1988; Wood et al., 2002).

The inclusion of the juvenile component makes the Siler model an attractive alternative to the Gompertz and Gompertz-Makeham models of adult mortality for researchers interested in including subadults in their analyses of risk of death in past populations. Examples of paleopathological and bioarchaeological research utilizing the Siler model include several studies of mortality risk in Dorset, England during the Roman period (Redfern & DeWitte, 2011a, 2011b; Redfern et al., 2015). For instance, to determine the effect of status on risk of mortality across the lifespan, Redfern and DeWitte (2011b) model burial type as a covariate affecting the parameters of the Siler model. The authors first model burial type as a covariate affecting the entire Siler model (i.e., proportional to the entire hazard and independent of age), then subsequently model burial type as a covariate affecting the juvenile and senescent components of the Siler model independently to allow the effect of status on risk of mortality to vary with age. Their findings promote further consideration of the age-dependent effects of status and other variables on risk of mortality in past populations, because, in the model with burial type specified as a covariate affecting the entire Siler model, the estimated value of the parameter representing the effect of the covariate was not significantly different from zero, suggesting that status had little or no effect on the risk of mortality across the entire lifespan. However, when burial type was modeled as a covariate affecting the juvenile and senescent components of the hazard independently, the estimated value of the parameter representing the effect of the burial type covariate on juvenile mortality was significantly less than zero, suggesting that higher status was associated with significantly reduced risks of mortality for subadult individuals, but not adult individuals. The results from this study and others confirm the potential of hazard models to explore the range and causes of variation in human mortality patterns in past populations.

Multistate Models

Multistate models, such as the one developed by Usher (2000), can incorporate a baseline hazard of mortality (such as the Siler or Gompertz models mentioned above) to explicitly examine heterogeneous frailty and selective mortality in past populations. Multistate models have been utilized in epidemiology and anthropology to study processes that involve multiple independent states, including research on malaria in children (Gottschau & Hogh, 1995) and fecundability (probability of becoming pregnant) and sterility in women from Taiwan, Sri Lanka, and the Amish (Wood et al., 1994). All multistate models of this type inherently assume that (1) each individual can only occupy one state at a time, (2) all individuals in the sample will occupy one of the states at any given time, and (3) movement from state to state is governed by specific parameters (transition rates) (Usher, 2000).

The multistate model of health and death developed and used by Usher (2000) is a three-state model composed of the nonoverlapping states of "well", "ill", and dead (Figure 4.1).[1] The "well" state (State 1) is defined as a living person who does not have a skeletal lesion. The "ill" state (State 2) is defined as a living person who does have a skeletal lesion. The final state is death (State 3). In brief, all individuals in this model are assumed to be "well" at birth, then they progress to the second state (i.e., they fall ill and develop a skeletal lesion) or they progress directly to the third state (i.e., they die). As mentioned above, the multistate model incorporates hazard functions (such as the Siler and Gompertz-Makeham models) to describe the likelihood of transitioning from one state to the next (transition rates). The risk of transitioning from State 1 ("well") to State 3 (death) is considered the baseline risk of death, and the risk of transitioning from State 2 ("ill") to State 3 (death) is assumed to be proportional to the baseline risk of death.

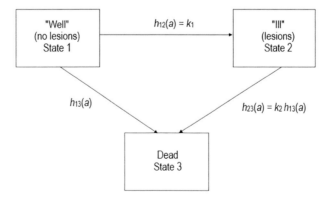

Figure 4.1 The multistate model of morbidity and mortality described by Usher (2000) and further applied by DeWitte and Wood (2008). Individuals are born into the "well" stage (State 1), and the transition between each stage is described by a Siler mortality function. The transition from "well" (State 1) to dead (State 3) follows the baseline Siler mortality function $h_{13}(a) = \alpha_1 \exp(-\beta_1 a) + \alpha_2 + \alpha_3 \exp(\beta_3 a)$, where a is age in years. The transition from "ill" (State 2) to dead (State 3) is proportional to the baseline rate because it is modified by k_2, which is the relative risk of dying associated with a given skeletal lesion. Modified from Usher (2000).

The Multistate Model in Paleopathology

Multistate models benefit paleopathological research because it directly addresses the issues of the Osteological Paradox mentioned above: hidden heterogeneity in frailty and selective mortality. Because the transitions between each of the living states ("well" and "ill") and the third state (dead) can vary, the model is able to determine differences in risk of death associated with lesion presence and absence. Therefore, this multistate model allows researchers to examine the relationship between skeletal lesions and risks of mortality (i.e., whether the presence of lesions impacts transition to the third state) by modeling skeletal lesions as a covariate affecting the baseline model of mortality estimated for each transition. In other words, the covariate included in Usher's (2000) model determines whether a skeletal indicator reduced or increased risks of mortality in a given context.

The multistate model developed by Usher has been successfully applied in multiple paleopathological studies to date. Following sufficient testing and simulation to determine whether it could be applied to bioarchaeological samples, Usher (2000) applied her own model on a skeletal sample from Tirup, an early medieval Danish cemetery. Specifically, the goal of Usher's study was to determine if the presence of observable skeletal indicators and traits (i.e., dental enamel hypoplasia (an indicator of childhood growth disruption), adult femur length, dental caries, osteolytic or proliferative changes on the femur and humerus, cribra orbitalia, porotic hyperostosis, metopic trait, and an erosive rhomboid fossa) had an effect on risk of death in the Tirup skeletal sample. The Siler or Gompertz-Makeham models were used to estimate the baseline risk of death, and these models were used to estimate the constants associated with getting each lesion (k_1) and the proportional difference in risk between individuals with a given skeletal lesion and individuals without the lesion (k_2) in each subsample. This second parameter contains the relevant information about selective mortality, such that when the estimated value of the parameter is greater than one, individuals with a lesion had an elevated risk of mortality compared to individuals of the same age without that lesion, and when the estimated value of the parameter is less than one, the individuals with a lesion had a reduced risk of mortality compared to individuals of the same age without that lesion. The results of Usher's study demonstrate that not all lesions were associated with increased risk of death among individuals in the Tirup skeletal sample. Although enamel hypoplasia on the first molar, cribra orbitalia, short femur length, and osteolytic or proliferative bony responses on the femur were all associated with increased risk of death, several traits were not associated with an increased risk of death or were associated with a reduced risk of death. In other words, the model developed by Usher (2000) examines the effect of lesion presence on risk of mortality in a given context, and her findings challenge the conventional paleopathological notion that all skeletal lesions indicate poor health.

A second use of Usher's multistate model is the study of the East Smithfield Black Death cemetery in London, England conducted by DeWitte and Wood (2008). The goal of the study was to determine if the Black Death (*c.* 1347–1351 AD) exhibited selective mortality despite being considered a catastrophic or indiscriminate killer. As in the original model developed by Usher (2000), DeWitte and Wood (2008) use a three-state model in which State 1 includes individuals with no detectable skeletal indicators, State 2 includes individuals with skeletal lesions, and State 3 includes all individuals who have died (i.e., entered the skeletal sample). Therefore, the age at death distributions and the presence or absence of skeletal lesions is used to estimate the parameters of the Siler mortality functions that govern the transition from one state to the next. As above, the parameter k_2 acts on the Siler function and

Table 4.1 Maximum likelihood estimates of k_2 with nominal standard error (SE) and likelihood ratio tests of the hypothesis that $k_2 = 1$ (i.e., no selectivity), in the study of Black Death mortality applying the multistate model produced by Usher (2000). Results indicate that each lesion was associated with increased risk of death (i.e., $k_2 > 1$) in both the epidemic (East Smithfield) and nonepidemic (Denmark) samples, suggesting that the Black Death was selective with respect to frailty

Skeletal lesion	East Smithfield (n = 490)		Denmark (n = 291)	
	k_2 (SE)	-2LLR	k_2 (SE)	-2LLR
Periosteal new bone (tibia)	1.5 (0.3)	27.80	5.3 (2.0)	61.74
Porotic hyperostosis	1.8 (0.3)	8.84	2.3 (0.7)	12.54
Cribra orbitalia	1.7 (0.4)	2.30	3.6 (2.1)	53.57
Linear enamel hypoplasia (mandibular canine)	2.9 (1.1)	13.16	7.6 (14.4)	11.96
Linear enamel hypoplasia (maxillary canine)	2.0 (0.5)	32.29	2.7 (3.0)	16.74
Femur length	1.2 (0.2)	0.12	2.7 (0.7)	0.09

Source: Reproduced from DeWitte and Wood (2008).

represents the proportional difference in risk between individuals with a given skeletal lesion and individuals without the lesion, thus describing the force of mortality associated with the presence of each lesion. If the k_2 parameter is greater than one, individuals with skeletal lesions faced an increased risk of dying compared to their peers who did not exhibit detectable skeletal lesions. In their study, DeWitte and Wood (2008) compare the East Smithfield skeletal sample with two nonepidemic (attritional) skeletal samples from the medieval Danish towns of Viborg and Odense, which were socially, economically, and demographically similar to the population in southern England at that time. They apply the Usher model to both the East Smithfield and Danish samples, then use likelihood ratio tests to determine if k_2 differs from one (i.e., if the skeletal lesions are associated with an elevated or reduced risk of dying in either sample). As seen in Table 4.1, every lesion type in both samples exhibited a k_2 estimate of greater than one, and most estimates were reasonably large (i.e., greater than two). These results indicate that the skeletal lesions studied (i.e., periosteal lesions on the tibia, porotic hyperostosis, cribra orbitalia, linear enamel hypoplasia on the mandibular and maxillary canines, and femur length) were all associated with an elevated risk of death for individuals in the East Smithfield and Danish samples. As a result, DeWitte and Wood (2008) are able to use Usher's multistate model to identify the degree to which mortality was selective with respect to frailty during the Black Death, as well as during nonepidemic periods. In sum, the multistate model produced and tested by Usher (2000) and further applied by DeWitte and Wood (2008) is capable of detecting the effects of selective mortality in skeletal samples using skeletal lesions routinely identified and recorded in paleopathological studies.

Logistic Regression

In epidemiological studies involving the analysis of risk of certain conditions, logistic regression may be used to describe the relationship between a categorical outcome of interest and multiple continuous or categorical predictor variables or covariates (Kleinbaum et al., 1982).

In paleopathological studies, logistic regression can be used to compare the risk for presence of a particular skeletal lesion (e.g., osteoarthritis) in multiple populations or population subgroups while simultaneously controlling for the effects of age, sex, time period, or other confounding variables (Baker & Pearson, 2006). The regression coefficients of the model can then be interpreted as the percent increase or decrease in risk as a covariate increases by one unit or changes factor levels. For example, a regression coefficient of 1.43 would suggest a 43% increase in risk for each unit of change in a covariate (or categorical change in factor level). Likewise, a regression coefficient of 0.55 would suggest a 45% decrease in risk for each unit of change in a covariate (or categorical change in factor level). Paleopathological studies incorporating logistic regression may find it useful to use the regression coefficients to compute odds ratios, which represent the ratio of the odds of an event occurring in one group to the odds of it occurring in another group. However, as noted elsewhere, odds ratios come with their own limitations and are susceptible to misinterpretation, and therefore they should be carefully considered and cautiously applied if they are utilized in paleoepidemiological studies (Klaus, 2013).

Logistic Regression in Paleopathology

Examples of paleopathological studies incorporating logistic regression are gradually becoming more common (e.g., Kemkes-Grottenthaler, 2005; Baker & Pearson, 2006; DeWitte & Bekvalac, 2011) and reflect a growing interest in incorporating techniques from epidemiology and biostatistics to measure prevalence and investigate questions of selective mortality in past populations. For example, a study by Yaussy and DeWitte (2019) investigated the mortality risks associated with dental calculus in a medieval skeletal sample using binary logistic regression and found significant negative associations between dental calculus and age. Given the relatively low frequencies of dental calculus among individuals over 60 years of age, the authors suggest that the results of the regression analyses may reflect the effects of selective mortality. That is, individuals without calculus were less frail and therefore more likely to survive to late adult ages, whereas frailer individuals with dental calculus died at younger adult ages.

Hierarchical Log-linear Analysis

A final analytical technique of interest to paleoepidemiological studies is hierarchical log-linear analysis, which is used to understand the associations between two or more categorical variables. Particularly, log-linear analysis is suited for investigations of whether a third (or fourth) variable impacts a two-way association indicated by cross-tabulations like chi-square analyses (Sloane & Morgan, 1996). That is, log-linear analyses can examine the separate main effects of variables included in the model, as well as higher-order interactions (i.e., associations among two or more variables). Although useful for identifying the most parsimonious, unsaturated model and determining the existence of associations between two variables that are independent of a third variable (e.g., the association between short femora and inclusion in famine burials independent of age), hierarchical log-linear analysis is not capable of determining the *direction* of any higher-order interactions. Therefore, in bioarchaeological studies of the associations among skeletal lesions and other variables of interest like sex, age, and status, hierarchical log-linear analysis must be combined with other statistical tests (e.g., chi-square tests) to investigate the nature of the interactions identified in the log-linear model.

Hierarchical Log-Linear Analysis in Paleopathology

Hierarchical log-linear analysis has been used in paleopathological studies of periodontal disease, periosteal lesions, linear enamel hypoplasia, cribra orbitalia, porotic hyperostosis, and femur length and their associations with variables of interest like age at death and sex (DeWitte & Bekvalac, 2011; Yaussy et al., 2016; DeWitte & Yaussy, 2017; Yaussy & DeWitte, 2018; Yaussy, 2019). In their study of periodontal disease in medieval London, DeWitte and Bekvalac (2011) found a significant association between periodontal disease and periosteal lesions that was independent of age. The authors suggest that their results may reflect an underlying susceptibility to infection (i.e., reduced immunocompetence), heightened proinflammatory responses, or exposure to an environmental factor capable of causing periodontal disease and periosteal lesions in individuals with both conditions. Thus, hierarchical log-linear analysis is one avenue by which paleopathological studies of health and disease can expose new and perhaps unexpected associations among pathological conditions and other variables of interest. Future paleoepidemiological and paleopathological studies incorporating hierarchical log-linear analysis may further expose the complex relationships among diseases, social and biological factors, and environmental conditions in past populations.

Conclusions and Future Directions

The approaches and mathematical models included in this chapter are far from comprehensive, as the field of paleoepidemiology continues to grow and evolve. Despite the challenges and limitations imposed by bioarchaeological data, paleopathologists and paleoepidemiologists demonstrate a firm resolve to develop an analytically rigorous field of study. Advances in various aspects of paleoepidemiological analysis, such as improvements in age and sex estimation (Milner & Boldsen, 2012a, 2012b), are particularly encouraging. For instance, advances in the estimation of age at death could enable paleoepidemiologists to capture patterns of morbidity and mortality at late adult ages, beyond the terminal age categories produced by traditional age estimation methods. Future paleoepidemiological studies of disease in past populations may also combine mathematical models of mortality risk with ancient DNA analysis and paleoproteomics to expand our understandings of disease susceptibility in the past, human–pathogen coevolution, and pathogen load in past populations (Dutour, 2008; Devault et al., 2014; Warinner et al., 2014; Harkins & Stone, 2015). Although currently limited by the cost of extracting ancient DNA from human skeletal remains in sufficiently large sample sizes, studies of ancient DNA and ancient biomolecules could be invaluable to future studies of the biocultural effects of specific diseases in the past and the coevolution of humans and pathogens over time.

Note

1 Usher (2000) also developed a four-state model consisting of "well" (no lesions), "ill" (active lesions), "healed" (healed lesions), and dead, but the four-state model is considered mathematically complicated, difficult to test, and hard to interpret. Therefore, the simplified three-state model is preferable for most bioarchaeological studies of selective mortality and is covered in detail here.

References

Angel, J. L. (1946). Skeletal change in ancient Greece. *American Journal of Physical Anthropology* 4(1):69–98. https://doi.org/10.1002/ajpa.1330040109

Angel, J. L. (1966). Porotic hyperostosis, anemias, malarias, and marshes in the prehistoric Eastern Mediterranean. *Science* 153(3737):760–763.

Angel, J. L. (1969). Paleodemography and evolution. *American Journal of Physical Anthropology* 31(3): 343–353. https://doi.org/10.1002/ajpa.1330310310

Armelagos, G. J. & Van Gerven, D. P. (2003). A century of skeletal biology and paleopathology: contrasts, contradictions, and conflicts. *American Anthropologist* 105(1):53–64.

Baker, B. J. & Kealhofer, L. (1996). *Bioarchaeology of Native American Adaptation in the Spanish Borderlands*. Gainesville, FL: University Press of Florida.

Baker, J. & Pearson, O. M. (2006). Statistical methods for bioarchaeology: applications of age-adjustment and logistic regression to comparisons of skeletal populations with differing age-structures. *Journal of Archaeological Science* 33(2):218–226.

Betsinger, T. K. & DeWitte, S. N. (2020). *The Bioarchaeology of Urbanization*. New York: Springer.

Bland, J. M. & Altman, D. G. (2004). The logrank test. *British Medical Journal* 328 (7447):1073.

Blondiaux, J., de Broucker, A., Colard, T., Haque, A., & Naji, S. (2015). Tuberculosis and survival in past populations: a paleo-epidemiological appraisal. *Tuberculosis* 95(Supplement 1):S93–S100. https://doi.org/10.1016/j.tube.2015.02.002

Bocquet-Appel, J. P. & Bar-Yosef, O. (Eds.) (2008). *The Neolithic Demographic Transition and its Consequences*. New York: Springer.

Bocquet-Appel, J.-P., Naji, S. & Bandy, M. (2008). Demographic and health changes during the transition to agriculture in North America. In Bocquet-Appel, J. P. (Ed.), *Recent Advances in Palaeodemography*, pp. 277–292. Dordrecht, The Netherlands: Springer.

Boldsen, J. L. (2005a). Analysis of dental attrition and mortality in the medieval village of Tirup, Denmark. *American Journal of Physical Anthropology* 126(2):169–176.

Boldsen, J. L. (2005b). Leprosy and mortality in the Medieval Danish village of Tirup. *American Journal of Physical Anthropology* 126(2):159–168.(15386293).

Boldsen, J. L. (2007). Early childhood stress and adult age mortality—A study of dental enamel hypoplasia in the medieval Danish village of Tirup. *American Journal of Physical Anthropology* 132(1):59–66. https://doi.org/10.1002/ajpa.20467

Boldsen, J. L. (2008). Leprosy in the early medieval Lauchheim community. *American Journal of Physical Anthropology* 135(3), 301–310.(18000890).

Boldsen, J. L., & Milner, G. R. (2012). An epidemiological approach to paleopathology. In Grauer, A. L. (Ed.), *A Companion to Paleopathology*, pp. 114–132. Oxford: Wiley-Blackwell.

Boldsen, J. L., Rasmussen, K. L., Riis, T., Dittmar, M. & Weise, S. (2013). Schleswig: Medieval leprosy on the boundary between Germany and Denmark. *Anthropologischer Anzeiger* 70(3): 273–287.

Buikstra, J. E. & Cook, D. C. (1980). Paleopathology: an American account. *Annual Review of Anthropology* 9:433–470.

Coale, A. & Demeny, P. (1983). *Regional Model Life Tables and Stable Populations*. Princeton, NJ: Princeton University Press.

Cohen, M. N. (1989). *Health and the Rise of Civilization*. New Haven: Yale University Press.

Cohen, M. N. & Armelagos, G. J. (Eds.) (1984). *Paleopathology at the Origins of Agriculture*. New York: Academic Press.

Cohen, M. N. & Crane-Kramer, G. (2003). The state and future of paleoepidemiology. In Greenblatt, C. L. & Spigelman, M. (Eds.), *Emerging Pathogens: The Archaeology, Ecology, and Evolution of Infectious Disease*, pp.79–91. Oxford: Oxford University Press.

Cohen, M. N. & Crane-Kramer, G. M. (2012). *Ancient Health: Skeletal Indicators of Agricultural and Economic Intensification* (Reprint edition). Gainesville, FL: University Press of Florida.

Devault, A. M., McLoughlin, K., Jaing, C., Gardner, S., Porter, T. M., Enk, J. M., … & Poinar, H. N. (2014). Ancient pathogen DNA in archaeological samples detected with a microbial detection array. *Scientific Reports* 4:4245. https://doi.org/10.1038/srep04245

DeWitte, S. N. (2009). The effect of sex on risk of mortality during the black death in London, A.D. 1349–1350. *American Journal of Physical Anthropology* 139:222–234.

DeWitte, S. N. (2010). Age patterns of mortality during the black death in London, A.D. 1349–1350. *Journal of Archaeological Science* 37(12):3394–3400. https://doi.org/10.1016/j.jas.2010.08.006

DeWitte, S. N. (2014a). Differential survival among individuals with active and healed periosteal new bone formation. *International Journal of Paleopathology* 7:38–44. https://doi.org/10.1016/j.ijpp.2014.06.001

DeWitte, S. N. (2014b). Health in post-black death London (1350–1538): age patterns of periosteal new bone formation in a post-epidemic population. *American Journal of Physical Anthropology* 155(2):260–267. https://doi.org/10.1002/ajpa.22510

DeWitte, S. N. (2014c). Mortality risk and survival in the aftermath of the medieval black death. *PLoS ONE* 9(5):e96513. https://doi.org/10.1371/journal.pone.0096513

DeWitte, S. N. (2015). Setting the stage for medieval plague: pre-black death trends in survival and mortality. *American Journal of Physical Anthropology* 158(3):441–451. https://doi.org/10.1002/ajpa.22806

DeWitte, S. N. & Bekvalac, J. (2011). The association between periodontal disease and periosteal lesions in the St. Mary Graces cemetery, London, England A.D. 1350–1538. *American Journal of Physical Anthropology* 146(4):609–618. https://doi.org/10.1002/ajpa.21622

DeWitte, S. N. & Hughes-Morey, G. (2012). Stature and frailty during the black death: the effect of stature on risks of epidemic mortality in London, A.D. 1348–1350. *Journal of Archaeological Science* 39(5):1412–1419. https://doi.org/10.1016/j.jas.2012.01.019

DeWitte, S. N., Hughes-Morey, G., Bekvalac, J. & Karsten, J. (2016). Wealth, health and frailty in industrial-era London. *Annals of Human Biology* 43(3):241–254. https://doi.org/10.3109/03014460.2015.1020873

DeWitte, S. N. & Stojanowski, C. M. (2015). The Osteological Paradox 20 years later: Past perspectives, future directions. *Journal of Archaeological Research* 23(4):397–450. https://doi.org/10.1007/s10814-015-9084-1

DeWitte, S. N. & Wood, J. W. (2008). Selectivity of black death mortality with respect to preexisting health. *Proceedings of the National Academy of Sciences of the United States of America* 105(5):1436–1441. https://doi.org/10.1073/pnas.0705460105

DeWitte, S. N. & Yaussy, S. L. (2017). Femur length and famine mortality in medieval London. *Bioarchaeology International* 1(3–4):171–182. https://doi.org/10.5744/bi.2017.1009

DeWitte, S. N. & Yaussy, S. L. (2020). Sex differences in adult famine mortality in medieval London. *American Journal of Physical Anthropology* 171(1):164–169.

Douglas, M. T. (2006). Subsistence change and dental health in the people of Non Nok Tha, northeast Thailand. In Oxenham, M. F. & Tayles, N. (Eds.), *Bioarchaeology of Southeast Asia*, pp. 191–219. Cambridge: Cambridge University Press.

Dutour, O. (2008). Archaeology of human pathogens: palaeopathological appraisal of palaeoepidemiology. In Raoult, D. & Drancourt, M. (Eds.), *Paleomicrobiology*, pp. 125–144. Berlin: Springer.

Finch, C. E. (1994). *Longevity, Senescence, and the Genome*. Chicago: University of Chicago Press.

Gage, T. B. (1988). Mathematical hazard models of mortality: an alternative to model life tables. *American Journal of Physical Anthropology* 76(4):429–441.

Gage, T. B. (1989). Bio-mathematical approaches to the study of human variation in mortality. *Yearbook of Physical Anthropology* 32:185–214.

Gage, T. B. & Dyke, B. (1986). Parameterizing abridged mortality tables: the siler three-component hazard model. *Human Biology* 58(2):275–291.

Gage, T. B. & Mode, C. J. (1993). Some laws of mortality: how well do they fit? *Human Biology* 65(3):445–461.

Goldstein, M. S. (1953). Some vital statistics based on skeletal material. *Human Biology* 25(1):3.

Goldstein, M. S. (1957). Skeletal pathology of early Indians in Texas. *American Journal of Physical Anthropology* 15(3):299–311. https://doi.org/10.1002/ajpa.1330150311.

Gompertz, B. (1825). On the nature of the function expressive of the law of human mortality, and on a new mode of determining the value of life contingencies. *Philosophical Transactions of the Royal Society of London* 115:513–583.

Goodman, A. H., Armelagos, G. J. & Rose, J. C. (1980). Enamel hypoplasias as indicators of stress in three prehistoric populations from Illinois. *Human Biology* 52(3):515–528. (7005071).

Goodman, A. H., Armelagos, G. J. & Rose, J. C. (1984). The chronological distribution of enamel hypoplasias from prehistoric Dickson Mounds populations. *American Journal of Physical Anthropology* 65(3):259–266. (6393775).

Gottschau, A. & Hogh, B. (1995). Interval censored survival data and multistate compartmental models in the analysis of first appearance of Plasmodium falciparum parasites in infants. *Statistics in Medicine* 14(24):2727–2736.

Harkins, K. M. & Stone, A. C. (2015). Ancient pathogen genomics: insights into timing and adaptation. *Journal of Human Evolution* 79:137–149. https://doi.org/10.1016/j.jhevol.2014.11.002

Harper, K. N. & Armelagos, G. J. (2013). Genomics, the origins of agriculture, and our changing microbe-scape: time to revisit some old tales and tell some new ones. *American Journal of Physical Anthropology* 152(S57):135–152.

Hooton, E. A. (1930). *The Indians of Pecos Pueblo: A Study of Their Skeletal Remains*. New Haven, CT: Yale University Press.

Hughes-Morey, G. (2016). Interpreting adult stature in industrial London. *American Journal of Physical Anthropology* 159(1):126–134. https://doi.org/10.1002/ajpa.22840

Jones, E. E. & DeWitte, S. N. (2012). Using spatial analysis to estimate depopulation for native American populations in northeastern North America, AD 1616–1645. *Journal of Anthropological Archaeology* 31(1):83–92. https://doi.org/10.1016/j.jaa.2011.10.004

Kaplan, E. L. & Meier, P. (1958). Nonparametric estimation from incomplete observations. *Journal of the American Statistical Association* 53(282):457–481.

Kelmelis, K. S. & Pedersen, D. D. (2019). Impact of urbanization on tuberculosis and leprosy prevalence in medieval Denmark. *88th Annual Meeting of the American Association of Physical Anthropologists* 168(68):56–56.

Kemkes-Grottenthaler, A. (2005). The short die young: the interrelationship between stature and longevity-evidence from skeletal remains. *American Journal of Physical Anthropology* 128(2):340–347. https://doi.org/10.1002/ajpa.20146

Klaus, H. D. (2013). Integrating pathophysiology, human biology, and epidemiology in studies of human remains: towards a clearer vision of stress and health in bioarchaeology. *American Journal of Physical Anthropology* 150(S56):168–169. https://doi.org/10.1002/ajpa.22247

Kleinbaum, D. G., Kupper, L. L. & Chambless, L. E. (1982). Logistic regression analysis of epidemiologic data: theory and practice. *Communications in Statistics-Theory and Methods* 11(5):485–547.

Kreger, M. B. (2010). *Urban Population Dynamics in a Preindustrial New World City: Morbidity, Mortality, and Immigration in Postclassic Cholula* (PhD). The Pennsylvania State University, University Park.

Lallo, J., Armelagos, G. J. & Rose, J. C. (1978). Paleoepidemiology of infectious disease in the Dickson Mounds Population. *Medical College of Virginia Quarterly* 14:17–23.

Lallo, J. W., Armelagos, G. J. & Mensforth, R. P. (1977). The role of diet, disease, and physiology in the origin of porotic hyperostosis. *Human Biology* 49:471–483.

Lambert, P. M. (2009). Health versus fitness: competing themes in the origins and spread of agriculture? *Current Anthropology* 50(5):603–608.

Larsen, C. S., Griffin, M. C., Hutchinson, D. L., Noble, V. E., Norr, L., Pastor, R. F., … & Schultz, M. (2001). Frontiers of contact: bioarchaeology of Spanish Florida. *Journal of World Prehistory* 15(1):69–123.

Lewis, M. E. (2002). Impact of industrialization: comparative study of child health in four sites from medieval and postmedieval England (A.D. 850–1859). *American Journal of Physical Anthropology* 119(3):211–223. https://doi.org/10.1002/ajpa.10126

Lewis, M. E. & Gowland, R. (2007). Brief and precarious lives: infant mortality in contrasting sites from medieval and post-medieval England (AD 850–1859). *American Journal of Physical Anthropology* 134(1):117–129. https://doi.org/10.1002/ajpa.20643

Makeham, W. (1860). On the law of mortality. *Journal of the Institute of Actuaries* 13:325–358.

McFadden, C. & Oxenham, M. F. (2020). A paleoepidemiological approach to the osteological paradox: Investigating stress, frailty and resilience through cribra orbitalia. *American Journal of Physical Anthropology* 173(2):205–217.

Milner, G. R. & Boldsen, J. L. (2012a). Estimating age and sex from the skeleton, a paleopathological perspective. In Grauer, A. (Ed.), *A Companion to Paleopathology*, pp. 268–284. Chichester, UK: Wiley.

Milner, G. R. & Boldsen, J. L. (2012b). Transition analysis: a validation study with known-age modern American skeletons. *American Journal of Physical Anthropology* 148(1):98–110. https://doi.org/10.1002/ajpa.22047

Milner, G. R. & Boldsen, J. L. (2017). Life not death: epidemiology from skeletons. *International Journal of Paleopathology* 17:26–39. https://doi.org/10.1016/j.ijpp.2017.03.007

Ortner, D. J. (1991). Theoretical and methodological issues in paleopathology. In Ortner, D. J. & Aufderheide, A. C. (Eds.), *Human Paleopathology: Current Syntheses and Future Options*, pp. 5–11. Washington, DC: Smithsonian Institution Press.

Pinhasi, R. & Stock, J. (Eds.). (2011). *Human Bioarchaeology at the Transition to Agriculture*. Chichester: Wiley-Blackwell.

Porta, M. (Ed.) (2016). *A Dictionary of Epidemiology* (sixth edition). New York: Oxford University Press.

Redfern, R. C. & DeWitte, S. N. (2011a). A new approach to the study of Romanization in Britain: A regional perspective of cultural change in Late Iron Age and Roman Dorset using the Siler and Gompertz-Makeham models of mortality. *American Journal of Physical Anthropology* 144(2):269–285. https://doi.org/10.1002/ajpa.21400

Redfern, R. C. & DeWitte, S. N. (2011b). Status and health in Roman Dorset: the effect of status on risk of mortality in post-conquest populations. *American Journal of Physical Anthropology* 146(2):197–208.

Redfern, R. C., DeWitte, S. N., Pearce, J., Hamlin, C. & Dinwiddy, K. E. (2015). Urban–rural differences in Roman Dorset, England: a bioarchaeological perspective on Roman settlements. *American Journal of Physical Anthropology* 157(1):107–120. https://doi.org/10.1002/ajpa.22693

Rich, J. T., Neely, J. G., Paniello, R. C., Voelker, C. C., Nussenbaum, B. & Wang, E. W. (2010). A practical guide to understanding Kaplan-Meier curves. *Otolaryngology—Head and Neck Surgery* 143(3):331–336.

Roney, J. G. (1959). Palaeopathology of a California archaeological site. *Bulletin of the History of Medicine* 33(2):97–109.

Siek, T. (2013). The osteological paradox and issues of interpretation in paleopathology. *Vis-à-Vis: Explorations in Anthropology* 13:92–101.

Siler, W. (1979). A competing-risk model for animal mortality. *Ecology* 60(4):750–757.

Singer, J. D., Willett, J. B. & Willett, J. B. (2003). *Applied Longitudinal Data Analysis: Modeling Change and Event Occurrence*. Oxford: Oxford University Press.

Sloane, D. & Morgan, S. P. (1996). An introduction to categorical data analysis. *Annual Review of Sociology* 22(1):351–375. https://doi.org/10.1146/annurev.soc.22.1.351

Souza, S. M., Carvalho, D. M. de. & Lessa, A. (2003). Paleoepidemiology: is there a case to answer? *Memórias Do Instituto Oswaldo Cruz* 98:21–27.

Steckel, R. H. & Rose, J. C. (2002). *The Backbone of History: Health and Nutrition in the Western Hemisphere*. Cambridge: Cambridge University Press.

Thomas, D. H. (1990a). *Columbian Consequences. Volume 1. Archaeological and Historical Perspectives on the Spanish Borderlands West*. Washington, DC: Smithsonian Institution Press.

Thomas, D. H. (1990b). *Columbian Consequences. Volume 2. Archaeological and Historical Perspectives on the Spanish Borderlands East*. Washington, DC: Smithsonian Institution Press.

Thomas, D. H. (1990c). *Columbian Consequences. Volume 3. The Spanish Borderlands in Pan-American Perspective*. Washington, DC: Smithsonian Institution Press.

Torino, M., Boldsen, J. L., Tarp, P., Rasmussen, K. L., Skytte, L., Nielsen, L., … & Ricci, P. (2015). Convento di san francesco a folloni: the function of a medieval Franciscan friary seen through the burials. *Heritage Science* 3(1):27.

Ubelaker, D. H. (1992). Patterns of demographic change in the Americas. *Human Biology* 64:361–379.

Usher, B. M. (2000). *A Multistate Model of Health and Mortality for Paleodemography: Tirup Cemetery* (PhD). Pennsylvania State University.

Vaupel, J. W., Manton, K. G. & Stallard, E. (1979). The impact of heterogeneity in individual frailty on the dynamics of mortality. *Demography* 16:439–454.

Vaupel, J. W. & Yashin, A. I. (1985). Heterogeneity's ruses: some surprising effects of selection on population dynamics. *American Statistician* 39:176–185. (BSSI86001847).

Verano, J. W. & Ubelaker, D. H. (1992). *Disease and Demography in the Americas*. Washington, DC: Smithsonian Institution Press.

Walter, B. S. & DeWitte, S. N. (2017). Urban and rural mortality and survival in Medieval England. *Annals of Human Biology* 44(4):338–348. https://doi.org/10.1080/03014460.2016.1275792

Warinner, C., Rodrigues, J. F. M., Vyas, R., Trachsel, C., Shved, N., Grossmann, J. & Cappellini, E. (2014). Pathogens and host immunity in the ancient human oral cavity. *Nature Genetics* 46(4):336–344. https://doi.org/10.1038/ng.2906.

Washburn, S. L. (1953). The strategy of physical anthropology. In Kroeber, A. L. (Ed.), Anthropology Today, pp. 714–27. Chicago: Univ. Chicago Press.

Weiss, K. M. (1973). *Demographic Models for Anthropology*. Washington, DC: Society for American Archaeology.

Wilson, J. J. (2010). *Modeling Life through Death in Late Prehistoric West-Central Illinois: An Assessment of Paleodemographic and Paleoepidemiological Variability*. (PhD). Binghamton University, SUNY, Binghamton, NY.

Wilson, J. J. (2014). Paradox and promise: Research on the role of recent advances in paleodemography and paleoepidemiology to the study of "health" in Precolumbian societies. *American Journal of Physical Anthropology* 155(2):268–280. https://doi.org/10.1002/ajpa.22601

Wood, J. W., Holman, D. J., O'Connor, K. A. & Ferrell, R. J. (2002). Mortality models for paleodemography. In Hoppa, R. D. & Vaupel, J. W. (Eds.), *Paleodemography: Age Distributions from Skeletal Samples*, pp. 129–168. Cambridge: Cambridge University Press.

Wood, J. W., Holman, D. J., Weiss, K. M., Buchanan, A. V. & LeFor, B. (1992a). Hazards models for human population biology. *American Journal of Physical Anthropology* 35(S15):43–87. https://doi.org/10.1002/ajpa.1330350604

Wood, J. W., Holman, D. J., Yashin, A. I., Peterson, R. J., Weinstein, M. & Chang, M.-C. (1994). A multistate model of fecundability and sterility. *Demography* 31(3):403–426.

Wood, J. W., Milner, G. R., Harpending, H. C. & Weiss, K. M. (1992b). The osteological paradox: Problems of inferring prehistoric health from skeletal samples. *Current Anthropology* 33(4):343–370.

Wright, L. E. & Yoder, C. J. (2003). Recent progress in bioarchaeology: approaches to the osteological paradox. *Journal of Archaeological Research* 11:43–70.

Yaussy, S. L. (2019). The intersections of industrialization: variation in skeletal indicators of frailty by age, sex, and socioeconomic status in 18th and 19th century England. *American Journal of Physical Anthropology* 170(1):116–130. https://doi.org/10.1002/ajpa.23881

Yaussy, S. L. & DeWitte, S. N. (2018). Patterns of frailty in non-adults from medieval London. *International Journal of Paleopathology* 22:1–7. https://doi.org/10.1016/j.ijpp.2018.03.008

Yaussy, S. L. & DeWitte, S. N. (2019). Calculus and survivorship in medieval London: the association between dental disease and a demographic measure of general health. *American Journal of Physical Anthropology* 168(3):552–565. https://doi.org/10.1002/ajpa.23772

Yaussy, S. L., DeWitte, S. N. & Redfern, R. C. (2016). Frailty and famine: patterns of mortality and physiological stress among victims of famine in medieval London. *American Journal of Physical Anthropology* 160(2):272–283. https://doi.org/10.1002/ajpa.22954

Zuckerman, M. K. (2014). *Modern Environments and Human Health: Revisiting the Second Epidemiological Transition* (first edition). Hoboken, NJ: Wiley-Blackwell.

5
PALEOHISTOPATHOLOGY
History, Technical Aspects, and Diagnostic Challenges

Sandra Assis and Hans H. de Boer

Introduction

Disease has accompanied and shaped humankind since times immemorial. Throughout history, many cultures and civilizations developed a variety of ideas and beliefs about diseases, their effect on an individual's health and well-being, and the best ways of managing them. Many early perceptions of disease combined "natural" and "supernatural" explanations, although a more "natural" interpretation of disease was already present in Hippocrates's writing (Hippocrates of Cos, physician, c. 460–c. 360 B.C.) (Hays, 2009). In absence of pathological or microbiological studies, the etiology of many diseases, however, remained uncertain (Davis, 2000).

The invention of the microscope in the 17th century marked a turning point and forever changed our perception of disease. The microscope unveiled an extraordinarily rich and previously unimaginable new world beneath the level of our ordinary perception (Burgess & Marten, 1990; Wilson, 1995). By showing intricate microstructures hidden in everyday objects and living organisms, the microscope replaced spiritual or "supernatural" entities explanations of macroscopic phenomena (Wilson, 1995). The invention of an optical instrument that outperformed natural vision also led to major scientific breakthroughs (Jacquette, 1997). Consequently, dominant philosophies and previous beliefs were reformed and a "recalibration of human knowledge" took place (Wilson, 1995: 41). Since its first application, the microscope became increasingly sophisticated (e.g., Hogg, 1854) and more frequently used. Consequently, its application surpassed the boundaries of biology and clinical medicine and found another useful application in paleopathology.

Although the microscope has been instrumental to the diagnosis and investigation of diseases for centuries, many paleopathologists still regard microscopy to be methodologically complex, difficult to interpret, and inaccessible when destructive techniques are prohibited. The microscope therefore remains a relatively little used analytical method. It is true that the microscopy of human remains, which are often in an advanced state of decomposition, presents specific and sometimes almost insurmountable challenges. Still, if applied in the appropriate context, microscopy can be a very valuable addition to the diagnostic toolkit.

The History of the Microscope, and Its Use in the Study of Disease

The invention of the microscope cannot be traced with accuracy before the year 1660. However, if we include instruments with a single lens, its history is far more ancient (Hogg, 1854). In fact, there are written records from the Greek author Aristophanes (4th century B.C.) that point to the existence of globular glasses, also called "burning spheres", used to increase visual perception (Hogg, 1854; Croft, 2006). The word microscope derives from the Greek terms "small" and "to view" and was introduced in 1625 by the Italian physician Johannes Faber (1574–1629) (Hajdu, 2002). A major contribution to microscopy was made by Robert Hooke (1635–1703, England) with the publication of his book "Micrographia" in 1665, in which the term "cell" was coined (Hogg, 1854; Croft, 2006; Wollman et al., 2015). In 1653, Petrus Borellus (1620–1689, France) published a report describing the first application of the microscope to medicine (Hajdu, 2002).

Remarkable achievements for understanding the world of microscopic organisms or "animalcula" were actually made by an amateur, the Dutch cloth merchant Antonie van Leeuwenhoek (1632–1723, the Netherlands) (Croft, 2006; Wollman et al., 2015). During his life, he produced increasingly better performing microscopes, with which he conducted ingenious experiments and developed new micrometry techniques to describe his findings (Allen, 2015; Davis, 2020). Van Leeuwenhoek added substantially to previous microscopic investigations; amongst others, he was the first to describe bacteria (Burgess & Marten, 1990; Money, 2014). He was also responsible for the identification of a variety of protists, yeast -from beer-, human spermatozoa, red blood cells (in 1695), and for the first microscopic observations of a bone-related tissue, namely the periosteum (Van Leeuwenhoek, 1720; Money, 2014; Allen, 2015).

All these new discoveries gave biology and medicine a new incentive for experimentation, observation, and comparative studies (Wilson, 1995; Hays, 2009). A more systematic use of the microscope, particularly in the late 18th century, allowed the advancement of anatomical dissection, since the microscope had unlocked anatomy beyond gross examination, enabling physicians better to examine the physiology of organs and to study the interaction of cells (Hogg, 1854; Stepney, 1990). Studies on the microstructure of bone tissue illustrate these early efforts. Rudimentarily, the histomorphology of bone was first portrayed in 1691 by Clopton Havers (1657–1702, United Kingdom) in his book *Osteologia Nova, or Some New Observations of the Bones, and the Parts Belonging to Them, With the Manner of Their Accretion and Nutrition* (Dobson, 1952). Havers identified the spaces or canals inside compact bone tissues, which now bear his name: Haversian canals (Dobson, 1952; Beasley, 1986).

Alongside anatomical studies, the microscope also contributed significantly to the study and diagnosis of disease (Hays, 2009). The foundations of histopathology can be traced back to 1799 when Xavier Bichat (1771–1802, France), a young pathologist, published a book entitled "*Traité des Membranes en General et de Diverses Membranes en Particulier*" in which, and for the first time, morbid anatomy and histopathological changes were described (Bichat, 1799). The 19th century subsequently saw a surge in the microscopic examination of disease. One of the most renowned medical scientists of that era, the German physician Rudolph Virchow (1821–1902), eventually stated that "every disease involves changes in normal cells, and that ultimately, all pathology is cellular pathology" (Schultz, 2008). This insight, amongst his many other contributions to medicine in general and anatomical pathology specifically, resulted in his moniker: the "father of modern pathology".

The microscope further contributed to the understanding of disease – particularly infectious disease – through the investigations of Louis Pasteur (1822–1895, France), Gerhard Hansen (1841–1912, Norway), and Robert Koch (1843–1919, Germany). Pasteur's discoveries revolutionized some fundamentals of biology and led to the foundation of microbiology as a distinct science. He showed experimentally that fermentation was caused by microorganisms, and not the result of chemical decomposition. Based on these observations, he hypothesized that many infectious diseases were most probably caused by microbes, a postulate that became known as the "germ theory of disease" (Smith, 2012). Guided by this, Joseph Lister (1827–1912), a British surgeon, developed a successful antiseptic technique (by means of carbolic and phenic acid solutions) (Lister, 1867). However, only after the experiments by the Prussian physician Robert Koch, was the "germ theory of disease" confirmed. Partly based on his microscopic examinations, Koch proposed a set of criteria (Koch's postulates) to assign a microbial origin of disease (Smith, 2012; Money, 2014). These postulates remain valid today. Koch is also renowned for the isolation of the organism that causes anthrax (1877, *Bacillus anthracis*), suppuration (1878, *Staphylococcus*), tuberculosis (1882, *Mycobacterium tuberculosis*), and cholera (1883, *Vibrio cholerae*) (Blevins & Bronze, 2010). Koch also dedicated time to improve the microscope and to developed techniques for specific staining of microbes (i.e., aniline dyes – eosin, fuchsin, safranin, and methyl violet) to enhance their visibility. The routine application of light microscopy for identifying bacteria is attributed largely to these efforts (Blevins & Bronze, 2010).

At the same time, Gerhard Hansen discovered the causative agent of leprosy, *Mycobacterium leprae*, in 1874. He based his discovery on the extensive collection and histological analysis of tissue specimens from infected individuals. This allowed him to confirm the contagious nature of leprosy, thereby debunking the then-accepted hereditary theory (Grzybowski et al., 2014). The realization that each infectious disease resulted from a specific pathogen gave rise to the idea that infectious diseases can be prevented and treated by prophylactic and therapeutic vaccination, respectively (Smith, 2012; Money, 2014).

The first half of the 20th century was characterized by considerable technical improvements in light and polarized microscopy, as well as by the development of new techniques for section production. For bone, methods for decalcification, paraffin wax embedding, and microtome sectioning were developed, alongside methods in which non-decalcified bone was ground down to translucent sections. This period was also marked by the development of the first transmission electron microscope (TEM), which occurred between 1929 and 1931, by Ernst Ruska (1906–1988, Germany) and Max Knoll (1897–1969, Germany) (Masters, 2009; Allen, 2015).

The History of Microscopy in Paleopathology

The first application of microscopy to the study of human remains can be traced back to the 19th century. In 1879, the Czech physician J. N. Czermak (1828–1873) used histology to describe a case of arteriosclerosis in an Egyptian mummy (Aufderheide & Rodríguez-Martín, 1998; Aufderheide, 2003; Denton, 2008). Histological techniques were also applied as early as 1889 by the French physician Daniel M. Fouquet (1850–1914) to examine mummified tissues (Ruffer, 1921; Sandison, 1967). With respect to the analysis of dry bone remains, one of the first histological examinations is attributed to the American pathologist Theophil Mitchell Prudden (1849–1924) who examined, in 1891, a possible case of syphilis from the prehistoric site of Animas River, Colorado (Garland, 1993). Another pioneering application of histology to the study of pathological skeletal remains is attributed to Carl Magnus Fürst

(1854–1935, Sweden) who diagnosed, in 1920, a case of periostitis ossificans in the tibia of King Magnus of Sweden, 13th century A.D. (Graf, 1949).

In spite of these advances, the application of histology to ancient samples posed challenges. Many investigations faced technical limitations dictated by the nature of the samples, namely its type (e.g., dry bone, teeth, or mummified remains), its preservation, and/or its size. Accordingly, the first applications of microscopy in paleopathology had to coincide with the re-adjustment of existing methods or the development of new methods.

An important contribution to overcome technical limitations in the study of mummified tissues was made by Sir Marc Armand Ruffer (1859–1917) in the beginning of the 20th century (Ruffer, 1921; Sandison, 1967; Swinton, 1981). In order to restore the flexibility of tissues for histological inspection, he embedded sectioned samples in several cycles of alkaline salts (sodium carbonate) mixed with alcohol or formol, followed by baths in alcohol, chloroform, and paraffin. This resulted in more pliable, easy-to-cut, and stainable sections. Ruffer's method was successfully used on sections of muscle, blood vessels, skin, intestine, stomach, liver, kidney, bone, mammary glands, and testicles, and as he predicted, the detection of various pathological conditions (Ruffer, 1909). *Schistosoma haematobium* bilharzia (schistosomiasis) in the kidneys of two Egyptian mummies (1250–1000 B.C.) (Ruffer, 1910); atherosclerosis in several mummified bodies (1090–945 B.C.) (Ruffer, 1911a); a possible case of smallpox in a male mummy (200–1100 B.C.) (Ruffer, 1911b); diffuse anthracosis in the lungs; and Pott's disease in Egyptian mummies (Ruffer & Chantre, 1911; Ruffer, 1921) are some of Ruffer's notable histological findings.

Ruffer was not alone. Almost at the same time, the American anatomist and zoologist Harris H. Wilder (1864 –1928) tested his own methods for rehydration of mummified tissue and studied samples from Peruvian, Cliff-dweller of Southern Utah, and Basketmaker American Indian bodies (Wilder, 1904). The British pathologist S. G. Shattock (1852–1924) also studied histological sections of an aorta from an Egyptian pharaoh (Shattock, 1909), further demonstrating the substantial contribution of histology to the paleopathology of mummified remains (see also: Reyman et al., 1976; Weinstein et al., 1981; Walker et al., 1987; Zimmerman, 1993; Zimmerman et al., 1998; Ciranni & Fornaciari, 2004; Fornaciari, 2018- to name a few).

The term "paleohistology" was coined, allegedly, in 1926 by Roy L. Moodie (1880–1934, USA) (Garland, 1993). Nevertheless, it was not until 1949 that an actual definition was proposed by Wilhelm Graf (Sweden), who described paleohistology as "(…) the examination of microscopic sections of ancient human beings and the recognition of tissues and cells in such sections" (Graf, 1949: 236). In the same publication, Graf presented the results of a study on tissue preservation in three Egyptian mummies and 15 Swedish skeletons, concluding that there were no parallels between the chronology and the histological preservation of tissues.

It was also in the 1950s that the electron microscope was first applied to the study of ancient bone remains. In 1950, Barbour compared ultrastructural differences between fresh and fossil bones (Barbour, 1950). Other studies followed (e.g., Macadam & Sandison, 1969). Meanwhile, new technical devices for cutting, embedding, and staining samples continued to be tested both in the study of living and fossilized bone (see further in this chapter). In addition to light, polarized, and electron microscopy, other microscopy techniques, such as the scanning electron microscopy (SEM), microscopic computerized tomography, or confocal laser scanning microscopy, were introduced and are currently in use, namely for the study of dry bone pathological changes (e.g., Bell Jones, 1991; Wakely et al., 1991; Eshed et al., 2002; Brickley et al., 2007; Rühli et al., 2007; Maggiano et al., 2009; Wade et al., 2011; Welsh et al., 2020).

Microscopy and the Preservation of Human Remains

The preservation of human remains is dependent on several intrinsic agents, such as age and sex of the individual; bone size, shape, mass, and density; and the presence of pathology and trauma. In addition, a plethora of extrinsic agents are of importance, such as burial assemblage, burial practice, and the duration of the inhumation; exposure to sunlight, temperature, water transportation, and humidity fluctuations; soil compaction and pH; animal activity; vegetation; fungal and bacterial invasion; and methods of archaeological excavation, analysis, and storage of remains (Galloway et al., 1997; Stodder, 2008; Jackes, 2011). The histological analysis of dry bone or mummified human remains is often substantially limited by these variables and processes, as they will affect the quantity and the quality of the data that can be retrieved at isotopic, molecular, biochemical, and structural levels (Hedges, 2002; Turner-Walker, 2008). It is of pivotal importance to consider these effects on paleohistopathological interpretations.

Despite the challenges, microscopy on taphonomically/diagenetically altered remains is by no means futile. As a matter of fact, histology has proven very useful to uncover diagenetic pathways in hard tissue remains (e.g., Stout, 1978; Hackett, 1981; Turner-Walker & Jans, 2008; Hollund et al., 2012; Dal Sasso et al., 2014; Turner-Walker, 2019). Also, it can be used as a means to differentiate between actual pathology and so-called "pseudo-pathology", induced by taphonomical and diagenetic alteration (Pinhasi & Bourbou, 2008).

The Effects of Mummification on Histological Analysis

Mummification describes the process of soft tissue preservation, when postmortem putrefaction or decay is arrested or substantially delayed (see Chapter 12, this volume for more information about mummified remains). The most well-known cause is desiccation, which is common in dry and arid climates, or in closed environments such as crypts and catacombs. Mummification may also occur by direct freezing and/or dehydration in very cold environments; after exposure to high concentrations of heavy metals such as mercury, arsenic, copper, and lead; or in environments that inhibit bacterial activity, such as peat bog waters or salty environments (Aufderheide, 2003; Lynnerup, 2007).

An aspect common to both natural and artificial (or anthropogenic) mummification is differential preservation. This differential preservation is not only visible macroscopically but also on a microscopic level, and must be kept in mind when considering the chances of successful histological analysis. Although many soft tissues survive remarkably well, tissues and organs with high enzymatic activity, such as the pancreas and liver, often appear decomposed or almost unrecognizable. Bone may or may not be well-preserved. In an acidic environment, demineralization may hamper the analysis substantially (Lynnerup, 2007, 2015; Aufderheide, 2011). In contrast, organs with more connective tissue are usually much better preserved. Examples of tissues that are usually well-preserved are the kidney, liver, heart, dermis, muscle fasciae, and tendons (Lynnerup, 2007; Fernández, 2012).

The preservation of tissues not only impacts the morphological and histological identification of tissues, but also the diagnosis of pathological conditions. For example, some histological artifacts produced by tissue decomposition can be mistakenly diagnosed as lesions; so-called pseudo-pathologies (Mekota & Vermehren, 2006).

The Effects of Taphonomy and Diagenesis on Skeletonized Remains

The skeleton is not impervious to taphonomic change and diagenesis. Diagenetic modification of bone will ensue especially after soft tissue decomposition (Grupe, 2007). The complex and hierarchical structure of bone initially confers a stabilizing effect that protects the tissue from early microbial and chemical degradation. The mineral fraction shields proteins from microbial enzymolysis and chemical hydrolysis, while the organic fraction inhibits mineral dissolution. However, in time, both the organic and inorganic components will deteriorate, and bone degradation will ensue (Turner-Walker, 2008).

The degradation of bone may occur either through chemical hydrolysis or through bioerosion (Collins et al., 2002; Hedges, 2002). Bioerosion refers to the microbial alteration of bones caused by bacteria, cyanobacteria, and fungi (Jans, 2008; Turner-Walker, 2019). On a histological level, microbial alteration of bone is recognized as "microscopic focal destruction", visible as tunnel-like structures in the cortical bone tissue. Various types of tunnels are recognized (Wedl or centrifugal, linear longitudinal, budded, and lamellate, for a review see: Jans, 2008), but these do not seem to relate to a specific type of microorganism or a specific phase of preservation. The existence of these tunnels is of particular importance, as they obscure the microstructure of the bone tissue and negatively alter the translucency of the histological section through diffraction.

The origin of these bacteria (either in the soil or endogenous within the gut) has been the subject of discussion. Jans and co-authors (2004) found that bones from complete burials presented more microbial degradation than bones subjected to dismemberment or butchering. This observation would suggest that microbial alteration is related to putrefaction, rather than soil bacteria. However, Turner-Walker (2019) recently showed that microbial tunneling may also be present in de-fleshed non-human remains buried in soil for a long period of time.

As soon as degradation sets in, the increase in bone porosity will facilitate further microbial degradation, which may subsequently increase the process of apatite dissolution and/or recrystallization (Nielsen-Marsh et al., 2000). Recrystallization is especially detrimental for histological analysis, as it obscures the original architecture. Apatite dissolution occurs more rapidly in acidic environments and in sites with active hydrology (Hedges, 2002). Burial places with repeated wet/dry cycles may therefore yield poorly preserved remains. The same may occur in highly conductive or well-drained soils that allow for the continuous flow of water through the bones (Hedges & Millard, 1995). Bone and teeth diagenesis furthermore depends on soil composition (e.g., pH, flora, and fauna), temperature and the presence of oxygen, soil pressure and drainage capabilities, groundwater chemistry and hydrological flow, microbial composition, and particle transport (Hedges, 2002; Grupe, 2007).

All in all, it is well-understood that bones from the same time period and assemblage may present extremely variable preservation, both on a macroscopic and a microscopic level. Further studies have revealed that the gross appearance of bones may bear no relation to the histological preservation of tissues (e.g., Garland, 1987; Bell & Jones, 1991; Guarino et al., 2006; Turner-Walker, 2008; Assis et al., 2015) and that bones belonging to the same individual may differ in preservation, especially histologically (e.g., Nielsen-Marsh et al., 2000, Assis et al., 2015). Hence, while poorly preserved bone will yield poorly preserved microstructure, the preservation of microarchitecture in well-preserved bone is almost impossible to predict.

A Primer on Bone Biology and Histomorphology

Interpretation of bone histology requires thorough knowledge of bone composition, macro- and microarchitecture, and cellular components. Bone tissue's basic response to physiological and pathological stimuli must also be understood. It goes beyond the scope of this chapter to provide an in-depth overview of these subjects, as they are readily available in standard anatomy, histology, and pathology textbooks (e.g., Väänänen et al., 2000; Jee, 2001; Marks & Odgren, 2002; Ott, 2002; Steiniche & Hauge, 2003; Young et al., 2006; Chappard et al., 2011; Allen & Burr, 2014; Burr & Akkus, 2014; Martin et al., 2015). However, a brief overview will be provided below (Table 5.1).

Bone is a multifunctional, physiologically dynamic, and self-repairing tissue, able to adjust its mass, shape, and properties to environmental and mechanical demands. The functions of bone are myriad. It provides strength and support to the body, protects major organs, supplies the framework for hematopoiesis, stores mineral salts, and serves as an attachment site for muscles. Bone is also recognized as an endocrine organ that, and through its hormones, helps to mediate phosphate metabolism and energy metabolism.

Different cells ensure distinct skeletal functions. While osteoblasts are responsible for the formation of osteoid – the unmineralized component of bone matrix that is subsequently mineralized to form bone, osteoclasts act on bone resorption, by solubilizing both its mineral and organic components. Osteoclastic resorption is a cyclical phenomenon – also called a resorption cycle – in which the cells converge on the target area, degrade the underlying matrix, detach and finally suffer apoptosis or return to their non-resorbing stage. During osteoid formation, some osteoblasts may become entrapped by their own matrix deposition and can differentiate into osteocytes. Others may be transformed into bone-lining cells (resting osteoblasts) or undergo apoptosis.

Bone is organized in a multiscale manner. At the macroscopic level, two distinct types of bone exist. Cortical or compact bone is a dense tissue that forms the outside shell of bones; while trabecular, cancellous, or spongy bone is a porous, mesh-like structure located within the medullary cavity. Bone tissue sits between two envelopes of condensed fibrous tissue: an external, the periosteum (periosteal surface); and an internal, the endosteum (endosteal or endocortical surface). When stimulated, the inner layer of the periosteum is capable of forming either highly organized lamellar bone or disorganized woven bone, as in certain pathologic situations. This accounts for the highly sensitive response of the periosteum to biomechanical stimulation, inflammation, infection, tumors, or trauma.

Histologically, cortical bone is composed of numerous osteons or Haversian systems. These cylindrical units of calcified bone are considered the "cornerstones" of the cortical bone (Steiniche & Hauge, 2003: 62) or their structural unit (BSU – bone structure unit) (Chappard et al., 2011: 2227). Osteons are formed by a neurovascular channel (Haversian canal) surrounded by layers of concentric lamellae. Between the lamellae, oval cavities (lacunae) for osteocytes are located, connecting to each other via canaliculi. From the Haversian canal, multiple vascular branches called perforating or Volkmann's canals spread at right angles to extend the system of nerves and vessels outward and inward through the cortical tissue, and between periosteal and endosteal spaces. In trabecular bone, the lamellae are arranged more or less parallel to the trabecular surface, and its BSUs are comparable to incomplete osteons (half osteons, or hemiosteons). BSUs in cancellous bone form two types of trabeculae: large plates (arranged along the stress lines), connected laterally by pillars, and rods that ensure cohesion, forming a honeycomb network structure.

Table 5.1 The hierarchical organization of bone*

Bone organization			Main features and functions
Macrostructure	**Types of bone**		
		Cortical bone	Compact or dense type of bone.
			Low porosity (5–10%).
			Shaft of long bones, around vertebral bodies and other cuboidal and flat bones.
		Trabecular bone	Reticulated type of bone.
			High porosity (75–95%) and low density.
			Epiphyses of long bones, bodies of vertebrae, and inside the flat bones of the pelvis and skull.
	Skeletal envelopes		
		Periosteum	Subdivided in two layers:
			An outer layer formed by a complex network of fibroblasts and collagenous fibers – Sharpey's fibers that anchor the membrane to the underlying bone; an inner layer (or cambium layer) that retains a highly osteogenic potential.
			Formed by a single layer of flattened cells.
		Endosteum	Covers all of the internal cavities within bone, including the trabeculae of spongy bone.
			Contains less connective tissue and is smaller than periosteum.
Microstructure	**Types of cells**		
		Osteoblasts	Bone-forming cells.
			Cuboidal shape with abundant basophilic cytoplasm (active cells).
			Flattened and "spindle-shaped" (inactive cells).
			Communicate with other cells (bone lining cells, osteocytes and bone marrow cells) by cellular processes that connect at intercellular channels or gap junctions.
		Osteocytes	Stellate cells, differentiated from osteoblasts.
			Correspond to 90–95% of all the cells in bone.
			Reside in oval cavities (lacunae).
			Possess long cytoplasmic extensions that spread through small channels (canaliculi) – to communicate with neighboring osteocytes, bone-lining cells, and osteoblasts.
			Key-role: regulation of calcium and phosphorus in the bone matrix and blood; mechano-sensors of bone – they orchestrate focal modeling and remodeling by detecting strain.

(Continued)

Bone organization		Main features and functions
	Bone-lining cells	Flat, elongated and inactive cells.
		Cover quiescent bone surfaces (e.g., Haversian canal wall).
		Seem to derive from inactive osteoblasts or osteoblast precursors.
		Key-role (not fully understood): bone resorption by removing surface osteoid and allowing osteoclast access to mineralized tissue; act on homeostatic, morphogenetic, and restructuring processes that constitute regulation of bone mineral, mass, architecture, and hematopoietic process.
	Osteoclasts	Bone-resorbing cells.
		Mobile, multinucleated giant cells.
		Reside in etched depressions – Howship's lacunae.
		Possess a "ruffled border" – a highly infolded area of the plasma membrane from where several organic acids and lysosomal proteolytic enzymes dissolve the underlying bone.
		Key-role: normal skeletal maturation and maintenance; tooth eruption; fracture healing; and maintenance of blood serum mineral levels.
Types of bone		
	Woven bone	Usually, but not exclusively, deposited "de novo", i.e., without any fibrous or cartilaginous precursor.
		Forms more rapidly and shows more osteocytes than other types of bone.
		Shows a random organization of the mineralized fibers (mostly type I collagen).
		It is replaced by lamellar bone (during growth).
		Reduced mechanical strength (weaker than lamellar bone).
		A primary type of bone.
		Forms more rapidly than other types of bone (except woven bone).
	Plexiform bone	Combines non-lamellar bone (woven type), which forms a trabecular network, and lamellar bone (the filled-in spaces).
		Contains rectilinear residual vascular spaces (brick-wall appearance).
		Stronger mechanical proprieties than woven bone.
		Reliable feature to differentiate human from non-human bone (e.g., bovines, pigs and horses).
		Reported in children with major growth spurts but considered extremely rare in humans.

	Primary lamellar bone	A primary type of bone.
		Forms more slowly than woven or plexiform bone.
		Composed of parallel and densely packed lamellae.
		Principal type of bone formed on the periosteal and endosteal surfaces (circumferential lamellae).
		Shows few vascular channels.
		Stronger mechanical proprieties.
	Primary osteons	A primary type of bone.
		Usually found within well-organized lamellar bone.
		Small diameter (50–100 μm) and small vascular canal than secondary osteons.
		Fewer concentric lamellae (circa of 10) in comparison with secondary osteons.
		No cement line (i.e., a well-defined boundary that separates osteons from the surrounding matrix).
	Secondary osteons	A secondary type of bone.
		Forms far more slowly than immature bone types.
		Bigger diameter (100–250 μm) and larger Haversian canals than primary osteons.
		Possess more concentric lamellae (circa of 20–25 lamellae) than primary osteons.
		Display a cement line.
		Predominant type of bone within adult cortical bone.
	Interstitial lamellae	A secondary type of bone.
		Remnants of primary lamellar bone or older osteons (partially resorbed during bone remodeling).
		Present cement lines.
Nanostructure and ultrastructure	**Components**	
	Organic matrix (20–25%)	Mostly type I collagen (90%).
		Other noncollagenous proteins (10%).
	Inorganic salts (65%)	Poorly crystalline hydroxyapatite tablets ($Ca_{10}[PO_4]_6[OH]_2$) with hydrogen phosphate (HPO_4) and carbonate (CO_3) groups.
	Water (10%)	Bound to the collagen-mineral components.
		Unbound water that flows through canalicular and vascular channels in bone.

*Based on Väänänen et al., 2000; Currey, 2001; Jee, 2001; Marks & Odgren, 2002; Nijweide et al., 2002; Ott, 2002; Steiniche & Hauge, 2003; Dittmann et al., 2006; Pfeiffer, 2006; Young et al., 2006; Chappard et al., 2011; Allen & Burr, 2014; Burr & Akkus, 2014; Martin et al., 2015.

At the microscopic level, bone is either classified as woven, plexiform, or lamellar. In the latter, a further subdivision between primary and secondary exists. These subdivisions relate to its morphology, but also to its mechanical and physiological properties and the manner in which it is deposited. While woven bone is a highly disorganized type of bone, lamellar bone is a densely packed tissue characterized by "regular parallel bands [or lamellae] of collagen arranged in sheets" (Young et al., 2006: 191). The haphazard appearance of woven bone is due to the rapid production of osteoid by osteoblasts, as normally observed during fetal bone development. Woven bone can also be found in adults, when rapid bone formation is induced. This can for instance be the case in tumors, some metabolic diseases (e.g., Paget's disease), and inflammatory processes, as well as during fracture repair. Lamellar bone is slowly formed. The lamellae may extend parallel to the endosteal or periosteal surfaces, composing the circumferential lamellar bone, within individual trabeculae, or may lie concentrically (concentric lamellae) around the Haversian canal of the osteon. Along the spectrum of woven and lamellar bone, plexiform bone, also called fibrolamellar bone, may be more or less regarded as an intermediate type.

Primary bone is defined as bone that is produced "de novo" (i.e., deposited directly) on an existing bone or cartilage surface by apposition, without resorption of pre-existing bone. In contrast, secondary bone is formed through "bone remodeling": the resorption of pre-existing bone, followed by its replacement with new, lamellar bone. Bone remodeling is essential to repair fatigue microdamage and contributes to mineral metabolism and ionic balance. It may occur at periosteal, endocortical, trabecular, and intracortical levels and is executed by so-called bone multicellular units (BMUs). BMUs are temporary units consisting of osteoclasts and osteoblasts that act in response to external signals or stimuli. Remodeling occurs simultaneously throughout the skeleton and follows a strict sequence: the remodeling cycle. This cycle broadly includes starting and organization of the BMU, resorption of pre-existing bone by osteoclasts, recruitment of osteoblasts, deposition of bone-precursor (osteoid), and mineralization. The resultant circular, lamellar structures are referred to as secondary osteons or Haversian systems. Hemiosteons (trabecular bone) and interstitial lamellae (cortical bone) are also the product of bone remodeling.

At the nanostructural level, bone consists of an organic and an inorganic fraction. Both have a well-defined function: the inorganic confers the rigidity and strength that characterizes bone, whereas the network of collagen fibers allows some degree of flexibility.

Methodology in Paleohistopathology

As mentioned above, the application of microscopy to paleopathology comes with significant technical challenges. Almost by definition, the samples are severely degraded by, for instance, mummification, skeletonization, thermal alteration, taphonomy, diagenesis, or a combination hereof. The destructive nature of microscopy, in combination with the historical value of the samples, often complicates matters more. Lastly, given the high resolution of microscopy, even the smallest methodological errors may hamper, or even preclude interpretation.

Many practitioners, therefore, not only focus on the actual interpretation of histomorphology but also consider the best ways in which the material under study should be processed. Although methods may differ, they are all derivatives of methods that are commonly used in pathology, biology, or geology laboratories. In clinical pathology laboratories, a lot of knowledge and experience exists on processing bone and soft tissue for histological analysis. Often within these laboratories, one or more technicians specialize in processing bone samples, as this is perceived to be a challenging process, even in clinical settings.

Choosing a method to process tissues depends on the nature of the material. Obviously, a distinction must be made between soft tissues (generally mummified remains) and hard tissue (bone, teeth). However, irrespective of the tissue or the processing method chosen, it is best practice to first undertake one or more "test runs" on material with less diagnostic potential. In that way, small alterations to the method can be made prior to processing the most valuable material.

Processing Mummified Tissue for Histology

Due to desiccation, mummified tissues are often hard, brittle, and difficult to process by conventional histology methods (Mekota & Vermehren, 2006). Without rehydration, it is likely that the material will either be impossible to section or the resultant sections will be non-diagnostic. Since rehydration techniques are specific to mummified tissues, a relatively large body of literature exists on the topic (e.g., Graf, 1949; Sandinson, 1955; Zimmerman, 1972; Turner & Holtom, 1981; Walker et al., 1987; Hess et al., 1998; Mekota & Vermehren, 2005; Collini et al., 2014; Grove et al., 2015).

For newcomers to the field, and as a starting point, the comprehensive review of Mekota and Vermehren in 2005 is probably the most informative. In this publication, the authors tested 13 different, well-known rehydration methods and three newly devised methods on various types of mummified remains from Egypt. They concluded that the diagnostic value of the sections depended mostly on preservation but was also dependent on the chosen rehydration method. Furthermore, the effectiveness of each rehydration method differed per tissue type. This again indicates that no uniform method exists and that testing methods prior to application are essential. Metkota and Vermehren also indicate that rehydration allows for the use of standard histochemical stains. However, again, the results depended on tissue preservation.

Methods for Dry Bone Material

The processing of skeletonized bone material presents a conundrum. Due to its hardness and brittleness, it is impossible to section by microtome without decalcification. However, since severely weathered bone no longer contains much protein, decalcification of badly preserved remains can result in total disintegration of the tissue. The obvious solution is to embed the material in a rigid matrix and to create undecalcified sections. However, the porosity of heavily weathered bone, in combination with the high viscosity of most embedding media, may complicate this. In addition, the production of non-decalcified sections through grinding (either by hand or automated) can be a laborious process that requires practice.

As such, when attempting to process bone material for histological examination, a practitioner should initially consider whether or not the material under study could be decalcified. Most recent textbooks state that, almost by definition, bone material for paleopathological study cannot be decalcified. However, as early as 1949, it was shown that the classical histopathological procedures of bone decalcification, paraffin-embedding and histochemical staining, can be applied to ancient bone (Graf, 1949). Also from our experience, ancient bone can be remarkably well-preserved.

To test if a bone contains enough organic matrix to retain its integrity after decalcification, a non-diagnostic sample can be processed. If, indeed, the material retains its integrity, it is best to process the material as standard histological slides, as practiced in clinical pathology. Not only will this allow more sections to be produced from a single piece of tissue, but it will also enable the use of standard histochemical stains, which renders comparison with clinical pathology specimens and textbooks easier.

In many instances, however, decalcification will not be possible and the material will have to be sectioned and ground down to translucency (approx. 100–50 μm). Ordinarily, given the brittleness of the material, this will require an embedding medium to provide support. However, if the bone material consists entirely of cortical bone, or if the cortex is the only region of interest (for instance when undergoing age-at-death estimation), embedding may not be necessary. In those instances, the method initially devised by Frost (1968) and revised and modified by Maat and co-authors (2001) can be used. This method is quick, easy to learn, and only uses materials that are commercially available (Beauchesne & Saunders, 2006; Martiniaková et al., 2006). The method also allows for the use of some histochemical staining (De Boer et al., 2012). A test by Haas and Stora (2015), however, showed that although the method is quick, easy, and cheap, it should only be used for well-preserved cortical bone. For more fragile material, using embedding media is preferred (see below).

Embedding bone for slide production has a long history, with one of the first methods developed by Axelrod (1947), who used a celloidin solution to embed fresh bone before cutting. In the 1950s, plastic embedding was introduced, with Arnold (1951) and Arnold and Jee (1954) using celloidin plasticized with diamyl phthalate and n-amyl sebacate, and Jowsey (1955) using a plastic substance (methyl methacrylate monomer). Other researchers, such as Kuhn and Lutz (1958), Pugh and Savchuck (1958), and Norris and Jenkins (1960), used synthetic resins (e.g., modified polyester resin, polyvinyl resin, and epoxy). Since then, most methods relied on polymeric resins, with different laboratories often publishing their own preferred methods. For example, Stout and Teitelbaum proposed a new method using methyl methacrylate in 1976, while Caropreso and colleagues presented a method based on epoxy resin embedding in 2000 (Caropreso et al., 2000). A year later, a method for the study of diagenetic changes in bone, combining resin embedding and staining techniques was presented by Dore et al. (2001). Later, publications refined these methods or developed their own specific method (e.g., Cho, 2012; Cooper et al., 2012; De Boer et al., 2013a).

Overall, it appears that every laboratory has found its favorite embedding medium and has developed its own method of cutting and grinding. Most of these methods, despite their differences, present excellent results. A common denominator in successful embedding methods is a low viscous embedding medium that has more or less the same hardness/elasticity as the bone material it must support. The embedding may be improved by applying one or more circles of vacuumization.

After embedding, the sections should be cut into "thick slices" of approximately 1–2 mm. Subsequently, they must be ground down to translucency. Hand-grinding is the cheapest method, as it only requires simple materials (De Boer et al., 2013a). However, it may be time-consuming and requires some practice, especially for larger sections. For large numbers of sections, automated grinding methods may be more suitable (Crowder et al., 2012). Also, in undecalcified and embedded sections, histochemical staining may increase the visibility of the microarchitecture (De Boer et al., 2013a)

Methods for Scanning Electron Microscopy

Scanning electron microscopy (SEM) is, within paleopathology, a relatively little used method to study bone microarchitecture. Its working principle is very different from the "ordinary" light microscope, but the resultant images can be comparable to light microscopy

(Bell, 1990; Wakely et al., 1991; De Boer et al., 2013b; De Boer & Van der Merwe, 2016; Van der Merwe et al., 2018; Welsh et al., 2020). The most important reason why practitioners do not use SEM is its limited availability, its expense, and the need for specialized technical knowledge.

The benefits of using an SEM are clear: it scans the surface of an object, rather than relying on translucency. Many of the technical limitations associated with light microscopy are therefore less of an issue in SEM. However, it still requires preparative steps, such as embedding and coating, which are impossible without the help of dedicated technicians. As a result, although SEM can be a valuable tool, it is generally still underutilized.

The Application of Histology to Paleopathology

Histology has been used to explore some of the most common research questions in paleopathology. For instance, a relatively large body of literature exists on the microscopic analysis of taphonomical processes (see above). Also, differentiation between human and non-human bone and histological age-at-death estimation has received attention, and, naturally, the diagnosis of diseases and the analysis of skeletal trauma. In the following sections, a summarizing overview of the latter three efforts is provided.

Human and Non-Human Remains

When a gross inspection fails to identify species-specific morphological landmarks, histology can be useful to distinguish between human and non-human bone material. This differentiation is possible because the microstructure of human bone is distinctly different from other animals as a result of different growth patterns, biomechanical stress, and nutritional requirements (Hillier & Bell, 2007; Mulhern & Ubelaker, 2012). At a microscopic level, human bone is characterized by a scattered distribution of cortical osteons and primary bone types, when compared with other mature mammals that have a plexiform pattern and show osteon banding (Cuijpers, 2006; Pfeiffer, 2006; Cattaneo et al., 2009; Mulhern & Ubelaker, 2012). However, histological features resembling "osteon banding" have also been reported in human bones (e.g., Cummaudo et al., 2018).

Besides qualitative morphological differences, several quantitative differences also exist. Of the numerous variables investigated (e.g., secondary osteon density, Haversian canal or secondary osteon diameter, bone perimeter or area), Haversian canal size is currently regarded as the most diagnostic feature differentiating human from non-human bone. The presence of small secondary osteons and Haversian canals may indicate a non-human origin (Mulhern & Ubelaker, 2012). Other than non-human primates, which share a similar bone microstructure and age-related changes, the quantitative analyses of bone microstructure may also allow for the taxonomic classification of zooarchaeological remains (e.g., Dittmann et al., 2006; Martiniaková et al., 2007).

Age-at-Death Estimation

Age-at-death estimation is fundamental for the reconstruction of a biological profile, both in archaeological and forensic contexts. Although histological age estimation is not frequently used in bioarchaeological studies since it is destructive, it can be useful for the study of burned or very fragmented and/or altered remains (Streeter, 2012). To this end, several histological methods have been developed in ancient and modern bone and in teeth.

Histological age estimation is based on the observation of age-dependent changes in bone tissue, most derived from the remodeling process in adult cortical bone (Streeter, 2012). During the aging process, the primary bone, which is mostly composed of circumferential lamellar bone, is gradually replaced by secondary bone, formed by intact osteons (Haversian systems) and osteons fragments. The latter are remnants of older osteons that were removed by new ones during cortical remodeling. Therefore, there is a relationship between age and the amount/density of osteons and osteon fragments (Robling & Stout, 2008). In addition to osteon population density, other microstructural variables have been explored for histomorphometric age estimation, namely the prevalence of non-Haversian canals/primary osteons, the amount of unremodeled lamellar bone, mean number of lamellae per osteon, and the size of osteons and of Haversian canals. For these analyses, different skeletal elements have been used, namely ribs and clavicle, long bones, and ilium (for a review see, e.g., Robling & Stout, 2008; Streeter, 2012). Most of the published literature rely upon regression formulae, with which a quantification of the remodeling can be used to estimate an age range. As with most age estimation techniques, accuracy diminishes with advanced age. The effects of intrinsic (sex and population variability) and extrinsic (adequate bone sampling) factors on age-at-death estimation, coupled with uncertainties regarding the use of weight-bearing bones, have also been noted and discussed (Robling & Stout, 2008).

Histological aging methods on teeth are based on the apposition of dentin, resulting in tooth cementum annulations (TCAs). Similarly, methods focusing on striae of Retzius in enamel and daily cross striations and root dentine translucency have also been proposed (e.g., Wittwer-Backofen et al., 2004; FitzGerald & Saunders, 2005; Roksandic et al., 2009; Guatelli-Steinberg & Huffman, 2012).

Disease Diagnosis

Overall, histology in paleopathology is mostly used for the study of disease. Consequently, a large body of literature is dedicated to the diagnosis of specific diseases, or the diagnostic potential of microscopy (De Boer & Maat, 2012; De Boer et al., 2013b; De Boer & Van der Merwe, 2016; De Boer & Maat, 2018). Although it falls outside the scope of this chapter to provide a detailed discussion of the histological changes associated with each disease, the benefits and limitations of histology for diagnosis are worth reviewing.

It is well-established that the histological analysis of human remains can provide a wide range of information regarding normal and pathological changes occurring in response to internal and external stimuli (Martin, 1991). More specifically, it offers a glimpse into cellular activity, such as excessive tissue mineralization, signs of abnormal bone resorption, and residual organics associated with past diseases (Bell & Piper, 2000; Ortner, 2003). However, it must be emphasized that bone tissue response to stimuli is extremely limited; it consists of bone resorption, bone apposition, or both. Furthermore, since resorption and apposition are intrinsically coupled; pure resorptive or pure appositional lesions almost never occur, further limiting researchers' ability to determine precise etiologies of lesions or bone changes. It is the pattern (i.e., net effect, location, extent, pace of change) of resorption and apposition that eventually provides the diagnostic clues needed for diagnosis. Hence, this is why understanding the dynamic interaction of bone cells to stimuli and the relation between bone type and speed of apposition is essential for differential diagnosis (Ragsdale & Lehmer 2012, and see Chapter 3, this volume).

It is also important to note that in clinical pathology, the histomorphology of bone tissue is seldomly regarded as diagnostic. Clinical pathologists rely more frequently on cytonuclear characteristics and patterns in the related soft tissues for diagnostic clues. Unfortunately, in paleopathological material, these hallmarks are seldomly preserved.

Understanding these limitations is pivotal in understanding the diagnostic potential of histology and furthermore emphasizes that this potential differs per case. It is currently accepted that a large number of diseases cannot be reliably diagnosed through histological analysis alone. For instance, comparative studies focusing on the microarchitecture of periosteal reactions have noted an absence of specific diagnostic traits (von Hunnius et al., 2006; Weston, 2009; Van der Merwe et al., 2010; Assis & Keenleyside, 2019). In fact, the lack of specificity of some pathological changes, in addition to the invasive nature of most histological techniques (Bell & Piper, 2000; Ortner, 2003; Turner-Walker & Mays, 2008; Pfeiffer & Pinto, 2012), along with the high level of scientific proficiency needed to process and interpret bone tissue at the microscopic level (Bell & Piper, 2000; Schultz, 2012) are factors frequently cited to justify the limited application of histology as a diagnostic technique in paleopathology.

In spite of these limitations, some diseases, such as hyperparathyroidism, Paget's disease, and primary osteosarcoma, may present with specific, "pathognomonic" histomorphological characteristics (e.g., Pfeiffer & Pinto, 2012, De Boer 2013b, 2016). Other diseases or conditions, such as scurvy, hypovitaminosis D, and non-specific infection or metastasis, may present a highly suggestive histomorphology (e.g., Schultz, 2012, Mays et al., 2015; De Boer & Maat, 2018), while the application of histology to trauma may also provide valuable results (e.g., Steyn et al., 2014; De Boer et al., 2015; Assis & Keenleyside, 2016; Paulis & Ali, 2018; Cappella et al., 2019). In all, the diagnostic value of histology, as with every diagnostic test, is highly dependent on the research question to which it is applied. In some instances, the addition of histological analysis may be of little value. In other cases, it may support, refute, or even prove a suspected diagnosis.

Concluding Remarks

Within paleopathology, the application of histology has a long history. Despite the technical and diagnostic challenges associated with the analytical method, it has proven to be a reliable and valuable diagnostic tool, both in mummified and skeletal remains. It is understandable that the application of microscopy is regarded as complex by many, as it requires methodological and technical knowledge, a firm theoretical foundation in human tissue histology and, most importantly, a thorough understanding of physiological and pathological bone tissue dynamics. However, if applied carefully and within an appropriate context, and in combination with other diagnostic means, it remains an extremely valuable component of the paleopathological toolkit.

References

Allen, M. R. & Burr, D. B. (2014). Bone modeling and remodeling. In Burr, D. & Allen, M. (Eds.), *Basic and Applied Bone Biology*, pp. 75–92. London: Academic Press.

Allen, T. (2015). *Microscopy: A Very Short Introduction*. Oxford: Oxford University Press.

Arnold, J. S. (1951). A method for embedding undecalcified bone for histologic sectioning, and its application to radioautography. *Science* 114(2955):178–180.

Arnold, J. S. & Jee, W. S. S. (1954). Embedding and sectioning undecalcified bone, and its application to radioautography. *Stain Technology* 29(5):225–239.

Assis, S. & Keenleyside, A. (2016). Below the callus surface: applying paleohistological techniques to understand the biology of bone healing in skeletonized human remains. *Pathobiology* 83(4):177–195.

Assis, S. & Keenleyside, A. (2019). The macroscopic and histomorphological properties of periosteal rib lesions and its relationship with disease development: evidence from the human identified skeletal collection of the Bocage Museum, Lisbon (Portugal). *Journal of Anatomy* 234:480–501.

Assis, S., Keenleyside, A., Santos, A. L. & Alves Cardoso, F. (2015). Bone diagenesis and its implication to disease diagnosis: the relevance of microstructure analysis in past human remains. *Microscopy and Microanalysis* 21(4):805–825.

Aufderheide, A. (2003). *The Scientific Study of Mummies*. Cambridge: Cambridge University Press.

Aufderheide, A. (2011). Soft tissue taphonomy: a paleopathology perspective. *International Journal of Paleopathology* 1: 75–80.

Aufderheide, A. & Rodríguez-Martín, C. (1998). *The Cambridge Encyclopedia of Human Paleopathology*. Cambridge: Cambridge University Press.

Axelrod, D. J. (1947). An improved method for cutting undecalcified bone sections and its application to radio-autography. *The Anatomical Record* 98(1):19–24.

Barbour, E. (1950). A study of the structure of fresh and fossil human bone by means of the electron microscope. *American Journal of Physical Anthropology* 8(3):315–330.

Beasley, A. (1986). Orthopaedics: evolution of the speciality. *Journal of the Royal Society of Medicine* 79(10):607–610.

Beauchesne, P. & Saunders, S. (2006). A test of the revised Frost's 'rapid manual method' for the preparation of bone thin sections. *International Journal of Osteoarchaeology* 16(1):82–87.

Bell, L. & Jones, S. (1991). Macroscopic and microscopic evaluation of archaeological pathological bone: backscattered electron imaging of putative pagetic bone. *International Journal of Osteoarchaeology* 1(3–4):179–184.

Bell, L. & Piper, K. (2000). An introduction to palaeohistopathology. In Cox, M. & Mays, S. (Eds.), *Human Osteology in Archaeology and Forensic Sciences*, pp. 255–274. London: Greenwich Medical Media, Ltd.

Bell, L. S. (1990). Palaeopathology and diagenesis: an SEM evaluation of structural changes using backscattered electron imaging. *Journal of Archaeological Science* 17(1):85–102.

Bichat, X. (1799). *Traité des Membranes en General et de Diverses Membranes en Particulier*. Paris: Richard, Caille et Ravier.

Blevins, S. M. & Bronze, M. S. (2010). Robert Koch and the 'golden age' of bacteriology. *International Journal of Infectious Diseases* 14:e744–e751.

Brickley, M., Mays, S. & Ives, R. (2007). An investigation of skeletal indicators of vitamin D deficiency in adults: effective markers for interpreting past living conditions and pollution levels in 18th and 19th century Birmingham, England. *American Journal of Physical Anthropology* 132(1):67–79.

Burgess, M. & Marten, M. (1990). Microcosms. In Burgess, J., Marten, M. & Taylor, R. (Eds.), *Under the Microscope: A Hidden World Revealed*, pp. 6–11. Cambridge: Cambridge University Press.

Burr, D. & Akkus, O. (2014). Bone morphology and organization. In Burr, D. & Allen, M. (Eds.), *Basic and Applied Bone Biology*, pp. 3–25. London: Academic Press.

Cappella, A., de Boer, H. H., Cammilli, P., De Angelis, D., Messina, C., Sconfienza, L. M., Sardanelli, F., Sforza, C. & Cattaneo, C. (2019). Histologic and radiological analysis on bone fractures: estimation of posttraumatic survival time in skeletal trauma. *Forensic Science International* 302:109909.

Caropreso, S., Bondioli, L., Capannolo, D., Cerroni, L., Macchiarelli, R. & Condo, S. (2000). Thin sections for hard tissue histology: a new procedure. *Journal of Microscopy* 199(3): 2 44–247.

Cattaneo, C., Porta, D., Gibelli, D. & Gamba, C. (2009). Histological determination of the human origin of bone fragments. *Journal of Forensic Sciences* 54:531–533.

Chappard, D., Baslé, M., Legrand, E. & Audran, M. (2011). New laboratory tools in the assessment of bone quality. *Osteoporosis International* 22(8):2225–2240.

Cho, H. (2012). The histology laboratory and principles of microscope instrumentation. In Crowder, C. & Stout, S. (Eds.), *Bone Histology: An Anthropological Perspective*, pp. 341–359. Boca Raton: CRC Press.

Ciranni, R. & Fornaciari, G. (2004). Juvenile cirrhosis in a 16th century Italian mummy. Current technologies in pathology and ancient human tissues. *Virchows Archiv* 445(6):647–650.

Collini, F., Andreola, S. A., Gentile, G., Marchesi, M., Muccino, E. & Zoja, R. (2014). Preservation of histological structure of cells in human skin presenting mummification and corification processes by Sandison's rehydrating solution. *Forensic Science International* 244:207–212.

Collins, M. J., Nielsen-Marsh, C. M., Hiller, J., Smith, C. I., Roberts, J. P., Prigodich, R. V., ... & Turner-Walker, G. (2002). The survival of organic matter in bone: a review. *Archaeometry* 44(3):383–394.

Cooper, D., Thomas, C. & Clement, J. (2012). Technological developments in the analysis of cortical bone histology. In Crowder, C. & Stout, S. (Eds.), *Bone Histology: An Anthropological Perspective*, pp. 361–375. Boca Raton: CRC Press.

Croft, W. (2006). *Under the Microscope: A Brief History of Microscopy*. New Jersey: World Scientific Publishing Co., Ltd.

Crowder, C., Heinrich, J. & Stout, S. D. (2012). Rib histomorphometry for adult age estimation. In Bell, L. S. (Ed.), *Forensic Microscopy for Skeletal Tissues* 2, pp. 109–127. Totowa, NJ: Humana Press.

Cuijpers, A. (2006). Histological identification of bone fragments in archaeology: telling humans apart horses and cattle. *International Journal of Osteoarchaeology* 16(6):465–480.

Cummaudo, M., Cappella, A., Biraghi, M., Raffone, C., Marquez-Grant, N. & Cattaneo, C. (2018). Histomorphological analysis of the variability of the human skeleton: forensic implications. *International Journal of Legal Medicine* 132:1493–1503.

Currey, J. D. (2001). Compact bone material proprieties. In Cowin, S.C. (Ed.), *Bone Mechanics Handbook*, pp. 191–196. Boca Raton: CRC Press LLC.

Dal Sasso, G., Maritan, L., Usai, D., Angelini, I. & Artioli, G. (2014). Bone diagenesis at the micro-scale: bone alteration patterns during multiple burial phases at Al Khiday (Khartoum, Sudan) between the early Holocene and the II century AD. *Palaeogeography, Palaeoclimatology, Palaeoecology* 416:30–42.

Davis, A. (2000). A historical perspective on tuberculosis and its control. In Reichman, L. B. & Hershfield, E. S. (Eds.), *Tuberculosis. A Comprehensive International Approach*, 2nd edition, pp. 3–54. New York: Marcel Dekker, Inc.

Davis, I. (2020). Antoni van Leeuwenhoek and measuring the invisible: the context of 16th and 17th century micrometry. *Studies in History and Philosophy of Science* 83:75–85.

De Boer, H. H., Aarents, M. & Maat, G. (2012). Staining ground sections of natural dry bone tissue for microscopy. *International Journal of Osteoarchaeology* 22(4):379–386.

De Boer, H., Aarents, M. & Maat, G. (2013a). Manual for the preparation and staining of embedded natural dry bone tissue sections for microscopy. *International Journal of Osteoarchaeology* 23(1):83–93.

De Boer, H. H. & Maat, G. J. (2012). The histology of human dry bone (a review). *Cuadernos de Prehistoria y Arqueología de la Universidad de Granada* 22:49–65.

De Boer, H. H. & Maat G. J. (2018). Dry bone histology of bone tumours. *International Journal of Paleopathology* 21:56–63.De Boer, H. H. & Van der Merwe, A. E. (2016). Diagnostic dry bone histology in human paleopathology. *Clinical Anatomy* 29(7):831–843.

De Boer, H. H., Van der Merwe, A. E. & Maat, G. J. (2013b).The diagnostic value of microscopy in dry bone palaeopathology: a review. *International Journal of Paleopathology* 3(2):113–121.

De Boer, H. H., Van der Merwe, A. E., Hammer, S., Steyn, M. & Maat G. J. (2015). Assessing post-traumatic time interval in human dry bone. *International Journal of Osteoarchaeology* 25(1):98–109.

Denton, J. (2008). Slices of mummy: a histologist's perspective. In David, R. (Ed.), *Egyptian Mummies and Modern Science*, pp.71–82. Cambridge: Cambridge University Press.

Dittmann, K., Grupe, G., Manhart, H., Peters, J. & Strott, N. (2006). Histomorphometry of mammalian and avian compact bone. In Grupe, G. & Peters, J. (Eds.), *Microscopic Examinations of Bioarchaeological Remains: Keeping a Close Eye on Ancient Tissues*, pp. 48–101. Leidorf: Verlag Marie Leidorf.

Dobson, J. (1952). Pioneers of osteogeny: Clopton Havers. *The Journal of Bone and Joint Surgery* 34 B(4):702–707.

Dore, B., Pavan, F. & Masali, M. (2001). Histological techniques and microscopic analysis of biological agents for preservation of human bone remains. *Biotechnic & Histochemistry* 76(2):89–95.

Eshed, V., Latimer, B., Greenwald, C., Jellema, L., Rothschild, B., Wish-Baratz, S. & Hershkovitz, I. (2002). Button osteoma: its etiology and pathophysiology. *American Journal of Physical Anthropology* 118(3): 217–230.

Fernández, P. (2012). Palaeopathology: the study of disease in the past. *Pathobiology* 79:221–227.

FitzGerald, C. & Saunders, S. (2005). Test of histological methods of determining chronology of accentuated striae in deciduous teeth. *American Journal of Physical Anthropology* 127(3):277–290.

Fornaciari, G. (2018). Histology of ancient soft tissue tumors: a review. *International Journal of Paleopathology* 21:64–76.

Frost, H. (1968). Tetracycline bone labeling in anatomy. *American Journal of Physical Anthropology* 29(2):183–195.

Galloway, A., Willwy, P. & Snyder, L. (1997). Human bone mineral densities and survival of bone elements: a contemporary sample. In Haglund, W. D. & Sorg, M. H. (Eds.), *Forensic Taphonomy: The Postmortem Fate of Human Remains*, pp. 295–318. Boca Raton: CRC Press LLC.

Garland, A. N. (1987). A histological study of archaeological bone decomposition. In Boddington, A., Garland, A. N. & Janaway, R. (Eds.), *Death, Decay and Reconstruction: Approaches to Archaeology and Forensic Science*, pp. 109–126. Manchester: Manchester University Press.

Garland, A. N. (1993). An introduction to the histology of exhumed mineralized tissue. In Grupe, G. & Garland, A. (Eds.), *Histology of Ancient Human Bone: Methods and Diagnosis*, pp.1–16. New York: Springer-Verlag.Graf, W. (1949). Preserved histological structures in Egyptian mummy tissues and ancient Swedish skeletons. *Acta Anatomica* 8(3):236–250.

Grove, C., Peschel, O. & Nerlich, A. G. (2015). A systematic approach to the application of soft tissue histopathology in paleopathology. *BioMed Research International* 631465:1–9.

Grupe, G. (2007). Taphonomic and diagenetic processes. In Henke, W. T., Attersall, I. & Hardt, T. (Eds.), *Handbook of Paleoanthropology*, pp. 241–259. New York: Springer-Verlag.

Grzybowski, A., Kluxen, G. & Pótorak, K. (2014). Gerhard Henrik Armauer Hansen (1841–1912) – 100 years anniversary tribute. *Acta Ophthalmologica* 92:296–300.

Guarino, F., Angelini, F., Vollono, C. & Orefice, C. (2006). Bone preservation in human remains from the Terme del Sarno at Pompeii using light microscopy and scanning electron microscopy. *Journal of Archaeological Science* 33(4):513–530.

Guatelli-Steinberg, D. & Huffman, M. (2012). Histological features of dental hard tissues and their utility in forensic anthropology. In Crowder, C. & Stout, S. (Eds.), *Bone Histology: An Anthropological Perspective*, pp. 91–107. Boca Raton: CRC Press.

Haas, K. & Storå, J. (2015). Different preparation techniques–similar results? On the quality of thin-ground sections of archaeological bone. *International Journal of Osteoarchaeology* 25(6):935–945.

Hackett, C. J. (1981). Microscopical focal destruction (tunnels in exhumed human bones). *Medicine, Science and Law* 21:243–265.

Hajdu, S. (2002). A note from history: the first use of the microscope. *Annals of Clinical & Laboratory Science* 32(3):309–310.

Hays, J. (2009). *The Burdens of Disease: Epidemics and Human Response in Western History*. New Brunswick: Rutgers University Press.

Hedges, R. E. M. (2002). Bone diagenesis: an overview of processes. *Archaeometry* 44:319–328.

Hedges, R. E. M. & Millard, A. R. (1995). Bones and groundwater: towards the modeling of diagenetic processes. *Journal of Archaeological Science* 22:155–164.

Hess, M., Klima, G., Pfaller, K., Künzel, K., & Gaber, O. (1998). Histological investigations on the Tyrolean Ice Man. *American Journal of Physical Anthropology* 106(4):521–532.

Hillier, M. & Bell, S. (2007). Differentiating human bone from animal bone: a review of histological methods. *Journal of Forensic Sciences* 52:249–263.

Hogg, J. (1854). *The Microscope: Its History, Construction and Applications*. London: The Illustrated London Library.

Hollund, H., Jans, M., Collins, M., Kars, H., Joosten, I. & Kars, S. (2012). What happened here? Bone histology as a tool in decoding the postmortem histories of archaeological bone from Castricum, The Netherlands. *International Journal of Osteoarchaeology* 22:537–548.

Jackes, M. (2011). Representativeness and bias in archaeological skeletal samples. In Agarwal, S. & Glencross, B. (Eds.), *Social Bioarchaeology*, pp. 107–146. Malden: Blackwell Publishing, Ltd.

Jacquette, D. (1997). The microscope in early modern science and philosophy. *Studies in History and Philosophy of Science* 28(2):377–386.

Jans, M. (2008). Microbial bioerosion of bone—A review. In Wisshak, M. & Tapanila, L. (Eds.), *Current Developments in Bioerosion*, pp. 397–413. New York: Springer-Verlag.

Jans, M., Nielsen-Marsh, C., Smith, C., Collins, M. & Kars, H. (2004). Characterization of microbial attack on archaeological bone. *Journal of Archaeological Science* 31:87–95.

Jee, W. S. S. (2001). Integrated bone tissue physiology: anatomy and physiology. In Cowin, S. C. (Ed.), *Bone Mechanics Handbook*, pp. 1–68. Boca Raton: CRC Press LLC.

Jowsey, J. (1955). The use of the milling machine for preparing bone sections for microradiography and microautoradiography. *Journal of Scientific Instruments* 32(5):159–163.

Kuhn, G. D. & Lutz, E. L. (1958). A modified polyester embedding medium for sectioning. *Stain Technology* 33(1):1–7.

Lister, J. (1867). On the antiseptic principle in the practice of surgery. *The British Medical Journal* 21:246–248.
Lynnerup, N. (2007). Mummies. *Yearbook of Physical Anthropology* 134(s45):162–190.
Lynnerup, N. (2015). Bog Bodies. *The Anatomical Record* 298(5):1007–1012.
Maat, G., Van Den Bos, R. & Aarents, M. (2001). Manual preparation of ground sections for the microscopy of natural bone tissue: update and modification of frost's 'rapid manual method'. *International Journal of Osteoarchaeology*, 11(5):366–374.
Macadam, R. & Sandison, T. (1969). The electron microscope in paleopathology. *Medical History* 13(1):81–85.
Maggiano, C., Dupras, T., Schultz, M. & Biggerstaff, J. (2009). Confocal laser scanning microscopy: a flexible tool for simultaneous polarization and three-dimensional fluorescence imaging of archaeological compact bone. *Journal of Archaeological Science* 36(10):2392–2401.
Marks, S. & Odgren, P. (2002). Structure and development of the skeleton. In Bilezikian, J., Raisz, L. & Rodan, G. (Eds.), *Principles of Bone Biology,* pp. 3–15. New York: Academic Press.
Martin, D. (1991). Bone histology and paleopathology: Methodological considerations. In Ortner, D. & Aufderheide, A. (Eds.), *Human Paleopathology: Current Syntheses and Future Options*, pp. 55–59. Washington, DC: Smithsonian Institution.
Martin, R. B., Burr, D. B., Sharkey, N. A. & Fyhrie, D. P. (2015). *Skeletal Tissue Mechanics,* 2nd edition. New York: Springer.
Martiniaková, M., Grosskopf, B., Omelka, R., Dammers, K., Vondráková, M. & Bauerová, M. (2007). Histological study of compact bone tissue in some mammals: a method for species determination. *International Journal of Osteoarchaeology* 17(1):82–90.
Martiniaková, M., Vondrakova, M. & Omelka, R. (2006). Manual preparation of thin sections from historical human skeletal material. *Timisoara Medical Journal* 56(1):15–17.
Masters, B. R. (2009). History of the electron microscope in cell biology. In *Encyclopedia of Life Sciences (ELS)*, pp.1–9. Chichester: John Wiley & Sons, Ltd. DOI: 10.1002/9780470015902.a0021539.
Mays, S., Brickley, M. & Ives, R. (2007). Skeletal evidence for hyperparathyroidism in a 19th century child with rickets. *International Journal of Osteoarchaeology* 17(1):73–81.
Mays, S., Maat, G. J. & De Boer, H. H. (2015). Scurvy as a factor in the loss of the 1845 Franklin expedition to the Arctic: a reconsideration. *International Journal of Osteoarchaeology* 25(3):334–344.
Mekota, A.-M. & Vermehren, M. (2005). Determination of optimal rehydration, fixation and staining methods for histological and immunohistochemical analysis of mummified soft tissues. *Biotechnic & Histochemistry* 80(1):7–13.
Mekota, A.-M. & Vermehren, M. (2006). Histological and immunohistochemical analysis of ancient mummies soft remains. In Grupe, G. & Peters, J. (Eds.), *Microscopic Examinations of Bioarchaeological Remains: Keeping a Close Eye on Ancient Tissues*, pp. 103–109. Rahden, Germany: Verlag Marie Leidorf.
Money, N. P. (2014). *Microbiology: A Very Short Introduction*. Oxford: Oxford University Press.
Mulhern, D. & Ubelaker, D. (2012). Differentiating human from non-human bone microstructure. In Crowder, C. & Stout, S. (Eds.), *Bone Histology: An Anthropological Perspective*, pp. 109–134. Boca Raton: CRC Press.
Nielsen-Marsh, C. M., Gernaey, A. M., Turner-Walker, G., Hedges, R. E. M., Pike, A. W. G. & Collins, M. J. C. (2000). The chemical degradation of bone. In Cox, M. & Mays, S. (Eds.), *Human Osteology: In Archaeology and Forensic Science,* pp.439–452. Cambridge: Greenwich Medical Media Limited.
Nijweide, P., Burger, E. & Klein-Nulend, J. (2002). The osteocyte. In Bilezikian, J., Raisz, L. & G. Rodan (Eds.), *Principles of Bone Biology*, pp. 93–107. New York: Academic Press.
Norris, W. P. & Jenkins, P. E. (1960). Epoxy resin embedding in contrast radioautography of bones and teeth. *Stain Technology* 35(5):253–260.
Ortner, D. (2003). *Identification of Pathological Conditions in Human Skeletal Remains*. Amsterdam: Academic Press.
Ott, S. (2002). Histomorphometric analysis of bone remodelling. In Bilezikian, J., Raisz, L. & Rodan, G. (Eds.), *Principles of Bone Biology*, 303–320. New York: Academic Press.
Paulis, M. G. & Ali, D. M. (2018). Antemortem, perimortem and postmortem bone fracture: could histopathology differentiate between them?. *The Egyptian Journal of Forensic Sciences and Applied Toxicology* 18(3):135–160.
Pfeiffer, S. (2006). Cortical bone in juveniles. In Grupe, G. & Peters J. (Eds.), *Microscopic Examinations of Bioarchaeological Remains: Keeping a Close Eye on Ancient Tissues*, pp. 15–28. Rahden, Germany: Verlag Marie Leidorf.

Pfeiffer, S. & Pinto, D. (2012). Histological analyses of human bone from archaeological contexts. In Crowder, C. & Stout, S. (Eds.), *Bone histology: An Anthropological Perspective*, pp. 297–311. Boca Raton, FL: CRC Press.

Pinhasi, R., & Bourbou, C. (2008). How representative are human skeletal assemblages for population analysis? In Pinhasi, R. & Mays, S. (Eds.), *Advances in Human Paleopathology*, pp. 31–44. London: John Wiley & Sons.

Pugh, M. & Savchuck, W. (1958). Suggestions on the preparation of undecalcified bone for microradiography. *Biotechnic & Histochemistry* 33(6):287–293.

Ragsdale, B. & Lehmer, L. (2012). A knowledge of bone at the cellular (histological) level is essential to paleopathology. In Grauer, A. (Ed.), *A Companion to Paleopathology*, pp. 227–249. London: Blackwell Publishing.

Reyman, T. A., Barraco, R. A. & Cockburn, A. (1976). Histopathological examination of an Egyptian mummy. *Bulletin of the New York Academy of Medicine* 52(4):506–516.

Robling, A. & Stout, S. (2008). Histomorphometry of human cortical bone: applications to age estimation. In Katzenberg, A. & Saunders, S. (Eds.), *Biological Anthropology of the Human Skeleton*, pp. 149–171. London: John Wiley Sons.

Roksandic, M., Vlak, D., Schillaci, M. & Voicu, D. (2009). Technical note: applicability of tooth cementum annulation to an archaeological population. *American Journal of Physical Anthropology* 140(2):583–588.

Ruffer, M. A. (1909). Preliminary note on the histology of Egyptian mummies. *The British Medical Journal* 24:1005.

Ruffer, M. A. (1910). Note on the presence of "Bilharzia haematobia" in Egyptian mummies of the twentieth dynasty (1250–1000 B.C.). *The British Medical Journal* 1:16.

Ruffer, M. A. (1911a). On arterial lesions found in Egyptian mummies (1580 B.C.—525 A.D.). *The Journal of Pathology and Bacteriology* 15(4):453–462.

Ruffer, M. A. (1911b). Note on an eruption resembling that of variola in the skin of a mummy of the twentieth dynasty (1200–1100 B.C.). *The Journal of Pathology and Bacteriology* 15(1):1–3.

Ruffer, M. A. (1921). *Studies in the palaeopathology of Egypt*. Chicago: The University of Chicago Press.

Ruffer, M. A. & Chantre, B. (1911). Histologie et anatomie pathologique des momies d'Egypte. *Bulletin de la Société d'Anthropologie de Lyon* 30:21–28.

Rühli, F., Kuhn, G., Evison, R., Müller, R. & Schultz, M. (2007). Diagnostic value of micro-CT in comparison with histology in the qualitative assessment of historical human skull bone pathologies. *American Journal of Physical Anthropology* 133(4):1099–1111.

Sandinson, A. (1955). The histological examination of mummified material. *Biotechnic & Histochemistry* 30(6):277–283.

Sandison, A. (1967). Sir Marc Armand Ruffer (1859–1917) pioneer of palaeopathology. *Medical History* 11(2):150–156.

Schultz, M. (2008). Rudolf Virchow. *Emerging Infectious Diseases* 14(9):1480–1481.

Schultz, M. (2012). Light microscopic analysis of macerated pathologically changed bones. In Crowder, C. & Stout, S. (Eds.), *Bone Histology: An Anthropological Perspective*, pp. 253–296. Boca Raton: CRC Press.

Shattock, S. G. (1909). A report upon the pathological condition of the aorta of King Menephtah, traditionally regarded as the Pharaoh of the Exodus. *Proceedings of the Royal Society of Medicine* 2:122–127.

Smith, K. A. (2012). Louis Pasteur, the father of immunology? *Frontiers in Immunology* 3(68):1–10. DOI: 10.3389/fimmu.2012.00068.

Steiniche, T. & Hauge, E. (2003). Normal structure and function of bone. In An, Y. & Martin, K. (Eds.), *Handbook of Histology Methods for Bone and Cartilage*, pp. 59–72. Totowa, NJ: Humana Press.

Stepney, R. (1990). Human body. In Burgess, J., Marten, M. R. & Taylor (Eds.), *Under the Microscope: A Hidden World Revealed*, pp. 12–41. Cambridge: Cambridge University Press.

Steyn, M., De Boer, H. H. & Van der Merwe, A. E. (2014). Cranial trauma and the assessment of posttraumatic survival time. *Forensic Science International* 244:e25–29.

Stodder, A. (2008). Taphonomy and the nature of archaeological assemblages. In Katzenberg, A. & Saunders, S. (Eds.), *Biological Anthropology of the Human Skeleton*, pp. 71–114. London: John Wiley & Sons.

Stout, S. & Teitelbaum, S. (1976). Histological analysis of undecalcified thin sections of archeological bone. *American Journal of Physical Anthropology* 44(2): 263–269.

Stout, S. (1978). Histological structure and its preservation in ancient bone. *Current Anthropology* 19:601–604.Streeter, M. (2012). Histological age-at-death estimation. In Crowder, C. & Stout, S. (Eds.), *Bone Histology: An Anthropological Perspective*, pp. 135–152. Boca Raton: CRC Press.

Swinton, W. E. (1981). Sir Marc Armand Ruffer: one of the first palaeopathologists. *The Canadian Medical Association Journal* 124:1388–1392.

Turner, P. & Holtom, D. (1981). The use of a fabric softener in the reconstitution of mummified tissue prior to paraffin wax sectioning for light microscopical examination. *Biotechnic & Histochemistry* 56(1):35–38.

Turner-Walker, G. (2008). The chemical and microbial degradation of bones and teeth. In. Pinhasi, R. & Mays, S. (Eds.), *Advances in Human Paleopathology*, pp. 3–29. London: John Wiley & Sons.

Turner-Walker, G. (2019). Light at the end of the tunnels? The origins of microbial bioerosion in mineralised collagen. *Palaeogeography, Palaeoclimatology, Palaeoecology* 529:24–38.

Turner-Walker, G. & Jans, M. (2008). Reconstructing taphonomic histories using histological analysis. *Palaeogeography, Palaeoclimatology, Palaeoecology* 266(3–4):227–235.

Turner-Walker, G. & Mays, S. (2008). Histological studies on ancient bones. In Pinhasi, R. & Mays, S. (Eds.), *Advances in Human Paleopathology*, pp. 121–146. London: John Wiley & Sons.

Väänänen, K., Zhao, H., Mulari, M. & Hallen, J. (2000). The cell biology of osteoclast function. *Journal of Cell Science* 113(3):377–381.

Van der Merwe, A., Maat, G. & Steyn, M. (2010). Ossified haematomas and infectious bone changes on the anterior tibia: histomorphological features as an aid for accurate diagnosis. *International Journal of Osteoarchaeology* 20(2):227–239.

Van der Merwe, A. E., Veselka, B., Van Veen, H. A., Van Rijn, R. R., Colman, K. L. & De Boer, H. H. (2018). Four possible cases of osteomalacia: The value of a multidisciplinary diagnostic approach. *International Journal of Paleopathology* 23:15–25.

Van Leeuwenhoek, F. (1720). Observations upon the bones and the periosteum, in a letter to the royal society. *Proceedings of the Royal Society of London. Philosophical Transactions of the Royal Society (1683–1775)* 31:91–97.

von Hunnius, T., Roberts, C., Boylston, A. & Saunders, S. (2006). Histological identification of syphilis in pre-Columbian England. *American Journal of Physical Anthropology* 129(4):559–566.

Wade, A., Holdsworth, D. & Garvin, G. (2011). CT and micro-CT analysis of a case of Paget's disease (osteitis deformans) in the grant skeletal collection. *International Journal of Osteoarchaeology* 21(2):127–135.

Wakely, J., Manchester, K. & Roberts, C. (1991). Scanning electron microscopy of rib lesions. *International Journal of Osteoarchaeology* 1(3–4):185–189.

Walker, R., Parsche, F., Bierbrier, M. & McKerrow, J. (1987a). Tissue identification and histologic study of six lung specimens from Egyptian mummies. *American Journal of Physical Anthropology* 72(1):43–48.

Walker, R., Parsche, F., Bierbrier, M. & McKerrow, J. H. (1987b). Tissue identification and histologic study of six lung specimens from Egyptian mummies. *American journal of physical anthropology* 72(1):43–48.

Weinstein, R., Simmons, D. & Lovejoy, C. (1981). Ancient bone disease in a Peruvian mummy revealed by quantitative skeletal histomorphometry. *American Journal of Physical Anthropology*, 54(3):321–326.

Welsh, H., Nelson, A. J., van der Merwe, A. E., de Boer, H. H. & Brickley, M. B. (2020). An investigation of Micro-CT analysis of bone as a new diagnostic method for paleopathological cases of osteomalacia. *International Journal of Paleopathology* 31:23–33.

Weston, D. (2009). Brief communication: paleohistopathological analysis of pathology museum specimens: can periosteal reaction microstructure explain lesion etiology? *American Journal of Physical Anthropology* 140(1):186–193.

Wilder, H. H. (1904). The restoration of dried tissues, with especial reference to human remains. *American Anthropologist* 6(1):1–17.

Wilson, C. (1995). *The Invisible World: Early Modern Philosophy and the Invention of the Microscope*. Princeton: Princeton University Press.

Wittwer-Backofen, U., Gampe, J. & Vaupel, J. (2004). Tooth cementum annulation for age estimation: results from a large known-age validation study. *American Journal of Physical Anthropology* 123(2):119–129.

Wollman, A. J. M., Nudd, R., Hedlund, E. G. & Leake, M. C. (2015). From Animaculum to single molecules: 300 years of the light microscope. *Open Biology* 5:150019.

Young, B., Lowe, J., Stevens, A. & Heath, J. (2006). *Wheater's Functional Histology: A Text and Colour Atlas*. London: Churchill Livingstone

Zimmerman, M. R. (1972). Histological examination of experimentally mummified tissues. *American Journal of Physical Anthropology* 37(2):271–280.

Zimmerman, M. R. (1993). The paleopathology of the cardiovascular system. *Texas Heart Institute Journal* 20:252–257.

Zimmerman, M. R., Brier, B. & Wade, R. (1998). Brief communication: twentieth-century replication of an Egyptian mummy. Implications for paleopathology. *American Journal of Physical Anthropology* 107(4):417–420.

6
PALEORADIOLOGY

Chiara Villa and Marie Louise Jørkov

Paleoradiology is a discipline that uses medical imaging techniques, such as X-ray radiography and computed tomography (CT), to study bioarchaeological materials (Chhem & Brothwell, 2008). These techniques are non-invasive and non-destructive and allow the visualization of the internal structures of the object of interest. They are important tools to study mummies, to assess skeletal development, and to help in the diagnosis of diseases. Another important role of radiography is the potential permanent documentation of diseases and conditions. In particular, CT scanning allows the creation of 3D virtual copies and can be accessible worldwide even when the actual material or individual is not physically available or can no longer be analyzed.

Radiographic techniques should be considered complementary tools to macroscopic analyses and used whenever possible. Fortunately, both X-ray machines and CT scanners are becoming more available to an increasing number of researchers. X-ray machines are definitively the most accessible equipment. Nonetheless, CT scanners have been recently introduced in many forensic departments (Rutty et al., 2008) and thus, biological anthropologists can have access to them for the analysis of human remains. Alternatively, imaging equipment in nearby hospitals may also be used.

This chapter is intended as an introduction to paleoradiology (for further information, please refer to Chhem and Brothwell (2008)). We provide a brief history of the radiography in paleopathology, some basic technical principles on X-ray radiography and CT scanning, and some general guidelines for interpreting pathological changes. Finally, we will provide an overview of other imaging modalities suitable for bioarchaeological applications and future prospective.

Brief History

It all started in 1895, when the German physicist Wilhelm Conrad Röntgen discovered X-rays (Röntgen, 1972; Thomas & Banerjee, 2013). The potential of this technique in archaeology and biological anthropology was immediately clear and a variety of specimens were subjected to X-ray examination. The first X-rays of mummies were performed only a few months after X-rays were discovered: "photographs with X-rays" of a child mummy's knee and the upper part of an Egyptian cat mummy were taken in 1896 by König (König,

1896). In the following years, many other "internal visualizations" of Egyptian mummies, bones, and fossils were carried out using X-rays (Böni et al., 2004). In 1931, Moodie performed the first systematic X-ray analysis of a large collection of Egyptian and Peruvian mummies housed at the Field Museum of Natural History in Chicago (Moodie, 1931). The entire collection of royal mummies at the Museum in Cairo, Egypt, was also radiographed in 1967 (Harris & Weeks, 1973, 1980).

The capability of radiology was greatly improved with the introduction of CT in the early 1970s. The invention of CT is generally attributed to the British engineer Godfrey Hounsfield in 1972, but the fundamentals of CT scanning were developed by the American physicist Alan Cormack in the 1960s (Kalender, 2011). The medical, as well scientific community, enthusiastically welcomed this new technology. As with X-ray machines, CT scanning was immediately used to study mummies. The first CT scan was performed in 1976 on a desiccated brain of an Egyptian mummy (Lewin & Harwood-Nash, 1977). Some years later, an entire mummy was CT scanned (Harwood-Nash, 1979). About ten years later, the first 3D visualizations from CT scanning data were carried out on a face (Marx & D'Auria, 1988) and on an entire skeleton (Magid et al., 1989). The quality of CT images and the reconstruction in 3D of any area of interest enabled a completely new kind of documentation. Not only bones, bodies, or internal organs can be virtually visualized, but also items such as amulets and clothing. Interestingly, CT scans can be used, for example, to estimate the quantity of textile used for mummification (Brandt et al., 2020). For a complete review of the early studies of ancient remains refer to Böni et al. (2004), Chhem (2008) and Lynnerup and Ruhli (2015), Cox (2015), and references therein.

Current Techniques

Radiographic techniques use X-rays to visualize the internal structures of an object. X-rays are electromagnetic waves, such as visible light, able to penetrate through materials that are opaque to visible light. X-rays can be absorbed or scattered by interaction with the atoms of the materials. The penetration depends on the density, thickness, and atomic number of the matter. The resultant reduction in X-ray intensity through materials is referred to as "attenuation". The remnant or the exit radiation has a pattern of intensity that reflects the absorption characteristics of the object. This pattern is recorded to form the image in the same way a photographic negative is formed by light. Different intensities correspond to different gray values. Dense materials, such as compact bone and metal objects, inhibit the passage of the X-rays and are visualized as white or light gray; such materials are defined as being radiodense or radiopaque. Less dense materials, such as soft tissues or bandages, allow a great number of X-rays to pass and are visualized in dark gray; such materials are defined as radiolucent. Empty spaces filled with air are visualized in black. For more details about the physics of X-rays, refer to Buzug (2008), Hsieh (2009), Seibert (2004), and Seibert and Boone (2005).

X-ray Radiography

Radiography equipment is composed of an X-ray source, called an X-ray tube, and a medium for recording the image, i.e. image detector. In conventional radiography, also known as film-screen radiography, photographic films are used to record the X-ray attenuation; while in digital radiography (DR) or computed radiography (CR) a digital plane is used. The advantages of images acquired with DR and CT are that they are digital and thus they can be readily stored and permanently archived.

A good radiograph can be defined as an image that has proper density, contrast, sharp outlines, and undistorted shape and size of the actual object. The **density** is the degree of darkening: black areas (air spaces) have maximum density, while white areas (bones, metal objects) have minimum density. Thus, air spaces and soft tissues appear as radiolucent area (black), while teeth, bones, and metal appear radiopaque (white). The **contrast** is defined as the difference in density (blackness) between various regions on a radiograph. Thus, the **resolution contrast** refers to the ability to distinguish structures with similar contrast, e.g. fat and muscle. A high contrast image shows both light and dark areas, while a low contrast image is only composed of light or gray zones. These features are regulated by the exposure parameters: the energy (kV – tube voltage) and the number of X-rays (mAs – X-ray dose). Low energy X-rays are more likely to be absorbed by the object and do not reach the detectors, while high energy X-rays easily pass through the material and are registered by the image detector. A good image is obtained when the most details of an object are visualized, thus a greater variation of X-rays should reach the image detector creating greater differences in shades of gray. Fortunately, brightness, contrast, and sharpness can be improved easily using modern radiography equipment (CR, DR) because a digital image is acquired and can be adjusted and manipulated.

To avoid distortions and magnifications of the X-ray of a bone, the relative position of the object, the X-ray beam, and image detector need to be considered. The center of object should be directly under the center of the X-ray beam, parallel and close to the image detector. If the object is poorly positioned in relation to the image detector, an elongated image is produced, while a foreshortened image is produced if the object is poorly positioned in relation to the X-rays beam. Magnification of artifacts is caused when the object is too far from the image detector: the greater the distance between the object and the image detector, the greater the magnification will be of the image (Seibert, 2004; Seibert & Boone, 2005; Saab et al., 2008). For more details about radiographic equipment, refer to Buzug (2008), Hsieh (2009), Seibert (2004) and Seibert and Boone (2005).

CT Scanning

A CT scanner can be defined as a "special X-ray machine" that produces hundreds of cross-sectional images of an object. Transverse projections are generated by mechanical movement of both the X-ray source and the image detector around the object. The cross-sectional images, called slices, are represented by a pixel matrix (usually 512×512 pixels), with each pixel representing the X-ray attenuation coefficient in a small volume (voxel) of the underlying anatomy. The x and y (pixel dimensions) of each slice in the transverse plane are determined by the matrix size and the fields of view (FoV). The third voxel dimension (z) is perpendicular to the transverse plane and corresponds to the slice thickness (Kalender, 2011).

There are many factors that can influence the quality of CT images, such as exposure parameters (in explained above for X-ray machines), the slice thickness, the slice increment, the pitch, and the reconstruction algorithm. For more technical details, please refer to Hsieh (2009), Kalender (2011) and Zollikofer and Ponce de Leon (2005). As a general guideline, we suggest scanning an object with the least thickness possible (0.6 or 0.75 mm) and with the pitch and slice increment values lower than the values used for the thickness in order to reduce possible artifacts. We also recommend scanning the entire object in order to have a permanent copy and then performing a focused scan of the area of interest, e.g. teeth or middle ear, to reach a better visualization of the details (i.e., to increase the spatial resolution).

In CT images, the X-ray attenuation coefficients of each voxel are expressed as Hounsfield Units (HU). The HU values are calibrated to the attenuation of the water and the air. Thus, water and all water-equivalent tissues have the value 0 HU. The attenuation produced by air corresponds to -1024 HU. Materials more radiopaque than water result in higher positive values of HU. The standard HU scale is from -1024 HU to + 3071 HU; extended HU can also be set at the time of the scanning, for example from -1024 to 30710, to better visualize metal, such as jewelry. A number of sources provide tables of typical HU ranges of human tissues for medical use (see Hounsfield, 1973; Buzug, 2008; Kalender, 2011). However, the clinical ranges of HU cannot be applied to paleopathological or bioarchaeological materials without some adjustment. Taphonomic alteration can change the composition of the tissues and, although the tissues are morphologically well preserved, they can display a different radiopaque response (Ruhli et al., 2004; Lynnerup, 2007, 2010; Villa & Lynnerup, 2012).

An important advantage of CT scanning is the possibility of creating 3D visualizations of single structures. Using post-processing software, such as Mimics (www.materialise.com/en/medical/software/mimics), Myriam (www.intrasense.fr), 3D slicer (www.slicer.org), or Osirix (www.osirix-viewer.com), it is possible to segment different structures inside an object using the process of segmentation. This process can be semi-automatic or requires manual extrapolation of the information from the CT images (Lynnerup, 2008). 3D models are also an important tool for diagnostic purposes. For instance, 3D visualizations of the skull and pelvis of a mummy have been used to confirm a possible fracture (Pickering et al., 1990) and 3D visualization of teeth have been used to assess dental disease (Melcher et al., 1997). Furthermore, 3D visualizations of the skull can be used for facial reconstruction. In the case of mummies and specimens no longer available, they are the only method to "look inside" and have a 3D overview of bones, internal organs, and foreign objects.

X-ray Radiography vs CT Scanning

Radiography has two main limitations. First, it produces a superimposed "shadow" of the internal structure of a specimen, providing a 2D image of a 3D object. This can cause difficulties in the visualization and interpretation of anatomical structures in bioarchaeological specimens, such as mummies. The superimposition of different body parts prevents a clear visualization of deep areas or structures (Lynnerup & Ruhli, 2015). For example, amulets, or other objects, will create radiopaque areas masking the structures beneath. Issues with superimposition are especially notable in bodies that have been extensively wrapped, such as Egyptian or Greenland mummies. Second, there is a low contrast difference among the soft tissues making spatial/tissue-specific discrimination challenging. Bones are generally well visualized due to the high attenuation, while soft tissues have almost identical attenuation coefficients and thus inhibit the ability to investigate pathological changes in the soft tissues.

CT scanning overcomes all these limitations by providing a 3D visualization of single structures in a body and better contrast between different tissues. However, X-ray radiography is still a common method of evaluation, as it is the most accessible and easy-to-use technology. There are even portable X-ray machines that can be used in the field (Conlogue et al., 2004; Nystrom et al., 2004). X-ray radiography is often used to assess dental development, since many of the existing methods were developed and calibrated from radiographs (see AlQahtani et al., 2010). It has also been used to evaluate the degree of pneumatization of the mastoid air cells of the temporal bone. The small pneumatized area of the temporal bones is strongly correlated with infections in middle ear diseases (Homoe & Lynnerup, 1991). Linear sclerotic foci within metaphyses or diaphyses, also known as Harris Lines or growth arrest lines, are commonly evaluated using X-rays (Brickley & McKinley, 2004).

Key Features for Interpreting Pathological Changes

Radiographic analyses are important diagnostic tools to study ancient diseases and should be performed whenever possible. However, their utility greatly varies based on the pathological changes under investigation. For instance, in some cases, radiographic analyses are indispensable to identify diseases that involve internal structures or are invisible by macroscopic examination of the bone: middle ear infection, osteoporosis, endosteal sclerosis, malignant neoplasms, and confirmation of suspected previous fractures (well-healed fractures), for example. However, small pathological changes, such as slight periosteal reaction, porous hypertrophic bone, or cribra orbitalia, are very difficult to detect, if at all, due to the limited spatial resolution.

The interpretation of pathological changes on radiographic images can be difficult and requires experience. An in-depth knowledge of normal anatomy, anatomical variation, and pathological conditions is essential. In general, pathological bone changes can be divided

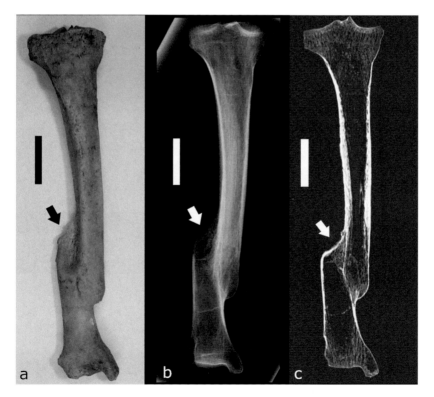

Figure 6.1 Healed malaligned fracture of a right tibia (a) photograph; (b) radiograph; (c) coronal CT scan. The photograph clearly shows gross morphological changes to the bone with minimal callous formation, while the radiograph clearly shows the degree of apposition of the two ends of the bone, along with the original cortical surfaces, especially visible on the CT image (arrows). Scale bar: 5 cm.

into abnormal bone size, abnormal bone shape, abnormal bone formation, and abnormal bone destruction.

Abnormal bone size and shape can easily be identified by macroscopic evaluation and radiographic analysis does not provide further information. However, CT scans of the sample provide a permanent documentation of the bones and should be performed, if possible. Some examples of diseases where imaging is not critical in order to reach a diagnosis are, for example, osteoarthritis, and lingual hyperostosis of the mandible (also known as tori mandibularis) and myositis ossificans traumatica. In other cases, such as bone tumors, healed malaligned fractures (Figure 6.1), and Pott's disease (Figure 6.2), the imaging allows visualization of internal bone structures, even though a diagnosis might be reached through macroscopic evaluation alone. For instance, in Figure 6.1, the photograph (macroscopic evaluation) clearly shows gross morphological changes to the bone with minimal callous formation. The radiograph, however, allows the researcher to clearly see the degree of apposition of the two ends of the bone, along with the original cortical surfaces, especially visible on the CT image.

Abnormal bone formation is visualized as whiter areas (radiodense) and can be associated with conditions such as osteochondroma, cartilaginous exostoses, and new bone formation (extraosseus and/or intraosseus). Abnormal bone destruction is visualized as darker areas (radiolucent) and can be associated with aneurysmal bone cysts, infectious diseases, treponemal diseases, metastatic carcinoma of bone, hematopoietic diseases, and severe osteoporosis.

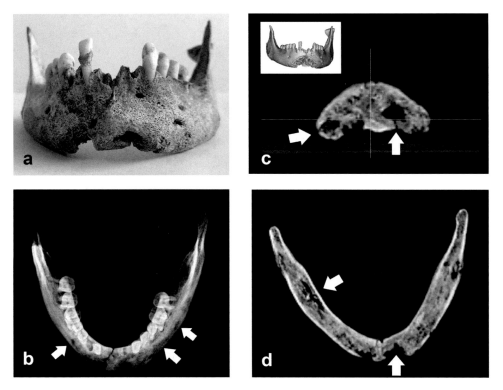

Figure 6.2 Mandible with pronounced destruction due to treponemal disease (syphilis): (a) photograph; (b) radiograph; (c) axial CT scan; (d) coronal CT scan. The photograph shows marked bone destruction, but the exact extent of this destruction can only be evaluated using radiograph and CT scanning (arrows).

Paleoradiology

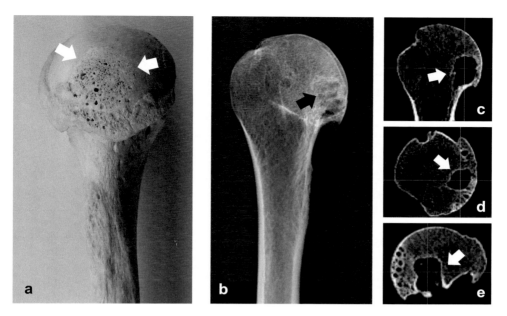

Figure 6.3 A right humerus showing sign of osteoarthritis on the head: (a) photograph; (b) lateral X-ray; (c) coronal CT scan; (d) axial CT scan; (e) sagittal CT scan. Periosteal reactions and microporosity along the margins of the joint and on the joint surface are visible on the photograph (macroscopic evaluation), while the X-ray shows the internal radiodense and radiolucent lesions, only CT scan images provide more details, revealing a cyst in the head of the humerus (arrows).

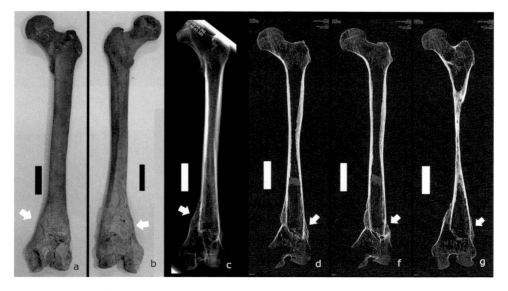

Figure 6.4 A right femur showing signs of osteomyelitis at the distal end due to a fracture: (a) photograph frontal view; (b) photograph posterior view; (c) X-ray; (d–f) coronal CT scans. The original cortical surface of the femur is not clearly seen macroscopically (photograph), but it is clearly visible on the radiograph and CT images (arrows). Scale bar: 5 cm.

In Figure 6.2, the photograph shows marked bone destruction due to treponemal disease (syphilis), but the exact extent of this destruction can only be evaluated using radiograph and CT scanning. In addition, the CT scan provides more information about the trabecular structure and the exact form of the destruction.

There are also some pathological conditions where both abnormal formation and bone destruction can be present, such as that found in septic arthritis, osteomyelitis, and osteosarcoma. Figures 6.3 and 6.4 show how macroscopic analysis, X-ray, and CT images are complementary tools. For instance, in Figure 6.3, macroscopic investigation reveals periosteal reaction and microporosity that are not visible on the imaging modalities, while the X-ray clearly shows internal radiodense and radiolucent lesions. However, only CT scan images provide more detail, revealing a cyst in the head of the humerus. In Figure 6.4, the original cortical surface of the tibia is not clearly seen macroscopically (photograph), but it is clearly visible on the radiograph and CT images.

Taphonomic Alterations

Taphonomic alteration needs to be taken into consideration when examining an archaeological specimen to avoid misinterpretation. For example, bones can contain soil intrusions that are visualized as radiopaque areas both on CT and X-rays and may be erroneously interpreted as sclerotic bone tumors (Mays, 2011). Similarly, soft tissues can drastically change their composition over time (Ruhli et al., 2004). Tissues from bodies preserved for centuries in anaerobic conditions, for instance, present similar HU values regardless of the tissue type (Villa & Lynnerup, 2012). Artificial or intentional mummification processes also have an effect on tissues, with embalming substances, such as resin, creating radiopaque areas that can be confused with pathological changes in Egyptian mummies (Ruhli et al., 2004; Villa et al., 2015). Finally, modern conservation techniques can also alter the sample, not necessarily macroscopically, but radiologically. For instance, the feet of the Tollund Man, a Danish bog body, showed a range of different HU values. The right foot was subjected to preservation and appeared more radiopaque than the left foot, which had naturally dried.

Other Imaging Modalities

Dual Energy CT Scanner

Dual energy CT scanner (DECT) is a particular type of scanner equipped with two X-ray sources and two detector array systems. The main purpose of using this equipment is to acquire two separate attenuation values (generally 80 and 140 KeV) of an object to extract material-specific information such as density, compositions of material, and effective atomic number (Coursey et al., 2010; Kalender, 2011). In a bioarchaeological context, it has been used, for example, on two ancient Egyptian cat mummies (Bewes et al., 2016). Here, the researchers could accurately differentiate desiccated soft tissues from low-density bone by the effective atomic number resulting from the scanning at two energy levels. DECT should be further investigated because the ability to differentiate low contrast tissues can improve the diagnosis in mummified remains.

Cone Beam CT Scanner

A cone beam CT scanner (CBCT) is a scanner optimized for dental scanning, used especially in oral and maxillofacial surgery, and in orthodontics. The field of view (FoV) is limited to the head region. The dose level in this scanner is almost an order of magnitude lower than in clinical CT scanning. However, reduced radiation also means a lower depth in gray values in the images. Thus, the difference between bones and soft tissue can easily be distinguished, while differences within soft tissues are more difficult to see (Dalstra et al., 2016). In an archaeological context, CBCT has been used to study human dentition from Early Bronze Age (Przystanska et al., 2017). The high contrast and the better resolution provided more precise information regarding individual teeth than clinical CT scanning.

Micro-CT

Micro-computed tomography (micro-CT or µCT) is a CT scanning technique that can visualize an object with very high spatial resolutions, i.e., a voxel size up to 1 µm. A micro-CT scan is produced by a CT scanner with a small FoV, around 1 to 100 mm, that renders high spatial resolution possible. The smaller the FoV the more details that can be visualized. A drawback is that it takes a long time for the acquisition of the images (from 10 to 300 minutes) (Kalender, 2011), and the quantity of generated data is very large (for example a micro-CT scan of lumbar vertebrae bodies with a spatial resolution of 50 µm occupy 1.8 terabits). Micro-CT has been used to study taphonomic changes in bones of bog bodies (Boel & Dalstra, 2007) and to investigate fossil teeth to evaluate ante-mortem treatment of dental pathology (Oxilia et al., 2017). In both cases, the images could provide details at micro levels (e.g., an accurate visualization of the structure of a tooth) that could not have been possible to obtain from the images from a clinical CT.

Magnetic Resonance Imaging

Magnetic resonance imaging (MRI) is a non-ionizing imaging technique, i.e., it does not use X-rays. MRI uses the properties of hydrogen atoms for visualizing the internal structures of a body (Rinck, 2001; Talbot et al., 2011). Hydrogen is the most abundant atom in a living body and is commonly found in water and fat. Thus, MRI provides detailed information of soft tissues. It is not suitable for investigating single dry bones, but it has been used to assess the development of bones such as the clavicle (Tangmose et al., 2014) or the knee (Kramer et al., 2014) on recently deceased or living patients.

In desiccated mummies, there are very few hydrogen atoms and, thus, the MRI technique is not suitable (Lewin & Notman, 1983; Notman et al., 1986 Hunt & Hopper, 1996). However, the first visualization of a mummy was possible after invasive rehydration of the tissues (Piepenbrink et al., 1986). This allowed researchers to visualize the soft tissues of ankle and wrist. Information of the state of the soft tissue can contribute to the identification of pathological changes and provide a better spectrum of a disease, not only on bones. For a comprehensive review, readers can refer to Ruhli (2015) and Giovannetti et al. (2016).

Propagation-Based Phase-Contrast CT

Propagation-based imaging allows the visualization of soft tissues with fine details. It enhances the contrast of soft tissues and, thus, facilitates better differentiation between tissues. Phase-contrast CT measures not only the absorption of X-rays but also the phase shift of X-rays as they pass through tissue. While MRI is also capable of capturing soft tissue, it is restricted to resolutions of approximately 1 mm. Alternatively, phase-contrast CT achieves resolutions of sub-0.01 mm (6 µm to 9 µm), which are ideal for identifying microscopic cell-sized features. The first scan was performed on the hand of an Egyptian mummy with incredible results (Romell et al., 2018): the scan differentiated and helped visualize linen, skin, tendons, ligaments, nerves, and arteries. The scan of the fingertip revealed additional features, including microvessels and tiny nerves in the nail bed, fat cells, and traces of bone marrow.

Terahertz Imaging

Terahertz (THz) imaging is another technique that uses non-ionizing radiation. THz waves are between microwave and infrared. Thus, they may provide complementary information to that obtained from X-rays, CT, and MRI. In addition, the imaging technique can be used on dry specimens since the presence of water in a specimen is a limitation for THz imaging. THz can be used to obtain structural and possibly spectroscopic information. Its full potential still needs to be explored in paleopathology. Only a few experiments have been carried out on bones and mummies. For more information, please refer to Ohrstrom et al. (2010) and Ohrstrom et al. (2015).

Future Prospects

The study of diseases in the past is fascinating and can contribute to our understanding of modern medicine. Knowing when a disease first appeared and how it manifested can provide essential information on its evolution and on the risk factors that cause it. An example of this is the study of atherosclerosis (an arterial disease caused by the deposition of cholesterol plaque on the inner walls of arteries) in past populations (Allam et al., 2011; Wann & Thomas, 2014). Using CT imaging, researchers demonstrated that ancient populations around the world, including ancient Egyptians and Peruvian populations, suffered from atherosclerosis. The study thereby dispelled claims that atherosclerosis was a modern disease. Recognizing its presence in the past can help paleopathologists recognize environmental, social, and biological factors contributing to the disease.

The study of skeletonized remains can provide important information to modern medicine, as it allows for a detailed view of pathological manifestations of a disease that are impossible to see in modern patients using radiological imaging (Ortner, 2005; Roberts & Manchester, 2007). Today's available treatments also prohibit diseases from developing into stages that might be seen in archaeological samples. Conversely, modern radiological imaging can help paleopathologists reach a diagnosis. As mentioned previously, it is not easy to interpret a pathological condition in ancient remains, especially when only the bones are left. Modern clinical imaging databases, however, can be used as a tool for comparison. Radiopaedia (https://radiopaedia.org) is an excellent example: it is a free resource with one of the internet's largest collections of radiological cases and reference articles.

Databases of paleopathological specimens should also be created and shared among experts around the world. A great example of this is "Digitized Diseases" (www.digitiseddiseases.org/) created and hosted by the University of Bradford, United Kingdom. Ideally, each bone should be investigated using a combination of different imaging modalities in order to provide information at different scales and of the different tissues. The creation of databases of images of ancient or modern pathological specimens provides a means to teach new generations of paleopathologists and provides means to monitor the evolution of the diseases throughout space and time.

References

Allam, A. H., Thompson, R. C., Wann, L. S., Miyamoto, M. I., Nur El-Din Ael, H., El-Maksoud, G. A., ... & Thomas, G. S. (2011). Atherosclerosis in ancient Egyptian mummies: the horus study. *JACC Cardiovasicular Imaging* 4(4):315–327. https://doi.org/10.1016/j.jcmg.2011.02.002

AlQahtani, S. J., Hector, M. P. & Liversidge, H. M. (2010). Brief communication: the London atlas of human tooth development and eruption. *American Journal of Physical Anthropology*, 142(3):481–490. https://doi.org/10.1002/ajpa.21258

Bewes, J. M., Morphett, A., Pate, F. D., Henneberg, M., Low, A. J., Kruse, L., Craig, B., Hindson, A. & Adams, E. (2016). Imaging ancient and mummified specimens: dual-energy CT with effective atomic number imaging of two ancient Egyptian cat mummies. *Journal of Archaeological Science: Reports 8*(Supplement C):173–177. https://doi.org/https://doi.org/10.1016/j.jasrep.2016.06.009

Boel, L. W. & Dalstra, M. (2007). Microscopical analyses of bone specimens: structural changes related to chronological age and possible diseases. In Asingh, P. & Linnerup, N. (Eds.), *Grauballe Man - An Iron Age Bog Body*, pp. 130–139. Jutland Archeological Society. Denmark: Aarhus University Press, Aarhus.

Böni, T., Ruhli, F. J. & Chhem, R. K. (2004). History of paleoradiology: early published literature, 1896–1921. *Canadian Association of Radiologists Journal-Journal De L Association Canadienne Des Radiologistes* 55(4): 203–210. WOS:000223586700003

Brandt, L. Ø., Hansen, A. H., Hussein, S. & C, V. (2020). Bandages for bastet: a study of three Egyptian cat mummies. In Strand, E. V., Grömer, K., Harlow, M., Malcolm-Davies, J. & Mannering, U. (Eds.), *Archeological Textile Review*, Vol. 62. Friends of ATN, hosted by the Centre for Textile Research. Copenhagen, Denmark: Grafisk University of Copenhagen, Copenhagen.

Brickley, M. L. & McKinley, J. I. (2004). *Guidelines to the Standards for Recording Human Remains*. Institute of Field Archaeologists - British Association For Biological Anthropology and Osteoarchaeology. Southhamptom, UK: University of Southampton; and Reading: University of Reading, Institute of Field Archaeologists, SHES.

Buzug, T. M. (2008). *Computed Tomography. From Photon Statistics to Modern Cone-Beam CT*. Berlin: Springer.

Chhem, R. K. (2008). Paleoradiology: History and new developments. In Chhem, R. K. & Brothwell, D. R. (Eds.), *Paleoradiology. Imaging Mummies and Fossils*. Berlin: Springer-Verlag.

Chhem, R. K. & Brothwell, D. R. (2008). *Paleoradiology. Imaging Mummies and Fossils*. Berlin: Springer-Verlag.

Conlogue, G., Nelson, A. J. & Guillen, S. (2004). The application of radiography to field studies in physical anthropology. *Canadian Association Radiology Journal* 55(4):254–257. https://www.ncbi.nlm.nih.gov/pubmed/15362349

Coursey, C. A., Nelson, R. C., Boll, D. T., Paulson, E. K., Ho, L. M., Neville, A. M., Marin, D., Gupta, R. T. & Schindera, S. T. (2010). Dual-energy multidetector CT: how does it work, what can it tell us, and when can we use it in abdominopelvic imaging? *Radiographics* 30(4):1037–1055. https://doi.org/10.1148/rg.304095175

Cox, S. L. (2015). A critical look at mummy CT scanning. *Anatomical Record-Advances in Integrative Anatomy and Evolutionary Biology* 298(6):1099–1110. https://doi.org/10.1002/ar.23149

Dalstra, M., Schulz, G., Dagassan-Berndt, D., Verna, C., Muller-Gerbl, M. & Muller, B. (2016). Hard X-ray micro-tomography of a human head post-mortem as a gold standard to compare X-ray modalities. *Developments in X-Ray Tomography X*:9967. https://doi.org/10.1117/12.2237655

Giovannetti, G., Guerrini, A., Carnieri, E. & Salvadori, P. A. (2016). Magnetic resonance imaging for the study of mummies. *Magnetic Resonance Imaging* 34(6):785–794. https://doi.org/10.1016/j.mri.2016.03.012

Harris, J. E. & Weeks, K. R. (1973). *X-Raying the Pharaohs*. New York: Charles Scribner and Sons.

Harris, J. E. & Weeks, K. R. (1980). *An X-Ray Atlas of the Royal Mummies*. Chicago: University of Chicago Press.

Harwood-Nash, D. C. (1979). Computed tomography of ancient Egyptian mummies. *Journal of Computer Assisted Tomography* 3:768–773.

Homoe, P. & Lynnerup, N. (1991). Pneumatization of the temporal bones in Greenlandic Inuit anthropological material. *Acta Oto-Laryngologica* 111(6):1109–1116. https://doi.org/10.3109/00016489109138458

Hounsfield, G. N. (1973). Computerized transverse axial scanning (tomography): description of system. *British Journal of Radiology* 46:1016–1022.

Hsieh, J. (2009). *Computed Tomography Principles, Design, Artifacts, and Recent Advances, Second Edition*. New York: Wiley.

Hunt, D. R. & Hopper, L. M. (1996). Non-invasive investigations of human mummified remains by radiographic techniques. In Spindler, K., Wilfing, H., Rastbichler-Zissernig, E., zur Nedden, D. & Nothdurfter, H. (Eds.), *Human Mummies. A Global Survey of their Status and the Techniques of Conservation*, pp. 15–31. Berlin: Springer.

Kalender, W. A. (2011). *Computed Tomography: Fundamentals, System Technology, Image Quality, Applications, 3rd Edition*. New York: Wiley.

König, W. (1896). *14 Photographien mit Röntgen-Strahlen, Aufgenommen im Physikalischen Verein Frankfurt A.M.* Leipzig: J.A. Barth.

Kramer, J. A., Schmidt, S., Jurgens, K. U., Lentschig, M., Schmeling, A. & Vieth, V. (2014). Forensic age estimation in living individuals using 3.0 T MRI of the distal femur. *International Journal of Legal Medicine* 128(3):509–514. https://doi.org/10.1007/s00414-014-0967-3

Lewin, P. K. & Harwood-Nash, D. C. (1977). Computerized axial tomography in medical archaeology. *Paleopathology Newsletter* 17:8–9.

Lewin, P. K. & Notman, D. N. H. (1983). Use of nuclear magnetic resonance imaging of archaeological specimens. *Paleopathology Newsletter* 43: 9.

Lynnerup, N. (2007). Mummies. *Yearbook of Physical Anthropology* 50:162–190. https://doi.org/10.1002/ajpa.20728

Lynnerup, N. (2008). Computed tomography scanning and three-dimensional visualization of mummies and bog bodies. In Pinhasi, R. & Mays, S. (Eds.), *Advances in Human Paleopathology*, pp. 101–119. Chichester: John Wiley and Sons, Ltd.

Lynnerup, N. (2010). Medical imaging of mummies and bog bodies - a mini-review. *Gerontology* 56(5):441–448. https://doi.org/10.1159/000266031

Lynnerup, N. & Ruhli, F. (2015). Short review: The use of conventional X-rays in mummy studies. *Anatomical Record-Advances in Integrative Anatomy and Evolutionary Biology* 298(6):1085–1087. https://doi.org/10.1002/ar.23147

Magid, D., Bryan, B. M., Drebin, R. A., Ney, D. & Fishman, E. K. (1989). Three-dimensional imaging of an Egyptian mummy. *Clinical Imaging* 13:239–240.

Marx, M. & D'Auria, S. H. (1988). Three-dimensional CT reconstructions of an ancient human Egyptian mummy. *American Journal of Roentgenology* 150:147–149.

Mays, S. (2011). The relationship between paleopathology and the clinical sciences. In Grauer, A. (Ed.), *A Companion to Paleopathology*, pp. 285–309. New York: Wiley-Blackwell. https://doi.org/10.1002/9781444345940.ch16

Melcher, A. H., Holowka, S., Pharoah, M. & Lewin, P. K. (1997). Non-invasive computed tomography and three-dimensional reconstruction of the dentition of a 2,800-year-old Egyptian mummy exhibiting extensive dental disease. *American Journal of Physical Anthropology* 103(3):329–340. https://doi.org/10.1002/(SICI)1096-8644(199707)103:3<329::AID-AJPA3>3.0.CO;2-L

Moodie, R. L. (1931). *Roentgenologic Studies of Egyptian and Peruvian Mummies*. Chicago: Field Museum of Natural History.

Notman, D. N., Tashjian, J., Aufderheide, A. C., Cass, O. W., Shane, O. C., 3rd, Berquist, T. H., Gray, J. E. & Gedgaudas, E. (1986). Modern imaging and endoscopic biopsy techniques in Egyptian mummies. *American Journal of Roentgenology* 146(1):93–96. https://doi.org/10.2214/ajr.146.1.93

Nystrom, K. C., Braunstein, E. M. & Buikstra, J. E. (2004). Field paleoradiography of skeletal material from the Early Classic Period of Copan, Honduras. *Canadian Association of Radiologists Journal* 55(4):246–253.

Ohrstrom, L., Bitzer, A., Walther, M. & Ruhli, F. J. (2010). Technical note: terahertz imaging of ancient mummies and bone. *American Journal of Physical Anthropology* 142(3):497–500. https://doi.org/10.1002/ajpa.21292

Ohrstrom, L., Fischer, B. M., Bitzer, A., Wallauer, J., Walther, M. & Ruhli, F. (2015). Terahertz imaging modalities of ancient Egyptian mummified objects and of a naturally mummified rat. *Anatomical Record (Hoboken)* 298(6):1135–1143. https://doi.org/10.1002/ar.23143

Ortner, D. J. (2005). Introduction. In Mann, R. W. & Hunt, D. R. (Eds.), *Photographic Regional Atlas of Bone Disease*. Springfield, IL: Charles C. Thomas.

Oxilia, G., Fiorillo, F., Boschin, F., Boaretto, E., Apicella, S. A., Matteucci, C., … & Benazzi, S. (2017). The dawn of dentistry in the late upper Paleolithic: an early case of pathological intervention at Riparo Fredian. *American Journal of Physical Anthropology* 163(3):446–461. https://doi.org/10.1002/ajpa.23216

Pickering, R. B., Conces, D. J. Jr., Braunstein, E. M. & Yurco, F. (1990). Three-dimensional computed tomography of the mummy Wenuhotep. *American Journal of Physical Anthropology* 83(1):49–55. https://doi.org/10.1002/ajpa.1330830106

Piepenbrink, H., Frahm, J., Haase, A. & Matthaei, D. (1986). Nuclear magnetic resonance imaging of mummified corpses. *American Journal of Physical Anthropology* 70(1):27–28. https://doi.org/10.1002/ajpa.1330700107

Przystanska, A., Lorkiewicz-Muszynska, D., Abreu-Glowacka, M., Glapinski, M., Sroka, A., Rewekant, A., Hyrchala, A., Bartecki, B., Zaba, C. & Kulczyk, T. (2017). Analysis of human dentition from early bronze age: 4000-year-old puzzle. *Odontology*: 105(1):13–22. https://doi.org/10.1007/s10266-015-0220-7

Rinck, P. A. (2001). *Magnetic Resonance in Medicine*. (4th edition). Chichester: Wiley-Blackwell.

Roberts, C. & Manchester, K. (2007). *The Archaeology of Disease*. Ithaca, NY: Cornell University Press.

Romell, J., Vagberg, W., Romell, M., Haggman, S., Ikram, S. & Hertz, H. M. (2018). Soft-tissue imaging in a human mummy: propagation-based phase-contrast CT. *Radiology* 289(3):670–676. https://doi.org/10.1148/radiol.2018180945

Ruhli, F. J. (2015). Short review: magnetic resonance imaging of ancient mummies. *Anatomical Record (Hoboken)* 298(6):1111–1115. https://doi.org/10.1002/ar.23150

Ruhli, F. J., Chhem, R. K. & Boni, T. (2004). Diagnostic paleoradiology of mummified tissue: interpretation and pitfalls. *Canadian Association of Radiologists Journal – Journal De L Association Canadienne Des Radiologistes* 55(4):218–227. WOS:000223586700005

Rutty, G. N., Morgan, B., O'Donnell, C., Leth, P. M. & Thali, M. (2008). Forensic institutes across the world place CT or MRI scanners or both into their mortuaries. *Journal of Trauma-Injury Infection and Critical Care*, 65(2):493–494. https://doi.org/10.1097/TA.0b013e31817de420

Röntgen, W. K. (1972). On a new kind of rays. *CA Cancer Journal for Clinicians* 22(3):153–157. https://www.ncbi.nlm.nih.gov/pubmed/4625566

Saab, G., Chhem, R. & Bohay, R. N. (2008). Paleoradiologic Techniques. In Chhem, R. K. & Brothwell, D. R. (Eds.), *Paleoradiology. Imaging Mummies and Fossils*, pp. 15–54. London: Springer.

Seibert, J. A. (2004). X-ray imaging physics for nuclear medicine technologists. Part 1: Basic principles of x-ray production. *Journal of Nuclear Medicine Technology* 32(3):139–147. https://www.ncbi.nlm.nih.gov/pubmed/15347692

Seibert, J. A. & Boone, J. M. (2005). X-ray imaging physics for nuclear medicine technologists. Part 2: X-ray interactions and image formation. *Journal of Nuclear Medicine Technology* 33(1):3–18. https://www.ncbi.nlm.nih.gov/pubmed/15731015

Talbot, J., Kaut Roth, C. & Westbrook, C. (2011). *MRI in Practice*. New York: John Wiley And Sons Ltd.

Tangmose, S., Jensen, K. E., Villa, C. & Lynnerup, N. (2014). Forensic age estimation from the clavicle using 1.0T MRI--preliminary results. *Forensic Science International* 234:7–12. https://doi.org/10.1016/j.forsciint.2013.10.027

Thomas, A. M. K. & Banerjee, A. K. (2013). *The History of Radiology*. Croydon: Oxford University Press. https://doi.org/10.1093/med/9780199639977.001.0001

Villa, C., Davey, J., Craig, P. J. G., Drummer, O. H. & Lynnerup, N. (2015). The advantage of CT scans and 3D visualizations in the analysis of three child mummies from the Graeco-Roman period. *Anthropologischer Anzeiger* 72(1):55–65. https://doi.org/10.1127/anthranz/2014/0330

Villa, C. & Lynnerup, N. (2012). Hounsfield Units ranges in CT-scans of bog bodies and mummies. *Anthropologischer Anzeiger*, 69(2):127–145. https://doi.org/10.1127/0003-5548/2012/0139

Wann, S. & Thomas, G. S. (2014). What can ancient mummies teach us about atherosclerosis? *Trends in Cardiovascular Medicine* 24(7):279–284. https://doi.org/10.1016/j.tcm.2014.06.005

Zollikofer, C. P. & Ponce de Leon, M. (2005). *Virtual Reconstruction: A Primer in Computer-Assisted Paleontology and Biomedicine*. New York: Wiley-Liss.

7
ISOTOPES IN PALEOPATHOLOGY

Chris Stantis and Ellen J. Kendall

Stable isotope analyses are simple; they are based on the very straightforward principle that when we are alive, we build the tissues of our bodies from the foods we eat and the water we drink. Or, as the famous adage goes, that we "are what we eat". Stable isotope analyses are also complex; they require knowledge of complicated, synergistic, and species-specific biological processes, as well as a comprehensive knowledge of the ecology and cultural practices of study regions.

As with all subfields of paleopathology and bioarchaeology, isotopic analyses benefit from a multidisciplinary approach, integrated with complementary knowledge from other disciplines to tackle the pressing questions in the wider field. Thus, paleopathologists seeking to integrate stable isotope data into their research interpretations should also understand some of the basic principles of this toolset. Destructive analyses, such as stable isotope analytical methods, must ethically seek to answer clear hypothesis-driven research questions and begin from a solid foundation of knowledge specific to period, region, and site. More detailed treatises on the principles of stable isotopes in biological systems are available elsewhere (e.g., Hoefs, 2009; Sharp, 2017), so we will touch upon them only briefly. This chapter focuses primarily on applications of isotopic analysis to paleopathological study. We also discuss the limitations inherent to isotopic analysis and suggest some future directions and opportunities for collaboration between paleopathologists and isotope researchers.

Principles of Isotopic Analysis

Isotopes are variants/forms of a chemical element that have the same number of protons and electrons but different numbers of neutrons. Isotopes of the same element behave differently during physical reactions due to their differences in atomic mass. As such, lighter isotopes preferentially diffuse out of a system, leaving the heavier isotope forms in the original source or reservoir. These differences in reaction rates between isotopes, also known as *kinetic isotope effects* or *fractionation*, dictate the ratio of isotopes in a sample. For example, evaporation of water creates water vapor (H_2O), which contains more ^{16}O than ^{18}O relative to its reservoir, because lighter oxygen isotopes more readily evaporate. While lighter ^{16}O preferentially evaporates, heavier ^{18}O more readily condenses and precipitates in such processes. This principle leads to enrichment in ^{18}O in low-latitude bodies of water, brewed beverages, and stewed foods, and greater representation of ^{16}O in cloud vapor and high-latitude rainfall. Understanding the dynamics of fractionation in organisms within ecosystems is valuable to researchers, as stable isotopes do not decay or change after death, providing an enduring biological record which is transferrable to the past.

Carbon (δ^{13}C), nitrogen (δ^{15}N), sulfur (δ^{34}S), strontium (^{87}Sr/^{86}Sr), and oxygen (δ^{18}O) stable isotopes—common isotopic systems utilized in bioarchaeological research—become integrated into the tissues of the body through consumption of water or food and thus become part of a body pool that is drawn upon for the synthesis of tissues. In theory, all human tissues are suitable for isotopic analysis, although different tissues require consideration of differing time resolution, metabolic processes, and analytical techniques. Due to the rarity of soft tissues surviving in the archaeological record, bone and teeth are the most frequently sampled tissue types.

Sampling of human tissues may be done either by bulk analysis or through incremental sectioning of target tissues. Many tissues in the body are subject to continuous maintenance and replacement through cellular turnover and thus do not have a spatial-temporal relationship if different sections are analyzed. Instead, these tissues (such as bone) are appropriate for bulk sampling, which provides time-averaged data covering the period it takes for the tissue to be completely replaced (Hedges et al., 2007). In contrast, tissues such as hair or dentine, which form incrementally, do not remodel once formed and preserve well-characterized relationships between formation time and their incremental microstructures (Smith & Tafforeau, 2008). For example, incremental sectioning of dentine allows investigation of diachronic dietary changes during tooth formation (Beaumont et al., 2014). This method is important for investigating connections between early life experiences in individuals and long-term population health, discussed in greater detail below.

Isotopic systems are often divided into "diet", "mobility", and "climate" isotopes to denote the type of information to be gained and the questions posed. While this terminology offers a convenient shorthand, caution in their use should be used, as isotope values are the product of complex, rather than single-input, systems. For instance, while ^{87}Sr/^{86}Sr ratios are correlated with local geology and used to identify non-local individuals (as they do not fractionate appreciably at increasing levels of the food chain), these isotopes make their way into human tissues through foods. In turn, the isotopes derive their ratios from the substrate on which foods are grown or raised. Consequently, a diet that includes substantial consumption of non-local foods can affect these values even if the individuals never left their local area (Kendall et al., 2013). Similarly, in analyses of oxygen stable isotopes, which enter the human body primarily through drinking water, δ^{18}O may be most frequently used to trace childhood origin and identify non-local individuals through geographic variation in the water cycle. However, δ^{18}O analyses are also used to characterize paleoclimatic variability, and further variation in local values from human tissues may occur through anthropogenic processes that produce isotope fractionation, such as brewing alcohol or boiling foods (Brettell et al., 2012). Conversely, "dietary" analyses of δ^{13}C, δ^{15}N, along with δ^{34}S values, have been used to identify non-local individuals in assemblages where "mobility" isotopes were not viable for differentiating movement due to spatial isotopic homogeneity (Stantis et al., 2016; Cheung et al., 2017). Isotopes are therefore often not clearly categorizable in discrete ways via function and need to be understood as belonging to interactive and dynamic systems.

Paleopathological Application of Isotopic Analyses

The *indirect* value of isotopic analyses to paleopathology has always been reasonably clear; diet and nutrition are known to be important mediators of immune function and overall health, and different types of subsistence strategy each provide their own set of risks and benefits. Likewise, isotopic analyses can provide important information about geographic mobility, which has important implications for the transmission of communicable disease and increased host susceptibility to disease. However, beyond paleodiet or paleomobility, stable isotope data also offer immense potential to better understand complex issues of human health. This can be done by one of two means, which will be addressed below: either by contributing to understanding of disease-mediating factors and disease ecologies or by providing direct evidence for the dynamics of diseases themselves.

Contributions to Understanding Disease-Mediating Factors

Contextualizing the information offered by isotopic analyses is perhaps the most familiar role of biogeochemistry to paleopathologists. This type of contribution does not offer direct evidence for disease. Instead, these analyses supplement wider knowledge of conditions relevant to disease ecology, such as early life development and diet, population-level trends in subsistence and social hierarchy, measurement of climatic fluctuation, and identification of migration and geographic mobility within and between populations. This can be accomplished through a range of analyses, and a range of applications, which will be discussed.

Early Life Diet and the Development of Disease in Adulthood

The first 1000 days of life, which includes both fetal development and the first two postnatal years, represent a crucial developmental window in which poor nutrition or exposure to physiological stress can create lifelong vulnerabilities to disease (Gluckman et al., 2008; Victora et al., 2008). Excessive levels of physiological stress in early life, particularly undernutrition or high pathogen exposure, may result in metabolic or immune dysfunction, with lasting effects. The propensity of fetal and infant physiology to adapt to adversity in ways that increase the risk of chronic disease in adulthood is known as the Developmental Origins of Health and Disease (DOHaD) hypothesis (Fleming et al., 2017; and see Chapter 28, this volume).

Even before development of the DOHaD hypothesis, archaeologists recognized the importance of early life health and nutrition to the short-term survival of young children and the reproductive patterns of their mothers. Consequently, infant feeding norms within past societies have long been a source of interest to bioarchaeologists and stable isotope researchers (e.g., Sillen & Smith, 1984; Fogel et al., 1989; Katzenberg & Pfeiffer, 1995). However, adoption of DOHaD as an interpretative lens by bioarchaeologists has endowed early childhood health and nutrition with an extra layer of significance. Several paleopathologists have explicitly applied or advocated a DOHaD model to their research, linking early life adversity with longer term morbidity and mortality, and even intergenerational effects (e.g., Armelagos et al., 2009; Gowland, 2015; Watts, 2015).

Through their ability to provide evidence for early life diet, isotopic analyses offer great potential to add to this growing understanding of formative influences on later life health. Detection and characterization of breastfeeding have formed the primary foci within infant feeding studies, as it represents the biological and historical norm and offers a range of developmental and immunological benefits to infants in addition to nutrition (Reynard & Tuross, 2015; Kendall et al., 2021). The introduction of complementary foods is an important milestone for nutritional sufficiency and modulation of growth. In particular, identifying the crucial phases in the transition between full dependence on human milk and final cessation of breastfeeding is critical to understanding early-life health (White et al., 2017).

The earliest isotopic applications to assess the role of infant diet in disease and mortality analyzed carbon and nitrogen stable isotopes in bone collagen. Synthesis of body tissues from diet creates fractionation, leading to an upward enrichment in $\delta^{15}N$ and $\delta^{13}C$ throughout the levels of the food chain. As infants consume human milk, synthesized by their mother's body, their tissues are thought to be nearly one step higher in the food chain (or one trophic level) while they are breastfed (approximately +2–3‰ for $\delta^{15}N$ and +1‰ for $\delta^{13}C$ in collagen), with decreases in tissue values as the infant transitions to full reliance on a family diet (Reynard & Tuross, 2015). Such studies have generally used a cross-sectional approach to create a snapshot of childhood diet and disease by aligning aggregate isotopic and paleopathological data (e.g., Dittmann & Grupe, 2000; Stantis et al., 2020b). This approach, however, carries interpretative limitations. Firstly, as mortality and disease risks are heterogenous and selective in nature, inferring wider childhood norms from the skeletal remains of individuals dying in early life may present bias (Wood et al., 1992). Secondly, in times of high physiological stress, the body may prioritize survival over growth and maintenance, disrupting rates of normal bone turnover (Szulc et al., 2000). In consequence, known parameters of bone turnover may be unreliable for a subpopulation that is likely to have suffered growth disruption due to stress or disease (Beaumont, 2020).

These pitfalls can be avoided through incremental sampling of adult teeth, particularly dentine. Teeth form during childhood and are not subject to growth arrest or remodeling. A reliable record of childhood diet is therefore preserved in the adult skeleton, and this may be aligned with adult paleopathological data. This shift in method has been driven by both methodological advances that enable a diachronic sampling approach (Fuller et al., 2003; Eerkens et al., 2011) and by theoretical developments that have prioritized a lifecourse approach and a focus on socially framed bioarchaeology (Gowland & Knüsel, 2006; Agarwal & Glencross, 2011). Use of a combined paleopathological and longitudinal isotopic approach may illuminate patterns not apparent in child skeletal remains alone, as recent scholarship has found meaningful differences in childhood diet based on age at death (Sandberg et al., 2014; Reitsema et al., 2016) and biological sex (Howcroft et al., 2012; Henderson et al., 2014).

Carbon and nitrogen stable isotope analyses currently dominate investigations of past infant feeding practices, with interpretation particularly relying on nitrogen data. Oxygen, sulfur, and hydrogen (δ^2H or sometimes δD) stable isotopes have also been explored as evidence for breastfeeding and early-life diet (Nehlich et al., 2011; Britton et al., 2015; Ryan et al., 2020). While none of the newer methods have made significant inroads to challenging the primacy of $\delta^{13}C$ and $\delta^{15}N$ analyses, they do offer promise, especially as the dietary and metabolic processes that alter these isotopic ratios during infancy and childhood become better understood.

Population Diet, Subsistence, and Social Inequality

As with analysis of early childhood diet, understanding wider population diet is an important application with implications for paleopathology. Processual questions regarding the role of subsistence strategies in nutrition and health were central concerns for early isotopic and paleopathological studies. Of particular interest was exploring reliance on different types of subsistence, such as North American maize agriculture or Pacific Northwest marine economies, often correlated with social inequality and complexity (Chisholm et al., 1982; Lynott et al., 1986). This approach was influenced predominantly by a theoretical emphasis on ecological determinism, wherein culture was perceived as an extra-somatic adaptation to ecosystem pressures, and particularistic explanations were spurned in favor of scientific methods and a search for universal laws of human behavior (Binford, 1987; Trigger, 1989).

Demineralization methods for human bone collagen—originally developed for radiocarbon (^{14}C) dating (Longin, 1971)—first permitted paleodietary reconstruction in archaeological populations. Some of the first paleodiet studies examined differences between the δ^{13}C value ranges of cultivated maize (*Zea mays*) or marine animals and other native terrestrial foods in the Americas, providing a means of differentiating between diets based on terrestrial hunting and foraging and those reliant on agriculture or marine hunting/fishing (Bender, 1968; Smith & Epstein, 1971). Paleodietary isotopic studies from the Americas, coupled with ^{14}C dating, were first used to demonstrate that adoption of maize-based agriculture correlated with changes in fertility and mortality patterns observed in paleopathological research (Vogel & Van Der Merwe, 1977; Van der Merwe & Vogel, 1978). Stable isotope analyses were subsequently applied more broadly to link agricultural subsistence with negative health outcomes, especially in terms of the association between maize consumption and skeletal markers of anemia (e.g., Cohen & Armelagos, 1984; Larsen, 1995; Hutchinson et al., 1998).

Beyond an early focus on agriculture, stable isotope data linking subsistence to disease risk have been used to inform paleopathological interpretation in a range of contexts. For example, Northwest Coast, Californian, and South American pre-contact cultures have shown similar skeletal evidence of anemias to those seen in maize agriculturalists (Cybulski, 1977; Walker, 1986; Pilloud & Schwitalla, 2020). Combining paleodietary data with paleoparasitological, archaeological, and ethnographic data from these contexts has helped to link the development of cribra orbitalia and porotic hyperostosis to anemias caused by parasite infection derived from heavily marine-dependent diets (Dickson et al., 2004; Bathurst, 2005; Suby, 2014). Other types of subsistence come with their own inherent hazards to health. In addition to risks to health posed by parasites or malnutrition associated with hunter-fisher or agricultural economies, pastoralism and other close contacts with livestock carry a risk of contracting zoonotic diseases. Some of these, such as tuberculosis or brucellosis, can become chronic and observable in skeletal remains (Ortner, 2003). While few studies have attempted to link zoonotic skeletal pathologies to paleodietary data (discussed in greater detail below), recent isotopic analyses of modern hair samples have distinguished dietary differences between individuals from pastoral, agricultural, and fishing communities (Cooper et al., 2019), representing a promising new avenue of research.

Substantial theoretical changes have occurred over the course of paleodietary discipline development, some of which are shared with paleopathology, and these have spurred changes to method. These changes have entailed a shift away from positivism and disembodied "societies" and toward a more descriptive, personalized social archaeology of diet. As post-processual and feminist archaeologies (e.g., Engelstad, 1991; Gero & Conkey, 1991; Hodder, 1991) fueled acknowledgment of the agency of women and children in the late 20th century, archaeological research began to integrate more nuanced interpretations of the social attributes that influence isotopic values (Kamp, 2001; Gilchrist, 2007). Identity-specific questions regarding access to different types of foods have also emerged, taking their place alongside the more structural aims of processualism (Twiss, 2012). Differential access to foods has become a major theme in isotopic research, exploring the relationship between social markers (such as grave goods and burial type) and biological factors such as age, sex, and pathology (e.g., Stantis et al., 2015; Colleter et al., 2019; Moreiras Reynaga et al., 2020; Stantis et al., 2021).

Mobility and Health

Human migration patterns are an important factor in the development and transmission of disease, as environment and interpersonal contact are key to modulating pathogenesis. Mobility analyses tie geographic origin to known spatial variation in geological or hydrological biochemistry, enabling a recognition of heightened vulnerability to unfamiliar pathogens for migrants, as well as the health impacts of potential socioeconomic marginalization—particularly when used as part of multi-isotope analyses, including diet. Researchers have also suggested that isotope analysis is an underused tool for exploring the role of migration in transmission pathways of infectious disease (Roberts & Buikstra, 2003; Millard et al., 2005).

The dual roles of migrants as both vulnerable subpopulation and unwitting vectors have been addressed by a wide range of paleopathological studies integrating mobility data. Major themes in health and infectious disease have included the geographic origins and global transmission routes of leprosy (Taylor et al., 2018; Roberts, 2018), treponemal diseases (Budd et al., 2004; Roberts et al., 2013), and tuberculosis (Okazaki et al., 2019; Snoddy et al., 2020a), among others. Environmental disequilibrium is another challenge facing migrant populations, as mobility isotopes have also been used to identify increased biological stress and susceptibility to disease among migrants (e.g., Redfern et al., 2018; Aronsen et al., 2019), as well as their vulnerability to interpersonal violence during periods of societal volatility (Pacheco-Forés et al., 2021). Paleogenomic analyses provide important information regarding the evolutionary history of infectious diseases, and these can also provide complementary data on the geographic source of pathogens. However, stable isotope analyses are unique in being able to provide histories of movement for people (rather than pathogens) during life, offering essential opportunities to align these data with other social and biological variables to better understand the complexities of human-disease interactions.

Direct Evidence for Disease Processes

In many regards, the type of evidence produced for disease-mediating factors has, in the past, lent itself to cross-sectional, big-picture approaches that have prioritized larger datasets, population averaging, and characterization of environmental conditions over the life experiences of the individuals who lived in them. However, individual and population-level data are not mutually exclusive, and individual-level data can be used to illuminate and enrich our understanding of wider population trends and lifeways. Nonetheless, the individual-specific direct evidence for disease that may be provided by isotopic analysis creates a natural pairing with an osteobiographical approach to paleopathology.

Sampling bones or teeth with observable pathologies has been warned against for paleodietary studies, as disease processes may create a shift in recorded values (Katzenberg & Lovell, 1999; Olsen et al., 2014; Plomp et al., 2020). However, strategic use of pathological bone or teeth can reveal pathophysiological biomarkers, which may, in turn, inform interpretation of anomalous isotopic values where these are not otherwise manifest in the observable morphological changes of disease.

Bone

Abnormal bone isotope values associated with physiological stress and altered metabolism have long been known, with these first observed as elevated $\delta^{15}N$ values in individuals with osteopenia (White & Armelagos, 1997). Similar results were found by Katzenberg and Lovell (1999) and were interpreted as catabolism—a breakdown and recycling of existing tissues to meet metabolic demands not being met by diet. Carbon has also been shown to be subject to pathological alteration, as comparison of anatomical bone samples with and without changes associated with syphilis showed small yet significant reductions in $\delta^{13}C$ values for syphilitic samples relative to healthy bone (Salesse et al., 2019). Olsen et al. (2014) observed localized effects associated with inflammation and new bone formation, finding altered $\delta^{13}C$ and $\delta^{15}N$ where healed fractures, osteoarthritis, and osteomyelitis or periostitis were present. Undernutrition may also alter bone $\delta^{15}N$ and $\delta^{13}C$ bone, with studies finding anomalous values for an individual with probable celiac disease (Scorrano et al., 2014) and victims of the Irish Famine (Beaumont et al., 2012; Beaumont & Montgomery, 2016). The potential for pathological states to alter protein metabolism and the amino acid composition of bone collagen has been supported by experimental work in human and animal subjects (D'Ortenzio et al., 2015; Warinner & Tuross, 2010). Nonetheless, pathophysiological effects on protein metabolism specific to each disease may produce mixed findings, as in a recent study that found no differences in $\delta^{13}C$ and $\delta^{15}N$ of bone collagen for lesions associated with chronic anemia (Carroll et al., 2018).

Oxygen stable isotope values in skeletal apatite (as opposed to collagen) may also be affected by disease processes or physiological stress. Depressed $\delta^{18}O$ values have been observed in archaeological skeletons with osteopenia (White et al., 2004) and also in transgenic mice with sickle cell disease (Reitsema & Crews, 2011), relative to healthy counterparts. Investigation of disease markers in bone is complicated by the fact that bone is a living tissue with imprecise rates of turnover, which may themselves be disrupted by disease or malnutrition (Weinbrenner et al., 2003). In consequence, while studies of bone have provided some tantalizing hints of the scope for studying disease through isotope biochemistry, it is not possible to be certain to what extent bone provides a reliable record of disease history.

Teeth

In contrast to bone, tooth enamel and primary dentine do not remodel once formed and provide a reliable and time-sensitive history of diet and health during formation, due to their incremental structures. The ability to offer a high-resolution record of health is limited only by the age range covered by dental development, which spans the late antenatal period to young adulthood (Al Qahtani et al., 2010). Teeth may be analyzed to detect systemic metabolic changes associated with nonspecific lesion-forming disease states (e.g., skeletal stress markers), or diseases which form specific lesions (e.g., neoplastic diseases) but which also have systemic effects not otherwise visible. While both dentine and enamel offer avenues for producing new data, the superior time resolution offered by incremental sampling of dentine makes it preferred to bulk enamel sampling. One of the strengths of isotopic applications to paleopathology in teeth is that, despite the timescales of teeth relating to infancy, childhood, and adolescence, childhood survivorship and differential frailty can be targeted as variables of interest through analysis of both adults and children.

A range of diseases and conditions have been explored through isotopic analysis of dental tissues in recent years, many of which have found evidence of nutritional stress (catabolism or disease-induced cachexia) in δ^{13}C and δ^{15}N data. Isotopic evidence for periods of starvation through famine or childhood poverty has been frequently noted in studies where historic documentation is available to supplement skeletal indicators of nonspecific stress (e.g., Henderson et al., 2014; Beaumont & Montgomery, 2016; Millard et al., 2020). More commonly still, for periods where supporting documentary context is unavailable, researchers report strong correlations between isotopic evidence of nutritional stress and skeletal markers of childhood stress, such as enamel hypoplasia or cribra orbitalia (e.g., Crowder et al., 2019; Adams et al., 2021).

Other studies have used stable isotopes alongside bony lesions (pathognomonic, or strongly linked to disease) to explore the pathophysiology of specific diseases, particularly where disease states induce nutritional stress. Linkage of cribra orbitalia in marshy areas to endemic malaria (Gowland & Western, 2012; Smith-Guzmán, 2015) prompted an investigation of childhood δ^{13}C and δ^{15}N incremental dentine data from early medieval English sites where high cribra orbitalia prevalence was linked to wetland residence (Kendall et al., 2020). Data produced were consistent with the known pathophysiology of chronic *Plasmodium vivax* infection in pregnancy and early childhood, presenting isotopic evidence of impaired fetal growth and catch-up, as well as episodic nutritional stress in infancy and early childhood (Kendall et al., 2020). The search for isotopic evidence of tuberculosis has found catabolic isotopic patterning associated with wasting, typical of active disease as appetite diminishes and energy needs rise (Goude et al., 2020; Snoddy et al., 2020a). Figure 7.1 shows a characteristic isotopic pattern associated with tuberculosis-induced catabolism in δ^{13}C and δ^{15}N dentine collagen data, in an adolescent of unknown sex from early medieval eastern England (Kendall, 2019). Following an isotopically uneventful early childhood, rising δ^{15}N and dropping δ^{13}C consistent with catabolism suggest that the onset of active disease occurred from around seven years of age. This individual was selected for isotopic analysis specifically due to exhibiting Pott's disease of the spine. More recently, a study by Mora et al. (2021) introduced single amino acid analysis of collagen serine δ^{13}C as a novel biomarker for tuberculosis infection in archaeological remains. Both bulk isotopic and amino acid-specific analytical approaches in bones and in teeth demonstrate the potential created by uniting paleopathological and isotopic data to produce direct evidence for disease.

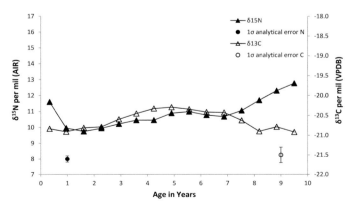

Figure 7.1 Carbon (δ^{13}C) and nitrogen (δ^{15}N) stable isotope incremental dentine collagen data for an adolescent with tuberculosis, showing the onset of wasting from around seven years of age.

Limitations of Current Methods, Ethical Concerns, and Future Directions

Despite the range of opportunities offered by advances in isotopic paleopathology, current methods carry some limitations and ethical concerns, and we will briefly outline these. Finally, we will discuss the range of future developments that offer most promise in addressing questions of health and disease in archaeology.

Confounders

Equifinality, the concept that an end state or value can be reached through multiple input scenarios, has long been a confounder in archaeology. Often blamed when unable to provide a confident provenance for artifacts or individuals (Torrence et al., 1992; Stantis et al., 2020a), equifinality is also a concern for isotopic paleopathology. In much the way that many skeletal lesions can represent nonspecific markers of stress, isotopic evidence of malnutrition or disequilibrium is also nonspecific. Thus, isotopic data must be interpreted tentatively, and with the aid of an often spotty range of contextual aids. Pathological conditions, in addition to having overlapping sequelae, may also be co-morbid, further complicating interpretation. Time resolution in incremental dentine analyses covers a period of several months at a minimum, which may fail to record isotopic shifts of insufficient duration or magnitude. Furthermore, the isotopic parameters of many disease processes are still unresearched or poorly understood. Reynard and Tuross (2015) wrote of the "known, unknown, and unknowable" regarding the parameters of fractionation in breastfeeding; this phrase also applies more generally. For example, thresholds of stress required to arrest bone turnover are not known, nor is the extent of stress-attributable isotopic fractionation prior to that threshold. Similarly, the magnitude of effects on isotopic values is still unknown for many diseases, as we lack the associated clinical studies. Future collaborative work with clinical researchers to document and characterize the isotopic impacts of specific diseases will resolve many of these difficulties and strengthen the interpretative power of isotopic paleopathology.

Though outside the strict bounds of a paleopathological lens, it is worth highlighting that differences in food preparation can result in isotopically similar foods having drastically different social perceptions. Staple foods could be prepared in elaborate and time-intensive ways, such as a simple homemade muffin having overlapping $\delta^{13}C$ and $\delta^{15}N$ values with an elaborate cake eaten at a large gathering. Similarly, isotopes cannot differentiate between the semiotic functions of the same foods served in particular contexts. The cake served at a large birthday party has the same isotopic values as the cake eaten for breakfast when we are sad.

Descendant Communities and the Ethics of Academic Privilege

Isotopic analysis of archaeologically derived human remains destroys a precious, nonrenewable resource. This reality creates a heavier moral responsibility for isotopic researchers than for those using less destructive morphological methods. Furthermore, for descendant groups—particularly Indigenous communities—human remains represent far more than a scientific resource. Outside of Western spirit-body dualities or linear conceptualizations of time, the dead may be viewed as family, equal in consequence to the living (Dumont, 2002). Thus, ancestors in many cultures represent more than links with the bygone past; they are central to the formation of narratives that direct present and future identities. Western objectification, depersonalization, and scientific commodification of ancestral human remains have been roundly criticized by Indigenous communities (Wilcox, 2010; Reardon & Tall-Bear, 2012). In this context, presumption of academic privilege and the imposition of Western ideologies have created significant friction and discord between descendant communities and some archaeologists.

Isotopic research should be global and diverse but should prioritize scientific opportunity below the needs of descendant communities. While isotopic analyses are not always at odds with Indigenous cultures and histories, which are not monolithic, long-term engagement and the creation of meaningful relationships will produce superior insights compared to "helicopter research" that involves sampling, analysis, and publication without the involvement of descendant communities. Such research is not only inherently exploitative but also often fails to understand the limitations of its understanding. Discussions around conflict between Western worldviews and descendant communities have tended to center on settler societies in North America, Australia, and Aotearoa but important questions are being asked by a multitude of voices (McNiven & Russell, 2008; Mehari et al., 2014; Pikirayi, 2015; Meihana & Bradley, 2018; Lans, 2021). Ethical, cooperative, and consensual partnerships must be forged with Indigenous communities, which acknowledge their cultural sovereignty and respect Indigenous knowledge.

Future Directions for Isotopic Paleopathology

Isotopic paleopathology presents a wealth of opportunity for future methodological and theoretical advances. Work to augment our existing knowledge of disease biodynamics among the isotopes in widespread use, particularly $\delta^{13}C$ and $\delta^{15}N$, through observational studies will greatly increase the range of questions that paleopathologists and isotope researchers are able to address using these methods.

Jaouen and Pons (2017) have suggested that analysis of newer, non-traditional isotope systems in archaeology—such as calcium, copper, iron, zinc, and magnesium — may provide more specific tracers of metabolic function and disease processes than the "classic" isotopes currently in use and could provide a useful supplementary tool. For instance, $\delta^{44/42}Ca$ may provide a means to investigate bone disorders, due to the fractionation occurring during bone mineralization (Tacail et al., 2020). Isotopes of copper and sulfur in blood have been used as a medical biomarker of cancer (Balter et al., 2015; Télouk et al., 2015), while isotopes of iron in blood have been used to detect iron deficiency (Van Heghe et al., 2013). Increasing knowledge of common and less commonly used isotopes, and the range of interpretations on health and disease that may be drawn from them, presents an exciting challenge.

The range of tissues that can be isotopically analyzed is also expanding. Analysis of dental calculus, for example, has been proposed as a dietary proxy that avoids destruction of bone or teeth (Poulson et al., 2013), but work must be done before a clear relationship between calculus and collagen values is evident (Salazar-García et al., 2014). Experimental research is also demonstrating that cremated remains, previously avoided over preservation concerns, may present a good analytical target for $^{87}Sr/^{86}Sr$ ratios (Snoeck et al., 2015). This expands options for the study of cultures in the past that routinely integrated cremation into their funerary practices (Snoeck et al., 2018; Grupe et al., 2020).

Isotopic research could be described as subject to theoretical lag. Nonetheless, we are increasingly seeing isotopic insights into understanding how social roles are formed and their subsequent consequences. Excitingly, some isotopic research explicitly incorporates intersectional models of social identity to interpret data on diet and health (e.g., Harvey, 2018; Redfern & Hefner, 2019; Reitsema et al., 2020). The uptake of social theory among paleopathologists and stable isotope researchers is encouraging and hopefully portends a theoretically richer future body of research.

As climate change and pandemic disease become ever greater threats to modern life, understanding the relationships between disease and climate through how they have interacted in the past supersedes mere academic interest. Climatic conditions such as temperature and rainfall are important factors in the transmission of infectious diseases, including bubonic plague and malaria (Tanser et al., 2003; Yue & Lee, 2018). Furthermore, severe climatic fluctuations have been implicated in several historic famines, with heavy impacts on short-term mortality and longer term frailty (McMichael, 2017; Helama et al., 2018).

Frustratingly, studies rarely fulfill the potential offered by explicit integration of paleopathological and paleoclimatic data. Archaeological interest in paleoclimate often relates to its potential role in the rise and fall of major empires, such as the fortunes of imperial Rome, the "collapse" of the Mayan civilization, or the decline of Mycenaean power (McCormick et al., 2012; Douglas et al., 2016; Finné et al., 2017), rather than effects on human health. Additionally, many of the diseases most heavily impacted by climatic fluctuations are acute infections (e.g., bubonic plague) and are usually not observable through traditional osteological methods. However, a small number of studies provide a tantalizing glimpse of the possibilities offered by directly aligning paleoclimatic and paleopathological data. These studies offer evidence for climate's modulating role in diseases such as tuberculosis (Nerlich & Lösch, 2009), micronutrient deficiencies (Koontz Scaffidi, 2020; Snoddy et al., 2020b), nonspecific respiratory disease (Davies-Barrett et al., 2020), and chronic malaria (Setzer, 2010; Bourbou, 2020). Future studies pairing biomolecular paleopathology with paleoclimate data will likely offer further valuable insights.

Conclusion

Isotopic analyses can provide a wealth of insights relevant to human health. Emerging research highlights ways in which isotopic analyses can not only provide evidence of contributory factors to disease such as early life experience, diet, or mobility but can provide direct evidence of disease itself. Interpretation of such evidence is complex, as metabolic, ecological, and cultural factors may add variables that all must be considered as contributing to the data produced. Experimental research continues to identify, isolate, and understand these many variables.

Diet, climate, and mobility continue to be major themes in isotopic research, with population and group-level data providing information on a larger scale. However, increasing emphasis on osteobiographies and longitudinal data provides a quantitative measure of each life in a way that enriches our understanding of the past as a dynamic and personal phenomenon. Although isotopic paleopathology is complex, with many unexplored and unknown parameters currently, this represents a challenge which should be viewed as an opportunity to expand and grow as a discipline. Increased knowledge of the interaction between disease processes and isotopic values not only ultimately aids understanding of past population structures but understanding of the lives of the people who lived in them.

References

Adams, A. B., Halcrow, S., King, C., Miller, M. J., Vlok, M., Millard, A. R. … & Oxenham, M. F. (2021). We're all in this together: accessing the maternal-infant relationship in prehistoric Vietnam. In Kendall, E. J. &. Kendall, R (Eds.), *The Family in Past Perspective: An Interdisciplinary Exploration of Familial Relationships Through Time*. London, United Kingdom: Routledge.

Agarwal, S. C. & Glencross, B. A. (2011). Building a social bioarchaeology. In Agarwal, S. C. & Glencross, B. A. (Eds.), *Social Bioarchaeology*, pp. 1–1. West Sussex, United Kingdom: Wiley-Blackwell.

AlQahtani, S. J., Hector, M. P., & Liversidge, H. M. (2010). The London atlas of human tooth development and eruption. *American Journal of Physical Anthropology* 142(3):481–490. DOI:10.1002/ajpa.21258

Armelagos, G. J., Goodman, A. H., Harper, K. N. & Blakey, M. L. (2009). Enamel hypoplasia and early mortality: bioarcheological support for the Barker hypothesis. *Evolutionary Anthropology: Issues, News, and Reviews* 18(6):261–271. DOI:10.1002/evan.20239

Aronsen, G. P., Fehren-Schmitz, L., Krigbaum, J., Kamenov, G. D., Conlogue, G. J., Warinner, C. ... & Bellantoni, N. F. (2019). "The dead shall be raised": multidisciplinary analysis of human skeletons reveals complexity in 19th century immigrant socioeconomic history and identity in New Haven, Connecticut. *PLoS ONE* 14(9):e0219279. DOI:10.1371/journal.pone.0219279

Balter, V., da Costa, A. N., Bondanese, V. P., Jaouen, K., Lamboux, A., Sangrajrang, S. ... & Gigou, M. (2015). Natural variations of copper and sulfur stable isotopes in blood of hepatocellular carcinoma patients. *Proceedings of the National Academy of Sciences* 112(4):982–985. DOI: 10.1073/pnas.1415151112

Bathurst, R. R. (2005). Archaeological evidence of intestinal parasites from coastal shell middens. *Journal of Archaeological Science* 32(1):115–123. DOI: 10.1016/j.jas.2004.08.001

Beaumont, J. (2020). The whole tooth and nothing but the tooth: or why temporal resolution of bone collagen may be unreliable. *Archaeometry* 62(3):626–645. DOI: 10.1111/arcm.12544

Beaumont, J., Geber, J., Powers, N., Wilson, A., Lee-Thorp, J. & Montgomery, J. (2012). Victims and survivors: stable isotopes used to identify migrants from the great Irish Famine to 19th century London. *American Journal of Physical Anthropology* 150(1):87–98. DOI: 10.1002/ajpa.22179

Beaumont, J., Gledhill, A. & Montgomery, J. (2014). Isotope analysis of incremental human dentine: towards higher temporal resolution. *Bulletin of the International Association for Paleodontology* 8(2): 212–223. DOI: 10.1073/pnas.1415151112

Beaumont, J. & Montgomery, J. (2016). The great Irish famine: Identifying starvation in the tissues of victims using stable isotope analysis of bone and incremental dentine collagen. *PloS One* 11(8):e0160065. DOI: 10.1371/journal.pone.0160065

Bender, M. M. (1968). Mass spectrometric studies of carbon 13 variations in corn and other grasses. *Radiocarbon* 10(2):468–472. DOI: 10.1017/S0033822200011103

Binford, L. R. (1987). Data, relativism and archaeological science. *Man* 22(3):391–404. DOI: 10.2307/2802497

Bourbou, C. (2020). Health and disease at the marshes: deciphering the human-environment interaction at Roman Aventicum, Switzerland (1st–3rd c. AD). In Robbins Schug, G. R. (Ed.), *The Routledge Handbook of the Bioarchaeology of Climate and Environmental Change*, pp. 141–155. Abingdon: Routledge.

Brettell, R., Montgomery, J. & Evans, J. (2012). Brewing and stewing: the effect of culturally mediated behaviour on the oxygen isotope composition of ingested fluids and the implications for human provenance studies. *Journal of Analytical Atomic Spectrometry* 27(5):778–785. DOI: 10.1039/C2JA10335D

Britton, K., Fuller, B. T., Tütken, T., Mays, S. & Richards, M. P. (2015). Oxygen isotope analysis of human bone phosphate evidences weaning age in archaeological populations. *American Journal of Physical Anthropology* 157(2):226–241. DOI: 10.1002/ajpa.22704

Budd, P., Millard, A., Chenery, C., Lucy, S. & Roberts, C. (2004). Investigating population movement by stable isotope analysis: a report from Britain. *Antiquity. A Quarterly Review of Archaeology* 78(299):127–141. DOI: 10.1017/S0003598X0009298X

Carroll, G. M., Inskip, S. A. & Waters-Rist, A. (2018). Pathophysiological stable isotope fractionation: assessing the impact of anemia on enamel apatite $\delta^{18}O$ and $\delta^{13}C$ values and bone collagen $\delta^{15}N$ and $\delta^{13}C$ values. *Bioarchaeology International* 2(2):117–146. DOI: 10.5744/bi.2018.1021

Cheung, C., Jing, Z., Tang, J., Weston, D. A. & Richards, M. P. (2017). Diets, social roles, and geographical origins of sacrificial victims at the royal cemetery at Yinxu, Shang China: new evidence from stable carbon, nitrogen, and sulfur isotope analysis. *Journal of Anthropological Archaeology* 48:28–45. DOI: 10.1016/j.jaa.2017.05.006

Chisholm, B. S., Nelson, D. E. & Schwarcz, H. P. (1982). Stable-carbon isotope ratios as a measure of marine versus terrestrial protein in ancient diets. *Science* 216(4550):1131–1132. DOI: 10.1126/science.216.4550.1131

Cohen, M. N. & Armelagos, G. J. (Eds.) (1984). *Paleopathology at the Origins of Agriculture*. Orlando: Academic Press, Inc.

Colleter, R., Clavel, B., Pietrzak, A., Duchesne, S., Schmitt, L., Richards, M. P. … & Jaouen, K. (2019). Social status in late medieval and early modern Brittany: insights from stable isotope analysis. *Archaeological and Anthropological Sciences* 11(3):823–837. DOI: 10.1007/s12520-017-0547-9

Cooper, C. G., Lupo, K. D., Zena, A. G., Schmitt, D. N. & Richards, M. P. (2019). Stable isotope ratio analysis (C, N, S) of hair from modern humans in Ethiopia shows clear differences related to subsistence regimes. *Archaeological and Anthropological Sciences* 11(7):3213–3223. DOI: 10.1007/s12520-018-0740-5

Crowder, K. D., Montgomery, J., Gröcke, D. R. & Filipek, K. L. (2019). Childhood "stress" and stable isotope life histories in Transylvania. *International Journal of Osteoarchaeology* 29(4):644–653. DOI:10.1002/oa.2760

Cybulski, J. S. (1977). Cribra orbitalia, a possible sign of anemia in early historic native populations of the British Columbia coast. *American Journal of Physical Anthropology* 47(1):31–39. DOI:10.1002/ajpa.1330470108

Davies-Barrett, A. M., Antoine, D. & Roberts C. A. (2020). Respiratory disease in the Middle Nile Valley: the impact of environment and aridification. In Robbins Schug, G. R. (Ed.), *The Routledge Handbook of the Bioarchaeology of Climate and Environmental Change*, pp. 122–140. Abingdon: Routledge.

Dickson, J. H., Richards, M. P., Hebda, R. J., Mudie, P. J., Beattie, O., Ramsay, S. … & Wigen, R. J. (2004). Kwäday Dän Ts'ìnchì, the first ancient body of a man from a North American glacier: reconstructing his last days by intestinal and biomolecular analyses. *The Holocene* 14(4):481–486. DOI:10.1191/0959683604hl742rp

Dittmann, K. & Grupe, G. (2000). Biochemical and palaeopathological investigations on weaning and infant mortality in the early middle ages. *Anthropologischer Anzeiger* 58(4):345–355.

D'Ortenzio, L., Brickley, M., Schwarcz, H. & Prowse, T. (2015). You are not what you eat during physiological stress: isotopic evaluation of human hair. *American Journal of Physical Anthropology* 157(3):374–388. DOI:10.1002/ajpa.22722

Douglas, P. M. J., Demarest, A. A., Brenner, M. & Canuto M. A. (2016). Impacts of climate change on the collapse of Lowland Maya civilization. *Annual Review of Earth and Planetary Sciences* 44(1):613–645. DOI:10.1146/annurev-earth-060115-012512

Dumont, C. (2002). Dead family or archaeological collections? On the significance of native dead. *Race, Gender & Class* 9(2):8–31.

Eerkens, J. W., Berget, A. G. & Bartelink, E. J. (2011). Estimating weaning and early childhood diet from serial micro-samples of dentin collagen. *Journal of Archaeological Science* 38(11):3101–3111. DOI:http://dx.doi.org/10.1016/j.jas.2011.07.010

Engelstad, E. (1991). Images of power and contradiction: Feminist theory and post-processual archaeology. *Antiquity* 65(248): 502–514. DOI:10.1017/s0003598x00080108

Finné, M., Holmgren, K., Shen, C.-C., Hu, H.-M., Boyd, M. & Stocker, S. (2017). Late Bronze Age climate change and the destruction of the Mycenaean Palace of Nestor at Pylos. *PLoS ONE* 12(12):e0189447. DOI:10.1371/journal.pone.0189447

Fleming, T. P., Eckert, J. J. & Denisenko, O. (2017). The role of maternal nutrition during the periconceptional period and its effect on offspring phenotype. *Advances in Experimental Medicine and Biology* 1014: 87–105.

Fogel, M. L., Tuross, N. & Owsley, D. W. (1989). Nitrogen isotope tracers of human lactation in modern and archaeological populations. *Carnegie Institution of Washington Yearbook* 88:111–117.

Fuller, B. T., Richards, M. P. & Mays, S. A. (2003). Stable carbon and nitrogen isotope variations in tooth dentine serial sections from Wharram Percy. *Journal of Archaeological Science* 30(12):1673–1684. DOI:http://dx.doi.org/10.1016/S0305-4403(03)00073-6

Gero, J. M. & Conkey, M. W. (Eds.) (1991). *Engendering Archaeology: Women and Prehistory*. Oxford: Wiley-Blackwell.

Gilchrist, R. (2007). Archaeology and the life course: a time and age for gender. In Meskell, L. & Preucel, R. W. (Eds.), *A Companion to Social Archaeology*, pp. 142–160. Malden, MA: Blackwell Publishing.

Gluckman, P. D., Hanson, M. A., Cooper, C. & Thornburg, K. L. (2008). Effect of in utero and early-life conditions on adult health and disease. *The New England Journal of Medicine* 359(1):61–73. DOI:10.1056/NEJMra0708473

Goude, G., Dori, I., Sparacello, V. S., Starnini, E. & Varalli, A. (2020). Multi-proxy stable isotope analyses of dentine microsections reveal diachronic changes in life history adaptations, mobility, and tuberculosis-induced wasting in prehistoric liguria (Finale Ligure, Italy, northwestern Mediterranean). *International Journal of Paleopathology* 28:99–111. DOI: 10.1016/j.ijpp.2019.12.007

Gowland, R. & Knüsel, C. (2006). *Social Archaeology of Funerary Remains*. Oxford: Oxbow.

Gowland, R. L. (2015). Entangled lives: implications of the developmental origins of health and disease hypothesis for bioarchaeology and the life course. *American Journal of Physical Anthropology* 158(4):530–540. DOI:10.1002/ajpa.22820

Gowland, R. L. & Western, A. G. (2012). Morbidity in the marshes: using spatial epidemiology to investigate skeletal evidence for malaria in Anglo-Saxon England (AD 410–1050). *American Journal of Physical Anthropology* 147(2):301–311. DOI:10.1002/ajpa.21648

Grupe, G., Klaut, D., Otto, L., Mauder, M., Lohrer, J., Kröger, P. & Lang, A. (2020). The genesis and spread of the early Fritzens-Sanzeno culture (5th/4th cent. BCE) – Stable isotope analysis of cremated and uncremated skeletal finds. *Journal of Archaeological Science: Reports* 29:102121. DOI: 10.1016/j.jasrep.2019.102121

Harvey, A. R. (2018). *An Analysis of Maya Foodways: Stable Isotopes and Oral Indicators of Diet in West Central Belize*. Doctoral Dissertation, University of Nevada: Reno.

Hedges, R. E. M., Clement, J. G., Thomas, C. D. L. & O'Connell, T. C. (2007). Collagen turnover in the adult femoral mid-shaft: modeled from anthropogenic radiocarbon tracer measurements. *American Journal of Physical Anthropology* 133(2):808–816. DOI:10.1002/ajpa.20598

Helama, S., Arppe, L., Uusitalo, J., Holopainen, J., Mäkelä, H. M., Mäkinen, H. ... & Oinonen, M. (2018). Volcanic dust veils from sixth century tree-ring isotopes linked to reduced irradiance, primary production and human health. *Scientific Reports* 8(1):1339. DOI:10.1038/s41598-018-19760-w

Henderson, R. C., Lee-Thorp, J. & Loe, L. (2014). Early life histories of the London poor using $\delta^{13}C$ and $\delta^{15}N$ stable isotope incremental dentine sampling. *American Journal of Physical Anthropology* 154(4):585–593. DOI:10.1002/ajpa.22554

Hodder, I. (1991). Interpretive archaeology and its role. *American Antiquity* 56(1):7–18.

Hoefs, J. (2009). *Stable Isotope Geochemistry* (6th ed.). Berlin, Germany: Springer-Verlag.

Howcroft, R., Eriksson, G. & Lidén, K. (2012). Conformity in diversity? Isotopic investigations of infant feeding practices in two Iron age populations from southern Öland, Sweden. *American Journal of Physical Anthropology* 149:217–230. DOI:10.1002/ajpa.22113

Hutchinson, D. L., Larsen, C. S., Schoeninger, M. J. & Norr, L. (1998). Regional variation in the pattern of maize adoption and use in Florida and Georgia. *American Antiquity* 63(3):397–416. DOI:10.2307/2694627

Jaouen, K. & Pons, M.-L. (2017). Potential of non-traditional isotope studies for bioarchaeology. *Archaeological and Anthropological Sciences* 9(7):1389–1404. DOI:10.1007/s12520-016-0426–9

Kamp, K. A. (2001). Where have all the children gone?: The archaeology of childhood. *Journal of Archaeological Method and Theory* 8(1):1–34.

Katzenberg, M. A. & Lovell, N. C. (1999). Stable isotope variation in pathological bone. *International Journal of Osteoarchaeology* 9(5):316–324.

Katzenberg, M. A. & Pfeiffer, S. (1995). Nitrogen isotope evidence for weaning age in a nineteenth century Canadian skeletal sample. In Grauer, A. L. (Ed.), *Bodies of Evidence: Reconstructing History Through Skeletal Analysis*, pp. 221–236. New York: Wiley-Liss.

Kendall, E. (2019). *An Isotopic Study of Environmental Influences on Early Anglo-Saxon Health and Nutrition*. Doctoral Dissertation. Durham University, Durham.

Kendall, E., Millard, A. & Beaumont, J. (2021). The "weanling's dilemma" revisited: evolving bodies of evidence and the problem of infant paleodietary interpretation. *American Journal of Physical Anthropology* 175 Suppl 72:57–78. DOI:10.1002/ajpa.24207

Kendall, E. J., Millard, A., Beaumont, J., Gowland, R., Gorton, M. & Gledhill, A. (2020). What doesn't kill you: early life health and nutrition in early Anglo-Saxon East Anglia. In. Gowland, R. & Halcrow, S. (Eds.), *The Mother-Infant Nexus in Anthropology: Small Beginnings, Significant Outcomes*, pp. 103–123. Cham: Springer International Publishing.

Kendall, E. J., Montgomery, J., Evans, J. A., Stantis, C. & Mueller, V. (2013). Mobility, mortality, and the Middle Ages: identification of migrant individuals in a 14th century black death cemetery population. *American Journal of Physical Anthropology* 150(2):210–222. DOI:10.1002/ajpa.22194

Koontz Scaffidi, B. (2020). Spatial paleopathology: a geographic approach to the etiology of cribrotic lesions in the prehistoric Andes. *International Journal of Paleopathology* 29:102–116. DOI: 10.1016/j.ijpp.2019.07.002

Lans, A. M. (2021). Decolonize this collection: integrating black feminism and art to re-examine human skeletal remains in museums. *Feminist Anthropology* 2(1): 130–142. DOI: 10.1002/fea2.12027

Larsen, C. S. (1995). Biological changes in human populations with agriculture. *Annual Review of Anthropology* 24(1):185–213. DOI:10.1146/annurev.an.24.100195.001153

Longin, R. (1971). New method of collagen extraction for radiocarbon dating. *Nature* 230(5291): 241–242. DOI:10.1038/230241a0

Lynott, M. J., Boutton, T. W., Price, J. E. & Nelson, D. E. (1986). Stable carbon isotopic evidence for maize agriculture in southeast Missouri and northeast Arkansas. *American Antiquity* 51(1):51–65.

McCormick, M., Büntgen, U., Cane, M. A., Cook, E. R., Harper, K., Huybers, P., ... & Tegel, W. (2012). Climate change during and after the Roman empire: reconstructing the past from scientific and historical evidence. *The Journal of Interdisciplinary History* 43(2):169–220. DOI:10.1162/JINH_a_00379

McMichael, A. (2017). *Climate Change and the Health of Nations: Famines, Fevers, and the Fate of Populations.* Oxford, United Kingdom: Oxford University Press.

McNiven, I. J. & Russell, L. (2008). Toward a postcolonial archaeology of Indigenous Australia. In Bentley, R. A., Maschner, H. D. G. & Chippendale, C. (Eds.), *Handbook of Archaeological Theories*, pp. 423–443. Lanham, Maryland: AltaMira Press.

Mehari, A. G., Schmidt, P. R. & Mapunda, B. B. (2014). Knowledge about archaeological field schools in Africa: the Tanzanian experience. *Azania: Archaeological Research in Africa* 49(2):184–202. DOI:10.1080/0067270X.2014.912492

Meihana, P. N. & Bradley, C. R. (2018). Repatriation, reconciliation and the inversion of patriarchy. *The Journal of the Polynesian Society* 127(3):307. DOI:10.15286/jps.127.3.307–324

Millard, A. R., Annis, R. G., Caffell, A. C., Dodd, L. L., Fischer, R., Gerrard, C. M.... & Speller, C. F. (2020). Scottish soldiers from the battle of Dunbar 1650: a prosopographical approach to a skeletal assemblage. *PLoS ONE* 15(12):e0243369. DOI:10.1371/journal.pone.0243369

Millard, A. R., Roberts, C. A. & Hughes, S. S. (2005). Isotopic evidence for migration in Medieval England: the potential for tracking the introduction of disease. *Society, Biology and Human Affairs* 70(1):9–13.

Mora, A., Pacheco, A., Roberts, C. A. & Smith, C. (2021). Palaeopathology and amino acid $\delta^{13}C$ analysis: investigating pre-Columbian individuals with tuberculosis at Pica 8, Northern Chile (1050–500 BP). *Journal of Archaeological Science* 129:105367. https://doi.org/10.1016/j.jas.2021.105367

Moreiras Reynaga, D. K., Millaire, J., García Chávez, R. E. & Longstaffe, F. J. (2020). Aztec diets at the residential site of San Cristobal Ecatepec through stable carbon and nitrogen isotope analysis of bone collagen. *Archaeological and Anthropological Sciences* 12:216. https://doi.org/10.1007/s12520-020-01174-3

Nehlich, O., Fuller, B. T., Jay, M., Mora, A., Nicholson, R. A., Smith, C. I. & Richards, M. P. (2011). Application of sulphur isotope ratios to examine weaning patterns and freshwater fish consumption in Roman Oxfordshire, UK. *Geochimica et Cosmochimica Acta* 75(17):4963–4977. DOI:10.1016/j.gca.2011.06.009

Nerlich, A. G. & Lösch, S. (2009). Paleopathology of human tuberculosis and the potential role of climate. *Interdisciplinary Perspectives on Infectious Diseases* 2009:437187. DOI:10.1155/2009/437187

Okazaki, K., Takamuku, H., Yonemoto, S., Itahashi, Y., Gakuhari, T., Yoneda, M. & Chen, J. (2019). A paleopathological approach to early human adaptation for wet-rice agriculture: the first case of Neolithic spinal tuberculosis at the Yangtze River Delta of China. *International Journal of Paleopathology* 24:236–244. DOI: 10.1016/j.ijpp.2019.01.002

Olsen, K. C., White, C. D., Longstaffe, F. J., von Heyking, K., McGlynn, G., Grupe, G. & Rühli, F. J. (2014). Intraskeletal isotopic compositions ($\delta^{13}C$, $\delta^{15}N$) of bone collagen: nonpathological and pathological variation. *American Journal of Physical Anthropology* 153(4):598–604. DOI:10.1002/ajpa.22459

Ortner, D. J. (2003). *Identification of Pathological Conditions in Human Skeletal Remains.* Washington, DC: Smithsonian Institution Press.

Pacheco-Forés, S. I., Morehart, C.T., Buikstra, J. E., Gordon, G. W. & Knudson, K. J. (2021). Migration, violence, and the "other": a biogeochemical approach to identity-based violence in the epiclassic basin of Mexico. *Journal of Anthropological Archaeology* 61:101263. https://doi.org/10.1016/j.jaa.2020.101263

Pikirayi, I. (2015). The future of archaeology in Africa. *Antiquity. A Quarterly Review of Archaeology* 89(345): 531–541. DOI: 10.15184/aqy.2015.31

Pilloud, M. A. & Schwitalla, A. W. (2020). Re-evaluating traditional markers of stress in an archaeological sample from central California. *Journal of Archaeological Science* 116:105102. DOI: 10.1016/j.jas.2020.105102

Plomp, E., von Holstein, I. C. C., Kootker, L. M., Verdegaal-Warmerdam, S. J. A., Forouzanfar, T. & Davies, G. R. (2020). Strontium, oxygen, and carbon isotope variation in modern human dental enamel. *American Journal of Physical Anthropology* 172(4):586–604. DOI:10.1002/ajpa.24059

Poulson, S. R., Kuzminsky, S. C., Scott, G. R., Standen, V. G., Arriaza, B., Muñoz, I. & Dorio, L. (2013). Paleodiet in northern Chile through the Holocene: extremely heavy $\delta15N$ values in dental calculus suggest a guano-derived signature? *Journal of Archaeological Science* 40(12):4576–4585. DOI:http://dx.doi.org/10.1016/j.jas.2013.07.009

Reardon, J. & TallBear, K. (2012). "Your DNA is our history": genomics, anthropology, and the construction of whiteness as property. *Current Anthropology* 53(S5):S233–S245. DOI:10.1086/662629

Redfern, R., DeWitte, S., Montgomery, J. & Gowland, R. (2018). A novel investigation into migrant and local health-statuses in the past: a case study from Roman Britain. *Bioarchaeology International*, 2(1):20–43. DOI: 10.5744/bi.2018.1014

Redfern, R. & Hefner, J. T. (2019). "Officially absent but actually present": bioarchaeological evidence for population diversity in London during the black death, AD 1348–1350. In Mant, M. L. & Holland, A. J. (Eds.), *Bioarchaeology of Marginalized People*, pp. 69–114. Cambridge, MA: Academic Press.

Reitsema, L. J. & Crews, D. E. (2011). Brief communication: oxygen isotopes as a biomarker for sickle-cell disease? Results from transgenic mice expressing human hemoglobin S genes. *American Journal of Physical Anthropology* 145(3):495–498. DOI:10.1002/ajpa.21513

Reitsema, L. J., Kyle, B. & Vassallo, S. (2020). Food traditions and colonial interactions in the ancient Mediterranean: stable isotope evidence from the Greek Sicilian colony Himera. *Journal of Anthropological Archaeology* 57:101144. DOI: 10.1016/j.jaa.2020.101144

Reitsema, L. J., Vercellotti, G. & Boano, R. (2016). Subadult dietary variation at Trino Vercellese, Italy, and its relationship to adult diet and mortality. *American Journal of Physical Anthropology* 160(4):653–664. DOI:10.1002/ajpa.22995

Reynard, L. M. & Tuross, N. (2015). The known, the unknown and the unknowable: Weaning times from archaeological bones using nitrogen isotope ratios. *Journal of Archaeological Science* 53(0):618–625. DOI:http://dx.doi.org/10.1016/j.jas.2014.11.018

Roberts, C. A. (2018). The bioarchaeology of leprosy: Learning from the past. In Scollard, D. M. & Gillis, T. P. (Eds.), *International Textbook of Leprosy,* American Leprosy Mission. https://internationaltextbook ofleprosy.org/chapter/bioarchaeology-leprosy-learning-skeletons

Roberts, C. A. & Buikstra, J. E. (2003). *The Bioarchaeology of Tuberculosis: A Global Perspective on a Re-emerging Disease*. Gainesville, Florida: University Press of Florida.

Roberts, C. A., Millard, A., Nowell, G. M., Gröcke, D. R., Macpherson, C. G., Pearson, D. G. & Evans, D. H. (2013).Isotopic tracing of the impact of mobility on infectious disease: the origin of people with treponematosis buried in hull, England, in the late medieval period. *American Journal of Physical Anthropology* 150(2):273–285. DOI:10.1002/ajpa.22203

Ryan, S. E., Reynard, L. M., Pompianu, E., van Dommelen, P., Murgia, C., Subirà, M. E. & Tuross, N. (2020). Growing up in Ancient Sardinia: infant-toddler dietary changes revealed by the novel use of hydrogen isotopes (δ^2H). *PloS One* 15(7):e0235080. DOI:10.1371/journal.pone.0235080

Salazar-García, D. C., Richards, M. P., Nehlich, O. & Henry, A. G. (2014). Dental calculus is not equivalent to bone collagen for isotope analysis: a comparison between carbon and nitrogen stable isotope analysis of bulk dental calculus, bone and dentine collagen from same individuals from the Medieval site of El Raval (Alicante, Spain). *Journal of Archaeological Science* 47(0):70–77. DOI:http://dx.doi.org/10.1016/j.jas.2014.03.026

Salesse, K., Kaupová, S., Brůžek, J., Kuželka, V. & Velemínský, P. (2019). An isotopic case study of individuals with syphilis from the pathological-anatomical reference collection of the national museum in Prague (Czech Republic, 19th century A.D.). *International Journal of Paleopathology* 25:46–55. DOI: 10.1016/j.ijpp.2019.04.001

Sandberg, P. A., Sponheimer, M., Lee-Thorp, J. & Van Gerven, D. (2014). Intra-tooth stable isotope analysis of dentine: a step toward addressing selective mortality in the reconstruction of life history in the archaeological record. *American Journal of Physical Anthropology* 155(2):281–293. DOI:10.1002/ajpa.22600

Scorrano, G., Brilli, M., Martínez-Labarga, C., Giustini, F., Pacciani, E., Chilleri, F.... & Rickards, O. (2014). Palaeodiet reconstruction in a woman with probable celiac disease: a stable isotope analysis of bone remains from the archaeological site of Cosa (Italy). *American Journal of Physical Anthropology* 154(3):349–356. DOI:10.1002/ajpa.22517

Setzer, T. J. (2010). *Malaria in Prehistoric Sardinia (Italy): An Examination of Skeletal Remains From the Middle Bronze Age*. Tampa: Doctoral Dissertation, University of South Florida

Sharp, Z. D. (2017). *Principles of Stable Isotope Geochemistry, Second Edition*. Published Online.

Sillen, A. & Smith, P. (1984). Weaning patterns are reflected in strontium-calcium ratios of juvenile skeletons. *Journal of Archaeological Science* 11(3):237–245. DOI:10.1016/0305–4403(84)90004-9

Smith-Guzmán, N. E. (2015). The skeletal manifestation of malaria: an epidemiological approach using documented skeletal collections. *American Journal of Physical Anthropology* 158(4):624–635. DOI:10.1002/ajpa.22819

Smith, B. N. & Epstein, S. (1971). Two categories of $^{13}C/^{12}C$ ratios for higher plants. *Plant Physiology* 47(3):380. DOI:10.1104/pp.47.3.380

Smith, T. M. & Tafforeau, P. (2008). New visions of dental tissue research: tooth development, chemistry, and structure. *Evolutionary Anthropology: Issues, News, and Reviews* 17(5):213–226. DOI:10.1002/evan.20176

Snoddy, A. M., Buckley, H., King, C., Kinaston, R., Nowell, G., Gröcke, D. ... & Petchey, P. (2020a). 'Captain of all these men of death': an integrated case study of tuberculosis in nineteenth-century Otago, New Zealand. *Bioarchaeology International* 3(4):217–237. DOI: 10.5744/bi.2019.1014

Snoddy, A. M., King, C. L., Halcrow, S. E., Millard, A. R., Buckley, H. R., Standen, V. G. & Arriaza, B. T. (2020b). Living on the edge: climate-induced micronutrient famines in the ancient Atacama desert? In Robbins Schug, G. R. (Ed.), *The Routledge Handbook of the Bioarchaeology of Climate and Environmental Change*, pp. 60–82. Abingdon: Routledge.

Snoeck, C., Lee-Thorp, J., Schulting, R., de Jong, J., Debouge, W. & Mattielli, N. (2015). Calcined bone provides a reliable substrate for strontium isotope ratios as shown by an enrichment experiment. *Rapid Communications in Mass Spectrometry* 29(1):107–114. DOI: 10.1002/rcm.7078

Snoeck, C., Pouncett, J., Claeys, P., Goderis, S., Mattielli, N., Parker Pearson, M. ... & Schulting, R. J. (2018). Strontium isotope analysis on cremated human remains from stonehenge support links with west wales. *Scientific Reports* 8(1):10790. DOI:10.1038/s41598-018-28969-8

Stantis, C., Buckley, H. R., Commendador, A. & Dudgeon, J. V. (2021). Expanding on incremental dentin methodology to investigate childhood and infant feeding practices on Taumako (southeast Solomon Islands). *Journal of Archaeological Science* 126:105294. DOI: 10.1016/j.jas.2020.105294

Stantis, C., Buckley, H. R., Kinaston, R. L., Nunn, P. D., Jaouen, K. & Richards, M. P. (2016). Isotopic evidence of human mobility and diet in a prehistoric/protohistoric Fijian coastal environment (c. 750–150 BP). *American Journal of Physical Anthropology* 159(3):478–495. DOI:10.1002/ajpa.22884

Stantis, C., Kharobi, A., Maaranen, N., Nowell, G. M., Bietak, M., Prell, S. & Schutkowski, H. (2020a). Who were the Hyksos? Challenging traditional narratives using strontium isotope ($^{87}Sr/^{86}Sr$) analysis of human remains from ancient Egypt. *PloS One* 15(7):e0235414. DOI:10.1371/journal.pone.0235414

Stantis, C., Kinaston, R. L., Richards, M. P., Davidson, J. M. & Buckley, H. R. (2015). Assessing human diet and movement in the Tongan maritime chiefdom using isotopic analyses. *PloS One* 10(3):e0123156. DOI:10.1371/journal.pone.0123156

Stantis, C., Schutkowski, H. & Sołtysiak, A. (2020b). Reconstructing breastfeeding and weaning practices in the bronze age near east using stable nitrogen isotopes. *American Journal of Physical Anthropology* 172(1):58–69. DOI:10.1002/ajpa.23980

Suby, J. A. (2014). Porotic hyperostosis and cribra orbitalia in human remains from southern Patagonia. *Anthropological Science* 122(2):69–79. DOI:10.1537/ase.140430

Szulc, P., Seeman, E. & Delmas, P. (2000). Biochemical measurements of bone turnover in children and adolescents. *Osteoporosis International* 11(4):281–294. DOI: 10.1007/s001980070116

Tacail, T., Le Houedec, S. & Skulan, J. L. (2020). New frontiers in calcium stable isotope geochemistry: perspectives in present and past vertebrate biology. *Chemical Geology* 537:119471. DOI: 10.1016/j.chemgeo.2020.119471

Tanser, F. C., Sharp, B. & le Sueur, D. (2003). Potential effect of climate change on malaria transmission in Africa. *The Lancet* 362(9398):1792–1798. DOI: 10.1016/S0140–6736(03)14898-2

Taylor, G. M., Murphy, E. M., Mendum, T. A., Pike, A. W. G., Linscott, B., Wu, H. ... & Stewart, G. R. (2018). Leprosy at the edge of Europe—Biomolecular, isotopic and osteoarchaeological findings from medieval Ireland. *PloS One* 13(12):e0209495. DOI:10.1371/journal.pone.0209495

Télouk, P., Puisieux, A., Fujii, T., Balter, V., Bondanese, V. P., Morel, A.-P. ... & Albarede, F. (2015). Copper isotope effect in serum of cancer patients. A pilot study. *Metallomics* 7(2):299–308. DOI: 10.1039/c4mt00269e

Torrence, R., Specht, J., Fullagar, R. & Bird, R. (1992). From Pleistocene to present: obsidian sources in West New Britain, Papua New Guinea. *Records of the Australian Museum* Supplement 15:83–98.

Trigger, B. G. (1989). *A History of Archaeological Thought*. Cambridge, United Kingdom: Cambridge University Press.

Twiss, K. (2012). The archaeology of food and social diversity. *Journal of Archaeological Research* 20(4):357–395. DOI:10.1007/s10814-012-9058-5

Van der Merwe, N. J. & Vogel, J. C. (1978). ^{13}C content of human collagen as a measure of prehistoric diet in Woodland North America. *Nature* 276(5690): 815–816.

Van Heghe, L., Delanghe, J., Van Vlierberghe, H. & Vanhaecke, F. (2013). The relationship between the iron isotopic composition of human whole blood and iron status parameters. *Metallomics* 5(11):1503–1509. DOI: 10.1039/c3mt00054k

Victora, C. G., Adair, L., Fall, C., Hallal, P. C., Martorell, R., Richter, L. ... & Child Undernutrition Study, G. (2008). Maternal and child undernutrition: consequences for adult health and human capital. *Lancet* 371(9609):340–357. DOI:10.1016/s0140-6736(07)61692-4

Vogel, J. C. & Van Der Merwe, N. J. (1977). Isotopic evidence for early maize cultivation in New York State. *American Antiquity* 42(2):238–242. DOI:10.2307/278984

Walker, P. L. (1986). Porotic hyperostosis in a marine-dependent California Indian population. *American Journal of Physical Anthropology* 69(3):345–354. DOI:10.1002/ajpa.1330690307

Warinner, C., & Tuross, N. (2010). Brief communication: Tissue isotopic enrichment associated with growth depression in a pig: implications for archaeology and ecology. *American Journal of Physical Anthropology* 141(3):486–493. DOI:10.1002/ajpa.21222

Watts, R. (2015). The long-term impact of developmental stress. evidence from later medieval and post-medieval London (AD1117–1853). *American Journal of Physical Anthropology* 158(4):569–580. DOI:10.1002/ajpa.22810

Weinbrenner, T., Zittermann, A., Gouni-Berthold, I., Stehle, P. & Berthold, H. K. (2003). Body mass index and disease duration are predictors of disturbed bone turnover in anorexia nervosa. A case–control study. *European Journal of Clinical Nutrition* 57:1262. DOI:10.1038/sj.ejcn.1601683

White, C. D. & Armelagos, G. J. (1997). Osteopenia and stable isotope ratios in bone collagen of Nubian female mummies. *American Journal of Physical Anthropology* 103(2):185–199.

White, C. D., Longstaffe, F. J. & Law, K. R. (2004). Exploring the effects of environment, physiology and diet on oxygen isotope ratios in ancient Nubian bones and teeth. *Journal of Archaeological Science* 31(2):233–250. DOI:10.1016/j.jas.2003.08.007

White, J. M., Bégin, F., Kumapley, R., Murray, C. & Krasevec, J. (2017). Complementary feeding practices: current global and regional estimates. *Maternal & Child Nutrition* 13(S2):e12505. DOI:10.1111/mcn.12505

Wilcox, M. (2010). Saving Indigenous Peoples from ourselves: separate but equal archaeology is not Scientific archaeology. *American Antiquity* 75(2):221–227.

Wood, J. W., Milner, G. R., Harpending, H. C. & Weiss, K. M. (1992). The osteological paradox: problems of inferring prehistoric health from skeletal samples. *Current Anthropology* 33(4):343–370.

Yue, R. P. H. & Lee, H. F. (2018). Climate change and plague history in Europe. *Science China Earth Sciences* 61(2):163–177. DOI:10.1007/s11430-017-9127-x

8
GENETICS AND GENOMICS

Susanna Sabin and Anne C. Stone

Introduction

The co-application of genetic data and traditional paleopathology to the study of human health through deep time opens pathways for increasing understanding of the human experience, human evolution, and pathogen evolution. Ancient DNA (aDNA) can offer direct molecular evidence of heritable conditions, cancers, individual microbes, and microbial communities from the past. With the acquisition of trustworthy aDNA, genetic data may supplement skeletal analysis by providing diagnosis with increased confidence or a window into health-related processes that did not leave skeletal changes. In this way, genetic and genomic approaches employed in paleopathology may strengthen and broaden its capacity for knowledge generation. Modern genomics also contributes to this capacity by providing genetic, temporal, and geographic context to ancient findings. aDNA research allows us to confirm not only the presence of a given pathogen, commensal microbe, or heritable condition in the long deceased but also to trace its relationship to humans through time and space and make inferences regarding human and pathogen evolution (see Box 8.1 for a glossary of common terms used in the field).

Box 8.1 Glossary of Terms

Bayesian phylogenetics: The application of Bayesian principles to phylogenetic inference (see **phylogenetics** below), in which "priors" in the form of model parameters are supplied and the posterior probability of each model can be calculated.

Capture/enrichment: The fishing-out of target DNA from a metagenomic sample, the washing-away of non-target DNA, and subsequent amplification of target DNA.

Contig: A unit of overlapping sequencing reads used in the computational assembly of a genomic sequence.

***De novo* assembly:** The computational reconstruction of a genomic sequence based on the assembly of overlapping sequencing reads into contigs and contigs into a contiguous sequence without the aid of a reference sequence.

Endogenous DNA: DNA that is (or is expected to be) directly from the sample under analysis, as opposed to exogenous, contaminant DNA.

Extract: DNA that has been isolated from other molecular components of the sample.

Library: A preparation of DNA extract in which overhangs have been removed from DNA fragments and universal sequencing adapters have been ligated to the ends of the fragments. Theoretically, libraries may be re-amplified (i.e., copied) *ad infinitum*.

Metagenomic: Containing numerous genetic sequences from different organisms.

Microbiome: The community of microorganisms occupying a specific ecological niche.

Paleofeces: Ancient fecal matter that has not fossilized.

Phylogenetics: The study of evolutionary relationships between groups of organisms based on molecular or morphological data.

Polymerase chain reaction (PCR): The process for enzymatically copying "template" DNA by separating DNA strands by heat (denaturation), activating a polymerase enzyme to read each strand and assemble a complementary strand, and recombining complementary DNA strands (annealing).

Single nucleotide polymorphism (SNP): A deviation of one nucleotide from the expected sequence, generally identified in comparison with a reference sequence. SNPs are the result of mutation.

Shotgun sequencing: The sequencing of all molecules in a DNA library without selective sample pre-processing, enrichment, or capture.

A Brief History of Ancient DNA

The first aDNA studies were published in 1984 and featured the cloning of DNA fragments from an ancient Egyptian mummy (Svante Pääbo, 1984) and the extinct quagga (Higuchi et al., 1984). Subsequently, the PCR method of DNA duplication was invented (Mullis & Faloona, 1987). This innovation opened the door to studying aDNA from pathogens (Pääbo, 1989). The resulting influx of studies garnered skepticism, and reproducibility became central to aDNA studies as the field grappled with how to authenticate findings (e.g., Roberts & Ingham, 2008). Gilbert and colleagues outlined a flexible, "cognitive" framework for authentication that takes into account the risk of contamination for different types of target organisms (Gilbert et al., 2005). Human and pathogen DNA had the first and second highest risk of contamination, respectively.

Next-generation sequencing (NGS) transformed the field of archaeogenetics, allowing data to be produced indiscriminately at high volumes (Mardis, 2008). NGS also allowed for routine identification and measurement of the chemical degradation of aDNA, which had previously been found to be correlated with time and environmental conditions (Lindahl, 1993). Depending on the size of the target genome, depth of sequencing, and proportion of target DNA in the sample, authentic whole genomes could be reconstructed from ancient remains using shotgun sequencing. For most cases where the amount of endogenous DNA was too low to reconstruct whole genomes or large swaths of a genome, capture methods emerged (Hodges et al., 2009; Burbano et al., 2010; Maricic et al., 2010) that allowed selective recovery of target DNA to sufficient levels for confident authentication and variant calling for genome analyses.

From Samples to Sequences

Sampling

A well-designed research project is particularly important for archaeogenetics, which is both destructive and expensive. Three important questions are as follows:

1. Have you consulted with rights holders and stakeholders such as descendant communities and museum curators about the project and obtained any required permits?
2. Could your research question be answered in full or in part by genetic data?
3. Would sampling for aDNA now eliminate the possibility of future additional analyses?

Prior to sampling, consultations with appropriate rights holders and descendant community members should occur, and required permissions should be obtained (Austin et al., 2019; Pálsdóttir et al., 2019). For rare samples, it is best to first assess whether DNA can be successfully obtained from faunal remains from the same site to determine the likelihood of preservation in more precious samples or by using non-destructive methods (Hofreiter et al., 2001; Bolnick et al., 2012). For pathogens found in specific locations in the body, it is useful to ask whether that tissue is preserved and available for sampling. Once an aDNA project begins, full documentation, including analysis by a skilled osteologist, photographs, and potentially X-rays or 3D scanning, is needed, as aDNA sampling is typically destructive (Fehren-Schmitz et al., 2016; Immel et al., 2016; Evin et al., 2020).

In the Laboratory

An aDNA laboratory should have separate designated areas for sample preparation, extraction, and other analyses. It should have a filtered, enclosed airflow system and ultraviolet (UV) lighting for use before and after laboratory use. Importantly, this space must be physically separate from any modern DNA laboratory to avoid contamination by modern or PCR-amplified DNA. Procedures for preparing samples and preventing contamination have been thoroughly discussed and tested in the aDNA community (e.g., Pilli et al., 2013). Surface contaminants should be removed from samples in a hood or other enclosure to prevent spread across the laboratory. The surface can be physically removed and/or sterilized by irradiating the surface with UV light or by briefly soaking the material in a hydrochloric acid or bleach solution (Kemp & Smith, 2005). The sample should then be pulverized into dust or small pieces. This step increases the surface area of the material, which improves the recovery of DNA during the extraction process.

DNA extraction releases and isolates DNA from other minerals and molecules (for a detailed review of aDNA methods see Orlando et al., 2021). The extraction method used can greatly affect the quality and quantity of DNA available for sequencing, and special considerations must be made for different types of samples. For paleopathology, bone, tooth, or other hard tissue samples are most commonly used due to their higher probability of preservation, though preserved soft tissue from mummified remains or medical specimens, hair, paleofeces, or sediments can also be used. These sample types have different chemical compositions and may require different extraction protocols.

Extraction protocols begin with a digestion stage, which breaks down the sample material. In the case of bone and dentine, digestion must (a) break down the protein component of the sample with a protease and (b) release the DNA from its bond to the hydroxyapatite component with EDTA. Following digestion, the DNA is separated from the other components of the sample either chemically (as in phenol-chloroform extraction) or physically (as in silica membrane extraction). Next, the extracted DNA is stabilized and "immortalized" through library preparation (Meyer & Kircher, 2010). Library preparation protocols involve the removal or filling-in of overhangs and ligation of adapters. The repair of strand overhangs and attachment of adapter sequences stabilize the strands for long term cold-storage, and the adapters allow all DNA fragments to be copied through PCR.

Following successful library preparation and indexing/barcoding, the sequencing library can be pooled with others and loaded into the sequencer. This method of sequencing a library without specific enrichment is also known as shotgun sequencing. In aDNA applications, the result is usually metagenomic data, meaning there are numerous taxa present. Especially when the target of the project is an infectious microorganism, identifying and authenticating the DNA of interest can resemble finding the proverbial needle in the haystack. Despite these challenges, shotgun sequencing can identify candidates for enrichment. It is also the optimal approach for the study of human microbiota (Ziesemer et al., 2015) and exploration of micro- (Sabin, Yeh, et al., 2020) or macro-ecologies (e.g., Slon et al., 2017) from sediments, coprolites, and dental calculus.

Several protocols exist for amplifying target DNA in a sequencing library. Though these methods vary, they are all fundamentally highly complex PCR reactions, variably referred to as hybridization, capture, or enrichment. They can be used to target and amplify DNA from any organism (e.g., the host or pathogens), including particular regions or the whole genome of a targeted species.

After the Laboratory

General Computational Biology

Preliminary treatment of sequencing data will generally depend on the sequencing platform used. What follows sequencing will also be dependent on the goals of the project, the computational resources available to the researchers, and the level of bioinformatics skills and experience available to the researchers. New computational tools are released regularly, increasing both accessibility and possible complexity of projects, and there are as many ways to analyze aDNA as there are aDNA projects.

As noted above, archaeological contexts typically involve sample infiltration by environmental water- or soil-borne microbes, and regardless of surface decontamination measures taken during sampling, it is safe to expect a busy microbial background. Numerous well-established taxonomic classifiers exist to assist researchers in sifting through shotgun-sequencing data, though all tools have pros and cons. Recent work investigated the efficacy of several popular taxonomic classifiers and found that ultimately, the best tool depends on the research question (Velsko et al., 2018).

The first step to producing a draft genome or calling SNPs from an organism is alignment of the data to a reference genome. In brief, aligners will find the best match for each read along a reference sequence, if possible. The results can then be used to assess DNA damage, which can contribute to the body of evidence supporting the data's authenticity.

An important component of genetic analyses is the accurate identification of SNPs and structural variants (indels) in the data. These can define the relationship between the sample sequence and existing data, which provides a crucial evolutionary context for interpretation. When attempting to call and authenticate SNPs for data taken from metagenomic contexts, issues of contamination by closely related organisms become a concern. Conserved sequences may attract contaminant reads despite measures to mitigate other effects of contamination, and careful detective work may be necessary to sort out erroneous calls.

Most aDNA studies relevant to questions in paleopathology will include a phylogeny. Broadly, phylogenies illustrate the relationship between different strains/samples based on nucleotide similarities and differences in a multiple sequence alignment. Bringing temporal and geographic metadata to the interpretation of phylogenies can reveal, for instance, the timing and location of a disease outbreak's origin. Bayesian phylogenetics, which compares the probabilities of possible tree topologies, substitution rates, and other parameter configurations, is frequently used to date the emergence of pathogens from their most recent common ancestor (MRCA) based on a set of existing facts and estimates. Including ancient samples in such trees enables more accurate MRCA estimates by calibrating the molecular clock through deep time and alleviating the time-dependency issue of molecular clocks that comes from sampling a short temporal window (Ho et al., 2015). Though the suitability of this analysis for certain species is under debate, as some rates of substitution do not behave in a clock-like manner (Duchêne et al., 2016), this form of analysis has offered important insights into the evolutionary history of some pathogens with the addition of aDNA (Bos et al., 2014).

An alternative to sequence alignment to a reference genome is *de novo* assembly, in which overlapping reads are computationally combined to create contigs, which can then be merged into a genomic assembly. *De novo* assembly is uncommon in aDNA due to the short fragment lengths and abundant contamination issues, though it is not impossible (Schuenemann et al., 2013). The advantage of this method is its elimination of reference bias from genomic reconstruction and its potential to reveal structural variants.

A crucial aspect of project design in paleogenetics is how the sequencing data are classified, stored, shared, and/or protected during and after completion of the project. Unlike human DNA from living subjects taken for research purposes, there are no clear protections for DNA taken from deceased individuals. To date, aDNA data management practices have varied by institution, but for a general rule that either raw data or alignments be made publicly available for the sake of data reproducibility. While this is an honorable objective, it does not account for the wishes of descendant communities or nations of origin. Currently, many calls exist for the development of data management conventions that include transparent agreements and ongoing communication with such parties (Wagner et al., 2020).

Box 8.2 Ethical Checkpoint: Data Management

At the initiation of a collaboration incorporating aDNA methods into a paleopathology project, the research team must consult and reach agreement with the local government and/or stakeholders regarding:

- The targeted data in the project (e.g., human DNA, pathogen DNA, *Mycobacterium leprae* DNA)
- Whether or not and in what ways discoveries outside the scope of the project may be pursued or reported (e.g., DNA from a different pathogen is identified; an individual happens to have a rare mitochondrial haplogroup for the time period and region)
- Who will act as steward over any resulting sequencing data

- What computational facilities will store the data
- How data storage and management will be funded
- The length of the storage term
- Who will have data sharing authority
- Under what conditions the data may be shared publicly or privately with other institutions/researchers

It is crucial that the research team be transparent with stakeholders at all points regarding the intent of the project and potential outcomes of data sharing. Once raw data is made publicly available, any resulting findings from an outside research group would fall outside the scope of the agreement. Possible sensitivities include the inadvertent discovery of stigmatizing pathogens or a different-than-expected ancestry group, either of which may lead to political and/or cultural consequences (see ETHICAL CHECKPOINT: Data Mining).

When the Project Is Over

The unique requirements of each project frequently result in the development of bespoke tools and scripts to assist in aDNA analysis. It is essential that the underlying code is made publicly available at the time of publication to ensure that results can be reproduced by other groups. Public code repositories such as Github allow easy code sharing.

At the project's conclusion, results should be communicated to descendant communities and/or other affected parties, and the reporting of results to the wider public should be undertaken collaboratively with those parties (e.g., Tsosie et al., 2020; Wagner et al., 2020). Depending on the agreements made prior to the start of research, this may include consultation prior to the publication of the research. Typically, upon publication, raw data are made available through repositories such as the NCBI Sequencing Read Archive or through permission from community representatives. It is important to discuss the potential uses of the raw data with the community (risks and benefits). In addition, any remaining samples and DNA (including libraries) should be returned to their source unless alternative arrangements are made. For high-impact/high-profile studies especially, a good-faith effort should be made to preempt inaccurate media coverage. This can be done through active engagement of researchers with social media platforms or press releases hosted by the research team.

Investigating Infectious Disease Through Ancient Genetic Data

Though there have been many "firsts" achieved over the past decade of ancient pathogen genomics, it remains a young subfield. Amid the universal challenges of aDNA work, each target organism poses a unique set of difficulties. Understanding the biology of each organism and the etiology of their infections is crucial for optimizing research design for successful DNA recovery and for authenticating and accurately interpreting the results. Furthermore, it is crucial to recognize the costs and benefits of conducting genetic analysis on human remains. While DNA may allow pathogen identification that skeletal analysis cannot in cases where an infection has left no specific changes to the remains (see example of *Y. pestis* below), its extraction is destructive. When choosing whether to incorporate a genetic component into a project, researchers face an ethical checkpoint, where they must balance the potential of discovery and knowledge generation with that of destroying or damaging a cultural resource and limiting opportunities for future knowledge generation (Figure 8.1).

> **Box 8.3 Ethical Checkpoint: Initiating a Genomics Project**
>
> When incorporating genetic methodologies into the study of human remains, it is important for the design of the sampling protocol that a research question is clearly defined and justified in light of existing biological, archaeological, and historical evidence. In addition, it is imperative that stakeholders, including descendant communities and institutions that curate human remains are consulted. Wagner et al. (2020) recommend that communities be formally involved during project planning and that cultural and ethical considerations be taken into account. Once a project is approved, the sampling should proceed in such a way that destruction of the sample is kept to the minimum necessary to answer the research question.
>
> - Is there a specific pathogen of interest?
> - Is there specific evidence of an infection from that pathogen in the bones?
> - Are there any skeletal changes suggesting an infection?
> - What would the benefit of genetic data be for that specific pathogen?
> - If a specific pathogen is targeted, do you or anyone on your current team have detailed knowledge about the biology of that pathogen and typical courses of infection it may follow? It may be valuable to consult an expert in that species or group of pathogens prior to conducting sampling, and certainly in the event of successfully producing data.
> - Is there agreement from stakeholders that the project is of interest and can proceed? Are there concerns or considerations (for example, regarding return of DNA extracts and remaining sample materials, data management, and future analyses) that have been discussed?

Once DNA has been extracted and sequenced, specific organisms must be identified amidst what is usually a busy metagenomic background. Many historically relevant and scientifically compelling pathogens have close, environmentally ubiquitous relatives. For instance, genetic sequences from environmental species in the genera *Mycolicibacterium* (formerly part of genus *Mycobacterium*) and *Mycobacterium* have been shown to easily misalign to sequences from pathogenic mycobacteria such as *M. tuberculosis*, leading to potential false-positive identifications (Warinner et al., 2017; Gupta et al., 2018). Though there are widely distributed guidelines to mitigate the possibility of false positives (Warinner et al., 2017), few are systematically adhered to throughout the aDNA community. The complexity of these issues and the accompanying authentication requirements differ according to the organism of interest and the context of the sample. Thus, scrutiny should be exercised when a particular organism has been identified. Important questions would include the following:

- Does the organism make geographical and/or historical sense in the context of the study?
- Were the samples handled according to protocols that limit contamination?
- Were the samples processed in a facility that also processes modern or aDNA from similar organisms?
- Were experts on that particular organism consulted and included in the research and publication process?

Ultimately, the mere presence or absence of an organism's DNA in an ancient sample means little. Absence of genetic evidence of a particular pathogen in a sample from skeletal remains

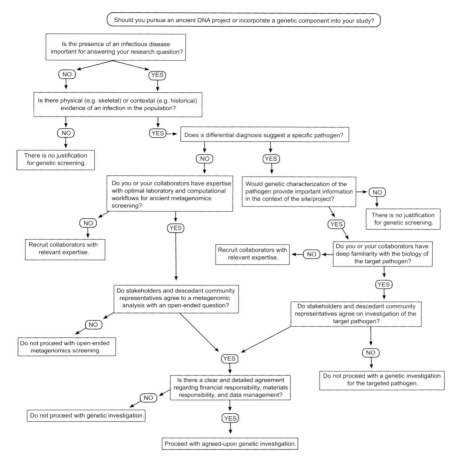

Figure 8.1 Decision tree for incorporating an ancient DNA component into a project. The destructive sampling inherent in most ancient DNA work, as well as the possible consequences of such analyses, requires careful consideration and discussion with stakeholders prior to initiation of the project.

provides no diagnostic information, because the fragility and stochastic preservation of DNA means it may be completely degraded. aDNA's contribution to questions of past human health largely depends on placing it in the context of modern genetic data. The availability of high-quality reference sequences of extant pathogens impacts our ability to successfully identify and authenticate ancient genetic sequences and provide meaningful interpretations.

Below, we provide a brief review of the aDNA work done so far pertaining to bacteria, viruses, and eukaryotes, discuss the genetic accessibility of different pathogens, and address specific methodological issues that arise when focusing on each organism type.

Bacteria

The first genomic reconstruction of an ancient bacterial pathogen, *Y. pestis* from the Black Death, was accomplished using genome-wide capture (Bos et al., 2011). Such techniques have led to the recovery of many other bacterial genomes, such as *Mycobacterium pinnipedii* from vertebrae (Bos et al., 2014), *M. tuberculosis* from a calcified lung nodule (Sabin, Herbig, et al., 2020), *M. leprae* from skeletal tissue and dental calculus (Schuenemann et al., 2013; Fotakis et al., 2020), *Salmonella enterica* from teeth (Vågene et al., 2018; Zhou et al., 2018; Key et al., 2020), *Treponema pallidum* from teeth (Schuenemann, Lankapalli, et al., 2018; Barquera et al., 2020; Giffin et al., 2020; Majander et al., 2020), *Vibrio cholerae* from preserved intestine (Devault et al., 2014), and *Helicobacter pylori* from mummified gastrointestinal tissue (Maixner et al., 2016). Shotgun sequencing alone, without any selective amplification of target DNA, has also yielded full bacterial genomes, such as in the case of *M. tuberculosis* and *M. leprae* from mummified remains (Chan et al., 2013; Kay et al., 2015; Neukamm et al., 2020), *Borrelia recurrentis* from teeth (Guellil et al., 2018), and *Brucella melitensis*, *Gardnerella vaginalis*, and *Staphylococcus saprophyticus* from calcified nodules (Kay et al., 2014; Devault et al., 2017).

For some bacterial pathogens, there are aspects of bacterial biology that favor the preservation and successful identification of DNA from archaeological and historical human remains. Bacterial infections that localize in the body and cause direct or immunologically mediated hard tissue changes, such as *M. tuberculosis*, provide ideal sampling sites for aDNA projects. Pathogens causing septicemic infections, though they do not necessarily leave evidence in the form of skeletal changes, can leave DNA preserved in the tooth pulp chamber, fed by blood flow during life, and protected to some degree from contamination and degradation by the tooth enamel after death (Drancourt et al., 1998). Dental calculus has been shown to be an excellent preservation environment for endogenous DNA of the oral microbiome (Warinner et al., 2014; Mann et al., 2018) and may offer a similar advantage for detecting pathogens that occupy the oral mucosa, as demonstrated for *M. leprae* (Fotakis et al., 2020). Some bacteria possess robust cell walls that may offer protection to DNA as well. Schuenemann and colleagues (2013) found that hydrolytic damage of *M. leprae* sequences extracted from human remains was less severe than that of the human sequences from the same sample, likely due to the lipid-rich cell wall found in *M. leprae*. Unlike many viruses, bacteria have a stable double-stranded DNA genome that is usually circular, and unlike eukaryotic pathogens, bacterial genomes are relatively compact.

Microbiome

Obligate pathogens are not the only organisms with an impact on human health. Studying human microbiota – the communities of microbes that inhabit the oral cavity, skin, gastrointestinal system, and vagina (Qin et al., 2010) – is essential for gaining a full understanding of human health. Indeed, the concept of humans, not as individual biological entities but as ecosystems with a eukaryotic foundation and multitudes of symbiotic microbes, or "holobionts," is becoming an increasingly valid perspective on human health (Gilbert et al., 2012). Associations between the oral microbiome and systemic disease have been identified in industrialized populations (Seymour et al., 2007). The gut microbiome is also increasingly being linked to mental health and neurological impacts through, for example, the production of 90% of the human body's serotonin (Dinan et al., 2015).

Researchers studying ancient human remains have optimal access to the oral microbiome through dental calculus, or calcified dental plaque, and, in some cases, from the pulp chamber, which may be due to a post-mortem colonization process (Mann et al., 2018). Dental calculus provides an excellent preservation environment for both host and oral microbiome DNA, across diverse climates and time periods (Ozga et al., 2016; Mann et al., 2018). The human gastrointestinal microbiome is less directly accessible than its oral counterpart but can be accessed through paleofeces (Borry et al., 2020), mummified tissues (Santiago-Rodriguez et al., 2015), or cesspit/latrine samples (Sabin, Yeh, et al., 2020).

Most studies thus far have addressed broad differences in taxonomic composition between modern and ancient microbiota and/or the presence of specific taxa (Adler et al., 2013; Warinner et al., 2014; Weyrich et al., 2017). For instance, a common aspect of ancient or historical oral microbiome studies is identification of the "Red Complex" bacteria *Treponema denticola, Tannerella forsythia*, and *Porphyromonas gingivalis*, associated with advanced periodontal disease in modern contexts (Warinner et al., 2014; Maixner et al., 2016; Orrù et al., 2017; Jensen et al., 2019; Achtman & Zhou, 2020; Bravo-Lopez et al., 2020; Eisenhofer et al., 2020; Jacobson et al., 2020). As modern microbiome sequencing has become increasingly sophisticated, with studies beginning to explore the uncultured constituents of human gastrointestinal microbiome through complex *de novo* assembly (Pasolli et al., 2019), and focus shifts toward the functional ecology of the human microbiome, we can expect to see analogous developments in aDNA (Jacobson et al., 2020).

Viruses

Viruses can pose special challenges in terms of DNA recovery and analysis based on their genetic composition. Double-stranded or partially double-stranded DNA viruses such as smallpox and hepatitis B virus (HBV), respectively, are comparable to bacteria in the stability of their genetic structure and, as a result, have been the focus of most virus-centered projects in paleogenetics. Both HBV and smallpox have been recovered from mummified and skeletal/dental remains (Duggan et al., 2016; Krause-Kyora et al., 2018; Ross et al., 2018; Barquera et al., 2020; Mühlemann et al., 2020; Neukamm et al., 2020), and both smallpox and measles virus have been recovered from antique medical specimens (Duggan et al., 2020; Düx et al., 2020; Ferrari et al., 2020). Single-stranded DNA and RNA viruses are less molecularly stable (Lindahl, 1993) and unlikely to be successfully recovered from archaeological human remains. However, RNA from measles virus has been successfully recovered from a formalin-fixed lung tissue sample (Düx et al., 2020), and historical RNA from the 1918 influenza pandemic was recovered from formalin-fixed lung tissue and human remains buried in permafrost (Tumpey et al., 2005). Thus, while our ability to recover historical human RNA viruses may be limited, it is not impossible.

Eukaryotes

Eukaryotic pathogens, single-celled or multicellular organisms in which the genetic material is contained within a nucleus, may also be studied through aDNA. Bloodborne and gastrointestinal parasites have been detected in data produced with NGS, though there have been no full-genome reconstructions to date. DNA from *Plasmodium falciparum*, a causative agent of malaria, has been recovered from skeletal remains dated to the 1st–2nd centuries CE (Marciniak et al., 2016), and from *P. falciparum* and *P. vivax* from early 20th-century blood slides (Gelabert et al., 2016). Genetic material from human intestinal parasites, including soil-transmitted helminths such as the giant roundworm (*Ascaris lumbricoides*) and foodborne tapeworms (*Taenia* spp., *Dibothriocephalus* spp.), has been recovered from coprolites and latrine sediments (e.g., Søe et al., 2018).

Among human pathogens, helminths are among the most poorly represented by curated reference sequences despite their broad impacts on human societies. This lack of diversity in genetic databases could lead to difficulties in identifying such organisms in ancient metagenomic datasets. However, researchers are actively working to remedy this (e.g., International Helminth Genomes Consortium, 2019). Difficulties for the production of high-quality reference data for many eukaryotic organisms are the size, content, and repetitiveness of eukaryotic genomes (Carlton et al., 2013), all of which can complicate the authentication of putatively ancient data as well. However, eukaryotic pathogens, like humans and other animals, possess relatively compact mitochondrial genomes. Enrichments for these smaller organellar genomes can be an effective way of extracting evidence for the presence of an organism from a highly metagenomic and/or highly eukaryotic background (e.g., from human tissue).

Investigating Heritable Diseases and Conditions through Ancient Genetic Data

Like today, people in the past were affected by heritable disorders including autosomal recessive disorders such as inborn errors of metabolism (like phenylketonuria), autosomal dominant disorders (de novo and inherited), as well as sex-linked disorders (like color-blindness or hemophilia). However, unless these result in clear morphological changes, the majority are not detected through paleopathological analysis. Whole genome analyses could be used to detect variants related to such heritable disorders; however, most published ancient human genome analyses have focused on questions related to population history and adaptation and not on the health of single individuals. The high coverage genomes available from Neandertals, for example, allow an examination of potential recessive conditions. Castellano et al. (2014) found that Neandertals carried more putatively deleterious alleles than modern humans and that those alleles causing amino acid changes that are at low frequency (i.e., only found in one heterozygous individual of the three Neandertals) were more likely to be predicted as functionally significant (and detrimental). They do not, however, identify specific genetic disorders affecting these individuals.

aDNA analyses focused on specific genes of individuals with morphological changes suggestive of a particular condition have been employed to confirm the diagnosis. For example, chronic anemia is associated with many causes both environmental and inherited, including genes involved in malarial resistance. aDNA assessments of such genes are discussed in the thalassemia example below. Some attempts have also been made to discern genetic causes of height extremes (Pusch et al., 2004; Boer et al., 2017). Beckers et al. (2017) investigated pituitary gigantism in a known individual whose clinical history suggested X-LAG syndrome, a genetic form of pituitary gigantism caused by duplications of the *GPR101* gene on the X chromosome. Beckers and colleagues (2017) extracted DNA from the petrous portion and used a quantification droplet digital PCR that allows a comparison of copy number at *GPR101* with another single copy gene, confirming increased copy number of *GPR101* as the likely cause.

Box 8.4 Ethical Checkpoint: Data Mining

Over the past decade, the amount of publicly available raw genetic data from ancient and historical human tissues has increased exponentially. The amount of privately held sequencing data in lab servers, from projects in progress or samples that were never used in a publication, has likely increased at a comparable level. This wealth of data can be seen as a treasure trove of potential discovery. As pathogen and gene marker screening processes are increasingly automated, many scientifically compelling findings may be mined from these data. However, it can also be seen as an ethical thicket, which requires transparent and empathetic dialogues with stakeholders to be navigated in a way that pays respect to and seeks to benefit, rather than harm, those who made the projects possible in the first place (e.g., local governments or descendant communities). Many national and international guidelines and regulations on living human subjects research require researchers to provide an assessment of potential harm. While there are few to no such guidelines for long-deceased persons and their descendants, and as of this writing such gestures and introspective practices can in many cases be the prerogative of the research team alone, we recommend research groups working with human remains adhere to ethical guidelines for the sake of common good as well as scientific discovery. Colonialist practices in anthropology, bioarchaeology, human genetics, and paleogenetics ultimately harm the impact of science as well as our ability to practice it. Listed below are some potential fallouts from data mining without appropriate consideration of stakeholder concerns or welfare:

- The discovery of stigmatizing pathogen may lead to discrimination against or defamation of descendant communities.
- The discovery of an individual or individuals with different ancestry than expected may lead to social, political, and/or economic consequences, such as the inflammation of property rights disputes or the questioning/countering of traditional beliefs.

Investigating Cancer through Ancient Genetic Data

Cancer is a group of diseases where both genetic and environmental factors affect risk for developing abnormal cell growth, resulting in a malignant neoplasm in some part of the body. In the archaeological record, cancer is visible primarily when it originates in bone or metastasizes to bone except where mummified remains are found (Hunt et al., 2018; Marques, 2019; Riccomi et al., 2019). Molecular analyses of ancient cancer cases have been limited and typically focus on known cancer genes, such as *p53* or *K-ras* or viruses linked to cancer, such as human papillomavirus (Nerlich, 2018). These may help identify the type of cancer or inherited susceptibility.

Case Studies

Thalassemia

As noted previously, chronic anemia can have environmental and inherited causes, and among the latter are conditions associated with malaria resistance alleles (such as those causing sickle cell anemia and thalassemia) (see Chapter 19, this volume, for more information on metabolic and endocrine disorders). These conditions are common in places that historically had malaria, and they can leave signs of chronic anemia in bone. Malaria resistance alleles are found in several genes involved in immune response and comprise red blood cell proteins such as hemoglobin (López et al., 2010; Leffler et al., 2017). Hemoglobin transports oxygen in the blood and is composed of α-globin and β-globin chains. Individuals with thalassemia or sickle cell anemia have a deficiency or complete lack of one of these two components. Filon et al. (1995) examined whether a child, excavated from a 3,800-year-old cemetery in

Israel, with skeletal pathologies consistent with severe anemia had beta thalassemia. They found that this child was homozygous for a two base pair (bp) deletion variant (*rs35497102*) that results in no production of the adult form of β-globin. Elevated levels of fetal hemoglobin production may have helped the child survive to age eight. Additional studies have searched for these variants at other sites in the Mediterranean (Sallares et al., 2004; Hughey et al., 2012).

Yersinia pestis

Y. pestis is the causative agent of plague. A descendant of the soil-dwelling bacterium *Yersinia pseudotuberculosis*, *Y. pestis* acquired two plasmids, and they, along with changes to its core genome, allowed it to infect mammalian hosts. These plasmids continue to act as genetic markers indicating the presence of pathogenic *Yersinia* in historical and ancient remains (Schuenemann et al., 2011). aDNA confirms that *Y. pestis* caused three major historical pandemics: the Justinianic Plague (6–8th centuries CE), the Black Death and its subsequent resurgences over a period of 400 years (14–18th centuries CE), and a third pandemic in the 19th and 20th centuries (Perry & Fetherston, 1997; Drancourt et al., 1998; Parkhill et al., 2001; Bos et al., 2011, 2016; Cui et al., 2013; Wagner et al., 2014) (see Chapter 31, this volume, for more information about plagues and pandemics).

As discussed earlier, *Y. pestis* was the first bacterial species for which an ancient genome was reconstructed in its entirety (Bos et al., 2011). Tooth samples from individuals in London's East Smithfield collection originally underwent PCR screening for the pPCP1 plasmid, one of the distinguishing features between *Y. pestis* and *Y. pseudotuberculosis* (Schuenemann et al., 2011). Subsequent genome enrichment led to reconstructions of *Y. pestis* from known plague victims concretely linking the species to the Black Death. Shortly thereafter, Wagner et al. (2014) successfully reconstructed genomes from an early medieval burial site in Germany associated with the Justinianic Plague. With these findings, questions regarding the Justinianic Plague and Black Death turned from their causal pathogen to their origins, dynamics, and how *Y. pestis* could have caused such devastation.

Importantly, *Y. pestis* does not leave specific signs in the skeleton over the course of infection. Identification of human remains of individuals who perished from plague is largely contextual. The remains sampled and sequenced in the Schuenemann et al. (2011) and Bos et al. (2011) studies came from a historically documented burial site for plague victims during the Black Death. When written documentation is lacking, inferences may be made regarding the likelihood of a burial being associated with acute infectious disease if, for example, it is a multiple burial of otherwise "healthy" adults with no skeletal indications of perimortem trauma (Blakely & Detweiler-Blakely, 1989; Rugg, 2000).

However, some of the most influential findings in archaeogenetics regarding plague have come from incidental identification of *Y. pestis* DNA in raw sequencing data from initially unrelated projects (Rasmussen et al., 2015; Rascovan et al., 2019). Though these data offered an unforeseen opportunity to the scientific community to gain a deeper understanding of the evolutionary history of *Y. pestis* and its impact on humanity, the use of genetic data for reasons other than the original project, and the release of raw sequencing data from human remains, is a practice that must be engaged in carefully.

In 2015, Rasmussen et al. reported the recovery of seven *Y. pestis* genomes from Bronze Age Eurasia, based on screening shotgun-sequencing data (from the pulp chambers of 101 individuals) originally generated as part of a human genetics paper (Allentoft et al., 2015). These were extraordinary results, reinforced by evidence that they were not the result of lab-based or environmental contamination. The results showed that *Y. pestis* had been infecting humans thousands of years prior to its first appearance in written records. Additionally, an in-depth genetic analysis revealed that the murine toxin gene (*ymt*) was present in only the most recent Bronze Age sample. The *ymt* gene was thought to be an early evolutionary acquisition since it allows the bacterium to survive inside the gut of the flea, the bubonic plague vector (Hinnebusch, 2005). While noting their limited sample size, Rasmussen et al. (2015) suggested that the *Y. pestis ymt* gene was acquired by horizontal gene transfer between 1686 and 951 BCE and spread quickly through the population. Prior to its acquisition, the flea route of transmission would not have been effective, and the primary forms of plague in humans were likely septicemic and pneumonic.

Andrades Valtueña et al. (2017) sequenced additional *Y. pestis* genome extending from the Late Neolithic to the Early Bronze age in Eurasia. All genomes fell on the same phylogenetic branch as those presented by Rasmussen et al. (2015), dubbed the Late Neolithic Bronze Age (LNBA) branch. None of the six genomes carried the *ymt* gene. Considering all available LNBA genomes and including human ancestry analyses from the infected individuals, they determined *Y. pestis* likely followed movements of people from the Central Asian steppe, into Europe, then back again. Soon however, a new publication presented two identical Late Bronze Age genomes from a double burial in present-day Russia (Spyrou et al., 2018). Compellingly, these genomes were distinct and contained the full genetic "package" necessary for flea-to-human transmission of plague (Spyrou et al., 2018). Based on the updated phylogeny, the new genomes appear to have ultimately given rise to strains linked to the Justinianic Plague, Black Death, and modern infections (Bos et al., 2011, 2016; Rasmussen et al., 2015; Feldman et al., 2016; Andrades Valtueña et al., 2017; Spyrou et al., 2018). This pushed the first potential cases of bubonic plague in humans back before 3,800 years before present.

A recent aDNA study may offer insight into why the Black Death lost momentum in the 18th century CE. Susat et al. (2020) reconstructed two *Y. pestis* genomes from a documented plague burial in 17th-century Riga (present-day Latvia). While historically these deaths would be associated with the Black Death (14th–18th centuries), the genomes shared a closer genetic relationship with post-Black Death genomes. Upon further inspection, the researchers found there were two pPCP1 plasmids, one of which contained the *pla* gene and the other of which did not. They discovered the same pattern in other genomes postdating the Black Death. Because the *pla* gene plays an important role in virulence, the authors suggest this depletion contributed to plague's decline.

Mycobacterium leprae

M. leprae is one of the bacterial species causing Hansen's disease or leprosy. Leprosy is recorded in ancient historical texts and skeletal evidence extends back to 4,000 years ago (Robbins et al., 2009) (see Chapter 17, this volume, for more information on mycobacterial infections). Unlike *Y. pestis*, *M. leprae* infections can cause distinct skeletal changes. This makes the selection of candidate samples for aDNA far more straightforward.

M. leprae was the second bacterial pathogen to undergo genomic reconstruction from aDNA in 2013. In this case, initial genetic screening was performed using a bead capture method targeting multiple genes and repeats (Schuenemann et al., 2013). Following sequencing of the capture products, a subset of the samples were selected for genome-wide sequencing. One sample was sufficiently rich in *M. leprae* DNA that it could undergo *de novo* assembly. To test the authenticity of the *M. leprae* DNA, the laboratory experiments were replicated between three additional laboratories with concordant results. Overall, in their phylogenetic analysis of *M. leprae* DNA, Schuenemann et al. (2013) found there to be little difference between the medieval and modern strains, indicating a lack of diversity over time. Mendum et al. (2014) presented further ancient genomes from a medieval leprosy hospital supporting the idea of *M. leprae* as highly clonal with limited diversity.

However, the case of *M. leprae* has demonstrated how limited data can skew our assumptions about the history and biology of a pathogen. In 2018, Schuenemann et al. presented ten additional genomes from medieval Europe. New, publicly available, modern *M. leprae* data were also included in the phylogenetic analysis, which showed the ancient genomes belonging to four different lineages. *M. leprae* is also a successful example of molecular dating with ancient genomes for clock calibration. Among the pathogens that have been studied genetically in ancient contexts, it has (to our knowledge) the strongest temporal signal (Duchêne et al., 2016), meaning there is a strong correlation between genetic divergence from the MRCA and the isolation date of the strain. In their 2013 paper, Schuenemann et al. estimated the MRCA of all *M. leprae* to be between 2,871 (95% HPD 1,350–5,078 years ago) and 3,126 (95% HPD 1,975–4,562 years ago) years old according to a relaxed and strict clock model, respectively. Later, with a more robust dataset, the estimate increased to 4,515 years ago (95% HPD 3,403–5,828) (Schuenemann, Avanzi, et al., 2018). Blevins et al. (2020), with the addition of modern samples from the Pacific Islands, estimated a date of 3,766 years ago (95% HPD 3,011–4,572). However, in the same year, Neukamm et al. (2020) presented the oldest *M. leprae* genome published to date, from mummified remains dated to 342–117 cal BCE. Using this genome, Neukamm et al. estimated the time to the MRCA to be 5,844 years (95% HPD 4,128–8,287). Though it is a dramatic extension of the oldest previous estimate, all estimates of the time to the MRCA of *M. leprae* have overlapping 95% HPD intervals.

Conclusion

The aDNA field remains relatively new and requires careful navigation of numerous challenges. Researchers must be conversant in a number of related fields including evolutionary biology, population genetics, biostatistics, human genetics, bioinformatics, and pathogen genetics. For example, understanding the evolutionary history of a pathogen requires comparative modern genetic data as well as an understanding of recombination and of compartmentalization (i.e. where the pathogen localizes in the body), while identifying inherited genetic conditions or cancers typically requires knowing which genes or pathways are involved. Much basic research of the life history and ecology of pathogens is still needed in modern genetics today, as is better understanding of genetic associations in the human genome with complex health traits and outcomes. Other challenges for the study of ancient pathogens include how to identify pathogens that affected people in the past but are extinct today (for example, the "sweating sickness" documented from 1485 to 1551 in England) and how to best model pathogen substitution rates. In the last ten years, the pace of aDNA research on disease has increased substantially and many studies have been discovery based. However, new research (or follow-up analyses following discovery) must include a clear research design with appropriate permissions. This will ensure the data obtained are informative from an anthropological and/or evolutionary perspective, facilitate the production of statistically robust results, and maintain interdisciplinary integrity for future collaborations and scientific advancement. Additionally, scholars in paleogenetics and paleomicrobiology must continue to work together to develop widely accepted standards and resources as the pace of research continues to accelerate (e.g., Fellows Yates et al., 2021). This standardization will also require editorial participation and compliance so it may be applied during peer review processes.

High-quality aDNA analyses are challenging, but in conjunction with paleopathology, they can help us gain deeper understanding of the underlying causes of conditions or provide evolutionary insight to a condition and its relationship to humans.

References

Achtman, M. & Zhou, Z. (2020). Metagenomics of the modern and historical human oral microbiome with phylogenetic studies on streptococcus mutans and streptococcus sobrinus. *Philosophical Transactions of the Royal Society B: Biological Sciences* 375(1812):20190573. https://doi.org/10.1098/rstb.2019.0573

Adler, C. J., Dobney, K., Weyrich, L. S., Kaidonis, J., Walker, A. W., Haak, W., ... & Cooper, A. (2013). Sequencing ancient calcified dental plaque shows changes in oral microbiota with dietary shifts of the neolithic and industrial revolutions. *Nature Genetics* 45(4):450–455. https://doi.org/10.1038/ng.2536

Allentoft, M. E., Sikora, M., Sjögren, K.-G., Rasmussen, S., Rasmussen, M., Stenderup, J., ... & Willerslev, E. (2015). Population genomics of bronze age Eurasia. *Nature* 522(7555):167–172. https://doi.org/10.1038/nature14507

Andrades Valtueña, A., Mittnik, A., Key, F. M., Haak, W., Allmäe, R., Belinskij, A., ... & Krause, J. (2017). The stone age plague and its persistence in Eurasia. *Current Biology* 27(23): 3683-3691.e8 https://doi.org/10.1016/j.cub.2017.10.025

Austin, R. M., Sholts, S. B., Williams, L., Kistler, L. & Hofman, C. A. (2019). Opinion: To curate the molecular past, museums need a carefully considered set of best practices. *Proceedings of the National Academy of Sciences* 116(5):1471–1474. https://doi.org/10.1073/pnas.1822038116

Barquera, R., Lamnidis, T. C., Lankapalli, A. K., Kocher, A., Hernández-Zaragoza, D. I., Nelson, E. A., ... & Krause, J. (2020). Origin and health status of first-generation Africans from early colonial Mexico. *Current Biology* 30(11):2078–2091.e11. https://doi.org/10.1016/j.cub.2020.04.002

Beckers, A., Fernandes, D., Fina, F., Novak, M., Abati, A., Rostomyan, L., ... & Daly, A. F. (2017). Paleogenetic study of ancient DNA suggestive of X-linked acrogigantism. *Endocrine-Related Cancer* 24(2):L17–L20. https://doi.org/10.1530/ERC-16-0558

Blakely, R. L. & Detweiler-Blakely, B. (1989). The impact of European diseases in the sixteenth-century southeast: a case study. *Midcontinental Journal of Archaeology* 14(1):62–89.

Blevins, K. E., Crane, A. E., Lum, C., Furuta, K., Fox, K. & Stone, A. C. (2020). Evolutionary history of mycobacterium leprae in the Pacific Islands. *Philosophical Transactions of the Royal Society B: Biological Sciences* 375(1812):20190582. https://doi.org/10.1098/rstb.2019.0582

Boer, L. L., Naue, J., de Rooy, L. & Oostra, R.-J. (2017). Detection of G1138A mutation of the *FGFR3* gene in tooth material from a 180-year-old museological achondroplastic skeleton. *Genes* 29;8(9):214.https://doi.org/10.3390/genes8090214

Bolnick, D. A., Bonine, H. M., Mata-Míguez, J., Kemp, B. M., Snow, M. H. & LeBlanc, S. A. (2012). Nondestructive sampling of human skeletal remains yields ancient nuclear and mitochondrial DNA. *American Journal of Physical Anthropology* 147(2):293–300. https://doi.org/10.1002/ajpa.21647

Borry, M., Cordova, B., Perri, A., Wibowo, M., Honap, T. P., Ko, J., ... & Warinner, C. (2020). CoproID predicts the source of coprolites and paleofeces using microbiome composition and host DNA content. *PeerJ* 8:e9001. https://doi.org/10.7717/peerj.9001

Bos, K. I., Harkins, K. M., Herbig, A., Coscolla, M., Weber, N., Comas, I., ... & Krause, J. (2014). Pre-Columbian mycobacterial genomes reveal seals as a source of new world human tuberculosis. *Nature* 514(7523):494–497. https://doi.org/10.1038/nature13591

Bos, K. I., Herbig, A., Sahl, J., Waglechner, N., Fourment, M., Forrest, S. A., Klunk, J., Schuenemann, V. J., Poinar, D. & Kuch, M. (2016). Eighteenth century *Yersinia pestis* genomes reveal the long-term persistence of an historical plague focus. *Elife* 5:e12994.

Bos, K. I., Schuenemann, V. J., Golding, G. B., Burbano, H. A., Waglechner, N., Coombes, B. K., ... & Krause, J. (2011). A draft genome of *Yersinia pestis* from victims of the black death. *Nature* 478(7370):506–510. https://doi.org/10.1038/nature10549

Bravo-Lopez, M., Villa-Islas, V., Rocha Arriaga, C., Villaseñor-Altamirano, A. B., Guzmán-Solís, A., Sandoval-Velasco, M., ... & Ávila-Arcos, M. C. (2020). Paleogenomic insights into the red complex bacteria *Tannerella forsythia* in Pre-hispanic and colonial individuals from Mexico. *Philosophical Transactions of the Royal Society B: Biological Sciences* 375(1812):20190580. https://doi.org/10.1098/rstb.2 019.0580

Burbano, H. A., Hodges, E., Green, R. E., Briggs, A. W., Krause, J., Meyer, M., ... & Pääbo, S. (2010). Targeted investigation of the Neandertal genome by array-based sequence capture. *Science* 328(5979):723–725. https://doi.org/10.1126/science.1188046

Carlton, J. M., Sullivan, S. A., Le Roch, K. G., Carlton, J. M., Perkins, S. L. & Deitsch, K. W. (2013). Plasmodium genomics and the art of sequencing malaria parasite genomes. In Carlton, J., Perkins, S. & Deitsch, K. (Eds.), *Malaria Parasites: Comparative Genomics, Evolution, and Molecular Biology*, pp. 35–58. Norfolk, UK: Caister Academic Press.

Castellano, S., Parra, G., Sánchez-Quinto, F. A., Racimo, F., Kuhlwilm, M., Kircher, M., ... & Pääbo, S. (2014). Patterns of coding variation in the complete exomes of three Neandertals. *Proceedings of the National Academy of Sciences* 111(18):6666–6671. https://doi.org/10.1073/pnas.1405138111

Chan, J. Z.-M., Sergeant, M. J., Lee, O. Y.-C., Minnikin, D. E., Besra, G. S., Pap, I., Spigelman, M., Donoghue, H. D. & Pallen, M. J. (2013). Metagenomic analysis of tuberculosis in a mummy. *New England Journal of Medicine* 369(3):289–290. https://doi.org/10.1056/NEJMc1302295

Cui, Y., Yu, C., Yan, Y., Li, D., Li, Y., Jombart, T., ... & Yang, R. (2013). Historical variations in mutation rate in an epidemic pathogen, *Yersinia pestis*. *Proceedings of the National Academy of Sciences* 110(2):577–582. https://doi.org/10.1073/pnas.1205750110

Devault, A. M., Golding, G. B., Waglechner, N., Enk, J. M., Kuch, M., Tien, J. H., ... & Poinar, H. N. (2014). Second-pandemic strain of *Vibrio cholerae* from the Philadelphia cholera outbreak of 1849. *New England Journal of Medicine* 370(4):334–340. https://doi.org/10.1056/NEJMoa1308663

Devault, A. M., Mortimer, T. D., Kitchen, A., Kiesewetter, H., Enk, J. M., Golding, G. B., ... & Pepperell, C. S. (2017). A molecular portrait of maternal sepsis from Byzantine Troy. *ELife* 6:e20983. https://doi.org/10.7554/eLife.20983

Dinan, T. G., Stilling, R. M., Stanton, C. & Cryan, J. F. (2015). Collective unconscious: how gut microbes shape human behavior. *Journal of Psychiatric Research* 63:1–9. https://doi.org/10.1016/j.jpsychires.2015.02.021

Drancourt, M., Aboudharam, G., Signoli, M., Dutour, O. & Raoult, D. (1998). Detection of 400-year-old *Yersinia pestis* DNA in human dental pulp: an approach to the diagnosis of ancient septicemia. *Proceedings of the National Academy of Sciences* 95(21):12637–12640. https://doi.org/10.1073/pnas.95.21.12637

Duchêne, S., Holt, K. E., Weill, F.-X., Le Hello, S., Hawkey, J., Edwards, D. J., Fourment, M. & Holmes, E. C. (2016). Genome-scale rates of evolutionary change in bacteria. *Microbial Genomics* 2(11) e000094. https://doi.org/10.1099/mgen.0.000094

Duggan, A. T., Klunk, J., Porter, A. F., Dhody, A. N., Hicks, R., Smith, G. L., ... & Poinar, H. N. (2020). The origins and genomic diversity of American civil war era smallpox vaccine strains. *Genome Biology* 21(1):175. https://doi.org/10.1186/s13059-020-02079-z

Duggan, A. T., Perdomo, M. F., Piombino-Mascali, D., Marciniak, S., Poinar, D., Emery, M. V., ... & Poinar, H. N. (2016). 17th century variola virus reveals the recent history of smallpox. *Current Biology* 26(24):3407–3412. https://doi.org/10.1016/j.cub.2016.10.061

Düx, A., Lequime, S., Patrono, L. V., Vrancken, B., Boral, S., Gogarten, J. F., Hilbig, A., ... & Calvignac-Spencer, S. (2020). Measles virus and rinderpest virus divergence dated to the sixth century BCE. *Science* 368(6497):1367–1370. https://doi.org/10.1126/science.aba9411

Eisenhofer, R., Kanzawa-Kiriyama, H., Shinoda, K. & Weyrich, L. S. (2020). Investigating the demographic history of Japan using ancient oral microbiota. *Philosophical Transactions of the Royal Society B: Biological Sciences* 375(1812):20190578. https://doi.org/10.1098/rstb.2019.0578

Evin, A., Lebrun, R., Durocher, M., Ameen, C., Larson, G. & Sykes, N. (2020). Building three-dimensional models before destructive sampling of bioarchaeological remains: A comment to Pálsdóttir et al. (2019). *Royal Society Open Science* 7(3):192034. https://doi.org/10.1098/rsos.192034

Fehren-Schmitz, L., Kapp, J., Ziegler, K. L., Harkins, K. M., Aronsen, G. P. & Conlogue, G. (2016). An investigation into the effects of X-ray on the recovery of ancient DNA from skeletal remains. *Journal of Archaeological Science* 76:1–8. https://doi.org/10.1016/j.jas.2016.10.005

Feldman, M., Harbeck, M., Keller, M., Spyrou, M. A., Rott, A., Trautmann, B., ... & Krause, J. (2016). A high-coverage *Yersinia pestis* genome from a 6th-century Justinianic plague victim. *Molecular Biology and Evolution* 33(11):2911-2923 https://doi.org/10.1093/molbev/msw170

Fellows Yates, J. A., Andrades Valtueña, A., Vågene, Å. J., Cribdon, B., Velsko, I. M., Borry, M., ... & Warinner, C. (2021). Community-curated and standardised metadata of published ancient metagenomic samples with AncientMetagenomeDir. *Scientific Data* 8(1):31. https://doi.org/10.1038/s41597-021-00816-y

Ferrari, G., Neukamm, J., Baalsrud, H. T., Breidenstein, A. M., Ravinet, M., Phillips, C., Rühli, F., Bouwman, A. & Schuenemann, V. J. (2020). Variola virus genome sequenced from an eighteenth-century museum specimen supports the recent origin of smallpox. *Philosophical Transactions of the Royal Society of London. Series B, Biological Sciences* 375(1812):20190572. https://doi.org/10.1098/rstb.2019.0572

Filon, D., Faerman, M., Smith, P. & Oppenheim, A. (1995). Sequence analysis reveals a β–thalassaemia mutation in the DNA from skeletal remains from the archaeological site of Akhziv, Israel. *Nature Genetics* 9(4):365–368. https://doi.org/10.1038/ng0495-365

Fotakis, A. K., Denham, S. D., Mackie, M., Orbegozo, M. I., Mylopotamitaki, D., Gopalakrishnan, S., ... & Vågene, Å. J. (2020). Multi-omic detection of *Mycobacterium leprae* in archaeological human dental calculus. *Philosophical Transactions of the Royal Society B: Biological Sciences* 375(1812):20190584. https://doi.org/10.1098/rstb.2019.0584

Gelabert, P., Sandoval-Velasco, M., Olalde, I., Fregel, R., Rieux, A., Escosa, R., ... & Lalueza-Fox, C. (2016). Mitochondrial DNA from the eradicated European *Plasmodium vivax* and *P. falciparum* from 70-year-old slides from the Ebro Delta in Spain. *Proceedings of the National Academy of Sciences* 201611017. https://doi.org/10.1073/pnas.1611017113

Giffin, K., Lankapalli, A. K., Sabin, S., Spyrou, M. A., Posth, C., Kozakaitė, J., ... & Bos, K. I. (2020). A treponemal genome from an historic plague victim supports a recent emergence of yaws and its presence in 15th century Europe. *Scientific Reports* 10(1):9499. https://doi.org/10.1038/s41598-020-66012-x

Gilbert, M. T. P., Bandelt, H. J., Hofreiter, M. & Barnes, I. (2005). Assessing ancient DNA studies. *Trends in Ecology & Evolution* 20(10):541–544. https://doi.org/10.1016/j.tree.2005.07.005

Gilbert, S. F., Sapp, J. & Tauber, A. I. (2012). A symbiotic view of life: we have never been individuals. *The Quarterly Review of Biology* 87(4):325–341. https://doi.org/10.1086/668166

Guellil, M., Kersten, O., Namouchi, A., Bauer, E. L., Derrick, M., Jensen, A. Ø., Stenseth, N. C. & Bramanti, B. (2018). Genomic blueprint of a relapsing fever pathogen in 15th century Scandinavia. *Proceedings of the National Academy of Sciences* 201807266. https://doi.org/10.1073/pnas.1807266115

Gupta, R. S., Lo, B. & Son, J. (2018). Phylogenomics and comparative genomic studies robustly support division of the genus *Mycobacterium* into an emended genus *Mycobacterium* and four novel genera. *Frontiers in Microbiology* 9:67. https://doi.org/10.3389/fmicb.2018.00067

Higuchi, R., Bowman, B., Freiberger, M., Ryder, O. A. & Wilson, A. C. (1984). DNA sequences from the quagga, an extinct member of the horse family. *Nature* 312: 282-284. http://www.nature.com/nature/journal/v312/n5991/abs/312282a0.html

Hinnebusch, B. J. (2005). The evolution of flea-borne transmission in *Yersinia pestis*. *Current Issues in Molecular Biology* 7(2):197–212.

Ho, S. Y. W., Duchêne, S., Molak, M. & Shapiro, B. (2015). Time-dependent estimates of molecular evolutionary rates: evidence and causes. *Molecular Ecology* 24(24):6007–6012. https://doi.org/10.1111/mec.13450

Hodges, E., Rooks, M., Xuan, Z., Bhattacharjee, A., Benjamin Gordon, D., Brizuela, L., Richard McCombie, W. & Hannon, G. J. (2009). Hybrid selection of discrete genomic intervals on custom-designed microarrays for massively parallel sequencing. *Nature Protocols* 4(6):960–974. https://doi.org/10.1038/nprot.2009.68

Hofreiter, M., Serre, D., Poinar, H. N., Kuch, M. & Pääbo, S. (2001). Ancient DNA. *Nature Reviews Genetics* 2(5):353–359.

Hughey, J. R., Du, M., Li, Q., Michalodimitrakis, M. & Stamatoyannopoulos, G. (2012). A search for β thalassemia mutations in 4000 year old ancient DNAs of Minoan cretans. *Blood Cells, Molecules, and Diseases* 48(1):7–10. https://doi.org/10.1016/j.bcmd.2011.09.006

Hunt, K. J., Roberts, C. & Kirkpatrick, C. (2018). Taking stock: a systematic review of archaeological evidence of cancers in human and early hominin remains. *International Journal of Paleopathology* 21:12–26. https://doi.org/10.1016/j.ijpp.2018.03.002

Immel, A., Le Cabec, A., Bonazzi, M., Herbig, A., Temming, H., Schuenemann, V. J., ... & Krause, J. (2016). Effect of X-ray irradiation on ancient DNA in sub-fossil bones – Guidelines for safe X-ray imaging. *Scientific Reports* 6(1):32969. https://doi.org/10.1038/srep32969

International Helminth Genomes Consortium, (2019). Comparative genomics of the major parasitic worms. *Nature Genetics* 51(1):163. https://doi.org/10.1038/s41588-018-0262-1

Jacobson, D. K., Honap, T. P., Monroe, C., Lund, J., Houk, B. A., Novotny, A. C., Robin, C., Marini, E. & Lewis, C. M. (2020). Functional diversity of microbial ecologies estimated from ancient human coprolites and dental calculus. *Philosophical Transactions of the Royal Society B: Biological Sciences*, 375(1812):20190586. https://doi.org/10.1098/rstb.2019.0586

Jensen, T. Z. T., Niemann, J., Iversen, K. H., Fotakis, A. K., Gopalakrishnan, S., Vågene, Å. J., … & Schroeder, H. (2019). A 5700 year-old human genome and oral microbiome from chewed birch pitch. *Nature Communications* 10(1):5520. https://doi.org/10.1038/s41467-019-13549-9

Kay, G. L., Sergeant, M. J., Giuffra, V., Bandiera, P., Milanese, M., Bramanti, B., Bianucci, R. & Pallen, M. J. (2014). Recovery of a medieval *Brucella melitensis* genome using shotgun metagenomics. *MBio* 5(4):e01337–14. https://doi.org/10.1128/mBio.01337-14

Kay, G. L., Sergeant, M. J., Zhou, Z., Chan, J. Z.-M., Millard, A., Quick, J., … & Pallen, M. J. (2015). Eighteenth-century genomes show that mixed infections were common at time of peak tuberculosis in Europe. *Nature Communications* 6:6717. https://doi.org/10.1038/ncomms7717

Kemp, B. M. & Smith, D. G. (2005). Use of bleach to eliminate contaminating DNA from the surface of bones and teeth. *Forensic Science International* 154(1):53–61. https://doi.org/10.1016/j.forsciint.2004.11.017

Key, F. M., Posth, C., Esquivel-Gomez, L. R., Hübler, R., Spyrou, M. A., Neumann, G. U., … & Krause, J. (2020). Emergence of human-adapted *Salmonella enterica* is linked to the neolithization process. *Nature Ecology & Evolution* 4(3):324–333. https://doi.org/10.1038/s41559-020-1106-9

Krause-Kyora, B., Susat, J., Key, F. M., Bosse, E., Immel, A., Rinne, C., Kornell, S.-C. & Yepes, D. (2018). Neolithic and medieval virus genomes reveal complex evolution of hepatitis B. *eLife* 2018(7):e36666. https://doi.org/10.7554/eLife.36666

Leffler, E. M., Band, G., Busby, G. B. J., Kivinen, K., Le, Q. S., Clarke, G. M., … & Network, M. G. E. (2017). Resistance to malaria through structural variation of red blood cell invasion receptors. *Science* 356(6343): eaam6393. https://doi.org/10.1126/science.aam6393

Lindahl, T. (1993). Instability and decay of the primary structure of DNA. *Nature* 362:709–715.

López, C., Saravia, C., Gomez, A., Hoebeke, J. & Patarroyo, M. A. (2010). Mechanisms of genetically-based resistance to malaria. *Gene* 467(1):1–12. https://doi.org/10.1016/j.gene.2010.07.008

Maixner, F., Krause-Kyora, B., Turaev, D., Herbig, A., Hoopmann, M. R., Hallows, J. L., Kusebauch, U., … & Zink, A. (2016). The 5300-year-old *Helicobacter pylori* genome of the Iceman. *Science* 351(6269):162–165. https://doi.org/10.1126/science.aad2545

Majander, K., Pfrengle, S., Kocher, A., Neukamm, J., du Plessis, L., Pla-Díaz, M., Arora, N., … & Schuenemann, V. J. (2020). Ancient bacterial genomes reveal a high diversity of *Treponema pallidum* strains in early modern Europe. *Current Biology* 30(19):3788–3803.e10. https://doi.org/10.1016/j.cub.2020.07.058

Mann, A. E., Sabin, S., Ziesemer, K., Vågene, Å. J., Schroeder, H., Ozga, A. T., … & Warinner, C. (2018). Differential preservation of endogenous human and microbial DNA in dental calculus and dentin. *Scientific Reports* 8(1):9822. https://doi.org/10.1038/s41598-018-28091-9

Marciniak, S., Prowse, T. L., Herring, D. A., Klunk, J., Kuch, M., Duggan, A. T., Bondioli, L., Holmes, E. C. & Poinar, H. N. (2016). *Plasmodium falciparum* malaria in 1st–2nd century CE southern Italy. *Current Biology* 26(23):R1220–R1222. https://doi.org/10.1016/j.cub.2016.10.016

Mardis, E. R. (2008). Next-generation DNA sequencing methods. *Annual Review of Genomics and Human Genetics* 9(1):387–402. https://doi.org/10.1146/annurev.genom.9.081307.164359

Maricic, T., Whitten, M. & Pääbo, S. (2010). Multiplexed DNA sequence capture of mitochondrial genomes using PCR products. *PLOS ONE* 5(11):e14004. https://doi.org/10.1371/journal.pone.0014004

Marques, C. (2019). Chapter 19—Tumors of Bone. In Buikstra, J. E. (Ed.), *Ortner's Identification of Pathological Conditions in Human Skeletal Remains (Third Edition)*, pp. 639–717. New York: Elsevier Science. https://doi.org/10.1016/B978-0-12-809738-0.00019-3

Mendum, T. A., Schuenemann, V. J., Roffey, S., Taylor, G. M., Wu, H., Singh, P., … & Stewart, G. R. (2014). *Mycobacterium leprae* genomes from a British medieval leprosy hospital: towards understanding an ancient epidemic. *BMC Genomics* 15(1):270. https://doi.org/10.1186/1471-2164-15-270

Meyer, M. & Kircher, M. (2010). Illumina sequencing library preparation for highly multiplexed target capture and sequencing. *Cold Spring Harbor Protocols* 2010(6):pdb.prot5448–pdb.prot5448. https://doi.org/10.1101/pdb.prot5448

Mühlemann, B., Vinner, L., Margaryan, A., Wilhelmson, H., Castro, C., de la F., Allentoft, M. E., ... & Sikora, M. (2020). Diverse variola virus (smallpox) strains were widespread in northern Europe in the Viking Age. *Science* 369(6502): eaaw8977. https://doi.org/10.1126/science.aaw8977

Mullis, K. B., & Faloona, F. A. (1987). Specific synthesis of DNA in vitro via a polymerase-catalyzed chain reaction. *Methods in Enzymology* 155:335–350. https://doi.org/10.1016/0076-6879(87)55023-6

Nerlich, A. G. (2018). Molecular paleopathology and paleo-oncology–state of the art, potentials, limitations and perspectives. *International Journal of Paleopathology* 21:77–82. https://doi.org/10.1016/j.ijpp.2017.02.004

Neukamm, J., Pfrengle, S., Molak, M., Seitz, A., Francken, M., Eppenberger, P., ... & Schuenemann, V. J. (2020). 2000-year-old pathogen genomes reconstructed from metagenomic analysis of Egyptian mummified individuals. *BMC Biology* 18(1):108. https://doi.org/10.1186/s12915-020-00839-8

Orlando L., Allaby R., Skoglund P., Der Sarkissian C., Stockhammer P.W., Avila-Arcos, M.C., ...& Warinner C., (2021) Ancient DNA analyses. *Nature Reviews Methods Primers* 1: 14 https://doi.org/10.1038/s43586-020-00011

Orrù, G., Contu, M. P., Casula, E., Demontis, C., Blus, C., Szmukler-Moncler, S., ... & Denotti, G. (2017). Periodontal microbiota of Sardinian children: comparing 200-year-old samples to present-day ones. *Journal of Pediatric and Neonatal Individualized Medicine (JPNIM)* 6(1):e060123–e060123. https://doi.org/10.7363/060123

Ozga, A. T., Nieves-Colón, M. A., Honap, T. P., Sankaranarayanan, K., Hofman, C. A., Milner, G. R., Lewis, C. M., Stone, A. C. & Warinner, C. (2016). Successful enrichment and recovery of whole mitochondrial genomes from ancient human dental calculus. *American Journal of Physical Anthropology* 160(2):220–228. https://doi.org/10.1002/ajpa.22960

Pääbo, Svante. (1984). Über den Nachweis von DNA in altägyptischen Mumien. *Das Altertum* 30:213 218.

Pääbo, S. (1989). Ancient DNA: Extraction, characterization, molecular cloning, and enzymatic amplification. *Proceedings of the National Academy of Sciences* 86(6):1939–1943. https://doi.org/10.1073/pnas.86.6.1939

Pálsdóttir, A. H., Bläuer, A., Rannamäe, E., Boessenkool, S. & Hallsson, J. H. (2019). Not a limitless resource: Ethics and guidelines for destructive sampling of archaeofaunal remains. *Royal Society Open Science* 6(10):191059. https://doi.org/10.1098/rsos.191059

Parkhill, J., Wren, B. W., Thomson, N. R., Titball, R. W., Holden, M. T. G., Prentice, M. B., ... & Barrell, B. G. (2001). Genome sequence of *Yersinia pestis*, the causative agent of plague. *Nature* 413(6855):523–527. https://doi.org/10.1038/35097083

Pasolli, E., Asnicar, F., Manara, S., Zolfo, M., Karcher, N., Armanini, F., ... & Segata, N. (2019). Extensive unexplored human microbiome diversity revealed by over 150,000 genomes from metagenomes spanning age, geography, and lifestyle. *Cell* 176(3):649–662.e20. https://doi.org/10.1016/j.cell.2019.01.001

Perry, R. D. & Fetherston, J. D. (1997). Yersinia pestis—etiologic agent of plague. *Clinical Microbiology Reviews* 10(1):35–66. https://doi.org/10.1128/CMR.10.1.35

Pilli, E., Modi, A., Serpico, C., Achilli, A., Lancioni, H., Lippi, B., Bertoldi, F., Gelichi, S., Lari, M. & Caramelli, D. (2013). Monitoring DNA contamination in handled vs. directly excavated ancient human skeletal remains. *PLOS ONE* 8(1):e52524. https://doi.org/10.1371/journal.pone.0052524

Pusch, C. M., Broghammer, M., Nicholson, G. J., Nerlich, A. G., Zink, A., Kennerknecht, I., Bachmann, L. & Blin, N. (2004). PCR-induced sequence alterations hamper the typing of prehistoric bone samples for diagnostic achondroplasia mutations. *Molecular Biology and Evolution* 21(11):2005–2011. https://doi.org/10.1093/molbev/msh208

Qin, J., Li, R., Raes, J., Arumugam, M., Burgdorf, K. S., Manichanh, C., Nielsen, T., ... & Wang, J. (2010). A human gut microbial gene catalogue established by metagenomic sequencing. *Nature* 464(7285):59. https://doi.org/10.1038/nature08821

Rascovan, N., Sjögren, K.-G., Kristiansen, K., Nielsen, R., Willerslev, E., Desnues, C. & Rasmussen, S. (2019). Emergence and spread of basal lineages of *Yersinia pestis* during the neolithic decline. *Cell* 176(1–2):295–305.e10. https://doi.org/10.1016/j.cell.2018.11.005

Rasmussen, S., Allentoft, M. E., Nielsen, K., Orlando, L., Sikora, M., Sjögren, K.-G., ... & Willerslev, E. (2015). Early divergent strains of *Yersinia pestis* in Eurasia 5,000 years ago. *Cell* 163(3):571–582. https://doi.org/10.1016/j.cell.2015.10.009

Riccomi, G., Fornaciari, G. & Giuffra, V. (2019). Multiple myeloma in paleopathology: a critical review. *International Journal of Paleopathology* 24:201–212. https://doi.org/10.1016/j.ijpp.2018.12.001

Robbins, G., Tripathy, V. M., Misra, V. N., Mohanty, R. K., Shinde, V. S., Gray, K. M. & Schug, M. D. (2009). Ancient skeletal evidence for leprosy in India (2000 B.C.). *PLOS ONE* 4(5):e5669. https://doi.org/10.1371/journal.pone.0005669

Roberts, C. & Ingham, S. (2008). Using ancient DNA analysis in palaeopathology: a critical analysis of published papers, with recommendations for future work. *International Journal of Osteoarchaeology* 18(6):600–613. https://doi.org/10.1002/oa.966

Ross, Z. P., Klunk, J., Fornaciari, G., Giuffra, V., Duchêne, S., Duggan, A. T., Poinar, D., Douglas, M. W., Eden, J.-S., Holmes, E. C. & Poinar, H. N. (2018). The paradox of HBV evolution as revealed from a 16th century mummy. *PLOS Pathogens* 14(1):e1006750. https://doi.org/10.1371/journal.ppat.1006750

Rugg, J. (2000). Defining the place of burial: what makes a cemetery a cemetery? *Mortality* 5(3):259–275. https://doi.org/10.1080/713686011

Sabin, S., Herbig, A., Vågene, Å. J., Ahlström, T., Bozovic, G., Arcini, C., Kühnert, D. & Bos, K. I. (2020). A seventeenth-century *Mycobacterium tuberculosis* genome supports a neolithic emergence of the mycobacterium tuberculosis complex. *Genome Biology* 21(1):201. https://doi.org/10.1186/s13059-020-02112-1

Sabin, S., Yeh, H.-Y., Pluskowski, A., Clamer, C., Mitchell, P. D. & Bos, K. I. (2020). Estimating molecular preservation of the intestinal microbiome via metagenomic analyses of latrine sediments from two medieval cities. *Philosophical Transactions of the Royal Society B: Biological Sciences* 375(1812):20190576. https://doi.org/10.1098/rstb.2019.0576

Sallares, R., Bouwman, A. & Anderung, C. (2004). The spread of malaria to southern Europe in antiquity: new approaches to old problems. *Medical History* 48(03):311–328. https://doi.org/10.1017/S0025727300007651

Santiago-Rodriguez, T. M., Fornaciari, G., Luciani, S., Dowd, S. E., Toranzos, G. A., Marota, I. & Cano, R. J. (2015). Gut microbiome of an 11th Century A.D. Pre-Columbian Andean mummy. *PLOS ONE* 10(9):e0138135. https://doi.org/10.1371/journal.pone.0138135

Schuenemann, V. J., Bos, K., DeWitte, S., Schmedes, S., Jamieson, J., Mittnik, A., … & Poinar, H. N. (2011). Targeted enrichment of ancient pathogens yielding the pPCP1 plasmid of *Yersinia pestis* from victims of the black death. *Proceedings of the National Academy of Sciences* 108(38):E746–E752. https://doi.org/10.1073/pnas.1105107108

Schuenemann, V. J., Avanzi, C., Krause-Kyora, B., Seitz, A., Herbig, A., Inskip, S., … & Krause, J. (2018). Ancient genomes reveal a high diversity of *Mycobacterium leprae* in medieval Europe. *PLOS Pathogens* 14(5):e1006997. https://doi.org/10.1371/journal.ppat.1006997

Schuenemann, V. J., Lankapalli, A. K., Barquera, R., Nelson, E. A., Hernández, D. I., Alonzo, V. A., Bos, K. I., Morfín, L. M., Herbig, A. & Krause, J. (2018). Historic *Treponema pallidum* genomes from colonial Mexico retrieved from archaeological remains. *PLOS Neglected Tropical Diseases* 12(6):e0006447. https://doi.org/10.1371/journal.pntd.0006447

Schuenemann, V. J., Singh, P., Mendum, T. A., Krause-Kyora, B., Jäger, G., Bos, K. I., … & Krause, J. (2013). Genome-wide comparison of medieval and modern *Mycobacterium leprae*. *Science* 341(6142):179–183. https://doi.org/10.1126/science.1238286

Seymour, G. J., Ford, P. J., Cullinan, M. P., Leishman, S. & Yamazaki, K. (2007). Relationship between periodontal infections and systemic disease. *Clinical Microbiology and Infection* 13:3–10. https://doi.org/10.1111/j.1469-0691.2007.01798.x

Slon, V., Hopfe, C., Weiß, C. L., Mafessoni, F., Rasilla, M., de la, Lalueza-Fox, C., … & Meyer, M. (2017). Neandertal and Denisovan DNA from Pleistocene sediments. *Science* eaam9695. https://doi.org/10.1126/science.aam9695

Søe, M. J., Nejsum, P., Seersholm, F. V., Fredensborg, B. L., Habraken, R., Haase, K., … & Kapel, C. M. O. (2018). Ancient DNA from latrines in Northern Europe and the middle east (500 BC–1700 AD) reveals past parasites and diet. *PLoS ONE* 13(4):e0195481. https://doi.org/10.1371/journal.pone.0195481

Spyrou, M. A., Tukhbatova, R. I., Wang, C.-C., Valtueña, A. A., Lankapalli, A. K., Kondrashin, V. V., … & Krause, J. (2018). Analysis of 3800-year-old *Yersinia pestis* genomes suggests Bronze Age origin for bubonic plague. *Nature Communications* 9(1):2234. https://doi.org/10.1038/s41467-018-04550-9

Susat, J., Bonczarowska, J. H., Petersone-Gordina, E.,Immel, A.. Nebel, A. Gerhards, G. & Krause-Kyora, B. (2020), *Yersinia pestis* strains from Latvia show depletion of the pla virulence gene at the end of the second plague pandemic. Sci Rep. 10(1):14628. https://doi.org/10.1038/s41598-020-71530-9

Tsosie, K. S., Begay, R. L., Fox, K. & Garrison, N. A. (2020). Generations of genomes: advances in paleogenomics technology and engagement for Indigenous people of the Americas. *Current Opinion in Genetics & Development* 62:91–96. https://doi.org/10.1016/j.gde.2020.06.010

Tumpey, T. M., Basler, C. F., Aguilar, P. V., Zeng, H., Solórzano, A., Swayne, D. E., Cox, N. J., Katz, J. M., Taubenberger, J. K., Palese, P. & García-Sastre, A. (2005). Characterization of the reconstructed 1918 Spanish influenza pandemic virus. *Science* 310(5745):77–80. https://doi.org/10.1126/science.1119392

Vågene, Å. J., Herbig, A., Campana, M. G., García, N. M. R., Warinner, C., Sabin, S., … & Krause, J. (2018). *Salmonella enterica* genomes from victims of a major sixteenth-century epidemic in Mexico. *Nature Ecology & Evolution* 2:520–528. https://doi.org/10.1038/s41559-017-0446-6

Velsko, I. M., Frantz, L. A. F., Herbig, A., Larson, G. & Warinner, C. (2018). Selection of appropriate metagenome taxonomic classifiers for ancient microbiome research. *MSystems* 3(4):e00080–18. https://doi.org/10.1128/mSystems.00080-18

Wagner, D. M., Klunk, J., Harbeck, M., Devault, A., Waglechner, N., Sahl, J. W., … & Poinar, H. (2014). *Yersinia pestis* and the plague of Justinian 541–543 AD: a genomic analysis. *The Lancet Infectious Diseases* 14(4):319–326. https://doi.org/10.1016/S1473-3099(13)70323-2

Wagner, J. K., Colwell, C., Claw, K. G., Stone, A. C., Bolnick, D. A., Hawks, J., Brothers, K. B. & Garrison, N. A. (2020). Fostering responsible research on ancient DNA. *The American Journal of Human Genetics* 107(2):183–195. https://doi.org/10.1016/j.ajhg.2020.06.017

Warinner, C., Herbig, A., Mann, A., Yates, J. A. F., Weiß, C. L., Burbano, H. A., Orlando, L. & Krause, J. (2017). A robust framework for microbial archaeology. *Annual Review of Genomics and Human Genetics* 18(1):321–356. https://doi.org/10.1146/annurev-genom-091416-035526

Warinner, C., Rodrigues, J. F. M., Vyas, R., Trachsel, C., Shved, N., Grossmann, J., … & Cappellini, E. (2014). Pathogens and host immunity in the ancient human oral cavity. *Nature Genetics* 46(4):336–344. https://doi.org/10.1038/ng.2906

Weyrich, L. S., Duchene, S., Soubrier, J., Arriola, L., Llamas, B., Breen, J., … & Cooper, A. (2017). Neanderthal behaviour, diet, and disease inferred from ancient DNA in dental calculus. *Nature* 544:357–361. https://doi.org/10.1038/nature21674

Zhou, Z., Lundstrøm, I., Tran-Dien, A., Duchêne, S., Alikhan, N.-F., Sergeant, M. J., … & Achtman, M. (2018). Pan-genome analysis of ancient and modern *Salmonella enterica* demonstrates genomic stability of the invasive para C lineage for millennia. *Current Biology* 28(15):2420–2428.e10. https://doi.org/10.1016/j.cub.2018.05.058

Ziesemer, K. A., Mann, A. E., Sankaranarayanan, K., Schroeder, H., Ozga, A. T., Brandt, B. W., … & Warinner, C. (2015). Intrinsic challenges in ancient microbiome reconstruction using 16S rRNA gene amplification. *Scientific Reports* 5:16498. https://doi.org/10.1038/srep16498

9
PARASITOLOGY AND PALEOPATHOLOGY

Aida R. Barbera, Morgana Camacho and Karl Reinhard

Introduction

Parasitology of archaeological remains, known as archaeoparasitology, is an interdisciplinary field that combines parasitology and archaeological methods to investigate specific patterns of ancient parasite infection in relation to environment, diets, behavior, and disease (Reinhard, 1992a; Reinhard & Araujo, 2012; Mitchell, 2015). The multifaceted nature of the discipline is reflected in the wealth of materials analyzed (e.g., ancient feces, burials, or refuse structures, among others), the variety of methods used, and the diverse research applications. Evolution of parasites related to subsistence, pathology, pharmacology, or human–animal interactions are some of the subjects investigated.

Since the beginning of the discipline in the early 20th century, there have been two bursts of interest in parasites derived from archaeological sites, and each began with exploration and innovation of methods. In the mid-20th century, research flourished in South America, North America, and Europe. Analytical methods were applied to coprolites, sediments, and mummies and were based on clinical and archaeological approaches. More recently, and especially after 2010, there was a second burst of interest associated with methodological innovation and critical evaluation.

Methods for coprolite and mummy study have been critically evaluated in historical context (Camacho et al., 2018) and within sediments (Camacho et al., 2020), while comparative methods addressing taphonomy have been developed for labs with limited facilities (Romera Barbera et al., 2020). This chapter explores a range of methods used to recover and evaluate parasites in archaeological contexts as well as highlights ways in which the analysis of parasites provides insights into disease in the past.

Recent Trends in Parasitology

Four collections of papers in peer-reviewed journals were published either dedicated or partly dedicated to archaeological/paleontological parasitology. These are the *Memórias do Instituto Oswaldo Cruz*, Volume 98 Supplement 1 (2003), the *International Journal of Paleopathology*, Volume 3, Issue 3 (2013), the *Korean Journal of Parasitology* 54, Issue 3 (2016), and the *Korean Journal of Parasitology,* Volume 57, issue 6 (2019). The collections represent an interest in critical assessment of laboratory methods, with particular interest in mummy studies and the analysis of sediments. However, they do not reflect the increased interest in molecular biology and parasitology. As summarized by Côté and Le Bailly (2018), over the past ten years, several papers focusing on molecular paleoparasitology have been published, and clearly the interest in aDNA techniques is increasing.

The diversification of the field, exemplified by these peer-reviewed volumes, included mummy studies. Mummy studies offered a unique opportunity, as they may preserve parasite remains as well as pathology derived from them, or in cases in which parasites cannot be recovered, immunological and molecular techniques can be applied. The potential for interdisciplinary and molecular studies on mummies has recently been summarized (Shin & Bianucci, 2020, and see Chapter 12, this volume). Coprolites (desiccated, mineralized, frozen feces, or stomach contents) have been a primary source of information throughout the 20th century (Reinhard, 2017); although, unless found in mummies, coprolites cannot be linked to a specific individual. However, ample sample sizes and diversification of the provenience within archaeological contexts can offer valuable epidemiological insights into the community.

Adopting an evolutionary perspective is also a recent trend within the field. For instance, Mitchell (2013) builds on the concept of souvenir and heirloom parasites. This concept originated with Sprent's (1969) assessment of the origin of zoonotic parasites and was established in paleoparasitology by Kliks (1990). Heirloom parasites evolved from ancestral species hosted by primate common pongid-hominid ancestors. Souvenir parasites are those acquired relatively recently in human prehistory through the breakdown of ecological-behavioral barriers between host and parasite species. Mitchell (2013) provides a review of souvenir and heirloom parasites for modern apes and sorts archaeological data into these classes to illustrate the evolutionary transitions in human–parasite relations. Molecular studies are also being used to comprehend the phylogeny of parasites. Recently, Ledger and Mitchell (2019) have summarized the data available to trace the emergence and re-emergence of parasitism through hominin evolution with special focus on zoonotic parasites.

Analytical Methods: Rigor and Interdisciplinarity

There are a number of methods used to evaluate the presence of parasites; all adopted in context of quantification and preservation. Regardless of the methods used, a primary goal is to reveal the presence or absence of parasites in samples. Equally important is quantification of parasite evidence for comparison between sites and features. In spite of these goals, Reinhard (2017) reveals emerging inadequacies in parasitology research. He asserts that during the first phases of research history, diagnostic rigor was maintained by interdisciplinary training of specialists in parasitology and archaeology sub-disciplines, including archaeobotany and archaeopalynology. Later, however, the parallel analysis of diet, pharmacology, and parasitology was lost. Confusion of sand, fungal spores, and pollen grains ensued and has been addressed in subsequent peer-reviewed publications (Camacho & Reinhard, 2019). Hence, Reinhard (2017) asserted that rigor was needed to develop in training, interdisciplinarity, sampling, archaeological control, quantification, and reproducibility. Collaborative work in molecular biology and biochemistry was also needed to verify human origins of samples. The value of this work has been underscored by McDonough (2019), Poshekhonova et al. (2020), and Teixeira-Santos et al. (2015). Archiving samples is also essential. As shown (Figure 9.1), laboratories can be designed to archive processed samples and unprocessed subsamples, allowing collaborative and future research. It appears that researchers rarely archive

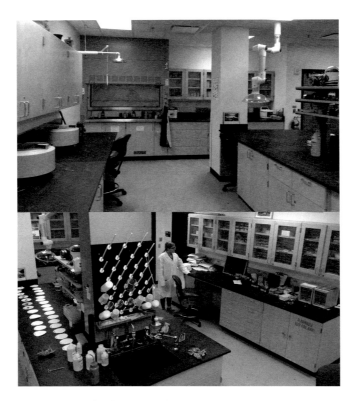

Figure 9.1 The Pathoecology Lab at the School of Natural Resources at the University of Nebraska-Lincoln is a multifunction facility designed to recover parasites from sediments, coprolites, and mummies. It is also designed for environmental and dietary analysis. The upper image shows the air handling system for processing remains. At the back of the image, there is a 1.83 meter fume hood for chemical processing of sediments. On the left of the image, the bench is used to concentrate samples after chemical processing with 12 ml or 50 ml tubes. On the right of the image is an island with microcentrifuge equipment on shelves. Over the island is a movable snorkel for capturing cave dust from sediments to prevent inhalation of infective spores. Underneath the image vantage point is a bench for final slide mounting and preparation of the samples in 2 dram vials for accession and storage. The lower image shows the coprolite processing space. On the left side of the island are coprolite macrofossils drying on blotter paper for analysis. The bench on the right is designed for organizing archived samples which are stored in three banks of cabinets, one of which is over the bench. The door to the microscope room is visible. In addition, the lab has an alcove with a laminar-flow hood to separate samples for molecular analysis at collaborative labs.

samples or, if they do, they do not include archive sources in published articles. Since reproducibility is a cornerstone of science, researchers have a responsibility to make samples available for other researchers.

To understand the current and future methodological approaches and to maintain rigor in analysis, it is useful to assess analytical methods. This section summarizes recent trends in the analysis of sediments, microscopy, the application of molecular techniques, and in quantification. Interestingly, in the analysis of ectoparasites, field methods and laboratory procedures have long been standardized (Kenward, et al., 1986; Bain, 2001; Reinhard, et al., 2020) and new imagining techniques have helped curate and preserve specimens for future aDNA tests (Reinhard, et al., 2020).

Sediment Analysis

Some of the most reliable methods of sediment analysis originated within the field of palynology, underscoring the importance of interdisciplinary work (Romera Barbera et al., 2020). The adoption of palynology methods for parasitological research was undertaken by Reinhard et al. (1986). Here, the authors subjected modern roundworm, tapeworm, and fluke eggs to hydrochloric acid and hydrofluoric acid baths, followed by acetolysis. Acetolysis involved treating samples in a solution of one part sulfuric acid to nine parts acetic anhydride. They found that fluke eggs were partly eliminated in the acetolysis solution, while roundworm and tapeworm eggs were preserved. Later, a formal application of palynology methods was proposed by Warnock and Reinhard (1992), which included hydrochloric acid and hydrofluoric acid baths to dissolve mineral components but followed by sonication rather than acetolysis. Eventually, the sonication stage was eliminated (Fisher et al., 2007). However, in a review of the historical connection between palynology and parasitology, Brinkkemper and van Haaster (2012) advocated the use of acetolysis in order to recover whipworm and ascarid eggs. Similarly, Florenzano and colleagues (2012) found that multistage processing of sediments enhanced egg recovery and quantification.

In our opinion, selecting palynological methods depends on assessing the nature of the soils when they arrive in the lab. For example, calcareous sediments may require hydrochloric acid, but perhaps less hydrofluoric acid. Sandy sediments might not require hydrochloric acid, but hydrofluoric acid will likely be necessary. Clay sediments might need extensive chemical, sedimentation, heavy density separation, and especially deflocculation. Peat sediments may need treatment in bases before acetolysis. Therefore, it is critical to assess the type of sediment collected from excavations in order to select the most efficient methods.

In Europe, a great number of studies have investigated sediments from cesspools, latrines, and other refuse pits that can contain human fecal matter (Mitchell, 2015). As latrines are used by a community of people over a period of time, the information obtained is at a population level. Sediment from habitation rooms has the potential to help understand the structure and use of the different areas within a household (Forbes et al., 2013). Sediment from the pelvic region of skeletonized burials has the advantage that reconstructions of host-parasite associations are possible (Rácz et al., 2015; Slepchenko et al., 2019). With large and diversified sample sizes, epidemiological questions and cultural behaviors can be evaluated (Flammer et al., 2020).

Microscope Methods

Microscopy is used to aid in taxonomic identification. It is conducted by looking at morphologic characteristics, ranging from shape to ornamentations and size. Basic knowledge of parasite lifecycles, morphology, as well as taphonomic processes that may have altered aspects of eggs is essential in this process (Dufour & Le Bailly, 2013; Camacho et al., 2018; Camacho et al., 2020; Romera Barbera et al., 2020). In addition, it is important to have basic knowledge of palynology and fungi spores that might be included within the archaeological sample. Some pollen grains appear similar to parasite eggs and can be misidentified. For instance, Camacho and Reinhard (2019) refute the identification of *Enterobius vermicularis* in sediments from a burial from Ancient Tehran, Iran, and assert that it is an *Ephedra* spp. pollen grain (Paknazhad et al., 2016).

Refined microscopy can assist with definitive diagnosis. Morrow and Elowsky (2019) explored the use of confocal laser scanning microscopy to generate detailed images of parasites within eggs with autofluorescence capture. This method allowed the imaging of diagnostic details of juvenile nematode eggs. The details are not visible using standard methods and allow for more secure diagnosis based on external egg morphology and internal juvenile structure. Refined processing also plays a role in revealing details of egg morphology.

Immunological and Molecular Methods

Microscopic examination of morphological features of parasite eggs is commonly used to identify eggs at the family and genus level but is rarely successful in classifying parasite eggs to the species level. Knowing the parasite's preferred or obligate host, however, can assist in species identification. For example, an heirloom parasite, like pinworm (*E. vermicularis*), is specific to the human species, hence it can be identified at the species level. However, most parasites found in ancient samples are not host specific, making the species diagnosis level difficult. For these cases, other techniques are necessary.

In the late 1980s, immunological techniques were implemented to aid with the detection and identification of parasite species (Mitchell, 2015). These techniques aim at identifying biomolecules that indicate the presence of an active infection (antigens) or a past exposure to the parasite that is no longer active (antibodies). There are three types of tests available to researchers, Enzyme-Linked Immunosorbent Assay (ELISA), Lateral-Flow Immunoassays (LFIA), and Immunofluorescence Assay (IFA). These techniques have been successfully applied in samples from the Middle East, Europe, and the Americas and have proven very useful in identifying intestinal protozoa that rarely survive in archaeological settings (Côté & Le Bailly, 2018).

Since the first reports of ancient parasite DNA from archaeological sites by Loreille and colleagues (2001), molecular techniques have been successfully used in sites from Europe (Myšková et al., 2014; Flammer et al., 2018; Søe et al., 2018; Tams et al., 2018; Roche et al., 2021), Asia (Oh et al., 2010; Shin et al., 2013; Hong et al., 2020), and South America (Jaeger & Iñiguez, 2014; Leles et al., 2014). Molecular investigation allows for the genetic differentiation of taxa that have similar egg morphology. The approach offers a more precise understanding of past parasite distribution and contributes to our knowledge of paleoepidemiology, parasite evolution, and cultural interactions. However, it has limitations. Ancient DNA damage resulting from taphonomic processes and laboratory extraction procedures have been identified (Côté et al., 2016) along with limitations of data sets used to compare the results (Sabin et al., 2020). Rigor, curation, and reporting of sample results have also recognized as problematic in aDNA analyses (Flammer et al., 2020). Therefore, careful aDNA extraction protocols are needed (Côté et al., 2016, and see Chapter 8, this volume). Hagan and colleagues (2020) compared five extraction and purification methods and applied them to three different samples from La Cueva de los Muertos Chiquitos, Mexico, dating from ~1,300 years ago. The study concluded that to recover aDNA, standardized methods developed for archaeological skeletal remains worked better than protocols developed for modern samples. Hence, it is recommended that molecular and immunological techniques developed for archaeological samples be used in conjunction with classical extraction procedures (Côté & Le Bailly, 2018; Sabin et al., 2020).

To target specific DNA fragments, especially in cases where microscopy is impossible or difficult, to assist with morphological identification, a number of techniques have been used, including polymerase chain reaction (PCR), molecular paleoparasitological hybridization (MPH), random amplified polymorphic (RAPD), and metagenomics next-generation sequencing (mNGS) (Côté & Le Bailly, 2018). For instance, Jaeger and Iñiguez

(2014) recovered pinworm aDNA in samples from 16th-century Brazil, verifying that paleogenetics can help identify eggs that are not durable in the soil. The mNGS approach has the advantage of analyzing all the genomic information of a sample, as well as allowing for the identification of the microbial composition and recognition of possible modern contamination (Søe et al., 2018; Tams et al., 2018; Borry, 2019; Borry et al., 2020; Chessa et al., 2020; Hagan et al., 2020; Sabin et al., 2020). Sabin and colleagues (2020), in an integrative study combining microscopy, metagenomics, and ELISA, explored the full microbiome of two latrines, one from medieval Riga (Latvia) and the other from Jerusalem (Israel). They found DNA traces of intestinal flora as well as eukaryotic parasites that were not seen under light microscopy such as *E. vermicularis* (pinworm). Similarly, Borba et al. (2019) used aDNA and light microscopy to reconstruct capillariid eggs phylogeny. Taking an evolutionary approach, Chessa et al. (2020) isolated a suite of intestinal parasites and offered the first description of aDNA of the human-specific *Trichuris trichiura* and *Ascaris* genus using next-generation sequencing from a 19th-century cesspit from an aristocratic palace in Sardinia.

Molecular techniques have also assisted in determining origins of coprolites, especially from humans. This is important, as it is essential to determine the original parasitic host when exploring the presence, transmission, and effects of parasitic diseases in the past. Differentiating dog from human feces, for instance, is especially important since dogs have lived close to humans and can consume similar diets and/or scavenge foods discarded by humans. This may result in aDNA transfer between humans and dogs (Guiry, 2012). For example, Shillito et al. (2020) recovered coprolites from Paisley Cave, a pre-Clovis site dating to 12,400^{14}C yr B.P., located in Oregon, and compared fecal biomarker data with mtDNA data. Fecal biomarkers include lipids that are produced by the organism, its diet, and biochemical processes occurring during digestion. In this study, of 21 coprolites recovered, two were determined to be from wild carnivores, eight samples had mtDNA and fecal biomarkers with human concordance, and two samples had dog concordance. Three samples had mtDNA and fecal biomarkers for both species, while six samples exhibited conflicting mtDNA and fecal biomarkers. Further research showed that human and dog signals can be recovered from the same coprolites. Hence, identifying fecal remains as human in origin and exploring the presence of human parasites is not a simple task. A second study conducted by Borry and colleagues (2020), combined two methods to determine the origin of the paleofeces from different archaeological sites: metagenomics and aDNA. The study used an open-sourced bioinformatics tool, known as coproID, to predict, differentiate, and authenticate the origin of human and dog coprolites (Borry, et al., 2020).

Quantitative Analysis

Interpretation of the presence and roles of parasites and their impact on health is dependent on the quantification of parasitic infestation. In the last few decades, diverse laboratory procedures have been adopted to include quantification analysis in order to facilitate comparability and to address epidemiological questions (Camacho and Reinhard, 2020). A simple method to quantify eggs per gram (EPG) is undertaken by adding a specific amount of *Lycopodium* spore tablets to samples after rehydration (Camacho et al., 2020). For sediment samples, Reinhard (1992a) counted a minimum of 25 *Lycopodium* spores and counted these along with parasite remains. The method was sufficient to identify infections and to indicate which samples were positive and which negative for parasite eggs. However, it failed to identify other less intense infections or provide a reasonable epidemiological picture and risks associated with parasitic infection. Morrow (2016), assessing coprolites, tested the technique of counting 25 *Lycopodium* or more and found that samples yielding between 25 and 200 spores offered different positive/negative results but between 200 and 500 spores, there were no significant differences. Therefore, it was established that quantification required counting a minimum of 200 *Lycopodium* spores (Morrow, 2016; Camacho & Reinhard, 2020). EPG counts are conducted following the pollen concentration formula $Concentration = [(p/m) \times a]/w$, where p is the number of parasite remains counted, m the number of spores counted, a the total number of spores added, and w weight of the sample.

While quantitative analyses allow for the examination of prevalence, they also assist in the evaluation of a parasitology principle known as overdispersion, a phenomenon also referred to as aggregation. We know in modern samples that parasite distribution is aggregated, meaning that most hosts have no or just a few parasites, while few hosts have most of them. To assess aggregated distribution in the past, it is essential to conduct biostatistical analyses that characterize and compare parasitic infections (Reiczigel et al., 2019). QPweb software facilitates this analysis by applying indices that evaluate prevalence, mean and median intensity, mean abundance, mean crowding, variance-to-mean ratio (VMR), and sex ratios (if applicable) of parasite infections, followed by appropriate statistical tests (Reiczigel et al., 2019). VMR calculation, used to verify aggregation indices, is the parameter by which past populations can be compared to modern ones (Camacho & Reinhard, 2020).

Through the use of quantification methods, highly infected individuals who would have been frailer and exposed to further health risks, when compared to the rest of the population, can be identified. Comparative studies looking at modern and ancient data have demonstrated that overdispersion was present in the past (Camacho et al., 2018). For instance, Camacho and Reinhard (2020), building upon over 50 years of research on pinworm infection in Southwest USA, used egg per count (EPG) and biostatistical analyses to explore parasitic burdens in the past. They concluded that previous studies underestimated parasitic burdens and offered two conclusions: (1) all sites under investigation showed aggregated distributions when compared to modern parasitism trends; and (2) the spread of pinworm infection reflected sociocultural habits, including activities undertaken in communal rooms and personal hygiene. They concluded that identifying habitation structures as infection catalyzers and the use of rock shelters enhancing transmission was inaccurate. Hence, understanding the theory of overdispersion contributes to rigorous interpretations that can aid in reconstructing scenarios for the emergence and re-emergence of infectious diseases (Camacho & Reinhard, 2020).

Taphonomy

It is extremely important to be mindful of taphonomic principles of preservation prior to conducting parasitology analysis. Morrow and colleagues (2016) identified five major factors affecting the taphonomy of endoparasite eggs. Abiotic factors include environmental conditions such as soil composition or temperature. Contextual factors involve the source of evidence analyzed (e.g., coprolites and latrines), as each influence the preservation and recovery of parasites. Organismal factors include biological characteristics of the parasite and the parasite egg, including life cycle, fecundity, and morphological structure. Ecological factors affect the interaction of the parasite with other microorganisms and decomposers, such as fungi or mites. Finally, anthropogenic factors include conditions that result from human manipulation of the parasite eggs, including excavation methods, storing and curation of the samples, or the extraction procedures in the laboratory. While the first four factors are beyond the control of the researcher, the anthropogenic factors are a direct consequence of researchers manipulating the samples. It is imperative, therefore, that parasitologists select laboratory methods that prioritize the recovery of eggs.

One of the first papers addressing taphonomy and methodology focused on preservation of helminth eggs from latrines and coprolites (Reinhard et al., 1986). Observations were drawn from archaeological samples and from experimental tests. The authors identified moist anaerobic conditions from latrines and desiccating environments as optimal environments for the preservation of eggs. Desiccated coprolites provided excellent preservation of eggs and larvae, although mechanical processes associated with desiccation, such as wrinkling, could alter the morphology of the egg. Sediments from latrines, despite being excellent sources for the recovery of parasites, offered variable taphonomic conditions. First, parasite eggs could be washed away by water and rainfall. Second, during the shift from aerobic to anaerobic soil, fungal proliferation could occur; fungi release enzymes and can digest eggs. The authors found that delicate morphological features, such as polar plugs in the eggs of *T. trichiura*, were favored by fungal mycelia. Third, mechanical processes such as freezing/thawing of the soils could alter egg morphology. Finally, soil conditions such as alkalinity could alter egg morphology and corrode diagnostic features that aid with the microscopic identification. Therefore, it is the responsibility of the researcher to take into account the different taphonomic factors that may have affected the egg preservation before deciding the laboratory procedure to analyze the samples.

Parasites, Parasitism, and Paleopathology

Parasites, broadly speaking, are divided into two main categories, endoparasites, if they live within the host, and ectoparasites, if they live on the surface of the host. Lifecycles can vary from organism to organism, some have simple life cycles developing and dying in a single host and others have complex systems requiring different hosts. The definitive host is that in which the adult parasite reproduces sexually and the intermediate host that in which the larvae and other non-sexual forms develop. Generally, the eggs, larvae, or juveniles are detected microscopically. Juvenile is the term to be used in reference to the developmental stages of nematodes. Other classes of worms have morphologically distinct larval stages. Molecular and chemical analyses can detect signals from all life stages.

Ectoparasites

Ectoparasites are parasites that live on the surface of the host from whom they obtain nutrients. Human louse, fleas, human lice, and, in less numbers, bedbugs and pubic lice are some of the most encountered ectoparasites in past human populations (Bain, 2004; Forbes et al., 2013; Reinhard et al., 2020). Health risks associated with heavy infestations and prevalence of ectoparasites in human populations in ancient times, like today, would have been very high regardless of the severity of the pathogenesis or their role as vectors. For instance, personal combs infested with head lice *Pediculus humanus capitis* were found in Israel dating from first century BC to eighth century AD, in Roman times, and in Chilean tombs (reviewed by Reinhard et al., 2020). Forbes and colleagues (2013) studied Polar Inuit communities of Greenland using ectoparasites to identify hygienic practices and activity areas within the habitation sites. Localized high concentrations of human flea *Pulex irritans*, human louse *P. humanus*, and the pubic louse *Phthirus pubis* in habitation areas likely corresponded to delousing practices. Reinhard and Buikstra's (2003) epidemiological investigation of head lice infestation among Chiribaya culture of southern Peru unveiled gendered social practices associated to braiding activities performed by males.

Some ectoparasites, beyond extracting nutrients from the host, can also be vectors for the transmission of other pathogens. Human body louse can be a vector of transmission for typhus, relapsing fever, or trench fever caused by *Bartonella quintana* (Bain, 2004; Forbes et al., 2013). Holck (2011) transcribed passages of Eyrbygg Icelandic saga from the 13th–14th century, describing what appears to be an epidemic outbreak of lice-transmitted typhus around the turn of the first millennium. Molecular analysis of teeth from soldiers of Napoleon's army identified a heavy burden of louse-borne pathogens including typhus and trench fever (Raoult et al., 2006). Fleas are also the vector for the transmission of *Yersinia pestis*, the bacterial causal agent of plague. Traditionally, the Oriental rat flea (*Xenopsylla cheopis*) has been identified as the vector of transmission; however, recent investigations have underscored the potential of the human flea for the human-human transmission (Dean et al., 2018).

Although bedbugs and mites have received less attention, their ubiquity in the past was noted in ancient texts from China, India, the Mediterranean, and the Middle East (Thomas et al., 2017). Scabies caused by parasitic mites was probably also ubiquitous in ancient and medieval Europe (Thomas et al., 2017). It has been reported in historical settings with deficient hygienic measures and overcrowding, such as during the Napoleonic wars and the American Civil War. Today, the main contributors to scabies are poverty and overcrowded living conditions (Mumcuoglu et al., 2009).

Protozoa

Protozoa are ephemeral, unicellular eukaryotic organisms that rarely survive in archaeological settings, although sometimes calcified cysts have been identified (Waters-Rist et al., 2014; Calleja et al., 2017). In these cases, immunological techniques combined with molecular analysis can help detect their presence (Côté & Le Bailly, 2018). Faulkner and colleagues (1989) conducted one of the earliest successful immunological tests to target *Giardia duodenalis* cysts in desiccated feces from prehistoric North America. In mummies, the identification of parasite DNA has been crucial to furthering the paleoparasitological investigation of protozoa (Aufderheide et al., 2005; Zink et al., 2006; Costa & Llagostera, 2014).

There are various classes of protozoa that infect humans. Parasitic protozoa that live in the intestines are often transmitted through the fecal-oral route by the unintentional ingestion of contaminated water or soil. Poor sanitation, overcrowded conditions, and lack of personal hygiene can trigger disease outbreaks. *Giardia* spp. has been identified using a combination of immunological tests and microscopic observations. So far, it has been found in the Europe and Asia (Le Bailly et al., 2008; Graff et al., 2020) and in the Americas (Gonçalves et al., 2004; Leles et al., 2019). Mitchell and colleagues (2008) identified *G. duodenalis* and *Entamoeba histolytica*, another intestinal protozoan, in medieval crusader latrines from Israel using ELISA.

In contrast, protozoa that live in the blood or in human tissue depend on a vector for its transmission, often arthropods such as mosquitos, fleas, or lice. An example is leishmaniasis, a disease caused by over 30 different organisms of the genus *Leishmania* and transmitted by flies *Phlebotomus* (Europe and Asia) and *Lutzomyia* (in the Americas) and with many mammals acting as a reservoir, is an example of protozoa. *Leishmania donovani*, a fatal form of the disease, was identified in Christian Nubian and Egyptian mummies dating 4,000 years ago (Zink et al., 2006) and *Leishmania tarentolae* from Brazilian mummies (Novo et al., 2015).

aDNA of *Plasmodium falciparum*, the protozoa agent of malaria transmitted by mosquitos of the genus *Anopheles*, has been found on skeletal remains from Roman deposits in Italy (Marciniak et al., 2016) and mummies from ancient Egypt (Lalremruata et al., 2013).

Trypanosoma cruzi, the causal agent for Chagas disease, and *Trypanosoma brucei*, behind African sleeping sickness, are two of the most-deadly vector-borne flagellate protozoa. The history and evolution of *T. brucei* in Africa have been summarized elsewhere with DNA suggesting it played an important role in hominid evolution (Steverding, 2020). Chagas disease is circumspect in Central and South America, transmitted by more than a dozen blood-sucking triatomines, of which the kissing bug (*Triatoma infestans*) is one of the most well-known; armadillos, rodents, dogs, and the domestic guinea pig are reservoir hosts (Aufderheide et al., 2005). The vectors usually feed on the host when they are sleeping, and infection occurs when the host is bitten by an infected vector that defecates on or near the bite. Scratching and rubbing the bite can help push the feces into the wound. *T. cruzi* does not leave traces in bones or coprolite remains, but during its chronic development, Chagastic megacolon and dilated hearts are common. Reinhard and colleagues (2003) described a case of megacolon in a mummy from Lower Pecos, US, dating from 1,150 BP whose diagnosis was later confirmed by the recovery of *T. cruzi* DNA (Dittmar et al., 2003). Since then, the paleoparasitological analysis of American trypanosomiasis has largely benefitted from molecular analysis (Guhl et al., 2014). Aufderheide and colleagues' (2005) extensive study of mummies from South America demonstrated that sylvatic (animal to human) Chagas disease was present at least 9,000 years ago.

Helminths

Parasitic worms, collectively known as helminths, tend to have complex life cycles with multiple intermediate hosts or may undergo free-living maturation stages requiring the presence of specific media (Lindquist and Cross, 2017). Helminth parasites are classified into three broad groups: trematodes (flukes), cestodes (tapeworms), and nematodes (roundworms). Some species produce resistant eggs that can be found archaeologically. For some species of helminths, high fecundity and highly resistant eggshells to taphonomic processes make them perdurable. Indeed, helminths are one of the most encountered types of parasite eggs in archaeological contexts. The egg production and durability make the soil-transmitted parasites (STH) *T. trichiura* and *Ascaris lumbricoides* especially easy to recover using a variety of methods. Up to 10,000 eggs are laid per day by *T. trichiura* and 200,000 eggs per day by *A. lumbricoides*. Therefore, tens of thousands of these eggs can be present per ml of latrine sediment. Because of this, simple methods such as the "squash" technique (Dainton, 1992) can be used to test for egg positivity. This method involves the use of light pressure to disperse small amounts of sediment in fluid across a microscope preparation. For samples with many eggs, this is a useful method for screening. These species' eggs distribution is also amenable to quantitative palynological and Stoll's dilution procedures. The researcher must choose a quantification method based on the archaeological context, time constraints, and laboratory facilities. A summary of what researchers may expect in relation to some of the most common helminth eggs is provided in Table 9.1.

Most cestodes and trematodes are food-borne parasites contracted by humans through consumption of undercooked contaminated meat and fish. For instance, a maturation stage of *Opisthorchis* liver flukes takes place in freshwater snails (first intermediate host) and then in freshwater fish or crustaceans (second intermediate host). Humans are definitive hosts and can become infected when they ingest uncooked or undercooked fish. *Opisthorchis felineus*

Table 9.1 Selected helminths of humans and their archaeological recovery potential. The potential for preservation is noted in the "Durability" column based on lifecycle and previous documentation from archaeological contexts

Type	Life stage released	Durability
Nematodes (Roundworm)		
Enterobius vermicularis	Thin-walled, nearly embryonated egg	Most eggs are not defecated but are laid on perianal folds by gravid female. Can be recovered in area with coprolites, but only two cases have been reported in sediments.
Ancylostoma duodenale, Necator americanus	Thin-walled, nearly embryonated egg	Eggs hatch shortly after defecation and larvae migrate from feces. Can be recovered from coprolites. Adults have been found in mummied remains.
Ascaris lumbricoides	Thick-walled, unembryonated	Eggs hatch weeks after defecation. Each female produces 100,000s of eggs per day. Durability and abundance allow recovery in mummies, coprolites, and sediments. Diagnosis must be based on the presence of the distinctive uterine layer.
Dioctophyme renale	Thick-walled, unembryonated	Eggs are passed in urine and require moist environments to survive. Found in sediments. Diagnosis must be based on the presence of a thick, uneven layer and bipolar plugs.
Strongyloides stercoralis	First stage larvae are released	The larvae migrate from feces. Found in coprolites.
Trichinella species	Infection occurs by consumption of muscle with cysts	Cysts have been discovered in mummified remains.
Trichuris trichiura	Thick-walled, unembryonated	Eggs embryonate weeks after defecation. Each female produces up to 10,000 eggs per day. Durability and abundance allow recovery from mummies, coprolites, and sediments.
Trematodes (Flukes)		
Clonorchis spp.	Thin-walled, resistant, unembryonated	Passed in feces. Eggs are operculated and often found without opercula in sediments, but intact in coprolites and mummies.
Fasciola spp.	"	"
Metagonimus yokogawai	"	"
Opisthorchis spp.	"	"
Paragonimus spp.	Medium-walled, unembryonated	"
Schistosoma japonicum, S. mansoni, and *S. intercalatum*	"	Passed in feces. Egg morphology varies between species. Reported in sediments, but best preservation in mummies and coprolites.
Schistosoma haematobium	"	Passed in urine. Eggs found in mummified remains.

Type	Life stage released	Durability
Echinostoma spp.	Medium-walled, unembryonated	Passed in feces. Eggs are operculated and often found without opercula in sediments, but intact in coprolites and mummies.
Cestodes (tapeworms)		
Diphyllobothrium spp.	Medium-walled, unembryonated	Passed in feces. Eggs are operculated and often found without opercula in sediments, but intact in coprolites and mummies.
Adenocephalus pacificus	"	"
Echinococcus spp.	Causes hydatid cyst disease	Cysts have been found in burial sediments.
Hymenolepis spp.	Medium-walled, embryonated	Passed in feces. Eggs loose outer layers leaving six-hooked oncospheres. Well preserved in coprolites.
Taenia spp.	Thick-walled, embryonated	Passed in feces. Radial, thick-walled eggs contain six-hooked oncospheres. Well preserved in coprolites and sediments.

has been identified in medieval to modern archaeological sites in Siberia (Slepchenko et al., 2019; Slepchenko, 2020). *Clonorchis sinensis*, endemic to East Asia, have been reported from Korean Joseon mummies (Shin et al., 2013) and in China from the Bronze Age to medieval times (Yeh & Mitchell, 2016). Other liver flukes, which are less common in archaeological samples, include *Fasciola hepatica* or *Paragonimus westermani*, both found in 15th-century Seoul (Cho et al., 2017). *Metagonimus yokogawai*, a minuscule intestinal fluke, was also reported by Cho and colleagues (2017) using molecular analysis from Joseon Korean mummies (Hong et al., 2020). Echinostomiasis, a diseased caused by intestinal flukes of the family *Echinostoma*, is contracted by ingesting poorly cooked contaminated snails or fish. Leles and colleagues (2014) corroborated echinostomiasis in a Peruvian mummy using microscopy and molecular amplification and suggested *Echinostoma paransei* as the pathogenic agent.

Schistosomiasis, also known as bilharzia, is caused by three species of blood flukes: *Schistosoma mansoni*, *Schistosoma haematobium*, and *Schistosoma japonicum*. Contrary to food-borne flukes, human schistosomes are acquired when cercariae released by the snail penetrate the skin of the host. Swimming, fishing, and other human activities that take place in contaminated waters are a risk factor. The first case of *S. haematobium* was reported by Ruffer (1910) from an Egyptian mummy dating to 5,200 years ago. Since then, more systematic analysis of Egyptian mummies' tissue has revealed a widespread occurrence (Kloos & David, 2002). In Asia, *S. japonicum* has been reported from China (Wei et al., 1981), and in Europe, findings of eggs of *S. mansoni* in a 15th-century private latrine from France indicated travel or migration from Africa where the snail host resides (Bouchet et al., 2002).

Tapeworms of genus *Taenia*, i.e., *Taenia saginata* (beef tapeworm), *Taenia solium* (pork tapeworm), and *Taenia asiatica* (Asian tapeworm, also in pigs), are contracted through close contact with respective domesticated animals and consumption of poorly processed meat. Taeniasis was reported from various deposits within the Chehrabad Salt Mine in Iran (Nezambadi et al., 2013a; 2013b). Søe and colleagues (2018), besides obtaining evidence of *T. solium* in latrines from Viking Denmark, found tapeworms for which different animals and not humans are definitive hosts, such as *T. hydatigena* (dog) and *T. suis* (pig), indicating that they lived in close proximity. Tams and colleagues (2018) arrived at similar conclusions in their investigation of Iron Age Denmark, where continuous finding of *T. saginata* suggested that cattle lived in the vicinity of humans. Taeniid-type eggs have also been reported from prehistoric North America, although the human origins of these is unclear (McDonough, 2019).

The accidental consumption of food, water, or soil contaminated with *Echinococcus granulosus* (hydatid tapeworm) can cause abdominal pain and vomiting if it affects the liver, or chest pain and chronic cough when affecting the lungs. Until the beginning of the 20th century, Iceland had the highest prevalence of echinococcosis in the world (Kristjánsdóttir & Collins, 2011). It is speculated that it arrived in Iceland sometime in the late 9th or early 10th century with the first settlers and became endemic by the 14th century. Kristjánsdóttir and Collins (2011) found calcified cysts in eight individuals from a medieval cemetery in Skriðuklaustur, Iceland. Cases of hydatid cysts have also been reported in the Middle East (Zias & Mumcuoglu, 1991), USA (Williams, 1985), Siberia (Waters-Rist et al., 2014), and Spain (Calleja et al., 2017).

Many species of the fish tapeworm (*Dibothriocephalus* spp. and *Diphyllobothrium* spp.) can parasitize humans if they consume infected freshwater fish undercooked or prepared in a manner that fails to kill the parasites. *Dibothriocephalus latus* (= *Diphyllobothrium latum*) has been reported from sites in Europe from Mesolithic times (Perri et al., 2018), Neolithic (Le Bailly et al., 2005; Maicher et al., 2017; 2019), and Roman through Medieval times (Mitchell, 2017; Søe et al., 2018; Sabin et al., 2020). Findings at Derragh Mesolithic Ireland provide a unique glimpse into the culinary and dietary customs of otherwise elusive hunter-gatherer bands, for which zooarchaeological and bioarchaeological data is lacking (Perri et al., 2018). Molecular and paleoparasitological investigation by Flammer et al. (2018) of the medieval city of Lübeck, in Germany, revealed surprising culinary trends involving the consumption of uncooked or poorly cooked red meat and freshwater fish. Eggs of *D. latus* and *T. saginata* were found in abundance in latrine deposits, with *D. latus* more abundant in earlier periods and *T. saginata* after 1,300 CE. The authors conclude that this change did not reflect a modification of culinary habits, but that the industry that grew along the river contaminated the waters resulting in the reduction of available first intermediate hosts. Multidisciplinary teams investigating diet and foodways in the Eurasian steppe have explored details of the community's culinary habits between seasons (Poshekhonova et al., 2020). In North America, *Dibothriocephalus* spp., found in an 18th-century urban colony of Nova Scotia, elucidated the culinary habits of fisherman and other seasonal habitants of the growing community of European origin (Fonzo et al., 2020). The prevalence of *Adenocephalus pacificus* (= *Diphyllobothrium pacificum*) acquired from eating infected saltwater fish among Chinchorro people in northern Chile has been widely discussed (Reinhard & Urban, 2003). Further investigations found a correspondence between the ENSO (El-Niño Southern Oscillations) events, the availability of intermediate fish, and parasitism among Chinchorro (Arriaza et al., 2010).

Among human intestinal helminths, STH are the most prevalent and widely distributed globally. It is estimated that 2.7 billion infections today are caused by nematodes of the species *T. trichiura* (whipworm), *A. lumbricoides* (roundworm) and hookworms (*Necator americanus* and *Ancylostoma duodenale*) (Linquist & Cross, 2017). Linked to poverty and access to clean water, STH are often spread through fecal contamination of food and poor urban and personal hygiene. Most STH infections can go undetected but heavy burdens can cause intestinal disorders, diarrhea, and in children can be associated with growth disruptions (Flammer & Smith, 2020). Of these, *A. lumbricoides* and *T. trichiura* are the most recovered species in archaeological contexts (Leles et al., 2010; Mitchell, 2015; Flammer et al., 2020).

Archaeoparasitology has contributed to a rich body of literature exploring the paleoepidemiology of STH as they intersect with health, hygiene, and other social practices. Leles and colleagues (2010) summarize data for both nematodes, unveiling very interesting temporal patterns. Co-infection of *T. trichiura* and *A. lumbricoides* around the world occurred in 59% of the cases, and in Europe over 78% and nearly 90% during Medieval times (Leles et al., 2010: 1511). This pattern has been confirmed by new investigations carried out by diverse teams exploring Neolithic Eurasia, which suggest that *A. lumbricoides* prevalence began only after urbanization (Le Bailly et al., 2005; Rácz et al., 2015; Maicher et al., 2017; 2019; Bergman, 2018; Perri et al., 2018; Slavinsky et al., 2018; Ledger et al., 2019; Slepchenko et al., 2019). Interestingly, all these sites were positive for fish tapeworm, unveiling past foodways and questions about human diphyllobothriid infections in the past. In the Americas, ascariasis is rare; population dispersion, higher mobility, and less pronounced urbanization, as well as findings of vermifuge plants, may explain this difference (Leles et al., 2010).

Parasitism at the brink of urbanization in Europe has been extensively reviewed with special attention to the Roman period (Mitchell, 2017; Williams et al., 2017; Ledger et al., 2018; Ledger et al., 2020) and the Middle Ages (Rocha et al., 2006; Florenzano et al., 2012; Rácz et al., 2015; Søe et al., 2018; Flammer et al., 2020; Graff et al., 2020; Sabin et al., 2020; Tams et al., 2018; Roche et al., 2021). Combining archaeology, historical sources, and paleoparasitology has informed us that even when sanitation was a priority during the planning of a city, if maintenance of latrines and other public buildings and personal hygiene was lacking, infection was prevalent (Knorr et al., 2019). Similar conclusions were made for Medieval and Renaissance Brussels, where findings of *T. trichiura*, *A. lumbricoides*, and protozoa that cause dysentery were found (Graff et al., 2020). The authors suggest that practices related to the manipulation of excrement, unsanitary conditions of markets, and a polluted river would have perpetuated parasitism. Co-infection following the construction of cities has also been reported in Asian contexts (Shin et al., 2018; Shin et al., 2020). For instance, in Korea, the practice of recycling nightsoil from the larger cities to use as fertilizers in agricultural lands may have facilitated the prevalence of STH (Kim et al., 2014). In North America, European colonialism and the development of cities brought a new epidemiological scenario and, despite the construction of latrines, heavy infestation rates persisted (Reinhard et al., 1986; Fisher et al., 2007; Trigg et al., 2017; Fonzo et al., 2020).

E. vermicularis (pinworm) causing an estimated 200 million infections today, is transmitted human-human when eggs are passed through direct contact, although contamination from contact with infected surfaces is also common. *E. vermicularis* have been extensively recovered from coprolites in the Americas (Camacho et al., 2018; Morrow & Reinhard, 2018; Valverde et al., 2020), mainly in association with agricultural communities. The authors of these studies looked at distribution and frequency of pinworm and reached two conclusions. On the one hand, fewer infections were found in pre-agricultural communities, which is explained by an increase of population in later times. On the other hand, habitation structures, such as rock shelters, were believed to have contributed to human-human spread. Recently, the application of statistical analysis has helped refine these hypotheses and, as mentioned in the discussion on quantification above, unveiled a much broader and complicated epidemiological scenario than previously thought (Camacho & Reinhard, 2020). Pinworm egg structure is, however, fragile and degrades easily in most taphonomic conditions. In Europe and Asia, only few cases have been reported (Horne, 2002; Shin et al., 2011; Paknazhad et al., 2016).

Emerging research in parasitism is helping us understand the synergistic relationship between infection, anemia, and bone pathology in light of diet and disease in the past. Porotic hyperostosis and *cribra orbitalia*, some of the most encountered pathological lesions noted by paleopathologists, have long been linked to anemia, but it has been suggested that these have more complicated etiologies than simple dietary deficiencies, including parasitism (Walker, et al., 2009; Lindquist & Cross, 2017). Diphyllobothriid infections can cause severe cases of anemia as the fish tapeworm competes for nutrients with its host, including B_{12} vitamin, causing megaloblastic anemia (Lindquist & Cross, 2017). Several remains of fish tapeworm eggs have been recovered in Eastern and Western Hemispheres from Paleolithic to Historical times, unveiling a history of infection and co-evolution. Bathurst (2005) suggests that the high occurrence of indicators of anemia in Northwestern North American pre-Columbian skeletons could be explained by the heavy burden of fish tapeworm. Reinhard (1992b) presented a case in which parasitism and dietary insufficiencies synergistically caused porotic hyperostosis. This is relevant to the newer hypotheses exploring the etiology of anemias (Walker et al., 2009; Lindquist & Cross, 2017). A similar approach was accomplished in the Lluta Valley, Chile, where an increase in *A. pacificus* parasitism occurred during the Inca Empire expansion exactly at the same time when the subsistence pattern was disrupted (Santoro et al., 2003; Vinton et al., 2009). Clearly, these studies emphasize the importance of interdisciplinarity in testing hypotheses.

Conclusion

Multi-proxy data obtained from multidisciplinary analysis of coprolites, sediments, and mummies can offer a wealth of information about health, diet, mobility, and social practices in the past. As reviewed, the impact of parasitological analysis on paleopathological assessments of past health and disease is tremendous. Parasitological analyses must follow rigorous methods that incorporate quantitative data and allow for interdisciplinary research in order to build comparable epidemiological data sets. Collaboration is a defining characteristic of parasitology. The development of methods and techniques specific to archaeoparasitology and fostered collaborations with other fields has expanded the scope of research in recent years. Researchers have been emphasizing the need for archaeologists and archaeoparasitologists to work together to integrate paleoenvironmental and paleoclimate perspectives (Dittmar, 2013), to incorporate cultural aspects (Dittmar et al., 2012) and historic resources and museum collections (Harmon et al., 2019; Pye, 2020) into our study of disease in the past, and to incorporate state-of-the-art techniques to unveil parasite ecologies in the past (Côté & Le Bailly, 2018; Flammer & Smith, 2020; Pye, 2020). It is our opinion that by maintaining rigor in the methods and techniques chosen, integrating multidisciplinary approaches, and grounding our research within archaeological contexts, we will advance the field and deepen our knowledge of disease in the past.

References

Arriaza, B. T., Reinhard, K. J., Araújo, A. G., Orellana, N. C & Standen, V. G. (2010). Possible influence of the ENSO phenomenon on the pathoecology of diphyllobothriasis and anisakiasis in ancient Chinchorro populations. *Memórias do Instituto Oswaldo Cruz* 105(1):66–72. https://doi.org/10.1590/S0074-02762010000100010

Aufderheide, A. C. Salo, W., Madden, M., Streitz, J., Dittmar de la Cruz, K., Buikstra, J., Arriaza, B. & Wittmers Jr., L. E. (2005). Aspects of ingestion transmission of Chagas disease identified in mummies and their coprolites. *Chungara: Revista de Antropología Chilena* 37(1):85–90. http://www.jstor.org/stable/27802409

Bain, A. (2001). *Archaeoentomological and Archaeoparasitological Reconstructions at Îlot Hunt (CeEt–110): New Perspectives in Historical Archaeology (1850–1900).* British Archaeological Reports S973. Oxford, UK: Archaeopress.

Bain, A. (2004). Irritating intimates: the archaeoentomology of lice, fleas, and bedbugs. *Northeast Historical Archaeology* 33(1):8. https://doi.org/10.22191/neha/vol33/iss1/8

Bathurst, R. R. (2005). Archaeological evidence of intestinal parasites from coastal shell middens. *Journal of Archaeological Science* 32(1):115–123. https://doi.org/10.1016/j.jas.2004.08.001

Bergman, J. (2018). Stone age disease in the north–human intestinal parasites from a Mesolithic burial in Motala, Sweden. *Journal of Archaeological Science* 96:26–32. https://doi.org/10.1016/j.jas.2018.05.008

Borba, V. H., Machado-Silva, J. R., Le Bailly, M. & Iñiguez, A. M. (2019). Worldwide paleodistribution of capillariid parasites: paleoparasitology, current status of phylogeny and taxonomic perspectives. *PLoS ONE* 14(4):e0216150. https://doi.org/10.1371/journal.pone.0216150

Borry, M. (2019). Sourcepredict: Prediction of metagenomic sample sources using dimension reduction followed by machine learning classification. *Journal of Open Source Software* 4(41):1540. https://doi.org/10.21105/joss.01540

Borry, M., Cordova, B., Perri, A., Wibowo, M., Honap, T. P., Ko, J., ... & Warinner, C. (2020). CoproID predicts the source of coprolites and paleofeces using microbiome composition and host DNA content. *PeerJ* 8:e9001 https://doi.org/10.7717/peerj.9001

Bouchet, F., Harter, S., Paicheler, J. C., Aráujo, A. & Ferreira, L. F. (2002). First recovery of *Schistosoma mansoni* eggs from a latrine in Europe (15–16th Centuries). *Journal of Parasitology* 88(2):404–405. https://doi.org/10.1645/0022-3395(2002)088

Brinkkemper, O. & van Haaster, H. (2012). Eggs of intestinal parasites whipworm (Trichuris) and mawworm (Ascaris): non–pollen palynomorphs in archaeological samples. *Review of Palaeobotany and Palynology* 186:16–21. https://doi.org/10.1016/j.revpalbo.2012.07.003

Calleja, Á. M. M., Sarkic, N., López, J. H., Antunes, W. D., Pereira, M. F., de Matos, A. P. A. & Santos, A. L. (2017). A possible *Echinococcus granulosus* calcified cyst found in a medieval adult female from the churchyard of Santo Domingo de Silos (Prádena del Rincón, Madrid, Spain). *International Journal of Paleopathology* 16:5–13. DOI: 10.1016/j.ijpp.2017.01.005.

Camacho, M., Araújo, A., Morrow, J., Buikstra, J. & Reinhard, K. (2018). Recovering parasites from mummies and coprolites: an epidemiological approach. *Parasites & Vectors* 11(1):1–17. https://doi.org/10.1186/s13071-018-2729-4

Camacho, M., Iñiguez, A. M. & Reinhard, K. J. (2018). Taphonomic considerations on pinworm prevalence in three Ancestral Puebloan latrines. *Journal of Archaeological Science: Reports* 20:791–798. https://doi.org/10.1016/j.jasrep.2018.06.024

Camacho, M. & Reinhard, K. J. (2019). Confusing a pollen grain with a parasite egg: an appraisal of "paleoparasitological evidence of pinworm (Enterobius Vermicularis) infection in a female adolescent residing in ancient Tehran". *The Korean Journal of Parasitology* 57(6):621–625. https://doi.org/10.3347/kjp.2019.57.6.621

Camacho, M. & Reinhard, K. J. (2020). Pinworm research in the Southwest USA: five decades of methodological and theoretical development and the epidemiological approach. *Archaeological and Anthropological Science* 12:63. https://doi.org/10.1007/s12520-019-00994-2

Camacho, M., Perri, A. & Reinhard, K. J. (2020). Parasite microremains: preservation, recovery, processing, and identification. In Henry, A. (Ed.), *Handbook for the Analysis of Micro-Particles in Archaeological Samples. Interdisciplinary Contributions to Archaeology*, pp.173–199. Cham: Springer. https://doi.org/10.1007/978-3-030-42622-4_8

Chessa, D., Murgia, M., Sias, E., Deligios, M., Mazzarello, V., Fiamma, M., ... & Rubino, S. (2020). Metagenomics and microscope revealed *T. trichiura* and other intestinal parasites in a cesspit of an Italian nineteenth century aristocratic palace. *Scientific Reports* 10(1):1–10. https://doi.org/10.1038/s41598-020-69497-8

Cho, P. Y., Park, J. M., Hwang, M. K., Park, S. H., Park, Y. K., Jeon, B. Y., Kim T. S. & Lee, H. W. (2017). Discovery of parasite eggs in archeological residence during the 15th century in Seoul, Korea. *The Korean Journal of Parasitology* 55(3):357–361. https://doi.org/10.3347/kjp.2017.55.3.357

Costa, M. A. & Llagostera, A. (2014). Leishmaniasis en coyo oriente: migrantes trasandinos en san pedro de atacama. *Estudios Atacameños* (47):5–18. http://dx.doi.org/10.4067/S0718-10432014000100002

Côté, N. M. L., Daligault, J., Pruvost, M., Bennett, E. A., Gorgé, O., Guimaraes, S., Capelli, N., Le Bailly, M., Geigl, E.-M. & Grange, T. (2016). A new high-throughput approach to genotype ancient human gastrointestinal parasites. *PLoS ONE* 11(1): e0146230. https://doi.org/10.1371/journal.pone.0146230

Côté, N. & Le Bailly, M. (2018). Palaeoparasitology and palaeogenetics: review and perspectives for the study of ancient human parasites. *Parasitology* 145(5):656–664. https://doi.org/10.1017/S003118201700141X

Dainton, M. A. (1992). Quick, semi-quantitative method for recording nematode gut parasite eggs from archaeological deposits. *Circaea Journal Association for Environmental Archaeology* 9:58–63.

Dean, K. R., Krauer, F., Walløe, L., Lingjærde, O. C., Bramanti, B., Stenseth, N. C. & Schmid, B. V. (2018). Human ectoparasites and the spread of plague in Europe during the second pandemic. *Proceedings of the National Academy of Sciences* 115(6):1304–1309. https://doi.org/10.1073/pnas.1715640115

Dittmar, K. (2013). Guest editorial. *International Journal of Paleopathology* 3:140–141. DOI: 10.1016/j.ijpp.2013.09.005

Dittmar, K., Jansen, A. M., Araújo, A. & Reinhard, K. (2003). *Molecular diagnosis of prehistoric Trypanosoma cruzi in the Texas-Coahuila Border Region*. Paper presented at the 13th Annual Meeting of the Paleopathology Association. Arizona (Suppl.)4:Tempe.

Dittmar, K., Araújo, A. & Reinhard, K. J. (2012). The study of parasites through time: archaeoparasitology and paleoparasitology. In Grauer, A. (Ed.), *A Companion to Paleopathology*, pp. 170–190. Oxford, UK: Blackwell Publishing Co. https://doi.org/10.1645/GE-1676.1

Dufour, B. & Le Bailly, M. (2013). Testing new parasite egg extraction methods in paleoparasitology and an attempt at quantification. *International Journal of Paleopathology* 3(3):199–203. https://doi.org/10.1016/j.ijpp.2013.03.008

Faulkner, C., Patton, S. & Johnson, S. (1989). Prehistoric parasitism in Tennessee: evidence from the analysis of desiccated fecal material collected from Big Bone Cave, Van Buren County, Tennessee. *The Journal of Parasitology* 75(3):461–463. DOI:10.2307/3282606

Fisher, C. L., Reinhard, K. J., Kirk, M. & DiVirgilio, J. (2007). Privies and parasites: the archaeology of health conditions in Albany, New York. *Historical Archaeology* 41(4):172–197. https://doi.org/10.1007/BF03377301

Flammer, P. G., Dellicour, S., Preston, S. G., Rieger, D., Warren, S., Tan, C. K. W., … & Smith, A. L. (2018). Molecular archaeoparasitology identifies cultural changes in the Medieval Hanseatic trading centre of Lübeck. *Proceeding of the Royal Society B* 28:520180991. https://doi.org/10.1098/rspb.2018.0991

Flammer, P. G. & Smith, A. L. (2020). Intestinal helminths as a biomolecular complex in archaeological research. *Philosophical Transactions of the Royal Society B* 375(1812):20190570. https://doi.org/10.1098/rstb.2019.0570

Flammer, P. G., Ryan, H., Preston, S. G., Warren, S., Přichystalová, R., Weiss, R., … & Smith, A. L. (2020). Epidemiological insights from a large-scale investigation of intestinal helminths in Medieval Europe. *PLoS Neglected Tropical Diseases* 14(8):e0008600. https://doi.org/10.1371/journal.pntd.0008600

Florenzano, A., Mercuri, A. M., Pederzoli, A., Torri, P., Bosi, G., Olmi, L., Rinaldi, R. & Bandini Mazzanti, M. (2012). The significance of intestinal parasite remains in pollen samples from medieval pits in the Piazza Garibaldi of Parma, Emilia Romagna, Northern Italy. *Geoarchaeology* 27(1):34–47. https://doi.org/10.1002/gea.21390

Fonzo, M., Scott, A. B. & Duffy, M. (2020). Eighteenth century urban growth and parasite spread at the Fortress of Louisbourg, Nova Scotia, Canada. In Betsinger, T. K. & DeWitte, S. N. (Eds.), *The Bioarchaeology of Urbanization. Bioarchaeology and Social Theory*, pp. 295–316. Cham: Springer. https://doi.org/10.1007/978-3-030-53417-2_12

Forbes, V., Dussault, F. & Bain, A. (2013). Contributions of ectoparasite studies in archaeology with two examples from the North Atlantic region. *International Journal of Paleopathology* 3(3):158–164. https://doi.org/10.1016/j.ijpp.2013.07.004

Gonçalves, M. L. C., da Silva, V. L., de Andrade, C. M., Reinhard, K., Da Rocha, G. C., Le Bailly, Bouchet, F., Ferreira, L. F. & Araújo, A. (2004). Amoebiasis distribution in the past: first steps using an immunoassay technique. *Transactions of the Royal Society of Tropical Medicine and Hygiene* 98(2):88–91. DOI: 10.1016/S0035–9203(03)00011-7.

Graff, A., Bennion-Pedley, E., Jones, A. K., Ledger, M. L., Deforce, K., Degraeve, A., Byl, S. & Mitchell, P. D. (2020). A comparative study of parasites in three latrines from Medieval and Renaissance

Brussels, Belgium (14th–17th centuries). *Parasitology* 147(13):1443–1451. https://doi.org/10.1017/S0031182020001298

Guhl, F., Aufderheide, A. & Ramírez, J. D. (2014). From ancient to contemporary molecular eco-epidemiology of Chagas disease in the Americas. *International Journal for Parasitology* 44(9):605–612. https://doi.org/10.1016/j.ijpara.2014.02.005

Guiry, E. J. (2012). Dogs as analogs in stable isotope-based human paleodietary reconstructions: a review and considerations for future use. *Journal of Archaeological Method and Theory* 19(3):351–376.

Hagan, R. W., Hofman, C. A., Hübner, A., Reinhard, K., Schnorr, S., Lewis, Jr., C. M., Sankanarayanan, K. & Warinner, C. G. (2020). Comparison of extraction methods for recovering ancient microbial DNA from paleofeces. *American Journal of Physical Anthropology* 171(2): 275–284. https://doi.org/10.1002/ajpa.23978

Harmon, A., Littlewood, D. T. J. & Wood, C. L. (2019). Parasites lost: using natural history collections to track disease change across deep time. *Frontiers in Ecology and the Environment* 17(3):157–166. https://doi.org/10.1002/fee.2017

Holck, P. (2011). Spotted typhoid fever in the Iceland of the sagas?. *Tidsskrift for den Norske Laegeforening: Tidsskrift for Praktisk Medicin, ny Raekke* 131(24):2504–2506. DOI: 10.4045/tidsskr.11.0830

Hong, J. H., Seo, M., Oh, C. S., Chai, J. Y. & Shin, D. H. (2020). Metagonimus yokogawai ancient DNA recovered from 16th- to 17th-century Korean mummy feces of the Joseon dynasty. *The Journal of Parasitology* 106(6):802–808. https://doi.org/10.1645/20-42

Horne, P. (2002). First evidence of enterobiasis in ancient Egypt. *The Journal of Parasitology* 88(5):1019–1021.DOI:10.2307/3285550

Jaeger, L. H. & Iñiguez, A. M. (2014). Molecular paleoparasitological hybridization approach as effective tool for diagnosing human intestinal parasites from scarce archaeological remains. *PLoS ONE* 9(8):e105910. https://doi.org/10.1371/journal.pone.0105910

Kenward, H. K., Hall, A. R. & Jones, A. K. G. (1986). Environmental evidence from a Roman well and Anglian pits in the legionary fortress. *The Archaeology of York* 14(5):241–288+fiche 2. London: Council for British Archaeology.

Kim, M. J., Ki, H. C., Kim, S., Chai, J., Seo, M., Oh, C. S. & Shin, D. H. (2014). Parasitic infection patterns correlated with urban–rural recycling of night soil in Korea and other East Asian countries: the archaeological and historical evidence. *Korean Studies* 38:51–74. https://www.muse.jhu.edu/article/594899.

Kliks, M. M. (1990). Helminths as heirlooms and souvenirs: A review of new world paleoparasitology. *Parasitology Today* 6(4):93–100. https://doi.org/10.1016/0169-4758(90)90223-Q

Kloos, H. & David, R. (2002). The paleoepidemiology of schistosomiasis in ancient Egypt. *Human Ecology Review* 9(1):14–25. http://www.jstor.org/stable/24707250

Knorr, D. A., Smith, W. P., Ledger, M. L., Peña-Chocarro, L., Pérez-Jordà, G., Clapés, R., Palma, M. F. & Mitchell, P. D. (2019). Intestinal parasites in six Islamic medieval period latrines from 10th–11th century Córdoba (Spain) and 12th–13th century Mértola (Portugal). *International Journal of Paleopathology* 26:75–83. https://doi.org/10.1016/j.ijpp.2019.06.004

Kristjánsdóttir, S. & Collins, C. (2011). Cases of hydatid disease in medieval Iceland. *International Journal of Osteoarchaeology* 21:479–486. https://doi.org/10.1002/oa.1155

Lalremruata, A., Ball, M., Bianucci, R., Welte, B., Nerlich, A. G., Kuhn, J. F. J. & Pusch, M. C. (2013). Molecular identification of falciparum malaria and human tuberculosis co-infections in mummies from the Fayum depression (Lower Egypt). *PLoS ONE* 8(4):e60307. https://doi.org/10.1371/journal.pone.0060307

Le Bailly, M., Leuzinger, U., Schlichtherle, H. & Bouchet, F.(2005). *Diphyllobothrium*: Neolithic Parasite? *The Journal of Parasitology* 91 (4): 957–959. https://doi.org/10.1645/GE-3456RN.1

Le Bailly, M., Gonçalves, M. L. C., Harter-Lailheugue, S., Prodéo, F., Araújo, A. & Bouchet, F. (2008). New finding of Giardia intestinalis (Eukaryote, Metamonad) in Old World archaeological site using immunofluorescence and enzyme-linked immunosorbent assays. *Memórias do Instituto Oswaldo Cruz*, 103(3):298–300. https://doi.org/10.1590/S0074-02762008005000018

Ledger, M. L., Grimshaw, E., Fairey, M., Whelton, H. L., Bull, I. D., Ballantyne, R., Knight, M. & Mitchell, P. D. (2019). Intestinal parasites at the Late Bronze Age settlement of must farm, in the fens of East Anglia, UK (9th century BCE). *Parasitology* 146(12):1583–1594. doi: 10.1017/S0031182019001021

Ledger, M. L. & Mitchell, P. D. (2019). Tracing zoonotic parasite infections throughout human evolution. *International Journal of Osteoarchaeology* 32(3): 553–564. https://doi.org/10.1002/oa.2786

Ledger, M. L., Rowan, E., Gallart Marques, F., Sigmier, J. H., Šarkić, N., Redžić, S., Cahill, N. D. & Mitchell, P. D. (2020). Intestinal parasitic infection in the Eastern Roman Empire during the

Imperial Period and Late Antiquity. *American Journal of Archaeology* 124(4):631–657. 10.3764/aja.124.4.0631

Ledger, M. L., Stock, F., Schwaiger, H., Knipping, M., Brückner, H., Ladstätter, S. & Mitchell, P. D. (2018). Intestinal parasites from public and private latrines and the harbour canal in Roman Period Ephesus, Turkey (1st c. BCE to 6th c. CE). *Journal of Archaeological Science: Reports* 21:289–297. https://doi.org/10.1016/j.jasrep.2018.07.013

Leles, D., Cascardo, P., dos Santos Freire, A., Maldonado, Jr, A., Sianto, L. & Araújo, A. (2014). Insights about echinostomiasis by paleomolecular diagnosis. *Parasitology International* 63(4): 646–649. https://doi.org/10.1016/j.parint.2014.04.005

Leles, D., Frías, F., Araújo, A., Brener, B., Sudré, A., Chame, M. & Laurentino, V. (2019). Are immunoenzymatic tests for intestinal protozoans reliable when used on archaeological material? *Experimental Parasitology* 205:107739. https://doi.org/10.1016/j.exppara.2019.107739.

Leles, D., Reinhard, K. J., Fugassa, M., Ferreira, L. F., Iñiguez, A. M. & Araújo, A. (2010). A parasitological paradox: why is ascarid infection so rare in the prehistoric Americas? *Journal of Archaeological Science* 37(7):1510–1520. https://doi.org/10.1016/j.jas.2010.01.011

Lindquist, H. D. & Cross, J. H. (2017). 195–Helminths. In Cohen, J., Opal, S. M. & Powderly, W. G. (Eds.), *Infectious Diseases* (Fourth Edition, Volume 2), pp. 1763–1779. Elsevier. https://doi.org/10.1016/B978-0-7020-6285-8.00195-7

Loreille, O., Roumat, E., Verneau, O., Bouchet, F. & Hänni, C. (2001). Ancient DNA from *Ascaris*: Extraction amplification and sequences from eggs collected in coprolites. *International Journal for Parasitology* 31(10):1101–1106. https://doi.org/10.1016/S0020-7519(01)00214-4

Maicher, C., Bleicher, N. & Le Bailly, M. (2019). Spatializing data in paleoparasitology: application to the study of the Neolithic lakeside settlement of zürich-parkhaus-opéra, Switzerland. *The Holocene* 29(7):1198–1205. DOI: 10.1177/0959683619838046

Maicher, C., Hoffmann, A., Côté, N. M., Palomo Pérez, A., Saña Segui, M. & Le Bailly, M. (2017). Paleoparasitological investigations on the Neolithic lakeside settlement of La Draga (Lake Banyoles, Spain). *The Holocene* 27(11):1659–1668. https://doi.org/10.1177/0959683617702236

Marciniak, S., Prowse, T. L., Herring, D. A., Klunk, J., Kuch, M., Duggan, A. T., Bondioli, L., Holmes, E. C. & Poinar, H. N. (2016). *Plasmodium falciparum* malaria in 1st–2nd century CE southern Italy. *Current Biology* 26(23):R1220–R1222. DOI: 10.1016/j.cub.2016.10.016

McDonough, K. (2019). Middle Holocene menus: dietary reconstruction from coprolites at the Connley Caves, Oregon, USA. *Archaeological and Anthropological Sciences*, 11:5963–5982.. DOI: 10.1007/s12520-019-00828-1.

Mitchell, P. D. (2013). The origins of human parasites: exploring the evidence for endoparasitism throughout human evolution. *International Journal of Paleopathology* 3(3):191–198. https://doi.org/10.1016/j.ijpp.2013.08.003

Mitchell, P. D. (2015). *Sanitation, Latrines and Intestinal Parasites in Past Populations*. London and New York: Routledge, Taylor and Francis Group.

Mitchell, P. D. (2017) Human parasites in the Roman world: health consequences of conquering an empire. *Parasitology* 1:48–58. DOI: 10.1017/S0031182015001651.

Mitchell, P. D., Stern, E. & Tepper, Y. (2008). Dysentery in the crusader kingdom of Jerusalem: an ELISA analysis of two medieval latrines in the city of Acre (Israel). *Journal of Archaeological Science* 35(7):1849–1853. https://doi.org/10.1016/j.jas.2007.11.017

Morrow, J. J. (2016). *Exploring Parasitism in Antiquity through the Analysis of Coprolites and Quids from La Cueva de los Muertos Chiquitos, Rio Zape, Durango, Mexico* (Publication No.10102325) Doctoral dissertation, The University of Nebraska-Lincoln. ProQuest Dissertations Publishing.

Morrow, J. J. & Elowsky, C. (2019). Application of autofluorescence for confocal microscopy to aid in archaeoparasitological analyses. *Korean Journal of Parasitology* 57(6):581–585. DOI: 10.3347/kjp.2019.57.6.581

Morrow, J. J., Newby, J., Piombino-Mascali, D. & Reinhard, K. J. (2016). Taphonomic considerations for the analysis of parasites in archaeological materials. *International Journal of Paleopathology* 13:56–64. https://doi.org/10.1016/j.ijpp.2016.01.005

Morrow, J. J. & Reinhard, K. J. (2018). The paleoepidemiology of *Enterobius vermicularis* (Nemata: Oxyuridae) among the Loma San Gabriel at la cueva de los muertos chiquitos (600–800 CE), Rio Zape Valley, Durango, Mexico. *Comparative Parasitology* 85(1):27–33. DOI: 10.1654/1525-2647-85.1.27

Mumcuoglu, K. Y., Gilead, L. & Ingber, A. (2009). New insights in pediculosis and scabies. *Expert Review of Dermatology* 4(3): 285–302. DOI: 10.1586/edm.09.18

Myšková, E., Ditrich, O., Sak, B., Kváč, M. & Cymbalak, T. (2014). Detection of ancient DNA of *Encephalitozoon intestinalis* (Microsporidia) in archaeological material. *The Journal of Parasitology* 100(3):356–359 DOI: 100. 10.1645/13–232.1.

Nezamabadi, M., Aali, A., Stöllner, T., Mashkour, M. & Le Bailly, M. (2013a). Paleoparasitological analysis of samples from the Chehrabad salt mine (Northwestern Iran). *International Journal of Paleopathology* 3(3):229–233. https://doi.org/10.1016/j.ijpp.2013.03.003

Nezamabadi, M., Mashkour, M., Aali, A., Stöllner, T. & Le Bailly, M. (2013b). Identification of *Taenia sp.* in a natural human mummy (Third Century BC) from the Chehrabad salt mine in Iran. *Journal of Parasitology* 99(3):570–572. https://doi.org/10.1645/12-113.1

Novo, S., Leles, D., Bianucci, R. & Araújo, A. (2015). *Leishmania tarentolae* molecular signatures in a 300 hundred-years-old human Brazilian mummy. *Parasites & Vectors* 8:72. DOI: 10.1186/s13071-015-0666-z

Oh, C. S., Seo, M., Chai, J. Y., Lee, S. J., Kim, M. J., Park, J. B. & Shin, D. H. (2010). Amplification and sequencing of *Trichuris trichiura* ancient DNA extracted from archaeological sediments. *Journal of Archaeological Science* 37(6):1269–1273. https://doi.org/10.1016/j.jas.2009.12.029

Paknazhad, N., Mowlavi, G., Dupouy Camet, J., Jelodar, M. E., Mobedi, I., Makki, M., … & Najafi, F. (2016). Paleoparasitological evidence of pinworm (*Enterobius vermicularis*) infection in a female adolescent residing in ancient Tehran (Iran) 7000 years ago. *Parasites & Vectors* 9:33. https://doi.org/10.1186/s13071-016-1322-y

Perri, A. R., Power, R. C., Stuijts, I., Heinrich, S., Talamo, S., Hamilton-Dyer, S. & Roberts, C. (2018). Detecting hidden diets and disease: zoonotic parasites and fish consumption in Mesolithic Ireland. *Journal of Archaeological Science* 97:137–146. https://doi.org/10.1016/j.jas.2018.07.010

Poshekhonova, O. E., Razhev, D. I., Slepchenko, S. M., Marchenko, Z. V. & Adaev, V. N. (2020). Reconstruction of dietary habits of a local Upper Taz Selkup group in the 18th and 19th centuries based on archaeoparasitology, osteology, stable isotope analysis, and archival documents. *Arctic Anthropology* 57(1):35–52. https://www.muse.jhu.edu/article/777305

Pye, J. W. (2020). "Unwanted guests": evidence of parasitic infections in archaeological mortuary contexts. *Historical Archaeology* 55:82–95. https://doi.org/10.1007/s41636-020-00271-3

Rácz, S. E., de Araújo, E. P., Jensen, E., Mostek, C., Morrow, J. J., Van Hove, M. L., … & Reinhard, K. J. (2015). Parasitology in an archaeological context: analysis of medieval burials in Nivelles, Belgium. *Journal of Archaeological Science* 53:304–315. https://doi.org/10.1016/j.jas.2014.10.023

Raoult, D., Dutour, O., Houhamdi, L., Jankauskas, R., Fournier, P. E., Ardagna, Y., … & Aboudharam, G. (2006). Evidence for louse-transmitted diseases in soldiers of Napoleon's grand army in Vilnius. *The Journal of Infectious Diseases* 193:112–120. https://doi.org/10.1086/498534

Reiczigel, J., Marozzi, M., Fabian, I. & Rozsa, L. (2019). Biostatistics for parasitologists – a primer to quantitative parasitology. *Trends in Parasitology* 35(4):277–281. https://doi.org/10.1016/j.pt.2019.01.003

Reinhard, K. J. (1992a). Parasitology as an interpretive tool in archaeology. *American Antiquity* 57(2):231–245. DOI: 10.2307/280729.

Reinhard, K. J. (1992b). The impact of diet and parasitism on Anemia in the prehistoric west. In Stuart-Macadam, P. & Kent, S. (Eds.), *Diet, Demography and Disease: Changing Perspectives of Anemia*, pp. 219–258. Aldine. New York.

Reinhard, K. J. (2017). Reestablishing rigor in archaeological parasitology. *International Journal of Paleopathology* 19:124–134. https://doi.org/10.1016/j.ijpp.2017.06.002

Reinhard, K. & Araujo, A. (2012). Synthesizing parasitology with archaeology in paleopathology. In Buikstra, J. & Roberts, C. (Eds.), *A Global History of Paleopathology*, pp. 751–764. New York: Oxford University Press.

Reinhard, K. J. & Buikstra, J. (2003). Louse infestation of the Chiribaya culture, southern Peru: variation in prevalence by age and sex. *Memórias do Instituto Oswaldo Cruz* 98:173–179. https://doi.org/10.1590/S0074-02762003000900026

Reinhard, K. J., Confalonieri, U. E., Herrmann, B., Ferreira, L. F. & de Araújo, A. J. (1986). Recovery of parasite remains from coprolites and latrines: Aspects of paleoparasitological technique. *Homo* 37(4):217–239.

Reinhard, K. J., de Araújo, E. P., Searcey, N. A., Buikstra, J. & Morrow, J. J. (2020). Automontage microscopy and SEM: a combined approach for documenting ancient lice. *Micron* 139:102931. https://doi.org/10.1016/j.micron.2020.102931

Reinhard, K., Fink, T. M. & Skiles, J. (2003). A case of megacolon in Rio Grande Valley as a possible case of Chagas disease. *Memórias do Instituto Oswaldo Cruz* 98:165–172. http://dx.doi.org/10.1590/S0074-02762003000900025

Reinhard, K., Mrozowski, S. & Orloski, K. (1986). Privies, pollen, parasites, and seeds: a biological nexus in historic archaeology. *Masca Journal* 4(1):31–36.

Reinhard, K. & Urban, O. (2003). Diagnosing ancient diphyllobothriasis from Chinchorro mummies. *Memórias do Instituto Oswaldo Cruz* 98(Suppl. 1):191–193. https://doi.org/10.1590/S0074-02762003000900028

Rocha, G. C., Harter-Lailheugue, S., Le Bailly, M., Araújo, A., Ferreira, L. F., Serra-Freire, N. M. & Bouchet, F. (2006). Paleoparasitological remains revealed by seven historic contexts from "Place d'Armes", Namur, Belgium. *Memórias do Instituto Oswaldo Cruz* 101(Suppl. 2):43–52. https://doi.org/10.1590/S0074-02762006001000008

Roche, K., Capelli, N., Pacciani, E., Lelli, P., Pallecchi, P., Bianucci, R. & Le Bailly, M. (2021). Gastrointestinal parasite burden in 4th–5th c. AD Florence highlighted by microscopy and paleogenetics. *Infection, Genetics and Evolution* 8:104713. https://doi.org/10.1016/j.meegid.2021.104713

Romera Barbera, A., Hertzel, D. & Reinhard, K. J. (2020). Attempting to simplify methods in parasitology of archaeological sediments: an examination of taphonomic aspects. *Journal of Archaeological Science: Reports* 33:102522. https://doi.org/10.1016/j.jasrep.2020.102522

Ruffer, M. A. (1910). Note on the presence of *Bilharzia haematobium* in Egyptian mummies of the twentieth dynasty (1250–1000 BC). *The British Medical Journal* 1:16. DOI: 10.1136/bmj.1.2557.16-a

Sabin, S., Yeh, H-Y., Pluskowski, A., Clamer, C., Mitchell, P. D. & Bos, K. I. (2020). Estimating molecular preservation of the intestinal microbiome via metagenomic analyses of latrine sediments from two medieval cities. *Philosophical Transactions of the Royal Society* B 375:20190576. http://dx.doi.org/10.1098/rstb.2019.0576

Santoro, C., Vinton, S. D. & Reinhard, K. J. (2003). Inca expansion and parasitism in the Lluta Valley: preliminary data. *Memórias do Instituto Oswaldo Cruz* 98(Suppl. 1):161–163. https://doi.org/10.1590/S0074-02762003000900024

Shillito, L. M., Whelton, H. L., Blong, J. C., Jenkins, D. L., Connolly, T. J. & Bull, I.D. (2020). Pre-Clovis occupation of the Americas identified by human fecal biomarkers in coprolites from Paisley Caves, Oregon. *Science Advances* 6(29):p.eaba6404. DOI: 10.1126/sciadv.aba6404

Shin, D. H. & Bianucci R. (Eds.) (2020). *The Handbook of Mummy Studies*. Singapore: Springer. https://doi.org/10.1007/978-981-15-1614-6

Shin, D. H., Oh, C. S., Chai, J. Y., Lee, H. J. & Seo, M. (2011). *Enterobius vermicularis* eggs discovered in coprolites from a medieval Korean mummy. *The Korean Journal of Parasitology* 49(3):323–326. https://doi.org/10.3347/kjp.2011.49.3.323

Shin, D. H., Oh, C. S., Lee, H. J., Chai, J. Y., Lee, S. J., Hong, D. W., Lee, S. D. & Seo, M. (2013). Ancient DNA analysis on *Clonorchis sinensis* eggs remained in samples from medieval Korean mummy. *Journal of Archaeological Science* 40(1):211–216. https://doi.org/10.1016/j.jas.2012.08.009

Shin, D. H., Kim, Y. J., Bisht, R. S., Dangi, V., Shirvalkar, P., Jadhav, N., Oh, C. S., Hong, J. H., Chai, J. Y., Seo, M. & Shinde, V. (2018). Archaeoparasitological strategy based on the microscopic examinations of prehistoric samples and the recent report on the difference in the prevalence of soil transmitted helminthic infections in the Indian Subcontinent. *Ancient Asia* 9:6. DOI: http://doi.org/10.5334/aa.166

Shin, D. H., Seo, M., Shim, S. Y., Hong, J. H. & Kim, J. (2020). Urbanization and parasitism: archaeoparasitology of South Korea. In Betsinger, T. B. & DeWitte, S. (Eds.), *The Bioarchaeology of Urbanization*, pp. 73–89. Cham: Springer. https://doi.org/10.1016/j.ijpp.2013.04.002

Slavinsky, V., Chugunov, K., Tsybankov, A., Ivanov, S., Zubova, A. & Slepchenko, S. (2018). *Trichuris trichiura* in the mummified remains of southern Siberian nomads. *Antiquity* 92(362):410–420. DOI:10.15184/aqy.2018.12

Slepchenko, S. (2020). *Opisthorchis felineus* as the basis for the reconstruction of migrations using archaeoparasitological materials. *Journal of Archaeological Science: Reports* 33:102548. https://doi.org/10.1016/j.jasrep.2020.102548

Slepchenko, S. M., Ivanov, S. N., Gusev, A. V., Svyatova, E. O. & Fedorova, N. V. (2019). Archaeoparasitological and palynological analysis of samples from the intestinal contents of a child mummy from the Zeleniy Yar Burial Ground (12–13th centuries AD). *Archaeological Research in Asia* 17:133–136. https://doi.org/10.1016/j.ara.2018.10.005

Slepchenko, S. M., Pererva, E. V., Ivanov, S. N., & Klepikov, V. M. (2019). Archaeoparasitological analysis of soil samples from Sarmatian Burial Ground Kovalevka I, 2nd–1st centuries BCE, Russia. *Journal of Archaeological Science: Reports* 26:101874. https://doi.org/10.1016/j.jasrep.2019.101874

Søe, M. J., Nejsum, P., Seersholm, F. V., Fredensborg, B. L., Habraken, R., Haase, K., ... & Kapel, C. M. O. (2018). Ancient DNA from latrines in Northern Europe and the Middle East (500 BC–1700 AD) reveals past parasites and diet. *PLoS ONE* 13(4):e0195481. https://doi.org/10.1371/journal.pone.0195481

Sprent, J. F. A. (1969). Evolutionary aspects of immunity in zooparasitic infections. *Immunity to Parasitic Animals* 1:3–62.

Steverding, D. (2020). The spreading of parasites by human migratory activities. *Virulence* 11(1):1177–1191. DOI: 10.1080/21505594.2020.1809963

Tams, K. W., Søe, J. M., Merkyte, I., Seersholm, F. V., Henriksen, P. S., Klingenberg, S., Willerslev, E., Kjær, K. H., Hansen, A. J. & Kapel, C. M. O. (2018). Parasitic infections and resource economy of Danish Iron age settlement through ancient DNA sequencing. *PLoS ONE* 13(6):e0197399. https://doi.org/10.1371/journal.pone.0197399.

Teixeira-Santos, I., Sianto, L., Araújo, A., Reinhard, K. J. & Chaves, S. A. M. (2015). The evidence of medicinal plants in human sediments from Furna do Estrago prehistoric site, Pernambuco State, Brazil. *Quaternary International* 377:112–117. https://doi.org/10.1016/j.quaint.2015.01.019

Thomas, J., Christenson, J. K., Walker, E., Baby, K. E. & Peterson, G. M. (2017). Scabies—an ancient itch that is still rampant today. *Journal of Clinical Pharmacy and Therapeutics* 42:793– 799. https://doi.org/10.1111/jcpt.12631

Trigg, H. B., Jacobucci, S. A., Mrozowski, S. A. & Steinberg, J. M. (2017). Archaeological parasites as indicators of environmental change in urbanizing landscapes: implications for health and social status. *American Antiquity* 82(3):517–535. DOI: 10.1017/aaq.2017.6.

Valverde, G., Ali, V., Durán, P., Castedo, L., Paz, J. L. & Martínez, E. (2020). First report in pre-Columbian mummies from Bolivia of *Enterobius vermicularis* infection and capillariid eggs: a contribution to paleoparasitology studies. *International Journal of Paleopathology* 31:34–37. https://doi.org/10.1016/j.ijpp.2020.08.002

Vinton, S. D., Perry, L., Reinhard, K. J., Santoro, C. M. & Teixeira-Santos, I. (2009). Impact of empire expansion on household diet: the Inka in Northern Chile's Atacama Desert. *PLoS ONE* 4(11):e8069. https://doi.org/10.1371/journal.pone.0008069

Walker, P. L., Bathurst, R. R., Richman, R., Gjerdrum, T. & Andrushko, V. A. (2009). The causes of porotic hyperostosis and *cribra orbitalia*: a reappraisal of the iron-deficiency-anemia hypothesis. *American Journal of Physical Anthropology* 139(2):109–125. https://doi.org/10.1002/ajpa.21031

Warnock, P. J. & Reinhard, K. J. (1992). Methods for extracting pollen and parasite eggs from latrine soils. *Journal of Archaeological Science* 19(3):261–264. https://doi.org/10.1016/0305-4403(92)90015-U

Waters-Rist, A. L., Faccia, K., Lieverse, A., Bazaliiskii, V. I., Katzenberg, M. A. & Losey, R. J. (2014). Multicomponent analyses of a hydatid cyst from an early neolithic hunter–fisher–gatherer from Lake Baikal, Siberia. *Journal of Archaeological Science* 50:51–62. https://doi.org/10.1016/j.jas.2014.06.015

Wei, D.W.Y., Huang, S., Lu, Y., Su, T., Ma, J., Hu, W. & Xie, N. (1981). Parasitological investigation on the ancient corpse of the Western Han Dynasty unearthed from tomb no. 168 on Phoenix Hill in Jiangling County. *Acta Academiae Medicinae Wuhan* 1:16–23. https://doi.org/10.1007/BF02857069

Williams, J. A. (1985). Evidence of hydatid disease in a Plains Woodland burial. *Plains Anthropologist* 30(107):25–28. DOI: 10.1080/2052546.1985.11909263

Williams, F. S., Arnold-Foster, T., Yeh, H. Y., Ledger, M. L., Baeten, J., Poblome, J. & Mitchell, P. D. (2017). Intestinal parasites from the 2nd–5th century AD latrine in the Roman Baths at Sagalassos (Turkey). *International Journal of Paleopathology* 19:37–42. https://doi.org/10.1016/j.ijpp.2017.09.002

Yeh, H. Y. & Mitchell, P. D. (2016). Ancient human parasites in ethnic Chinese populations. *Korean Journal of Parasitology* 54(5):565–572. DOI: 10.3347/kjp.2016.54.5.565

Zias, J. & Mumcuoglu, K. Y. (1991). Case reports on paleopathology: calcified hydatid cysts. *Paleopathology Newsletter* 73:7–8.

Zink, A. R., Spigelman, M., Schraut, B., Greenblatt, C. L., Nerlich, A. G. & Donoghue, H. D. (2006). Leishmaniasis in ancient Egypt and upper Nubia. *Emerging Infectious Diseases* 12(10):1616. DOI: 10.3201/eid1210.060169

10
HISTORICAL SOURCES, HISTORIOGRAPHY, AND PALEOPATHOLOGY

Piers D. Mitchell

Introduction

Paleopathologists investigate the diseases that affected past populations in order to better understand the lives of those who existed before us. The vast majority of research in this field is focused on archaeological sources of evidence in the form of skeletons, mummies, latrine sediment, and other excavated materials (Mitchell, 2015; Nystrom, 2018; Mays, 2021). For populations living prior to the development of writing by the Sumerians in Mesopotamia in the 4th millennium BC (Black & Spada, 2008), archaeological approaches are the only ways in which we can investigate past disease experiences. However, once the many textual forms spread across the world, valuable records created by many different societies became available for analysis. Here, we investigate the role that historical sources can play in the field of paleopathology. In the process, we will shine a light on key steps that have been taken to explore disease in the past using textual evidence, and the debates that have developed within this field.

There are two main ways in which historical texts can be useful in the study of disease in the past. The first is when texts provide sufficiently clear descriptions of past disease events that may identify the cause of illness. This approach is often referred to by historians as "retrospective diagnosis" (Arrizabalaga, 1999; Karenberg & Moog, 2004; Foxhall, 2014); although, in fact, all subfields of paleopathology involve retrospective diagnosis. This approach is important, as analyzing written evidence might be the only way to identify conditions that do not leave any evidence in human remains. If we only studied disease from skeletonized individuals and archaeological materials, we would have no understanding of mental illness, nor of diseases that only affected soft tissues other than in areas of the world where remains are mummified (either culturally or naturally) (Mitchell, 2011a). If symptoms and signs of a disease are provided in a text, we may be able to equate the condition to our modern understanding of the disease, referred to as "modern biological diagnosis". This also helps us to better understand the diagnostic labels used for disease in the past, referred to as the "social diagnosis", which are frequently very different to those used today. For instance, for the Hmong people of China, the modern biological diagnosis of epilepsy is better understood as the social diagnosis *quag dab peg*, which translates as "the spirit catches you and you fall down" (Khalil et al., 2021). However, not all forms of epilepsy lead to a person falling down, and not all causes of falling down are due to epilepsy, so these biological and social diagnoses overlap but do not mean exactly the same thing. Furthermore, we must recognize that every time a past diagnostic label is used within historical sources, we cannot assume that it was routinely applied by different authors to the same condition or set of symptoms.

Textual sources can offer insight into how a disease was thought to have occurred; its etiology. For instance, medical texts from ancient Greece typically described illnesses as resulting from an imbalance of the four humors (black bile, yellow bile, blood, and phlegm) or corruption of one of those humors (Mann, 2012). The texts may also provide information about how common a disease was or what proportion of the population had developed it over a certain period of time. Some texts contain illustrations, which may attempt to display some of the more visible signs of a disease (such as skin lesions), or the impact upon the population (such as dead lying in the streets). However, we must bear in mind that most illustrations in early manuscripts were not created by physicians or individuals who had ever seen a person with the disease being represented. Many illustrations in early manuscripts are stylized images that coincide with the accompanying text but would not by any means serve as a realistic representation of a person with that illness (Jones and Nevell, 2016).

The second way that textual sources can be helpful in paleopathology is to provide context that improves our interpretation of pathological lesions in excavated human remains (Mitchell, 2011b, 2017). For example, textual descriptions of marshes, biting insects, and fevers can help with the interpretation of skeletal lesions, such as those often associated with anemia, since these lesions on skeletons found in geographically low-lying areas could indicate the presence of malaria (Gowland & Western, 2012). Reading texts on surgery, pathology, and anatomy enables us to interpret tool marks on excavated bones created during surgery, autopsy, or anatomical dissection for teaching medical practitioners (Dittmar & Mitchell, 2015). An understanding of the kinds of illness described in written sources allows us to flag specific diseases within a population that are worthy of more targeted investigation using tests that we might not use routinely due to their cost, such as aDNA analysis (Spyrou et al., 2019). Medical texts can also highlight treatments used in the past. This allows us to actively search for evidence of these treatments using laboratory tests, such as measuring mercury levels in individuals who might have undergone treatment for syphilis or ectoparasites (Parascandola, 2009; Fornaciari et al., 2011).

The Types of Textual Evidence Recording Disease in the Past

If we wish to understand the diseases that affected a particular population, it might seem most logical to start with medical texts written by physicians. This is where we could potentially find both diagnostic labels, along with the symptoms and signs of each condition. This could, in theory, provide a form of dictionary for social diagnostic terms. However, the medical texts of the past were not necessarily a summary of the medical understanding of that society, but rather, depended upon the distinct needs and expectations of the intended audience (Rosa, 2006). Texts in early medical traditions, for example in ancient Mesopotamia and Egypt, were not detailed regarding symptoms and signs of disease (Nunn, 1996; Geller, 2010). Some texts can be a real challenge to translate if the medical terms are only found in medical works, so we may never be able to understand what they mean. A further problem is that medical traditions may include descriptions of diseases or treatments from earlier texts to ensure the author appeared knowledgeable and scholarly, even if those diseases or treatments were no longer present in that society (Savage-Smith, 2000). Therefore, if we are to use medical texts from past societies as evidence for disease in those populations, we need to do so cautiously by studying them with medical historians who have expertise in interpreting those texts and the culture that created them.

Other documentary evidence that can record disease episodes in past populations include personal letters, biographies and autobiographies, diaries, wills, hospital records, customs documents, death registers, chronicles, and histories (Mitchell, 2011a). Not all of these textual forms will be available for all societies, as some only developed in recent centuries. However, when eyewitness observation of people with diseases is recorded in a clear manner, without the constraints of the medical perspectives of that time period, then fascinating descriptions of illness can be preserved (Mitchell, 2004; Wagner & Mitchell, 2011). In the following section, some of the challenges associated with historical evidence used within paleopathology are discussed. Rather than exhaustively listing all known sources and issues, exemplars are offered to highlight the complex task of using historical sources to understand disease in the past.

Historiography and Paleopathology

Historiography can be thought of as the study of the writing of history and of written histories. Historiography differs from history, as history is the study of the past, while historiography is the study of historical writing. Historiography asserts that over time there will be changing perceptions of past events that make up history. Current views of history and how it should be studied differ from those of a century ago, and will no doubt change over the next century. In order to better understand the historiography of methods and techniques used in paleopathological research, we will explore some thought-provoking examples from the past two centuries.

Charles Creighton – 1890s

Creighton (1847–1927) was a Scottish physician who was appointed demonstrator of anatomy at the University of Cambridge in 1876. He resigned in 1881 and focused on writing his most significant work, *A History of Epidemics in Britain* (Creighton, 1891–1894). He compiled the first comprehensive evidence for written descriptions of disease outbreaks throughout British history, using Anglo-Saxon, medieval, and early modern textual sources. Although not a trained historian, the book's footnotes and references indicate that he gathered his information from printed editions of these texts in their original languages, and he did include some relevant quotes from the sources. This monumental task presented a number of challenges. These included how to translate the identity of disease from many centuries in the past, written in different languages, and try to allocate a term that was understood in the 1890s. He categorized the records into disease groups that we would recognize today, such as the plague, leprosy, influenza, smallpox, measles, whooping cough, diphtheria, dysentery, and cholera. However, he also categorized some outbreaks using terms we would not use today, such as gaol fevers, epidemic agues, continued fevers, sweating sickness, and the French pox. This was because in the 1800s, there were a wide range of terms used for infectious diseases, some of which appear to have symptoms from a number of distinct conditions present in the same patient. For example, medical practitioners did not realize that "gaol fever" was not a distinct disease linked to a single cause, but rather, appears to have been a suite of symptoms shared by prisoners in unsanitary jails who were prone to infection from a range of different pathogens. Hence, Creighton's diagnostic label of "diphtheria" may not be the same disease as diphtheria diagnosed today. For these reasons, the work must be viewed within the context of its time.

Another key point to contend with is the inclusion of opinion in Creighton's work. Creighton abided by widespread early 18th-century beliefs on disease causality, which were obsolete by the late 1800s, when he was writing. He rejected germ theory and the concept of vaccination, instead explaining the spread of infections as due to malnutrition and bad smells emanating from the ground. He argued that "for the next seven centuries, the pestilences of Britain are mainly the results of famine and therefore of indigenous origin" (Creighton, 1891, vol.1:8) and that "plague had its habitat in the soil, from which it rose in emanations" (Creighton, 1894, vol.2:35). For this, he was ridiculed by his contemporaries in the medical profession. A review of his book published in the journal *Nature* applauds him for the detailed compilation of historical evidence but cuts to shreds his credibility as a clinician with phrases such as, "It may be that much studying of the records of the past begets a tendency to a medieval frame of mind" (Anonymous, 1895). It has also been noted that Creighton appears to have deliberately omitted examples of epidemic outbreaks that would support the germ theory of infectious diseases, in order to support his preferred miasma theory (Roberts, 1971:38–40). Hence, while Creighton can be commended as an early trail blazer in the use of historical texts, by not placing them in a context that was acceptable to his contemporaries and by massaging his data to support his beliefs, the result fell far short of the acclaim for which he had hoped.

Jean-Noël Biraben – 1970s

Biraben was a French physician who compiled a database of textual evidence for outbreaks of plague in Europe from the 1300s to the 1800s (Biraben, 1975–1976). Although he restricted himself to one disease (unlike Creighton), he would have needed to consult textual sources from across an entire continent to do this well. This raises questions regarding the range of languages required and the challenges faced when gathering data for eastern Europe, which remained behind the Iron Curtain throughout the 1970s. Key criticisms of Biraben centre on the lack of justification for the sources used and the brief and incomplete referencing provided for his original documents. It appears that he acquired data from secondary works without referencing them. A further criticism is that Biraben did not explain his criteria for identifying plague within the texts. It is quite possible that some were epidemics of other infectious diseases and not bubonic plague (Roosen & Curtis, 2018).

A more recent problem has developed from the digitization of the Biraben database (Büntgen et al., 2012). Although this has allowed data mining by epidemiologists and statisticians, the data is often treated as if this is reliable, comprehensive, and reflective of the whole of Europe (Schmid et al., 2015; Yue et al., 2016; Yue et al., 2017). Biraben's data on outbreaks is most detailed for France, and fairly detailed for Britain, moderately detailed for other parts of western Europe, and very thin for eastern Europe. This could suggest that plague was most severe and recurrent in France than elsewhere, but more likely reflects Biraben's access to French libraries (Roosen & Curtis, 2018). Similarly, the relative paucity of outbreak records for eastern Europe is unlikely to indicate that plague was rare in this region, but rather that he never had access to libraries behind the Iron Curtain. While digitizing Biraben's data in 2012 seemed promising, the process dissociated the data from its limitations and, thus, led to its later use by well-meaning researchers who perhaps did not all fully understand the nature of the data with which they were working (Schmid et al., 2015; Yue et al., 2016; Yue et al., 2017).

Death Registers

Registers of deaths, especially church registers, began to be collected by governments in Europe from the 1700s and 1800s. This would seem to be a logical place to gather data about diseases in the past, or at least those diseases that killed people. While the absolute numbers of deaths recorded over time may well be a reasonable focus of study, it has been noted that the stated cause of death is frequently unreliable. Most stated cause of death recorded by the clergy were based on information from relatives of the deceased, not from a diagnosis by a physician, and often included vernacular descriptions that emphasized the most visible symptoms. Some entries in church registers were used commonly for several decades and then fell out of use, representing either the preferred terms of a specific clergyman or preferred terms for that region and time (Radtke, 2002). Similarly misleading is the fact that cause of death in registers could sometimes be declared by the family who did not want a stigmatizing label for their loved one. A death labeled as "plague" in 17th century Italy might result in anonymous burial within a mass grave, while stating another cause of death might allow burial in consecrated ground alongside a church with a gravestone. Consequently, some death certificates are known to have been falsified (Arrizabalaga, 1999). While study of how social diagnostic terms were used in the past is valid, we can see that equating those terms directly to modern biological diagnoses is not.

Modern Examples and Cautionary Tales

Issues concerning the rigor and interpretation of historical sources are not limited to past authors, practitioners, and scholars. Many problems exist in work presented by modern researchers. For instance, a number of medical practitioners and paleopathologists have studied diseases in famous people from the past. They move from one well-known figure to another without necessarily having adequate expertise in the time period or culture within which the person lived. These authors have become "serial publishers" of case reports in medical journals. As editors of most medical journals cannot identify appropriate historical experts to serve as reviewers, the peer review process becomes an ineffective tool to ensure that rigorous science is being conducted. The result is a plethora of conflicting opinions being published on the same topic in different clinical journals by different authors. One paper raising concerns about targeting diseases of famous historical figures aptly used the title, "Next Emperor, Please!" (Karenberg & Moog, 2004). Although there is logic in becoming a specialist in a particular disease or one time period, specializing simply in famous people who happen to have any disease is scientifically problematic. As an example, there are deep concerns regarding publications about the cause of death of one well-known religious figure, Jesus of Nazareth (Maslen & Mitchell, 2006). At least ten causes of death for Jesus have been proposed by different authors, ranging from heart failure and hypovolaemic shock to pulmonary embolism and asphyxia. If there are so many different opinions, it seems likely that there is not enough evidence for anyone to convincingly propose a single probable cause of death. It is possible that the reason so many papers have been published on the cause of death of famous people is because famous people had more written about them and so their diseases were described in more detail, or that journal editors may be more likely to publish articles about the famous, rather than the unknown or obscure. Whatever the cause, the large number of case reports published in clinical journals has contributed significantly to disdain for retrospective diagnosis among many medical historians.

There are a number of reasons why some of these publications lack credibility. One key issue of concern is that authors base their conclusions upon textual sources that were not eyewitness accounts, but potentially written hundreds of years after the events occurred. This is even more problematic if those texts were read in translation and not in the original source language. For example, interpretation of the cause of death of Alexander the Great as being from carotid artery dissection following a blow from a sling stone (Williams & Arnott, 2004) has been criticized for relying on evidence from texts written 400 years after the event (York & Steinberg 2004). As time passes and eyewitnesses die, the stories told about famous people can become embellished and evolve to the point where they are no longer a reliable source of evidence from which to diagnose disease.

Equally essential to consider is the nature of the original textual source. For example, some researchers have interpreted fictitious accounts in novels as indicative of true examples of disease, assuming that the authors must have seen a particular disease in real life in order to have included it in the novel (Toscano et al., 2016). While it is possible that the author did recount a genuine disease episode, it is equally plausible that the true event was modified to make the story more exciting, or even that it was an entirely fictional scenario created for dramatic effect.

The next issue is how much evidence is needed before it is possible to identify past disease episodes. A study of the writings of William Shakespeare (1564–1616) by a clinician led to a publication suggesting that Shakespeare had syphilis (Ross, 2005). The diagnosis was based upon the premise that Shakespeare wrote often about sexually transmitted diseases, such as "the pox", he lived apart from his wife and had mistresses, and that due to mercury poisoning in his older years, his literary productivity declined and he developed a tremor, memory loss, and hair loss. No actual symptoms of syphilis (such as rashes or ulcers) appear to have been used in their argument, nor was there a record of Shakespeare receiving mercury treatment, which would be important for such a claim. Furthermore, many people develop loss of memory, loss of hair, and tremor as they age. A medical historian responded to this publication and commented how reference to "the pox" was widespread throughout English literature at that time, and if the author had worked with a historian when researching this topic, the author would have realized that Shakespeare was in no way unusually fixated on the disease (McGough, 2005). It is possible that Shakespeare did have syphilis, but it is also quite possible he did not and was just a wealthy man who did not get on with his wife and developed a range of degenerative conditions associated with old age. The declaration that Shakespeare suffered from syphilis appears to be another attempt at retrospective diagnosis that does not meet the threshold for rigorous disease identification. Readers must clearly be shown that symptoms and signs of a disease that are unique to, or highly suggestive of, a particular condition are present before retrospective diagnosis is offered.

Illustrations in textual sources have the potential to provide insight into past diseases that might not be captured by the written word alone (Grmek & Gourvitch, 1998). However, hand-drawn illustrations will not necessarily be clear or accurate. Some past artists were technically deft and looking at their art can give the impression of absolute accuracy and clarity. However, if an artist was being paid to make their patron more attractive, taller, or more "noble" in appearance, we as a viewer are deceived. The same applies to potential diseases recorded in art, as disease might potentially be erased from the image or be added in at the artist's discretion, especially if the client wished their wonky leg to appear straight or a war wound added to appear heroic.

A further concern is the interpretation of historic illustrations by modern medical clinicians as if they were clinical photos. They ignore the fact that illustrations can be stylized drawings by an artist who may not even have seen the original pathology that they were commissioned to draw. A number of physicians who have published papers describing the appearance of cancers in historical portraits have been accused of only seeing what they want to see (Wagner, 2017). Sadly, such publications frequently do not include a textual historian and art historian among the list of co-authors. Subsequent historical investigation may show that the individual being painted lived many years after the portrait was created, rendering the diagnosis of malignancy, such as breast cancer, highly unlikely.

Beyond the issue of whether an artistic representation is accurate, we face challenges introduced by modern technology. Similar to the case of digitizing Biraben's plague database, discussed above, images from historical texts and paintings are now widely found on the internet. However, they are often disassociated from their original context, such as the page of text on which there were originally placed. Use of illustrations from medieval texts in the absence of original adjacent text frequently results in poor and inaccurate interpretations of disease. It has been noted that a good number of 12th–15th-century images labelled on websites as representing bubonic plague actually originated on pages discussing leprosy (Green et al., 2014; Jones & Nevell 2016; King & Green, 2018). Furthermore, these images are often greatly stylized and do not match the visual effects of diseases known today. It takes training in history to understand these complexities.

Historiography: Changing Attitudes

In the 1980s, Charles Rosenberg asserted that the concept of disease is difficult to define and is interpreted differently by different people. His key points are that "the act of diagnosis itself becomes a key event in the experience of illness" and "in some ways, disease does not exist until we have agreed that it does – by perceiving, naming, and responding to it" (Rosenberg, 1989:2,10). There is great merit in Rosenberg's approach, especially when looking at disease from the perspective of the person experiencing it. Clearly, this is a social interpretation of disease and is appropriate when looking at questions of interest to medical historians. However, it is inappropriate when investigating issues of interest to paleopathologists. Social diagnoses ignore the fact that bacteria or cancer cells caused disease regardless of whether a human has detected it. This poses a fundamental challenge for paleopathologists. Researchers examining archaeological material (bioarchaeologists) are taught to approach disease from a biological viewpoint. However, for those who use written texts to study historical events, a different approach is taken. Although anecdotal, my impression from decades working in this field is that most historians believe that using textual evidence to identify disease in the past is reasonable (whether or not they themselves have an interest in the topic). In contrast, this is not common amongst medical historians. A surprising proportion of medical historians regard the concept of retrospective diagnosis as insulting to their field and argue that those engaged in it are amateurs from other fields who dabble in history without appropriate expertise or skills, and who pose inappropriate questions of historical records (Cunningham, 2002; Karenberg & Moog, 2004). Many medical historians, therefore, support the views of Rosenberg.

Andrew Cunningham, a British medical historian, has also contributed to the discourse on retrospective diagnosis. He holds, perhaps, the most adamant opinion on retrospective diagnosis based on textual analysis, which I refer to as the "Cunningham debate" (Mitchell, 2011a). He argues that diagnosis of past disease is inappropriate because in the past "people died of what their doctor (or bystander) says they died of, and that's that" and "once we understand the sources of our unjustified assumption about the validity of retrospective diagnosis, we can stop trying to do it" (Cunningham, 2002: 15, 34). The fundamental premise expressed by Cunningham is that a disease does not exist without the act of diagnosing. A simple analogy is that if a tree falls in the forest and no one hears the fall, did it really fall? From an anthropocentric perspective, then, it only matters if humans hear it. From the point of the planet, it is of no consequence whether one particular species heard that incident. I would argue that disease occurred in the past regardless of whether any human recognized or knew the disease was there. Bacteria were present or cancerous cells were dividing regardless of the individual's knowledge or social response. Therefore, the act of *diagnosis* at the time of the past disease event becomes irrelevant to whether or not that disease genuinely existed. Cunningham's argument can only be made if we rely on past social diagnostic labels when making modern biological diagnoses. I agree entirely with him that this should not be done. If we, instead, aim for a modern biological diagnosis based upon textual descriptions of past symptoms and signs (and not social diagnostic labels), then the diagnostic concerns Cunningham expressed are avoided.

Jon Arrizabalaga, a Spanish medical historian, has published further on this topic. He highlights the challenges in using texts to identify past disease episodes (which I term social diagnosis). In the late 1990s, he studied the medical causes of death in pre-industrial Europe, writing, "It is difficult to imagine that any medical label of disease can be fully understood outside its relevant representational framework", "There is no avoiding the fact that the practice of retrospective diagnosis – at least grosso modo – is indispensable, from a methodological viewpoint, to the study of the biological and ecological history of human kind and of its diseases", and "retrospective diagnosis plays an important role in research fields like paleopathology, historical epidemiology, and historical demography" (Arrizabalaga, 1999: 252, 258). Hence, while Arrizabalaga wrote with a much more optimistic tone than Cunningham, he warns against linking past diagnostic labels to modern ones that happen to incorporate similar wording (Arrizabalaga, 2002). This view represents the sector of medical historians who are open to using texts to investigate past disease, as long as we view those diseases within socio-cultural contexts and are wary of past diagnostic labels.

Osamu Muramoto, based in the US, raises a number of important ethical considerations regarding diagnosing disease in the past, especially in those who are famous (Muramoto, 2014). One point made is that diagnosis of famous people can tarnish their reputation and/or offend their descendants. How far back in time can we go before these concerns fade and disappear? Perhaps the question holds for any historical assessment, regardless of whether it is about the health or the actions of people from the past. If it is acceptable for historians to highlight and evaluate controversial behaviour by living notable individuals, then many would argue that it is of less ethical concern to highlight and evaluate diseases experienced by people who are no longer living (so cannot be impacted). Muramoto also notes that diagnosing a disease that carries a stigma can tarnish reputations. For example, diagnosing alcoholic liver disease could imply that the person was an alcoholic, or recognizing the new onset of venereal disease in a married person could be used to infer that one partner in the marriage was having extra-marital sex. In some societies, either or both these scenarios could lead to stigmatization. However, if we are sensitive to the social tendencies toward stigmatizing certain conditions, the presence or absence of disease in itself might not be interpreted as tarnishing, but merely provides information about that individual. Muramoto also makes the ethical argument that diagnoses of disease in famous people must be completed for the purpose of understanding how that disease affected their work or behavior, to provide insight into what it was like to live with the disease in the past, or how untreated diseases progressed without modern treatment, and not to sensationalize the condition. Muramoto proposes that when descriptions are unclear or unspecific, then a label of a clinical syndrome (i.e., a group of symptoms commonly found together) should be applied, and not a specific diagnosis. In other words, retrospective diagnosis could stop with the label of a "chest infection" without proposing the organism responsible. These steps ensure that researchers are open and transparent about the degree of confidence they have in their diagnostic certainty.

Conclusion

So, what can we learn from past work using textual evidence to study disease in past populations? We need to have the skills of a historian to read and interpret the source texts in their original languages. Knowing who wrote the text, when, and why it was written are key aspects to evaluate when interpreting the reliability of the details. There must be a clear understanding of how terms to describe disease have changed over time. The use of a diagnostic term in one century does not necessarily mean that the same disease was present when the term is used again hundreds of years later. Thus, we should avoid directly equating social diagnostic labels of the past with modern biological diagnoses.

We need clear descriptions of symptoms and signs of disease from eyewitnesses of the disease episode if we are to propose a modern biological diagnosis. If a goal is to equate past textual descriptions of disease with our modern biological view of disease, then the expertise of a physician is also essential. When studying epidemic disease outbreaks across a large geographical area, we must consult a high percentage of all the sources available to ensure the data gathered is representative of the geographic region and centuries of interest. We must restrict ourselves to using information in a manner that is justified by the nature of the sources, and not regard data as a 100% complete, reliable scientific dataset. When large datasets are investigated, then the expertise of statisticians and epidemiologists is clearly important. If illustrations from texts are studied, then the input of an art historian is essential.

Regardless of the approach used, it is good practice to qualify our level of confidence in the proposed modern biological diagnosis when interpreting a disease based on description in a historical text. Listed by increasing certainty, we can use terms such as "possible example of", "is compatible with", "a probable example of", or "very likely to represent" the disease we propose. It is also sensible to consider a differential diagnosis, where other conditions that share some of the relevant symptoms are systematically discussed and considered. All these points argue that we should diagnose past disease only if the evidence is sufficiently robust, the procedure is performed by those with the relevant expertise, and if the interpretation and conclusions are appropriately framed within a suitable social context.

Future Prospects

I hope that with increasing awareness of this complex topic, we can foster interdisciplinary collaboration between paleopathologists and historians, to the point where collaboration becomes the standard. In this way, we can improve the contextualization of archaeological evidence for disease in past populations and utilize written records of disease to provide evidence for the large number of medical conditions that leave no archaeological trace. Several steps are needed to enable this. The first is for paleopathologists to seek out and collaborate with medical historians who see the constructive benefit of interweaving archaeological and textual evidence to understand conditions in past populations. The second is to avoid the publication (and readers' acceptance) of papers in clinical journals where doctors dip into medical history to make uninformed diagnoses in famous people. This will involve journal editors seeking out appropriate reviewers, historical reviewers explaining to authors ways in which the research might be unreliable, and authors to accept this feedback and end the cycle of resubmission of their work to multiple journals until a less informed editor accepts and publishes the paper. These changes might bolster the confidence and trust within medical historians who currently argue that identifying disease in past populations from textual evidence is unreliable or inappropriate. When textual evidence is used carefully and rigorously, by researchers with the appropriate training and expertise, then the fields of paleopathology and history will both benefit immensely.

References

Anonymous. (1895). Review of: A history of epidemics in Britain, by Charles Creighton. *Nature* 51:579–580. https://doi.org/10.1038/051579a0

Arrizabalaga, J. (1999). Medical causes of death in preindustrial Europe: some historiographical considerations. *Journal of the History of Medicine* 54(2):241–260. doi: 10.1093/jhmas/54.2.241

Arrizabalaga, J. (2002). Problematizing retrospective diagnosis in the history of disease. *Asclepio* 54(1):51–70. DOI:10.3989/asclepio.2002.v54.i1.135

Biraben, J.-N. (1975–1976). *Les Hommes et la Peste en France et dans les Pays Méditerranéens*. 2 vols. Paris: Mouton.

Black, J. E. & Spada, G. (2008). *Texts from Ur, kept in the Iraq Museum and the British Museum*. Messina: Di.Sc.A.M.

Büntgen, U., Ginzler, C., Esper, J., Tegel, W. & McMichael, A. J. (2012). Digitizing historical plague. *Clinical Infectious Diseases* 55(11):1586–1588. doi:.org/10.1093/cid/cid723

Creighton, C. (1891–1894). *A History of Epidemics in Britain from A.D. 664 to the Extinction of Plague*. 2 vols. Cambridge: Cambridge University Press.

Cunningham, A. (2002). Identifying disease in the past: cutting the Gordian knot. *Asclepio,* 54(1): 13–34. https://doi.org/10.3989/asclepio.2002.v54.i1.133

Dittmar, J. M. & Mitchell, P. D. (2015). A new method for identifying and differentiating human dissection and autopsy in archaeological human skeletal remains. *Journal of Archaeological Science: Reports* 3:73–79. https://doi.org/10.1016/j.jasrep.2015.05.019

Fornaciari, G., Marinozzi, S., Gazzaniga, V., Giuffra, V., Picchi, M. S., Giusiani, M. & Masetti, M. (2011). The use of mercury against pediculosis in the renaissance: the case of Ferdinand II of Aragon, king of Naples, 1467–1491. *Medical History* 55(1):109e115. https://doi.org/10.1017/S0025727300006074

Foxhall, K. (2014). Making modern migraine medieval: men of science, Hildegard of Bingen and the life of a retrospective diagnosis. *Medical History* 58:354–374. DOI: 10.1017/mdh.2014.28

Geller, M. J. (2010). *Ancient Babylonian Medicine: Theory and Practice*. Chichester: Wiley-Blackwell.

Gowland, R. L. & Western, A. G. (2012). Morbidity in the marshes: using spatial epidemiology to investigate skeletal evidence for malaria in Anglo-Saxon England (AD 410–1050). *American Journal of Physical Anthropology* 147(2):301–311. DOI: 10.1002/ajpa.21648

Green, M. H., Walker-Meikle, K. & Müller, W. P. (2014). Diagnosis of a "Plague" image: a digital cautionary tale. *The Medieval Globe* 1(1):article 13.

Grmek, M. D. & Gourvitch, D. (1998). *Les Maladies dans l'Art Antique*. Paris: Fayard.

Jones, L. & Nevell, R. (2016). Plagued by doubt and viral misinformation: the need for evidence-based use of historical disease images. *The Lancet Infectious Diseases* 16(10):e235–240. DOI: 10.1016/S1473-3099(16)30119-0

Karenberg, A. & Moog, F. P. (2004). Next emperor please! No end to retrospective diagnostics. *Journal of the History of the Neurosciences* 13(2):143–149. https://doi.org/10.1080/0964704049052158

Khalil, N., McMillan, S., Benbadis, S. R. & Robertson, D. (2021). Fish soup for the falling sickness: tracing epilepsy through Hmong and Western beliefs. *Epilepsy and Behaviour* 115:107725.

King, H. & Green, M. H. (2018). On the misuses of medical history. *The Lancet* 391:1354–1355. https://doi.org/10.1016/s0140–6736(18)30490-2

Mann, J. E. (2012). *Hippocrates, on the Art of Medicine*. Brill: Leiden.

Maslen, M. & Mitchell, P. D. (2006). Medical theories on the cause of death in crucifixion. *Journal of the Royal Society of Medicine* 99(4):185–188. DOI: 10.1258/jrsm.99.4.185

Mays, S. (2021). *The Archaeology of Human Bones*. 3rd edition. Abingdon: Routledge.

McGough, L. J. (2005). Syphilis in history: a response to 2 articles. *Clinical Infectious Diseases* 41(4):573–575. DOI: 10.1086/432127

Mitchell, P. D. (2004). *Medicine in the Crusades: Warfare, Wounds and the Medieval Surgeon*. Cambridge: Cambridge University Press ISBN 0–521–84455 x.

Mitchell, P. D. (2011a). Retrospective diagnosis, and the use of historical texts for investigating disease in the past. *International Journal of Paleopathology* 1(2):81–88. DOI: 10.1015/j.ijpp.2011.04.002

Mitchell, P. D. (2011b). Integrating historical sources with paleopathology. In Grauer, A. (Ed.), *Companion to Paleopathology*, pp. 310–323. New York: Wiley-Blackwell.

Mitchell, P. D. (Ed.) (2015). *Sanitation, Latrines and Intestinal Parasites in Past Populations*. Farnham: Ashgate.

Mitchell, P. D. (2017). Improving the use of historical written sources in paleopathology. *International Journal of Paleopathology* 19:88–95. https://doi.org/10.1016/j.ijpp.2016.02.005

Muramoto, O. (2014). Retrospective diagnosis of a famous historical figure: ontological, epistemic and ethical considerations. *Philosophy, Ethics and Humanities in Medicine* 9:10. https://doi.org/10.1186/1747–5341–9–10

Nunn, J. F. (1996). *Ancient Egyptian Medicine*. London: British Museum Press.

Nystrom, K. (2018). *The Bioarchaeology of Mummies*. London: Routledge.

Parascandola, J. (2009). From mercury to miracle drugs: syphilis therapy over the centuries. *Pharmacy in History* 51(1):14–23.

Radtke, A. (2002). Rethinking the medical causes of infant death in early modern Europe: a closer look at church registers and medical terminology. *History of the Family* 7(4):505–514. https://doi.org/10.1016/S1081–602X(02)00123-9

Roberts, R. S. (1971). The use of literary and documentary evidence in the history of medicine. In Clarke, E. (Ed.), *Modern Methods in the History of Medicine*, pp. 36–56. London: Athlone Press.

Roosen, J. & Curtis, D. R. (2018). Dangers of noncritical use of historical plague data. *Emerging Infectious Diseases* 24(1):103–110. DOI:10.3201/eid2401.170477

Rosa, M. C. (2006). Ancient medical texts, modern reading problems. *Memorias do Instituto Oswaldo Cruz* 101(suppl.2):147–150. DOI: 10.1590/s0074–02762006001000022

Rosenberg, C. E. (1989). Disease in history: Frames and framers. *The Millbank Quarterly* 67(S1):1–15. https://doi.org/10.2307/3350182

Ross, J. J. (2005). Shakespeare's chancre: did the bard have syphilis? *Clinical Infectious Diseases* 40(3):399–404. doi:10.1086/427288

Savage-Smith, E. (2000). The practice of medicine in Islamic lands myth and reality. *Social History of Medicine* 13(2):307–321. https://doi.org/10.1093/shm/13.2.307

Schmid, B. V., Büntgen, U., Easterday, W. R., Ginzler, C., Walløe, L., Bramanti, B. & Stenseth, N. C. (2015). Climate-driven introduction of the black death and successive plague reintroductions into Europe. *Proceedings of the National Academy of Sciences* 112(10):3020–3025. https://doi.org/10.1073/pnas.1412887112

Spyrou, M. A., Bos, K. I., Herbig, A. & Krause, J. (2019). Ancient pathogen genomics as an emerging tool for infectious disease research. *Nature Reviews Genetics* 20:323–340. https://doi.org/10.1038/s41576-019-0119-1

Toscano F., Spani, G., Papio, M., Rühli F. J. & Galassi, F. M. (2016). A case of sudden death in Decameron IV.6: aortic dissection or atrial myxoma? *Circulation Research* 119(2):187–189. https://doi.org/10.1161/circresaha.116.309113

Wagner, T. G. & Mitchell, P. D. (2011). The illnesses of king Richard and king Philippe on the third crusade: an understanding of Arnaldia and Leonardie. *Crusades* 10:23–44. ISBN 9781315271576

Wagner, W. (2017). Cancer and the arts: how often do doctors only see what they want to see? Or: the case of an 'epidemic of breast cancer among famous artists'. *ESMO Open* 2(3):e000249. DOI: 10.1136/esmoopen-2017–000249

Williams, A. N. & Arnott, R. (2004). A stone at the siege of cyropolis and the death of Alexander the great. *Journal of the History of the Neurosciences* 13(2):130–137. DOI: 10.1080/0964704049052156

York G. K. & Steinberg, D. A. (2004). Commentary: The diseases of Alexander the great. *Journal of the History of the Neurosciences* 13(2):153–156. DOI: 10.1080/0964704049052160

Yue, R. P. H., Lee, H. F. & Wu, C. Y. H. (2016). Navigable rivers facilitated the spread and recurrence of plague in pre-industrial Europe. *Scientific Reports* 6:34867. https://doi.org/10.1038/srep34867

Yue, R. P. H., Lee, H. F. & Wu, C. Y. H. (2017). Trade routes and plague transmission in pre-industrial Europe. *Scientific Reports* 7:12973. https://doi.org/10.1038/s41598-017-13481-2

11
OSTEOBIOGRAPHY AND CASE STUDIES

Alexis T. Boutin

This chapter reviews paleopathological research that uses osteobiography or case studies of individuals to investigate health and disease in the past. Vis-à-vis traditional paradigms of bioarchaeology, osteobiographies are sometimes "dismissed as simply a tool for engaging the public in a popular book or museum exhibition through human interest stories; the most rigidly quantitative practitioners may see it as unscientific, as a sample size of one cannot 'prove' a general point" (Hosek & Robb, 2019:2). Case studies of individuals are often tarred with the same brush. Yet, case studies have been a standard mode of inquiry in paleopathology since its inception, and osteobiography is becoming an increasingly popular way to engage with health status and disease experiences in the past. This chapter investigates the persistence, and even growth, of these models, ultimately arguing that they have earned their place in paleopathological research.

I begin by reviewing the role that research on individuals played in the origins of paleopathology as a discipline. Then, I turn to current applications of case studies and osteobiography, respectively, in paleopathology and recommend best practices for each of them. Next, research themes in paleopathology that have benefitted from exploration via case study and osteobiography are discussed, and emerging research directions identified. Due to space constraints, this review of case studies and osteobiographies in paleopathology research is far from exhaustive. Mummy studies, for example, are beyond the scope (but receive excellent coverage in Lynnerup, 2019; Nystrom, 2019; and see Chapter 12, this volume). It is also limited to scholarship in English because of the author's own language (in)abilities. For reviews of traditions of paleopathological case studies and osteobiographies by scholars in Latin America, Europe, Asia, and Oceania, see Buikstra and Roberts (2012). Nevertheless, even this brief overview will demonstrate that, when carried out rigorously, systematically, and according to best practices, case studies and osteobiographies can provide unique insights on past health and disease experiences that traditional population-scale paleopathological research cannot.

Historical Background

Since the 1892 coining of the term "paleopathology" to describe the study of ancient disease, case studies have been common in the scholarly literature (Grauer, 2018:904). Following the tradition of the medical sciences, where case studies of individuals are a standard publication form in clinical literature, physicians were some of the most frequent authors of paleopathological case studies through the 1970s (e.g., Henri Denninger and Saul Jarcho in the United States [see Cook & Powell, 2006], Calvin Wells in the United Kingdom [see Roberts, 2006]). However, these early case studies, as well as those written by contemporary physical anthropologists and archaeologists, frequently focused on qualitative descriptions and diagnoses of pathological lesions, neglecting the human remains' contexts (archaeological, historical, social) and failing to relate this "evidence of disease to broader problems of human adaptation" (Buikstra & DeWitte, 2019:12).

Hooton (1930) is widely recognized as one of the first scholars to employ a population approach to paleopathology with his analysis of the remains of Ancestral Puebloans from Pecos Pueblo, New Mexico. Whereas some of his peers might only have made incidental mention of pathological conditions, Hooton recognized that analyzed collectively and contextually, they could lead to major insights on population dynamics (Beck, 2006). Thus, Hooton is often lauded as an early practitioner of epidemiology in studying past human health; although the "racial typological approach" he employed is another legacy that should not be ignored (Armelagos & van Gerven, 2003:56). Paleopathological research on populations has since flourished, in the second half of the 20th century shifting away from the medical paradigm of disease toward a holistic, biocultural approach to population health that encompasses a wide span of physiological, psychological, and social factors (Grauer, 2018:905).

What has this meant for paleopathological research at the scale of the individual? Reflecting on the British tradition of paleopathology, Roberts (2006:424) contrasts case studies with "hypothesis and question-driven approaches." In this sense, she echoes Mays's (1997) argument that the population-based approach maximizes the relevance of paleopathological research and thus represents the discipline's future. Mays (2012a, b) further cites the diminishing role of case study publications in the clinical sciences, and the reduced frequency of their citation in the paleopathological literature, to support his argument that case studies should "have a lesser role than they do at present" (Mays, 2012a:303) in order for paleopathology to mature as a discipline. However, Mays (2012b:84) does allow that case studies should not completely disappear, provided they have "some wider significance" for paleopathological, archaeological, or historical research. For example, a recent bibliometric and altmetric analysis of the paleopathological literature concludes that case studies that propose and/or exemplify the application of a novel methodological, theoretical, or analytical frameworks are cited as frequently as population studies (Boutin et al., 2022). Fortunately, many paleopathologists—even those who themselves employ population-scale epidemiological or biocultural approaches (e.g., Grauer et al., 2016; Buikstra & DeWitte, 2019)—agree with Mays' latter (2012b) sentiment. The result has been an abundance of broadly relevant, well-contextualized case studies, and more recently osteobiographies, over the last two decades, as demonstrated below.

Best Practices for Case Studies in Paleopathological Research

Recent explorations of multi-scalar approaches to bioarchaeology (Bradbury et al., 2016; Torres-Rouff & Knudson, 2017), which integrate individual- and population-level analyses and interpretations, demonstrate the continuing relevance of the case study. Yet, ongoing discussions about the need to increase the rigor of paleopathological research (Buikstra et al., 2017; Grauer, 2018) are especially germane to the case study approach. Yin (2018: xx) argues that case study research is a distinctive "mode of inquiry" with its own formal methodologies. While efforts are now being made in the medical sciences to formalize guidelines for case studies to ensure their rigor and relevance (Crowe et al., 2011; Riley et al., 2017), comparable efforts in paleopathology are incipient. It should go without saying that paleopathological case study research must employ standardized data collection practices and terminology and interpret the osteological evidence for a given individual in the context of the sample (if available) to which it belongs. One of the most popular venues for publishing case studies is *International Journal of Paleopathology*, whose Guide for Authors specifies that they must be "justified in terms of disease, temporal, and/or locational uniqueness. IMPORTANTLY, a case study must clearly explain how it significantly contributes to understanding disease in the past" (original emphasis; IJPP, 2021). It is this last charge that could benefit most from formalized guidelines and best practices. While the creation of standards for case study research in paleopathology is beyond the scope of this chapter, a preliminary attempt at identifying best practices follows.

Two approaches to case studies in paleopathology have consistently produced high-quality scholarship that makes important contributions to modern understandings of health and disease in the past: contextualization of osteological data with all available lines of evidence (e.g., archaeological, historical, ethnographic, iconographic, clinical, etc.) and engagement with social theory, such as a life course model (cf. Cheverko, 2021), which acknowledges the iterative nature of health and disease throughout an individual's life and even across generations. Three case studies are offered here: their use of both of these approaches maximizes their disciplinary impact.

Knüsel's (2002) case study of the adult female buried in an elaborate Iron Age chamber grave at Vix, France interprets the pathological conditions evident in her skeleton alongside a thorough stylistic analysis of grave goods and mortuary context and close consideration of ethnohistoric sources and ethnographic evidence. Applying a life course approach that begins with birth complications, Knüsel (2002:294) explores how her resulting bodily non-normativity (including "diminutive size, unusual gait and twisted face") may have combined with her elevated social status to result in her role as a ritual specialist.

An Ancestral Puebloan adult female from Arroyo Hondo, New Mexico is the subject of a case study by Palkovich (2012). Although this female survived a severe bout of rickets during infancy, bowing deformities of all limbs impaired her mobility during the remainder of her life. Buried in the same part of the settlement as several other individuals who suffered from vitamin D deficiency, Palkovich (2012:249) speculates that a combination of "dietary problems compounded by child-care practices" can be inferred for some community members. Interpreted in the context of archaeological, ethnographic, and iconographic evidence, this type of impairment was a salient category of difference but not necessarily a source of stigma.

The third example is a multi-phase analysis of an individual from Umm an-Nar period Tell Abraq, U.A.E. This young adult female was first described by Martin and Potts (2012), who preliminarily diagnosed her with a neuromuscular condition and speculated about its functional and social implications based on clinical evidence and her unusual mortuary context. Next, Schrenk et al. (2016) employed stable isotope analysis to explore this female's residential mobility across her life course. The discovery that she had migrated to Tell Abraq as an adolescent supported paralytic poliomyelitis as the likely etiology of her pathological conditions. Finally, the Index of Care method (discussed below) was applied by Schrenk and Martin (2017) to investigate this female's disease experience and the care that she may have required due to paraplegia. Thus, adherence to the two best practices described above has helped these case studies in paleopathological research make a significant contribution to the discipline.

Best Practices for Osteobiography in Paleopathological Research

Osteobiography represents a more recent development in paleopathological research. The original concept of osteobiography, as is well known, originated with Saul (1972), who described this approach as aiming to reconstruct life histories recorded in bone, at both individual and population scales, and emphasized the interpretation of osteological evidence in relation to archaeological, ecological, and socio-cultural contexts. Saul and Saul (1989) then applied this model to investigate Maya lifeways, including the effects of disease on population health and social organization. The first bioarchaeologist to engage with osteobiography as a conceptual model grounded in social theory was Robb (2002). He understands osteobiography to be the biography of human skeletons as a "cultural narrative" that reflects the cultural interpretation of biological phenomena and life events (including death) (Robb, 2002:160–161). Thus, Robb's model incorporates the best practices identified above for case studies: contextualization of osteological data with all available lines of evidence, and use of social theory (here, a life course model). On the other hand, forensic anthropologist Snow articulates a concept of osteobiography that is largely synonymous with the biological profile used in his discipline to achieve personal identification of human remains (Weizman & Snow, 2011). Geller (2019:89) argues that Snow's notion of osteobiography as "singular life histories" has become "popularized and for this reason possibly more influential" than the one promulgated by Robb. In the context of paleopathological research, she seems to be correct. The term "osteobiography" is frequently used *sensu* Snow by studies that document the first osteological evidence for a disease (Merrett et al., 2019), identify a novel context for a disease's appearance (Hardy et al., 2019), or describe health status along with many other aspects of identity gleaned from a skeleton (e.g., Couoh, 2015; Melton et al., 2010). However, I believe that osteobiography has the potential to make a more significant contribution to paleopathology when it is employed according to Robb's (2002) understanding; accordingly, that is the model to which the rest of the chapter will be devoted.

Hosek and Robb (2019:2) have recently elaborated on Robb's (2002) definition of osteobiography by offering a more rigorous and "explicit theorization and methodology." They argue that, compared to traditional, population-level approaches to bioarchaeology, osteobiography is the most effective way to explore past lived experiences, as well as the historical contingency and social construction of life courses. In this sense, osteobiography builds upon the best practices for case study research described above, now applying them in a more critical, experiential fashion, and at multiple scales. As Saul (1972:8) originally explained, osteobiography can be applied at the level of both the individual and the population. In fact, according to Hosek and Robb (2019:11), one of the strengths of osteobiography is its ability to "humanize population statistics." In their now canonical *The Bioarchaeology of Individuals*, Stodder and Palkovich (2012) described this volume's life histories of 16 past individuals as osteobiographies. Since then, the individual scale of analysis has become the most common way to deploy the osteobiography model in paleopathological research, although osteobiographies of populations have also represented important contributions. Moreover, the utility of an osteobiographical approach for understanding the health and disease experiences of past individuals, as a complement to population-scale biocultural and paleoepidemiological research, is now widely recognized (e.g., Grauer & Buikstra, 2019, Mennear, 2017; Stodder & Byrnes, 2020). Four bioarchaeological examples are reviewed here to illustrate the effectiveness of the osteobiography model promulgated by Robb (2002) and Hosek and Robb (2019) in paleopathology research, at both individual and population levels.

Although it predates either of the latter publications, Hawkey's (1998) osteobiography of a severely disabled Ancestral Puebloan adult male from Gran Quivira Pueblo, New Mexico has influenced many scholars. Her complementary use of osteological, archaeological, and ethnographic evidence to investigate this male's lived experience and the social construction of impairment and disability, due to juvenile-onset rheumatoid arthritis, across his life course set the standard toward which future osteobiographical analyses of past individuals' health and disease would aspire.

More recently, Alfaro Castro, Waters-Rist, and Zborover (2017) created an osteobiography for a pre-modern Chontal female from Oaxaca, Mexico. Although health status represents only one component of her osteobiography, the authors' use of osteological evidence, archaeological evidence, and stable isotope analysis facilitates a nuanced reconstruction of this adolescent's culturally mediated nutritional deficiencies and disease experience across her life course.

Robb (2019) uses a sample from Classical period Pontecagnano, Italy to study the potential of "comparative osteobiography," in which individual human life courses in one society are studied in aggregate. "Moments" in the life course for members of this community (Robb, 2019:62) were typified by pathological lesions (e.g., non-specific stress indicators, trauma, dental disease, osteoarthritis), which reflect conditions such as impairment and habitual, intensive physical labor.

Millard and colleagues start with Robb's (2019) approach and expand it by means of "prosopography, an approach to the study of multiple partial biographies used by historians" (Millard et al., 2020:10) to investigate the health of Scottish soldiers captured at the Battle of Dunbar (1650 CE). They analyze the skeletal remains via a wide array of sophisticated techniques, then carefully interpret them in the context of historical evidence, producing fine-grained individual- and population-level reconstructions of these males' diet, health, and disease experiences across the life course.

These four examples of osteobiography prove the effectiveness of this approach for exploring past lived experiences of health and disease, as well as in examining the historical contingency and social construction of past life courses. In the next section, I review thematically some of the important contributions to paleopathological research made by case studies and osteobiographies.

Research Themes in Paleopathological Case Studies and Osteobiography

Trauma and Violence

Osteobiographies and case studies of individuals with traumatic injuries have productively explored the roles of interpersonal violence and warfare in past societies (see Chapters 13 and 27, this volume). An adult male from Iron Age IIB Israel, studied by Cohen et al. (2015), exhibits multiple cranial and post-cranial perimortem sharp trauma wounds. The authors interpret these injuries as the first osteological evidence to support written and iconographic accounts of the violence deployed by Assyrians against defeated enemy soldiers, as part of their imperial strategy. Hosek's (2019) osteobiography of an elite male warrior in the early medieval Czech Republic recounts sharp force perimortem trauma and the inclusion of multiple weapons as grave goods. Her "microhistorical" approach discloses "how a warrior personhood might be embodied through a life history," and how this man participated in "macroscale narratives of political violence and Christianization" (Hosek, 2019:53). Walker et al. (2012) also reconstruct the life course of an adult male, this time from Viking Age Iceland, whose cranium exhibits perimortem wounds caused by sharp trauma. The researchers argue that his grisly injuries corroborate frequent accounts of interpersonal violence in the Icelandic sagas. The life course of a pre-modern Chamorro man from the Pacific island of Tinian is traced in a comprehensive osteobiography written by Heathcote and colleagues (2012). A significant biographical event was his survival of sharp trauma to the face, which the researchers interpret with the help of archaeological evidence for weaponry, historical evidence for the Spanish-Chamorro Wars, and ethnographic and ethnohistoric evidence for Chamorro healing practices.

Etiology, Epidemiology, and Social Organization

Research on past individuals with pathological conditions has shed light on the etiology and epidemiology of diseases and has revealed new facets of past social organization. Solari and colleagues (2020) employ the Bioarchaeology of Care model (discussed below, and see Chapter 25, this volume) to interpret the remains of an infant who suffered from a systemic, severe health condition in Middle Holocene Brazil. The researchers assert that caregiving may have been a community effort, based on the composition of foraging groups. Unique and elaborate mortuary treatment suggests that this infant received "special attention" during death, as well as in life (Solari et al., 2020:489).

Across the world in Russia, an adult male also living in the Middle Holocene suffered from diffuse idiopathic skeletal hypertrophy (DISH). Faccia et al. (2016) arrive at this conclusion via rigorous differential diagnosis; they also infer low social status based on his mortuary treatment. When his activity patterns and diet are compared with other members of his community, DISH does not seem to have resulted in any impairment. Nevertheless, this rare instance of DISH in a lower status member of a foraging community allows the authors to argue that the correlation between DISH, elite status, and protein- and calorie-rich diets presumed by many other authors is due for reconsideration.

Two individuals with treponemal disease in Neolithic Vietnam studied by Vlok et al. (2020) seem to have suffered from scurvy. The researchers interpret this co-morbidity in the social and biological contexts of transitions in demography and subsistence in Mainland Southeast Asia, explaining that increased sedentism and rapid population growth associated with the adoption of agriculture may have accelerated infectious disease transmission and led to nutritional deficiencies.

Cerezo-Román and Tsukamoto (2021) employ a life course model to reconstruct the osteobiography of an elite male standard-bearer who lived in a Late Classic period Maya society. Healed porotic hyperostosis suggests that he suffered from childhood disease and/or nutritional deficiency—health challenges that were apparently common for residents of contemporary urban centers. The light to moderate degenerative joint disease of his arm, hand, leg, and foot joints may be attributed to his occupation: Maya standard-bearers were known to play "the role of ambassador in negotiating political alliances" between regional rulers, which required them to travel long distances over uneven terrain while carrying a banner (Cerezo-Román and Tsukamoto, 2021:276).

One thousand years later, the remains of two infants who suffered from scurvy and other metabolic diseases shed light on rapid urbanization and social and religious reform movements in early 19th century CE New York City. Ellis (2016) explores the implications of this condition for the subadults' life courses, which she ties to deficiencies in maternal and weaning diets. Notably, these two infants' remains derive from a large commingled assemblage, indicating that burials need not be recovered individually to permit a productive case study or osteobiographical analysis.

Social Perception and Stigma

Social perceptions of pathological conditions can also be inferred from case studies and osteobiographies. Many of them deviate from normative perceptions in modern Western societies, revealing the contingent and constructed nature of stigma. An Early Iron Age adult male from Athens, Greece who suffered antemortem cranial trauma is the subject of a case study by Little and Papadopoulos (1998). Based on the clinical literature, the authors argue that his depression fracture could have caused "post-traumatic neurologic impairment," including epilepsy (Little & Papadopoulos, 1998:376). Contemporary medical and literary texts reveal that epilepsy carried a social stigma, and this male was indeed buried in a non-normative fashion (in a well)—but he was deposited intentionally and carefully, and accompanied by a grave good, revealing the complexity of stigma. Slon and colleagues (2013) describe an adult male from Byzantine Israel with achondroplastic dwarfism. Textual evidence from early Christian societies around the Mediterranean indicates that responses to people with dwarfism were mixed. But this individual's normative mortuary treatment suggests to the researchers that he was treated as "an ordinary member of society" (Slon et al., 2013:587). Baker and Bolhofner (2014) investigate a young adult female with leprosy in medieval Cyprus. Skeletal evidence for activity patterns, including "long-term participation in textile work" and her burial "within the sanctified space of the church," indicates that she was well-integrated into society, leading them to argue that leprosy may not have been stigmatized in medieval Cyprus like it is in many societies today (Baker & Bolhofner, 2014: 22–23).

Disability and Impairment

Investigations of disability and impairment in the past have frequently drawn upon osteobiographies and case studies. Although this body of literature is covered comprehensively and effectively by Tilley (Chapter 25, this volume), three publications are reviewed here (in addition to those mentioned elsewhere in this chapter, e.g., Hawkey, 1998; Palkovich, 2012; Boutin, 2016). Lovell (2016) describes an older adult male who lived in Roman period Erculam, Italy. He would have had a conspicuously unusual gait, due to a well-healed fracture of the right femoral neck, with severe osteoarthritis of the knee developing secondarily. Based on mention of a similar condition in the Roman medical literature, and his normative mortuary treatment, Lovell (2016:94) infers that "while he may have been identified as mobility impaired, he was not socially identified as disabled."

Two adult females from medieval Poland—one with leprosy, the other with gigantism—are the subjects of Matczak and Kozłowski's (2017) osteobiographical analysis. By comparing clinical data with ethnographic, historical, and archaeological evidence, they evaluate each woman's relative level of disability. The researchers conclude that the woman with leprosy likely was perceived as disabled and received a great deal of care in life and death, while the woman with gigantism probably was not considered disabled and received care periodically during life but little after death.

Zakrzewski, Evelyn-Wright, and Inskip (2017) argue that creating and synthesizing osteobiographies of populations can lead to improved understanding of disability in Anglo-Saxon England. Applying this model involves a careful mortuary and taphonomic analysis of burials, coupled with paleopathological analysis of skeletons, in order to evaluate whether each individual "was able to act and live as a *social person* in their own society" across the life course (original emphasis; Zakrzewski et al., 2017:285). A pilot study, focused on a cluster of individuals with pathologies buried at Great Chesterford, leads the authors to conclude that the central location of the cluster in the cemetery "does not reflect a desire to exclude or marginalize these individuals, but perhaps to represent them as a group identity" (Zakrzewski et al., 2017:276).

Personhood

Social theories other than, or in addition to, the life course model have also proven productive for framing inquiries into the health and disease experiences of past individuals. The utility of the osteobiography model for exploring the relationality, dividuality, and partibility of personhood in past populations—and as a means of interrogating the primacy of the Western model of individualism—has been discussed by several authors (Boutin, 2011; Geller, 2012; Appleby, 2019). One emerging direction for this scholarship is the interface of personhood between animals and humans, particularly with regard to disease and health status. Hosek's (2019) exploration of warrior personhood for a medieval Czech male (discussed above) relies, in part, on analysis of a trauma pattern consistent with injuries having been suffered on horseback. The "bodily consequences" that result from "articulations of weapons, horse, and human" are central to her reconstruction of his lived experience (Hosek, 2019:53).

Zooarchaeological research on the paleopathology of animals has recently drawn on the osteobiographical model, as well. These studies include osteobiographies of a domesticated cat with age-related pathologies from early medieval Kazakhstan (Haruda et al., 2020), a domesticated dog from 19th century CE Toronto, Canada whose pathologies would have caused great pain (Tourigny et al., 2016), and a wild caribou with disabilities from early 20th century CE Alberta, Canada (Hull, 2020). By investigating human-animal relationships in the context of health and disease, and the conditions of care and emotion that can result, this scholarship represents an intriguing movement toward using cross-species paleopathological analysis to explore past personhoods.

Biohistorical Research

Paleopathological case studies and osteobiographies periodically fall into the realm of biohistorical research by focusing on individuals who "have a pre-existing connection to public consciousness and historical imagination" (Stojanowski & Duncan, 2016:4). Some of them compare the named person's historically documented health status or cause of death with the pathological lesions on their skeleton (Belcastro et al., 2011; Bianucci et al., 2012). Others start from a similar premise, then go further by contextualizing their findings within relevant social and historical contexts. For example, Bruwelheide et al. (2016) were tasked by the family of Smithsonian naturalist Robert Kennicott with determining his cause of death. The researchers concluded that he died of cardiac arrest, but their multi-disciplinary analysis also shed new light on mortuary practices and the therapeutic use of toxins such as strychnine for a variety of conditions, including mental health disorders, in the mid-19th-century CE United States.

Paleopathological research formed a primary line of inquiry into the remains of 15th century CE English King Richard III. A research team led by Appleby sheds light on his life and death by conducting detailed investigations of his scoliosis (Appleby et al., 2014) and traumatic injuries (Appleby et al., 2015). Mitchell (2017) uses Richard III as a case study for how historical evidence can be ground-truthed by paleopathological analysis. He concludes that the rich documentary and literary record associated with the English king may need to be critically reevaluated, based on the findings of Appleby and colleagues. Despite the comprehensive and multi-disciplinary research conducted on Richard III's remains prior to reburial, Appleby (2019) demonstrates that novel opportunities for exploring his life course still exist. Namely, she explores the future potential of applying an osteobiographical model to Richard III, arguing that doing so would attend to his body as a "both a product of elite local biologies and a unique response to the biological and social circumstances of his life" (Appleby, 2019:39). This might include reconstructing his royal diet, exploring the psycho-social stress he potentially experienced due to scoliosis, and documenting the genetic and embodied effects of a family tree filled with consanguineous marriages.

Reconstructing the health status and disease experiences of historic-era individuals who were not themselves historical personages can also be enhanced by comparing textual records with bioarchaeological analysis (see Chapter 10, this volume). Snoddy et al.'s (2019) osteobiography of an English-born male resident of 19th century CE Aotearoa/New Zealand corroborates his documented cause of death as tuberculosis. This diagnosis becomes a jumping-off point for reconstructing his life course via multiple analytical techniques. The researchers also explore his health status via the Index of Care method (discussed below), which allows them to draw conclusions about "community, provision of care, and quality of life in rural colonial New Zealand" (Snoddy et al., 2019:219).

Robb et al. (2019) compare two contemporary males in medieval England—one known through historical records, the other through archaeologically recovered skeletal remains. Their findings lead the authors to argue that "osteobiography provides a more detailed, reliable, and insightful life story than textual biography" (Robb et al., 2019:18), especially with regard to understanding each man's experiences of health and disease. Mant, de la Cova, and Brickley (2021) present two case studies to illustrate the utility of employing social theory in trauma analysis: the remains of a male who died in early 20th century CE Missouri are interpreted with the help of abundant demographic and newspaper evidence for his life; while only general historical records are available to contextualize the remains of a female from mid-19th century CE London. But by drawing on the concept of intersectionality to interpret traumatic injury recidivism for each individual, they are able to explore substance abuse, impoverishment, and social marginalization in the recent past. Thus, case studies and osteobiographies of prehistoric and historical individuals and populations have made significant contributions to paleopathological research on topics including violence, social organization, stigma, disability and impairment, and the use of written records to investigate health and disease in the past.

New Directions in Applications of Case Studies and Osteobiography to Paleopathology

Paleopathology, as a discipline, has matured tremendously over the past century. But Buikstra et al. (2017) believe that further refinement is possible, calling for rigorous, standards-based approaches to paleopathology that marry methods and theories from the biomedical sciences, social sciences, and humanities. According to some researchers, the life course and osteobiography models are, themselves, humanistic (Hosek & Robb, 2019; Stodder & Byrnes, 2020). More recently, additional humanistic perspectives—which engage with care and emotion, among other topics—have emerged in paleopathological research; these hold great promise for broadening the relevance of bioarchaeological research and producing richer interpretations of the health and disease experiences of past people.

Case studies of three individuals were (in)famously cited by Dettwyler (1991) to assert that survival of pathological conditions is not sufficient to infer the existence of compassion and caregiving in the past. This argument has been challenged by the Bioarchaeology of Care model, its associated Index of Care methodology, and the recent surge of publications that utilize them (e.g., Tilley & Schrenk, 2017; and see Chapter 26, this volume). Tilley (2015) critically reevaluates the same case studies cited by Dettwyler and reviews many others to convincingly argue that the systematic, contextualized analysis of past individuals' health across the life course can indeed reveal caregiving and the presence of emotions, including compassion, in the past. Boutin (2016) applies the Index of Care in writing a fictive osteobiographical narrative to explore how pathological conditions evident in the skeleton of a young woman with disabilities from the Early Dilmun period in Bahrain were experienced personally and perceived socially. Osteobiographical narratives such as this one have proven effective at connecting modern readers emotionally with the past subjects whose skeletal remains are being interpreted (Boutin & Callahan, 2019). Emotions in the past are likewise explored by Robbins Schug (2020) in the context of Harappa, India during the Mature Period. Here, five-year-old putative twins with deformational plagiocephaly likely evoked powerful emotional responses, both within their family and in the community at large, during their short lives and after violent deaths due to perimortem trauma.

Martin and Harrod (2016) agree that bioarchaeologists can engage with the emotional and sensory experiences of suffering and pain by using tools such as the Index of Care and osteobiography. They present the osteobiography of an Ancestral Puebloan woman who suffered massive, and possibly debilitating, antemortem cranial trauma and speculate that her gender and non-local status made her vulnerable to social inequality and physical violence. Their work builds upon that of de la Cova (2012), Klaus (2012), Stone (2012), and Nystrom (2014), some of the first bioarchaeologists to write about the unique insights that human remains can shed on structural violence in the past. These authors emphasize that the origins of modern systemic social inequities and injustice can be discerned from skeletal evidence of nutritional deficiency, disease, habitual activity, chronic stress caused by body modifications, traumatic injuries, and dissection and autopsy in past bodies. Recent studies illustrate how paleopathological research on past individuals contributes to these efforts.

Lans argues that the pathologizing of Black women's bodies by American society made them more vulnerable to accession into collections after their deaths. She draws on Black feminist theory, and archival and bioarchaeological evidence, to reconstruct the life course of a woman whose name was recorded as Lizzie when her remains became part of the Huntington Collection (Lans 2018). Utilizing the medical records that list Lizzie's cause of death as tuberculosis, evaluating her skeleton for signs of this disease, and drawing on historical evidence, Lans explores her lived experience as a Black woman who migrated northward to New York City at the turn of the 20th century CE and worked as a domestic laborer, inferring the many social challenges—and associated health impacts—that would have resulted. Another Black woman whose story Lans (2020:42) recounts is Annie, whose death of eclampsia made her remains "highly desirable to anatomists and medical doctors."

Doubek and Grauer (2019) create an osteobiography of a now-nameless man of Asian ancestry whose skeleton was added to the collections of Chicago's Field Museum in the late 19th century CE. Although all records associated with the accession of his remains to the museum have been lost, his bones were permanently labeled with a racial epithet (Doubek & Grauer,

2019:207). Likely an immigrant to the United States during a time of anti-Asian sentiment, the effects of structural violence during life (enamel hypoplasia, dental disease, antemortem trauma) and after death (autopsy or dissection and, later, display) are evident in his bones.

As discussed above, Snoddy et al. (2019) also produced an osteobiography of a migrant, in this case from England to Aotearoa/New Zealand during a period of European colonization. However, this man's body was buried after death, and his first and last name are known today. The authors acknowledge that his descendants granted them permission to "share part of his story" (Snoddy et al., 2019:235). Sadly, this is an opportunity that the descendants of the anonymized people studied by Lans (2018) and Doubek and Grauer (2019) could not be afforded—yet another manifestation of the structural violence embodied by anatomical collections.

Recently, Watkins (2020) and Blakey (2020) have drawn on their extensive research with human skeletal remains to argue that normative (namely, White) anthropological scholarship will continue to perpetuate racism and colonialism unless concerted efforts are made to reckon with our discipline's legacy and to become more inclusive (see Chapter 22, this volume). Indeed, Geller (2019) recounts how the multi-disciplinary analysis of the remains of Kennewick Man/Ancient One, which included identification of his pathological conditions, took place against the wishes of tribal claimants. The "epistemological and ethical concerns" (Geller, 2019:88) raised by this process have led her to begin the process of developing a bioethos for osteobiography. In this regard, the need for contextualized paleopathological research on past individuals that is built around collaboration with descendant communities and other stakeholder groups (LaRoche & Blakey, 1997), that involves local scholars (for bioarchaeologists working outside of their own country), and that supports and promotes the research of scholars who identify as Black, Indigenous, and People of Color (BIPOC), is more acute than ever. Two recent examples of important contributions to such scholarship follow.

Littleton and Wallace (2019) apply an osteobiographical perspective to the traumatic injuries suffered by a prehistoric Australian Aboriginal woman in the late stages of pregnancy. The original interpretation of this burial, which dated to the early 1980s, sensationally proposed that she may have been the victim of a "mercy killing" during a "difficult childbirth" (Littleton & Wallace, 2019:105). Littleton and Wallace's updated analysis questions the assumptions that past women's lives should primarily be interpreted via their reproductive functions, and that hunter-gatherer societies are poorly equipped to deal with the challenges of childbirth. Their re-analysis carefully attends to all available archaeological and taphonomic evidence and extensively consults ethnographic and historical evidence for Aboriginal birthing and midwifery practices and cultural patterns of violence. They conclude that while the woman did suffer perimortem trauma, it was likely due to the "intracommunal violence" that was not uncommon in these societies (Littleton & Wallace 2019:113); further, she was unlikely to have been in labor at the time of her death. The authors also emphasize that modern interpretations of past lives are prone to erasing ambiguity and complexity, in favor of reductive explanations. Their re-analysis of this burial is part of a larger project conducted "with traditional owners represented by the River Murray and Mallee Aboriginal Corporation...to address both academic and community interests in the site and its people" (Littleton & Wallace, 2019:104). The authors are careful to acknowledge that community violence is a sensitive subject, and they thank community members for discussing this burial with them and sharing insights.

Fleskes and colleagues pair population-scale osteobiography with a community-engagement model to reconstruct "the health, ancestry, and lived experience among African or African-descended persons" buried in 18th century CE Charleston, South Carolina

(Fleskes et al., 2021:4). This research project occurred at the behest of The Gullah Society and other members of Charleston's African American community, who "expressed keen interest in understanding the lives of each individual, as well as the history of the burial ground" (Fleskes et al., 2021:5). The authors provide an ethics statement that describes multiple stages of community collaboration and culturally sensitive data collection, analysis, interpretation, and reburial. The resulting synthesis of bioarchaeological, isotopic, and genomic evidence sheds light on the ways that maternal ancestry, mobility, and health shaped the lives of the "Anson Street Ancestors," who had likely been enslaved. The authors also emphasize that an osteobiographical approach facilitates a "deeper investigation into, and remembrance of, the lives of the deceased" (Fleskes et al., 2021:20). Joining Fleskes in reporting on this research project are 11 other authors, several of whom are community members and BIPOC scholars. Similarly, Vlok et al.'s (2020) research (discussed above) is notable because it resulted from a productive collaboration between 11 scholars in five countries, including four from the Institute of Archaeology in Hanoi, Vietnam.

Paleopathological projects such as these demonstrate how case study research and osteobiography can help decolonize disciplinary praxis. Research questions posed and answered by BIPOC and local scholars, and with the consent and collaboration of descendant communities and stakeholders, are more likely to generate interpretations that are meaningful to diverse publics, thus enhancing the broader relevance of paleopathology. The small scale of case studies and osteobiographies, and the use of multiple lines of evidence, also make them more amenable to exploring the ambiguity and contingency that characterize not only individual life courses but also the production of scientific knowledge about health and disease in the past.

Osteobiographies and case studies of past individuals' health and disease experiences also are effective means of harnessing the public outreach potential of bioarchaeology. O'Donnabhain and Murphy (2014:160) report that in Ireland, the publication of paleopathology case studies in "general-reader journals, particularly *Archaeology Ireland*" have helped "raise the profile" of bioarchaeological research both among the general public and in Irish archaeology. Similarly, for three of the years that Killgrove (2016, 2017, 2018) produced her bioarchaeology blog on Forbes.com, she wrote an annual post on the most "fascinating" skeletons highlighted that year. In her 2018 post, Killgrove explained that, while bioarchaeologists have "produced countless articles on diet, activities, and health of populations around the world, the work showcased [here] demonstrates how these techniques can also produce poignant pictures of diverse lives." Notably, of the 22 stories featured in these three annual posts, 13 of them were about skeletons of individuals who stood out due to their pathological conditions. Just the 2018 post alone has been viewed 53,246 times since publication (as of 1/14/21; K. Killgrove, personal communication), demonstrating the level of public interest in the personal stories produced by osteobiography and case study approaches to paleopathological research. Given the ability of osteobiographical narratives to elicit empathy and reduce prejudice in readers (Boutin & Callahan, 2019), widely disseminated stories about past individuals with pathological conditions—especially if they involve community collaboration and BIPOC and local scholars—could potentially have a transformative social impact.

Conclusion

The publications reviewed in this chapter demonstrate how the use of case study approaches and osteobiographical models grounded in best practices enhances paleopathologists' ability to explore health and disease in the past. For case studies, these best practices include drawing on multiple lines of contextual evidence to interpret human remains and the use of social theory, such as a life course model. Scholars creating osteobiographies would do well to employ the model espoused by Hosek and Robb (2019), which explores past health and disease in terms of lived experience, and the historical contingency and social construction of life courses. Case study and osteobiography approaches are also excellent ways to "breathe new life" into extant skeletal remains. For example, scholars can: reinterpret an existing case study via an osteobiographical model (cf. Appleby, 2019) or by deploying recently developed analytical techniques (cf. Millard et al., 2020; Schrenk et al., 2016); apply a humanistic lens to remains in anatomical collections (cf. Lans, 2018, 2020) or a life course approach to an individual whose remains have been reburied (cf. Palkovich, 2012); or question assumptions about already-analyzed remains in collaboration with descendant communities and stakeholder groups (cf. Littleton & Wallace, 2019). All the while, authors of case studies and osteobiographies must be mindful of the ethical implications of their work, to avoid perpetrating further harm on individuals and populations who already were victims of structural violence in the past (cf. Boutin, 2019; Geller, 2019). Uniquely significant contributions to paleopathological research will result, in the form of richer, more meaningful, and more inclusive interpretations about the lived experiences of individuals and the social construction of health and disease in the past.

Acknowledgments

Many thanks to Anne Grauer for inviting me to be part of this volume, and for her support along the way. I am also grateful to Kristina Killgrove for kindly providing me with the impressive statistics for her Forbes posts. Helpful feedback on the first draft of this manuscript was provided by my graduate students, Victoria Calvin, Sandy Durden, Leslie Hoefert, and Taylor Love.

References

Alfaro Castro, M. E., Waters-Rist, A. L. & Zborover, D. (2017). An osteobiography of a Oaxacan late adolescent female. *Journal of Archaeological Science: Reports* 13:759–772. DOI:10.1016/j.jasrep.2016.12.016

Appleby, J. (2019). Osteobiographies: local biologies, embedded bodies, and relational persons. *Bioarchaeology International* 3:32–43. DOI:10.5744/bi.2019.1004

Appleby, J., Mitchell, P. D., Robinson, C., Brough, A., Rutty, G. & Harris, R. A. (2014). The scoliosis of Richard III, last plantagenet king of England: diagnosis and clinical significance. *The Lancet* 383:1944.

Appleby, J., Rutty, G., Hainsworth, S. V., Woosnam-Savage, R. C., Morgan, B. & Brough, A. (2015). Perimortem trauma in King Richard III: a skeletal analysis. *The Lancet* 385:253–259. DOI:10.1016/S0140-6736(14)60804-7

Armelagos, G. J. & Van Gerven, D. P. (2003). A century of skeletal biology and paleopathology: contrasts, Contradictions, and Conflicts. *American Anthropologist* 105:53–64.

Baker, B. J. & Bolhofner, K. L. (2014). Biological and social implications of a medieval burial from Cyprus for understanding leprosy in the past. *International Journal of Paleopathology* 4:17–24. Doi:10.1016/j.ijpp.2013.08.006

Beck, L. A. (2006). Kidder, Hooton, Pecos, and the birth of bioarchaeology. In Buikstra, J. E. & Beck, L. A. (Eds.), *Bioarchaeology: The Contextual Analysis of Human Remains*, pp. 83–94. Burlington, Mass: Elsevier.

Belcastro, M. G., Todero, A., Fornaciari, G. & Mariotti, V. (2011). Hyperostosis frontalis interna (HFI) and castration: the case of the famous singer Farinelli (1705–1782). *Journal of Anatomy* 219:632–637. DOI:10.1111/j.1469-7580.2011.01413.x

Bianucci, R., Giuffra, V., Bachmeier, B. E., Ball, M., Pusch, C. M., Fornaciari, G…. & Nerlich, A. G. (2012). Eleonora of Toledo (1522–1562): evidence for tuberculosis and leishmaniasis co-infection in Renaissance Italy. *International Journal of Paleopathology* 2:231–235. DOI:10.1016/j.ijpp.2012.11.002

Blakey, M. L. (2020). Archaeology under the blinding light of race. *Current Anthropology* 61:S183–S197. Doi:10.1086/710357

Boutin, A. T. (2011). Crafting a bioarchaeology of personhood: osteobiographical narratives from Alalakh. In Baadsgaard, A., Boutin, A. T. & Buikstra, J. E. (Eds.), *Breathing New Life Into the Evidence of Death: Contemporary Approaches to Bioarchaeology*, pp. 109–133. Santa Fe: School for Advanced Research Press.

Boutin, A. T. (2016). Exploring the social construction of disability: an application of the bioarchaeology of personhood model to a pathological skeleton from ancient Bahrain. *International Journal of Paleopathology* 12:17–28. DOI:10.1016/j.ijpp.2015.10.005

Boutin, A. T. & Callahan, M. P. (2019). Increasing empathy and reducing prejudice: an argument for fictive osteobiographical narrative. *Bioarchaeology International* 3:78–87. DOI:10.5744/bi.2019.1001

Boutin, A. T., Longo, C. M. & Lehnhard, R. (2022). The role of case studies in recent paleopathological literature: an argument for continuing relevance. *International Journal of Paleopathology* 38:45–54. DOI:10.1016/j.ijpp.2022.06.002

Bradbury, J., Davies, D., Jay, M., Philip, G., Roberts, C. & Scarre, C. (2016). Making the dead visible: problems and solutions for "big" picture approaches to the past, and dealing with large "mortuary" datasets. *Journal of Archaeological Method and Theory* 23:561–591. DOI:10.1007/s10816-015-9251-1

Bruwelheide, K. S., Schlachtmeyer, S. S., Owsley, D. W., Simon, V. E., Aufderheide, A. C. & Cartmell, L. W. (2016). Unearthing Robert Kennicott: Naturalist, explorer, Smithsonian scientist. In Stojanowski, C. M. & Duncan, W. N. (Eds.), *Studies in Forensic Biohistory: Anthropological Perspectives*, pp. 92–123. Cambridge: Cambridge University Press.

Buikstra, J. E. & Roberts, C. A. (Eds.) (2012). *The Global History of Paleopathology: Pioneers and Prospects*. Oxford: Oxford University Press.

Buikstra, J. E. & DeWitte, S. (2019). A brief history and 21st century challenges. In Buikstra, J. E. (Ed.), *Ortner's Identification of Pathological Conditions in Human Skeletal Remains* (3rd ed.), pp. 11–19. London: Elsevier.

Buikstra, J. E., Cook, D. C. & Bolhofner, K. L. (2017). Introduction: scientific rigor in paleopathology. *International Journal of Paleopathology* 19:80–87. DOI:10.1016/j.ijpp.2017.08.005

Cerezo-Román, J. I. & Tsukamoto, K. (2021). The life course of a standard-bearer: a nonroyal elite burial at the archaeological site of El Palmar, Mexico. *Latin American Antiquity* 32:274–291. DOI:10.1017/laq.2020.96.

Cheverko, C. M. (2021). Life course approaches and life history theory: synergistic perspectives for bioarchaeology. In Cheverko, C. M., Prince-Buitenhuys, J. R. & Hubbe, M. (Eds.), *Theoretical Approaches in Bioarchaeology*, pp. 59–75. London: Routledge.

Cohen, H., Slon, V., Barash, A., May, H., Medlej, B. & Hershkovitz, A. (2015). Assyrian attitude towards captive enemies: a 2700-year-old paleo-forensic study. *International Journal of Osteoarchaeology* 25:265–280. DOI:10.1002/oa.2288

Cook, D. C. & Powell, M. L. (2006). The evolution of American paleopathology. In Buikstra, J. E. & Beck, L. A. (Eds.), *Bioarchaeology: The Contextual Analysis of Human Remains*, pp. 281–322. Burlington, Mass: Elsevier.

Couoh, L. R. (2015). Bioarchaeological analysis of a royal burial from the oldest Maya tomb in Palenque, Mexico. *International Journal of Osteoarchaeology* 25:711–721. DOI:10.1002/oa.2338

Crowe, S., Cresswell, K., Robertson, A., Huby, G., Avery, A. & Sheikh, A. (2011). The case study approach. *BMC Medical Research Methodology* 11:100. DOI:10.1186/1471–2288-11–100

de la Cova, C. (2012). Patterns of trauma and violence in 19th-century-born African American and Euro-American females. *International Journal of Paleopathology* 2:61–68.

Dettwyler, K. A. (1991). Can paleopathology provide evidence for "compassion"? *American Journal of Physical Anthropology* 84:375–384.

Doubek, S. L. & Grauer, A. L. (2019). Exploring the effects of structural inequality in an individual from 19th-century Chicago. In Mant, M. L. & Holland, A. J. (Eds.), *Bioarchaeology of Marginalized People*, pp. 205–221. London: Elsevier.

Ellis, M. A. B. (2016). Presence and absence: an exploration of scurvy in the commingled subadults in the Spring Street Presbyterian Church Collection, Lower Manhattan. *International Journal of Osteoarchaeology* 26:759–766.

Faccia, K., Waters-Rist, A. L., Lieverse, A. R., Bazaliiskii, V. I., Stock, J. T. & Katzenberg, M. A. (2016). Diffuse idiopathic skeletal hyperostosis (DISH) in a middle Holocene forager from Lake Baikal, Russia: potential causes and the effect on quality of life. *Quaternary International* 405:66–79. DOI:10.1016/j.quaint.2015.10.011

Fleskes, R. E., Ofunniyin, A. A., Gilmore, J. K., Poplin, E., Abel, S. M., Bueschgen, W. D.… & Schurr, T. G. (2021). Ancestry, health, and lived experiences of enslaved Africans in 18th century Charleston: an osteobiographical analysis. *American Journal of Physical Anthropology* 175(1):3–24. DOI:10.1002/ajpa.24149

Geller, P. L. (2012). Parting (with) the dead: body partibility as evidence of commoner ancestor veneration. *Ancient Mesoamerica* 23(1):115–130. DOI:10.1017/S0956536112000089

Geller, P. L. (2019). The bioethos of osteobiography. *Bioarchaeology International* 3:88–101. doi:10.5744/bi.2019.1000

Grauer, A. L. (2018). A century of paleopathology. *American Journal of Physical Anthropology* 165:904–914. DOI:10.1002/ajpa.23366

Grauer, A. L. & Buikstra, J. E. (2019). Themes in Paleopathology. In Buikstra, J. E. (Ed.), *Ortner's Identification of Pathological Conditions in Human Skeletal Remains* (3rd ed.), pp. 21–33. London: Elsevier.

Grauer, A. L., Williams, L. A. & Bird, M. C. (2016). Life and death in nineteenth-century Peoria, Illinois: taking a biocultural approach towards understanding the past. In Zuckerman, M. K. & Martin, D. L. (Eds.), *New Directions in Biocultural Anthropology*, pp. 201–217. Hoboken: John Wiley & Sons, Inc.

Hardy, E., Merrett, D. C., Zhang, H., Zhang, Q., Zhu, H. & Yang, D. Y. (2019). Possible case of pressure resorption associated with osteoarthritis in human skeletal remains from ancient China. *International Journal of Paleopathology* 24:1–6. DOI:10.1016/j.ijpp.2018.07.005

Haruda, A. F., Ventresca Miller, A. R., Paijmans, J. L. A., Barlow, A., Tazhekeyev, A., Bilalov, S., … & Arzhantseva, I. (2020). The earliest domestic cat on the Silk Road. *Scientific Reports* 10:11241. doi:10.1038/s41598-020-67798-6

Hawkey, D. E. (1998). Disability, compassion and the skeletal record: using musculoskeletal stress markers (MSM) to construct an osteobiography from early New Mexico. *International Journal of Osteoarchaeology* 8:326–340.

Heathcote, G. M., Diego, V. P., Ishida, H. & Sava, V. J. (2012). An osteobiography of a remarkable protohistoric Chamorro man from Taga, Tinian. *Micronesica* 4:131–213.

Hooton, E. A. (1930). *The Indians of Pecos Pueblo: A Study of Their Skeletal Remains.* New Haven: Yale University Press.

Hosek, L. (2019). Osteobiography as microhistory: writing from the bones up. *Bioarchaeology International* 3:44–57. DOI:10.5744/bi.2019.1007

Hosek, L. & Robb, J. (2019). Osteobiography: a platform for bioarchaeological research. *Bioarchaeology International* 3:1–15. doi:10.5744/bi.2019.1005

Hull, E. H. (2020). Love and death: theoretical and practical examination of human-animal relations in creating wild animal osteobiography. *Society & Animals* (early view):1–21. DOI:10.1163/15685306-BJA10012

International Journal of Paleopathology, (2021). Guide for authors. Last accessed at: https://www.elsevier.com/journals/international-journal-of-paleopathology/1879-9817/guide-for-authors

Killgrove, K. (2016, December 21). The 10 most intriguing skeletons of 2016. Last accessed at: https://www.forbes.com/sites/kristinakillgrove/2016/12/21/the-10-most-intriguing-skeletons-of-2016/?sh=1a9edac96c1a

Killgrove, K. (2017, December 29). The 5 most fascinating skeletons of 2017. Last accessed at: https://www.forbes.com/sites/kristinakillgrove/2017/12/29/the-5-most-fascinating-skeletons-of-2017/?sh=1e5487a95ea1

Killgrove, K. (2018, December 31). The 7 most fascinating skeletons of 2018. Last accessed at: https://www.forbes.com/sites/kristinakillgrove/2018/12/31/the-7-most-fascinating-skeletons-of-2018/?sh=445813ae2510

Klaus, H. D. (2012). The bioarchaeology of structural violence: a theoretical model and a case study. In Martin, D. L. & Harrod, R. P. (Eds.), *The Bioarchaeology of Violence*, pp. 29–62. Gainesville: University Press of Florida.

Knüsel, C. J. (2002). More Circe than Cassandra: the princess of Vix in ritualized social context. *European Journal of Archaeology* 5:275–308.

Lans, A. (2018). "Whatever was once associated with him, continues to bear his stamp": articulating and dissecting George S. Huntington and his anatomical collection. In. Stone, P. K (Ed.), *Bioarchaeological Analyses and Bodies: New Ways of Knowing Anatomical and Archaeological Skeletal Collections*, pp. 11–26. Cham: Springer.

Lans, A. M. (2020). Embodied discrimination and "mutilated historicity": archiving black women's bodies in the Huntington Collection. In Tremblay, L. A. & Reedy, S. (Eds.), *The Bioarchaeology of Structural Violence: A Theoretical Framework for Industrial Era Inequality*, pp. 31–52. Cham: Springer.

La Roche, C. J. & Blakey, M. L. (1997). Seizing intellectual power: the dialogue at the New York African burial ground. *Historical Archaeology* 31(3):84–106.

Little, L. M. & Papadopoulos, J. K. (1998). A social outcast in Early Iron Age Athens. *Hesperia* 67:375–404.

Littleton, J. & Wallace, S. (2019). Ambiguity in the bioarchaeological record: the case of "euthanasia" at Roonka, South Australia. *Bioarchaeology International* 3:103–117. DOI:10.5744/bi.2019.1003

Lovell, N. C. (2016). Tiptoeing through the rest of his life: a functional adaptation to a leg shortened by femoral neck fracture. *International Journal of Paleopathology* 13:91–95. DOI:10.1016/j.ijpp.2016.03.001

Lynnerup, N. (2019). Mummies and paleopathology. In Buikstra, J. E. (Ed.), *Ortner's Identification of Pathological Conditions in Human Skeletal Remains* (3rd ed.), pp. 799–807. London: Elsevier.

Mant, M., de la Cova, C. & Brickley, M. B. (2021). Intersectionality and trauma analysis in bioarchaeology. *American Journal of Physical Anthropology* 174:583–594. DOI:10.1002/ajpa.24226

Martin, D. L. & Harrod, R. P. (2016). The bioarchaeology of pain and suffering: human adaptation and survival during troubled times. In Hegmon, M. (Ed.), *Archaeology of the Human Experience*, pp. 161–174. Washington, DC: American Anthropological Association.

Martin, D. L. & Potts, D. T. (2012). Lesley: a unique Bronze Age individual from southeastern Arabia. In Stodder, A. L. W. & Palkovich, A. M. (Eds.), *The Bioarchaeology of Individuals*, pp. 113–126. Gainesville: University Press of Florida.

Matczak, M. D. & Kozłowski, T. (2017). Dealing with difference: using the osteobiographies of a woman with leprosy and a woman with gigantism from medieval Poland to identify practices of care. In Tilley, L. & Schrenk, A. (Eds.), *New Developments in the Bioarchaeology of Care*, pp. 125–151. Cham: Springer.

Mays, S. A. (1997). A perspective on human osteoarchaeology in Britain. *International Journal of Osteoarchaeology* 7:600–604.

Mays, S. (2012a). The relationship between paleopathology and the clinical sciences. In Grauer, A. L. (Ed.), *A Companion to Paleopathology*, pp. 285–309. Chichester: Blackwell Publishing Ltd.

Mays, S. (2012b). The impact of case reports relative to other types of publication in paleopathology. *International Journal of Osteoarchaeology* 22:81–85. DOI:10.1002/oa.1186

Melton, N., Montgomery, J., Knüsel, C. J., Batt, C., Needham, S., Parker Pearson, M., … & Wilson, A. (2010). Gristhorpe man: an Early Bronze Age log-coffin burial scientifically defined. *Antiquity* 84:796–815. DOI:10.1017/S0003598X00100237

Mennear, D. (2017). Highlighting the importance of the past: public engagement and bioarchaeology of care research. In Tilley, L. & Schrenk, A. (Eds.), *New Developments in the Bioarchaeology of Care*, pp. 343–364. Cham: Springer.

Merrett, D. C., Sawatzky, R. M. & Meiklejohn, C. (2019). Possible case of glanders in a late-nineteenth- or early-twentieth-century Mennonite woman in Manitoba, Canada. *Bioarchaeology International* 3:240–261. DOI:10.5744/bi.2019.1015

Millard, A. R., Annis, R. G., Caffell, A. C., Dodd, L. L., Fischer, R., Gerrard, C. M., … & Speller, C. F. (2020). Scottish soldiers from the Battle of Dunbar 1650: a prosopographical approach to a skeletal assemblage. *PLoS ONE* 15(12):e0243369. doi:10.1371/journal.pone.0243369

Mitchell, P. D. (2017). Improving the use of historical written sources in paleopathology. *International Journal of Paleopathology* 19:88–95. DOI:10.1016/j.ijpp.2016.02.005

Nystrom, K. C. (2019). *The Bioarchaeology of Mummies*. New York: Routledge.

O'Donnabhain, B. & Murphy, E. (2014). The development of the contextual analysis of human remains in Ireland. In. O'Donnabhain, B. & Lozada. M. C. (Eds.), *Archaeological Human Remains: Global Perspectives*, pp. 155–164. Cham: Springer.

Palkovich, A. M. (2012). Reading a life: a fourteenth-century Ancestral Puebloan woman. In Stodder, A. L. W. & Palkovich, A. M. (Eds.), *The Bioarchaeology of Individuals*, pp. 242–254. Gainesville: University Press of Florida.

Riley, D. S., Barber, M. S., Kienle, G. S., Aronson, J. K., von Schoen-Angerer, T., Tugwell, P., ... & Gagnier, J. J. (2017). CARE guidelines for case reports: explanation and elaboration document. *Journal of Clinical Epidemiology* 89:218–235. DOI:10.1016/j.jclinepi.2017.04.026

Roberts, C. A. (2006). A view from afar: bioarchaeology in Britain. In Buikstra, J. E. & Beck, L. A. (Eds.), *Bioarchaeology: The Contextual Analysis of Human Remains*, pp. 417–439. Burlington, Mass: Elsevier.

Robb, J. (2002). Time and biography: osteobiography of the Italian Neolithic lifespan. In Hamilakis, Y., Pluciennik, M. & S. Tarlow (Eds.), *Thinking Through the Body: Archaeologies of Corporeality*, pp. 153–171. New York: Kluwer Academic/Plenum Publishers.

Robb, J. (2019). Beyond individual lives: using comparative osteobiography to trace social patterns in Classical Italy. *Bioarchaeology International* 3:58–77. doi:10.5744/bi.2019.1007

Robb, J., Inskip, S. A., Cessford, C., Dittmar, J., Kivisild, T., Mitchell, P. D., ... & Scheib, C. (2019). Osteobiography: the history of the body as real bottom-line history. *Bioarchaeology International* 3:16–31. DOI:10.5744/bi.2019.1006

Robbins Schug, G. (2020). Touching the surface: biological, behavioral, and emotional aspects of plagiocephaly at Harappa. In Halcrow, S. & Gowland, R. (Eds.), *The Mother-Infant Nexus in Anthropology: Small Beginnings, Significant Outcomes*, pp. 235–256. Cham: Springer.

Saul, F. P. (1972). *The Human Skeletal Remains of Altar de Sacrificios: An Osteobiographic Analysis*. Cambridge, Mass: The Peabody Museum.

Saul, F. P. & Saul, J. M. (1989). Osteobiography: a Maya example. In İşcan, M. Y. & Kennedy, K. A. R. (Eds.), *Reconstruction of Life from the Skeleton*, pp. 287–302. New York: Alan R. Liss, Inc.

Schrenk, A. A. & Martin, D. L. (2017). Applying the Index of Care to the case study of a Bronze Age teenager who lived with paralysis: moving from speculation to strong inference. In Tilley, L. & Schrenk, A. (Eds.), *New Developments in the Bioarchaeology of Care*, pp. 47–64. Cham: Springer.

Schrenk, A., Gregoricka, L. A., Martin, D. L. & Potts, D. T. (2016). Differential diagnosis of a progressive neuromuscular disorder using bioarchaeological and biogeochemical evidence from a Bronze Age skeleton in the UAE. *International Journal of Paleopathology* 13:1–10. DOI:10.1016/j.ijpp.2015.12.004

Slon, V., Nagar, Y., Kuperman, T., & Hershkovitz, I. (2013). A case of dwarfism from the Byzantine city Rehovot-in-the-Negev, Israel. *International Journal of Osteoarchaeology* 23:573–589. DOI:10.1002/oa.1285

Snoddy, A. M. E., Buckley, H. R., King, C. L., Kinaston, R. L., Nowell, G., Gröcke, D. R., ... & Petchey, P. (2019). "Captain of all these men of death": an integrated case study of tuberculosis in nineteenth-century Otago, New Zealand. *Bioarchaeology International* 3:219–239. DOI:10.5744/bi.2019.1014

Solari, A., da Silva, S. F. S. M., Pessis, A. M., Martin, G. & Guidon, N. (2020). Applying the bioarchaeology of care model to a severely diseased infant from the Middle Holocene, north-eastern Brazil: a step further into research on past health-related caregiving. *International Journal of Osteoarchaeology* 30:482–491. DOI:10.1002/oa.2876

Stodder, A. L. W. & Palkovich, A. M. (Eds.) (2012). *The Bioarchaeology of Individuals*. Gainesville: University Press of Florida.

Stodder, A. L. W. & Byrnes, J. F. (2020). (Re)discovering paleopathology: integrating individuals and populations in bioarchaeology. In Willermet, C. & Lee, S.-H. (Eds.), *Evaluating Evidence in Biological Anthropology: The Strange and the Familiar*, pp. 103–125. Cambridge: Cambridge University Press.

Stojanowski, C. M. & Duncan, W. N. (2016). Defining an anthropological biohistorical research agenda: the history, scale, and scope of an emerging discipline. In Stojanowski, C. M. &. Duncan, W. N (Eds.), *Studies in Forensic Biohistory: Anthropological Perspectives*, pp. 1–28. Cambridge: Cambridge University Press.

Stone, P. K. (2012). Binding women: Ethnology, skeletal deformations, and violence against women. *International Journal of Paleopathology* 2:53–60. DOI:10.1016/j.ijpp.2012.09.008

Tilley, L. (2015). *Theory and Practice in the Bioarchaeology of Care*. Cham: Springer.

Tilley, L. & Schrenk, A. (Eds.) (2017). *New developments in the Bioarchaeology of Care*. Cham: Springer.

Torres-Rouff, C. & Knudson, K. J. (2017). Integrating identities: an innovative bioarchaeological and biogeochemical to analyzing the multiplicity of identities in the mortuary record. *Current Anthropology* 58:381–409. DOI:10.1086/692026

Tourigny, E., Thomas, R., Guiry, E., Earp, R., Allen, A., Rothenburger, J. L., ... & Nussbaumer, M. (2016). An osteobiography of a 19th-century dog from Toronto, Canada. *International Journal of Osteoarchaeology* 26:818–829. DOI:10.1002/oa.2483

Walker, P. L., Byock, J., Eng, J. T., Erlandson, J. M., Holck, P., Schwarcz, H., ... & Zori, D. (2012). The axed man of Mosfell: skeletal evidence of a Viking Age homicide, the Icelandic sagas, and feud. In Stodder, A. L. W. & Palkovich, A. M. (Eds.), *The Bioarchaeology of Individuals*, pp. 26–43. Gainesville: University Press of Florida.

Watkins, R. J. (2020). An alter(ed)native perspective on historical bioarchaeology. *Historical Archaeology* 54:17–33. DOI:10.1007/s41636-019-00224-5

Weizman, E. & Snow, C. (2011). Osteobiography: An interview with Clyde Snow. *Cabinet* 43:68–74.

Vlok, M., Oxenham, M. F., Domett, K., Minh, T. T., Huong, N. T. M., Matsumura, H., ... & Buckley, H. R. (2020). Two probable cases of infection with Treponema pallidum during the Neolithic period in northern Vietnam (ca. 2000–1500 B.C.). *Bioarchaeology International* 4:15–36. DOI:10.5744/bi.2020.1000

Yin, R. K. (2018). *Case Study Research and Applications: Design and Methods* (6th ed.). Thousand Oaks: SAGE Publications, Inc.

Zakrzewski, S., Evelyn-Wright, S. & Inskip, S. (2017). Anglo-Saxon concepts of dis/ability: placing disease at Great Chesterford in its wider context. In Byrnes, J. F. & Muller, J. L. (Eds.), *Bioarchaeology of Impairment and Disability*, pp. 269–289. Cham: Springer.

12
MUMMIFIED REMAINS

*Ken Nystrom, Dario Piombino-Mascali, Jane E. Buikstra
and Lucía Watson Jiménez*

Introduction

The study of health and disease is a dominant theme of mummy studies, especially prominent since the early 20th-century pioneering research of scholars such as Sir Marc Armand Ruffer and Grafton Elliot Smith. Indeed, this disciplinary emphasis is explicitly set center-stage in a recent special issue of *The Anatomical Record*, where the editors stated that "The *raison d'être* for the scientific study of mummies is to gain an understanding of the evolution of health and disease in previous or extinct populations of humans" (Monge & Rühli, 2015: 936). This comment also highlights the fact that though not strictly synonymous, the study of soft tissue paleopathology is such a significant component of the broader field of mummy studies that it is hard to divorce the discussion of one from the other.

The fact that there is a chapter specifically devoted to the paleopathology of mummies in this volume reveals two important points. First, although the paleopathological investigation of a mummy has the potential to reveal both soft tissue and osseous evidence of health and disease, most likely, when people read "the paleopathology of mummified remains" they will naturally think about evidence drawn from soft tissue. It is axiomatic in our discipline that bone tissue has a limited range of responses to any disruption of homeostasis – the main responses being the deposition and/or destruction of bone tissue. In contrast, the preservation of soft tissue potentially provides more opportunities to observe a wider range of morphological changes stemming from homeostatic disruption in a wider range of tissues, including eye sclera and the optic nerve (Esteban et al., 2015), the spleen (O'Neill et al., 2016), mammary gland (Ventura et al., 2014), the skin (Diana et al., 2014), liver (Ciranni & Fornaciari, 2004), lung tissue (Salo et al., 1994), thyroid tissue (Gerszten et al., 1976), and nervous tissue (Prats-Muñoz et al., 2012). Further, the environmental conditions and factors associated with soft tissue preservation also raise the possibility that other biological materials, such as coprolites and intestinal contents, could be preserved and thus offer insight into health and disease (Searcey et al., 2013).

Of course, this potential is offset by the fact that soft tissue is much more susceptible to postmortem changes stemming from autolysis and decomposition than osseous tissue. The rate of decomposition is influenced by metabolic activity – those cells and tissues that have high turnover rates or that have secretory/absorption functions (e.g., epithelial) decay more quickly than connective tissues such as collagen and cartilage. Thus, while organs such as the liver and kidneys decay rapidly, seemingly delicate structures like the lungs can be well preserved (Aufderheide, 2003). Therefore, while the preservation of soft tissue offers the promise of identifying a wider range of pathological conditions, caution must be exercised. In fact, although there are notable exceptions (e.g., Gill-Frerking & Healey, 2011; Prats-Muñoz et al., 2013), taphonomic research that specifically addresses how cellular and tissue morphology may be impacted by post-depositional forces has been very limited.

Secondly, having a separate chapter devoted to the paleopathology of mummies acknowledges, at least implicitly, that there is a certain degree of "academic distance" from skeletal paleopathology and by extension bioarchaeology/biological anthropology. In a truly integrated, holistic paleopathology, mummy research *should not* warrant its own chapter. Ideally, research based solely on the examination of soft tissue could be seamlessly integrated into most (if not all) of the chapters contained in the second section of this volume (e.g., Trauma: Nerlich et al., 2009; Congenital and Developmental Disorders: Hershkovitz et al., 2014; Tumors and Neoplasms: Fornaciari, 2018). From a historical perspective, mummy studies has always been somewhat separate from these sister disciplines. This likely stems, at least in part, from the academic background and training of researchers. Researchers from the biomedical-aligned fields have always been drawn to mummy studies. Indeed, many of the key figures in the development of the modern incarnation of mummy studies were medical doctors, pathologists, and medical imaging experts. Somewhat ironically, the dissection of two mummies organized by Aidan Cockburn, an epidemiologist, spurred the development of the Paleopathology Association (Powell, 2012), which is now one of the main venues for the presentation of skeletal paleopathology research. While this clearly ties the fields together, another academic group, the Paleopathology Club, formed during the late 1970s. Established by Enrique Gerszten and Marvin Allison that group meets annually in association with the United States and Canadian branch of the International Academy of Pathology.

This "academic distance" is also reflected in journal publications. In his review of publication patterns in mummy studies, Nystrom (2018) found that in a sample of 1,063 journal articles, the majority were published in journals more closely aligned with biomedicine (e.g., *The Lancet, The Prostrate, Canadian Medical Association Journal*) than with anthropology (e.g., *American Journal of Physical Anthropology, Journal of Archaeological Science*). Further, there is a lack of interdisciplinary projects that integrate the social and biological perspective, from an understanding of the cosmovision of the area where the material was found (Watson, 2019).

In this chapter, we will discuss three topics as they provide insight into the state of the discipline; autopsy, paleoimaging, and paleogenetics. Transposed from its biomedical home, the autopsy has served as the *sine qua non* method in mummy paleopathology since the birth of the discipline in the first decades of the 20th century. Although the centrality of the autopsy has waned since the 1980s, it is still an important aspect of mummy paleopathology. The last two topics are areas where it is possible to observe significant advances in the identification and documentation of soft tissue disease. We will end by considering some of the recent critiques of mummy studies and soft tissue paleopathology and what they may portend for the future of the discipline.

Autopsies and Morphology

Whether it was through direct observation of organs and tissues via autopsy (Pettigrew, 1834; Gaeta et al., 2019), radiography (Beckett & Conlogue, 2020), or through the lens of a microscope (Ruffer, 1921; Fornaciari, 2018), the methodological core of the discipline has been and continues to be grounded in anatomical morphology (Aufderheide, 2003).

Autopsy has served as a methodological core of mummy studies since the field began to crystalize. In his discourse on the history of mummy studies, Aufderheide (2003) linked the earliest scientific investigation of mummies to advances in normal and pathological anatomy during the Renaissance. It was not until the first decades of the 20th century, however, that the scientific study of mummies truly began to develop and the autopsy was a principal means of investigation. After a period of quiescence during the mid-1900s, the modern manifestation of the field began to form in the 1970s with the dissection of the mummies known as PUM I (Zimmerman, 1974), PUM II (Cockburn et al., 1975), and ROM I (Hart et al., 1977). These investigations involved gross observations (e.g., Scott et al., 1977) and extensive tissue sampling for histological analyses (e.g., Horne & Lewin, 1977). Although gross visual observation of morphology remained the principal method of investigation during the 1970s and into the 1980s, the field began to increasingly incorporate imaging modalities and non- or minimally invasive methods based on immunology, molecular, and biochemical methods (Nystrom, 2018). Even as the methodological toolkit has expanded, however, the autopsy has remained a significant feature of the discipline and continues to be employed, though less frequently (e.g., Dedouit et al., 2010; Kim et al., 2015; Slepchenko et al., 2019; Nerlich et al., 2021).

Aufderheide identified several goals of the mummy dissection: generating cultural data (e.g., description of wrappings, material artifacts), health and disease, demographic data, taking tissues samples (i.e., for radiometric dating, biochemical analyses), and basic research. Today, many of these goals may be accomplished through "virtual" autopsies based on computed tomography (CT). Three-dimensional (3-D) volume rendering provides researchers the opportunity to document and describe material culture that may be enclosed by mummy wrappings, granting them the ability to manipulate virtual, and 3-D printed, representations of these objects (e.g., Sutherland et al., 2014, Nelson et al., 2021; and see Chapter 6, this volume). Given these alternatives, and the legal and ethical issues (e.g., principles of consent and right of bodily integrity – Lynnerup, 2007; Kaufmann & Rühli, 2010; Kreissl Lonfat et al., 2015; Mytum, 2021) that surround autopsies, the decision to perform an autopsy should be carefully considered and firmly grounded within a clearly defined, hypothesis-driven research framework. Although recommendations for new international protocols have been advanced (e.g., Moissidou et al., 2015), no concrete progress has been made (Piombino-Mascali & Gill-Frerking, 2019). Additional issues related to mummy studies that should be taken into account may include data anonymization and the diffusion of photographs, which certainly pose new challenges for those working in this field (Harries et al., 2018; Piombino-Mascali & Beckett, 2021).

Paleoimaging

With the recognition that destructive analyses should be avoided, the field has become increasingly reliant on advances in paleoimaging for detecting pathological morphology (see Chapter 6, this volume). Broadly speaking, the term "paleoimaging" refers to all imaging techniques that can be applied to mummified remains for documentation and study, assessing not only pathology, but postmortem mortuary behavior, as well. Paleoimaging includes multiple modalities such as photography, endoscopy, X-ray fluorescence, to infrared and ultraviolet lighting, as well as 3-D surface scanning (Beckett, 2014). More specifically, it is paleoradiology, a term first used by Notman and colleagues (1987) in their examination of the frozen bodies of two sailors from the Franklin expedition, that is most commonly employed to assess the presence of disease in mummified remains. Modalities in paleoradiology include X-ray, CT, micro-CT, and even terahertz (THz) radiation.

Medical imaging modalities were employed in a bioarchaeological context shortly after their discovery, with the study of a child and a cat mummy carried out in Germany by Walter König in 1896 (Böni et al., 2004). It was not until 1988 that data on health and disease were published (Braunstein et al., 1988; Chhem & Brothwell, 2008; Lynnerup & Rühli, 2015). Initially developed as an advanced imaging technique in 1975, CT became a preferred method for mummy investigation starting in 1985 (Lynnerup, 2009; Cox, 2015). In contrast to two-dimensional conventional radiography, CT imaging offers several advantages (Beckett, 2014; Cox, 2015; Nelson et al., 2021, Sydler et al., 2015; Wann et al., 2015). Micro-CT, which employs a pixel size of the cross-sections in the micrometer range, has been successfully utilized to investigate mummified remains such as ancient Egyptian animals (Johnston et al., 2020). Use of terahertz (THz) radiation (which falls on the opposite end of the electromagnetic spectrum from X-rays) has been limited to date, although it could be used to detect *in situ* material artifacts (e.g., amulets, jewelry) as well as the chemical identification of embalming substances (Öhrström et al., 2010, 2015).

At first, the application of nuclear magnetic resonance imaging (MRI) to mummy studies seemed ill-fated as the method relies upon the magnetizing of water molecules within the human body, given that desiccation is one of the principal ways in which soft tissue may come to be preserved. Indeed, while Piepenbrink and colleagues (1986) produced usable images in rehydrated tissue samples from an 11th–13th-century AD Peruvian mummy, they were not able to produce good images from desiccated remains. Nevertheless, advances in MRI, particularly with the advent of fast imaging techniques (Rühli et al., 2007), have produced good results. Still, MRI will likely remain as a complementary modality to CT, providing information on features such as anatomical parts or substances that may be hardly discernible with the latter alone (Münnemann et al., 2007).

How researchers visualize, and therefore interpret data has also improved significantly. Advances in software and post-imaging processing have expanded on the "virtual autopsy" (e.g., Dedouit et al., 2010; Borrini et al., 2012; Pedersen et al., 2021). Further, 3-D volume rendered reconstructions are being increasingly common in the visualization of mummified remains, aiding in the documentation of pathologies (Thompson et al., 2014; Davey & Drummer, 2016). These advances have also impacted the reconstruction of mortuary behavior, the identification of artifacts (e.g., Sutherland et al., 2014), museum conservation (e.g., Fantini et al., 2005), and even attempts to reconstruct long dead voices (Avanzini et al., 2017; Howard et al., 2020). Still, there remain some important features of mummies and mummy bundles that remain elusive to CT visualization, such as the color and manufacture technique of textiles and artifacts, details for the identification of certain organic species, and the presence or absence of facial painting or tattoos (Watson, 2019).

The potential of 3-D models produced from CT was first discussed in the 1990s (zur Nedden et al., 1994; Hjalgrim et al., 1995). Later, Lynnerup and colleagues (2007a, 2007b) used a 3-D model to help in differentiating between taphonomy and trauma. Similarly, Olszewski and colleagues (2019) have suggested that 3-D models could serve as a diagnostic and training aid in paleopathology. Printed 3-D models have also been used in morphometric analysis (Hughes et al., 2005), facial reconstruction (Gill-Robinson et al., 2006; Marić et al., 2020), museography (Pickering et al., 1990; Conlogue, 2015), and the creation of CT-scan digital collections which could provide researchers around the world with access to virtual material (Nelson & Wade, 2015). Two important examples of these types of virtual collections are the work of the HORUS group (Thompson et al., 2013; Sutherland et al., 2014) and the project Mummies as Microcosms (Nelson et al., 2021).

Although there are limitations (Conlogue, 2015), CT-based analyses have led to the identification and diagnosis of a range of pathologies that do not leave bony traces, including atherosclerosis (e.g., Thompson et al., 2013; Piombino-Mascali et al., 2014), hypoplastic left heart syndrome (Haas et al., 2015), congenital diaphragmatic hernia (Kim et al., 2014), prostatic hyperplasia (Fornaciari et al., 2001), pulmonary (Friedrich et al., 2010) and renal tuberculosis (Prates et al., 2015), Chagas disease (Panzer et al., 2014), and neurofibromatosis type 1 (Panzer et al., 2017). Further, CT imaging can facilitate the analysis of skeletal material that might otherwise be inaccessible, such as within conserved mummy bundles (e.g., Melcher et al., 1997; Sutherland et al., 2014).

Paleogenetics

The ability to extract and amplify ancient DNA has been one of the most significant methodological developments impacting the course and direction of mummy studies, being used to investigate long-distance migration and population history (e.g., Francalacci, 1995), kinship and within-site analyses (e.g., Gilbert et al., 2007; Gamba et al., 2011), and even the reconstruction of mortuary ritual (e.g., Hanna et al., 2012). Still, it is in the reconstruction of health and disease where paleogenetics has had the biggest impact on mummy studies (see Chapter 8 for more information on the use of DNA).

Pathogenic DNA

Bacterial DNA

DNA from several pathogenic bacteria has been isolated and identified in mummified remains, including *Escherichia coli* (e.g., Zink et al., 2000), members of the *Corynebacterium* genus (Zink et al., 2001), and *Bordetella pertussis* (Thèves et al., 2011). While the skeletal paleopathological literature on treponemal diseases is extensive (see discussion by Baker et al., 2020 and Chapter 16, this volume), research that has attempted to isolate treponemal DNA has been largely unsuccessful. Although there have been some recent successes based on sampling from bone, there has been only one study that attempted to isolate treponemal DNA from soft tissue samples. Based on immunological, histological, and ultrastructural analyses of the mummified remains of Maria of Aragon, Gino Fornaciari and colleagues (1989) concluded that she had tertiary stage venereal syphilis. Several years later, Marota and colleagues (1996) successfully amplified short fragments of the 16S ribosomal rRNA gene of *Treponema pallidum*. Sequencing of one of the fragments (95 bp) demonstrated close similarity (85%) with reference samples (Marota et al., 1996; Rollo & Marota, 1999). Sequencing of cloned amplicons, however, resulted in no *T. pallidum* sequence. Instead, the authors found sequences from a variety of oral bacteria (e.g., *Propionibacterium*, *Peptostreptococcus*, *Clostridium*, and *Capnocytophaga*) and *Mycobacterium*.

Salo and colleagues (1994) produced one of the first studies that successfully extracted *Mycobacterium tuberculosis* DNA from a large calcified nodule recovered from the lung of female from the Chiribaya culture of southern Peru (1000–1300 AD). *M. tuberculosis* DNA has also been successfully extracted from mummified remains from prehistoric Chile (Arriaza et al., 1995), 16th- to 19th-century Eastern Siberia (Dabernat et al., 2014), prehispanic Brazil (Sotomayor et al., 2004), 18th-century Hungary (Fletcher et al., 2003), and ancient Egypt

(Zink et al., 2007). Although case studies certainly establish the presence of a specific disease, there have also been larger scale studies that facilitate paleoepidemiological reconstructions (Zink et al., 2003; Donoghue et al., 2011).

Viral DNA and RNA

Studies that have successfully amplified viral DNA from mummified remains are not common. Nonetheless, the viruses that have been identified are significant human pathogens and therefore provide implications for our understanding of viral evolution.

Soft tissue evidence of smallpox (*Variola major* or *Variola minor*) infection is rare. Ruffer and Ferguson (1911) identified skin lesions thought to represent smallpox in Ramses V (1200–1100 BC), but this has not been confirmed histologically (Aufderheide, 2003). Fornaciari and Marchetti (1986: 625) identified "egg-shaped, dense virus-like particles" from skin lesions as evidence of smallpox from a 16th-century AD mummy from Italy, though it was not possible to recover any variola DNA (Marennikova et al., 1989). Further research actually suggests that the child suffered from Gianotti-Crosti syndrome (one clinical manifestation of which is skin lesions) caused by hepatitis B infection (Ross et al., 2018).

Biagini and colleagues (2012) were able to amplify three segments of the *Variola* genome from Siberian mummies dating to the 17th to 19th century. Additionally, based on phylogenetic analysis, the researchers concluded that the isolated strain is distinct from modern clades and "could be a direct progenitor of modern viral strains or a member of an ancient lineage that did not cause outbreaks in the 20th century" (Biagini et al., 2012: 2059). Recent research based on soft tissue samples from a 17th-century Lithuanian mummy suggests that the evolution of the major lineages of smallpox may have been more recent than previously thought (Duggan et al., 2016).

Hepatitis is an infection of the liver caused by one of five different viruses – A, B, C, D, and E – each with its own mode of transmission, symptoms, and outcomes. Today, HBV and HCV are the main sources of mortality, responsible for 96% of an estimated 1.34 million deaths in 2015 (WHO Report, 2017). There are two examples in the mummy paleopathological literature where researchers have documented hepatitis infection. Using the same samples scraped from the bandage from the mummified remains of Maria of Aragon, Marota et al. (1998) amplified a 24-bp complementary DNA sequence for one segment of the E hepatitis virus RNA genome. Given that HEV is composed solely of RNA, the authors (1998: 57) admit that this "cannot be explained easily." One idea is that Maria of Aragon was infected by HEV *and* a retrovirus, the latter being responsible for the production of the complementary DNA sequence. Alternatively, the authors suggest that the sequence represents a "normal component of the human genome present since very ancient times" (Marota et al., 1998: 58).

The other example comes from the Korean Joseon Dynasty (1392–1910 AD). Researchers examining the mummified remains of a young male child (4.5–6.6 years of age at death) identified nodules on the surface of the liver, though no diagnosis was suggested (Kim et al., 2006; Shin et al., 2003). Genetic analysis of liver samples later confirmed the presence of HBV genotype C2 DNA (Bar-Gal et al., 2012). Unlike the other hepatitis viruses, HBV is composed of partially double-stranded circular DNA. There are several different genotypes and subgenotypes of the virus, and modern clinical data indicates that HBV genotype C is a more aggressive and virulent strain (Kao et al., 2002). Given the estimated age of the individual, the most likely mode of virus transmission was from the mother during birth which increases the likelihood (>90%) that this child would have developed a chronic form of the infection (Araujo et al., 2011).

During the course of their examination of the mummified remains of Maria of Aragon, Gino Fornaciari and colleagues (2003: 1160) also observed "a large pedunculated branching skin neoformation" in the "right paravulvar region" which they suggest was an anogenital wart. They were able to amplify DNA that targeted a 141 bp sequence from several different types of human papillomavirus (HPV). There are five major genera of HPV with 174 different types with manifestations ranging from benign epithelial lesions to cancer (Bzhalava et al., 2013). Twelve HPV types are responsible for 99.7% of all cervical cancers, with HPV 16 and HPV 18 alone accounting for 70% of cases worldwide (Ault, 2006). Hybridization and subsequent sequencing of the amplified DNA from Maria of Aragon indicated the presence of HPV 18 as well as JC9813.

In contrast to the above examples, the paleogenetic research conducted by Li et al. (1999) and Sonoda et al. (2000) does not seem to have been based on the gross observation of soft tissue pathology. Rather, their research was attempting to reconstruct the evolutionary history of the human T lymphotropic virus (HTLV-1) in Japan and South America. Based on bone marrow samples taken from mummies from northern Chile, the researchers were able to identify two regions of HTLV-1, and when compared to modern Chilean and Japanese HTLBv-1, concluded that the virus had an Asian origin and was introduced during initial New World colonization. These publications were followed by a short series of responses that questioned the antiquity of the strain identified by Li and colleagues (Gessain et al., 2000; Vandamme et al., 2000). A more recent phylogenetic analysis of the sequences led Coulthart et al., (2006: 95) to conclude that "the ancient versus modern status of the putatively mummy-derived HTLV-1 LTR sequences of Li et al. (1999) and Sonoda et al. (2000) remains open…"

Parasitic DNA

The mummy studies literature documenting parasitic infection is extensive. This research has predominantly been predicated upon morphological or immunological evidence (e.g., Deelder et al., 1990; Bianucci et al., 2008). Paleogenetic evidence of infection by *Plasmodium falciparum* (Nerlich et al., 2008; Hawass et al., 2010), *Leishmania donovani* (Zink et al., 2006) and *Leishmania tarentolae* (Novo et al., 2015), *Enterobius vermicularis* (Iñiguez et al., 2003), *Clonorchis sinensis* (Liu et al., 2007; Shin et al., 2013), *Ascaris* sp. (Loreille et al., 2001; Leles et al., 2008), and *Pulex* sp. has also been published. Although the epidemiology of schistosomiasis in Egypt has been extensively examined (e.g., Kloos & David, 2002) only more recently has the question been approached using DNA (Matheson et al., 2014). To date, the most extensive paleogenetic research on parasitic infection has focused on Chagas' disease.

Chagas' disease is caused by the *Trypanosoma cruzi*, a protozoan parasite that is passed onto a host when bitten by triatomine bugs. While more common in Latin American countries, some six to seven million people are infected worldwide. One of the signature features of Chagas' disease is enlargement of the heart, esophagus, and colon resulting from damage to the peripheral autonomic nervous system. Evidence of megalopathies has been identified in mummified remains from northern Chile (Rothhammer et al., 1985), Peru (Fornaciari et al., 1992), and the North American Southwest (Reinhard et al., 2003).

Guhl and colleagues (1997, 1999) were able to amplify a segment of *T. cruzi* DNA from soft tissue samples collected from 27 northern Chilean/southern Peruvian mummies (2000 BC to 1400 AD). Several subsequent studies have expanded upon these results (Ferreira et al., 2000; Madden et al., 2001). In the broadest study, Aufderheide and colleagues (2004) tested tissue samples from 283 mummies ranging in time from 7050 BC to 1850 AD. Based on their results, the authors estimated a 40.6% prevalence rate of Chagas, with no significant differences between the different cultural periods sampled.

Researchers have also explored the presence of *T. cruzi* and Chagas' disease in prehistoric Brazil based on parasitic DNA. Lima and colleagues (2008) took rib samples from a 7,000–4,500-year-old mummy from the site known as Abrigo do Malhador in the Peruaçu Valley. Fernandes and colleagues (2008) took both bone and soft tissue samples from a 560 ± 40-year-old mummy, also from the Peruaçu Valley, that exhibited evidence of megacolon.

Human DNA

Perhaps one of the most significant advances, and by extension the area with the most potential, in paleopathology is in linking observations based on gross morphological changes with paleogenetics (see Chapter 8, this volume and Maixner et al., 2021). The potential exists not only for diagnosing genetic disorders linked to genomic abnormalities (e.g., mutations, abnormalities in chromosomal reproduction) but also for identifying genetic risk factors associated with other disease processes.

Paleopathological evidence of genetic disorders is rare. Despite this, there have been several recent successes in identifying their causative genomic roots, including the identification of mutations associated with achondroplastic dwarfism (Boer et al., 2017) and Paget's disease (Shaw et al., 2019), as well as documenting trisomy 21 (Cassidy et al., 2020). Although the preservation of soft tissue seemingly increases the potential for observing genetic disorders, there is only a single published example. Hershkovitz et al. (2014) described a case of cherubism observed in the mummified remains of a young adult female from the Joseon Dynasty of Korea. Cherubism is an autosomal dominant disease resulting from the mutation of the *SH3BP2* gene on chromosome 4p16.3 (Li & Yu, 2006). A benign childhood disease, it typically manifests as hypertrophy of the maxilla and mandible and replacement of the bone with fibrous tissue cysts. This hypertrophy leads to encroachment on the orbits, and when coupled with depression of the maxillae, makes it appear as if the eyes gaze upward. Though the morphological results support this diagnosis, the researchers were unable to confirm it through DNA analyses.

Paleogenetics also offers the potential for identifying genetic predisposition to disease. This has the potential to expand the paleopathological conversation by providing the basis for the discussion of risk factors, lifestyle, and genotype-environment interaction. The following discussion will highlight three instances in which researchers used DNA evidence to facilitate the discussion of genetic predisposition and disease risk.

Atherosclerosis is a chronic immunoinflammatory disease of medium and large arteries and is the most common cause of coronary artery disease, carotid artery disease, and peripheral arterial disease. There are environmental and behavioral risk factors associated with atherosclerosis as well as several single nucleotide polymorphisms (SNPs) that increase risk. The documentation of atherosclerosis in mummified remains actually has a fairly deep history, the first reported observation based on Johann Nepomuk Czermak's examination of two Egyptian mummies in 1852 (Thompson et al., 2013). More recently, there have been many more reported examples, with reports from Egypt, Italy, Korea, Lithuania, North America, and South America (Nerlich et al., 1997; Abdelfattah et al., 2013; Thompson et al., 2013; Piombino-Mascali et al., 2014; Kim et al., 2015; Gaeta et al., 2019; Madjid et al., 2019). In the oldest example, Murphy et al. (2003) observed several calcifications in the Tyrolean Iceman that indicated atherosclerosis. These run counter to the general understanding of the etiology of atherosclerosis being associated with modern risk factors (e.g., diet and stress).

Subsequently, in the course of sequencing the Tyrolean Iceman's genome, researchers were able to determine that he was homozygous for allele *rs10757274*, located in chromosomal region 9p21, which would have doubled his risk of cardiac heart disease (Zink et al., 2014). They also identified several other SNPs that would have predisposed him to cardiovascular diseases.

In 1994, Gino Fornaciari and colleagues identified a mucinous adenocarcinoma in the colon of King Ferrante I of Aragon. Today, colorectal cancers are the third most commonly diagnosed cancer and are the second leading cause of cancer-related death in the United States (American Cancer Society, 2021). In addition to a number of behavioral and diet-related risk factors (e.g., high red meat consumption, lack of physical activity, alcohol consumption), there are also several genetic factors that increase risk, including mutation at the microsatellite loci BAT 25 and BAT26 and point mutations at codon 12 of the oncogene *K-Ras* and at V599E on the *BRAF* gene (Oliveira et al., 2007). Molecular analyses all report that although there were no changes in the BAT25 microsatellite or the BRAF V599E, the codon 12 mutation on the *K-Ras* gene was present (Marchetti et al., 1996; Falchetti et al., 2006; Ottini et al., 2011).

Rheumatoid arthritis (RA) is an autoimmune disease resulting in chronic inflammation and fibrosis of joint capsules. There are more than 30 genomic regions thought to be associated with the condition (Scott et al., 2010) with alleles of the *HLA-DRB1* gene considered to be a major contributor to RA susceptibility (Barton & Worthington, 2009). In 2002, Ciranni and colleagues examined a late 16th-century mummy dubbed the "Braids Lady"; a 50–55-year-old woman buried in the San Francis Church in Arezzo, Italy. These authors documented several lesions that indicated a severe form of arthritis including erosions of the joint surfaces, deviation of the toes, and "z" deformation of the second ray of the left hand, ultimately leading them to conclude that the Braids Lady suffered from RA. Fontecchio et al. (2006a, b, 2012) were able to extract and amplify DNA from this individual and identified the presence of the DRB1★0101 allele – one of the main genetic risk factors of AR.

Discussion: Critiques and Looking Forward

The study of soft tissue paleopathology is a small, specialized aspect of paleopathology. It is specialized in that engaging in this type of research requires experience and training in soft tissue pathophysiology – something more commonly associated with biomedical training than most bianthropologists and skeletal paleopathologists receive. It is a small field not only because mummies are relatively rare, but also because documenting pathological changes in soft tissue morphology that have survived the vagaries of time and environment is especially challenging. Despite this, soft tissue paleopathology has the potential to significantly improve our understanding of health and disease in the past. Indeed, Michael Zimmerman (2011: 164) has stated that new developments in paleoimaging, paleoserology, and paleogenetics will expand "our knowledge of the life stories and fate of ancient individuals, their relationships to others, ancient migrations, the evolution of disease, and the role of ancient disease in human evolution and social history…" To balance this promise, it is also important to consider several challenges facing the discipline, some that are technical and methodological in nature and some that are broader and more fundamental.

Some challenges reflect the nature and longevity of the discipline. For instance, the editors of the *Yearbook of Mummy Studies* have stated that the field lacking a dedicated journal has hampered its development into a strong independent discipline (Gill-Frerking et al., 2011). Aufderheide (2013: 134) voiced a similar concern when he said that it is "…unlikely that the field of mummy studies will ever be large enough to be an independent scientific discipline. Thus, to survive and flourish, the field will need to join a related discipline."

A related concern pertains to training. Aufderheide (1981: 867) noted three decades ago that one of the problems facing soft tissue paleopathology was "a paucity of interested physicians (especially pathologists)." Biomedical training, particularly training in pathology, clearly provides the foundational knowledge necessary for engaging in mummy research. This knowledge base, however, cannot be applied uncritically, as time and taphonomy can dramatically change soft tissue morphology. On the other hand, while graduate training in biological anthropology does commonly teach about taphonomy, there commonly is not any coursework in pathophysiology or opportunities for experiential learning in pathology. Although there have been some training workshops for those interested in mummy research and by extension soft tissue pathology, they are infrequent. As the training and expertise of the observer is key to determine the accuracy and detail of the findings, this is something that the field must address.

From a methodological perspective, the most significant issue facing the discipline relates to standardization. This covers a broad range of topics, including soft tissue differentiation and artifact identification (Villa & Lynnerup, 2012), quantification of soft tissue preservation (e.g., Panzer, et al., 2015; Wittmers, et al., 2011), and establishing research protocols (e.g., Ikram, 2015; Moissidou, et al., 2015). Given the centrality of paleoimaging in mummy studies, and even more so in terms of documenting soft tissue pathology, it is particularly important that the field address these significant issues.

Several authors have provided "state-of-the-art" reviews of different paleoimaging modalities, including THz imaging (Öhrström et al., 2015), radiography (Lynnerup & Rühli, 2015), MRI (Rühli, 2015; Posh, 2015), CT (Conlogue, 2015; Cox, 2015), and endoscopy (Beckett, 2015). This type of methodological exploration and experimentation is a natural part of any discipline. The issue that is facing mummy studies and soft tissue paleopathology is that there is inconsistency in the reporting of imaging protocols (Beckett & Conlogue, 2010; Cox, 2015; Nelson & Wade, 2015). As the literature is dominated by isolated "case studies," this makes comparative studies difficult if not impossible and thus limits our ability to generate broader interpretations (Nelson & Wade, 2015). The IMPACT database was established to explicitly address this issue, fostering standardization as well as serving as a centralized archive for imaging data and thus facilitates the development of large-scale comparative studies (Nelson & Wade, 2015).

This latter point is also reflected in the results of O'Brien and colleagues' (2009) analysis of CT use in mummy studies. Of 31 articles published between 1979 and 2005, only three articles (9.7%) were explicitly hypothesis-driven, and in 65% of the articles, CT was used "for curiosity and without specific intent…" There is no doubt that medical imaging technology has had a profound impact on the development and expansion of mummy studies. Arguably, however, it is the evolution of the technology itself that has driven the field, rather than the development and elaboration of research questions. Such points are raised in order to emphasize the fact that while the fields of mummy studies, paleopathology, and bioarchaeology were at roughly the same time period (1970s and 1980s), the former is now experiencing some of the critical methodological and goal-oriented discussions that occurred earlier in bioarchaeology and paleopathology.

In 1980, two reviews presented contrasting views of soft tissue paleopathology. Aufderheide (1981) noted the potential and promise of the application of biomedical methods to the study of soft tissue paleopathology, while Dastugue (1980) struck a much more pessimistic note, effectively dismissing the potential contribution of mummy studies to paleopathology.

A decade later Donald Ortner and Arthur Aufderheide (1991: 1) provided another glimpse into the development of paleopathology and discussed two key areas where the field has "reached a plateau beyond which significant further progress cannot be made without major changes in the type of research we do and the methods we use to do it." Specifically, they note the lack of theoretical development and the need to focus on the biocultural context of disease itself, rather than just on description. In his review of Ortner and Aufderheide's 1991 edited volume, George Armelagos (1994: 239) argued that the editors "ally paleopathology with medicine rather than with anthropological science with its biocultural perspective." Further, Armelagos (1994: 240) states that "the delayed development in paleopathology is also due to the lack of a problem orientation and a reliance on the newest technology to drive the research."

More recently, Zuckerman and colleagues (2012: 37), referring specifically to skeletal paleopathology, contend that the field has developed from a principally descriptive, case-study–driven discipline to "an interpretive, interrogative, and independent one" that increasingly adopted a population-based, hypothesis-driven approach that incorporated consideration of sociocultural and environmental/ecological factors." A biocultural approach to paleopathology facilitates the examination of the impact of social roles, social status, the living environment, activity patterns, infectious disease, diet, injuries, and trauma on the interpretation of paleopathological data (Buzon, 2012). Indeed, paleopathological data should be "interpreted in an adaptive context" considering how cultural strategies may buffer, or fail to buffer, in the face of social/cultural and environmental/ecological factors (Zuckerman et al., 2012: 35).

From this perspective, while it is obvious that as it stands the study of soft tissue paleopathology contributes significantly to our understanding of health and disease in the past, the field is also primed for growth. Indeed, researchers have not only documented the existence of rare diseases (e.g., cherubism, carcinoma) but also have contributed significantly to our knowledge of the evolutionary history and paleoepidemiology of worldwide scourges (e.g., tuberculosis, schistosomiasis). No doubt researchers will continue to address the methodological issues discussed above while also expanding the methodological toolkit, bringing to light new evidence of disease in the past. We contend, however, that it is equally important that such efforts be coupled with greater elaboration and incorporation of bioculturally informed interpretative frameworks. The treatment of the mummy as part of a larger environmental and social context and not as an isolated object provides information that is indispensable to fully understand the factors that affect the evolution of health and disease. This would not only draw soft tissue paleopathology and mummy studies closer to skeletal paleopathology and bioarchaeology, but it would also enrich the narrative we can construct social dynamics related to life and health in the past.

References

Abdelfattah, A., Allam, A. H., Wann, S., Thompson, R. C., Abdel-Maksoud, G., Badr, I., … & Thomas, G. S. (2013). Atherosclerotic cardiovascular disease in Egyptian women: 1570 BCE–2011 CE. *International Journal of Cardiology* 167(2):570–574.

American Cancer Society, (2021). www.cancer.org (accessed November 13, 2021).

Araujo, N. M., Waizbort, R. & Kay, A. (2011). Hepatitis B virus infection from an evolutionary point of view: how viral, host, and environmental factors shape genotypes and subgenotypes. *Infection, Genetics and Evolution* 11(6):1199–1207.

Armelagos, G. J. (1994). Review of human paleopathology: current syntheses and future options. *Journal of Field Archaeology* 21(2):239–243.

Arriaza, B. T., Salo, W., Aufderheide, A. C. & Holcomb T. A. (1995). Pre-Columbian tuberculosis in northern Chile: molecular and skeletal evidence. *American Journal of Physical Anthropology* 98:37–45.

Aufderheide, A. C. (1981). Soft tissue paleopathology - an emerging subspecialty. *Human Pathology* 12(10):865–867.

Aufderheide, A. C. (2003). *The Scientific Study of Mummies*. Cambridge: Cambridge University Press.

Aufderheide, A. C. (2013). A brief history of soft tissue paleopathology. In Lozada Cerna, M. C. & O'Donnabhain, B. (Eds.), *The Dead Tell Tales: Essays in Honor of Jane E. Buikstra*, pp. 130–135. Los Angeles: Cotsen Institute of Archaeology Press.

Aufderheide, A. C., Salo, W., Madden, M., Streitz, J., Buikstra, J. E., Guhl, F., … & Allison, M. (2004). A 9,000-year record of Chagas' disease. *Proceedings of the National Academy of Sciences of the United States of America* 101:2034–2039.

Ault, K. A. (2006). Epidemiology and natural history of human papillomavirus infections in the female genital tract. *Infectious Diseases in Obstetrics and Gynecology* 2006:Article ID:040470.

Avanzini, F., Cosi, P., Füstös, R. & Sandi, A. (2017). When fantasy meets science: an attempt to recreate the voice of ötzi the "iceman". *Associazione Italiana Scienze della Voce (AISV)* 3:425–431.

Baker, B. J., Crane-Kramer, G., Dee, M. W., Gregoricka, L. A., Henneberg, M., Lee C., Lukehart, S. A., Mabey, D. C., Roberts, C. A. & Stodder, A. L. (2020). Advancing the understanding of treponemal disease in the past and present. *American Journal of Physical Anthropology* 171:5–41.

Bar-Gal, G. K., Kim, M. J., Klein, A., Shin, D. H., Oh, C. S., Kim, J. W., … & Shouval, D. (2012). Tracing hepatitis B virus to the 16th century in a Korean mummy. *Hepatology* 56(5):1671–1680.

Barton, A. & Worthington, J. (2009). Genetic susceptibility to rheumatoid arthritis: an emerging picture. *Arthritis Care & Research* 61(10):1441–1446.

Beckett, R. G. (2014). Paleoimaging: a review of applications and challenges. *Forensic Science, Medicine & Pathology* 10:423–436.

Beckett, R. G. (2015). Application and limitations of endoscopy in anthropological and archaeological research. *The Anatomical Record* 298(6):1125–1134.

Beckett, R. G. & Conlogue, G. J. (2010). *Paleoimaging: Field Applications for Cultural Remains and Artifacts*. Boca Raton: CRC Press.

Beckett, R. G. & Conlogue G. J. (2020). *Advances in Paleoimaging: Applications for Paleoanthropology, Bioarchaeology, Forensics, and Cultural Artifacts*. Boca Raton: CRC Press.

Biagini, P., Thèves, C., Balaresque, P., Géraut, A., Keyser, C., Nikolaeva, D., … & Crubézy, E. (2012). Variola virus in a 300-year-old Siberian mummy. *New England Journal of Medicine* 367(21):2057–2059.

Bianucci, R., Mattutino, G., Lallo, R., Charlier, P., Jouin-Spriet, H., Peluso, A., Higham, T., Torre, C. & Rabino Massa, E. (2008). Immunological evidence of *Plasmodium falciparum* infection in an Egyptian child mummy from the early dynastic period. *Journal of Archaeological Science* 35(7):1880–1885.

Boer, L. L., Naue, J., De Rooy, L. & Oostra, R.-J. (2017). Detection of G1138A mutation of the *FGFR3* gene in tooth material from a 180-year-old museological achondroplastic skeleton. *Genes* 8(9):214.

Böni, T., Rühli, F. J. & Chhem, R. K. (2004). History of paleoradiology: early published literature, 1896–1921. *Canadian Association of Radiologists Journal* 55(4):203–210.

Borrini, M., Mariani, P. & Rosati, G. (2012). Virtual autopsy of two Egyptian mummies from the florentine collection: a preliminary anthropological analysis. *Journal of Biological Research* 85(1):183–185.

Braunstein, E., White, S., Russell, W. & Harris, J. (1988). Paleoradiologic evaluation of the Egyptian royal mummies. *Skeletal Radiology* 17(5):348–352.

Buzon, M. R. (2012). The bioarchaeological approach to paleopathology. In Grauer, A. L. (Ed.) *A Companion to Paleopathology*, pp. 58–75. Chichester: Wiley-Blackwell.

Bzhalava, D., Guan, P., Franceschi, S., Dillner, J. & Clifford, G. (2013). A systematic review of the prevalence of mucosal and cutaneous human papillomavirus types. *Virology* 445(1–2):224–231.

Cassidy, L. M., Ó Maoldúin, R., Kador, T., Lynch, A., Jones, C., Woodman, P. C., … & Bradley, D. G. (2020). A dynastic elite in monumental Neolithic society. *Nature* 582(7812) 384–388.

Chhem, R. K. & Brothwell, D. R. (2008). *Paleoradiology: Imaging Mummies and Fossils*. Berlin: Springer.

Ciranni, R. & Fornaciari, G. (2004). Juvenile cirrhosis in a 16th century Italian mummy: current technologies in pathology and ancient human tissues. *Virchows Archiv* 445(6):647–650.

Ciranni, R., Garbini, F., Neri, E., Melai, L., Giusti, L. & Fornaciari, G. (2002). The "braids lady" of Arezzo: a case of rheumatoid arthritis in a 16th century mummy. *Clinical and Experimental Rheumatology* 20:745–752.

Cockburn, A., Barraco, R. A., Reyman, T. A. & Peck, W. H. (1975). Autopsy of an Egyptian mummy. *Science* 187(4182):1155–1160.

Conlogue, G. (2015). Considered limitations and possible applications of computed tomography in mummy research. *The Anatomical Record* 298(6):1088–1098.

Coulthart, M. B., Posada, D., Crandall, K. A. & Dekaban, G. A. (2006). On the phylogenetic placement of human T cell leukemia virus type 1 sequences associated with an Andean mummy. *Infection, Genetics and Evolution* 6(2):91–96.

Cox, S. L. (2015). A critical look at mummy CT scanning. *The Anatomical Record* 298(6):1099–1110.

Dabernat, H., Thèves, C., Bouakaze, C., Nikolaeva, D., Keyser, C., Mokrousov, I., … & Ludes, B. (2014). Tuberculosis epidemiology and selection in an autochthonous Siberian population from the 16th –19th century. *PLoS One* 9(2):e89877.

Dastugue, J. (1980). Possibilities, limits and prospects in paleopathology of the human skeleton. *Journal of Human Evolution* 9(1):3–8.

Davey, J. & Drummer, O. H. (2016). The use of forensic radiology in determination of unexplained head injuries in child mummies – Cause of death or mummification damage? *Journal of Forensic Radiology and Imaging* 5:20–24.

Dedouit, F., Géraut, A., Baranov, V., Ludes, B., Rougé, D., Telmon, N. & Crubézy, E. (2010). Virtual and macroscopical studies of mummies - Differences or complementarity? Report of a natural frozen Siberian mummy. *Forensic Science International* 200:e7–e13.

Deelder, A. M., Miller, R. L., de Jonge, N. & Kerijger, F. W. (1990). Detection of schistisome antigen in mummies. *The Lancet* 335(8691):724.

Diana, E., Maupas, E., Boano, R., Rabino Massa, E. & Arriaza, B. (2014). Spectroscopic characterization of ancient human tissue from the Chinchorro mummies. *Yearbook of Mummy Studies* 2:175–180.

Donoghue, H. D., Pap, I., Szikossy, I. & Spigelman, M. (2011). Detection and characterization of *Mycobacterium tuberculosis* DNA in 18th-century Hungarians with pulmonary and extra-pulmonary tuberculosis. *Yearbook of Mummy Studies* 1:51–56.

Duggan, A. T., Perdomo, M. F., Piombino-Mascali, D., Marciniak, S., Poinar, D., Emery, M. V., … & Poinar, H. N. (2016). 17th-century variola virus reveals the recent history of smallpox. *Current Biology* 26(24):3407–3412.

Esteban, J., Cases-Mérida, S., Tortosa, M., Marzal, B., Fernández, A., Gálvez, C., Franco, R. & Fernández, P. L. (2015). Histopathological study of a mummified eye and optic nerve from a strangled Peruvian mummy. *Pathobiology* 82(2):90–93.

Falchetti, M., Lupi, R. & Ottini, L. (2006). Molecular analysis of a colorectal carcinoma from a mummy of the XVth century. *Medicina nei Secoli* 18(3):943–951.

Fantini, M., Benazzi, S., De Crescenzio, F., Persiani, F. & Gruppioni, G. (2005). Virtual reconstruction of a dismembered Andean mummy from CT data. *Short & Project Papers Proceedings VAST* 2005:61–66.

Fernandes, A., Iñiguez, A. M., Lima, V. S., Souza, S. M., Ferreira, L. F., Vicente, A. C. P. & Jansen, A. M. (2008). Pre-Columbian chagas disease in Brazil: *Trypanosoma cruzi* I in the archaeological remains of a human in Peruaçu Valley, Minas Gerais, Brazil. *Memórias do Instituto Oswaldo Cruz* 103(5):514–516.

Ferreira, L. F., Britto, C., Cardoso, M. A., Fernandes, O., Reinhard, K. & Araújo, A. (2000). Paleoparasitology of Chagas disease revealed by infected tissues from Chilean mummies. *Acta Tropica* 75(1):79–84.

Fletcher, H. A., Donoghue, H. D., Taylor, G. M., van der Zanden, A. G. & Spigelman, M. (2003). Molecular analysis of *Mycobacterium tuberculosis* DNA from a family of 18th century Hungarians. *Microbiology* 149(1):143–151.

Fontecchio, G., Fioroni, M., Azzarone, R., Battistoni, C., Cervelli, C., Ventura, L., Mercurio, C., Fornaciari, G. & Papola, F. (2006a). Genetic predisposition to rheumatoid arthritis in a Tuscan (Italy) ancient human remain. *International Journal of Immunopathology and Pharmacology* 20(1):103–109.

Fontecchio, G., Ventura, L., Azzarone, R., Fioroni, M., Fornaciari, G. & Papola, F. (2006b). HLA-DRB genotyping of an Italian mummy from the 16th century with signs of rheumatoid arthritis. *Annals of the Rheumatic Diseases* 65(12):1676–1677.

Fontecchio, G., Ventura, L. & Poma, A. M. (2012). Further genomic testing and histological examinations confirm the diagnosis of rheumatoid arthritis in an Italian mummy from the 16th century. *Annals of the Rheumatic Diseases* 71(4):630.

Fornaciari, G. (1994). Malignant tumor in the mummy of Ferrante 1st of Aragon, King of Naples (1431–1494). *Medicina nei Secoli* 6:139–146.

Fornaciari, G. (2018). Histology of ancient soft tissue tumors: a review. *International Journal of Paleopathology* 21:64–76.

Fornaciari, G., Castagna, M., Tognetti, A., Tornaboni, D. & Bruno, J. (1989). Syphilis in a renaissance Italian mummy. *The Lancet* 334(8663):614.

Fornaciari, G., Castagna, M., Viacava, P., Tognetti, A. & Bevilacqua, G. (1992). Chagas' disease in Peruvian Inca mummy. *The Lancet* 399(8785):128–129.

Fornaciari, G., Ciranni, R. & Ventura, L. (2001). Paleoandrology and prostatic hyperplasia in Italian mummies (XV–XIX centuries). *Medicina nei Secoli* 13:269–284.

Fornaciari, G. & Marchetti, A. (1986). Intact smallpox virus particles in an Italian mummy of sixteenth century. *The Lancet* 328(8507):625.

Fornaciari, G., Zavaglia, K., Giusti, L., Vultaggio, C. & Ciranni, R. (2003). Human papillomavirus in a 16th century mummy. *The Lancet* 362(9396):1160.

Francalacci, P. (1995). DNA analysis of ancient desiccated corpses from Xinjiang. *Journal of Indo-European Studies* 23(3–4):385–398.

Friedrich, K. M., Nemec, S., Czerny, C., Fisher, H., Plischke, S., Gahleitner, A., Viola, T. B., Imhof, H., Seidler, H. & Guillen, S. (2010). The story of 12 Chachapoyan mummies through multidetector computed tomography. *European Journal of Radiology* 76: 143–150.

Gaeta, R., Fornaciari, A., Izzetti, R., Caramella, D. & Giuffra, V. (2019). Severe atherosclerosis in the natural mummy of Girolamo Macchi (1648–1734), "major writer" of Santa Maria della Scala Hospital in Siena (Italy). *Atherosclerosis* 280:66–74.

Gamba, C., Fernández, E., Tirado, M., Pastor, F. & Arroyo-Pardo, E. (2011). Ancient nuclear DNA and kinship analysis: the case of a medieval burial in San Esteban church in Cuellar (Segovia, Central Spain). *American Journal of Physical Anthropology* 144(3):485–491.

Gerszten, E., Allison, M., Pezzia, A. & Klurfeld, D. (1976). Thyroid disease in a Peruvian mummy. *Medical College of Virginia Quarterly* 12:52–53.

Gessain, A., Pecon-Slattery, J., Meertens, L. & Mahieux, R. (2000). Origins of HTLV-1 in South America. *Nature Medicine* 6(3):232.

Gill-Frerking, H. & Healey, C. (2011). Experimental archaeology for the interpretation of taphonomy related to bog bodies: lessons learned from two projects undertaken a decade apart. *Yearbook of Mummy Studies* 1:69–74.

Gill-Frerking, H., Rosendahl, W., Zink, A. & Piombino-Mascali, D. (2011). Editorial: the yearbook of mummy studies. *Yearbook of Mummy Studies* 1:5.

Gill-Robinson, H., Elias, J., Bender, F., Allard, T. T. & Hoppa, R. D. (2006). Using image analysis software to create a physical skull model for the facial reconstruction of a wrapped Akhmimic mummy. *Journal of Computing and Information Technology* 14(1):45–51.

Gilbert, M. T. P., Djurhuus, D., Melchior, L., Lynnerup, N., Worobey, M., Wilson, A. S., Andreasen, C. & Dissing, J. (2007). mtDNA from hair and nail clarifies the genetic relationship of the 15th century Qilakitsoq Inuit mummies. *American Journal of Physical Anthropology* 133(2):847–853.

Guhl, F., Jaramillo, C., Yockteng, R., Vallejo, G. A. & Cárdenas-Arroyo, F. (1997). *Trypanosoma cruzi* DNA in human mummies. *The Lancet* 349(9062):1370.

Guhl, F., Jaramillo, C., Vallejo, G. A., Yockteng, R., Cárdenas-Arroyo, F., Fornaciari, G., Arriaza, B. & Aufderheide, A. C. (1999). Isolation of *Trypanosoma cruzi* DNA in 4,000-year-old mummified human tissue from northern Chile. *American Journal of Physical Anthropology* 108(4):401–407.

Haas, N. A., Zelle, M., Rosendahl, W., Zink, A., Preuss, R., Laser, K. T., Gostner, P., Arens, S., Domik, G. & Burchert, W. (2015). Hypoplastic left heart in the 6500-year-old detmold child. *The Lancet* 385(9985):2432.

Hanna, J., Bouwman, A. S., Brown, K. A., Pearson, M. P. & Brown, T. A. (2012). Ancient DNA typing shows that a bronze age mummy is a composite of different skeletons. *Journal of Archaeological Science* 39(8):2774–2779.

Harries, J., Fibiger, L., Smith, J., Adler, T. & Szöke, A. (2018). Exposure: the ethics of making, sharing and displaying photographs of human remains. *Human Remains & Violence* 4(1):3–24.

Hart, G. D., Cockburn, A., Millet, N. B. & Scott, J. W. (1977). Lessons learned from the autopsy of an Egyptian mummy. *Canadian Medical Association Journal* 117:415–418.

Hawass, Z., Gad, Y. Z., Ismail, S., Khairat, R., Fathalla, D., Hasan, N., … & Pusch, C. M. (2010). Ancestry and pathology in King Tutankhamun's family. *Journal of the American Medical Association* 303(7):638–647.

Hershkovitz, I., Spigelman, M., Sarig, R., Lim, D.-S., Lee, I. S., Oh, C. S., ... & Shin, D. H. (2014). A possible case of cherubism in a 17th-century Korean mummy. *PLoS One* 9(8):e102441.

Hjalgrim, H., Lynnerup, N., Liversage, M. & Rosenklint, A. (1995). Stereolithography: potential applications in anthropological studies. *American Journal of Physical Anthropology* 97(3):329–333.

Horne, P. D. & Lewin, P. K. (1977). Autopsy of an Egyptian mummy. 7. Electron microscopy of mummified tissue. *Canadian Medical Association Journal* 117:472–473.

Howard, D. M., Schofield, J., Fletcher, J., Baxter, K., Iball, G. R. & Buckley, S. A. (2020). Synthesis of a vocal sound from the 3,000 year old mummy, Nesyamun 'true of voice'. *Scientific Reports* 10(1):1–6.

Hughes, S., Wright, R. & Barry, M. (2005). Virtual reconstruction and morphological analysis of the cranium of an ancient Egyptian mummy. *Australasian Physical and Engineering Sciences in Medicine* 28:122–127.

Ikram, S. (2015). Studying Egyptian mummies in the field. In Ikram, S., Kaiser, J. &Walker, R. (Eds.), *Egyptian Bioarchaeology: Humans, Animals, and the Environment*, pp. 67–76. Leiden: Sidestone Press.

Iñiguez, A. M., Araújo, A., Ferreira, L. F. & Vicente, A. C. P. (2003). Analysis of ancient DNA from coprolites: a perspective with random amplified polymorphic DNA-polymerase chain reaction approach. *Memórias do Instituto Oswaldo Cruz* 98:63–65.

Johnston, R., Thomas, R., Jones, R., Graves-Brown, C., Goodridge, W. & North, L. (2020). Evidence of diet, deification, and death within ancient Egyptian mummified animals. *Scientific Reports* 10:14113.

Kao, J.-H. & Chen, D.-S. (2002). Global control of hepatitis B virus infection. *The Lancet Infectious Diseases* 2(7):395–403.

Kaufmann, I. M. & Rühli, F. J. (2010). Without 'informed consent'? Ethics and ancient mummy research. *Journal of Medical Ethics* 36:608–613.

Kim, M. J., Kim, Y.-S., Oh, C. S., Go, J.-H., Lee, I. S., Park, W.-K., Cho, S.-M., Kim, S.-K. & Shin, D. H. (2015). Anatomical confirmation of computed tomography-based diagnosis of the atherosclerosis discovered in 17th-century Korean mummy. *PLoS One* 10(3):e0119474.

Kim, S. B., Shin, J. E., Park, S. S., Bok, G. D., Chang, Y. P., Kim, J., ... & Kim, M. J. (2006). Endoscopic investigation of the internal organs of a 15th-century child mummy from Yangju, Korea. *Journal of Anatomy* 209:681–688.

Kim, Y.-S., Lee, I. S., Jung, G.-U., Kim, M. J., Oh, C. S., Yoo, D. S., Lee, W.-J., Lee, E., Cha, S. C. & Shin, D. H. (2014). Radiological diagnosis of congenital diaphragmatic hernia in 17th-century Korean mummy. *PLoS One* 9(7):e99779.

Kloos, H. & David, R. (2002). The paleoepidemiology of schistosomiasis in ancient Egypt. *Human Ecology Review* 9(1):14–25.

Kreissl Lonfat, B. M., Kaufmann, I. M. & Rühli, F. J. (2015). A code of ethics for evidence-based research with ancient human remains. *The Anatomical Record* 298:1175–1181.

Leles, D., Araújo, A., Ferreira, L. F., Vicente, A. C. P. & Iñiguez, A. M. (2008). Molecular paleoparasitological diagnosis of *Ascaris sp.* from coprolites: new scenery of ascariasis in pre-Colombian South America times. *Memórias do Instituto Oswaldo Cruz* 103(1) 106–108.

Li, C.-Y. & Yu, S.-F. (2006). A novel mutation in the *SH3BP2* gene causes cherubism: case report. *BMC Medical Genetics* 7(1):84.

Li, H.-C., Fujiyoshi, T., Lou, H., Yashiki, S., Sonoda, S., Cartier, L., Nunez, L., Munoz, I., Horai, S. & Tajima, K. (1999). The presence of ancient human T-cell lymphotropic virus type I provirus DNA in an Andean mummy. *Nature Medicine* 5(12):1428–1432.

Lima, V. S., Iñiguez, A. M., Otsuki, K., Ferreira, L. F., Araújo, A., Vicente, A. C. P. & Jansen, A. M. (2008). Chagas disease in ancient hunter-gatherer population, Brazil. *Emerging Infectious Diseases* 14(6):1001–1002.

Liu, W.-Q., Liu, J., Zhang, J.-H., Long, X.-C., Lei, J.-H. & Li, Y.-L. (2007). Comparison of ancient and modern *Clonorchis sinensis* based on ITS1 and ITS2 sequences. *Acta Tropica* 101(2):91–94.

Loreille, O., Roumat, E., Verneau, O., Bouchet, F. & Hänni, C. (2001). Ancient DNA from Ascaris: extraction amplification and sequences from eggs collected in coprolites. *International Journal for Parasitology* 31(10):1101–1106.

Lynnerup, N. (2009). Medical imaging of mummies and bog bodies - A mini-review. *Gerontology* 56:441–448.

Lynnerup, N., Dalstra, M. & Hansen, R. B. (2007a). The making of the replica of Grauballe Man's skull. In Asingh, P. & Lynnerup, N. (Eds.), *Grauballe Man: An Iron Age Bog Body Revisited*, pp. 122–123. Aarhus: Aarhus University Press.

Lynnerup, N., Jurik, A. G. & Dalstra, M. (2007b). CT scanning, 3D visualization and stereolithography. In Asingh, P. & Lynnerup, N. (Eds.), *Grauballe Man: An Iron Age Bog Body Revisited,* pp. 111–121. Aarhus: Aarhus University Press.

Lynnerup, N. & Rühli, F.J. (2015). Short review: the use of conventional X-rays in mummy studies. *The Anatomical Record* 298(6):1085–1087.

Madden, M., Salo, W. L., Streitz, J., Aufderheide, A. C., Fornaciari, G., Jaramillo, C., Vallejo, G. A., Yockteng, F., Arriaza, B. T., Cárdenas-Arroyo, F. & Guhl, F. (2001). Identification of *Trypanosoma cruzi* DNA in ancient human Chilean mummies. *Biotechniques* 30(1):102–109.

Madjid, M., Safavi-Naeini, P. & Lodder, R. (2019). High prevalence of cholesterol-rich atherosclerotic lesions in ancient mummies: a near-infrared spectroscopy study. *American Heart Journal* 216:113–116.

Maixner, F., Gresky, J. & Zink, A. (2021). Ancient DNA analysis of rare genetic bone disorders. *International Journal of Paleopathology* 33:182–187.

Marchetti, A., Pellegrini, S., Bevilacqua, G. & Fornaciari, G. (1996). K-RAS mutation in the tumour of Ferrante I of Aragon, King of Naples. *The Lancet* 347(9010):1272.

Marennikova, S., Shelukhina, E., Zhukova, O., Yanova, N. & Loparev, V. (1989). Smallpox diagnosed 400 years later: results of skin lesions examination of 16th-century Italian mummy. *Journal of Hygiene, Epidemiology, Microbiology, and Immunology* 34(2):227–231.

Marić, J., Bašić, Ž., Jerković, I., Mihanović, F., Anđelinović, Š. & Kružić, I. (2020). Facial reconstruction of mummified remains of Christian Saint-Nicolosa Bursa. *Journal of Cultural Heritage* 42:249–254.

Marota, I., Fornaciari, G. & Rollo, F. (1996). La sifilide nel rinascimento: identificazione di sequenze ribosomali batteriche nel DNA isolato dalla mummia di Maria d'Aragona (XVI secolo). *Antropologia Contemporanea* 19:157–174.

Marota, I., Fornaciari, G. & Rollo, U. (1998). Hepatitis E Virus (HEV) RNA sequences in the DNA of Maria of Aragon (1503–1563): paleopathological evidence or anthropological marker? *Journal of Paleopathology* 10(2): 53–58.

Matheson, C. D., David, R., Spigelman, M. & Donoghue, H. D. (2014). Molecular confirmation of schistosoma and family relationship in two ancient Egyptian mummies. *Yearbook of Mummy Studies* 2:39–47.

Melcher, A., Holowka, S., Pharoah, M. & Lewin, P. (1997). Non-invasive computed tomography and three-dimensional reconstruction of the dentition of a 2,800-year-old Egyptian mummy exhibiting extensive dental disease. *American Journal of Physical Anthropology* 103:329–340.

Moissidou, D., Day, J., Shin, D. H. & Bianucci, R. (2015). Invasive versus non invasive methods applied to mummy research: will this controversy ever be solved? *Biomed Research International* 2015:192829.

Monge, J. M. & Rühli, F. J. (2015). The anatomy of the mummy: mortui viventes docent – When ancient mummies speak to modern doctors. *The Anatomical Record* 298:935–940.

Münnemann, K., Böni, T., Colacicco, G., Blümich, B. & Rühli, F. (2007). Noninvasive ^{1}H and ^{23}Na nuclear magnetic resonance imaging of ancient Egyptian human mummified tissue. *Magnetic Resonance Imaging* 25(9):1341–1345.

Murphy Jr, W. A., zur Nedden, D., Gostner, P., Knapp, R., Recheis, W. & Seidler, H. (2003). The Iceman: discovery and imaging. *Radiology* 226(3):614–629.

Mytum, H. (2021). Ethics and practice in the excavation, examination, analysis, and preservation of historical mummified human remains. *Historical Archaeology* 55:96–109.

Nelson, A., Watson, L., Williams, J., Gauld, S., Motley, J., Poeta, L., Seston, D., Gomez, E., Baldeos, J., Fuentes, S. & Pozzi-Escot, D. (2021) Análisis de los fardos funerarios de pachacamac: Aplicación sistemática de rayos X y tomografía computarizada en el contexto arqueológico. In Neyra Sánchez, A. A. (Ed.), *Actas VI Congreso Nacional de Arqueología,* Vol. 2, pp. 293–308. Lima: Ministerio de Cultura del Perú.

Nelson, A. J. & Wade, A. D. (2015). Impact: development of a radiological mummy database. *The Anatomical Record* 298(6):941–948.

Nerlich, A. G., Kirchhoff, S. M., Panzer, S., Lehn, C., Bachmeier, B. E., Bayer, B., Anslinger, K., Röcker, P. & Peschel, O. K. (2021). Chronic active non-lethal human-type tuberculosis in a high royal Bavarian officer of Napoleonic times – a mummy study. *PLoS One* 16(5):e0249955.

Nerlich, A. G., Peschel, O. & Egarter Vigl, E. (2009). New evidence for Ötzi's final trauma. *Intensive Care Medicine* 35:1138–1139.

Nerlich, A. G., Schraut, B., Dittrich, S., Jelinek, T. & Zink, A. R. (2008). *Plasmodium falciparum* in ancient Egypt. *Emerging Infectious Diseases* 14(8):1317–1319.

Nerlich, A. G., Wiest, I. & Tubel, J. (1997). Coronary arteriosclerosis in a male mummy from ancient Egypt. *Journal of Paleopathology* 9(2):83–89.

Notman, D. N. H., Anderson, L., Beattie, O. B. & Amy, R. (1987). Arctic paleoradiology: portable radiographic examination of two frozen sailors from the Franklin Expedition (1845–1848). *American Journal of Roentgenology* 149:347–350.

Novo, S. P. C., Leles, D., Bianucci, R. & Araújo, A. (2015). *Leishmania tarentolae* molecular signatures in a 300 hundred-years-old human Brazilian mummy. *Parasites & Vectors* 8:72.

Nystrom, K. C. (2018). *The Bioarchaeology of Mummies*. New York: Routledge.

O'Brien, J. J., Battista, J. J., Romagnoli, C. & Chhem, R. K. (2009). CT imaging of human mummies: a critical review of the literature. *International Journal of Osteoarchaeology* 19:90–98.

Öhrström, L., Bitzer, A., Walther, M. & Rühli, F. J. (2010). Terahertz imaging of ancient mummies and bone. *American Journal of Physical Anthropology*, 142(3):497–500.

Öhrström, L., Fischer, B. M., Bitzer, A., Wallauer, J., Walther, M. & Rühli, F. (2015). Terahertz imaging modalities of ancient Egyptian mummified objects and of a naturally mummified rat. *The Anatomical Record* 298(6):1135–1143.

Oliveira, C., Velho, S., Moutinho, C., Ferreira, A., Preto, A., Domingo, E., … & Seruca, R. (2007). KRAS and BRAF oncogenic mutations in MSS colorectal carcinoma progression. *Oncogene* 26:158–163.

Olszewski, R., Tilleux, C., Hastir, J.-P., Delvaux, L. & Danse, E. (2019). Holding eternity in one's hand: first three-dimensional reconstruction and printing of the heart from 2700 years-old Egyptian mummy. *The Anatomical Record* 302(6):912–916.

O'Neill, K., Banning, J., Chow, W. & Gersztén, E. (2016). Paleopathology of spleens in South American mummies. *Pathobiology* 83: 196–200.

Ortner, D. J. & Aufderheide, A. C. (1991). Introduction. In Ortner, D. J. & Aufderheide, A. C. (Eds.), *Human Paleopathology: Current Syntheses and Future Options*, pp. 1–2. Washington: Smithsonian Institution Press.

Ottini, L., Falchetti, M., Marinozzi, S., Angeletti, L. R. & Fornaciari, G. (2011). Gene-environment interactions in the pre–Industrial Era: the cancer of King Ferrante I of Aragon (1431–1494). *Human Pathology* 42(3):332–339.

Panzer, S., Mc Coy, M. R., Hitzl, W., Piombino-Mascali, D., Jankauskas, R., Zink, A. R. & Augat, P. (2015). Checklist and scoring system for the assessment of soft tissue preservation in CT examinations of human mummies. *PloS One* 10(8):e0133364.

Panzer, S., Peschel, O., Hass-Gebhard, B., Bachmeier, B. E., Pusch, C. M. & Nerlich, A. G. (2014). Reconstructing the life of an unknown (ca. 500 years old South American Inca) mummy - Multidisciplinary study of a Peruvian Inca mummy suggests severe Chagas disease and ritual homicide. *PLoS One* 9(2):e89528.

Panzer, S., Wittig, H., Zesch, S., Rosendahl, W., Blache, S., Müller-Gerbl, M. & Hotz, G. (2017). Evidence of neurofibromatosis type 1 in a multi-morbid Inca child mummy: a paleoradiological investigation using computed tomography. *PLoS One*, 12(4):e0175000.

Pedersen, C. C. E., Asingh, P., Thali, M. J. & Gascho, D. (2021). Looking deep into the past – Virtual autopsy of a Mongolian warrior. *Forensic Imaging* 25:200455.

Pettigrew, T. J. (1834). *A History of Egyptian Mummies*. London: Longman et al.

Pickering, R. B., Conces, D. J., Braunstein, E. M. & Yurco, F. (1990). Three-dimensional computed tomography of the mummy Wenohotep. *American Journal of Physical Anthropology* 83(1):49–55.

Piepenbrink, H., Frahm, J., Haase, A. & Matthaei, D. (1986). Nuclear magnetic resonance imaging of mummified corpses. *American Journal of Physical Anthropology* 70(1):27–28.

Piombino-Mascali, D. & Beckett, R. G. (2021). Respecting the dead. *Forensic Imaging* 25: 200448.

Piombino-Mascali, D. & Gill-Frerking, H. (2019). The mummy autopsy: some ethical considerations. In Squires, K., Errickson, D. & Márquez-Grant, N. (Eds.), *Ethical Approaches to Human Remains*, pp. 605–625. Cham: Springer.

Piombino-Mascali, D., Jankauskas, R., Tamošiūnas, A., Valančius, R., Thompson, R. C. & Panzer, S. (2014). Atherosclerosis in mummified human remains from Vilnius, Lithuania (18th–19th centuries AD): a computed tomographic investigation. *American Journal of Human Biology* 26:676–681.

Posh, J. C. (2015). Technical limitations on the use of traditional magnetic resonance imaging in the evaluation of mummified remains: a view from a hands-on radiologic technologist's perspective. *The Anatomical Record* 298(6):1116–1124.

Powell, M. L. (2012). The history of the paleopathology association. In Buikstra, J. E. & Roberts, C. A. (Eds.), *The Global History of Paleopathology: Pioneers and Prospects*, pp. 667–677. Oxford: Oxford University Press.

Prates, C., Oliveira, C., Sousa, S. & Ikram, S. (2015). A kidney's ingenious path to trimillennar preservation: renal tuberculosis in an Egyptian mummy? *International Journal of Paleopathology* 11:7–11.

Prats-Muñoz, G., Galtés, I., Armentano, N., Cases, S., Fernández, P. L. & Malgosa, A. (2013). Human soft tissue preservation in Cova des Pas site (Minorca Bronze Age). *Journal of Archaeological Science* 40:4701–4710.

Prats-Muñoz, G., Malgosa, A., Armentano, N., Galtés, I., Esteban, J., Bombi, J. A., ... & Fernández, P. L. (2012). A paleoneurohistological study of 3,000-year-old mummified brain tissue from the Mediterranean Bronze Age. *Pathobiology* 79:239–246.

Reinhard, K., Fink, T. M. & Skiles, J. (2003). A case of megacolon in Rio Grande Valley as a possible case of Chagas disease. *Memórias do Instituto Oswaldo Cruz* 98:165–172.

Rollo, F. & Marota, I. (1999). How microbial ancient DNA, found in association with human remains, can be interpreted. *Philosophical Transactions of the Royal Society of London* 354:111–119.

Ross, Z. P., Klunk, J., Fornaciari, G., Giuffra, V., Duchêne, S., Duggan, A. T., Poinar, D., Douglas, M. W., Eden, J.-S., Holmes, E. C. & Poinar H. N. (2018). The paradox of HBV evolution as revealed from a 16th-century mummy. *PLoS Pathogens* 14(1):e1006750.

Rothhammer, F., Allison, M. J., Núñez, L., Standen, V. & Arriaza, B. (1985). Chagas' disease in pre-Columbian South America. *American Journal of Physical Anthropology* 68(4):495–498.

Rühli, F. J. (2015). Short review: magnetic resonance imaging of ancient mummies. *The Anatomical Record* 298(6):1111–1115.

Rühli, F. J., Böni, T., Perlo, J., Casanova, F., Baias, M., Egarter Vigl, E. & Blumich, B. (2007). Non-invasive spatial tissue discrimination in ancient mummies and bones in situ by portable nuclear resonance. *Journal of Cultural Heritage* 8:257–263.

Ruffer, M. A. (1921). *Studies in the Palaeopathology of Egypt*. Chicago: University of Chicago Press.

Ruffer, M. A. & Ferguson, A. (1911). Note on an eruption resembling that of variola in the skin of a mummy of the twentieth dynasty (1200–1100 BC). *The Journal of Pathology and Bacteriology* 15(1):1–3.

Salo, W. L., Aufderheide, A. C., Buikstra, J. E. & Holcomb, T. A. (1994). Identification of *Mycobacterium tuberculosis* DNA in a pre-Columbian peruvian mummy. *Proceedings of the National Academy of Sciences of the United States of America* 91(6):2091–2094.

Scott, D. L., Wolfe, F. & Huizinga, T. W. J. (2010). Rheumatoid arthritis. *The Lancet* 376(9746): 1094–1108.

Scott, J. W., Horne, P. D., Hart, G. D. & Savage, H. (1977). Autopsy of an Egyptian mummy. 3. Gross anatomic and miscellaneous studies. *Canadian Medical Association Journal* 117:464–469.

Searcey, N., Reinhard, K. J., Egarter Vigl, E., Maixner, F., Piombino-Mascali, D., Zink, A. R., van der Sanden, W., Gardner, S. L. & Bianucci, R. (2013). Parasitism of the Zweeloo Woman: dicrocoeliasis evidenced in a Roman period bog mummy. *International Journal of Paleopathology* 3:224–228.

Shaw, B., Burrell, C. L., Green, D., Navarro-Martinez, A., Scott, D., Daroszewska, A., ... & Layfield, R. (2019). Molecular insights into an ancient form of Paget's disease of bone. *Proceedings of the National Academy of Sciences of the United States of America* 116(21):10463–10472.

Shin, D. H., Choi, Y. H., Shin, K. J., Han, G. R., Youn, M., Kim, C., Han, S. H., Seo, J. C., Park, S. S., Cho, Y. & Chang, B. S. (2003). Radiological analysis on a mummy from a medieval tomb in Korea. *Annals of Anatomy* 185:377–382

Shin, D. H., Oh, C. S., Lee, H. J., Chai, J. Y., Lee, S. J., Hong, D. W., Lee, S. D. & Seo, M. (2013). Ancient DNA analysis on *Clonorchis sinensis* eggs remained in samples from medieval Korean mummy. *Journal of Archaeological Science* 40(1): 211–216

Slepchenko, S. M., Gusev, A. V., Svyatova, E. O., Hong, J. H., Oh, C. S., Lim, D. S. & Shin, D. H. (2019). Medieval mummies of Zeleny Yar burial ground in the Arctic zone of Western Siberia. *PLoS One* 14(1):e0210718.

Sonoda, S., Li, H.-C., Cartier, L., Nunez, L. & Tajima, K. (2000). Ancient HTLV type 1 provirus DNA of Andean mummy. *AIDS Research and Human Retroviruses* 16(16):1753–1756.

Sotomayor, H., Burgos, J. & Arango, M. (2004). Demonstration of tuberculosis by DNA ribotyping of mycobacterium tuberculosis in a Colombian prehispanic mummy. *Biomedica: Revista del Instituto Nacional de Salud* 24:18–26.

Sutherland, M. L., Cox, S. L., Lombardi, G. P., Watson, L., Vallodolid, C. M., Finch, C. E., … & Sutherland, J. D. (2014). Funerary artifacts, social status, and atherosclerosis in ancient Peruvian mummy bundles. *Global Heart* 9(2):219–228.

Sydler, C., Öhrström, L., Rosendahl, W., Woitek, U. & Rühli, F. (2015). CT-based assessment of relative soft-tissue alteration in different types of ancient mummies. *The Anatomical Record* 298:1162–1174.

Thèves, C., Senescau, A., Vanin, S., Keyser, C., Ricaut, F. X., Alekseev, A. N., Dabernat, H., Ludes, B., Fabre, R. & Crubézy, E. (2011). Molecular identification of bacteria by total sequence screening: determining the cause of death in ancient human subjects. *PLoS One* 6(7):e21733.

Thompson, R. C., Allam, A. H., Lombardi, G. P., Sutherland, M. L., Sutherland, J. D., Soliman, A.-T. M., … & Thomas, G. S. (2013). Atherosclerosis across 4000 years of human history: the Horus study of four ancient populations. *The Lancet* 381:1211–1222.

Thompson, R. C., Allam, A. H., Zink, A., Wann, L. S., Lombardi, G. P., Cox, S. L., … & Thomas, G. S. (2014). Computed tomographic evidence of atherosclerosis in the mummified remains of humans from around the world. *Global Heart* 9(2):187–196.

Wittmers, L. E., Aufderheide, A. C. & Buikstra, J. (2011). Soft tissue preservation system: applications. *International Journal of Paleopathology* 1:150–154.

World Health Organization, (2017). *Global Hepatitis Report 2017*. Geneva: World Health Organization.

Vandamme, A.-M., Hall, W. W., Lewis, M. J., Goubau, P. & Salemi, M. (2000). Origins of HTLV-1 in South America (letter 2). *Nature Medicine* 6(3):232–233.

Ventura, L., Gaeta, R., Giuffra, V., Mercurio, C., Pistoia, M. L., Ciccozzi, A., Castagna, M. & Fornaciari, G. (2014). Breast pathology in ancient human remains. An approach to mummified mammary gland by modern investigation methods. *Pathologica* 106:216–218.

Villa, C. & Lynnerup, N. (2012). Hounsfield units ranges in CT-scans of bog bodies and mummies. *Anthropologischer Anzeiger* 69(2):127–145.

Wann, S., Lombardi, G., Ojeda, B., Benfer, R., Rivera, R., Finch, C., Thomas G. & Thompson, R. (2015). The Tres Ventanas mummies of Peru. *The Anatomical Record* 298:1026–1035.

Watson, L. (2019). *Los fardos de Ancón-Perú (800 d.C–1532 d.C). Una Perspectiva Bioarqueológica de Los Cambios Sociales en la Costa Central del Perú*. Oxford: BAR Publishing.

Zimmerman, M. R. (1974). PUM I autopsy report. *Paleopathology Newsletter* 7:6–7.

Zimmerman, M. R. (2011). The analysis and interpretation of mummified remains. In Grauer, A. L. (Ed.), *A Companion to Paleopathology*, pp. 152–169. Chichester: Wiley-Blackwell.

Zink, A. R., Molnár, E., Motamedi, N., Pálfy, G., Marcsik, A. & Nerlich, A. G. (2007). Molecular history of tuberculosis from ancient mummies and skeletons. *International Journal of Osteoarchaeology* 17(4):380–391.

Zink, A., Reischl, U., Wolf, H. & Nerlich, A.G. (2000). Molecular evidence of bacteremia by gastrointestinal pathogenic bacteria in an infant mummy from ancient Egypt. *Archives of Pathology and Laboratory Medicine* 124:1614–1618.

Zink, A., Reischl, U., Wolf, H., Nerlich, A. G. & Miller, R. (2001). Corynebacterium in ancient Egypt. *Medical History* 45:267–272.

Zink, A., Wann, L. S., Thompson, R. C., Keller, A., Maixner, F., Allam, A. H., … & Krause, J. (2014). Genomic correlates of atherosclerosis in ancient humans. *Global Heart* 9(2):203–209.

Zink, A. R., Sola, C., Reischl, U., Grabner, W., Rastogi, N., Wolf, H. & Nerlich, A. G. (2003). Characterization of mycobacterium tuberculosis complex DNAs from Egyptian mummies by spoligotyping. *Journal of Clinical Microbiology* 41(1):359–367.

Zink, A. R., Spigelman, M., Schraut, B., Greenblatt, C. L., Nerlich, A. G. & Donoghue, H. D. (2006). Leishmaniasis in ancient Egypt and upper Nubia. *Emerging Infectious Diseases* 12(10):1616–1617.

Zuckerman, M. K., Turner, B. L. & Armelagos, G. J. (2012). Evolutionary thought in paleopathology and the rise of the biocultural approach. In Grauer, A. L. (Ed.), *A Companion to Paleopathology*, pp. 34–57. Chichester: Wiley-Blackwell.

zur Nedden, D., Knapp, R., Wicke, K., Judmaier, W., Murphy, W. A. Jr, Seidler, H. & Platzer, W. (1994). Skull of a 5,300-year-old mummy: reproduction and investigation with CT-guided stereolithography. *Radiology* 193(1):269–272.

PART II

Investigating Diseases and Conditions of the Past

13
"STICKS AND STONES MAY BREAK MY BONES"
Traumatic Injuries in Paleopathology

Jennifer F. Byrnes and Katherine Gaddis

An osteologist's rhyme may go something like this: "sticks and stones may have broken their bones, but without social theory what's the point?" If you were unlucky enough to have suffered a severe traumatic injury during childhood, then you may painfully remember the injury, as well as the social repercussions that followed. Although taphonomy and bone remodeling can obscure osteological traces of past injuries, many types of traumatic injuries remain inscribed in the bones. Skillful application of paleopathological methods allows anthropologists to identify and interpret the evidence of these potentially life-altering events. This chapter provides an overview of traumatic injuries, including how they are interpreted through skeletal changes and the ways to apply paleopathological and theoretical frameworks to datasets.

Trauma – An Overview

Trauma can be defined as the application of an external force to a living organism that causes tissue damage, resulting in injury (Lovell, 1997). Traumatic injuries are common, particularly in humans, due to our mode of locomotion (i.e., bipedalism) putting us at risk of falling more often than our quadrupedal relatives (Latimer, 2005). Additionally, individuals and groups can be marginalized by their societies and face increased risk of violence (Martin & Harrod, 2015, and see Chapter 27, this volume). For example, child and elder abuse target specific age demographics that are vulnerable in human society (e.g., Wheeler et al., 2013; Gowland, 2016). Paleopathologists commonly observe traumatic injuries in higher frequencies than other pathological conditions (Lovell & Grauer, 2019; Redfern & Roberts, 2019). Traumatic injuries continue to be one of the most common causes of morbidity and mortality around the world (Haagsma et al., 2016), suggesting that a holistic anthropological paradigm can yield insights into this painful human experience.

Skeletal Biomechanics

Thorough paleopathological analyses of trauma should be guided by an understanding of the basic principles of skeletal biomechanics. When a force is applied to bone, energy is transferred, which has the potential to cause deformation and, ultimately, damage (Turner,

2006). Like all physical materials, the mechanical properties of bone determine its resistance to deformation under the application of force. These properties are related to both the macrostructure and microstructure of the particular skeletal element involved (Currey, 2013). At the microscopic level, bone is a composite material consisting of both organic and inorganic components. Specifically, bone is made up of a combination of collagen and calcium hydroxyapatite, each contributing to bone's unique properties. Collagen fibers allow the bone to be more resistant to force by increasing the amount of energy that the bone can absorb prior to deformation, while the mineral inorganic component of bone contributes to its strength and rigidity (Pathria et al., 2016).

The mechanical properties of bone change over an organism's life course. Intrinsic factors such as age, sex (e.g., Ensrud, 2013), and pathological history (e.g., Weiss et al., 2010; Bonafede et al., 2016) make certain individuals disproportionately susceptible to traumatic injury. For example, older individuals with osteoporosis have bones that are more brittle and prone to fracture than those of younger individuals (Agarwal et al., 2004; Turner, 2006). This means that while the bones of younger individuals may require significant force to reach the point of failure (i.e., fracture), the bones of elderly individuals or those with significant pathological changes in bone quality may fracture as the result of relatively minor mechanical loading, such as the result of everyday activities. Additionally, different bones will respond to external forces differently depending upon their composition, geometry, and cross-sectional area (Claes et al., 2012). These factors may vary by population, depending on genetics and/or environmental conditions (Cho et al., 2006). Therefore, it is important to consider demographic factors when interpreting skeletal trauma.

The biomechanical properties of bone can be understood in terms of the relationship between stress and strain. Stress refers to the intensity of force being exerted upon the bone, and strain refers to the bone's capacity for deformation prior to fracture. The application of force to a material, which causes stress, is referred to as mechanical loading. Under normal loading conditions, the relationship between stress and strain can be represented graphically by a stress-strain curve, in which stress is the load applied per unit area and strain is a measurement of the relative deformation of the material (Currey, 2013; Pathria et al., 2016; Turner, 2006). The slope of this curve is referred to as the elastic modulus, otherwise known as Young's modulus. The elastic modulus represents a material's ability to resist deformation under the application of force (Turner, 2006). The area beneath the curve represents a bone's toughness or ability to absorb energy. Elasticity refers to a material's ability to return to its original shape after an applied force has been removed, without permanent deformation (Symes et al., 2012). Bone will initially react to an applied force elastically. However, it will eventually reach a point at which it is no longer able to do so. The point at which a material is no longer able to resist permanent deformation is referred to as the yield point (Turner, 2006). After this, the bone will enter a state of plasticity. Plastic deformation results in structural damage that compromises the integrity of the bone and will result in failure if the load is not removed. Fracture occurs when bone is loaded beyond its strength or the capacity at which it can absorb energy without sustaining structural damage (Pathria et al., 2016).

Biomechanical forces may be classified by the direction in which the load is applied. The primary directional forces that affect bone are compression, tension, and shear (Pathria et al., 2016). Compressive forces act to squeeze bone, while tensile forces pull bone apart, and shear forces slide parts of a bone against one another. Directional forces often occur in combination. Bending and torsion are examples of directional forces acting in unison. Bending occurs when one side of a bone is under tension while the opposite side is under compression. Torsion occurs when shear forces are combined with a rotational or twisting motion. Bone is an anisotropic material, meaning that its strength varies depending upon the direction of the applied force. For example, bone is stronger under compressive forces than tensile forces and is most resistant to bending (Currey, 2013).

The way a bone will fracture is influenced by both the magnitude of the force and the rate at which it is applied. Greater magnitudes of force typically result in more severe fractures (Blau, 2017). Bone is more resistant to deformation if a force is applied over a larger surface area than if the same force is applied to a smaller surface area. This difference is due to the distribution of the force(s) through the bone/material, in which magnitude increases when surface area decreases. When referring to the rate of force application, forces that are applied suddenly and at a high rate of speed are referred to as dynamic, while forces that are applied slowly are referred to as static. Skeletal material is better able to resist deformation under static forces compared to dynamic forces because the bone will be better able to absorb the energy from the slow-loading static force (Blau, 2017). For example, while repetitive loading from ill-fitting footwear may eventually result in weakening of the bones of the feet over time, suddenly dropping a heavy load onto your foot is more likely to result in a fracture.

Recording Trauma – Methods

The methods used to record trauma have been standardized several times over the years (e.g., Buikstra & Ubelaker, 1994; Osteoware, 2011; Steckel et al., 2002). However, many researchers develop site-specific recording methods depending on their research foci and the resources available to them (Lovell, 1997; Redfern & Roberts, 2019). Typically, the most common approach to recording traumatic injuries in human skeletal remains involves macroscopic observation at minimum and medical imaging, such as radiography, if the technology/resources are available and feasible to utilize (Roberts & Manchester, 2005; Roberts, 2006). Redfern and Roberts (2019: Table 9.4) provide a 12-step fracture recording method encompassing demographics, specific location of the trauma on the bone, as well as the trauma type and characteristics to maximize the level of detail. Arguably, researchers should strive for a high level of detailed documentation of each traumatic injury by keeping detailed notes alongside quantitative data, drawings, photographs, and radiographs. These details can subsequently be used towards estimating the degree of physical impairment and possible disability (see models presented by Tilley & Cameron, 2014; Stodder, 2017; and Chapter 25, this volume).

Most antemortem traumatic injuries can be easily observed by the trained eye, especially if they are not well-healed or well-aligned. Comparison with the bone's antimere can usually assist with identifying hard calluses (i.e., the result of fracture healing), as well as malunions. Once the bone or joint segment displaying trauma is identified, the next step is to determine the type of trauma (e.g., fracture, dislocation) as well as the possible type of fracture or dislocation (e.g., transverse fracture, partial dislocation). These data can help in the interpretation of the cause of trauma (e.g., fall from a height). If the individual survived, these data could further inform the subsequent sociocultural effects.

The primary categories of hard tissue traumatic injuries are soft tissue ossification (e.g., myositis ossificans), abnormal shape or deformity, dislocation, and fracture (Lovell & Grauer, 2019; Redfern & Roberts, 2019). It is notable that most paleopathologists do not usually include traumatic enthesopathy with these categories, even though these are hard tissue reactions from soft tissue injuries. While enthesopathies resulting from trauma are usually considered trauma complications, they can also occur without an associated fracture or dislocation (Villotte et al., 2010; Villotte & Knüsel, 2013).

Trauma Classification

There are several distinct ways in which the application of force can affect the skeleton, including fracture and displacement or dislocation of a joint. There is some debate among paleopathologists as to whether artificial changes to the shape or contour of bone, such as those induced by cultural body modifications or surgical procedures, should be considered alongside trauma. These occurrences, while certainly important and worthy of study, will not be included in this chapter. In the following sections, we focus on the description of fractures, dislocations, various mechanisms of injury, and potential complications associated with trauma.

Dislocations

The application of force to a joint surface may result in either subluxation or dislocation. Subluxations are incomplete dislocations in which some contact remains between the articular surfaces (Lovell, 1997). Dislocations most often occur in the upper limb, as noted by a recent study that calculated the annual treatment incidence of orthopedic dislocation in Taiwan (Yang et al., 2011).

Dislocations happen most commonly in young and middle-aged adults (Nabian et al., 2017). In subadults, it is more common for epiphyseal separation to occur than for the joint to dislocate (refer to Lewis, 2018 for details on physeal fractures in children). In older adults, the joints are less stable due to the associated ligaments having lost elasticity, making it possible for joint dislocations to occur with less force (de Beer & Bhatia, 2010). However, it is also likely that the bones of elderly adults will fracture rather than dislocate (de Beer & Bhatia, 2010). For dislocations to be recognizable in skeletal remains, they must have remained unreduced long enough for bony changes to occur. If the dislocation was reduced, then the injury is likely to go undetected in skeletal analyses.

Fractures

Fractures are produced when bone is loaded beyond its capacity for elastic deformation, resulting in failure. Traumatic forces result in different fracture patterns depending upon the type of force that is applied (e.g., shear) and the magnitude of the applied force (e.g., small or large area) (Moraitis & Spiliopoulu, 2006). Although it is not always possible to determine the types of force involved in the production of an antemortem fracture due to remodeling, this type of information may lend important context to the injury. For example, certain injury patterns may be more indicative of interpersonal violence than others, such as fractures to the cranium or mandible (Martin & Harrod, 2015, and see Chapter 27, this volume). Careful and detailed description of traumatic bone injuries during the analysis of skeletal material is essential to determining the mechanism of injury in any case (Raul et al., 2008).

Several classification systems for skeletal fractures exist. Typically, fractures are characterized by the degree of fragmentation (e.g., comminuted), the location of the fracture (e.g., cranial vs. long bone fracture), its geometric properties, the completeness of the break, and the position of the fracture on the affected bone (e.g., proximal epiphysis) (Raul et al., 2008) (see Figure 13.1). Fractures are referred to as simple when they result in a single break in the bone (e.g., Figure 13.1 a, b, f) and are referred to as complex, or comminuted, when they result in multiple fragments (Lovell, 1997) (see Figure 13.1c). Fractures may be further described based upon the direction in which they propagate. Radiating fractures

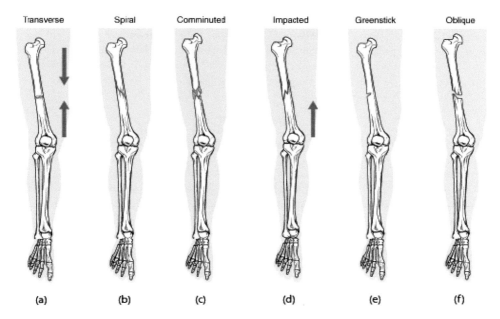

Figure 13.1 Illustrations of fracture types. (A) Transverse fracture; (B) Spiral fracture; (C) Comminuted fracture; (D) Impacted fracture; (E) Greenstick fracture; and (F) Oblique fracture. Image reproduced from Betts et al. (2013), OpenStax under Creative Commons Attribution License 4.0 license

will typically extend outward from the point of impact, while concentric fractures will occur circumferentially around this point (Raul et al., 2008). Linear fractures follow the longitudinal axis of the bone, whereas transverse fractures (e.g., Figure 13.1a) run perpendicular to this axis (Müller & Nazarian, 2010). Torsional loading causes the bone to twist around its longitudinal axis, resulting in fracture. Spiral fractures (e.g., Figure 13.1b) are caused when torque is applied to bone, which results in the application of both tensile and shear forces (Pierce et al., 2004). This results in a winding fracture line following rotational downward stress on the longitudinal axis of a bone (Müller & Nazarian, 2010). Oblique fracture lines (e.g., Figure 13.1f) angle across the longitudinal axis of the bone (Müller & Nazarian, 2010). When they are well-healed, oblique fractures are often confused with spiral fractures (Lovell, 1997).

Complete fractures are those in which the fractured ends are completely separated, whereas incomplete fractures maintain some continuity. Incomplete fractures occur more commonly in children than adults (Lewis, 2018). Common types of incomplete fractures include greenstick fractures, buckle (or torus) fractures, vertical fractures, and depression fractures. Greenstick fractures (e.g., Figure 13.1e) are incomplete transverse fractures that are caused when bending forces place one side of a bone under compression and the other under tension (Atanelov & Bentley, 2018). Torus fractures are a type of greenstick fracture that involves a buckling of the bone cortex (Allison, 2008). Finally, depression fractures are caused by direct force and appear as a concave area of the bone cortex (Hossai et al., 2008). They commonly occur in the skull, although they may also occur on the tibial plateau (Raul et al., 2008; Kfuri & Schatzker, 2018).

Other types of traumatic injuries include impact, avulsion, and burst fractures (Lovell, 1997). Impacted fractures (e.g., Figure 13.1d) are those in which the broken ends of a bone are pushed into each other by force. Avulsion fractures are caused when bone is pulled away by a joint capsule, ligament, or tendon. Burst fractures are located in the spine and occur when vertical compressive forces rupture the intervertebral disc, forcing tissue through the vertebral endplate into the vertebral body. This type of injury may be minor and present as a small depression on the endplate known as a "Schmorl's node" (Faccia & Williams, 2008).

Stress Fractures

Injuries to bone may be the result of either a single traumatic event or cumulative mechanical stress over time (Pathria et al., 2016). Bone can tolerate moderate stress and strain prior to failure, although the capacity at which it is able to do so varies depending on the skeletal element involved (Pathria et al., 2016). Stress (or fatigue) fractures are caused by repetitive force placed on a skeletal element (Matcuk et al., 2016). They are particularly common in the lower limbs, specifically the tibiae, metatarsals, and calcanei, as these bones are subject to mechanical loading related to locomotion (e.g., Martin-Francés et al., 2015; Meardon et al., 2015; Beck et al., 2000). Stress fracture lines typically occur perpendicular to the longitudinal axis of the bone, which may complicate differentiating them from transverse fractures. Stress fractures typically appear as non-displaced lines or cracks in bones, which are commonly referred to as hairline fractures. For example, spondylolysis, a fracture of the *pars interarticularis* of the vertebra, is attributed to repetitive stress on the spinal column leading to unilateral or bilateral fracturing (Berger & Doyle, 2019; Merbs, 2002).

Pathological Fractures

Some pathological conditions may affect the structural integrity of bone and reduce its ability to resist deformation under stress (De Mattos et al., 2012; Canavese et al., 2016). Certain metabolic conditions (e.g., osteoporosis), congenital diseases (e.g., osteogenesis imperfecta), infections, or neoplasms can contribute to an increased fracture risk by altering the normal biomechanical properties of bone (Brickley & Ives, 2008; Cope & Dupras, 2011; De Mattos et al., 2012). For example, in modern clinical contexts, childhood pathological fractures most often occur secondary to benign neoplasms (Canavese et al., 2016). As mentioned above, diseases that result in abnormal bone loss or quality, such as osteopenia and osteoporosis, increase the risk of fracture from even relatively normal loading conditions (Kanis et al., 2005). Vertebral compression fractures are particularly common secondary to osteoporosis (Freedman et al., 2008) as are fractures of the femoral neck (e.g., Lovell, 2016).

Fracture Mechanisms

Bony defects that result from blunt force, sharp force, or high-velocity projectile (HVP) trauma leave distinct signatures that allow the researcher to determine which mechanism(s) were responsible. Determining the fracture mechanism(s) relates to how the force was applied to the bone (e.g., small area and static load versus small area dynamic load).

Blunt force trauma (BFT) is the most commonly encountered bone injury when conducting skeletal analyses (Symes et al., 2012). The forces that cause blunt force injuries, such as a fall from a height, travel at relatively slow speeds and affect a comparatively large area of bone (Passalacqua & Fenton, 2012). How a bone responds to BFT depends on the intrinsic factors involved (Smith et al., 2003). For example, a long bone (e.g., femur) will be able to sustain certain forces and loading rates better than a flat bone (e.g., cranial bone) due to their intrinsic morphological differences. Similarly, a post-menopausal woman's vertebrae may be more susceptible to fracturing than a young child's vertebrae based on bone density and morphological differences. The bony margins of a BFT fracture will be deformed permanently as a result of passing the plastic deformation of bone. This is one key characteristic to distinguish between BFT versus HVP trauma (Table 13.1).

In some instances, fracture directionality can be determined by examining the margins of fractures for signs of tensile or compressive forces that acted upon the bone (see Christensen et al., 2018 for a detailed analysis of this fracture propagation process). Failure typically occurs on the bone surface under tension. In some instances, an impression from a tool may be left on the bone surface. Although this is more commonly observed in forensic contexts (Symes et al., 2012), it may occasionally be observed in paleopathological contexts when preservation permits. Lastly, based on bone properties and response to BFT, the number and sequence of impacts might be detectable (Madea & Staak, 1988). This is important in potentially distinguishing trauma associated with violence or the result of an accident

Table 13.1 Summary of characteristics of fracture mechanisms and fracture timing

Blunt force	*Sharp force*	*High-velocity projectile*
Slow load applied to large area	Slow load applied to small area	Rapid load application
Plastic deformation	Plastic deformation	Minimal to no plastic deformation
Cranial delamination	Elliptical or straight-line incised alteration	Entrance/exit wound traits (beveling, plug-and-spall fracturing)
Internal beveling of concentric fractures (Hart, 2005)	Punctures or gouges	External beveling of concentric fractures (Hart, 2005)
Tool marks/impressions of impact site(s)	Kerfs[a]	Gunshot residue (Berryman et al., 2010) and radiopaque bullet wipe (Lukefahr et al., 2021)
Antemortem	*Perimortem*	*Postmortem*
Osteogenic reaction (healing/healed)	No bony reaction or signs of healing or infection	No bony reaction or signs of healing or infection
	Smooth fracture surfaces (Wheatley, 2008)	Rough/jagged fracture surfaces (Wheatley, 2008)
	Acute fracture angle to bone surface (Villa & Mahieu, 1991)	Right-angle breaks, perpendicular fracturing (Villa & Mahieu, 1991)
	Fracture edges will be similar in color as surrounding bone (hematoma staining)	Broken edges of bone different colors than surrounding bone
	Bony hinging and greenstick fractures	No plastic deformation

[a]Kerfs are the base of a cut mark and vary in shape from V- to W-shaped based on the tool that produced the defect (e.g., knives versus saws).

(see Chapter 27, this volume). For a more detailed examination of BFT types by body region, see Wedel and Galloway (2014).

Sharp force trauma (SFT) is similar to BFT in that the rate of applied force is slow and dynamic; however, it is the relative surface area impacted (i.e., magnitude) that changes (Symes et al., 2012) (see Table 13.1). All SFT marks are produced by an instrument with a beveled edge or a point (Symes et al., 1998; Symes et al., 2002). These include machetes and axes (i.e., knives) and saws. Depending on the instrument, distinctive marks can be left on bone, assisting in determining the type or class of instrument causing the bony defect(s). It is possible that the instrument may be embedded in the bone, providing more information on the type of instrument used and context (e.g., Flohr et al., 2015). SFT in paleopathology is most likely to be observed in instances of conflict or warfare (e.g., Knüsel, 2005), ritual processing (e.g., Osterholtz, 2020a), as well as anatomical dissection (e.g., Nystrom, 2017). Detailed analysis of cut mark morphology may help paleopathologists to distinguish between acts of violence and cultural practices (Pérez, 2012). For more details, we refer the reader to Symes et al. (2010).

Paleopathologically, HVP trauma injuries do not appear until the historic period. In a review by Crist (2006) of 50+ bioarchaeological instances of gunshot wounds, he found that the majority appeared in adults post-1850 CE. While there are earlier instances of gunshot wounds (e.g., Larsen et al., 1996; Kim et al., 2013), they are rare. HVP trauma is the result of a fast-loaded force to a small surface area of bone, most often caused by a bullet. The force acting on the bone typically causes beveling on the internal surface of the entrance wound, as well as on the external surface of an exit wound. Typically, entrance wounds, depending on the angle of entry, will be smaller than exit wounds. While both BFT and HVP can produce radiating and concentric fractures in crania, the fracture margins differ. This is due to the projectile traveling through the brain leading to intracranial pressure that produces heaving forces from internal to external (Hart, 2005). As with BFT, there are instances where the trajectory of the projectile, the number of entrance/exit wounds, and the trauma sequence can be determined. A review and descriptions of HVP trauma in human remains can be found in Berryman et al. (2012).

Injury Timing

Injury timing can be discerned by noting signs of bony reaction or healing (i.e., osteogenic reaction) (Sauer, 1998). The healing process is typically divided into three stages (Hankenson et al., 2014; Frick, 2015) (see Figure 13.2). The first phase is the inflammatory phase, which typically lasts a few days depending upon the extent of the injury (Ghiasi et al., 2019). Traumatic forces severe enough to fracture bone will often damage the surrounding soft tissue, causing hemorrhage around the fracture site (Symes et al., 2012). This initiates the formation of a hematoma, which triggers an inflammatory immune response and provides a framework for the subsequent formation of a fibrocartilaginous callus (Marsell & Einhorn, 2011; Frick, 2015; Clark et al., 2017).

The second phase of the healing process is reparative (Frick, 2015). This phase involves the initiation of repair to damaged blood vessels and the beginning of cartilage formation at the injury site. As blood supply returns to the area, the cartilaginous (soft) callus will eventually be replaced by a callus of woven bone. During this phase, clinical union of the fractured ends takes place, meaning that the bony (hard) callus successfully joins the fracture and gives stability back to the bone. The final phase of the healing process is the remodeling phase. During this phase, the woven bone callus is remodeled into mature lamellar bone

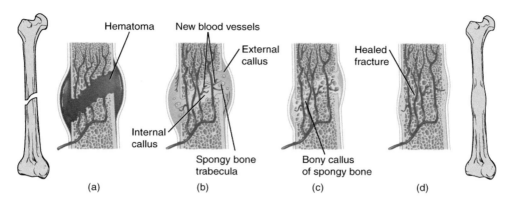

Figure 13.2 Illustration of fracture healing process. (a) Hematoma formation; (b) Soft callus formation; (c) Hard callus formation; (d) Remodeling of hard callus. Image reproduced from Betts et al. (2013), OpenStax under Creative Commons Attribution License 4.0 license

(Mirhadi et al., 2013). Remodeling is a lengthy process that takes place over several months or longer (Kalfas, 2001). This phase is characterized by secondary bone formation, which lends to restoration of the overall mechanical and biological functions of the bone (Hankenson et al., 2014).

Understanding the healing process allows paleopathologists to recognize the presence of perimortem trauma – trauma that occurs at or around the time of death. However, distinguishing between perimortem trauma and postmortem damage is challenging. Table 13.1 provides common characteristics associated with injury timing events in bone. Importantly, Wieberg and Wescott (2008) caution that no single factor provides accurate injury timing due to the prolonged appearance of "green" characteristics after death.

Recognizing the stages of healing can also assist in determining the timeline of multiple fracture events. In instances of child abuse, for instance, multiple traumatic events can occur over the course of their short lives. Patterns of healing can also help determine the presence of elder abuse (Gowland, 2017a). If no sign of healing is detected in a fractured bone, then perimortem trauma or postmortem alterations should be considered (White & Toth, 1989; Frayer, 1997).

Complications of Traumatic Injury

Fracture healing is a complex process that takes time to complete but commences immediately after the injury occurs (Doblare et al., 2004). However, the rate at which a bone heals depends upon several factors, including the location and properties of the fracture, associated comorbidities, and the age of the individual (Claes et al., 2012). Clinical research has shown that age complicates all stages of the healing process and increases the likelihood that associated complications will develop (Clark et al., 2017).

Proper healing of skeletal fractures requires three components: repositioning and realignment of the fractured ends, temporary immobilization of the injury, and maintenance of circulation to the affected area. While the process is fairly straightforward, there can be complications. Instances in which the fractured ends are not set properly, but still unite, are referred to as malunions and can result in deformity and possible impairment of the individual. Occasionally, a fractured bone will not unite and the ends will heal separately, resulting in non-union. Infection may also ensue, especially in cases of open or compound fractures.

Penetration of the skin leaves the injury site vulnerable to infectious pathogens. In most cases, when an infection occurs, it is caused by the bacteria *Staphylococcus aureus* (Waldron, 2009).

Traumatic injuries may also contribute to the development of osteoarthritis (OA). Post-traumatic OA may develop secondary to joint injuries, including injuries to the bone, cartilage, or associated ligaments (Wang et al., 2020). Damage to the joint surface and surrounding soft tissues may result in joint instability and acute inflammatory responses that contribute to the development of post-traumatic OA (Loeser, 2013). The presence of post-traumatic OA may be indicated by the observation of trauma in the affected bone and bilateral asymmetry in the pattern or severity of OA (Resnick, 2002). Post-traumatic OA has the potential to result in severe physical impairment (e.g., ankylosis of a joint) (Delco et al., 2017; Redfern & Austin, 2020).

Myositis ossificans traumatica (MOT) is another potential complication that may arise secondary to traumatic injury. Myositis ossificans involves the ossification of soft tissue and typically affects skeletal muscle; although, it may also affect subcutaneous fat, tendons, or nerves (Walczak et al., 2015). Although this condition may also be hereditary and sometimes occurs in relation to systemic conditions, it most commonly occurs secondary to trauma (Gindele et al., 2000). MOTs are often painful and may result in limited mobility of the affected area (Smith & Liston, 2020). MOTs are frequently described in paleopathological literature. Smith and Liston (2020) present an interesting case of spinal MOT and the development of associated pseudarthroses from a Late Bronze Age site in Athens, Greece that affected the lumbar vertebrae.

Proximate versus Ultimate Cause

The first step in reconstructing the sociocultural and behavioral context of traumatic injuries is the establishment of proximate and ultimate cause (Walker, 2001). Proximate cause refers to the direct, mechanical cause of the trauma, such as a weapon or object. The ultimate cause, by contrast, refers to the biological and sociocultural factors that led to the injury taking place. Traumatic injuries should be considered from the perspective of both the individual and population (Martin & Harrod, 2015). Patterns of traumatic injuries at the population level may suggest unique interpretations that might otherwise be obscured at the level of the individual (Walker, 2001).

Accidental versus Intentional Injury

Determining if injuries are the result of an accident or violent intent can be difficult to determine based on (available) skeletal evidence. The interpretation of bony injuries needs to be framed within a biocultural perspective (Goodman et al., 1988; Klaus, 2012), not just the context of the remains. For example, considering the age, sex, and ethnicity of an individual within a particular time frame can elucidate potential occupational hazards, as well as the relative prevalence of violence within that time and space. This is particularly important in instances of child and elder abuse, in which certain types of fractures or fracture patterns may not normally occur in that particular age group unless it was intentionally inflicted (e.g., Love et al., 2011; Wheeler et al., 2013; Gowland, 2016). Thus, considering trauma recidivism alongside demographic factors can paint a more complete picture in cases of intentional violent injury (Judd, 2017).

As Walker (2001) cautions, it can be difficult to make the distinction between accidental versus intentional injuries due to the limited contextual information we have on past peoples' lives and cultures. Paleopathologists are urged to be cautious with their interpretations of injuries resulting from violent intent and to reserve these calls only in instances in which there is overwhelming evidence of violent intent such as SFT or embedded projectiles. Walker provided a guide to help researchers through the interpretation of trauma in skeletal remains (2001: Figure 2). Koziol (2017) used archaeological and ethnographic case studies to caution inherent Western bias when interpreting violence, behavior, and their intersection with sex and gender in the past. Koziol specifically warned against casting females as noncombatants and victims based on Western stereotypes and assumed norms instead of combatants or perpetrators, especially in past cultures that may have recognized more than two gender identities.

Social and Cultural Interpretations

Paleopathologists and bioarchaeologists actively engage with sociocultural theories. This high-level theoretical contextualization of data provides a nuanced interpretation of disease in the past. Being cognizant of the vast array of human difference across time and space is important in the careful interpretation of how traumatic injuries may have occurred, as well as how the individuals who survived those injuries may have been treated within their society.

A number of theoretical paradigms have been used to interpret trauma in the archaeological record. These include violence theories (e.g., Martin et al., 2012; Pérez 2016), feminist and queer theories (e.g., Geller, 2017), the life course approach (e.g., Glencross, 2011; Redfern, 2016: 83–125), ethnogenesis (e.g., Osterholtz, 2020b), care in the past (e.g., Tilley, 2015; Tilley & Schrenk, 2017), personhood (e.g., Boutin, 2016), and race theory (e.g., de la Cova, 2017). Additionally, specific facets of social identities have been explored over the last 20 years (e.g., Knudson & Stojanowski, 2020). These include works on how trauma intersects and interacts with gender (e.g., Martin & Tegtmeyer, 2017; Stone, 2020), age (e.g., Gowland, 2017b; Toyne, 2018), disability and impairment (e.g., Redfern, 2016: 168–204; Byrnes, 2017), race (e.g., de la Cova, 2020), ethnicity (e.g., Johnson, 2020), socioeconomic status (e.g., Mant et al., 2021), immigration (e.g., Byrnes, 2017), slavery and captivity (e.g., Martin et al., 2010), and sexuality (e.g., Geller, 2017). For example, Hollimon (2017) argued that, by utilizing a biocultural approach, it is possible to reveal non-binary genders (e.g., third and fourth genders) through the observation of patterns of traumatic injuries in skeletal remains. Hollimon (2000, 2001) found trauma patterns in female-sexed skeletons from pre-contact California and protohistoric Northern Plains that are consistent with male patterns of injury, suggesting the presence of more than two gender identities. As well, Martin et al. (2010) embed their skeletal data in archaeological and ethnographic contexts to explore how "outsider" female captives from the La Plata site (AD 1000–3000) experienced different patterns of traumatic injuries, disease, impairment, and disability.

Researchers have more recently applied intersectionality theory to understand social identity. DeWitte and Yaussy (2020) evaluate how intersectionality theory (see Crenshaw, 1989, 1991), has or has not been applied fully within bioarchaeology, while Mant et al. (2021) provide an overview of bioarchaeological work on intersectionality and traumatic injuries. Through the lens of intersectionality theory, researchers are able to amplify axes of power (Farmer, 2004) that result in discrimination, marginalization, and social inequality (e.g., Mant & Holland, 2019; Watkins, 2020). Trauma analyses, through an intersectional lens, can provide a nuanced and powerful approach to examining structural violence and other forms of socially sanctioned forms of violence against people in the past.

Placing intentional trauma into cultural contexts is complex, as it may manifest as cultural body modifications. Waist training from a corset with tight lacing, for instance, while not intending to break bones, left skeletal structures permanently deformed. Foot binding in Chinese culture, however, fractured bones in order to modify the shape and size of the foot. This practice may also result in an increased risk of fracture related to falls (Lee, 2019). Ultimately, the result of these body modifications can be detected in bone and are the result of socially sanctioned structural violence. Stone (2020) demonstrated through her exploration of corseting, foot binding, and neck elongation practices, the beauty expectations of girls and women in specific times and cultures do not simply inflict trauma on female bodies but may be enforced by women to maintain gender roles (i.e., mothers).

Limitations and Opportunities

The paleopathological analysis of trauma has the potential to elucidate our understanding of the lives and lifestyles of past individuals and societies. Paleopathological analyses of trauma have developed significantly in both theory and methodology over the course of the field's history. However, there is still work to be done if we are to overcome gaps that persist in our knowledge of traumatic injuries, past and present. Challenges related to the identification and interpretation of trauma may be overcome through interdisciplinary collaboration and the development of standardized methods for data collection and trauma classification.

There remains some disagreement in the literature as to what constitutes trauma, and more uncommon classifications are often under-researched (Murphy & Juengst, 2020). For example, little attention has been paid to the analysis and interpretation of post-cranial fractures, joint dislocations, and accidental injuries in the paleopathological literature (Murphy & Juengst, 2020).

Fracture patterns are often difficult to interpret. Taking an interdisciplinary perspective by drawing from forensic anthropology, the National Institute of Standards and Technology (NIST), Organization of Scientific Area Committees for Forensic Science (OSAC), highlights difficulties in interpreting BFT injuries, specifically in regard to the number and location of impacts (OSAC, 2016). They encourage collaboration with biomechanical engineers to facilitate controlled experimental studies focused on understanding how variables such as bone geometry and morphology play a role in the initiation and propagation of fractures. This may help to identify points of impact and potentially the instrument and type of force involved. This research focus overlaps with our own methodological approaches and demonstrates that synergistic collaboration with other disciplines may help to address known gaps in the literature.

Recording procedures remain problematic in that they lack consistency from one researcher to the next, complicating comparisons between different sites and studies. The introduction of a consistently utilized standard system for the classification of traumatic injuries would lend significantly to more consistent identification, which would in turn facilitate collaborative and comparative research. Paleopathological research has become increasingly interdisciplinary, but it stands to benefit from further incorporation of clinical, forensic, and zooarchaeological literature. In doing so, we open doors to opportunities for new advancements in trauma research and fresh perspectives on shared problems. As an example, studies of childhood trauma remain scarce in paleopathological literature, although there has been progress made over the last decade to combat challenges related to the identification and interpretation of different types of childhood injuries (Mays et al., 2017). This may in part be due to the difficulties associated with the analysis of subadult skeletal remains, including poor preservation (Lewis, 2018 DeWitte & Stojanowski, 2015; Mays et al., 2017). However, the exclusion of certain age groups leads to significant gaps in our understanding of traumatic injuries throughout the life course.

Conclusion: Future Considerations

While the field of paleopathology has progressed significantly both methodologically and theoretically over the last several decades, there is still much work to be done. Future avenues for research include the reassessment of existing osteological collections from new theoretical perspectives. For example, attention should be paid to the possible presence of non-binary individuals, as evidenced by observed patterns of trauma (Hollimon, 2017). Additionally, collections should be reexamined for potential occurrences of interpersonal violence that could be interpreted through a different biocultural framework. For example, Walker (1997) interpreted intimate partner violence ("wife beating") through the trauma patterns he observed in female-sexed skeletons. However, this was reinterpreted by de la Cova (2010, 2012) as interpersonal and structural violence related to practices in early mental institutes, and not due to domestic abuse. Additionally, distinguishing between trauma caused by assaults versus sports (e.g., boxing causing non-lethal trauma to the skull) should be considered particularly for historic skeletal remains (e.g., Torres Colón & Smith, 2020).

References

Agarwal, S. C., Dumitriu, M., Tomlinson, G. A. & Grynpas, M. D. (2004). Medieval trabecular bone architecture: the influence of age, sex, and lifestyle. *American Journal of Physical Anthropology* 124(1):33–44.

Allison, S. G. (2008). Paediatric torus fracture. *Emergency Nurse* 16(6):22–25. DOI: 10.7748/en2008.10.16.6.22.c6780

Atanelov, Z. & Bentley, T. P. (2018). *Greenstick fracture*. Treasure Island: StatPearls Publishing.

Beck, T. J., Ruff, C. B., Shaffer, R. A., Betsinger, K., Trone, D. W. & Brodine, S. K. (2000). Stress fracture in military recruits: gender differences in muscle and bone susceptibility factors. *Bone* 27(3):437–444. https://doi.org/10.1016/s8756-3282(00)00342-2

Berger, R. G. & Doyle, S. M. (2019). Spondylolysis 2019 update. *Current Opinion in Pediatrics* 31(1):61–68.

Berryman, H. E., Kutyla, A. K. & Davis, J. R. (2010). Detection of gunshot primer residue on bone in an experimental setting—an unexpected finding. *Journal of Forensic Sciences* 55(2):488–491.

Berryman, H. E., Lanfear, A. K. & Shirley, N. R. (2012). The biomechanics of gunshot trauma to bone: research considerations within the present judicial climate. In Dirkmaat, D. (Ed.), *A Companion to Forensic Anthropology*, pp. 390–399. Chichester: Blackwell Publishing.

Betts, J. G., Young, K. A., Wise, J. A., Johnson, E., Poe, B., Kruse, D. H., Korol, O., Johnson, J. E., Womble, M. & DeSaix, P. (2013). *Anatomy and Physiology*. Houston, Texas: OpenStax. https://openstax.org/books/anatomy-and-physiology/pages/6-5-fractures-bone-repair.

Blau, S. (2017). How traumatic: a review of the role of the forensic anthropologist in the examination and interpretation of skeletal trauma. *Australian Journal of Forensic Sciences* 49(3):261–280.

Bonafede, M., Shi, N., Barron, R., Li, X., Crittenden, D. B. & Chandler, D. (2016). Predicting imminent risk for fracture in patients aged 50 or older with osteoporosis using US claims data. *Archives of Osteoporosis* 11(1):1–7.

Boutin, A. T. (2016). Exploring the social construction of disability: an application of the bioarchaeology of personhood model to a pathological skeleton from ancient Bahrain. *International Journal of Paleopathology* 12:17–28.

Brickley, M. & Ives, R. (2008). *The Bioarchaeology of Metabolic Bone Disease*. Amsterdam: Elsevier.

Buikstra, J. E. & Ubelaker, D. (1994). *Standards for Data Collection from Human Skeletal Remains*. Fayetteville: Arkansas Archaeological Survey Research Series, 44.

Byrnes, J. F. (2017). Injuries, impairment, and intersecting identities: the poor in Buffalo, NY 1851–1913. In Byrnes, J. F. & Muller, J. L. (Eds.), *Bioarchaeology of Impairment and Disability,* pp. 201–222. New York: Springer Cham.

Canavese, F., Samba, A. & Rousset, M. (2016). Pathological fractures in children: diagnosis and treatment options. *Orthopaedics & Traumatology: Surgery & Research* 102(1):S149–S159.

Cho, H., Stout, S. D. & Bishop, T. A. (2006). Cortical bone remodeling rates in a sample of African American and European American descent groups from the American Midwest: comparisons of age and sex in ribs. *American Journal of Physical Anthropology* 130(2):214–226.

Christensen, A. M., Hefner, J. T., Smith, M. A., Webb, J. B., Bottrell, M. C. & Fenton, T. W. (2018). Forensic fractography of bone: a new approach to skeletal trauma analysis. *Forensic Anthropology* 1(1):32–51.

Claes, L., Recknagel, S. & Ignatius, A. (2012). Fracture healing under healthy inflammatory conditions. *National Review of Rheumatology* 8:133–143.

Clark, D., Nakamura, M., Miclau, T. & Marcucio, R. (2017). Effects of aging on fracture healing. *Current Osteoporosis Report*s 15(6):601–608.

Cope, D. J. & Dupras, T. L. (2011). Osteogenesis imperfecta in the archeological record: an example from the Dakhleh Oasis, Egypt. *International Journal of Paleopathology* 1(3–4):188–199.

Crenshaw, K. (1989). Demarginalizing the intersection of race and sex: a black feminist critique of antidiscrimination doctrine, feminist theory and antiracist politics. *University of Chicago Legal Forum* 8(1):139–167.

Crenshaw, K. (1991). Mapping the margins: intersectionality, identity politics, and violence against women of color. *Stanford Law Review* 43(6):1241–1299.

Crist, T. (2006). The good, the bad, and the ugly: bioarchaeology and the modern gun culture debate. *Historical Archaeology* 40(3):109–130.

Currey, J. D. (2013). *Bones: Structure and Mechanics*. Princeton: Princeton University Press.

de Beer, J. & Bhatia, D. (2010). Shoulder instability in the middle-aged and elderly patients: pathology and surgical implications. *International Journal of Shoulder Surgery* 4(4):87.

de la Cova, C. (2010). Cultural patterns of trauma among 19th-century-born males in cadaver collections. *American Anthropologist* 112(4):589–606.

de la Cova, C. (2012). Patterns of trauma and violence in 19th century-born African American and Euro-American females. *International Journal of Paleopathology* 2:61–68.

de la Cova, C. (2017). Fractured lives: Structural violence, trauma, and recidivism in urban and institutionalized 19th-century-born African Americans and Euro-Americans. In Tegtmeyer, C. E. & Martin, D. L. (Eds.), *Broken Bones, Broken Bodies: Bioarchaeological and Forensic Approaches for Accumulative Trauma and Violence*, pp. 153–180. New York: Lexington Books.

de la Cova, C. (2020). Making silenced voices speak: restoring neglected and ignored identities in anatomical collections. In Cheverko, C. M., Prince-Buitenhuys, J. R. & Hubbe, M. (Eds.), *Theoretical Approaches in Bioarchaeology*. London: Routledge.

Delco, M. L., Kennedy, J. G., Bonassar, L. J. & Fortier, L. A. (2017). Post-traumatic osteoarthritis of the ankle: a distinct clinical entity requiring new research approaches. *Journal of Orthopaedic Research* 35(3):440–453.

De Mattos, C. B. R., Binitie, O. & Dormans, J. P. (2012). Pathological fractures in children. *Bone & Joint Research* 1(10):272–280.

DeWitte, S. N. & Stojanowski, C. M. (2015). The osteological paradox 20 years later: past perspectives, future directions. *Journal of Archaeological Research* 23(4):397–450.

DeWitte, S. & Yaussy, S. (2020). Bioarchaeological applications of intersectionality. In Cheverko, C. M., Prince-Buitenhuys, J. R. & Hubbe, M. (Eds.), *Theoretical Approaches in Bioarchaeology*, pp. 45–58. London: Routledge.

Doblare, M., Garcia, J. M. & Gomez, M. J. (2004). Modelling bone tissue fracture and healing: a review. *Engineering Fracture Mechanics* 71:1809–1840.

Ensrud, K. E. (2013). Epidemiology of fracture risk with advancing age. *The Journals of Gerontology: Series A* 68(10): 1236–1242.

Faccia, K. J. & Williams, R. C. (2008). Schmorl's nodes: clinical significance and implications for the bioarchaeological record. *International Journal of Osteoarchaeology* 18(1):28–44.

Farmer, P. H. (2004). *Pathologies of Power: Health, Human Rights, and the New War on the Poor.* Los Angeles: University of California Press.
Flohr, S., Brinker, U., Schramm, A., Kierdorf, U., Staude, A., Piek, J., Jantzen, D., Hauenstein, K. & Orschiedt, J. (2015). Flint arrowhead embedded in a human humerus from the Bronze Age site in the Tollense Valley, Germany – a high-resolution micro-CT study to distinguish antemortem from perimortem projectile trauma to bone. *International Journal of Paleopathology* 9:76–81.
Frayer, D. W. (1997). Ofnet: evidence for a mesolithic massacre. In Martin, D. L. & Frayer, D. W. (Eds.), *Troubled Times: Violence and Warfare in the Past,* pp. 181–216. Netherlands: Gordon and Breach Publishers.
Freedman, B. A., Potter, B. K., Nesti, L. J., Giuliani, J. R., Hampton, C. & Kuklo, T. R. (2008). Osteoporosis and vertebral compression fractures—continued missed opportunities. *The Spine Journal* 8(5):756–762.
Frick, S. L. (2015). Skeletal growth, development, and healing as related to pediatric trauma. In Mencio, G. A. & Swiontkowski, M. F. (Eds.), *Green's Skeletal Trauma in Children* (5th edition), pp. 1–15. Amsterdam: Elsevier. https://doi.org/10.1016/B978-0-323-18773-2.00001-9
Geller, P. L. (2017). *The Bioarchaeology of Socio-Sexual Lives: Queering Common Sense about Sex, Gender, and Sexuality.* New York: Springer.
Ghiasi, M. S., Chen, J. E., Rodriguez, E. K., Vaziri, A. & Nazarian, A. (2019). Computational modeling of human bone fracture healing affected by different conditions of initial healing stage. *BMC Musculoskeletal Disorders* 20:1–14. https://doi-org.ezproxy.library.unlv.edu/10.1186/s12891-019-2854-z
Gindele, A., Schwamborn, D., Tsironis, K. & Benz-Bohm, G. (2000). Myositis ossificans traumatica in young children: report of three cases and review of the literature. *Pediatric Radiology* 30(7):451–459.
Glencross, B. A. (2011). Skeletal injury across the life course: towards understanding social agency. In Agarwal, S. C. & Glencross, B. A. (Eds.), *Social Bioarchaeology,* pp. 390–409. New York: Blackwell Publishing.
Goodman, A. H., Brooke Thomas, R., Swedlund, A. C. & Armelagos, G. J. (1988). Biocultural perspectives on stress in prehistoric, historical, and contemporary population research. *American Journal of Physical Anthropology* 31(S9):169–202.
Gowland, R. L. (2016). Elder abuse: evaluating the potentials and problems of diagnosis in the archaeological record. *International Journal of Osteoarchaeology* 26:514–523.
Gowland, R. L. (2017a). That 'tattered coat upon a stick' the ageing body: evidence for elder marginalisation and abuse in Roman Britain. In Powell, L., Southwell-Wright, W. & Gowland, R. (Eds.), *Care in the Past: Archaeological and Interdisciplinary Perspectives,* pp. 71–90. Oxford: Oxbow Books.
Gowland, R. L. (2017b). Growing old: Biographies of disability and care in later life. In Tilley, L. & Schrenk, A. A. (Eds.), *New Developments in the Bioarchaeology of Care: Further Case Studies and Expanded Theory,* pp. 237–251. New York: Springer Cham. DOI:10.1007/9783-319-39901-0_12.
Haagsma, J. A., Graetz, N., Bolliger, I., Naghavi, M., Higashi, H., Mullany, E. C. & et al. (2016). The global burden of injury: incidence, mortality, disability-adjusted life years and time trends from the global burden of disease study 2013. *Injury Prevention* 22(1):3–18. https://doi.org/10.1136/injuryprev-2015-041616
Hankenson, K. D., Zimmerman, G. & Marcucio, R. (2014). Biological perspectives of delayed fracture healing. *Injury* 45:S8–S15.
Hart, G. O. (2005). Fracture pattern interpretation in the skull: differentiating blunt force from ballistics trauma using concentric fractures. *Journal of Forensic Sciences* 50(6):1276–1281.
Hollimon, S. E. (2017). Bioarchaeological approaches to nonbinary genders. In Agarwal, S. C. & Wesp, J. K. (Eds.), *Exploring Sex and Gender in Bioarchaeology,* pp. 51–69. Albuquerque: University of New Mexico Press.
Hollimon, S. E. (2000). Sex, health, and gender roles among the Arikara of the Northern Plains. In Rautman, A. E. (Ed.), *Reading the Body: Representations and Remains in the Archaeological Record,* pp. 25–37. Philadelphia: University of Pennsylvania Press.
Hollimon, S. E. (2001). Warfare and gender in the Northern Plains: osteological evidence of trauma reconsidered. In Arnold, B. & Wicker, N. L. (Eds.), *Gender and the Archaeology of Death,* pp. 179–193. Walnut Creek, CA: AltaMira.
Hossain, M. Z., Mondle, M. S. & Hoque, M. M. (2008). Depressed skull fracture: outcome of surgical treatment. *TAJ: Journal of Teachers Association* 21(2):140–146.

Johnson, K. M. (2020). Exploring family, ethnic, and regional identities among Tiwanaku-affiliated communities in Moquegua, Peru. In Knudson, K. J. & Stojanowski, C. M. (Eds.), *Bioarchaeology and Identity Revisited*, pp. 20–55. Gainesville: University Press of Florida.

Judd, M. (2017). Injury recidivism revisited. Clinical research, limitations, and implications for bioarchaeology. In Tegtmeyer, C. E. & Martin, D. L. (Eds.), *Broken Bones, Broken Bodies: Bioarchaeological and Forensic Approaches for Accumulative Trauma and Violence*, pp. 1–23. New York: Lexington Books.

Kalfas, I. H. (2001). Principles of bone healing. *Neurosurgical focus* 10(4):1–4.

Kanis, J. A., Borgstrom, F., De Laet, C., Johansson, H., Johnell, O., Jonsson, B., … & Khaltaev, N. (2005). Assessment of fracture risk. *Osteoporosis International* 16(6):581–589.

Kfuri, M. & Schatzker, J. (2018). Revisiting the Schatzker classification of tibial plateau fractures. *Injury* 49(12):2252–2263.

Kim, Y.-S., Kim, M. J., Yu, T.-Y., Lee, I. S., Yi, Y. S., Oh, C. S. & Shin, D. H. (2013). Bioarchaeological investigation of possible gunshot wounds in 18th century human skeletons from Korea. *International Journal of Osteoarchaeology* 23(6):716–722.

Klaus, H. D. (2012). The bioarchaeology of structural violence: a theoretical model and a case study. In Martin, D. L. & Harrod, R. P. (Eds.), *The Bioarchaeology of Violence*, pp. 29–62. Gainesville: University Press of Florida.

Knudson, K. J. & Stojanowski, C. M. (Eds.) (2020). *Bioarchaeology and Identity Revisited*. Gainesville: University Press of Florida.

Knüsel, C. J. (2005). The physical evidence of warfare: a subtle stigmata? In Parker Pearson, M. & Thorpe, I. J. N. (Eds.), *Warfare, Violence and Slavery in Prehistory*, pp. 49–66. Oxford: British Archaeological Reports, International Series 1374.

Koziol, K. M. (2017). Shattered mirrors: gender, age, and westernized interpretations of war (and Violence) in the Past. In Martin, D. L. & Tegtmeyer, C. (Eds.), *Bioarchaeology of Women and Children in Times of War: Case Studies from the Americas*, pp. 15–26. New York: Springer Cham.

Larsen, C. S., Huynh, H. P. & McEwan, B. G. (1996). Death by gunshot: biocultural implications of trauma at Mission San Luis. *International Journal of Osteoarchaeology* 6(1):42–50.

Latimer, B. (2005). The perils of being bipedal. *Annals of Biomedical Engineering* 33(1):3–6.

Lee, C. (2019). A bioarchaeological and biocultural investigation of Chinese footbinding at the Xuecun archaeological site, Henan Province, China. *International Journal of Paleopathology* 25:9–19.

Lewis, M. (2018). *Paleopathology of Children: Identification of Pathological Conditions in the Human Skeletal Remains of Non-Adults*. New York: Academic Press.

Loeser, R. F. (2013). Osteoarthritis year in review 2013: biology. *Osteoarthritis and Cartilage* 21(10):1436–1442.

Love, J. C., Derrick, S. M. & Wiersema, J. M. (2011). *Skeletal Atlas of Child Abuse*. Totowa, NJ: Humana Press.

Lovell, N. (1997). Trauma analysis in paleopathology. *Yearbook of Physical Anthropology* 40:139–170.

Lovell, N. (2016). Tiptoeing through the rest of his life: a functional adaptation to a leg shortened by femoral neck fracture. *International Journal of Paleopathology* 3:91–95.

Lovell, N. & Grauer, A. (2019). Analysis and interpretation of trauma in skeletal remains. In Katzenberg, M. A. & Grauer, A. L. (Eds.), *Biological Anthropology of the Human Skeleton,* 3rd edition, pp. 335–384. London: Wiley Blackwell.

Lukefahr, A., Vollner, J., Anderson, B. & Winston, D. (2021). Radiodense bullet wipe around osseous entrance gunshot wounds. *Journal of Forensic Sciences* 66(1):229–235.

Madea, B. & Staak, M. (1988). Determination of the sequence of gunshot wounds of the skull. *Journal of the Forensic Science Society* 28(5–6):321–328. https://doi.org/10.1016/S0015-7368(88)72858-3

Mant, M., de la Cova, C. & Brickley, M. B. (2021). Intersectionality and trauma analysis in bioarchaeology. *American Journal of Physical Anthropology* 174(4):1–12.

Mant, M. L. & Holland, A. J. (Eds.) (2019). *Bioarchaeology of Marginalized People*. New York: Academic Press.

Marsell, R. & Einhorn, T. A. (2011). The biology of fracture healing. *Injury* 42(6):551–555.

Martin, D., Harrod, R. & Fields, M. (2010). Beaten down and worked to the bone: bioarchaeological investigations of women and violence in the ancient southwest. *Landscapes of Violence* 1(1):Article 3.

Martin, D. L., Harrod, R. P. & Pérez, V. P. (2012). *The Bioarchaeology of Violence*. Gainesville: University Press of Florida.

Martin, D. L. & Harrod, R. P. (2015). Bioarchaeological contributions to the study of violence. *American Journal of Physical Anthropology* 156:116–145.

Martin, D. L. & Tegtmeyer, C. (Eds.) (2017). *Bioarchaeology of Women and Children in Times of War: Case Studies from the Americas.* New York: Springer Cham.

Martin-Francés, L., Martinon-Torres, M., Gracia-Téllez, A. & Bermúdez de Castro, J. M. (2015). Evidence of stress fracture in a *Homo antecessor* metatarsal from Gran Dolina site (Atapuerca, Spain). *International Journal of Osteoarchaeology* 25(4):564–573.

Matcuk, G. R., Mahanty, S. R., Skalski, M. R., Patel, D. B., White, E. A. & Gottsegen, C. J. (2016). Stress fractures: pathophysiology, clinical presentation, imaging features, and treatment options. *Emergency Radiology* 23(4):365–375.

Mays, S., Gowland, R., Halcrow, S. & Murphy, E. (2017). Child bioarchaeology: perspectives on the past 10 years. *Childhood in the Past* 10(1):38–56.

Meardon, S. A., Willson, J. D., Gries, S. R., Kernozek, T. W. & Derrick, T. R. (2015). Bone stress in runners with tibial stress fracture. *Clinical Biomechanics* 30(9):895–902.

Merbs, C. F. (2002). Asymmetrical spondylolysis. *American Journal of Physical Anthropology* 119(2):156–174.

Mirhadi, S., Ashwood, N. & Karagkevrekis, B. (2013). Factors influencing fracture healing. *Trauma* 15(2):140–155.

Moraitis, K. & Spiliopoulou, C. (2006). Identification and differential diagnosis of perimortem blunt force trauma in tubular long bones. *Forensic Science, Medicine, and Pathology* 2(4):221–229.

Müller, M. E. & Nazarian, S. K. P. (2010). *Müller AO classification of fractures—long bones.* Pamphlet. Last accessed at: https://kkh-hagen.de/wp-content/uploads/dokumente/Traumazentrum/mueller_ao_class.pdf

Murphy, M. S. & Juengst, S. L. (2020). Patterns of trauma across Andean South America: new discoveries and advances in interpretation. *International Journal of Paleopathology* 29:35–44.

Nabian, M. H., Zadegan, S. A., Zanjani, L. O. & Mehrpour, S. R. (2017). Epidemiology of joint dislocations and ligamentous/tendinous injuries among 2,700 patients: five-year trend of a tertiary center in Iran. *The Archives of Bone and Joint Surgery* 5(6):426–434.

Nystrom, K. (Ed.) (2017). *The Bioarchaeology of Dissection and Autopsy in the United States.* New York: Springer International Publishing.

Organization of Scientific Area Committees for Forensic Science (OSAC), Anthropology Subcommittee, (2016). *Controlled Experimental Bone Trauma Studies.* National Institute of Science and Technology. Last accessed at: https://www.nist.gov/osac/osac-research-and-development-needs

Osteoware [computer program]. (2011). *Osteoware: Standardized Skeletal Documentation Software.* Washington, DC: Smithsonian Institute National Museum of Natural History; https://osteoware.si.edu/

Osterholtz, A. (Ed.) (2020a). *The Poetics of Processing: Memory Formation, Identity, and the Handling of the Dead.* Louisville, CO: University Press of Colorado.

Osterholtz, A. (2020b). Collective bodies, collective identities: the development of identity in Bronze-Age Cyprus. In Knudson, K. J. & Stojanowski, C. M. (Eds.), *Bioarchaeology and Identity Revisited,* pp. 107–135. Gainesville: University Press of Florida.

Passalacqua, N. V. & Fenton, T. W. (2012). Developments in skeletal trauma: blunt-force trauma. In Dirkmaat, D. (Ed.), *A Companion to Forensic Anthropology,* pp. 400–411. New York: Blackwell Publishing.

Pathria, M. N., Chung, C. B. & Resnick, D. L. (2016). Acute and stress-related injuries of bone and cartilage: pertinent anatomy, basic biomechanics, and imaging perspective. *Radiology* 280(1):21–38.

Pérez, V. R. (2012). The taphonomy of violence: recognizing variation in disarticulated skeletal assemblages. *International Journal of Paleopathology* 2(2–3):156–165.

Pérez, V. R. (2016). The poetics of violence in bioarchaeology: integrating social theory with trauma analysis. In: Zuckerman, M. K. & Martin, D. L. (Eds.), *New Directions in Biocultural Anthropology,* pp. 453–469. New York: Wiley & Sons.

Pierce, M. C., Bertocci, G. E., Vogeley, E. & Moreland, M. S. (2004). Evaluating long bone fractures in children: a biomechanical approach with illustrative cases. *Child Abuse & Neglect* 28(5):505–524.

Raul, J. S., Ludes, B. & Willinger, R. (2008). Differential diagnosis of skeletal injuries. In Kimmerle, E. H. & Baraybar, J. P. (Eds.), *Skeletal Trauma: Identification of Injuries Resulting from Human Rights Abuse and Armed Conflict,* pp. 21–93. Boca Raton, FL: CRC press.

Redfern, R. (2016). *Injury and Trauma in Bioarchaeology: Interpreting Violence in Past Lives.* Cambridge: Cambridge University Press. doi:10.1017/9780511978579

Redfern, R. & Roberts, C. A. (2019). Trauma. In Buikstra, J. E. (Ed.), *Ortner's Identification of Pathological Conditions in Human Skeletal Remains,* 3rd edition, pp. 211–284. New York: Academic Press.

Redfern, R. C. & Austin, A. (2020). Ankylosis of a knee joint from medieval London: trauma, congenital anomaly or osteoarthritis? *International Journal of Paleopathology* 28:69–87.

Resnick, D. (2002). Degenerative disease of extraspinal locations. In Resnick, D. (Ed.), *Diagnosis of Bone and Joint Disorders*, 3rd edition, pp. 1271–1381. Philadelphia: Saunders.

Roberts, C. A. & Manchester, K. (2005). *Archaeology of Disease*. Stroud: Sutton Publishing.

Roberts, C. A. (2006). Trauma in biocultural perspective: past, present and future work in Britain. In Cox, M. & Mays, S. (Eds.), *Human Osteology in Archaeology and Forensic Science*, pp. 337–356. Cambridge: Cambridge University Press.

Sauer, N. (1998). The timing of injuries and manner of death: distinguishing among antemortem, perimortem, and postmortem trauma. In Reichs, K. (Ed.), *Forensic Osteology: Advances in the Identification of Human Remains*, 2nd edition, pp. 321–332. Springfield, IL: Charles C Thomas.

Smith, S. K. & Liston, M. A. (2020). Myositis ossificans traumatica with associated pseudarthroses in an adult from late Bronze Age Athens, Greece. *International Journal of Osteoarchaeology* 30(3):410–414.

Smith, O. E., Pope, E. E. & Symes, S. A. (2003). Look until you see: identification of trauma in skeletal material. In Steadman, D.W. (Ed.), *Hard Evidence: Case Studies in Forensic Anthropology*, pp. 138–154. Old Tappan, NJ: Pearson Education,

Steckel, R. H., Rose, J. C., Larsen, C. S. & Walker, P. L. (2002). Skeletal health in the Western Hemisphere from 4000 B.C. to the present. *Evolutionary Anthropology* 11:142–155.

Stodder, A. L. (2017). Quantifying impairment and disability in bioarchaeological assemblages. In Byrnes, J. F. & Muller, J. L. (Eds.), *Bioarchaeology of Impairment and Disability*, pp.183–200. New York: Springer, Cham.

Stone, A. (2020). Bound to please: the shaping of female beauty, gender theory, structural violence, and bioarchaeological investigations. In Sheridan, S. G. & Gregoricka, L. A. (Eds.), *Purposeful Pain: The Bioarchaeology of Intentional Suffering*, pp. 39–62. New York: Springer, Cham.

Symes, S. A., Berryman, H. E. & Smith, O. C. (1998). Saw marks in bone: Introduction and examination of residual kerf contour. In Reichs, K. J. (Ed.), *Forensic Osteology: Advances in the Identification of Human Remains*, 2nd edition, pp. 389–409. Springfield IL: Charles C. Thomas.

Symes, S. A., Williams, J. A., Murray, E. A., Hoffman, J. M., Holland, T. D., Saul, J. M., Saul, F. P. & Pope, E. J. (2002). Taphonomic context of sharp force trauma in suspected cases of human mutilation and dismemberment. In Haglund, W. D. & Sorg, M. H. (Eds.), *Advances in Forensic Taphonomy*, pp. 403–434. New York: CRC Press.

Symes, S. A., Chapman, E. N., Rainwater, C. W., Cabo, L. L. & Myster, S. M. (2010). *Knife and Saw Toolmark Analysis in Bone: A Manual Designed for the Examination of Criminal Mutilation and Dismemberment*. Pennsylvania: Mercyhurst College.

Symes, S. A., L'Abbé, E. N., Chapman, E. N., Wolff, I. & Dirkmaat, D. C. (2012). Interpreting traumatic injury to bone in medicolegal investigations. In Dirkmaat, D. C. (Ed.), *A Companion to Forensic Anthropology*, pp. 340–389. New York: Blackwell Publishing.

Tilley, L. (2015). *Theory and Practice in the Bioarchaeology of Care*. New York: Springer, Cham.

Tilley, L. & Cameron, T. (2014). Introducing the index of care: a web-based application supporting archaeological research into health-related care. *International Journal of Paleopathology* 6:5–9.

Tilley, L. & Schrenk, A. A. (2017). *New Developments in the Bioarchaeology of Care*. New York: Springer, Cham.

Torres Colón, G. A. & Smith, S. (2020). Meaningful play, meaningful pain: learning the purpose of injury in sport. In. Sheridan, S. G & Gregoricka, L. A. (Eds.), *Purposeful Pain: The Bioarchaeology of Intentional Suffering*, pp. 63–77. New York: Springer, Cham.

Toyne, J. M. (2018). A childhood of violence: a bioarchaeological comparison of mass death assemblages from ancient Peru. In Beauchesne, P. & Agarwal, S. C. (Eds.), *Children and Childhood in Bioarchaeology*, pp. 171–203. Gainesville: University Press of Florida.

Turner, C. H. (2006). Bone strength: current concepts. *Annals of the New York Academy of Sciences* 1068(1):429–446.

Villa, P. & Mahieu, E. (1991). Breakage patterns of human long bones. *Journal of Human Evolution* 21(1):27–48.

Villotte, S., Castex, D., Couallier, V., Dutour, O., Knüsel, C.J. & Henry-Gambier, D. (2010). Enthesopathies as occupational stress markers: evidence from the upper limb. *American Journal of Physical Anthropology* 142(2):224–234.

Villotte, S. & Knüsel, C.J. (2013). Understanding entheseal changes: definition and life course changes. *International Journal of Osteoarchaeology* 23(2):135–146.

Walczak, B. E., Johnson, C. N. & Howe, B. M. (2015). Myositis ossificans. *JAAOS-Journal of the American Academy of Orthopaedic Surgeons* 23(10):612–622.

Waldron, T. (2009). *Paleopathology*. Cambridge Manuals in Archaeology. Paleopathology: Cambridge Manuals in Archaeology.

Walker, P. L. (1997). Wife beating, boxing, and broken noses: skeletal evidence for the cultural patterning of violence. In Martin, D. L. & Frayer, D. W. (Eds.), *Troubled times: Violence and Warfare in the Past*, pp. 145– 179. Amsterdam: Gordon and Breach.

Walker, P. (2001). A Bioarchaeological perspective on the history of violence. *Annual Review of Anthropology* 30: 573–596.

Watkins, R. J. (2020). An alter(ed)native perspective on historical bioarchaeology. *Historical Archaeology* 54:17–33. doi:10.1007/s41636-019-00224-5

Wang, L. J., Zeng, N., Yan, Z. P., Li, J. T. & Ni, G. X. (2020). Post-traumatic osteoarthritis following ACL injury. *Arthritis Research & Therapy* 22:1–8.

Wedel, V. L. & Galloway, A. (2014). *Broken Bones: Anthropological Analysis of Blunt Force Trauma*, 2nd edition. Springfield, IL: CC Thomas.

Weiss, R. J., Wick, M. C., Ackermann, P. W. & Montgomery, S. M. (2010). Increased fracture risk in patients with rheumatic disorders and other inflammatory diseases—a case-control study with 53,108 patients with fracture. *The Journal of Rheumatology* 37(11):2247–2250.

Wheatley, B. P. (2008). Perimortem or postmortem bone fractures? An experimental study of fracture patterns in deer femora. *Journal of Forensic Sciences* 53(1):69–72.

Wheeler, S. M., Williams, L., Beauchesne, P. & Dupras, T. L. (2013). Shattered lives and broken childhoods: evidence of physical child abuse in ancient Egypt. *International Journal of Paleopathology* 3:71–82.

White, T. D. & Toth, N. (1989). Engis: preparation damage, not ancient cutmarks. *American Journal of Physical Anthropology* 78:361–368.

Wieberg, D. A. & Wescott, D. J. (2008). Estimating the timing of long bone fractures: correlation between the postmortem interval, bone moisture content, and blunt force trauma fracture characteristics. *Journal of Forensic Sciences* 53(5):1028–1034.

Yang, N. P., Chen, H. C., Phan, D. V., Yu, I. L., Lee, Y. H., Chan, C. L., … & Renn, J. H. (2011). Epidemiological survey of orthopedic joint dislocations based on nationwide insurance data in Taiwan, 2000–2005. *BMC Musculoskeletal Disorders* 12(1):1–7.

14
DEVELOPMENTAL CONDITIONS IN PALEOPATHOLOGY

Anne R. Titelbaum, Scott E. Burnett and D. Troy Case

Introduction

Variations in skeletal morphology arise from factors that affect growth and development. Such factors include single gene mutations, chromosomal abnormalities, teratogens, or multifactorial etiologies arising from the interactions of intrinsic (i.e., genetic) and extrinsic (i.e., environmental) influences (Hobbs et al., 2002). Although some skeletal variations may compromise an individual's longevity, the majority do not. And while some variations may be outwardly obvious in a living person, most are only discovered by accident, if at all (e.g., via medical imaging). Paleopathologists benefit from the ability to observe a skeleton in its entirety, and as a result, variations of skeletal development are frequently encountered, ranging from common and minor to rare and, at least occasionally, incompatible with life.

In the paleopathological literature, numerous terms have been used to refer to skeletal morphology that differs from the standard range of expression (Table 14.1). Some of these terms, however, convey negative connotations. As Turkel (1989:109) noted, the term "malformation" is derived from the Latin *malus* meaning evil, which conveys a pejorative sense, and similarly, "defect" derives from the Latin *deficere* meaning "to fail", which suggests that

Table 14.1 Terms used in the paleopathological literature to describe variations of skeletal morphology

Inborn anomaly
Congenital anomaly
Developmental anomaly
Congenital defect
Developmental defect
Congenital abnormality
Developmental abnormality
Congenital condition
Developmental condition
Congenital malformation
Developmental deviation
Anatomical variant

an individual did not form successfully, or has a shortcoming or deficiency. "Abnormal" too, generally refers to an undesirable deviation from the norm. Therefore, to avoid loaded terminology, we prefer to utilize developmental anomaly, developmental variant, or developmental condition to refer to skeletal morphology that differs from what is expected and is not life-threatening. We reserve malformation for those variations that are potentially life-threatening or present major structural or functional differences from the hypothetical norm.

The terms "developmental" and "congenital" are often used interchangeably, but their meanings are not precisely the same. A congenital condition is one with a prenatal origin that is perceptible at birth. Developmental conditions include these, as well as conditions that arise after birth as the skeleton matures (Barnes, 1994:1–2). Thus, the term "developmental" is more inclusive.

Many descriptions of developmental conditions in the published paleopathological literature consist of case reports, which can be valuable additions, particularly for rare and poorly documented conditions. That said, more systematic and population-based studies are necessary to improve our understanding of the frequencies and geographic and temporal distribution of developmental conditions. Fortunately, the past two decades have seen a significant increase in these kinds of studies.

The following pages will briefly address the etiology of developmental conditions and methodological considerations pertaining to their analysis. A synopsis of the past 20 years of paleopathological research concerning anomalies will then be presented, followed by a discussion that considers the observed differences in clinical versus archaeological frequencies.

The Etiology of Anomalies

Genetic and chromosomal disorders have the potential to affect growth and development from the time of conception. Examples of conditions that arise from spontaneous or inherited single gene mutations include achondroplasia, Marfan syndrome, osteogenesis imperfecta, and some forms of brachydactyly. Some even follow the classic Mendelian inheritance pattern. Conditions that arise from chromosomal abnormalities include Turner syndrome and the trisomies (e.g., Down syndrome). Chromosomal assays, pedigree and twin studies, and histological studies of embryos and fetuses were once the primary ways to identify developmental skeletal conditions that were likely genetic in origin. More recently, direct molecular analysis has identified specific genes linked to skeletal changes, such as the Indian hedgehog gene with fifth finger brachydactyly (Gao et al., 2001), and the *GDF6* gene with segmentation errors of vertebrae associated with Klippel-Feil syndrome (Tassabehji et al., 2008).

Beyond genes, the developing embryo and fetus are subject to the conditions of the maternal environment. Teratogens include toxins, infections, and medications that can pass from a pregnant mother to the developing embryo or fetus. For example, tobacco use or excessive consumption of alcohol while pregnant can cause developmental problems such as cleft palate, among others (Lorente et al., 2000). Infections such as syphilis can pass to the fetus and lead to dental anomalies in the child (e.g., Hutchinson teeth) (Hillson et al., 1998). The most infamous example is the drug thalidomide. It was widely prescribed during the 1950–1960s to treat nausea in pregnant women but tragically led to severe malformations including phocomelia in which the arms and/or legs are mostly or completely absent (Kim & Scialli, 2011).

Similarly, maternal health affects the developing offspring, as has been shown in both animals and humans. Diseases that produce high fever during pregnancy, such as tuberculosis, have been associated with major skeletal malformations among offspring (e.g., Graham & Edwards, 1998). And maternal nutritional deficiency, particularly in folate, vitamin A, and riboflavin, has been implicated as the cause of various developmental anomalies, including neural tube defects (e.g., spina bifida cystica and anencephaly), hypoplasia of the vertebral arch, coalitions between ribs and among bones of the hands and feet, club foot, the proportionate lengths of certain bones, and hypoplasia of the nasal area, ribs, or sternebrae (Warkany & Nelson, 1941; McDonald, 1961; Seller, 1987; See et al., 2008; Clagett-Dame & Knutson, 2011; Li et al., 2012).

Beyond the maternal environment, some anomalies may arise from mechanical stress during youth, prior to epiphyseal closure. The os acromiale, for example, is an accessory bone resulting from the failure of the acromial epiphysis to fuse to the scapula. Based on investigations that observed population, sex, and laterality differences in the frequencies of this trait, it appears that there may be a threshold level for the genetic expression that is exacerbated by physical activity (Case, Burnett, & Nielsen, 2006; Hunt & Bullen, 2007).

By understanding the etiology of specific developmental conditions, paleopathologists can begin to use them to better interpret lifeways in the past. For example, many genetic conditions that are directly inherited provide the potential for tracing relationships in archaeological cemeteries under the right circumstances (Stojanowski & Schillaci, 2006). When several skeletons in a cemetery share a single genetic anomaly, or when fewer skeletons share the anomaly but are buried in the same grave or discrete burial cluster, the probability of a shared genetic relationship is heightened (Sjovold, 1977). And if multiple traits are shared in common, the likelihood further increases (Alt et al., 1996). Rare developmental conditions can also play an important role in forensic investigations, by providing a unique trait that can assist in skeletal identification (Hunt & Bullen, 2007; Duncan & Stojanowski, 2008).

Methodological Considerations Concerning Developmental Conditions

Developmental conditions reported by paleopathologists are typically identified and studied visually through macroscopic analysis, with osteometric, imaging, and molecular techniques used as supporting evidence or diagnostic aids. Due to the rarity of major malformations and complex conditions such as syndromes and dysplasias, most of the focus is on minor and often asymptomatic anomalies.

Many of the specific methodological concerns surrounding the study of developmental variants are similar to those faced in other studies of morphological features. Some anomalies show age and/or sex bias, and so attention to sample composition may be needed. Clear definitions and descriptions of conditions improve intra- and inter-observer consistency and are essential for valid frequency comparisons. The morphogenetic approach, advocated by Barnes (1994, 2008, 2012a, 2012b), focuses on disturbances within developmental fields to best explain structural malformations in the skeleton and has proven useful for classification. It is often helpful to report frequencies explicitly by both element count and by individual to maximize potential comparisons, particularly as some bioarchaeological contexts may contain discrete individuals, while disturbed contexts and ossuaries may not. The affected side(s) should be noted with a description of whether the condition is bilateral, unilateral, or laterality unknown when the condition is present but only observable on one side.

Differential fragmentation and preservation may further reduce the potential for recovering or identifying conditions characterized by bone fragility such as osteogenesis imperfecta

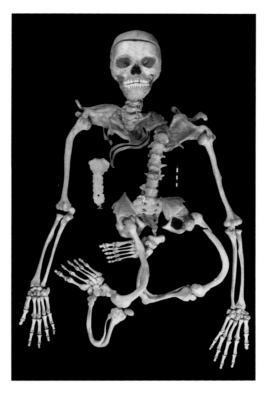

Figure 14.1   Osteogenesis imperfecta in a 20th c. young adult female (see Burnett, 2005:198). Note: most ribs were not pictured here. Raymond A. Dart Collection of Modern Human Skeletons. Photo by S. E. Burnett.

(Figure 14.1) or in compromised elements, such as cleft palate. In the case of serious malformations or conditions that may contribute to early death, the fragility of perinate or other non-adult remains can inhibit analysis. In other cases, careful attention is necessary to identify aplasia of elements, particularly in disarticulated remains; for example, missing facets on normally articulating elements can be seen in aplasia of the patella (Patrick & Waldron, 2003), and ulna (Mann et al., 1998).

Misidentification is a potential concern since developmental anomalies may be rare and, by definition, represent some departure from perceived normal morphology. Affected elements may not be easy to recognize, as is seen in carpal or tarsal bipartitions (Burnett & Case, 2011; Burnett et al., 2015), and may even resemble non-human species, as noted for the short, robust limbs seen in some dwarfing dysplasias (Hoffman, 1976). Indeed, the potential confusion between human and non-human should be considered, as demonstrated by Cook (2013) who described the misattribution of a hydrocephalic calf cranial vault as human hydrocephaly. More rarely, anomalies may be misidentified as a different element altogether, as seen in the erroneous identification of osseous lunate-triquetral coalition in the La Ferrassie II Neandertal as a scaphoid (Oberlin & Sakka, 1989).

A primary concern is misdiagnosis, as many developmental anomalies may mimic other forms of pathology in some way. Segmentation errors of the vertebrae, ribs, and long, short, and irregular bones of the appendicular skeleton can result in blocks of elements that are normally distinct and may be confused with ankylosis secondary to arthritis, trauma, or other conditions. Conversely, a failure of separate components to properly unite during development may be confused with trauma, as seen in smaller accessory bones of the hands or feet (Mann & Hunt, 2019), or os odontoideum (e.g., Titelbaum & Uceda Castillo, 2015; Wang et al., 2015). Stewart (1975) noted multiple cases where cranial dysraphism was misdiagnosed as trephination.

A related concern is that developmental conditions are not being recognized among skeletal remains. This issue is particularly relevant for syndromic conditions such as trisomy 21, where many skeletal findings may not be pathognomonic (e.g., brachydactyly). Revisiting collections where individual congenital anomalies have already been recorded may prove fruitful for the identification of conditions that may have eluded prior researchers. Identifying the co-occurrence of multiple variants, even relatively minor ones, might indicate specimens that are worthy of another look in the search for syndromes (Burnett, 2005).

Ultimately, we agree with Oostra and colleagues (2016) who point out the importance of paleopathologists recognizing atypical development in archaeological contexts but acknowledge the limited value of developing a thorough understanding of the myriad developmental conditions given their expected low rate of occurrence. Indeed, diagnosis of complex developmental conditions can be particularly difficult due to our reliance on skeletal remains in the absence of soft tissue, as well as preservation issues and other factors noted earlier. To best understand developmental conditions in the bioarchaeological record, it is important to take a broader analytical perspective that considers developmental aberration throughout the entire skeleton instead of a sole focus on particular elements or parts of the body (Spitery, 1983). It is also important to consider remains from all age groups, and we are particularly encouraged by the increased focus on subadults within paleopathology (e.g., Lewis, 2018a, 2018b).

Developmental Anomalies in Paleopathology

A survey of the recent paleopathological literature reveals that research on developmental anomalies includes case studies, population-based investigations, and studies that apply scientific and cultural perspectives to augment our understanding about anomalies and what their presence may indicate about prehistoric lifeways. Overall, it appears that research is trending away from case studies toward either informative problem-based investigations that address larger questions or ones based on quantitative research.

Case Studies

On a basic level, case studies present a detailed description of a developmental anomaly that was observed among skeletal remains. However, beyond simply expanding the temporal and geographic ranges of identified anomalies, it is important for these reports to incorporate robust differential diagnoses, meaningfully contribute to our ability to identify and understand the skeletal manifestation of anomalies, deliver new information by describing anomalies that have rarely been observed and reported, situate an anomaly in the context of the entire skeleton, and consider anomalies among subadult remains.

Case studies of rarely identified conditions are informative in that they present an opportunity to closely examine altered skeletal morphology (e.g., Palacios C. & Sierpe G., 2019). For example, Palamenghi et al. (2021) recently presented the first detailed description of a fetus with holoprosencephaly and cyclopia. This study documented in detail the severe malformations of the midline facial skeleton, premature fusion of cranial elements, and the single orbit. As a subtler example, Curate (2008) presented one of the first paleopathological descriptions of congenital os odontoideum, an anomaly where the odontoid process forms as an ossicle separate from the second cervical vertebra. Without a clear description of this condition, its presence could go unrecognized, the ossicle might be missed during archaeological excavation, and if recovered, the ossicle could easily be miscategorized.

Studies that include the examination of an entire skeleton of an individual enable paleopathologists to consider anomalies holistically and identify any co-occurring or associated pathologies. In one investigation, Usher and Christiansen (2000) presented a comprehensive analysis of a young adult who demonstrated numerous anomalies of the axial skeleton. By considering the suite of developmental errors, the authors were able to deduce that an initial anomaly occurred early during development and led to a cascade of subsequent anomalies during the developmental sequence. In the case of anomalies that affect the functioning of joints, such as radioulnar synostosis, it is important to acknowledge that individuals adapt by employing compensatory motions to overcome functional limitations (Antón & Polidoro, 2000), evidence of which may be observable through osteoarthritis and/or entheseal robusticity. Such observations provide information about the life and behavior of an individual affected by a long-term condition and underscore the importance of viewing the entire skeleton as a biomechanical unit.

Analyses that consider anomalies among subadult remains are relatively few, likely due to challenges of identification among bones that have not reached skeletal maturity. Such challenges are particularly true of dwarfism, since diagnostic features are often not macroscopically visible in subadult skeletons. One investigation, however, presented the morphological features of a subadult with Madelung's deformity and Leri-Weill dyschondrosteosis, a rarely reported form of mesomelic dysplasia characterized by shortened bones of the forearm and leg, short stature, and misaligned wrist joints (Whitmore & Buzon, 2019). Identification of the condition was made through comparative observations of an adult skeleton with the same condition and through age-matched measurement comparisons with subadult remains from the same site. Another investigation considered microscopic indications of dwarfism in perinates by examining trabecular bone microarchitecture with micro-computerized tomography (CT) (Colombo et al., 2018). This study was able to detect microarchitectural changes indicating a functional deficit of the growth plate that can be used to identify genetic dwarfism. These cases are particularly informative for understanding the expression of anomalies over the life course and how they may be identified in subadult skeletal remains.

Population-Based Investigations

Population-based investigations shift the analytical focus from an individual to a sample, or to multiple samples. To conduct population studies, the presence and absence of developmental anomalies are tabulated for each skeleton in a sample, excluding those that could not be observed for the condition. This approach is the only way that an estimated population frequency of anomalies can be calculated. Once calculated, it is possible to compare the frequency between and within populations, as well as over time through diachronic analysis.

Population studies via direct skeletal analysis have some important functions. First, they have the potential to provide better estimates of the population frequency of developmental conditions than are found in the clinical literature, because clinical samples typically rely on medical imaging done for non-research purposes. Second, population data can identify if variations in frequency exist for a particular anomaly, which is a strong clue that there may be genetic or environmental factors involved in its expression. It is not uncommon to find only minor differences in frequency between populations of the same ancestry, even when separated by a considerable distance and hundreds of years of time, while major differences are seen between populations with a more distant relationship (e.g., Tenney, 1991; Case & Burnett, 2012; Case et al., 2016). Finally, population studies provide the reference frequency against which an archaeological sample can be compared in order to assess whether the condition is unusually concentrated in a cemetery or larger region, suggesting a heightened frequency due to genetic relatedness or environmental insult.

Interpopulation Comparisons: Single Anomalies

While population studies involving simple nonmetric traits of the cranium and dentition have been common for many decades (e.g., Spence, 1974; Corruccini, 1982; Bondioli et al., 1986), population studies involving developmental conditions did not gain traction until the late 1980s and early 1990s. In 1988, for example, Cybulski studied brachydactyly, a condition characterized by one or two disproportionately short digital bones, in a skeletal series representing eight prehistoric archaeological sites in British Columbia (Figure 14.2a). This study was one of the first to document variation in the population frequency of a developmental condition, and in doing so, was able to identify clustering of two or more cases at several of the sites. Evidence of the heritability of brachydactyly in family and pedigree studies (Bell, 1951; Temtamy & Aglan, 2008) supports the possibility of genetic connections between the sites.

Other studies have considered single developmental anomalies among multiple samples as a way to gauge the variability present in human populations and to better understand the etiology. Accessory bones such as os intermetatarseum (Case et al., 1998) and accessory navicular (Offenbecker & Case, 2012), both heritable conditions, have demonstrated frequency variation among populations. Bipartitions, where a normally single bone develops as two separate elements, have been studied as well. Examples include the bipartite medial cuneiform in the foot (Burnett & Case, 2011), and bipartite trapezoid in the hand (Burnett et al., 2015). Such studies provide information on the relative frequency of these conditions in different populations and may help clinicians distinguish developmental conditions from trauma.

One of the better studied developmental conditions is tarsal coalition. Tarsal coalition is a segmentation error that occurs when two tarsal bones fail to separate properly during the first trimester of development. Most often, there is a band of cartilaginous or fibrous tissue that joins the two bones together, resulting in matching skeletal lesions where the two bones were connected (Figure 14.2b). Coalitions have been shown to be quite variable in frequency in different populations (Burnett & Wilczak, 2012; Case & Burnett, 2012), likely due to a strong genetic component to their etiology (Leonard, 1974). Population research into these conditions suggests that the most common intertarsal coalitions involve the calcaneus among individuals of European heritage, and the midfoot tarsals in populations of African ancestry (Burnett & Case, 2005; Case & Burnett, 2012; Albee, 2020).

Data on population variation in frequencies of coalitions throughout the foot have been used by Burnett and Wilczak (2012) to highlight frequency similarities between East Asian and Native American populations. East Asians tend to show the highest frequencies of

Developmental Conditions in Paleopathology

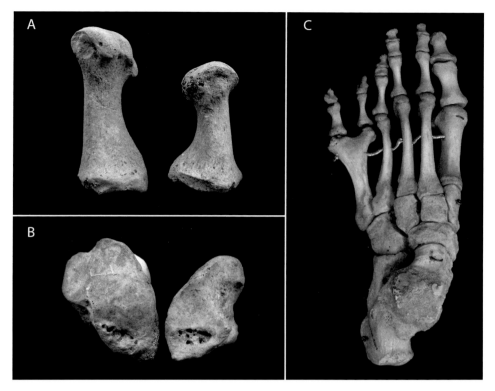

Figure 14.2 Anomalies of the foot: (a) Brachydactylous right first metatarsal (on the right), compared with a nonbrachydactylous left first metatarsal. Note the short length but comparatively thick diaphysis with relatively large proximal and distal ends. *Chullpa* 7, Marcajirca, Ancash, Peru. Photo by A. R. Titelbaum; (b) Nonosseous coalition of a right navicular and first cuneiform. The lesions on the articular surfaces indicate the location where the cartilaginous or fibrous band connected the two bones. *Chullpa* 26, Marcajirca, Ancash, Peru. Photo by A. R. Titelbaum; (c) Postaxial polydactyly, left foot. NMHM 1996.0017, National Museum of Health and Medicine, Silver Spring, MD. Photo by S. E. Burnett.

interbone coalitions throughout the foot, and some of these high frequencies date back to the Neolithic in Siberia. The presence of calcaneonavicular and third metatarsal-third cuneiform coalitions in Kennewick Man speaks to their antiquity in the New World as well (Case, 2014). Carpals have also been studied for coalitions (Burnett, 2011), but they are much less common in most populations than coalitions of the foot, and population data from skeletons have yet to be published.

Interpopulation Comparisons: Multiple Anomalies

Several population studies have focused on multiple developmental anomalies of the axial skeleton, variably including those affecting the vertebrae, ribs, and the sternum (Merbs, 2003; Masnicova & Benus, 2003; Sarry El-Din & El Banna, 2006; Hussein et al., 2009; Tague, 2018; Molto et al., 2019; Titelbaum, 2020; Smith-Guzman, 2021). These studies are important because they not only establish regional frequency baselines that will be useful for future comparative investigations, they also consider congenital variations that have been associated with severe nutritional stress in laboratory studies of animals and therefore have the potential to be markers of such developmental stress in humans when considered together as a group.

Interestingly, three studies were conducted on different populations from ancient Egypt showing a wide range of variation in the frequency of clefting of the sacral neural arch. Frequencies at Giza, near the Nile river, are quite low, while frequencies at Dakhleh Oasis are reported to be four times higher, and those at Bahriyah Oasis are nearly 19 times higher (Sarry El-Din & El Banna, 2006; Hussein et al., 2009; Molto et al., 2019). Scoring differences may account for some of this variation, but the two studies with the lowest and highest frequencies included some of the same authors. Such a high degree of variation suggests the possibility that genetic and/or nutritional differences during early development might be a contributing factor to these frequencies (see Mutlu et al., 2020).

Another study focused on Medieval individuals from two sites in Slovakia and found sacral clefting, sternal apertures, and segmentation errors of the vertebrae to be among the most common developmental anomalies (Masnicova & Benus, 2003) (Figure 14.3). Lumbar ribs were quite common at one of the two sites but absent from the other. More recently, two studies focused on Pre-Columbian South America. One considered a sample of

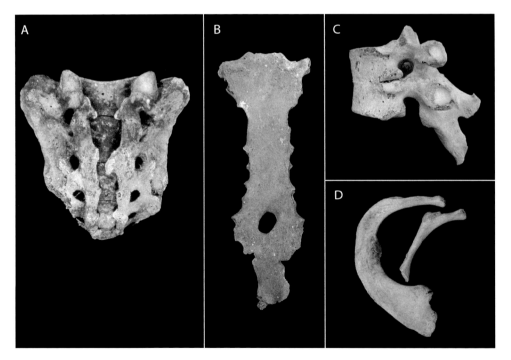

Figure 14.3 Developmental anomalies of the axial skeleton: (a) Sacral clefting, posterior view, Raymond A. Dart Archaeological Human Remains Collection. Photo by S. E. Burnett; (b) Sternal aperture, anterior view, *Chullpa* 7, Marcajirca, Ancash, Peru. Photo by A. R. Titelbaum; (c) Segmentation error of adjacent thoracic vertebrae (block vertebrae), left lateral view, Raymond A. Dart Collection of Modern Human Skeletons. Photo by S. E. Burnett; (d) Cervical rib with articular facet on the body of the first rib, superior view, Raymond A. Dart Collection of Modern Human Skeletons. Photo by S. E. Burnett.

Panamanian remains from 12 sites and reported frequencies for several conditions including cleft neural arches and segmentation errors of the vertebrae and ribs (Smith-Guzman, 2021). Another took a diachronic approach, by considering vertebral, rib, and sternal anomalies among successive prehistoric Peruvian populations that utilized the same geographic location, discussed further below (Titelbaum, 2020).

Intrapopulation Comparisons

Because some anomalies are inherited through autosomal dominance, their presence in multiple individuals in a cemetery may reveal familial relationships. Nevertheless, only a limited amount of research has been conducted utilizing developmental conditions to answer questions about intracemetery genetic relationships. While biological distance studies focusing on cranial or dental nonmetric traits have been common in anthropology for several decades, the rarity of most developmental conditions means that traditional multivariate analyses are less effective because the absence of rarer traits is common, and sharing that absence in common would cause two groups to appear more genetically similar than is actually the case. Therefore, univariate statistical approaches are still common. Generally, individual variant frequencies are compared with a reference sample from related sites or from a population with a similar genetic background to identify cemeteries or burial clusters with unusually high frequencies of a given anomaly. Individuals sharing a trait with a higher frequency than expected based on the reference sample are hypothesized relatives (Alt & Vach, 1992, 1995). If they share a second trait in common, the probability of a relationship increases.

One example is a study by Case et al. (2016) that considered ten developmental anomalies of the feet to identify possible genetic relatives in three archaeological cemeteries – two from medieval Denmark and one from 17th century London. Using reference samples from the same place and time period to compare frequencies, the authors were able to identify a high frequency of tarsal coalition affecting the calcaneus in one of the medieval Danish cemeteries. All affected individuals were male. Unfortunately, none of the males shared any other uncommon foot anomalies that might have bolstered the case for a relationship, though they did all seem to date to the early half of the cemetery's period of use and may have lived within a few generations of each other. Tur et al. (2019) used a similar approach to identify two probable relatives among a sample of 59 burials based on presence of a rare transverse basilar cleft at a site in the Altai Mountains of Russia. As another example, Titelbaum et al. (2015) identified two individuals with Madelung's deformity and possible Leri-Weill dyschondrosteosis within one of six commingled multi-individual tombs at a prehispanic cemetery in the Peruvian Andes. Given the rarity of this condition, it is likely that the two individuals were related, which suggests that tombs were used for familial interment. Not long after, excavation at the same site revealed three individuals with brachydactyly but from two different tombs (Titelbaum et al., 2021). As brachydactyly is also a rare condition, two individuals with this anomaly in one tomb further support the suggestion that tombs were used for familial interment, and the third individual in a different tomb may reflect postmarital residence.

Diachronic Population Comparisons

A few investigations have considered developmental anomalies among successive populations, offering insight into how genetic relationships, cultural behavior, or environmental factors change over time. For example, by considering the fluctuating frequency of the palatine torus among 12 Anatolian populations ranging from the Early Bronze Age to the early

20th century, Eroğlu & Erdal (2008) were able to document changes in gene flow associated with the recurring invasions and migrations along the Silk Road during Medieval times. In another investigation, Titelbaum (2020) examined axial anomalies among three populations that successively occupied the same location on the littoral of Peru. Though the types of anomalies were similar among the groups, the pattern of frequencies differed, which raises the possibility for genetic drift, in-migration, and/or cultural changes (e.g., postmarital residence, elite endogamy).

Research Inquiries

Some recent investigations have turned toward clarifying diagnostic criteria for the identification of developmental anomalies, incorporating a myriad of novel analytical techniques to augment macroscopic analyses, and testing hypotheses regarding the etiology of anomalies. These research foci improve paleopathological analysis, reveal the potential of technological applications, and improve our understanding about anomalies.

A number of studies have presented diagnostic criteria for identifying developmental anomalies. These publications include the compendia of axial and appendicular anomalies by Barnes (1994; 2012a) and articles that focus on specific anomalies, such as spina bifida (Molto et al., 2019), cranial dysraphism (Halling & Seidemann, 2018), tarsal coalitions (Case & Burnett, 2012; Albee, 2020), and hip dysplasia (Mitchell & Redfern, 2008, 2011). With their detailed morphological descriptions and images, these investigations constitute an important resource for paleopathologists, particularly since they provide a standardized set of criteria to be followed. These publications not only improve diagnoses, they also promote consistent observations among researchers and enable findings to be compared.

Other studies of developmental anomalies have incorporated a variety of analytical techniques to diagnose conditions and their effects on the individual. Such approaches go beyond standard observations by utilizing imaging technology, histology, stable isotope analysis, and molecular techniques. For example, one multidisciplinary investigation considered spina bifida occulta, a developmental anomaly whose phenotype is related to genetic and environmental factors including maternal dietary intake of folate. This investigation explored how genetic and dietary information could create an overall picture of health in the population through a combination of molecular analysis, paleoethnobotanical and zooarchaeological analyses, and stable isotope analysis (Armstrong et al., 2013).

Imaging technology (e.g., radiography, CT) is particularly useful as a diagnostic tool, as it enables nondestructive and noninvasive observations of an individual that goes beyond what is visible through macroscopic observation. For example, Panzer et al. (2018) performed a full-body CT examination of an artificially mummified body of a young adult male from the Capuchin Catacombs of Palermo, Sicily. Not only were skeletal features and anomalies observable, this technology enabled the visualization of soft tissue structures, and together, the findings contributed to a diagnosis of Marfan syndrome. Specifically, it was possible to observe a proximal aortic dissection which is a life-threatening condition uncommonly observed in young individuals but a characteristic finding among individuals with Marfan syndrome.

Since it is not always clear why skeletal variants arise, several studies have investigated etiological factors of anomalies including os acromiale, as described above. As another example, it has previously been suggested that supracondylar processes of the humerus are related to mechanical stress, however, Palamenghi et al. (2020) were able to challenge this suggestion by observing supracondylar processes in newborn individuals. Observing this trait in newborns suggests a congenital origin and does not support the idea that it results from biomechanical factors associated with day-to-day activities. Similar investigations have focused on the etiology of sutural ossicles of the cranium (O'Laughlin, 2004; Wilczak & Ousley, 2009).

Insight into Prehistoric Cultural Behavior

The presence of developmental anomalies may provide insight into prehistoric cultural behavior. Such insight is gained by considering the effects of the anomaly on the individual's quality of life, in terms of functionality, health, and treatment in society. Further, how an individual's body was treated after death provides important cultural insights, as do artistic renderings of anomalous traits. Developmental anomalies may therefore offer insight into prehistoric lifeways.

Individuals with severe developmental conditions may be faced with functional limitations in daily activities that may limit their ability to access resources (Cormier & Buikstra, 2017). The survival of these individuals may therefore depend on care and assistance from the community (Oxenham et al., 2009; Tilley & Oxenham, 2011). Palma Málaga and Makowski (2019) described a case of an older adult female from Pachacamac, Peru with severe osteoarthritic destruction of the right shoulder and multiple anomalies including bilateral cervical ribs. Cervical ribs may cause thoracic outlet syndrome, a chronic form of neurovascular impingement that affects the motor functioning of the upper extremity and may lead to progressive nerve damage. The authors therefore suggested that the individual likely required assistance, direct support, and accommodation by the community.

Beyond the limitations imposed by the anomaly itself, co-occurring pathological observations provide information about cultural behavior. For example, relative health and evidence of traumatic injury may reflect access to resources and potentially how the individual was treated. How the individual was treated is also expressed by the archaeological context in which the individual was found. Burial location, burial treatment, and grave offerings can provide insight into how the individual and ostensibly their anomaly was regarded by their community. By contextualizing developmental conditions, it is therefore possible to gain insight into the challenges that the individual faced, as well as prehistoric cultural behavior (Vairamuthu & Pfeiffer, 2018).

Interestingly, depictions of developmental anomalies have been identified in prehistoric art. For example, Egyptian iconography includes dwarfs (Dasen, 1988), and polydactyly (where an individual has an extra finger or toe, see Figure 14.2c) has been depicted in rock art, pottery figurines, and lithic stelae among pre-Columbian societies in the Americas (Case, Hill et al., 2006; Standen et al., 2018). Although the renderings are subject to a variety of interpretations, they do suggest that the anomalies were present in the community and did not go unnoticed. Polydactylism is a relatively rare condition, and while the number of archaeological cases is few, the anomaly has been depicted relatively frequently. What accounts for this frequency is unclear; however, rather than represent an artistic cannon, it appears that the renderings likely represent observations of the condition. It is also plausible that the frequency of depictions reflects a special status conferred to polydactylous individuals, which appears to be supported by differential burial treatment given to those with the trait (Case, Hill et al., 2006; Titelbaum et al., 2017).

Developmental anomalies may also provide clues about population dynamics (Barnes, 1994, Merbs, 2003; Offenbecker & Case, 2012; Case & Burnett, 2012; Case et al., 2017; Titelbaum, 2020). Unusually high frequencies of an otherwise uncommon anomaly may suggest that the population experienced genetic isolation with low gene flow (Barnes, 1994; Merbs, 2004; Titelbaum, 2020; Smith-Guzmán, 2021) and may reveal information about evolutionary relationships and trends (Le Minor & Trost, 2004; Williams et al., 2016). For example, Tocheri et al. (2016) observed that while coalitions were infrequently observed among western gorillas, they were present in relatively high frequencies among the hands and feet of two eastern gorilla subspecies. The authors suggest that the anomalies likely became common due to a founder effect and subsequent reproductive isolation after the eastern gorillas diverged from the western during the early to middle Pleistocene.

Frequency of Developmental Conditions

Compared to other topics such as trauma and infectious disease, developmental anomalies have been reported relatively infrequently in the paleopathological literature. And when developmental conditions are reported, it appears that there is a discrepancy between the frequencies reported for clinical and paleopathological contexts (e.g., Burnett, 2005). In some cases, frequencies may seem to be higher among archaeological samples, as seen in some cases of brachydactyly (e.g., Cybulski, 1988; Titelbaum et al., 2021) or tarsal coalitions (Case & Burnett, 2012). In other cases, conditions that are relatively common in a clinical context are rarely seen archaeologically, such as trisomy 21 (e.g., Rivollat et al., 2014) or cleft palate (e.g., Phillips & Sivilich, 2006).

To begin to understand the differences in numbers, it is worth reiterating that neither clinical nor paleopathological samples can be assumed to be representative of the populations from which they derive (e.g., Jackes, 2011; Sellier, 2011). In the medical context, clinicians are generally limited to observing individuals who seek medical attention, and even then, less apparent anomalous traits may not be identified during visual inspection. Indeed, it is not uncommon for developmental anomalies to be found incidentally during clinical consult for a different reason. In the paleopathological context, it is important to note that archaeological sites are rarely excavated in full, and an individual's burial location and treatment may vary by demographic factors such as age or sex, status, or cause of death, among others. Furthermore, even when present, developmental conditions may not be recognized or published for many reasons – ranging from sample size, representativeness, and taphonomic factors to those that relate to the professional training and research foci of the analyst. The published medical and paleopathological literature therefore reflect a subset of potential developmental anomalies, with significant results and highly unusual cases or frequencies more likely to be reported than minor cases or those with insignificant results.

What Accounts for Higher Frequencies of Developmental Conditions Among Archaeological Samples?

As noted above, paleopathological reports concerning developmental conditions are few, which may underscore their overall rarity. That said, when rare anomalies are reported, the paleopathological frequencies may be higher than those reported in the clinical literature. When higher archaeological frequencies occur, it may be due to the genetic relatedness among the sample; indeed, small population sizes, low gene flow, and factors of endogamy may lead to higher frequencies of rare heritable traits, especially if it is a kin group that is represented in a burial context (Alt & Vach, 1992, 1995; Stojanowski & Schillaci, 2006; Case et al., 2017).

What Accounts for Lower Frequencies of Developmental Conditions Among Archaeological Samples?

Several factors may account for the overall low incidence of developmental conditions across the paleopathological record. One relevant possibility is that infanticide was practiced prehistorically, as historical cases of infanticide have been noted (e.g., Hrdlicka, 1908; Gregg et al., 1981) and cross-cultural studies of infanticide have found that the birth of malformed or ill neonates is one of the primary motivations for the practice (Daly & Wilson, 1984; Scrimshaw, 1984). Because infanticide is typically committed at or around the time of birth in ways that may not leave skeletal manifestations (Scrimshaw, 1984) archaeological identification of infanticide has focused on mortality profiles and context (e.g., Smith & Kahila, 1992; Mays, 1993; Mays & Evers, 2011). However, interpretations of possible infanticide have been contested (e.g., Gowland & Chamberlain, 2002; Gilmore & Halcrow, 2014).

Another reason that may account for the rarity of anomalies is that individuals with observable conditions may have received differential mortuary treatment that removed them from typical burial locations. Although atypical burials of individuals with developmental conditions have not frequently been observed (see Lewis, 2016), examples include a human fetus with anencephaly that was found among mummified monkeys and ibises at Hermopolis (Egypt) (Geoffroy Saint-Hilaire, 1832–1837). While the nonnormative treatment of this individual may have occurred due to their morphology, various interpretations have been drawn with respect to ancient Egyptian attitudes toward developmental conditions (Dasen & Leroi, 2005).

Another potential explanation that can account for the rarity is that individuals with developmental conditions may not have survived to adulthood, and it tends to be more challenging to identify conditions in subadult skeletons that have not yet developed more visible characteristics associated with the conditions. However, as research concerning the remains of subadults has increased in recent years (see Halcrow & Tayles, 2018), it has been found that many developmental conditions are observable among fetuses, infants, and children (Lewis, 2016; 2018a; 2018b). Indeed, developmental conditions have been found to be the most common paleopathological observations made in perinatal skeletal remains from archaeological contexts (Lewis, 2018a). Certainly, the archaeological occurrence of severe conditions in older individuals (e.g., Hawkes & Wells, 1978; Mann et al., 1992) implies that they should also be present in subadults and also suggests that infanticide should not be assumed even when physical differences would have been apparent at the time of birth.

A related possibility is that developmental conditions are going unrecognized during paleopathological analysis. As an example, trisomy 21 (Down syndrome) is one of the most commonly occurring genetic syndromes in modern humans, occurring in roughly 1 out of 700 live births in the United States (Mai et al., 2019), but is rarely reported in the paleopathological literature. Usually arising from chromosomal non-disjunction, individuals with trisomy 21 display intellectual deficiencies, developmental delays, increased risk of cardiac and digestive tract issues, and skeletal manifestations including brachycephaly, depressed nasal bridge, micrognathia, dental agenesis, tooth transposition, tooth crowding, and digital hypoplasia (e.g., Aufderheide & Rodriguez-Martin, 1998; Rivollat et al., 2014). The predicted risk of a trisomy 21 birth increases with maternal age: from ~1/1500 for pregnant women at 20 years of age, to ~1/350 at 35 years of age, and ~1/25 in women at 50 years of age (Morris et al., 2002). Despite these elevated frequencies, only a few cases have been proposed in the paleopathological literature (e.g., Brothwell, 1960; Charlier, 2008; Halle et al., 2019;

Rivollat et al., 2014). In fact, recent aDNA testing of two of the three individuals proposed to be trisomy 21 from Germany, revealed diploidy for the 21st chromosome, conclusively rejecting a Down syndrome diagnosis in both (Halle et al., 2019).

While infanticide, differential burial treatment, or lower maternal age at pregnancy may contribute to the general paucity of trisomy 21 cases in the paleopathological record, these do not seem to wholly account for the disparity in frequencies (Spitery, 1983; Halle et al., 2019). Indeed, it seems more likely that paleopathologists may not be recognizing trisomy 21 through skeletal analysis, since the morphology associated with trisomy 21 is not pathognomonic. It is therefore likely that cases have been missed, and it may be that the reanalysis of skeletons that demonstrated the combination of some characteristics in prior studies, such as reduced stature and hyperbrachycephaly for example, may yield additional morphological traits that occur at higher rates in trisomy 21, such as tooth transposition (Shapira et al., 2000). Such targeted reanalysis may prove productive in narrowing the disparity between expected and observed frequencies.

Conclusions

While there is still room for case studies that describe atypical skeletal morphology, the literature over the past 20 years demonstrates that research concerning developmental anomalies has moved toward population-based investigations that consider relationships within and between populations, revealing population histories and migration patterns, and identifying familial linkages within cemeteries. Other studies have identified individual behavior and adaptation to long-term conditions and have interpreted cultural behavior toward individuals with developmental differences. It is only through population-based investigations however, that frequencies of traits will be revealed, permitting inter- and intrapopulation comparisons, and a better understanding of the differences between clinical and archaeological frequencies. As such, research concerning developmental anomalies represents a growth area in paleopathology, particularly for population-based research.

Acknowledgments

SEB would like to acknowledge those whose bodies were donated for study in the Raymond A. Dart Collection, and the assistance of Brendon Billings and Anja Meyer – both of the University of Witwatersrand – and Kristen Pearlstein of the National Museum of Health and Medicine (Silver Spring, MD). ART would like to thank the students and staff of the 2013–2017 seasons of the Huari-Ancash Bioarchaeological Field School. The pictured human skeletal remains from Marcajirca were excavated by the field school and curated in Ancash.

References

Albee, M. E. (2020). Diagnosing tarsal coalition in medieval Exeter. *International Journal of Paleopathology* 28:32–41. https://doi.org/10.1016/j.ijpp.2019.11.005

Alt, K. W., Pichler, S., Vach, W., Huckenbeck, W. & Stloukal, M. (1996). Early Bronze Age family burial from Velke Pavlovice. Verification of kinship hypothesis by odontologic and other nonmetric traits. *Homo* 46:256–266.

Alt, K. W. & Vach, W. (1992). Non-spatial analysis of "genetic kinship" in skeletal remains. In Schader, M. (Ed.), *Analyzing and Modeling Data and Knowledge: Proceedings of the 15th Annual Conference of the "Gesellschaft für Klassifikation e.V"*, pp. 247–256. Berlin: Springer-Verlag.

Alt, K. W. & Vach, W. (1995). Odontologic kinship analysis in skeletal remains: concepts, methods, and results. *Forensic Science International* 74(1–2):99–113. https://doi.org/10.1016/0379-0738(95)01740-a

Antón, S. C. & Polidoro, G. M. (2000). Prehistoric radio-ulnar synostosis: implications for function. *International Journal of Osteoarchaeology* 10:189–197. https://doi.org/10.1002/1099-1212 (200005/06)10:3<189::AID-OA521>3.0.CO;2-G

Armstrong, S., Cloutier, L., Arredondo, C., Roksandic, M. & Matheson, C. (2013). Spina bifida in a pre-Columbian Cuban population: a paleoepidemiological study of genetic and dietary risk factors. *International Journal of Paleopathology* 3:19–29. https://doi.org/10.1016/j.ijpp.2013.01.004

Aufderheide, A. C. & Rodriguez-Martin, C. (1998). *The Cambridge Encyclopedia of Human Paleopathology*. Cambridge: Cambridge University Press.

Barnes, E. (1994). *Developmental Defects of the Axial Skeleton in Paleopathology*. Niwot: University of Colorado Press.

Barnes, E. (2008). Congenital anomalies. In Pinhasi, R. & Mays, S. (Eds.), *Advances in Human Paleopathology*, pp. 329–362. Chichester: John Wiley & Sons Ltd.

Barnes, E. (2012a). *Atlas of Developmental Field Anomalies of the Human Skeleton: A Paleopathology Perspective*. New York: Wiley-Blackwell. https://doi.org/10.1002/9781118430699

Barnes, E. (2012b). Developmental disorders in the skeleton. In Grauer, A. L. (Ed.), *A Companion to Paleopathology*, pp. 380–400. New York: Wiley-Blackwell. https://doi.org/10.1002/9781444345940.ch21

Bell, J. (1951). On brachydactyly and symphalangism. In Penrose, L. S. (Ed.), *Treasury of Human Inheritance*, Vol. 5, pp. 1–31. London: Cambridge University Press.

Bondioli, L., Corruccini, R. S. & Macchiarelli, R. (1986). Familial segregation in the iron age community of Alfedena, Abruzzo, Italy, based on osteodental trait analysis. *American Journal of Physical Anthropology* 71:393–400.

Brothwell, D. R. (1960). A possible case of mongolism in a Saxon population. *Annals of Human Genetics* 24:141–150. https://doi.org/10.1111/j.1469-1809.1959.tb01727.x

Burnett, S. E. (2005). *Developmental Variation in South African Bantu: Variant Co-Occurrence and Skeletal Asymmetry* (Unpublished doctoral dissertation). Arizona State University, Tempe, Arizona.

Burnett, S. E. (2011). Hamate-pisiform coalition: morphology, clinical significance, and a simplified classification scheme for carpal coalition. *Clinical Anatomy* 24:188–196. https://doi.org/10.1002/ca.21086

Burnett, S. E. & Case, D. T. (2005). Naviculo-cuneiform I coalition: evidence of significant differences in tarsal coalition frequency. *The Foot* 15:80–85. https://doi.org/10.1016/j.foot.2005.02.006

Burnett, S. E. & Case, D. T. (2011). Bipartite medial cuneiform: new frequencies from skeletal collections and a meta-analysis of previous cases. *Homo* 62:109–125. https://doi.org/10.1016/j.jchb.2011.01.002

Burnett, S. E., Stojanowski, C. M. & Mahakkanukrauh, P. (2015). Six new examples of the bipartite trapezoid bone: morphology, significant population variation, and an examination of pre-existing criteria to identify bipartition of individual carpal bones. *Annals of Anatomy-Anatomischer Anzeiger* 198:58–65. https://doi.org/10.1016/j.aanat.2014.11.002

Burnett, S. E. & Wilczak, C. A. (2012). Tarsal and tarsometatarsal coalitions from mound C (Ocmulgee Macon Plateau site, Georgia): implications for understanding the patterns, origins, and antiquity of pedal coalitions in native American populations. *Homo* 63:167–181. https://doi.org/10.1016/j.jchb.2012.03.004

Case, D. T. (2014). Bones of the hands and feet. In Owsley, D. W. & Jantz, R. L. (Eds.), *Kennewick Man: The Scientific Investigation of an Ancient American Skeleton*, pp. 249–278. College Station: Texas A&M University Press.

Case, D. T. & Burnett, S. E. (2012). Identification of tarsal coalition and frequency estimates from skeletal samples. *International Journal of Osteoarchaeology*, 22:667–684. https://doi.org/10.1002/oa.1228

Case, D. T., Burnett, S. E. & Nielsen, T. (2006). Os acromiale: population differences and their etiological significance. *Homo* 57(1):1–18. https://doi.org/10.1016/j.jchb.2005.11.001

Case, D. T., Hill, R. J., Merbs, C. F., M. & Fong, M. (2006). Polydactyly in the prehistoric American Southwest. *International Journal of Osteoarchaeology* 16:221–235. https://doi.org/10.1002/oa.820

Case, D. T., Jones, L. B. & Offenbecker, A. M. (2016). Skeletal kinship analysis using developmental anomalies of the foot. *International Journal of Osteoarchaeology* 27:192–205. https://doi.org/10.1002/oa.2529

Case, D. T., Ossenberg, N. S. & Burnett, S. E. (1998). Os intermetatarseum: a heritable accessory bone of the human foot. *American Journal of Physical Anthropology* 107:199–209. https://doi.org/10.1002/(SICI)1096-8644(199810)107:2<199::AID-AJPA6>3.0.CO;2-Q

Charlier, P. (2008). The value of palaeoteratology and forensic pathology for the understanding of atypical burials: two Mediterranean examples from the field. In Murphy, E. M. (Ed.), *Deviant Burial in the Archaeological Record*, pp. 57–70. Oxford: Oxbow Books.

Clagett-Dame, M. & Knutson, D. (2011). Vitamin A in reproduction and development. *Nutrients* 3(4):385–428. https://doi.org/10.3390/nu3040385

Colombo, A., Hoogland, M., Coqueugniot, H., Dutour, O. & Waters-Rist, A. (2018). Trabecular bone microarchitecture analysis, a way for an early detection of genetic dwarfism? Case study of a dwarf mother's offspring. *International Journal of Paleopatholog* 20:65–71. https://doi.org/10.1016/j.ijpp.2017.12.002

Cook, D. C. (2013). Normal goat or diseased human? Disciplinary boundaries and methodological traps in the analysis of fragmentary remains at Franchthi Cave, Greece. In Osterholtz A. J., Baustian, K. M. & Martin, D. L. (Eds.), *Commingled and Disarticulated Human Remains: Working Toward Improved Theory, Method, and Data*, pp. 255–263. New York: Springer.

Cormier, A. A. & Buikstra, J. E. (2017). Impairment, disability, and identity in the Middle Woodland period: life at the juncture of achondroplasia, pregnancy, and infection. In Byrnes, J. F. & Muller, J. L. (Eds.), *Bioarchaeology of Impairment and Disability: Theoretical, Ethnohistorical, and Methodological Perspectives*, pp. 225–248. Champaign, IL: Springer.

Corruccini, R. S., Handler, J. S., Mutaw, R. J. & Lange, F. W. (1982). Osteology of a slave burial population from Barbados, West Indies. *American Journal of Physical Anthropology* 59:443–459. https://doi.org/10.1002/ajpa.1330590414

Curate, F. (2008). A case of os odontoideum in the palaeopathological record. *International Journal of Osteoarchaeology* 18:100–105. https://doi.org/10.1002/oa.915

Cybulski, J. S. (1988). Brachydactyly, a possible inherited anomaly at prehistoric Prince Rupert Harbour. *American Journal of Physical Anthropology* 76:363–376. https://doi.org/10.1002/ajpa.1330760309

Dasen, V. (1988). Dwarfism in Egypt and classical antiquity: iconography and medical history. *Medical History* 32:253–276. https://doi.org/10.1017/s0025727300048237

Dasen, V. & Leroi, A. M. (2005). Homme ou bête? Le dieu caché de l'anencéphale d'hermopolis. In Bertrand, R. & Carol, A. (Eds.), *Le "Monstre" Humain, Imaginaire et Société*, pp. 21–44. Aix-en-Provence: Presses Universitaires de Provence.

Daly, M. & Wilson, M. (1984). A sociobiological analysis of human infanticide. In Hausfater, G. & Hrdy, S. B. (Eds.), *Infanticide: Comparative and Evolutionary Perspectives*, pp. 487–502. New York: Aldine Publishing Co.

Duncan, W. N. & Stojanowski, C. M. (2008). A case of squamosal craniosynostosis from the 16th century Southeastern United States. *International Journal of Osteoarchaeolog*, 18:407–420. https://doi.org/10.1002/oa.943

Eroğlu, S. & Erdal, Y. S. (2008). Why did the frequency of palatine torus increase in the ancient Anatolian populations? *HOMO* 59(5):365–382. https://doi.org/10.1016/j.jchb.2008.06.005

Gao, B., Guo, J., She, C., Shu, A., Yang, M., Tan, Z., Yang, X., Guo, S., Feng, G. & He, L. (2001). Mutations in IHH, encoding Indian hedgehog, cause brachydactyly type A–1. *Nature Genetics* 28:386–388. https://doi.org/10.1038/ng577

Geoffroy Saint-Hilaire, I. (1832–1837). *Histoire Générale et Particulière des Anomalies de l'Organisation chez l'Homme et les Animaux, Ouvrage Comprenant des Recherches sur les Caractères, la Classification, l'Influence Physiologique et Pathologique, les Rapports Généraux, les Lois et les Causes des Monstruosités, des Variétés et des Vices de Conformation, ou Traité de Tératologie*. Paris: J-B. Baillière.

Gilmore, H. F. & Halcrow, S. E. (2014). Sense or sensationalism? Approaches to explaining high perinatal mortality in the past. In Thompson, J. L., Alfonso-Durruty, M. P. & Crandall, J. J. (Eds.), *Tracing Childhood: Bioarchaeological Investigations of Early Lives in Antiquity*, pp. 123–138. Gainesville: University Press of Florida.

Gowland, R. L. & Chamberlain, A. T. (2002). A Bayesian approach to ageing perinatal skeletal material from archaeological sites: implications for the evidence for infanticide in Roman-Britain. *Journal of Archaeological Science* 29:677–685. https://doi.org/10.1006/jasc.2001.0776

Graham Jr, J. M. & Edwards, M. J. (1998). Teratogen update: gestational effects of maternal hyperthermia due to febrile illnesses and resultant patterns of defects in humans. *Teratology* 58(5):209–221. DOI: https://doi.org/10.1002/(SICI)1096-9926(199811)58:5<209::AID-TERA8>3.0.CO;2-Q

Gregg, J. B., Zimmerman, L., Clifford, S. & Gregg P. S. (1981). Craniofacial anomalies in the upper Missouri River basin over a millennium: archaeological and clinical evidence. *Cleft Palate Journal* 18(3):210–222. PMID: 7018741

Halcrow, S., Tayles, N. & Elliott, G. E. (2018). The bioarchaeology of fetuses. In Han, S., Betsinger, T. K. & Scott, A. B. (Eds.), *The Anthropology of the Fetus: Biology, Culture, and Society*, pp. 83–111. New York: Berghahn Books.

Halle, U., Hähn, C., Krause, S., Krause-Kyora, B., Nothnagel, M., Drichel, D. & Wahl, J. (2019). Die unsichtbaren. Menschen mit trisomie 21 in archäologie und anthropologie. *Archäologische Informationen* 42:219–235. https://doi.org/10.11588/ai.2019.0.69361

Hawkes, S. C. & Wells, C. (1978). Absence of the left upper limb and pectoral girdle in a unique Anglo-Saxon burial. *Bulletin of the New York Academy of Medicine* 52:1229–1235. PMID: 793658

Halling, C. L. & Seidemann, R. M. (2018). A probable example of cranial dysraphism from New Orleans, Louisiana. *International Journal of Osteoarchaeology* 28:470–474. https://doi.org/10.1002/oa.2672

Hillson, S., Grigson, C. & Bond, S. (1998). Dental defects of congenital syphilis. *American Journal of Physical Anthropology* 107:25–40. https://doi.org/10.1002/(SICI)1096-8644(199809)107:1<25::AID-AJPA3>3.0.CO;2-C

Hobbs, C. A., Cleves, M. A. & Simmons, C. J. (2002). Genetic epidemiology and congenital malformations: from the chromosome to the crib. *Archives of Pediatrics & Adolescent Medicine* 156:315–320. https://doi.org/10.1001/archpedi.156.4.315

Hoffman, J. M. (1976). An achondroplastic dwarf from the Augustine site (CA–Sac 127). *Contributions of the University of California Archaeological Research Facility* 30:65–119.

Hrdlicka, A. (1908). *Physiological and Medical Observations Among the Indians of the Southwestern United States and Northern Mexico. Bureau of Ethnology Bulletin 34*. Washington, DC: Government Printing Office.

Hunt, D. R. & Bullen, L. (2007). The frequency of os acromiale in the Robert J. Terry collection. *International Journal of Osteoarchaeology* 17:309–317. https://doi.org/10.1002/oa.877

Hussein, F. H., El-Din, A. S., Kandeel, W. E. S. & Banna, R. E. S. E. (2009). Spinal pathological findings in ancient Egyptians of the Greco-Roman period living in Bahriyah Oasis. *International Journal of Osteoarchaeology* 19:613–627. https://doi.org/10.1002/oa.984

Jackes, M. (2011). Representativeness and bias in archaeological skeletal samples. In Agarwal, S. C. & Glencross, B. A. (Eds.), *Social Bioarchaeology*. Chichester: Blackwell Publishing.

Kim, J. H. & Scialli, A. R. (2011). Thalidomide: the tragedy of birth defects and the effective treatment of disease. *Toxicological Sciences* 122:1–6. https://doi.org/10.1093/toxsci/kfr088

Leonard, M. A. (1974). The inheritance of tarsal coalition and its relationship to spastic flat foot. *Journal of Bone and Joint Surgery* 56B:520–526. PMID: 4421359.

Le Minor, J.-M. & Trost, O. (2004). Bony ponticles of the atlas (C1) over the groove for the vertebral artery in humans and primates: polymorphism and evolutionary trends. *American Journal of Physical Anthropology* 125:16–29. https://doi.org/10.1002/ajpa.10270

Lewis, M. (2016). Childcare in the past: the contribution of paleopathology. In Powell, L., Gowland, R. & Southwell-Wright, W. (Eds.), *Care in the Past Archaeological and Interdisciplinary Perspectives*, pp. 23–37. Oxford: Oxbow Books.

Lewis, M. (2018a). Fetal paleopathology: an impossible discipline? In Han, S., Betsinger, T. K. & Scott, A. B. (Eds.), *The Anthropology of the Fetus: Biology, Culture, and Society*, pp. 112–131. New York: Berghahn Books.

Lewis, M. (2018b). *Paleopathology of Children: Identification of Pathological Conditions in the Human Skeletal Remains of Non-Adults*. London: Academic Press.

Li, Z., Shen, J., Wu, W. K. K., Wang, X., Liang, J., Qiu, G. & Liu, J. (2012). Vitamin A deficiency induces congenital spinal deformities in rats. *PloS ONE* 7(10):e46565. https://doi.org/10.1371/journal.pone.0046565

Lorente, C., Cordier, S., Goujard, J., Aymé, S., Bianchi, F., Calzolari, E., De Walle, H. E. & Knill-Jones, R. (2000). Tobacco and alcohol use during pregnancy and risk of oral clefts. Occupational exposure and congenital malformation working group. *American Journal of Public Health* 90(3):415. https://doi.org/10.2105/ajph.90.3.415

Mai, C. T., Isenburg, J. L., Canfield, M. A., Meyer, R. E., Correa, A., Alverson, C. J., ... & National Birth Defects Prevention Network, (2019). National population-based estimates for major birth defects, 2010–2014. *Birth Defects Research* 111:1420–1435. https://doi.org/10.1002/bdr2.1589

Mann, R. W. & Hunt, D. R. (2019). Non-metric traits and anatomical variants that can mimic trauma in the human skeleton. *Forensic Science International* 301:202–224. https://doi.org/10.1016/j.forsciint.2019.05.039

Mann, R. W., Thomas, M. D. & Adams, B. J. (1998). Congenital absence of the ulna with humeroradial synostosis in a prehistoric skeleton from Moundville, Alabama. *International Journal of Osteoarchaeology* 8:295–299. https://doi.org/10.1002/(SICI)1099-1212(199807/08)8:4<295::AID-OA424>3.0.CO;2-N

Mann, R. W., Wiercinska, A. & Scheffrahn W. (1992). Distal phocomelia of the forearm in a thirteenth-century skeleton from Poland. *Teratology* 45(2):139–143. https://doi.org/10.1002/tera.1420450207

Masnicová, S. & Beňuš, R. (2003). Developmental anomalies in skeletal remains from the Great Moravia and Middle Ages Cemeteries at Devín (Slovakia). *International Journal of Osteoarchaeology* 13:266–274. https://doi.org/10.1002/oa.684

Mays, S. (1993). Infanticide in Roman Britain. *Antiquity* 67:883–888. https://doi.org/10.1017/S0003598X00063900

Mays, S. & Eyers, J. (2011). Perinatal death at the Roman villa site at Hambleden, Buckinghamshire, England. *Journal of Archaeological Science* 38:1931–1938. https://doi.org/10.1016/j.jas.2011.04.002

McDonald, A. D. (1961). Maternal health in early pregnancy and congenital defect: final report on a prospective inquiry. *British Journal of Preventive & Social Medicine* 15:154.

Merbs, C. F. (2004). Sagittal clefting of the body and other vertebral developmental errors in Canadian Inuit skeletons. *American Journal of Physical Anthropology* 123:236–249. https://doi.org/10.1002/ajpa.10264

Mitchell, P. D. & Redfern, R. C. (2008). Diagnostic criteria for developmental dislocation of the hip in human skeletal remains. *International Journal of Osteoarchaeology* 18:61–71. https://doi.org/10.1002/oa.919

Mitchell, P. D. & Redfern, R. C. (2011). Brief communication: developmental dysplasia of the hip in medieval London. *American Journal of Physical Anthropology* 144:479–484. https://doi.org/10.1002/ajpa.21448

Molto, J. E., Kirkpatrick, C. L. & Keron, J. (2019). The paleoepidemiology of sacral spina bifida occulta in population samples from the Dakhleh Oasis, Egypt. *International Journal of Paleopathology* 26:93–103. https://doi.org/10.1016/j.ijpp.2019.06.006

Morris, J. K., Mutton, D. E. & Alberman, E. (2002). Revised estimates of the maternal age specific live birth prevalence of Down's syndrome. *Journal of Medical Screening* 9:2–6. https://doi.org/10.1136/jms.9.1.2

Mutlu, H., Kızgut, B., Sözer, Ç. S., Ürker, K., Açar, O. & Erol, A. S. (2020). Sacral spina bifida occulta rare occurrence in Byzantine Belentepe population in Muğla, Turkey: a possible case for adequate folic acid intake. *Homo* 71:175–188. https://doi.org/10.1127/homo/2020/1233

Oberlin, C. & Sakka, M. (1989). Le plus ancien cas de synostose du carpe: la synostose pyramido-lunaire de la Ferrassie. *Annales de Chirurgie de la Main* 8:269–272. https://doi.org/10.1016/S0753-9053(89)80066-3

Offenbecker, A. M. & Case. D. T. (2012). Accessory navicular: a heritable accessory bone of the human foot. *International Journal of Osteoarchaeology* 22:158–167. https://doi.org/10.1002/oa.1193

O'Loughlin, V. D. (2004). Effects of different kinds of cranial deformation on the incidence of wormian bones. *American Journal of Physical Anthropology* 123:146–155. https://doi.org/10.1002/ajpa.10304

Oostra, R.-J., Boer, L. & Van Der Merwe, A. E. (2016). Paleodysmorphology and paleoteratology: diagnosing and interpreting congenital conditions of the skeleton in anthropological contexts. *Clinical Anatomy* 29:878–891. https://doi.org/10.1002/ca.22769

Oxenham, M. F., Tilley, L., Matsumura, H., Nguyen, L. C., Nguyen, K. T., Nguyen, K. D., Domett, K. & Huffer, D. (2009). Paralysis and severe disability requiring intensive care in Neolithic Asia. *Anthropological Science* 117:107–112. https://doi.org/10.1537/ase.081114

Palacios, C. C. & Sierpe, G. V. (2019). Análisis bioarqueológico de un feto anencefálico del sitio arqueológico cueva de los niños (provincia de última esperanza, Región de Magallanes, Chile): a 29 años de su hallazgo. *Magallania* 47(2):107–124. https://doi.org/10.4067/S0718-22442019000200107

Palamenghi, A., Biehler-Gomez, L., Mattia, M., Breda, L. & Cattaneo, C. (2021). A probable case of holoprosencephaly with cyclopia in a full-term fetus from a modern skeletal collection. *International Journal of Paleopathology* 33:25–29. https://doi.org/10.1016/j.ijpp.2020.12.003

Palamenghi, A., Cinti, A., Mann, R. W., Viano, G., Girotti, M., Garanzini, F., Fulcheri, E. & Rosa Boano, R. (2020). The supracondylar process in subadult skeletal remains from Northern

Italy (15th–18th century A.D.). *International Journal of Osteoarchaeology* 30:575–579. https://doi.org/10.1002/oa.2882

Palma Málaga, M. R. & Makowski, K. (2019). Bioarchaeological evidence of care provided to a physically disabled individual from Pachacamac, Peru. *International Journal of Paleopathology* 25:139–149. https://doi.org/10.1016/j.ijpp.2018.08.002

Panzer, S., Thompson, R. C., Hergan, K., Zink, A. R. & Piombino-Mascali, D. (2018). Evidence of aortic dissection and Marfan syndrome in a mummy from the capuchin catacombs of Palermo, Sicily. *International Journal of Paleopathology* 22:78–85. https://doi.org/10.1016/j.ijpp.2018.05.002

Patrick, P. & Waldron, T. (2003). Congenital absence of the patella in an Anglo-Saxon skeleton. *International Journal of Osteoarchaeology* 13:147–149. https://doi.org/10.1002/oa.668

Phillips, S. M. & Sivilich, M. (2006). Cleft palate: a case study of disability and survival in prehistoric North America. *International Journal of Osteoarchaeology* 16:528–535. https://doi.org/10.1002/oa.847

Rivollat, M., Castex, D., Hauret, L. & Tillier, A.-M. (2014). Ancient down syndrome: an osteological case from Saint-Jean-des-Vignes, northeastern France, from the 5–6th century AD. *International Journal of Paleopathology* 7:8–14. https://doi.org/10.1016/j.ijpp.2014.05.004

Sarry El-Din, A. M. & El Banna, R. A. E.-S. (2006). Congenital anomalies of the vertebral column: a case study on ancient and modern Egypt. *International Journal of Osteoarchaeology* 16:200–207. https://doi.org/10.1002/oa.816

See, A. W. M., Kaiser, M. E., White, J. C. & Clagett-Dame, M. (2008). A nutritional model of late embryonic vitamin A deficiency produces defects in organogenesis at a high penetrance and reveals new roles for the vitamin in skeletal development. *Developmental Biology* 316(2):171–190. https://doi.org/10.1016/j.ydbio.2007.10.018

Seller, M. J. (1987). Nutritionally induced congenital defects. *Proceedings of the Nutrition Society* 46(2):227–235. https://doi.org/10.1079/pns19870030

Scrimshaw, S. (1984). Infanticide in human population: societal and individual concerns. In Hausfater, G. & Hrdy, S. B. (Eds.), *Infanticide: Comparative and Evolutionary Perspectives,* pp. 439–462. New York: Aldine Publishing Co.

Sellier, P. (2011). Tous les morts? Regroupement et sélection des inhumés: les deux pôles du « recrutement funéraire. In Castex, D., Courtaud, P., Duday, H., Le Mort, F. & Tillier, A.-M. (Eds.), *Le Regroupement des Morts: Genèse et Diversité Archéologique,* pp. 83–94. Bordeaux: Maison des Sciences de l'Homme d'Aquitaine.

Shapira, J., Chaushu, S. & Becker, A. (2000). Prevalence of tooth transposition, third molar agenesis and maxillary canine impaction in individuals with Down syndrome. *The Angle Orthodontist* 70(4):290–296. https://doi.org/10.1043/0003-3219(2000)070<0290:POTTTM>2.0.CO;2

Sjovold, T. (1976/77). A method for familial studies based on minor skeletal variants. *Ossa* 3/4:97–107.

Smith, P. & Kahila, G. (1992). Identification of infanticide in archaeological sites: a case study from the late Roman-early Byzantine periods at Ashkelon, Israel. *Journal of Archaeological Science* 19:667–675. https://doi.org/10.1016/0305-4403(92)90036-3

Smith-Guzmán, N. E. (2021). An isthmus of isolation: the likely elevated prevalence of genetic disease in ancient Panama and implications for considering rare diseases in paleopathology. *International Journal of Paleopathology* 33:1–12. https://doi.org/10.1016/j.ijpp.2021.01.002

Spence, M. W. (1974). Residential practices and the distribution of skeletal traits in Teotihuacan, Mexico. *Man* 9:262–273. https://doi.org/10.2307/2800077

Spitery, E. (1983). *La Paleontologie des Maladies Osseuses Constitutionelles. Paleoecologie de L'Homme Fossile No. 6.* Paris: Editions du Centre National de la Recherche Scientifique.

Standen, V. G., Santoro, C. M., Arriaza, B., Valenzuela, D., Coleman, D. & Monsalve, S. (2018). Prehistoric polydactylism: biological evidence and rock art representation from the Atacama Desert in northern Chile. *International Journal of Paleopathology* 22:54–65. https://doi.org/10.1016/j.ijpp.2018.05.005

Stewart, T. D. (1975). Cranial dysraphism mistaken for trephination. *American Journal of Physical Anthropology* 42:435–437. https://doi.org/10.1002/ajpa.1330420310

Stojanowski, C. M. & Schillaci, M. A. (2006). Phenotypic approaches for understanding patterns of intracemetery biological variation. *Yearbook of Physical Anthropology* 49:49–88. https://doi.org/10.1002/ajpa.20517

Tague, R. G. (2018). Proximate cause, anatomical correlates, and obstetrical implication of a supernumerary lumbar vertebra in humans. *American Journal of Physical Anthropology* 165:444–456. https://doi.org/10.1002/ajpa.23361

Tassabehji, M., Fang, Z. M., Hilton, E. N., McGaughran, J., Zhao, Z., de Bock, C. E., ... & Clarke, R. A. (2008). Mutations in GDF6 are associated with vertebral segmentation defects in Klippel-Feil syndrome. *Human Mutation* 29:1017–1027. https://doi.org/10.1002/humu.20741

Temtamy, S. A. & Aglan, M. S. (2008). Brachydactyly. *Orphanet Journal of Rare Diseases* 3(1):1–16. https://doi.org/10.1186/1750-1172-3-15

Tenney, J. M. (1991). Comparison of third metatarsal and third cuneiform defects among various populations. *International Journal of Osteoarchaeology* 1:169–172. https://doi.org/10.1002/oa.1390010305

Tilley, L. & Oxenham, M. F. (2011). Survival against the odds: modeling the social implications of care provision to seriously disabled individuals. *International Journal of Paleopathology* 1:35–42. https://doi.org/10.1016/j.ijpp.2011.02.003

Titelbaum, A. R. (2020). Developmental anomalies and South American paleopathology: a comparison of block vertebrae and co-occurring axial anomalies among three skeletal samples from the El Brujo archaeological complex of northern coastal Peru. *International Journal of Paleopathology* 29:76–93. https://doi.org/10.1016/j.ijpp.2019.07.001

Titelbaum, A. R., Fresh, S., McNeil, B. E. & Asencios, B. (2021). Three cases of brachydactyly type E from two commingled tombs at the Late Intermediate period - Late Horizon site of Marcajirca, Ancash, Peru. *International Journal of Paleopathology* 33:146–157. https://doi.org/10.1016/j.ijpp.2021.04.006

Titelbaum, A. R., Ibarra, B. & Naji, S. (2015). Madelung's deformity and possible Leri-Weill dyschondrosteosis: two cases from a Late Intermediate period tomb, Ancash, Peru. *International Journal of Paleopathology* 9:8–14. https://doi.org/10.1016/j.ijpp.2014.11.004

Titelbaum, A. R., Querevalú, J., Rios, N. & Chirinos, R. (2017). An analysis of human remains from an Inca ushnu: polydactylism, infection, blunt force trauma, and sharp force trauma at Soledad de Tambo, Huachis, Ancash Peru. *American Journal of Physical Anthropology* 162 (S64):382. https://doi.org/10.1002/ajpa.23210

Titelbaum, A. R. & Uceda Castillo, S. (2015). A rare case of os odontoideum from an early intermediate tomb at the Huacas de Moche, Peru. *International Journal of Paleopathology* 11:23–29. https://doi.org/10.1016/j.ijpp.2015.08.001

Tocheri, M. W., Dommain, R., McFarlin, S. C., Burnett, S. E., Case, D. T., Orr, C. M., ... & Jungers, W. L. (2016). The evolutionary origin and population history of the Grauer gorilla. *Yearbook of Physical Anthropology* 159:S4–S18. https://doi.org/10.1002/ajpa.22900

Tur, S. S., Svyatko, S. V. & Rykun, M. P. (2019). Transverse basilar cleft: two more probable familial cases in an archaeological context. *International Journal of Osteoarchaeology* 29:144–148. https://doi.org/10.1002/oa.2692

Turkel, S. J. (1989). Congenital abnormalities in skeletal populations. In İşcan, M. Y. & Kennedy, K. A. R. (Eds.), *Reconstruction of Life from a Skeleton*, pp. 109–127. New York: Alan R. Liss.

Usher, B. M. & Christensen M. N. (2000). A sequential developmental field defect of the vertebrae, ribs, and sternum, in a young woman of the 12th century AD. *American Journal of Physical Anthropology* 111:355–367. https://doi.org/10.1002/(SICI)1096-8644(200003)111:3<355::AID-AJPA5>3.0.CO;2-9

Vairamuthu, T. & Pfeiffer, S. (2018). A juvenile with compromised osteogenesis provides insights into past hunter-gatherer lives. *International Journal of Paleopathology* 20:1–9. https://doi.org/10.1016/j.ijpp.2017.11.002

Wang, A. R., Nasrallah, I. M. & Wardak, K. S. (2015). Os odontoideum mimicking acute odontoid peg fracture: case report. *Academic Forensic Pathology* 5:699–706. https://doi.org/10.23907/2015.074

Warkany, J. & Nelson, R. C. (1941). Skeletal abnormalities in the offspring of rats reared on deficient diets. *The Anatomical Record* 79(1):83–100. https://doi.org/10.1002/ar.1090790109

Whitmore, K. M. & Buzon, M. R. (2019). Two cases of skeletal dysplasia from New Kingdom (c. 1400–1050 BCE) Tombos, Sudan. *International Journal of Paleopathology* 26:135–144. https://doi.org/10.1016/j.ijpp.2019.07.006

Wilczak, C. A. & Ousley, S. D. (2009). Test of the relationship between sutural ossicles and cultural cranial deformation: results from Hawikuh, New Mexico. *American Journal of Physical Anthropology* 139:483–493. https://doi.org/10.1002/ajpa.21005

Williams, S. A., Middleton, E. R., Villamil, C. I. & Shattuck, M. R. (2016). Vertebral numbers and human evolution. *Yearbook of Physical Anthropology* 159:S19–S36. https://doi.org/10.1002/ajpa.22901

15
TUMORS AND NEOPLASTIC DISEASES
Assessing Antiquity and Pondering Prevalence

Casey L. Kirkpatrick

Introduction

Historically, paleopathologists have given little attention to the investigation of tumors and neoplastic diseases unless they have stumbled upon visible evidence. With respect to benign tumors, this lack of research interest is largely due to the fact that most benign tumors are asymptomatic and therefore do not significantly affect the lives of those affected (Siek, 2020). Cancerous (malignant) tumors and neoplastic diseases, however, often contribute to significant morbidity and mortality. Nevertheless, many early paleopathologists did not search for malignancies due to the popular belief that cancers are modern diseases, largely linked to man-made carcinogens that were introduced during the Industrial Revolution. This belief was supported by the apparent paucity of evidence in examined remains (Micozzi, 1991; Capasso, 2005; David & Zimmerman, 2010); however, most primary tumors occur in rarely preserved soft tissues and many neoplastic lesions in bone are invisible without radiological analysis. Therefore, the visible evidence of cancers in biological remains does not accurately represent cancer rates in past populations.

The past prevalence of neoplastic diseases, and cancers in particular, continues to be debated within, and beyond, the field of paleopathology. However, paleopathologists are in a unique position to expand the known history of cancers and investigate their origins, evolution, natural causes, natural progression, and their effects on the skeleton. This chapter will summarize the challenges associated with existing paleopathological methods for the detection and diagnosis of neoplastic diseases, the known history and evolutionary hypotheses of cancer, and the ongoing debate over the past prevalence of cancers.

What are Tumors and Neoplastic Diseases?

In normal tissues, cell growth, division, and death are regulated in accordance with the needs of the organism. Tumors, or neoplasms (Greek: neo = new, plasm = formation), are abnormal masses of tissues in which cells multiply excessively independent of physiologic growth signals (Kumar et al., 2015).

Benign tumors are mostly slow-growing solitary masses with clear boundaries and well-differentiated cells (meaning: the tumor cells closely resemble the normal cells from which they originate). They also remain localized without spreading (i.e., metastasizing) to other locations or tissues. Although benign tumors are generally harmless, they can sometimes affect normal body processes and/or grow to block or press on nerves, blood vessels, or organs, resulting in significant complications, or even death (Siek, 2020, e.g., Weiss et al., 1983, Ryder et al., 1986, Fukiyama et al., 1993). Additionally, some benign tumors contain so-called 'atypical' or 'pre-cancerous' cells that are benign but have undergone abnormal cancer-like changes. These cell lines may remain atypically benign, return to normal, or become malignant through further mutation (Burnett, 2020).

Cancerous (malignant) tumors often grow quickly and have the potential to spread (i.e., metastasize) to secondary locations or tissues. Their cells are poorly differentiated or dedifferentiated, meaning that they have lost the specialized structure and function of the normal cell from which the cancer originated. Malignant tumors have a deleterious effect on the body and, depending on their size, location, speed of growth, and stage of spread, can contribute to significant morbidity and/or mortality (Mohan, 2019).

Although all malignant and benign tumors can be classified as neoplastic diseases, not all neoplastic diseases are tumors. For example, there are hereditary neoplastic syndromes that produce multiple growths (e.g., neurofibromatosis, Von Hippel-Lindau disease) and/or predispose the affected individual to malignancy (e.g., Li-Fraumeni syndrome). There are also malignant neoplastic diseases, so-called blood cancers, that are not characterized by the growth of tumors at all, although their malignant cells can sometimes cluster together; namely, leukemias (cancers of the myeloid and lymphoid hematopoietic cell lines), lymphomas (cancers of lymphocytes), and multiple myeloma (cancer of plasma cells) (Rosmarin, 2019).

Paleo-Oncological Methods and Their Limitations

Paleo-oncology is the study of the origins, evolution, and history of neoplastic diseases. It is a growing multidisciplinary field that often integrates historical, archaeological, oncological, and paleopathological information. Most discussions of the past prevalence of neoplastic diseases revolve around paleopathological data because historical records are limited and they are heavily influenced by cancer stigmas and the poor diagnostic methods of the past. Consequently, an understanding of the limitations of current paleo-oncological methods (i.e., macroscopic visual analysis, radiology, histology, and biomolecular analysis) is necessary to consider the antiquity and past prevalence of neoplastic diseases.

As a whole, it should be acknowledged that issues of preservation heavily affect all paleo-oncological methods for the detection and diagnosis of neoplastic diseases. All methods of paleo-oncological diagnosis are also based on an assumption that modern diseases affect the body in the same manner as their ancient counterparts (Kirkpatrick, 2020). The assumption of cancer's rarity also biases differential diagnoses, likely contributing to an underestimation of cancers (Marques et al., 2021). Furthermore, modern clinical literature must be used with caution in paleo-oncological research as clinical studies rarely describe skeletal reactions to neoplastic disease or the entire natural (untreated) progression of a disease (Ragsdale et al., 2018). In addition to these limitations, method-specific challenges impact the recognition and analysis of neoplastic disease in the past.

Macroscopic Visual Analysis

Methods for the detection and diagnosis of neoplastic diseases through macroscopic visual analysis (hereafter, visual analysis) are severely limited by the rarity of soft-tissue preservation and the paucity of pathognomonic skeletal reactions allowing for specific diagnosis. When soft-tissue tumors are not preserved, they are evident only from the rarely observed pressure defects in bone (i.e., direct pressure from a tumor or secondary pressure from fluids, such as in hydrocephalus), soft-tissue calcifications, new bone or dental tissue inclusions (e.g., teratomas), hormone-related abnormalities of growth or bone density, skeletal deformities linked with hereditary neoplastic syndromes (e.g., neurofibromatosis, Gorlin syndrome), or more commonly, metastatic (secondary) bone lesions (McGinnis & Parham, 1978; Morandi et al. 2006; Muzio, 2008; Elefteriou et al., 2009; Mohamadi & Salvatori, 2012). Although metastatic lesion morphology and distribution patterns, along with age and sex estimates, can be used to narrow down the differential diagnoses for the responsible primary tumor, these characteristics are far from pathognomonic and it is possible that patterns and rates of metastasis varied in the past (Ragsdale et al., 2018; Marques et al., 2021). Given that there are over 100 types of cancers alone (National Cancer Institute, 2015) and bony reactions to any disease are limited to osteoblastic (bone forming) and/or osteoclastic (bone resorbing) processes, even the diagnoses of primary bone cancers can be difficult to ascertain. See Table 15.1 for an overview of the different types of neoplastic diseases that can affect the skeleton. Differential diagnoses must therefore consider a wide spectrum of conditions with similar presentations, including developmental abnormalities, cysts, rheumatic diseases, trauma, infectious diseases, and even normal skeletal variation (Aufderheide & Rodriguez-Martin, 1998; Ragsdale et al., 2018).

Given the difficulties involved in the differential diagnosis of neoplastic diseases, paleopathologists using visual and/or radiologic analysis more accurately assign skeletal lesions to one of the seven basic categories of disease (VITAMIN – Vascular, Innervation/mechanIcal, Trauma/repair, Anomaly, Metabolic, Inflammatory/Immune, Neoplastic) than to specific diagnoses (Ragsdale et al., 2018). At times, this categorization is as specific as one can get without sacrificing accuracy (Miller et al., 1996; Marques et al., 2013). Using visual analysis alone, neoplastic lesions in bone are also often overlooked if they are not visible on the surface, and cancers (or other conditions) can kill the individual before spreading to bone, leaving no visible skeletal evidence at all (Rothschild & Rothschild, 1995; Marques et al., 2018). These problems were demonstrated by Marques et al. (2018) who found in their study of a skeletal collection composed of individuals known to have succumbed to cancer that only 17.6% of the individuals had indisputable visual evidence of cancer, while 45% had non-pathognomonic lesions, and 37.4% had no visible skeletal lesions.

Challenges to the visual detection and diagnosis of neoplastic diseases are further complicated by the fact that bones are rendered more vulnerable to post-mortem damage and decay by lytic malignant lesions and/or osteoporosis, which often affects older adults – the most cancer-prone demographic group (Mays, 1998; Pinhasi & Bourbou, 2007). Additionally, fragmentary or incomplete remains, anthropogenic modifications (e.g., trephination), or taphonomic processes can easily be mistaken for evidence of neoplastic disease or mask it (Miller et al., 1996; Aufderheide & Rodriguez-Martin, 1998; Halperin, 2004; Brothwell, 2012; Ragsdale et al., 2018; Kirkpatrick, 2020). Consequently, any conclusions based on visual analysis alone – the most commonly used paleo-oncological method – should be made cautiously.

Radiological Analysis

Paleo-radiological methods include plain X-rays, digital radiography, computed tomography, microCT, and three-dimensional (3D) image rendering techniques (see Chapter 6

Table 15.1 Types of neoplastic diseases that can affect the skeleton

Neoplasm type	Brief description	Effect on the skeleton
Carcinoma	Malignancies originating in epithelial cells (e.g., skin or tissues lining other organs or glands)	• Can metastasize to bone, forming osteoblastic and/or osteoclastic lesions depending on type • Even in predominantly osteolytic metastasis, osteoblastic response is common • Different carcinomas have different patterns and rates of metastasis; however, metastases are most commonly found in parts of the skeleton with hematopoietic marrow • Depending on size and location, tumors can cause pressure defects on bone • On rare occasions, may also produce calcifications (e.g. urinary bladder carcinoma)
Sarcoma	Malignancies originating in bone or in soft tissues such as muscle, fat, blood vessels, fibrous tissue, cartilage, or other connective or supportive tissues	• Can manifest as primary bone lesions (osteoblastic and/or osteoclastic) • Location and morphology of lesions differ depending on the type of sarcoma • Less likely than carcinomas to metastasize to bone from other tissues • Different sarcomas have different patterns and rates of metastasis • On rare occasions, tumors may cause pressure defects on bone • May produce calcifications (e.g., chondrosarcoma)
Melanoma	Malignancy of melanocytes (melanin-forming cells in the skin).	• Can metastasize to bone in late stages, generally presenting as osteolytic lesions with poorly defined limits, usually in the axial skeleton • Atypically, metastatic melanoma may present as mixed, or very rarely osteoblastic lesions • On occasion, osteolytic lesions may contribute to pathological fracture
Leukemia	Malignancies of the myeloid and lymphoid hematopoietic cell lines. May be acute or chronic in nature.	• Skeletal involvement varies according to type and is more common in acute childhood leukemias • Can present as fields of small, well-defined, smooth-walled pores/pits without marginal inflammation or reactive bone • Often occur in and around areas of hematopoietic tissue and near vascular foramina, which may be enlarged • May result in periosteal reaction, osteopenia, and sometimes pathological fractures (including joint compression or vertebral collapse). Widespread subperiosteal bone deposits may also be found on thinned cortices of long bones and ribs • In acute childhood leukemia, narrow radiolucent metaphyseal bands may be observed radiographically and exaggerated grooving and porosity may be seen on the metaphyseal cortical surface

Lymphoma	Malignancies of lymphocytes found primarily in the glands or nodes of the lymphatic system. Extranodal lymphomas can sometimes occur in specific organs, such as the stomach, breast, brain, or in bone	• Tends to involve bones with hematopoietic marrow, lesion patterns differ depending on the type of lymphoma • Most commonly present with multiple osteolytic lesions in motheaten, poorly defined, or permeative patterns, sometimes involving endosteal scalloping • May sometimes manifest as solitary lesions • Lesions may contribute to pathological fracture • Periosteal bone formation and/or localized or diffuse osteosclerosis may also be present • May be associated with rheumatoid arthritis, gout, or hypertrophic arthropathy
Multiple myeloma	Malignancy of plasma cells found primarily in hematopoietic bone marrow May begin as a solitary lesion (solitary plasmacytoma), but quickly progresses to multiple myeloma	• Appears as diffuse osteoclastic 'punched out' or 'motheaten' lesions (usually 5–20 mm in diameter) and/or endosteal scalloping without reactive bony margins • Lesions appear in highly vascularized bones. Hands and feet are usually spared • In advanced stages, pathologic fractures may occur, in some cases resulting in vertebra plana • In rare cases, lesion margins are sclerotic and/or the skeleton may present with generalized osteopenia • Skeletal evidence is difficult to differentiate from metastatic carcinoma.
Blastoma	Tumors (benign or malignant) originating in precursor cells (blasts). Most commonly found in children	• Depending on the tumor type, blastomas can affect bone primarily (e.g., osteoblastoma, chondroblastoma) or may metastasize to bone, often in areas with hematopoietic bone marrow (e.g., neuroblastoma). • Bone metastases are predominantly osteolytic, though osteoblastic lesions and/or periosteal reactions may also occur
Germ cell tumors	Rare tumors (benign or malignant) originating in germ cells	• On rare occasions, malignant germ cell tumors can metastasize to bone manifesting in lytic and/or sclerotic bone lesions, often in areas with hematopoietic bone marrow • Rarely, pathological fracture and spinal cord compression can occur.

(Continued)

Neoplasm type	Brief description	Effect on the skeleton
Mixed tumor	Rare tumors (benign or malignant) affecting more than one type of tissue (e.g., carcinosarcoma, adenosquamous carcinoma, mixed mesodermal tumor, teratoma)	• Depending on the type of tumor, bone may be affected primarily and/or by metastasis (e.g., carcinosarcoma) • Teratomas may present with new abnormal growths of bone or teeth
Benign/atypical tumor	Benign tumors generally do not: 1. spread to distant tissues; 2. invade adjacent tissues; 3. proliferate quickly; 4. become undifferentiated Atypical cells have at least one sign of malignancy, but not all of them. Benign and atypical tumors have the potential to advance to malignancy	• Benign tumors may affect bone primarily (e.g., osteoma) or secondarily (e.g., pressure defects, hydrocephaly, hormonally linked skeletal abnormalities resulting from pressure on endocrine glands) • Some benign tumors may also produce calcifications (e.g., enchondroma) • [See "Mixed Tumor", "Endocrine and Neuroendocrine Tumor", "Central Nervous System Tumor", and "Hereditary Neoplastic Syndrome" in this table for more information on the effects of benign tumors]
Endocrine and neuroendocrine tumor	Any tumors (benign or malignant) that affect the endocrine or neuroendocrine system (e.g., pituitary sarcoma, papillary thyroid carcinoma, carcinoid tumors). In some cases, tumors may secrete hormones. [These tumors can originate in various cells/tissues but are grouped together here because of their shared potential effects on the skeleton]	• Depending on the type of tumor and location, may cause a pressure defect and/or metastasize to bone • Some tumors may secrete hormones or suppress hormone secretion from a gland • Depending on hormones affected, changes to skeleton may include bone density abnormalities, gigantism/acromegaly, pituitary dwarfism

Tumors and Neoplastic Diseases

Central nervous system tumor	Any tumors (benign or malignant) affecting the brain and/or spinal cord (e.g., ependymoma, glioblastoma, pituitary adenoma) Some tumors affecting the CNS may not originate in brain or spinal cord tissues (e.g., chordoma, meningioma, primary CNS lymphoma) [These tumors can originate in various cells/tissues, but are grouped together here because of their shared potential effects on the skeleton]	• Depending on type of tumor, may metastasize to bone • Meningiomas sometimes erode, invade, or metastasize to bone • Some bone tumors affect the CNS (e.g. chordoma) • Depending on tumor size and location, may cause pressure defects in bone, hydrocephaly, musculoskeletal atrophy, and/or paralysis • Pituitary tumors may result in hormonally linked skeletal abnormalities. [see "Endocrine and Neuroendocrine Tumor" above]
Hereditary neoplastic syndrome	Inherited genetic abnormalities that result in the formation of tumors (benign or malignant) and/or predispose the affected individual to malignancy. [May be considered a precursor to neoplasia in some cases]	• Depending on the syndrome, neoplastic disease may develop and affect the skeleton • Some syndromes have genetically linked skeletal abnormalities (e.g., neurofibromatosis, Gorlin syndrome)
Langerhans' cell hystiocytosis (aka hystiocytosis X)	Uncontrolled clonal proliferation (along with increased mobility and phagocytic activity) of Langerhans' cells. It predominantly affects children but can also develop in adults. [It has been debated for decades whether LCH is a true neoplastic disease or an immune response disease]	• Generally presents with isolated or multiple osteolytic lesions, round or oval, that may coalesce to create irregularly shaped, map-like lesions • Occasionally associated with sclerotic margins or reactive bone formation • Type and location(s) of the lesion(s) is dependent on the type of LCH • Pathological fracture and vertebra plana may be observed in some cases.

for more information on imaging in paleopathology). All of these methods are vulnerable to misdiagnosis due to post-mortem treatments, taphonomy, or foreign matter inclusions (Aufderheide & Rodriguez-Martin, 1998; Ragsdale et al., 2018). However, in a study by Rothschild & Rothschild (1995) comparing visual and radiographic detection methods in a collection of skeletonized individuals known to have succumbed to cancers, radiologic analysis revealed three times more individuals with evidence of cancer than visual analysis alone. Biehler-Gomez et al. (2019) have since shown that visual and radiographic analyses are complementary and should be applied together to screen for neoplastic diseases and improve differential diagnoses. To this end, Ragsdale et al. (2018) published a useful guide for the differential diagnosis of neoplastic diseases through macroscopic and radiographic analysis of dry bones. Nevertheless, the diagnostic indicators used in both visual and radiographic methods are somewhat subjective and benefit from consensus-led diagnosis (Ragsdale et al., 2018). Furthermore, although radiographic analysis significantly improves the detection and diagnosis of paleo-oncological evidence, it should be remembered that radiographic information can still be obscured by faults in the scope, focus, angle, quality, or processing of the X-ray (Kirkpatrick, 2020). Radiological methods also differ in their sensitivity, with plain radiographs only detecting a loss of bone density exceeding 40% (Western & Bekvalac, 2020). MicroCT is more sensitive and it can better identify bone lesions due to its 3D nature, though many of the aforementioned radiological limitations still apply (Odes et al., 2016, 2018; Mitchell et al., 2021). Regardless of the radiological methods used, without the aid of a trained radiologist, there is a significant risk of overlooking many subtle, but important, diagnostic indicators (Ragsdale et al., 2018; Kirkpatrick, 2020).

Histological Analysis

Histological analysis can be invaluable for the specific diagnosis of neoplastic diseases, particularly if soft tissues are preserved (Fornaciari, 2018, and see Chapter 5, this volume). Although there are few published paleo-oncological studies in which this method has been used, Fornaciari (2018) has noted that methods for rehydration, staining, and microscopy varied among them. Although Zimmerman (1977) demonstrated that desiccation and subsequent rehydration does not affect the histological diagnosis of cancers, caution is still warranted, as little is known about the effects of post-mortem treatments or taphonomic processes on soft-tissue histological analyses.

In addition to soft-tissue histology, De Boer and Maat (2018) recently demonstrated that the histological study of bone lesions can be used to define the biological behavior of a tumor and to differentiate between benign tumors, high-grade conventional osteosarcomas, and other unspecified malignant tumors. Although this method may be useful for distinction between high-grade osteosarcomas and malignancies with similar macroscopic morphology, it is limited by the fact that the delicate lace-like bone depositions of high-grade osteosarcomas are vulnerable to destruction. Further studies of bony reactions that mimic neoplastic diseases are also required to ensure that they can be differentiated histologically.

Biomolecular Analysis

Lastly, biomolecular methods for the detection and diagnosis of neoplastic diseases include the analysis of ancient DNA (aDNA analysis) and proteins (paleo-proteomic analysis). aDNA analysis is useful for investigating genetic biomarkers for cancers, and these may be used to narrow a differential diagnosis (see Chapter 8, this volume, for more information on aDNA).

However, due to the epigenetic nature of cancers, the detection of aDNA biomarkers for cancer can often only indicate that an individual had a higher risk of developing cancer, unless physical evidence of the cancer was preserved (Nerlich, 2018). This method is also limited to recognized genetic biomarkers for neoplastic diseases (e.g., oncogenes and cancer suppressor genes); a list that is still growing.

In addition to human biomarkers, pathogen aDNA can be used to identify carcinogenic viral, bacterial, and parasitic infections (e.g., Fornaciari et al., 2003). These studies may be useful in the assessment of the risk of cancers in past populations; however, they are limited to carcinogenic pathogens that have been recognized in modern populations. Furthermore, although the oncogenes of several pathogens (e.g., *EBV, HHV-8, HTLV-1*) have been shown to predate *Homo sapiens* (Ewald, 2018), phylogenetic analyses are still required to determine when some pathogens became carcinogenic to humans. In both human and pathogen aDNA analysis, preservation and contamination are among the greatest challenges; however, next-generation sequencing has enabled the reconstruction of genomes from more fragmentary aDNA than was previously possible and molecular authentication methods are being increasingly used to confirm that DNA samples are indeed ancient (Jónsson et al., 2013; Key et al., 2017). Unfortunately, the destructive nature of aDNA analysis, its cost, and the need for specialized knowledge continue to limit the use of this method.

Paleo-proteomic analysis is showing great promise for the detection of tissue-specific protein biomarkers from better-differentiated soft-tissue tumors that still resemble their tissue of origin. Like histology, paleo-proteomic analysis can be used to diagnose preserved soft-tissue tumors; however, it can also be used to identify primary tumors from bone metastases (Nerlich, 2018). Schultz et al. (2007) have shown that even miniscule amounts of tumor tissue collected from within osteoblastic bone metastases can provide paleo-proteomic data. Unfortunately, this analytical method is limited by accessibility, cost, its destructive nature, and the need for at least a minute amount of uncontaminated preserved tissue. Furthermore, it can only be used to recognize known tissue-specific proteins and it is not useful in the assessment of poorly differentiated or dedifferentiated tumors. Moreover, research is still needed to determine whether tissue-specific proteins are affected by taphonomic processes (Nerlich, 2018).

Combining Forces

It is clear that there are many challenges associated with the detection and diagnosis of neoplastic diseases in ancient remains. However, the accuracy and specificity of paleo-oncological analyses can be improved through multidisciplinary collaboration and consensus-led diagnosis with the use of multiple analytical methods. Hunt and colleagues (2018) revealed a need for increased application of advanced diagnostic methods in their systematic review of published cancers in ancient remains. They discovered that although all of the studies that provided methodological information incorporated macroscopic visual analysis (n = 211), only 58.3% (123/211) of the cases were examined radiologically, a mere 22.3% (47/211) underwent histological analysis, and a scant 2.8% (6/211) were analyzed with biomolecular methods. Nevertheless, even when multiple diagnostic methods are used, researchers must remain aware of the limitations of each method and the possible impact that these limitations may have on paleo-oncological data. Furthermore, when synthesizing the existing paleo-oncological data, it is necessary to acknowledge that many of the aforementioned methodological recommendations and standards have been variably applied and early studies preceded the introduction of advanced diagnostic methods. Issues of accessibility, affordability, and the need for specialized training and destructive processes also continue to prevent widespread use of advanced diagnostic methods. Moreover, documentation of the applied analytical methods, descriptions of lesions, associated population data, and other relevant contextual information also vary widely in published paleo-oncological literature, hindering comparative studies (Hunt et al., 2018).

A Brief Summary of the Paleo-Oncological Data

Despite the many limitations of paleo-oncological methods, the evidence that has been collected to date demonstrates the long history of neoplastic diseases (cf. Capasso, 2005). For example, an Upper Devonian armored fish, dating to approximately 350 million years ago (mya), yields perhaps the earliest evidence of a benign tumor, though this diagnosis is not certain (Scheele, 1954; Capasso, 2005). The earliest unequivocally diagnosed benign tumor, an osteoma, was found in a fossilized fish, *Phanerosteon mirabile*, from the Lower Carboniferous Period (approx. 300 mya) (Moodie, 1927; Capasso, 2005). The relative rarity of malignant tumors, and particularly those affecting bone, may be one of the reasons that the earliest known evidence of cancer dates to around 60 million years later than the earliest unequivocal evidence of a benign tumor. This ancient malignancy, an osteosarcoma, was found in a Triassic Period (approx. 240 mya) stem turtle (Haridy et al., 2019). Following the Triassic Period, the known evidence of neoplastic diseases, both benign and malignant, increases over time with the greater preservation of vertebrate remains, and can be found in many extinct species, including dinosaurs (see Capasso, 2005; Kirkpatrick et al., 2018 for more detailed summaries). This rise in paleo-oncological evidence may be attributable to larger organisms having larger, more easily preserved neoplasms; however, comparative studies of modern species have shown that cancers are most prevalent in the biological Kingdom Animalia, and in vertebrates in particular. It is also worth noting that among vertebrates, cancers appear to affect mammals more frequently than birds, reptiles, amphibians, or fish, but more research is necessary (Aktipis et al., 2015). Furthermore, current data indicate that non-human primates have orthologues for each human cancer gene and that cancers are more prevalent in non-human primates than previously believed; however, some human cancers remain rare in non-human primates (Albuquerque et al., 2018).

At the time of this publication, six early hominin individuals have been diagnosed with a benign neoplastic disease. Specifically, osteomata were found in an *Australopithecus sediba*, *Homo naledi*, and three Middle Pleistocene hominins including the famous Florisbad skull (Pérez et al., 1997; Curnoe & Brink, 2010; Randolph-Quinney et al., 2016; Odes et al., 2018). Additionally, a *Homo neanderthalensis* individual has been diagnosed with a benign intraosseous neoplasm (Colella et al., 2012).

There are only three possible cases of malignant neoplastic diseases found in early hominins. The earliest and most diagnostically secure case is a probable osteosarcoma found on a 1.7-million-year-old unspecified hominin metatarsal from the South African Swartkrans Cave site (Odes et al., 2016). The other two cases are famously controversial; the Kanam mandible and the Trinil femur. The taxonomy of the Kenyan Kanam mandible was originally debated because of its apparent chin-like protrusion, despite its Lower Pleistocene date (Leakey, 1935). However, in addition to recent skepticism regarding its dating, it is now known that the chin-like protrusion is a pathological growth (Oakley et al., 1977). This growth has been variously attributed to infection, trauma, and several malignant neoplastic diseases (Lawrence, 1935; Brothwell, 1967; Stathopoulos, 1975; Tobias, 1994). However, it now seems most likely that the growth is a result of trauma-related osteomyelitis

(Tobias, 1962; Phelan et al., 2007). Compared to the Kanam mandible, a diagnostic consensus for the abnormal bony growth on the Trinil femur seems far more elusive. This specimen was discovered at the Trinil site in Java, Indonesia along with a *Homo erectus* skullcap (Dubois, 1894; Semah et al., 1981; Van den Bergh et al., 1996). Since its excavation, diagnoses considered for the bony mass have included: infection (Virchow, 1895; Julien, 1965), fluorosis (Soriano, 1970), osteosarcoma (Day & Molleson, 1973), hereditary multiple exostoses (Day & Molleson, 1973), and myositis ossificans traumatica (Day & Molleson, 1973; Ortner, 2003). This case is further complicated by the ongoing debate about whether the Trinil femur belonged to an *H. erectus* individual, or if it is an intrusive deposit from an *H. sapiens* burial (Day & Molleson, 1973; Bartstra, 1982; Kennedy, 1983; Bartsiokas & Day, 1993).

Turning to *H. sapiens*, to date, there has not yet been a systematic review or meta-analysis of published benign tumors in ancient human remains. However, a cursory search of the literature reveals bony or calcified evidence of osteoma, osteoid osteoma, meningioma, ossifying fibroma, calcified myoma, hemangioma, osteochondroma, mature teratoma, and ameloblastoma in human remains. Siek (2020) also reports cases of osteoblastoma, chondroblastoma, enchondroma, enostosis, and giant cell tumor among the paleo-oncological data. Additionally, Fornaciari (2018) has described squamous papilloma, vesical papilloma, verruca vulgaris, histiocytoma, condyloma acuminatum, angiokeratoma circumscriptum, mammary fibroadenoma, ovarian cystadenoma, neurilemmoma, and lipoma as benign soft-tissue tumors that have been histologically diagnosed. Evidence of neurofibromatosis has also been found in ancient human remains, though it has not been studied histologically (Panzer et al., 2017; Ruggieri et al., 2018).

Unlike benign tumors, the paleopathological evidence for malignant neoplastic diseases has been synthesized multiple times. A recent systematic review of ancient cancers resulted in the establishment of the open access CRAB (Cancer Research in Ancient Bodies) database, which is keeping a tally of published evidence of cancers in humans and early hominins. At the time of writing this chapter, the CRAB database has collected 299 published cases of cancer in human remains from around the world that predate 1900 CE, with the earliest evidence of cancer in *H. sapiens* currently dating to 4000 BCE (Hunt et al., 2018, 2022; cf. Strouhal & Kritscher, 1990). According to these data, the most prevalent malignant diagnosis in ancient human remains is metastatic cancer (6.9%, 178/313), followed by multiple myeloma (17.3%, 54/313), osteosarcoma (12.1%, 38/313), and nasopharyngeal cancer (2.9%, 9/313). In addition to these diagnoses, there are 15 other types of cancer represented in ancient remains and there are four individuals with unspecified malignancies. All of this paleo-oncological evidence was discovered in human remains from 38 different countries, with England, Egypt, Germany, Hungary, and Peru contributing more than half of all the data. Of course, this does not necessarily indicate higher rates of cancer in these populations, as these countries tend to have relatively well-preserved organic remains and long histories of bioarchaeological research (Hunt et al., 2018). As the pool of paleo-oncological data continues to grow, we are learning much more about the history of cancers in *H. sapiens*, our vulnerability to malignant diseases prior to the introduction of many anthropogenic carcinogens, and the natural progression and skeletal manifestations of neoplastic diseases.

Evolutionary Hypotheses of Cancer

As previously mentioned, cancer rates vary widely among different vertebrate species, with mammals showing the highest rates. At first glance, one might assume that larger organisms are more commonly affected by cancers due to a greater potential for malignant transformation resulting from their larger number of cells and relatively long lifespans. However, Peto and colleagues (1975) demonstrated that larger vertebrates do not show an increased risk for the development of cancer, particularly when compared to humans (a principle now known as Peto's Paradox). A recent study supports the 'life history theory', which attributes this paradox to long-lived animals with low fecundity (that are typically larger) investing more energy in cancer defenses to prolong their reproductive and care-giving period, while short-lived animals invest more energy into their high rate of reproduction (Boddy et al., 2015; Boddy et al., 2020). However, other factors such as differences in metabolic rate or number of activated tumor suppressor genes among species may also explain the observed differences in cancer susceptibility between species (Caulin & Maley, 2011).

On a larger scale, some researchers have developed evolutionary hypotheses to explain the greater vulnerability of complex organisms to cancers. For example, Robert (2010) has hypothesized that the more sophisticated immune responses in complex organisms have contributed to the natural selection for more invasive and aggressive neoplastic diseases, and therefore higher rates of cancer, in vertebrates. Davies (2004) has proposed that recently evolved organs (e.g., those found in mammals) are more vulnerable to oncogenesis, perhaps due, in part, to an 'inherent instability characteristic of recently-evolved differentiation states' (Davies, 2004:60). Meanwhile, Kozlov (2010) has taken the relationship between cancers and complex multicellular organisms a step further by suggesting that neoplasms may have had a role in the evolution of the affected species by introducing and nurturing newly evolved genes to the gene pool. Although detailed discussions of these and other hypotheses are beyond the scope of this chapter, see Ujvari et al. (2017) for a deep dive into the evolution of cancer.

In addition to the proposed evolutionary origins of cancers, evolutionary principles have been used to explain human vulnerability to cancer. These explanations include mismatch with the modern environment due to the slow pace of natural selection, co-evolution with quickly evolving pathogens, constraints on selection for mechanisms that suppress cancer, disease defense trade-offs, reproductive success at the cost of health, and the costs of evolved capacities for defense (Aktipis & Nesse, 2013). These and other evolutionary hypotheses of cancer are valuable, as they provide new frameworks for investigating and understanding the (paleo-)epidemiology of cancers, and perhaps neoplastic diseases more generally.

Past Prevalence of Neoplastic Diseases

A hotly debated topic within human paleo-oncology is the past prevalence of neoplastic diseases, especially cancers. Despite the abundance of benign tumors observed in the archaeological record, there is no systematic review or meta-analysis of this data. While this might be due to the generally asymptomatic nature of benign neoplasms, compiling benign neoplastic data is significantly complicated by inconsistent reporting and the ubiquity of some benign neoplasms (e.g., osteomata) that become buried within larger bioarchaeological studies. To date, only two published paleo-epidemiological studies of osteomata, the most common benign bone tumor, have been conducted. Siek et al. (2020) investigated the age- and sex-specific intra-population prevalence of osteomata, and Eshed et al. (2002) compared frequencies of osteomata in past (41%) and present (37.6%) population samples. Nevertheless, a systematic review of ancient benign neoplasms would be a valuable contribution, especially since there is little clinical data on the prevalence, distribution, or etiologies of many of these growths. Paleo-epidemiological studies might reveal interesting relationships between the prevalence of benign and malignant neoplastic diseases in different populations.

The antiquity and past prevalence of cancers has been discussed far more frequently than that of benign tumors. Some researchers attribute the paucity of evidence in physical remains and historical documents to the rarity of cancer in the past and have deemed cancers to be modern diseases. Proponents of this hypothesis believe that cancer rates have drastically risen due to anthropogenic carcinogens in the diet and environment, longer life expectancy, increasing time indoors/sedentary, and an increase in the transmission of oncogenic infectious diseases in growing populations (e.g., Micozzi, 1991; Capasso, 2005; David & Zimmerman, 2010). Given that evidence of cancer has been found as far back as the Triassic Period and continues to be found in most modern vertebrates, it is clear that "cancer" (if we take this reductionist view of cancer as a single entity) is not a strictly modern human disease. However, it is difficult to deny the relatively recent increase in anthropogenic carcinogens or the modern statistical data showing increases in certain types of cancer (e.g., tobacco-related lung cancer). Furthermore, cancer rates have risen in comparison with infectious diseases since the introduction of vaccines and antibiotics. As a result of these medical interventions, more individuals survive infectious diseases and live long enough to develop cancer. Consequently, it is important to consider population demographics when comparing past and present cancer rates (Waldron, 1996; Nerlich et al., 2006; Faltas, 2011; Zuckerman et al., 2016; Hunt et al., 2018). However, some modern populations have also experienced an increase in cancer rates despite little change in overall life expectancy, pointing to the great complexity of the issue (Capasso, 2005).

Paleo-epidemiological studies of cancers seem to indicate that there was a relatively lower prevalence of cancer in antiquity; however, caution should be taken in declaring its rarity since "rare disease" is an epidemiological term that is variably defined according to prevalence threshold statistics (Kirkpatrick et al., 2018). The average prevalence threshold for defining rare diseases rests between 40 and 50 cases/100,000 people, or between rates of 0.04% and 0.05% (Richter et al., 2015). Paleo-epidemiological studies of cancer have shown that the visible evidence of cancers in archaeological remains alone exceeds this threshold. For example, Nerlich and Bianucci (2020) calculated the mean relative frequency of cancers in ancient Egyptians as 0.5% through their meta-analysis of eight paleo-epidemiological studies conducted through visual analyses of ancient Egyptian population samples (frequency ranged from 0.2% to 2.8%). Marques et al. (2021) expanded on this idea and calculated a crude prevalence of 0.5% and a mean frequency of 1.2% from 180 published studies of cancer with population data for 20 or more individuals (altogether 32,353 skeletons and 151 cases of cancer). These authors argued that overall cancers were not rare in the ancient past, though the ability to identify specific cancer types (and therefore their specific rates) is limited. They also noted that the number of individuals with evidence of cancer was positively correlated with the size of the population sample, demonstrating that sample size is a limiting factor in paleo-oncological studies. Of course, it is also important to consider sample biases such as those resulting from taphonomic changes that can destroy, mask or mimic pathology. Importantly, even well-preserved skeletons from cemeteries are not representative of the once-living populations. Additionally, selection biases associated with skeletal collections (e.g., collection of specific skeletal elements or pathological bones) can heavily influence paleo-epidemiological studies of neoplastic diseases.

Molto and Sheldrick (2018) have recommended that paleo-epidemiological cancer data be compared with lifetime cancer risk (LTCR) statistics to accommodate for the cross-sectional nature of paleo-epidemiological data and the inability to ascertain specific cancer diagnoses in most cases. If we are to compare the LTCR of British males (53.5%) and females (47.5%) born in 1960 (Ahmad et al., 2015) to the estimated mean relative frequency of cancers in ancient Egyptians (0.5%, Nerlich & Bianucci, 2020), it is clear that there is an extreme discrepancy between ancient and modern cancer rates. However, it should be remembered that the paleo-epidemiological data are based only on cases that have survived in the archaeological record and that most cancers affect the rarely preserved soft tissues. It should also be considered that the LTCR of British males and females born in 1930 was only 38.5% and 36.7%, respectively, and a comparison of LTCR and cumulative risk statistics for the 1930 and 1960 cohorts indicated that this drastic increase in the LTCR was largely due to increased longevity rather than an increase in environmental or dietary carcinogens (Ahmad et al., 2015). Of course, this increase in human longevity did not begin in 1930 and likely extends deeper into the human past, further contributing to differences between past and present cancer rates.

With the introduction of the first vaccines, antibiotic, and life-extending medications like insulin, increasing human longevity likely factored into the rise in cancer rates between 1900 and 1930. However, the rising popularity of cigarettes since the end of the 19th century also contributed to a drastic change in cancer rates during this time (Proctor, 2012). Consequently, Waldron (1996) proposed that ancient cancer rates should be compared with age- and sex-specific cancer data from the early 20th century, which feature extremely low rates of tobacco-related lung cancer and relatively accurate statistical data resulting from improved reporting methods and increasing detection through surgery or autopsy. With this in mind, Waldron (1996) presented a method that used historic (1901–1905 CE) British cancer mortality and metastasis data to calculate the expected number of metastatic bone lesions based on an ancient population's age and sex demographics. When applied to archaeological population samples, this method is assumed to underestimate the prevalence of cancer because the statistics on which it is based do not include many types of cancers that can affect bone. Furthermore, although these historic data are more accurate than earlier reports, the 1901–1905 CE cancer statistics are likely an underestimation themselves, due to the diagnostic limitations and lingering cancer stigmas of the time. Nevertheless, when Waldron (1996) applied this method to an 18th–19th-century skeletal collection, the number of individuals with observable skeletal evidence of cancer fell within the calculated confidence intervals of the expected number. This suggested that the frequency of cancers in the observed 18th–19th-century population sample was similar to that of the early 20th-century reference population. This method was later applied to an ancient Egyptian population sample in which the number of individuals with observed cancerous lesions was higher than the estimated frequency of cancers based on the 20th century reference population but still lower than modern cancer rates (Zink et al., 1999). Another study expanded this ancient Egyptian data while also considering a historic Southern German population. This study revealed that the number of individuals with visible evidence of cancer in both of these populations fell within the cancer frequency range estimated using the age- and sex-specific 20th-century reference population data (Nerlich et al., 2006). Nerlich et al. (2006) interpreted these age-adjusted results as proof that human longevity is the greatest contributor to the increasing prevalence of cancers over time, not anthropogenic carcinogens.

Marques et al. (2021) have, however, argued that factors other than human longevity must be considered as contributors to the rise in cancers. They note that the human longevity hypothesis is weakened by the probability that despite changes in population demographics, many ancient individuals would have lived at least until middle adulthood when many cancers manifest, and there is no evidence that maximum lifespan has changed over time. They also note that paleo-demographics are limited by current osteological methods for estimating age-at-death, issues of preservation, and the current paucity of age- and sex-specific paleo-epidemiological studies of cancer. In a novel attempt to assess the rarity of cancers, Marques et al. (2021) also compared paleo-epidemiological data for metastatic bone lesions and skeletal evidence of tuberculosis in two post-Medieval European populations. Despite preconceived notions regarding the rarity of cancers and the ubiquity of tuberculosis during this time period, these studies showed that the amount of skeletal evidence for both conditions is very similar. However, the age-adjusted rates of metastatic cancers exceeded those for tuberculosis in the UK populations, while the opposite was true for the Portuguese populations. Consequently, this study further challenged the assumed rarity of cancers and the authors reiterated the need for age-adjusted paleo-epidemiological studies of cancers.

In another novel study, Western and Bekvalac (2020) conducted a visual and digital radiographic survey of 2241 middle-aged and old adult skeletons from pre-Industrial (before 1066–1750 CE) and Industrial (1750–1900 CE) Period populations in England. This survey showed an overall rate of 0.51% for metastatic cancers; however, more cases were found in the Industrial Period London population (0.71%) than the combined data from pre-Industrial Londoners (0%), and pre-Industrial (0.36%) and Industrial populations (0.21%) from outside of London. Multiple myeloma was also only seen in Industrial Period Londoners (four cases/1371 individuals), prompting the authors to conclude that cancer rates had risen as a result of industrial developments and the urbanization of London. As the first attempt to radiologically screen for cancers in a large skeletal population sample, this study represents a great stride in paleo-oncological methodology. However, until further research is completed, it remains unclear if these data are typical for all urban and rural populations transitioning from pre-Industrial to Industrial periods.

Most recently, Mitchell et al. (2021) analyzed 143 adult skeletons from 6 cemeteries in the Cambridge area (6th–16th centuries) through visual inspection, plain radiographs, and microCT. They reported that visual inspection revealed that only around 1% of the population had skeletal evidence of cancer, while radiography raised this rate to 3.5% (five individuals). This percentage is significantly higher than the aforementioned rates Western and Bekvalac (2020) observed in pre-Industrial British populations. Similar to Waldron (1996), Mitchell et al. (2021) used estimated overall rates of metastasis to bone to calculate a more accurate representation of the past cancer rate from the prevalence of skeletal evidence. Additionally, they considered the sensitivity of computed tomography for the detection of bone metastases to estimate a more accurate minimum prevalence of cancer in the population. These calculations estimated the minimum prevalence of all cancers in adults in this population to be between 9% and 14%.

It must be noted that none of the aforementioned studies applied radiographic screening to all skeletal elements and most only used radiographic analysis to study visually detected lesions. Considering this and issues of preservation, it is probable that the true prevalence of cancer in these archaeological collections was higher than reported. Furthermore, these paleo-epidemiological studies are largely based on cemetery populations, which are not true representations of the associated living population – a point raised prominently in the 'Osteological Paradox', which emphasizes the effects of demographic nonstationarity, selective mortality, and hidden heterogeneity in risks on paleo-epidemiological data (Wood et al., 1992). Additionally, remains can be differentially preserved and/or recovered from a cemetery, cemeteries may not include all local individuals and/or may include foreigners, and some populations may choose to bury stigmatized individuals (e.g., individuals with disfiguring cases of cancer) separately from the rest of the population (Milner et al., 2008).

Consequently, although paleo-epidemiological studies may provide important information about the history of neoplastic diseases, they are not a direct representation of the health of their associated living populations. Moreover, due to the limitations of paleo-oncological diagnosis, most studies assess cancers as a single disease group, despite there being over 100 different diseases with different etiologies and frequencies (National Cancer Institute, 2015). This is an important consideration since some types of cancer that are considered rare in the modern world are well represented in the archaeological record. For example, multiple myeloma (modern incidence rate = approx. 0.007%, Padala et al., 2021) is the second most commonly diagnosed malignancy in past populations (17.3%, 54/313, Hunt et al. 2022). Primary bone cancers also make up an uncharacteristically large proportion (15.0%, 47/313, Hunt et al. 2022) of the paleo-oncological data despite their present-day rarity (modern incidence rate = approx. 0.0009%, Cancer Research UK, 2020). Furthermore, given that some types of cancer are clinically rare and it seems that past populations had lower cancer rates overall, it can be assumed that some types of cancer could have been considered "rare diseases" in the past. Unfortunately, such declarations could only be made with an extremely large, perfectly preserved paleo-epidemiological dataset and the ability to detect and diagnose all cancers from human remains. In contrast, it has been stated that some cancers may have been more prevalent in some past populations compared to their modern counterparts. For example, Whitley and Boyer (2018) demonstrated the devastating effect of radon on a pit-house-dwelling pre-Columbian population in which 4/82 (5%) individuals developed the aforementioned rare disease, multiple myeloma. Likewise, improvements in food hygiene and advances in vaccines and antibiotics have contributed to sharp decreases in the rates of pathogen-linked stomach and liver cancers in the modern world (Ewald, 2018).

Although the aforementioned paleo-epidemiological studies of cancer have contributed significantly to our collective understanding of the past prevalence of cancers, they do not represent all of the regional differences and temporal fluctuations of cancer rates that surely extended deep into the human past. Further research is needed to determine if the observed cancer rates in these population studies are typical for most ancient populations. Unfortunately, in addition to the methodological limitation of paleo-oncological detection and diagnosis, current paleo-oncological data is largely composed of small case studies without associated population data, preventing any attempt to estimate population cancer prevalence. Furthermore, curated skeletal collections are often geographically and temporally diverse and are heavily affected by preservation and selection biases (e.g., cranial collections, pathology collections) (Hunt et al., 2018). Consequently, new paleo-epidemiological data are needed.

Conclusion

Future paleo-epidemiological studies of cancers may bring estimates closer to the true frequency of neoplastic diseases; however, due to the many limitations of paleo-oncology, we may never truly know their past prevalence. Consequently, comparisons of past and present cancer rates should be conducted with an abundance of caution. Nevertheless, paleopathological studies of neoplastic diseases, benign and malignant, continue to provide important information about the history of neoplastic diseases and their impact on humans. These studies also have the potential to reveal new paleo-epidemiological patterns and risk factors and they can inspire new understandings of how neoplastic diseases develop and evolve in the human body. Given the growing interest in evolutionary medicine, particularly with regard to cancers, it is important that paleo-oncological data continue to grow and improve. To this end, "7 S's" for continued progress in the field of paleo-oncology have been recommended: (1) **Stay current**, (2) **Standardize methods**, (3) **Scrutinize** existing data and give a **Second Opinion**, (4) **Search** for new evidence in situ, (5) **Screen** for evidence with advanced methods, (6) **Share** your data, and (7) **Synthesize** paleo-oncological data to find meaningful patterns (see Kirkpatrick et al., 2018 for a more comprehensive explanation of these principles). Through these actions, the accuracy and amount of paleo-oncological data will increase, enabling more meaningful conclusions to be reached in the future.

References

Ahmad, A., Ormiston-Smith, N. & Sasieni, P. (2015). Trends in the lifetime risk of developing cancer in Great Britain: comparison of risk for those born from 1930 to 1960. *British Journal of Cancer* 112(5):943–947. https://doi.org/10.1038/bjc.2014.606.

Aktipis, C. A., Boddy, A. M., Jansen, G., Hibner, U., Hochberg, M. E., Maley, C. C. & Wilkinson, G. S. (2015). Cancer across the tree of life: cooperation and cheating in multicellularity. *Philosophical Transactions of the Royal Society B: Biological Sciences* 370(1673):20140219. https://doi.org/10.1098/rstb.2014.0219.

Aktipis, C. A. & Nesse, R. M. (2013). Evolutionary foundations for cancer biology. *Evolutionary Applications* 6(1):144–159. https://doi.org/10.1111/eva.12034.

Albuquerque, T. A., Drummond do Val, L., Doherty, A. & de Magalhaes, J. P. (2018). From humans to hydra: patterns of cancer across the tree of life. *Biological Reviews* 93(3):1715–1734. https://doi.org/10.1111/brv.12415.

Aufderheide, A. C. & Rodriguez-Martin, C. (1998). Neoplastic conditions. In Aufderheide, A. & Rodríguez-Martín, C. (Eds.), *The Cambridge Encyclopedia of Human Paleopathology*, pp. 371–392. Cambridge: Cambridge University Press.

Bartsiokas, A. & Day, M. H. (1993). Electron probe energy dispersive x-ray microanalysis (EDXA) in the investigation of fossil bone: the case of Java Man. *Proceedings of the Royal Society of London. Series B: Biological Sciences* 252(1334):115–123. https://doi.org/10.1098/rspb.1993.0054.

Bartstra, G. -J. (1982). The river-laid strata near Trinil, site of *Homo erectus erectus*, Java, Indonesia. *Modern Quaternary Research in Southeast Asia* 7:97–130.

Biehler-Gomez, L., Tritella, S., Martino, F., Campobasso, C. P., Franchi, A., Spairani, R., Sardanelli, F. & Cattaneo, C. (2019). The synergy between radiographic and macroscopic observation of skeletal lesions on dry bone. *International Journal of Legal Medicine* 133(5):1611–1628. https://doi.org/10.1007/s00414-019-02122-0.

Boddy, A. M., Abegglen, L. M., Pessier, A. P., Aktipis, A., Schiffman, J. D., Maley, C. C. & Witte, C. (2020). Lifetime cancer prevalence and life history traits in mammals. *Evolution, Medicine, and Public Health* 2020(1):187–195. https://doi.org/10.1093/emph/eoaa015.

Boddy, A. M., Kokko, H., Breden, F., Wilkinson, G. S. & Aktipis, C. A. (2015). Cancer susceptibility and reproductive trade-offs: a model of the evolution of cancer defences. *Philosophical Transactions of the Royal Society B: Biological Sciences* 370(1673):20140220. https://doi.org/10.1098/rstb.2014.0220.

Brothwell, D. (1967). The evidence for neoplasms. In Brothwell, D. R. & Sandison, A. (Eds.), *Diseases in Antiquity*, pp. 320–345. Springfield: CC Thomas.

Brothwell, D. (2012). Tumors: problems of differential diagnosis in paleopathology. In Grauer, A. (Ed.), *A Companion to Paleopathology*, pp. 420–433. Oxford: Wiley-Blackwell. https://doi.org/10.1002/9781444345940.ch23.

Burnett, T. (2020). Atypical cells: are they cancer? https://www.mayoclinic.org/diseases-conditions/cancer/expert-answers/atypical-cells/faq-20058493.

Cancer Research UK. (2020, March 11). Bone sarcoma incidence statistics. Retrieved February 15, 2021, from https://www.cancerresearchuk.org/health-professional/cancer-statistics/statistics-by-cancer-type/bone-sarcoma/incidence#heading-Zero.

Capasso, L. L. (2005). Antiquity of cancer. *International Journal of Cancer* 113(1):2–13. https://doi.org/10.1002/ijc.20610.

Caulin, A. F. & Maley, C. C. (2011). Peto's paradox: evolution's prescription for cancer prevention. *Trends in Ecology & Evolution* 26(4):175–182. https://doi.org/10.1016/j.tree.2011.01.002.

Colella, G., Cappabianca, S., Gerardi, G. & Mallegni, F. (2012). *Homo neanderthalensis*; first documented benign intraosseous tumor in maxillofacial skeleton. *Journal of Oral and Maxillofacial Surgery* 70(2):373–375. https://doi.org/10.1016/j.joms.2011.03.022.

Curnoe, D. & Brink, J. (2010). Evidence of pathological conditions in the Florisbad cranium. *Journal of Human Evolution* 59(5):504–513. https://doi.org/10.1016/j.jhevol.2010.06.003.

David, A. R. & Zimmerman, M. R. (2010). Cancer: an old disease, a new disease or something in between? *Nature Reviews Cancer* 10(10):728–733. https://doi.org/10.1038/nrc2914.

Davies, J. A. (2004). Inverse correlation between an organ's cancer rate and its evolutionary antiquity. *Organogenesis* 1(2):60–63. https://doi.org/10.4161/org.1.2.1338.

Day, M. H. & Molleson, T. (1973). The Trinil femora. In Day, M. H. (Ed.), *Human Evolution*, pp. 127–154. London: Taylor and Francis.

De Boer, H. H. & Maat, G. G. (2018). Dry bone histology of bone tumours. *International Journal of Paleopathology* 21:56–63. https://doi.org/10.1016/j.ijpp.2016.11.005.

Dubois, M. E. F. T. (1894). *Pithecanthropus Erectus: Eine Menschenähnliche Übergangsform aus Java*. Batavia: Landesdruckerei.

Elefteriou, F., Kolanczyk, M., Schindeler, A., Viskochil, D. H., Hock, J. M., Schorry, E. K., … & Stevenson, D. A. (2009). Skeletal abnormalities in neurofibromatosis type 1: approaches to therapeutic options. *American Journal of Medical Genetics Part A* 149A:2327–2338. https://doi.org/10.1002/ajmg.a.33045.

Eshed, V., Latimer, B., Greenwald, C. M., Jellema, L. M., Rothschild, B. M., Wish-Baratz, S. & Hershkovitz, I. (2002). Button osteoma: its etiology and pathophysiology. *American Journal of Physical Anthropology* 118(3):217–230. https://doi.org/10.1002/ajpa.10087.

Ewald, P. W. (2018). Ancient cancers and infection-induced oncogenesis. *International Journal of Paleopathology* 21:178–185. https://doi.org/10.1016/j.ijpp.2017.08.007.

Faltas, B. (2011). Cancer is an ancient disease: the case for better palaeoepidemiological and molecular studies. *Nature Reviews Cancer* 11(1):76–76. https://doi.org/10.1038/nrc2914-c1.

Fornaciari, G. (2018). Histology of ancient soft tissue tumors: a review. *International Journal of Paleopathology* 21:64–76. https://doi.org/10.1016/j.ijpp.2017.02.007.

Fornaciari, G., Zavaglia, K., Giusti, L., Vultaggio, C. & Ciranni, R. (2003). Human papillomavirus in a 16th century mummy. *The Lancet* 362(9390):1160. https://doi.org/10.1016/S0140-6736(03)14487-X.

Fukiyama, J., Nao-I, N., Maruiwa, F. & Sawada, A. (1993). Two cases of benign lacrimal gland tumors. In Till, P. (Ed.), *Ophthalmic Echography* 13. Documenta Ophthalmologica Proceedings Series, vol 55. Dordrecht: Springer. https://doi.org/10.1007/978-94-011-1846-0_10.

Halperin, E. C. (2004). Paleo-oncology: the role of ancient remains in the study of cancer. *Perspectives in Biology and Medicine* 47(1):1–14. https://doi.org/10.1353/pbm.2004.0010.

Haridy, Y., Witzmann, F., Asbach, P., Schoch, R. R., Fröbisch, N. & Rothschild, B. M. (2019). Triassic cancer—osteosarcoma in a 240-million-year-old stem-turtle. *JAMA Oncology* 5(3):425–426. https://doi.org/10.1001/jamaoncol.2018.6766.

Hunt, K., Kirkpatrick, C. L., Campbell, R. & Willoughby, J. (2022). Cancer research in ancient bodies (C.R.A.B.) database. Retrieved February 1, 2022, from https://www.cancerantiquity.org/crabdatabase.

Hunt, K. J., Roberts, C. & Kirkpatrick, C. L. (2018). Taking stock: a systematic review of archaeological evidence of cancers in human and early hominin remains. *International Journal of Paleopathology* 21:12–26. https://doi.org/10.1016/j.ijpp.2018.03.002.

Jónsson, H., Ginolhac, A., Schubert, M., Johnson, P. L. & Orlando, L. (2013). mapDamage2.0: fast approximate Bayesian estimates of ancient DNA damage parameters. *Bioinformatics* 29(13):1682–1684.

Julien, R. (1965). *Les Hommes Fossiles de la Pierre Taillée*. Paris: Boubée et Cie.

Kennedy, G. (1983). Some aspects of femoral morphology in *Homo erectus*. *Journal of Human Evolution* 12(7):587–616. https://doi.org/10.1016/S0047-2484(83)80001-3.

Key, F. M., Posth, C., Krause, J., Herbig, A. & Bos, K. I. (2017). Mining metagenomic data sets for ancient DNA: recommended protocols for authentication. *Trends in Genetics* 33(8):508–520.

Kirkpatrick, C. L. (2020). Neoplasm or not? Considering the limitations of palaeo-oncology. *ΑΚΑΔΗΜΙΑ ΑΘΗΝΩΝ. Special Issue on Palaeo-oncology: Proceedings of the 2nd International Symposium of the European Society of Oncology History*, pp. 49–66.

Kirkpatrick, C. L., Campbell, R. A. & Hunt, K. J. (2018). Paleo-oncology: taking stock and moving forward. *International Journal of Paleopathology* 21:3–11. https://doi.org/10.1016/j.ijpp.2018.02.001.

Kozlov, A. (2010). The possible evolutionary role of tumors in the origin of new cell types. *Medical Hypotheses* 74(1):177–185. https://doi.org/10.1016/j.mehy.2009.07.027.

Kumar, V. L., Abbas, A. K. & Aster, J. C. (2015). *Robbins and Cotran Pathologic Basis of Disease*. Philadelphia, PA: Saunders.

Lawrence, J. (1935). A note on the pathology of the Kanam mandible. In Leakey, L. (Ed.), *The Stone Age Races of Kenya*, pp. 139. Oxford: Oxford University Press.

Leakey, L. S. B. (1935). *The Stone Age Races of Kenya*. Oxford: Oxford University Press.

Marques, C., Matos, V., Costa, T., Zink, A. & Cunha, E. (2018). Absence of evidence or evidence of absence? A discussion on paleoepidemiology of neoplasms with contributions from two Portuguese human skeletal reference collections (19th–20th century). *International Journal of Paleopathology* 21:83–95. https://doi.org/10.1016/j.ijpp.2017.03.005.

Marques, C., Roberts, C., Matos, V. M. & Buikstra, J. E. (2021). Cancers as rare diseases: terminological, theoretical, and methodological biases. *International Journal of Paleopathology* 32:111–122. https://doi.org/10.1016/j.ijpp.2020.12.005.

Marques, C., Santos, A. L. & Cunha, E. (2013). Better a broader diagnosis than a misdiagnosis: the study of a neoplastic condition in a male individual who died in early 20th century (Coimbra, Portugal). *International Journal of Osteoarchaeology* 23(6):664–675. https://doi.org/10.1002/oa.1294.

Mays, S. (1998). *The Archaeology of Human Bones*. London: Routledge.

McGinnis Jr, J. P. & Parham, D. M. (1978). Mandible-like structure with teeth in an ovarian cystic teratoma. *Oral Surgery, Oral Medicine, Oral Pathology* 45(1):104–106.

Micozzi, M. S. (1991). Disease in antiquity. *Archives of Pathology & Laboratory Medicine* 115(8): 838–844.

Miller, E., Ragsdale, B. D. & Ortner, D. J. (1996). Accuracy in dry bone diagnosis: a comment on palaeopathological methods. *International Journal of Osteoarchaeology* 6(3):221–229. https://doi.org/10.1002/(SICI)1099-1212(199606)6:3<221::AID-OA267>3.0.CO;2-2.

Milner, G. R., Wood, J. W. & Boldsen, J. L. (2008). Advances in paleodemography. In Katzenberg, M. A. & Saunders, S. R. (Eds.), *Biological Anthropology of the Human Skeleton* (2nd ed.), pp. 561–600. Hoboken: John Wiley & Sons, Inc.

Mitchell, P. D., Dittmar, J. M., Mulder, B., Inskip, S., Littlewood, A., Cessford, C. & Robb, J. E. (2021). The prevalence of cancer in Britain before industrialization. *Cancer* 127(17):3054–3059. https://doi.org/10.1002/cncr.33615.

Mohamadi, A. & Salvatori, R. (2012). Neuroendocrine growth disorders–dwarfism, gigantism. In Fink, G., Pfaff, D. W. & Levine, J. E. (Eds.), *Handbook of Neuroendocrinology*, pp. 707–721. London: Academic Press. https://doi.org/10.1016/B978-0-12-375097-6.10032-0.

Mohan, H. (2019). *Textbook of Pathology*. St. Louis: Jaypee Brothers Medical Publishers (P) Ltd.

Molto, E. & Sheldrick, P. (2018). Paleo-oncology in the Dakhleh Oasis, Egypt: case studies and a paleoepidemiological perspective. *International Journal of Paleopathology* 21:96–110. https://doi.org/10.1016/j.ijpp.2018.02.003.

Moodie, R. L. (1927). Tumors in the lower carboniferous. *Science* 66(1718):540–540. https://doi.org/10.1126/science.66.1718.540-a.

Morandi, X., Amlashi, S. F. & Riffaud, L. (2006). A dynamic theory for hydrocephalus revealing benign intraspinal tumours: tumoural obstruction of the spinal subarachnoid space reduces total CSF compartment compliance. *Medical Hypotheses* 67(1):79–81.

Muzio, L. L. (2008). Nevoid basal cell carcinoma syndrome (Gorlin syndrome). *Orphanet Journal of Rare Diseases* 3(1):1–16. https://link.springer.com/article/10.1186/1750-1172-3-32.

National Cancer Institute. (2015, February 9). What is cancer? Retrieved February 15, 2021, from https://www.cancer.gov/about-cancer/understanding/what-is-cancer#types.

Nerlich, A. G. (2018). Molecular paleopathology and paleo-oncology–state of the art, potentials, limitations and perspectives. *International Journal of Paleopathology* 21:77–82. https://doi.org/10.1016/j.ijpp.2017.02.004.

Nerlich, A. G. & Bianucci, R. (2020). Paleo-oncology and mummies. In Shin, D. H. & Bianucci, R. (Eds.), *The Handbook of Mummy Studies: New Frontiers in Scientific and Cultural Perspectives*, pp. 1–16. Singapore: Springer Nature. https://doi.org/10.1007%2F978-981-15-1614-6_38-1.

Nerlich, A. G., Rohrbach, H., Bachmeier, B. & Zink, A. (2006). Malignant tumors in two ancient populations: an approach to historical tumor epidemiology. *Oncology Reports* 16(1):197–202. https://doi.org/10.3892/or.16.1.197.

Oakley, K. P., Campbell, B. G. & Molleson, T. I. (1977). *Catalogue of Fossil Hominids*. London: British Museum.

Odes, E. J., Delezene, L. K., Randolph-Quinney, P. S., Smilg, J. S., Augustine, T. N., Jakata, K. & Berger, L. R. (2018). A case of benign osteogenic tumour in *Homo naledi*: evidence for peripheral osteoma in the UW 101–1142 mandible. *International Journal of Paleopathology* 21:47–55. https://doi.org/10.1016/j.ijpp.2017.05.003.

Odes, E. J., Randolph-Quinney, P. S., Steyn, M., Throckmorton, Z., Smilg, J. S., Zipfel, B., Augustine, T. N., De Beer, F., Hoffman, J. W. & Franklin, R. D. (2016). Earliest hominin cancer: 1.7-million-year-old osteosarcoma from Swartkrans Cave, South Africa. *South African Journal of Science* 112(7–8):1–5. https://doi.org/10.17159/sajs.2016/20150471.

Ortner, D. J. (2003). Tumors and tumor-like lesions in bone. In Ortner, D. J. (Ed.), *Identification of Pathological Conditions in Human Skeletal Remains*, pp. 503–543. San Diego, CA: Academic Press.

Padala, S. A., Barsouk, A., Barsouk, A., Rawla, P., Vakiti, A., Kolhe, R., Kota, V. & Ajebo, G. H. (2021). Epidemiology, staging, and management of multiple myeloma. *Medical Sciences* 9(1):3. https://doi.org/10.3390/medsci9010003.

Panzer, S., Wittig, H., Zesch, S., Rosendahl, W., Blache, S., Müller-Gerbl, M. & Hotz, G. (2017). Evidence of neurofibromatosis type 1 in a multi-morbid Inca child mummy: a paleoradiological investigation using computed tomography. *PLoS ONE* 12(4):e0175000. https://doi.org/10.1371/journal.pone.0175000.

Pérez, P. -J., Gracia, A., Martínez, I. & Arsuaga, J. -L. (1997). Paleopathological evidence of the cranial remains from the Sima de los Huesos Middle Pleistocene site (Sierra de Atapuerca, Spain). Description and preliminary inferences. *Journal of Human Evolution* 33(2–3):409–421. https://doi.org/10.1006/jhev.1997.0139.

Peto, R., Roe, F., Lee, P., Levy, L. & Clack, J. (1975). Cancer and ageing in mice and men. *British Journal of Cancer* 32(4):411–426. https://doi.org/10.1038/bjc.1975.242.

Phelan, J., Weiner, M., Ricci, J., Plummer, T., Gauld, S., Potts, R. & Bromage, T. (2007). Diagnosis of the pathology of the Kanam mandible. *Oral Surgery, Oral Medicine, Oral Pathology, Oral Radiology and Endodontology* 4(103):e20. https://doi.org/10.1016/j.tripleo.2006.12.041.

Pinhasi, R. & Bourbou, C. (2007). How representative are human skeletal assemblages for population analysis? In Pinhasi, R. & Mays, S. (Eds.), *Advances in Human Palaeopathology*, pp. 31–44. https://doi.org/10.1002/9780470724187.ch2.

Proctor, R. N. (2012). The history of the discovery of the cigarette–lung cancer link: evidentiary traditions, corporate denial, global toll. *Tobacco Control* 21(2):87–91. https://doi.org/10.1136/tobaccocontrol-2011-050338.

Ragsdale, B. D., Campbell, R. A. & Kirkpatrick, C. L. (2018). Neoplasm or not? General principles of morphologic analysis of dry bone specimens. *International Journal of Paleopathology* 21:27–40. https://doi.org/10.1016/j.ijpp.2017.02.002.

Randolph-Quinney, P. S., Williams, S. A., Steyn, M., Meyer, M. R., Smilg, J. S., Churchill, S. E., Odes, E. J., Augustine, T., Tafforeau, P. & Berger, L. R. (2016). Osteogenic tumour in *Australopithecus sediba*: earliest hominin evidence for neoplastic disease. *South African Journal of Science* 112(7–8):1–7. https://doi.org/10.17159/sajs.2016/20150470.

Richter, T., Nestler-Parr, S., Babela, R., Khan, Z. M., Tesoro, T., Molsen, E. & Hughes, D. A. (2015). Rare disease terminology and definitions—a systematic global review: report of the ISPOR rare disease special interest group. *Value in Health* 18(6):906–914. https://doi.org/10.1016/j.jval.2015.05.008.

Robert, J. (2010). Comparative study of tumorigenesis and tumor immunity in invertebrates and non-mammalian vertebrates. *Developmental & Comparative Immunology* 34(9):915–925. https://doi.org/10.1016/j.dci.2010.05.011.

Rosmarin, A. (2019). Leukemia, lymphoma, and myeloma. In Stein, G. S. & Luebbers, K. P. (Eds.), *Cancer: Prevention, Early Detection, Treatment and Recovery*, pp. 299–316. New York: John Wiley and Sons. https://doi.org/10.1002/9781119645214.ch16.

Rothschild, B. M. & Rothschild, C. (1995). Comparison of radiologic and gross examination for detection of cancer in defleshed skeletons. *American Journal of Physical Anthropology* 96(4):357–363. https://doi.org/10.1002/ajpa.1330960404.

Ruggieri, M., Praticò, A. D., Catanzaro, S., Palmucci, S. & Polizzi, A. (2018). Did Cro-Magnon 1 have neurofibromatosis type 2? *The Lancet* 392(10148):632–633. https://doi.org/10.1016/S0140-6736(18)31544-7.

Ryder, J. W., Kleinschmidt-DeMasters, B. K., and Keller, T. S. (1986). Sudden deterioration and death in patients with benign tumors of the third ventricle area. *Journal of Neurosurgery* 64(2):216–223. https://doi.org/10.3171/jns.1986.64.2.0216.

Scheele, W. E. (1954). *Prehistoric Animals*. Cleveland: World Publishing Co.

Schultz, M., Parzinger, H., Posdnjakov, D. V., Chikisheva, T. A. & Schmidt-Schultz, T. H. (2007). Oldest known case of metastasizing prostate carcinoma diagnosed in the skeleton of a 2,700-year-old Scythian king from Arzhan (Siberia, Russia). *International Journal of Cancer* 121(12):2591–2595. https://doi.org/10.1002/ijc.23073.

Semah, F., Semah, A., Sartono, S., Zaim, Y. & Djubiantono, T. (1981). Age and environment of *Homo erectus* in Java – new paleomagnetic and pollen analytic results. *Anthropologie* 85(3):509–516.

Siek, T. (2020). In defence of the osteoma: the relevance of benign tumours in bioarchaeology and palaeo-oncology. *International Journal of Osteoarchaeology* 30(2):281–283. https://doi.org/10.1002/oa.2839.

Siek, T., Rando, C., Cieślik, A., Spinek, A. & Waldron, T. (2020). A palaeoepidemiological investigation of osteomata, with reference to Medieval Poland. *International Journal of Osteoarchaeology* 31(2):154–161. https://doi.org/10.1002/oa.2935.

Soriano, M. (1970). The fluoric origin of the bone lesion in the *Pithecanthropus erectus* femur. *American Journal of Physical Anthropology* 32(1):49–57. https://doi.org/10.1002/ajpa.1330320107.

Stathopoulos, G. (1975). Kanam mandible's tumour. *The Lancet* 305(7899):165. https://doi.org/10.1016/S0140-6736(75)91462-2.

Strouhal, E. & Kritscher, H. (1990). Neolithic case of a multiple myeloma from Mauer (Vienna, Austria). *Anthropologie* 28(1):79–87.

Tobias, P. (1994). The pathology of the Kanam mandible. *Journal of Paleopathology* 6(3):125–128.

Tobias, P. V. (1962). A re-examination of the Kanam mandible. *Actes du IVe Congrès Panafricain de Préhistoire et de l'Étude du Quaternaire, Sections I and II. Tervuren, Belgique: Annales Ser. Qu-80, Sciences Humaines* 40:341–350.

Ujvari, B., Roche, B. & Thomas, F. (2017). *Ecology and Evolution of Cancer*. London: Academic Press.

van den Bergh, G. D., Mubroto, B., Aziz, F., Sondaar, P. Y. & de Vos, J. (1996). Did *Homo erectus* reach the island of Flores? *Bulletin of the Indo-Pacific Prehistory Association* 14:27–36.

Virchow, R. (1895). Exostosen und hyperostosen von extremitäten-knochen des menschen, im hinblick auf den pithecanthropus. *Zeitschrift für Ethnologie* 27:787–793.

Waldron, T. (1996). What was the prevalence of malignant disease in the past? *International Journal of Osteoarchaeology* 6(5):463–470. https://doi.org/10.1002/(SICI)1099-1212(199612)6:5<463::AID-OA304>3.0.CO;2-Y.

Weiss, M. H., Teal, J., Gott, P., Wycoff, R., Yadley, R., Apuzzo, M. L. J., Giannotta, S. L., Kletzky, O. & March, C. (1983). Natural history of microprolactinomas: six-year follow-up. *Neurosurgery* 12(2):180–183. https://doi.org/10.1227/00006123-198302000-00008.

Western, G. & Bekvalac, J. (2020). Cancer. In Western, G. & Bekvalac, J. (Eds.), *Manufactured Bodies: The Impact of Industrialisation on London Health*, pp. 194–246. Oxford: Oxbow Books.

Whitley, C. B. & Boyer, J. L. (2018). Assessing cancer risk factors faced by an Ancestral Puebloan population in the North American southwest. *International Journal of Paleopathology* 21:166–177. https://doi.org/10.1016/j.ijpp.2017.06.004.

Wood, J. W., Milner, G. R., Harpending, H. C., Weiss, K. M., Cohen, M. N., Eisenberg, L. E., Hutchinson, D. L., Jankauskas, R., Cesnys, G. & Česnys, G. (1992). The osteological paradox: problems of inferring prehistoric health from skeletal samples [and comments and reply]. *Current Anthropology* 33(4):343–370. https://doi.org/10.1086/204084.

Zimmerman, M. R. (1977). An experimental study of mummification pertinent to the antiquity of cancer. *Cancer* 40(3):1358–1362. https://doi.org/10.1002/1097-0142(197709)40:3<1358::AID-CNCR2820400354>3.0.CO;2-J.

Zink, A., Rohrbach, H., Szeimies, U., Hagedorn, H., Haas, C., Weyss, C., Bachmeier, B. & Nerlich, A. (1999). Malignant tumors in an ancient Egyptian population. *Anticancer Research* 19(5B):4273–4277.

Zuckerman, M. K., Harper, K. N. & Armelagos, G. J. (2016). Adapt or die: three case studies in which the failure to adopt advances from other fields has compromised paleopathology. *International Journal of Osteoarchaeology* 26(3):375–383. https://doi.org/10.1002/oa.2426.

16
TREPONEMAL INFECTION

Brenda J. Baker

Treponemal infection produces disease in humans that is clinically categorized as pinta, yaws, bejel (endemic syphilis), and syphilis. The origin and evolution of treponemal infection have been contested for several centuries. The primary focus of this debate concerns whether treponemal infection existed in Europe and other parts of the eastern hemisphere before the Columbian voyages of the late 1400s (the pre-Columbian hypothesis) or whether it was carried to Europe by Columbus's crew (the Columbian hypothesis). The emphasis on sexually transmitted syphilis has been shaped by colonialist views that stress the centrality of European conquest and colonization of the Americas to change over time. This perspective has masked the significance of other questions about the origin and spread of treponemal infection and inhibited the thorough consideration of other hypotheses. For instance, in the alternative Unitarian hypothesis, pinta, yaws, bejel, and syphilis are viewed as one disease caused by a single organism with a zoonotic origin that shows different clinical manifestations depending on climatic (e.g., arid, tropical, or temperate environment), socio-cultural (e.g., sanitation), and demographic (e.g., population density, age of onset) factors. The related Evolutionary hypothesis, proposed by Hackett (1963), presented alternative phylogenies for divergence of the treponemal variants that affect humans but are not supported by recent genetic research (Baker et al., 2020:10–12).

Addressing questions about treponemal disease that go beyond the fascination with the geographic origin of syphilis is best pursued through interdisciplinary and collaborative research involving expertise in bioarchaeology and paleopathology, genetics, evolutionary medicine, immunology, absolute dating methods, and medical history, as advocated by Baker et al. (2020), and more generally by Buikstra et al. (2017). Paleopathology can contribute considerably to elucidating the co-evolution of the genus *Treponema* (*T. pallidum*, in particular), and human populations. Paleopathologists should be involved actively in collaborative research investigating this complex host/pathogen relationship.

Persistent Problems in Unraveling the Impact of Treponemal Disease in the Past

To improve our understanding of treponemal infection and the disease it produced in past populations, several issues must be confronted. Persistent problems include, but are not limited to, difficulties in our ability to diagnose treponemal disease in human skeletal remains; gaps in both modern and ancient DNA (aDNA) sampling for reconstructing *T. pallidum* phylogeny and its co-evolution with *Homo sapiens*; and a focus on Western historical documentation that has led to a biased perspective for understanding disease transmission and responses to it. Traction recently has been gained on some fronts, with more work required in other areas, as discussed in subsequent sections.

Difficulties in Differential Diagnosis

The causative organism of syphilis (*T. pallidum* subsp. *pallidum*) was discovered in March 1905 by Fritz Richard Schaudinn, a protozoologist who directed the Protozoan Laboratory of the Kaiserlichen Gesundheitsamtes in Berlin (Thorburn, 1971; Waugh, 2005). Initially named *Spirochaeta pallida*, the discovery was published in April 1905 by Schaudinn and Erich Hoffmann, a dermatologist and syphilologist (Schaudinn & Hofmann, 1905b; Thorburn, 1971; Waugh, 2005) and elaborated upon a month later (Schaudinn & Hoffmann, 1905a). The etiological agent of yaws (*T. pallidum* subsp. *pertenue*) was discovered quickly thereafter and designated *Spirochaeta pertenuis* by Aldo Castellani, a physician working with yaws patients in Sri Lanka (Castellani, 1905; Stamm, 2015b). These diseases, along with congenital syphilis and an array of other maladies such as leprosy, skin ulcers, and even lice, were treated with mercury in various forms since the Middle Ages, continuing into the early 20th century (Parker, 1860; Rosebury, 1971; Quétel, 1986/1990; O'Shea, 1990; Sartin & Perry, 1995; Demaitre, 2007:264; Norn et al., 2008; Swiderski, 2008; Fornaciari et al., 2011; Obladen, 2013; Lanzirotti et al., 2014:204; Tampa et al., 2014; Baker et al., 2020:16). In 1884, bismuth salts, which were less toxic, began to be used to treat syphilis (Tampa et al., 2014). Salvarsan (compound 606) was developed in 1910, with other less toxic arsenicals following, and treatment of treponemal disease with penicillin began in 1943 (Sartin & Perry, 1995; Obladen, 2013; Tampa et al., 2014; Stamm, 2015b).

The impact of mercury- and arsenic-based treatments on the course of disease, and their potential effects on the skeleton and dentition of those treated, is one factor that may complicate differential diagnosis in paleopathology (Box 16.1). Alterations arising from repeated doses of mercury are most recognizable in dentitions of those treated in infancy and childhood due to the impact on amelogenesis and resulting enamel defects (Ioannou et al., 2015; Radu & Soficaru, 2016; Baker et al., 2020:26). Presence of such severely hypoplastic permanent teeth is strongly suggestive of congenital treponemal infection but requires other supporting evidence because mercury treatments were widely used (Baker et al., 2020:16, 26). While arsenical treatments may cause tooth abrasion and linear enamel hypoplasia, and bismuth may lead to enamel pigmentation, particularly on the cervical area of incisors, they do not produce severe enamel defects like those related to mercury (Ioannou & Henneberg, 2017:457; Baker et al., 2020:26). With sufficient sampling, including controls from surrounding soil matrix and careful bioarchaeological contextualization as discussed by Baker and colleagues (2020:16–17; see also Lanzirotti et al., 2014, and Walser et al., 2018, for examples), use of various analytical techniques for identifying mercury and arsenic in skeletal tissues may aid the differential diagnosis of treponemal disease and its identification even in individuals without pathological lesions.

Differential diagnosis is a principal goal of paleopathology but only the most severe cases that display pathognomonic lesions (i.e., those lesions that occur only in a single condition) are typically identified. Pinta is a skin condition that does not affect the skeletal system, although it potentially may be evident in desiccated or mummified individuals with preserved

> **Box 16.1 Current Issues in the Paleopathological Diagnosis of Treponemal Disease**
>
> 1. Effects of treatments with toxins including mercury and arsenic must be distinguished from bony alterations caused by the disease process and not used as a proxy for the presence of treponemal disease (though strongly suggestive of treatment for it) without careful bioarchaeological contextualization.
> 2. Early stages of skeletal involvement are not diagnostic/recognized so reliance on pathognomonic criteria will only identify the most severely affected individuals in skeletal samples.
> 3. Persistence in attributing a modern clinically defined variant (yaws, bejel, or syphilis) as the cause of skeletal lesions in archaeological remains.
> 4. Standardized descriptions/criteria are needed for investigating presence/absence of treponemal disease globally.
> 5. Systematic investigations of skeletal collections for patterns of lesions consistent with, strongly suggestive of, or diagnostic of treponemal disease are needed on a broader scale with contextualization of entire site/sample.

skin. For untreated yaws, bejel, and syphilis, the course of disease is similar, progressing from the initial lesion at the site of infection (primary stage), followed by a secondary stage that resolves after several weeks and enters a latent stage. Approximately 10–12% subsequently advance to a tertiary stage (Gjestland, 1955:148; Steinbock, 1976:143; Giacani & Lukehart, 2014:93). Skeletal manifestations occur in approximately 10–24% of those with untreated secondary and tertiary stages of treponemal disease (Hackett, 1951; Grin, 1952:19; Steinbock, 1976:109, 142), but diagnostic lesions are found only in the tertiary stage of disease. The initial stages of skeletal involvement may include non-specific lesions such as periosteal new bone formation or lesions shared with one or more other specific conditions (e.g., dactylitis is also found in tuberculosis).

Congenital infection occurs in all forms of treponemal disease (Akrawi, 1949:118; Grin, 1952:31–32; Román & Román, 1986) so its presence in a skeleton cannot be used unequivocally as an indicator of sexually transmitted syphilis (Baker et al., 2020:19; see also Schuenemann et al., 2018, discussed in the next section). Pathognomonic dental lesions of congenital treponemal disease—Hutchinson's incisors and Moon's molars—are found in 10–30% of those afflicted (Hillson et al., 1998), whereas Fournier's (mulberry) molars are consistent with congenital treponemal disease but also occur in other conditions (Hillson et al., 1998; Ioannou et al., 2015, 2017). Most skeletal lesions of both early and late stages of congenital treponemal disease are identical to those in other forms, except for certain ephemeral radiological lesions and Higoumenakis's sign of the clavicle (see Baker et al., 2020:19, Table 1; Frangos et al., 2011).

Clinical studies demonstrate that the tertiary skeletal manifestations of yaws, bejel, and syphilis are extremely similar (e.g., Akrawi, 1949; Hackett, 1951:181–182; Grin, 1952:19*ff*.), with gummatous lesions producing gangosa (perforated palate and nasal area changes including saddle nose), goundou (periosteal new bone formation of the rhinomaxillary region), and saber shins (new bone formation principally on the anterior aspects of tibiae). Pathognomonic lesions include caries sicca of the skull, first described by Virchow

(1858, 1896) and further elaborated by Hackett (1976) as discrete and contiguous series. For infracranial bones, Hackett (1976:93–97) determined that focal destructive lesions (superficial cavitation) that penetrate the periosteal new bone deposition to the original cortex are diagnostic of treponemal disease. Hackett's (1976) thorough work provides a sequence of lesions from initial occurrence to late and healed appearance for both cranial and infracranial pathology. For the caries sicca sequence, Hackett's (1976:31, 42) initial and discrete changes (numbered 1–5) are strongly suggestive of treponemal disease, while the contiguous series of changes (6–8) are pathognomonic (see Baker et al., 2020: Table 1). In long bones, saber shin tibiae as well as bone apposition with striae and rippling are also strongly suggestive (Baker et al., 2020: Table 1). Hackett (1976) proposed that several of these changes were likely diagnostic but required further testing using other documented skeletal collections from different regions of the world. These criteria, if confirmed through further testing, would help identify earlier manifestations of skeletal involvement in treponemal disease (Baker et al., 2020:19). Additionally, with developments in aDNA recovery from archival and archaeological samples (discussed below), potential diagnostic lesions like Hackett's "on trial" criteria or newly proposed skeletal changes also may be supported in the future.

Clinicians and paleopathologists have long recognized that the lesions produced in yaws, bejel, and syphilis are indistinguishable and the form of disease may shift under differing environmental and social conditions even in the same area (e.g., Hudson, 1965:889; Willcox, 1974; Hackett, 1976; Steinbock, 1976:111, 139, 143; Baker & Armelagos, 1988:705; Heathcote et al., 1998). Paleopathologists, however, frequently continue to attribute lesions in archaeological remains to a particular clinically defined variant that exists today based on the geographical location of the site and the archaeological contextualization of demographic and social factors (e.g., Cole & Waldron, 2010; Rissech et al., 2011; Hernandez & Hudson, 2015; Lopez et al., 2017; Betsinger & Smith, 2019; Vlok et al., 2020; Zhou et al., 2022). Narrowing the diagnosis to an extant form of treponemal infection in human remains that are hundreds or thousands of years old ignores the co-evolution of the pathogen and human hosts that is demonstrable even very recently (see next section on Gaps in Genetic Data). The approach taken in Powell & Cook's (2005b) *Myth of Syphilis* more cautiously directed contributors to describe the skeletal pathology indicative of treponemal disease along with contextualization of the sites and samples demographically, ecologically, and culturally, recognizing that the disease identified may not equate to the modern forms of treponemal disease (Powell & Cook, 2005a:7). While many contributors to that volume identified yaws-like or bejel-like patterns, my own examination of skeletal samples from the northeastern United States found a pattern unlike that of any of the modern forms (Baker, 2005:73), a finding echoed by Hutchinson et al. (2005:111) for Georgia and Florida.

Several paleopathologists advocate increased standardization and rigor in differential diagnosis with description of lesion sensitivity and specificity that can be categorized as consistent with, strongly suggestive of, or pathognomonic for particular conditions, including treponemal disease (e.g., Baker et al., 2020:20, Table 1; Powell & Cook, 2005a:6). Categorization of lesions in this way stresses the probability of a diagnosis similar to the modified Istanbul Protocol (Office of The United Nations High Commissioner for Human Rights, 2004) recommended by Appleby et al. (2015) and Buikstra et al. (2017). This protocol includes five criteria (not consistent, consistent with, highly consistent, typical of, and diagnostic). Collapsing the categories of highly consistent (the lesion could have been caused by the condition) and typical of (the lesion is usually found with this condition but there are other possible causes) into a single category of "strongly suggestive" avoids potential difficulty in classifying lesions. Skeletal lesions that are consistent with, strongly suggestive, or pathognomonic for treponemal disease are illustrated copiously in other works, including Hackett (1976), Steinbock (1976), and Roberts & Buikstra (2019).

Using more rigorous and standardized criteria for diagnosis, with detailed descriptions, images of lesions, and thorough differential diagnoses, systematic investigations of skeletal collections focused specifically on treponemal disease are needed on a much broader scale (Baker et al., 2020:22, 27–28) and particularly in underrepresented regions of the world. In order to understand its distribution, such studies must consider climate changes that may have affected the expression of disease rather than projecting today's environment into the past (see Cook, 2005, for an example of an apparent temporal shift in disease pattern in a single area).

Additionally, focusing more on the lived experiences of those afflicted with treponemal disease will enrich our understanding of its impact on those individuals and their communities. Investigating the distribution of disease demographically, geospatially, and temporally in particular regions provides far more insight into changes in the relationship among people and treponemal pathogens, rather than prioritizing evidence for sexual transmission. For example, Baker & Armelagos (1988:719) postulated that high rates of treponemal disease in certain parts of North America reflect population nucleation and sociopolitical organization that allowed widespread exchange of material goods as well as infectious disease. Indeed, the summary data provided by Cook & Powell (2005:466, Table 20.3) demonstrated an increase in treponemal disease in settled villagers, beginning c. 1000 BCE, compared with earlier and more mobile Archaic groups, and showed that both temperate and subtropical groups in coastal and interior areas were equally affected. Further research in the Southeastern and Midwestern United States (see summary in Baker et al., 2020:21–22) relates treponemal disease frequency not only to population size, density, and degree of sedentism but also to sociopolitical organization, settlement organization, and ethnic differences (Betsinger et al., 2017).

Gaps in Genetic Data

To date, no isolate of the causative organism of pinta (currently designated a separate species, *T. carateum*) has been available due to a lack of surveillance for this disease for more than 20 years and an absence of archived samples (Baker et al., 2020:8), although some researchers suggested it may still exist in remote areas where it was previously known to be endemic (Salazar & Bennett, 2014; Stamm, 2015a). Indeed, a sample obtained from a recent clinically diagnosed case in Brazil (Rosa et al., 2021) will provide an opportunity to sequence its genome (Stevie Winingear, personal communication, February 11, 2022). Doing so will help determine its relationship to *T. pallidum* and fill a significant void in the *Treponema* phylogeny.

The recent breakthrough in culturing *T. pallidum* in vitro (Edmondson et al., 2018) has led to rapid progress in research on this spirochete. As of late October 2021, 368 *T. pallidum* genomes are available to researchers on the National Center for Biotechnology Information (2021) database. This number more than doubles the 150 full genomes that were accessible in late 2019 (Baker et al., 2020:8). Additional genomes are available in the European Nucleotide Archive. Recent work by Beale et al. (2021) and Lieberman et al. (2021) has added significantly to the accumulation of *T. pallidum* genomes, though almost all are from recent (post-1950) *T. pallidum* subsp. *pallidum,* with research geared mainly toward understanding genetic diversity within the modern strains of this subspecies. For example, of the 196 near-complete genomes of *T. pallidum* sequenced by Lieberman et al. (2021) from patient samples representing eight countries on six continents, 191 were subspecies *pallidum*. Beale et al. (2021)

examined 726 clinical and laboratory samples of *T. pallidum* genomes from Africa, Asia, South America, Europe, and North America. Of the 726 genomes with sufficient coverage for primary lineage classification (Nichols or SS14), 593 were new (Beale et al., 2021:1550). Beale et al. (2021:1556) suggested a population bottleneck in the late 1990s to early 2000s to explain the substantial change in genetic diversity, which the authors connected to changes in sexual behavior associated with the HIV/AIDS pandemic. Additionally, point mutations conferring resistance to macrolides (e.g., azithromycin) have arisen since the 1980s (Beale et al., 2019). Differences in the presence or absence of pathogenicity islands, which carry genes related to virulence, and genomic islands among the *T. pallidum* subspecies have also been identified (Jaiswal et al., 2020). Specifically, certain gene clusters related to amino acid and lipid biosynthesis in a pathogenicity island of *T. pallidum* subsp. *pallidum* are not found in either the *endemicum* or *pertenue* subspecies (Jaiswal et al., 2020). Such studies hold promise for investigating differences in virulence of subspecies and strains found in older samples, particularly recovery of archaeological genomes. Significantly, Beale and coworkers (2021:1556) conclude that *T. pallidum* of today differs from that of just 30 years ago, with extinction of ancestral sublineages and replacement by new ones that spread rapidly with the substantial increase in syphilis in the United States and Europe in the early 21st century.

Dating divergences and timing of the most recent common ancestor (MRCA) of *T. pallidum* subspecies and strains of each subspecies is another goal of the genetic research recently published, but dates do not always coincide. This timing is of interest in relation to the apparent European epidemic in the late 1400s to early 1500s. Using 520 samples and 883 variable sites, Beale et al. (2021:1553) found a median date of 1534 (95% highest posterior density [HPD] 1430–1621) for the divergence of the Nichols and SS14 lineages of *T. pallidum* subsp. *pallidum*. Lieberman et al. (2021), however, dated the MRCA of the Nichols and SS14 clades to 1717 (95% HPD 1543–1869). Prior work by Beale et al. (2019) on a smaller sample dated the separation of the Nichols and SS14 lineages to 1662 (95% HPD 1517–1791). The addition of historical European samples places the MRCA of all *T. pallidum* before 2000 BCE with divergence of the *endemicum* and *pertenue* subspecies between the 4th century BCE and 12th century CE, although the MRCA of *T. pallidum* subsp. *endemicum* was positioned between the 14th and 16th centuries CE (Majander et al., 2020:3792, 3794). Giffin et al. (2020), however, indicate a more recent emergence of *T. pallidum* subsp. *pertenue* between the 12th and 14th centuries CE. It is clear that sampling differences and estimated clock rates have substantial effects on these reconstructions (Beale & Lukehart, 2020:R1094; Majander et al., 2020:3789). For example, Lieberman et al. (2021) used a smaller sample of DNA obtained directly from patients between 1998 and 2020, with many samples from Madagascar (85 of 196, or 43%). In contrast, Beale et al. (2021) had a far larger sample size that dated from 1951 to 2019 (though 96% were from 2000 or later) with Europe and North America disproportionately represented. Therefore, caution must be observed in using molecular data to interpret the timing of divergence and MCRAs among treponemal subspecies and strains and must take sampling biases into consideration. Far more DNA samples are needed from underrepresented regions and from older samples, including those from archaeological human remains, to provide more secure phylogenetic reconstructions and timing of divergences (Baker et al., 2020:12).

These findings have several implications for investigating *T. pallidum* in the past. Could changes like those observed in recent *T. pallidum* genomes have occurred at other points in time, affecting their virulence and spread? Clearly, this possibility must be considered. New breakthroughs suggest we may soon be able to explore such questions. Kolman et al. (1999) used PCR to target a single nucleotide polymorphism (SNP) diagnostic of *T. pallidum* subsp.

pallidum from a 240-year-old Easter Island skeleton. Such success was not repeated until Montiel et al. (2012) obtained *T. pallidum* DNA from two of the four neonates with lesions suggestive of congenital syphilis interred in a crypt in southwestern Spain dating to the 16th to 17th centuries. Recovery of *T. pallidum* DNA genomes from archaeological remains that permit identification of subspecies, however, has only recently occurred, thus far extending only to the 15th century.

Using DNA hybridization capture methods and high-throughput sequencing, Schuenemann et al. (2018) reconstructed *T. pallidum* genomes from a perinate and two infants with skeletal manifestations consistent with congenital treponemal disease who were interred at a convent in Mexico City that operated between 1681 and 1861. This study was the first to provide genome-level data for *T. pallidum* from archaeological remains. Surprisingly, the DNA from one infant was identified as *T. pallidum* subsp. *pertenue*, while the other two were *T. pallidum* subsp. *pallidum*. The discovery of the yaws-producing subspecies in an infant showing evidence of congenital infection demonstrates the fallacy of equating such lesions to the presence of syphilis in archaeological contexts. The two historic *T. pallidum* subsp. *pallidum* strains recovered are most closely related to the modern SS14 strain, while the *T. pallidum* subsp. *pertenue* strain branches with the modern yaws strains (Schuenemann et al., 2018).

Building on this study, Majander et al. (2020) investigated treponemal aDNA from four northern European individuals—two adults, an adolescent, and a perinate—dating from the early 15th century to the 17th century. The adult from Turku, Finland, displays treponemal skeletal lesions, while the others exhibit no lesions or non-diagnostic pathology (Majander et al., 2020:3789). The genomes recovered by Majander and coworkers include two strains related to subspecies *pallidum*, one (from Turku) related to *pertenue*, plus a previously unknown *T. pallidum* lineage from an individual interred between 1494 and 1631 at Gertrude's Infirmary in Kampen, the Netherlands. Phylogenetically, this newly discovered *T. pallidum* genome is basal, and likely ancestral, to both the *pertenue* and *endemicum* subspecies (Beale & Lukehart, 2020:R1094; Majander et al., 2020:3796–3797) and establishes the presence of a now extinct variant. This discovery emphasizes the need to refrain from overdiagnosis of treponemal disease by narrowing it to a modern variant as the cause of past infection.

Giffin et al. (2020) also identified *T. pallidum* subsp. *pertenue* in an adult female plague victim in Vilnius, Lithuania, with a calibrated radiocarbon date between 1447 and 1616 (95% confidence interval). Therefore, two independent analyses demonstrate the occurrence of the causative agent of yaws well outside the tropical regions where this clinically defined variant is found today (Giffin et al., 2020; Majander et al., 2020:3796). These results reinforce the danger of mapping modern distributions of yaws, bejel, and syphilis onto past occurrences of treponemal disease and ignore past migration. The presence of yaws in the 15th to 16th centuries in northern Europe suggests that the importation of enslaved Africans was a significant source of treponemal infection (Giffin et al, 2020; Majander et al., 2020). The relationship of the Lithuanian genome to extant West African yaws genomes noted by Giffin et al. (2020) supports the hypothesis that the African slave trade played a significant role in the global dissemination of treponemal infection as originally proposed by Thomas Sydenham in the 17th century (Paugh, 2014:240) and elaborated more recently by E. H. Hudson (1964).

Holes in Historical Documentation

The burgeoning descriptions of a new disease in Europe in the late 15th century coincided with the expansion of the voyages of Columbus, the Atlantic slave trade, and spread of the Gutenberg printing press. Historical documentation in Latin and common Western European languages (Italian, Portuguese, Spanish, French, German, and English) has provided protracted discussion of the origin of this perceived epidemic that was blamed on various nationalities or groups of people. The epidemic, often declared to be caused by venereal syphilis, has captured the attention of researchers and the public imagination, alike, for decades and led to the creation of the four hypotheses (pre-Columbian, Columbian, Unitarian, and Evolutionary, discussed earlier in this chapter) posited to explain the origin of the disease. Non-Western literature and oral history, however, continue to be largely ignored as sources of evidence. Their inclusion undoubtedly would contribute considerably to unraveling the history of treponemal infection (for example, see Lee, 2021, for insight into the potential of African source material and Zhou et al., 2022, for early Chinese literary evidence and its application).

With the recent recovery of historic *T. pallidum* subsp. *pertenue* genomes in both northern Europe and Mexico described in the preceding section, it is abundantly clear that attention must be paid to the role of the Atlantic and trans-Atlantic African slave trade in disseminating treponemal infection rather than focusing only on a Columbian importation from the Americas. Western European exploration and colonization of the West African coast began in the 1300s, with enslaved African people soon exploited for labor in gold operations on the "Gold Coast" and on sugar plantations on Madeira and the Canary Islands. Enslaved Africans were first transported to Iberia by the Portuguese Lagos Company in 1444 (Newson & Minchin, 2007:3; Ferreira et al., 2019). Significantly, the Lisbon customs house alone recorded the arrival of 442 African slaves per year between 1486 and 1493 (Curtin, 1969:18), with more entering Lagos. By the middle of the 16th century, up to 10% of the population of Lisbon, Evora, and the Algarve, was of African descent, and formed about 3% of the total Portuguese population (Saunders, 1982). Excavations in 2009 at Valle da Gafaria in Lagos, Portugal, revealed skeletons of 158 individuals in a trash deposit dated from the 15th to 17th centuries who were identified as enslaved Africans (Wasterlain et al., 2015; Ferreira et al., 2019). Although no pathology diagnostic of treponemal disease has been reported in these remains, preadults showed high rates of non-specific stress markers including linear enamel hypoplasia, porotic lesions, and stunted growth (Cardoso et al., 2018; Wasterlain et al., 2018). Importation of enslaved Africans into Europe, however, was certainly established far earlier due to Roman imperialism and was continued by Arab traders in the circum-Mediterranean region, particularly through trans-Saharan routes in North Africa (Hudson, 1964). Nonetheless, little is known about the state of health in the areas from which slaves were abducted or in which they were forcibly relocated. This gap may be due in part to a paucity of research on non-Western and Arab medical sources and partly to missing records that might shed light on health status. For example, medical examinations of enslaved Africans forcibly shipped to Cartagena, Colombia, were conducted at the market to set the sale price and, beginning in 1663, were performed upon arrival to determine the customs duty to be paid; however, few such records have survived (Newson & Minchin, 2007:261–262).

Enslaved Blacks were transported from Iberia to the Americas immediately and, by 1518, Africans were being forcibly shipped directly to Portuguese and Spanish colonial holdings in the Caribbean and Americas with substantial impact on health during prolonged voyages and subsequent treatment in slavery (Kiple, 1984). The French and English soon also began transporting enslaved Africans, followed by the Dutch (Newson & Minchin, 2007:4). Alongside the devastating effects on the health of the enslaved Africans, this trans-Atlantic human trafficking has been recognized as a source of repeated introductions of infectious disease, including smallpox, leprosy, malaria, and yellow fever (e.g., Scott, 1943; Kiple, 1984; Alden & Miller, 1987; Cooper & Kiple, 1993; Gilmore, 2008; Hammond, 2020:105–153-16, 356–358). The African slave trade was a likely source of yaws, as well (Scott, 1943:183; Kiple, 1984; Paugh, 2014).

An African practice transmitted to the Caribbean with the slave trade involved prophylactic yaws inoculation—the deliberate transfer of yaws matter (e.g., pus from a yaws sore) from one person to another to produce mild illness—much like smallpox inoculation, which was brought to the attention of Cotton Mather by his enslaved African, Onesimus, in Boston in 1706 (Kiple, 1984:154; Paugh, 2014). Paugh (2014) discusses a slave owner's account of his interview in the late 18th century with his slave called Clara, who hailed from the Gold Coast area (now Ghana). Clara described this practice in her homeland in which an incision was made on the thigh for the introduction of infectious yaws matter. Afro-Caribbean women were sometimes seen practicing yaws inoculation and it was used in infants to produce mild illness that did not affect their bones (Paugh, 2014:226). Physicians in Jamaica recognized the familiarity that Afro-Caribbean people had with the course of the disease and the need to limit its severity through inoculation (Paugh, 2014:236). This thorough understanding suggests a long acquaintance with yaws and its effects, potentially originating before the slave trade began. Additional traditional African remedies using an array of natural medications were also reported for treating yaws in the Caribbean (Kiple, 1984:154; Paugh, 2014). Occasionally, these medicaments were developed by Europeans as a treatment for syphilis, yet the opinion of some physicians that yaws and syphilis were the same disease was a threat to the profitable slave trade and the economic reliance upon forced labor, so those who emphasized that they were distinct conditions prevailed (Paugh, 2014). In fact, syphilis was viewed as a white man's disease, while yaws was considered a source of disfigurement among enslaved Africans and African Americans, a distinction that contributed to scientific racism (Kiple, 1987:8, 22; see also Kiple, 1984:139, 178, 244–245 note 29).

The above example illustrates how medical historians contribute to unraveling the complicated spread of treponemal infection and how it was interpreted by different groups of people at different times. Such work demonstrates the need to reorient questions that paleopathologists ask and review received wisdom and persistent assumptions that may be veiled by colonialism.

Conclusion

Recent emphasis on testing hypotheses concerning the origin and spread of *T. pallidum*, the causative organism and its subspecies, has allowed rejection of at least two hypotheses (the Evolutionary and Columbian hypotheses) concerning its origin and also identified gaps in genetic data that need to be filled for reconstructing its phylogeny (Baker et al., 2020). Much progress has been made on the latter problem yet sampling still disproportionately represents recent (post-1950) *T. pallidum* subsp. *pallidum* from Europe and North America. Breakthroughs in obtaining genome-level *T. pallidum* from archaeological remains promise to disentangle the complicated evolutionary history of this pathogen. Additionally, both Giffin et al. (2020) and Majander et al. (2020), obtained historic treponemal genomes from adult individuals for the first time—a promising development.

The increasing calls for rigor and standardization in paleopathology, along with the inherent interdisciplinarity of bioarchaeology, promise to advance our understanding of treponemal disease in the future. Macroscopic and archaeological biogeochemistry methods are providing insight into treatments with toxic compounds. Shifting research on treponemal disease away from the colonialist-centered question of whether Columbus and his crew carried it to Europe from the Americas to issues of its temporal and spatial patterning (e.g., coastal/inland, rural/urban, lowland/upland) and environment has already proven fruitful in several studies. The need to delve into non-Western historical documentation and oral traditions is imperative to understanding this temporal and spatial patterning, along with variant skeletal manifestations that may differ from those expected in modern clinically defined treponemal disease. Investigating how different groups (e.g., demographic, socio-economic, religious, ethnic) were affected and responded to treponemal disease sheds light on disease burdens and the lived experiences of affected individuals and communities in the past. The time depth provided by such studies may help inform current responses to the resurgence of treponemal infection in both developed and developing countries today.

Acknowledgments

I thank Anne Grauer for inviting me to contribute this chapter. Information provided by Sheila Lukehart and Stevie Winingear has been extremely helpful in interpreting recent DNA data. I also appreciate discussions with Katherine Paugh and her comments on an earlier version of this chapter.

References

Akrawi, F. (1949). Is bejel syphilis? *British Journal of Venereal Diseases* 25:115–123. https://doi.org/10.1136/sti.25.3.115.

Alden, D. & Miller, J. C. (1987). Out of Africa: the slave trade and the transmission of smallpox to Brazil, 1560–1831. *Journal of Interdisciplinary History* 18:195–224. https://doi.org/10.2307/204281.

Appleby, J., Thomas, R. & Buikstra, J. (2015). Increasing confidence in paleopathological diagnosis – Application of the Istanbul terminological framework. *International Journal of Paleopathology* 8:19–21. https://doi.org/10.1016/j.ijpp.2014.07.003.

Baker, B. J. (2005). Patterns of pre- and post-Columbian treponematosis in the northeastern United States. In Powell, M. L. & Cook, D. C. (Eds.), *The Myth of Syphilis*, pp. 63–76. Gainesville, FL: University Press of Florida.

Baker, B. J. & Armelagos, G. J. (1988). The origin and antiquity of syphilis: paleopathological diagnosis and interpretation. *Current Anthropology* 29:703–738. https://doi.org/10.1086/203691.

Baker, B. J., Crane-Kramer, G., Dee, M. W., Gregoricka, L. A., Henneberg, M., Lee, C., Lukehart, S. A., ... & Winingear, S. (2020). Advancing the understanding of treponemal disease in the past and present. *Yearbook of Physical Anthropology* 171(Suppl. 70):5–41. https://doi.org/10.1002/ajpa.23988.

Beale, M. A. & Lukehart, S. A. (2020). Archaeogenetics: what can ancient genomes tell us about the origin of syphilis? *Current Biology* 30(19):R1092–R1095. https://doi.org/10.1016/j.cub.2020.08.022.

Beale, M. A., Marks, M., Cole, M. J., Lee, M. -K., Pitt, R., Ruis, C., ... & Thomson, N. R. (2021). Global phylogeny of *Treponema pallidum* reveals recent expansion and spread of contemporary syphilis. *Nature Microbiology* 6:1549–1560. https://doi.org/10.1038/s41564-021-01000-z.

Beale, M. Marks, M., Sahi, S. K., Tantalo, L. C., Nori, A., French, P., Lukehart, S. Marra, C. M. & Thomson, N. R. (2019). Genomic epidemiology of syphilis reveals independent emergence of macrolide resistance across multiple circulating lineages. *Nature Communications* 10(3255):1–9. https://doi.org/10.1038/s41467-019-11216-7.

Betsinger, T. K. & Smith, M. O. (2019). A singular case of advanced caries sicca in a pre-Columbian skull from East Tennessee. *International Journal of Paleopathology* 24:245–251. https://doi.org/10.1016/j.ijpp.2019.01.003.

Betsinger, T. K, Smith, M. O., Helms Thorson, L. J. & Williams, L. L. (2017). Endemic treponemal disease in late pre-Columbian prehistory: new parameters, new insights. *Journal of Archaeological Science: Reports* 15:252–261. https://doi.org/10.1016/j.jasrep.2017.07.033.

Buikstra, J. E., Cook, D. C. & Bolhofner, K. L. (2017). Introduction: scientific rigor in paleopathology. *International Journal of Paleopathology* 19:80–87. https://doi.org/10.1016/j.ijpp.2017.08.005.

Cardoso, H. F. V., Spake, L., Wasterlain, S. N. & Ferreira, M. T. (2018). The impact of social experiences of physical and structural violence on the growth of African enslaved children recovered from Lagos, Portugal (15th–17th centuries). *American Journal of Physical Anthropology* 168(2019):209–221. https://doi.org/10.1002/ajpa.23741.

Castellani, A. (1905). On the presence of spirochaetes in some cases of parangi (yaws, framboesia tropica) preliminary note. *Journal of the Ceylon Branch of the British Medical Association* 2:54.

Cole, G, & Waldron, T. (2010). Apple Down 152: a putative case of syphilis from sixth century AD Anglo-Saxon England. *American Journal of Physical Anthropology* 144(2011):72–79. https://doi.org/10.1002/ajpa.21371.

Cook, D. C. (2005). Syphilis? Not quite. Paleoepidemiology in an evolutionary context in the Midwest. In Powell, M. L. & Cook, D. C. (Eds.), *The Myth of Syphilis*, pp. 177–199. Gainesville, FL: University Press of Florida.

Cook, D. C. & Powell, M. L. (2005). Piecing the puzzle together: North American treponematosis in overview. In Powell, M. L. & Cook, D. C. (Eds.), *The Myth of Syphilis*, pp. 442–479. Gainesville, FL: University Press of Florida.

Cooper, D. B. & Kiple, K. F. (1993). Yellow fever. In Kiple, K. F. (Ed.), *The Cambridge World History of Human Disease*, pp. 1100–1107. Cambridge: Cambridge University Press.

Curtin, P. D. (1969). *The Atlantic Slave Trade: A Census*. Madison: University of Wisconsin Press.

Demaitre, L. (2007). *Leprosy in Premodern Medicine: A Malady of the Whole Body*. Baltimore, MD: Johns Hopkins University Press.

Edmondson, D. G., Hu, B. & Norris, S. J. (2018). Long-term *in vitro* culture of the syphilis spirochete *Treponema pallidum* subsp. *pallidum*. *mBio* 9(3):e01153-18. https://doi.org/10.1128/mBio.01153-18.

Ferreira, M. T., Coelho, C. & Wasterlain, S. N. (2019). Discarded in the trash: burials of African enslaved individuals in Valle da Gafaria, Lagos, Portugal (15th–17th centuries). *International Journal of Osteoarchaeology* 29:670–680. https://doi.org/10.1002/oa.2747.

Fornaciari, G., Marinozzi, S., Gazzaniga, V., Giuffra, V., Piccchi, M. S., Giusiani, M. & Masetti, M. (2011). The use of mercury against pediculosis in the Renaissance: the case of Ferdinand II of Aragon, King of Naples, 1467–1496. *Medical History* 55:109–115. https://doi.org/10.1017/S0025727300006074.

Frangos, C. C., Lavranos, G. M. & Frangos, C. C. (2011). Higoumenakis' sign in the diagnosis of congenital syphilis in anthropological specimens. *Medical Hypotheses* 77:128–131. https://doi.org/10.1016/j.mehy.2011.03.044.

Giacani, L. & Lukehart, S. A. (2014). The endemic treponematoses. *Clinical Microbiology Reviews* 27(1):89–115. https://doi.org/10.1128/CMR.00070-13.

Gilmore, J. K. (2008). Leprosy at the lazaretto on St Eustatius, Netherlands Antilles. *International Journal of Osteoarchaeology* 18:72–84. https://doi.org/10.1002/oa.929.

Giffin, K., Lankapalli, A. K., Sabin, S., Spyrou, M. A., Posth, C., Kozakaitė, J., … & Bos, K. I. (2020). A treponemal genome from an historic plague victim supports a recent emergence of yaws and its presence in 15th century Europe. *Scientific Reports* 10:9499. https://doi.org/10.1038/s41598-020-66012-x.

Gjestland, T. (1955). *The Oslo Study of Untreated Syphilis*. Acta Dermato-Venereologica 55(S34). Oslo, Norway: Akademisk Forlag.

Grin, E. I. (1952). Endemic syphilis in Bosnia: clinical and epidemiological observations on a successful mass-treatment campaign. *Bulletin of the World Health Organization* 7:1–74.

Hackett, C. J. (1951). *Bone Lesions of Yaws in Uganda*. Oxford, UK: Blackwell.

Hackett, C. J. (1963). On the origin of the human treponematoses. *Bulletin of the World Health Organization* 29:7–41.

Hackett, C. J. (1976). *Diagnostic Criteria of Syphilis, Yaws and Treponarid (Treponematoses) and Some Other Diseases in Dry Bones*. Berlin and Heidelberg, Germany, and New York, NY: Springer-Verlag.

Hammond, M. L. (2020). *Epidemics and the Modern World*. Toronto: University of Toronto Press.

Heathcote, G. M., Stodder, A. L. W., Buckley, H. R., Hanson, D. B., Douglas, M. T., Underwood, J. H., Taisipic, T. F. & Diego, V. P. (1998). On treponemal disease in the Western Pacific: corrections and critique. *Current Anthropology* 39:359–368. https://doi.org/10.1086/204745.

Hernandez, M. & Hudson, M. J. (2015). Diagnosis and evaluation of causative factors for the presence of endemic treponemal disease in a Japanese sub-tropical island population from the Tokugawa period. *International Journal of Paleopathology* 10:16–25. https://doi.org/10.1016/j.ijpp.2015.04.001.

Hillson, S., Grigson, C., & Bond, S. (1998). Dental defects of congenital syphilis. *American Journal of Physical Anthropology* 107: 25-40. https://doi:10.1002/(SICI)1096-8644(199809)107:1%3C25::AID-AJPA3%3E3.0.CO;2-C.

Hudson, E. H. (1964). Treponematosis and African slavery. *British Journal of Venereal Diseases* 40:43–52. https://doi.org/10.1136/sti.40.1.43.

Hudson, E. H. (1965). Treponematosis and man's social evolution. *American Anthropologist* 67(4):885–901. https://doi.org/10.1525/aa.1965.67.4.02a00020.

Hutchinson, D. L., Larsen, C. S., Williamson, M. A., Green-Clow, V. D. & Powell, M. L. (2005). Temporal and spatial variation in the patterns of treponematosis in Georgia and Florida. In Powell, M. L. & Cook, D. C. (Eds.), *The Myth of Syphilis*, pp. 92–116. Gainesville, FL: University Press of Florida.

Ioannou, S. & Henneberg, M. (2017). Dental signs attributed to congenital syphilis and its treatments in the Hamann-Todd skeletal collection. *Anthropological Review* 80:449–465. https://doi.org/10.1515/anre-2017-0032.

Ioannou, S., Henneberg, R. J. & Henneberg, M. (2017). Presence of dental signs of congenital syphilis in pre-modern specimens. *Archives of Oral Biology* 85(2018):192–200. https://doi.org/10.1016/j.archoralbio.2017.10.017.

Ioannou, S., Sassani, S., Henneberg, M. & Henneberg, R. J. (2015). Diagnosing congenital syphilis using Hutchinson's method: differentiating between syphilitic, mercurial, and syphilitic-mercurial dental defects. *American Journal of Physical Anthropology* 159(2016):617–629. https://doi.org/10.1002/ajpa.22924.

Jaiswal, A. K., Tiwari, S., Jamal, S. B., Oliveira, L. de, C., Alves, L. G., Azevedo, V., Ghosh, P., Oliveira, C. J. F. & Soares, S. C. (2020). The pan-genome of *Treponema pallidum* reveals differences in genome plasticity between subspecies related to venereal and non-venereal syphilis. *BMC Genomics* 21:33. https://doi.org/10.1186/s12864-019-6430-6.

Kiple, K. F. (1984). *The Caribbean Slave: A Biological History*. Cambridge & New York: Cambridge University Press.

Kiple, K. F. (1987). A survey of recent literature on the biological past of the Black. In Kiple, K. F. (Ed.), *The African Exchange: Toward a Biological History of Black People*, pp. 7–34. Durham, NC: Duke University Press.

Kolman, C. J., Centurion-Lara, A., Lukehart, S. A., Owsley, D. W. & Tuross, N. (1999). Identification of *Treponema pallidum* subspecies *pallidum* in a 200-year-old skeletal specimen. *The Journal of Infectious Diseases* 180:2060–2063. https://doi.org/10.1086/315151.

Lanzirotti, A., Bianucci, R., LeGeros, R., Bromage, T. G., Giuffra, V., Ferroglio, E., Fornaciari, G. & Appenzeller, O. (2014). Assessing heavy metal exposure in Renaissance Europe using synchrotron microbeam techniques. *Journal of Archaeological Science* 52:204–217. https://dx.doi.org/10.1016/j.jas.2014.08.019.

Lee, R. (2021). *Health, Healing, and Illness in African History*. London: Bloomsbury.

Lieberman, N. A. P., Lin, M. J., Xie, H., Shrestha, L., Nguyen, T., Huang, M.-L., ... & Greninger, A. L. (2021). *Treponema pallidum* genome sequencing from six continents reveals variability in vaccine candidate genes and dominance of Nichols clade strains in Madagascar. *PLoS Neglected Tropical Diseases* 15(12):e0010063. https://doi.org/10.1371/journal.pntd.0010063.

Lopez, B., Lopez-Garcia, J. M., Costilla, S., Garcia-Vazquez, E., Dopico, E. & Pardiñas, A. F. (2017). Treponemal disease in the Old World? Integrated palaeopathological assessment of a 9th–11th century skeleton from north-central Spain. *Anthropological Science* 125:101–114. https://doi.org/10.1537/ase.170515.

Majander, K, Pfrengle, S. Kocher, A., Neukamm, J., du Plessis, L., Pia-Díaz, M., ... & Schuenemann, V. (2020). Archaeogenetics: what can ancient genomes tell us about the origin of syphilis? *Current Biology* 30(19):3788–3803. https://doi.org/10.1016/j.cub.2020.08.022.

Montiel, R., Solórzano, E., Díaz, N., Álvarez-Sandoval, B. A., González-Ruiz, M., Cañada, M. P., Simões, N., Isidro, A. & Malgosa, A. (2012). Neonate human remains: a window of opportunity to the molecular study of ancient syphilis. *PLoS ONE* 7(5):e36371. https://doi.org/10.1371/journal.pone.0036371.

National Center for Biotechnology Information (2021, October 26). Genomes datasets. *U.S. National Institutes of Health, National Library of Medicine.* https://www.ncbi.nlm.nih.gov/datasets/genomes/?taxon=160&utm_source=assembly&utm_medium=referral&utm_campaign=KnownItemSensor:taxname.

Newson, L. A. & Minchin, S. (2007). *From Capture to Sale: The Portuguese Slave Trade to Spanish South America in the Early Seventeenth Century*. Leiden and Boston, MA: Brill.

Norn, S., Permin, H., Kruse, E. & Kruse, P. R. (2008). Mercury – a major agent in the history of medicine and alchemy. *Dansk Medicinhistorisk Arbog* 36:21–40.

Obladen, M. (2013). Curse on two generations: a history of congenital syphilis. *Neonatology* 103:274–280. https://doi.org/10.1159/000347107.

Office of the United Nations High Commissioner for Human Rights. (2004). Istanbul protocol: manual on the effective investigation and documentation of torture and other cruel, inhuman or degrading treatment or punishment. Professional Training Series No. 8/Rev.1. United Nations, New York and Geneva. https://www.ohchr.org/documents/publications/training8rev1en.pdf.

O'Shea, J. G. (1990). 'Two minutes with Venus, two years with mercury' – mercury as an antisyphilitic chemotherapeutic agent. *Journal of the Royal Society of Medicine* 83(6):392–395. https://doi.org/10.1177/014107689008300619.

Parker, L. (1860). *The Modern Treatment of Syphilitic Diseases, Both Primary and Secondary* (4th ed.). London, UK: John Churchill.

Paugh, K. (2014). Yaws, syphilis, sexuality, and the circulation of medical knowledge in the British Caribbean and the Atlantic world. *Bulletin of the History of Medicine* 88:225–252. https://doi.org/10.1353/bhm.2014.0029.

Powell, M. L. & Cook, D. C. (2005a). Introduction. In Powell, M. L. & Cook, D. C. (Eds.), *The Myth of Syphilis*, pp. 1–8. Gainesville, FL: University Press of Florida.

Powell, M. L. & Cook, D. C. (Eds.). (2005b). *The Myth of Syphilis*. Gainesville: University Press of Florida.

Quétel, C. (1990). *History of Syphilis*. (J. Braddock & B. Pike, Trans). Baltimore, MD: The Johns Hopkins University Press. (Original work published 1986).

Radu, C., & Soficaru, A. D. (2016). Dental developmental defects in a subadult from 16th-19th centuries Bucharest, Romania. *International Journal of Paleopathology* 15:33–38. http://dx.doi.org/10.1016/j.ijpp.2016.08.001.

Rissech, C., Roberts, C., Tomás-Batlle, X., Tomás-Gimeno, X., Fuller, B., Fernandez, P. L. & Botella, M. (2011). A Roman skeleton with possible treponematosis in the north-east of the Iberian Peninsula: a morphological and radiological study. *International Journal of Osteoarchaeology* 23(2013):651–653. https://doi.org/10.1002/oa.1293.

Roberts, C. A. & Buikstra, J. E. (2019). Bacterial infections. In Buikstra, J. E. (Ed.), *Ortner's Identification of Pathological Conditions in Human Skeletal Remains* (3rd ed.), pp. 321–439. New York, NY: Academic Press.

Román, G. C. & Román, L. N. (1986). Occurrence of congenital, cardiovascular, visceral, neurologic, and neuro-ophthalmologic complications in late yaws: a theme for future research. *Reviews of Infectious Diseases* 8:760–770. https://doi.org10.1093/clinids/8.5.760.

Rosa, R. V. da, Souza, D. D. R. de, Cartell, A. & Souza, P. R. M. (2021). Correspondence: mal de pinta, first autochthonous case from south of Brazil. *International Journal of Dermatology* 60:e19–e20. https://doi.org/10.1111/ijd.15264.

Rosebury, T. (1971). *Microbes and Morals*. New York, NY: Viking.

Salazar, J. C. & Bennett, N. J. (2014). Endemic treponematosis including yaws and other spirochaetes. In Farrar, J., Hotez, P. J., Junghanss, T., Kang, G., Lalloo, D. & White, N. J. (Eds.), *Manson's Tropical Diseases* (23rd ed.), pp. 421–432.e3. Philadelphia, PA: Saunders/Elsevier. https://doi.org/10.1016/B978-0-7020-5101-2.00037-6.

Sartin, J. S. & Perry, H. O. (1995). From mercury to malaria to penicillin: the history of the treatment of syphilis at the Mayo Clinic. *Journal of the American Academy of Dermatology* 32:255–261.https://doi.org/10.1016/0190-9622(95)90136-1.

Saunders, A. C. de C. M. (1982). *A Social History of Black Slaves and Freedmen in Portugal, 1441–1555*. Cambridge and New York: Cambridge University Press.

Schaudinn, F. & Hoffmann, E. (1905a). Ueber Spirochaetenbefunde im Lymph-drüsensaft Syphilitischer. *Deutsche Meizinishe Wochenschrift* 18:711–714.

Schaudinn, F. & Hoffmann, E. *(1905b). Vorläufiger Bericht über das Vorkommen von Spirochaeten in syphilitischen Krankheitsprodukten und bei Papillomen. Arbeiten aus dem Kaiserlichen Gesundheitsamte* 22:527–534.

Schuenemann, V. J., Kumar Lankapalli, A., Barquera, R., Nelson, E. A., Iraíz Hernández, D., Acuña Alonzo, V., Bos, K. I., Márquez Morfín, L., Herbig, A. & Krause, J. (2018). Historic *Treponema pallidum* genomes from colonial Mexico retrieved from archaeological remains. *PLoS Neglected Tropical Diseases* 12(6):e0006447. https://doi.org/10.1371/journal.pntd.0006447.

Scott, H. H. (1943). The influence of the slave-trade in the spread of tropical disease. *Transactions of the Royal Society of Tropical Medicine and Hygiene* 37(3):169–188.

Stamm, L. V. (2015a). Pinta: Latin America's forgotten disease? *American Journal of Tropical Medicine and Hygiene* 93(5):901–903. https://doi.org/10.4269/ajtmh.15-0329.

Stamm, L. V. (2015b). Yaws: 110 Years after Castellani's discovery of *Treponmena pallidum* subspecies *pallidum*. *American Journal of Tropical Medicine and Hygiene* 93:4–6. https://doi.org/10.4269/ajtmh.15-0147.

Steinbock, R. T. (1976). *Paleopathological Diagnosis and Interpretation*. Springfield, IL: Charles C. Thomas.

Swiderski, R. M. (2008). *Quicksilver: A History of the Use, Lore and Effects of Mercury*. London: McFarland & Co.

Tampa, M., Sarbu, I., Matei, C., Benea, V. & Georgescu, S. R. (2014). Brief history of syphilis. *Journal of Medicine and Life* 7(1):4–10.

Thorburn, A. L. (1971). Fritz Richard Schaudinn, 1871–1906: protozoologist of syphilis. *British Journal of Venereal Diseases* 47:459–461. https://doi.org.10.1136/sti.47.6.459.

Virchow, R. (1858). Ueber die Natur der constitutionell-syphilitischen affectionen. *Archiv für pathologische Anatomie und Physiologie und für klinische Medicin* 15:217–336. https://doi.org/10.1007/BF01914843.

Virchow, R. (1896). Beitrag zur Geschichte der Lues. *Dermatologische Zeitschrift* 3:1–9.

Vlok, M., Oxenham, M. F., Domett, K., Tran, T. M., Nguyen, T. M. H., Mastumura, H., ... & Buckley, H. R. (2020). *Bioarchaeology International* (4):15–36. https://doi.org/10.5744/bi.2020.1000.

Walser, J. W. III, Kristjánsdóttir, S., Gowland, R., & Desnica, N. (2018). Volcanoes, medicine, and monasticism: investigating mercury exposure in medieval Iceland. *International Journal of Osteoarchaeology*, 29(2019):48–61. https://doi.org/10.1002/oa.2712.

Wasterlain, S. N., Costa, A. & Ferreira, M. T. (2018). Growth faltering in a skeletal sample of enslaved nonadult Africans found at Lagos, Portugal (15th–17th centuries). *International Journal of Osteoarchaeology* 28:162–169. https://doi.org/10.1002/oa.2643.

Wasterlain, S. N., Neves, M. J. & Ferreira, M. T. (2015). Dental modifications in a skeletal sample of enslaved Africans found at Lagos (Portugal). *International Journal of Osteoarchaeology* 26(2016):621–632. https://doi.org/10.1002/oa.2453.

Waugh, M. (2005). The centenary of *Treponema pallidum*: on the discovery of *Spirochaeta pallida*. *International Journal of STD & AIDS* 16:594–595.

Willcox, R. R. (1974). Changing patterns of treponemal disease. *British Journal of Venereal Diseases* 50:169–178. http://dx.doi.org/10.1136/sti.50.3.169.

Zhou, Y., Gao, G. Zhang, X, Gao, B., Duan, C. Zhu, H., Barbera, A. R., Halcrow, S., & Pechenkina, K. 2022. Identifiying treponemal disease in early East Asia. *American Journal of Biological Anthropology* 178:530–543. https://doi.org/10.1002/ajpa.24526.

17

HERE AND NOW, THERE AND THEN

Two Mycobacterial Diseases Still with Us Today

Charlotte A. Roberts, Kelly E. Blevins, Kori Lea Filipek and Aryel Pacheco Miranda

Introduction: Mycobacterial Diseases That Are Pertinent to Paleopathology

Mycobacteria are aerobic gram-positive bacilli that have a waxy cell wall (Lucas, 2008), with the majority being environmental saprophytes, living on dead or decaying matter and in the soil and water. The genus Mycobacterium contains over 100 species, with species within the Mycobacterium tuberculosis complex (MTBC), along with *Mycobacterium leprae*, being parasitic bacteria (Pin et al., 2014). Members of the MTBC include *M. bovis, M. africanum, M. microti, M. orygis, M. caprae, M. pinnipedii, M. mungi, M. suricattae,* and *M. canettii* (Wilson, 2021). The most relevant species of mycobacteria for humans are *Mycobacterium leprae* (along with the more recently discovered *M. lepromatosis*), *M. tuberculosis*, and *M. bovis*, although all of these species can be transmitted between animals and humans, and potentially vice versa. Leprosy and tuberculosis (TB) are two of the very few infections identified in paleopathological study where the specific causative organisms are known (as opposed to non-specific infections), and where bone changes can be linked to them (Roberts & Buikstra, 2019).

Fine (1984) usefully documented commonalities between leprosy and TB: they are diseases of poverty, transmitted by the respiratory route; they have long and variable incubation periods; and they can have subclinical infection phases. In the 1980s, they were both declining in developing countries (more so for TB) and becoming resistant to the drugs used for treatment (also more so for TB). Their responses to the Bacillus Calmette-Guérin (TB) vaccine vary, maybe because of the presence of environmental mycobacteria, but latitude appears to be relevant, too. Importantly, both diseases are stigmatized.

Of the 17 United Nations' Sustainable Development Goals established in 2017 (https://www.un.org/en/), there are four that are particularly relevant to this chapter: (1) No poverty (both leprosy and TB are associated with poverty today); (2) Good health and well-being (without these infections people's health benefits); (3) Clean water and sanitation (necessary to prevent transmission via respiratory droplets or animals and their products); (4) Reduced inequalities (equality promotes health for all today and would have in the past). In thinking about leprosy and TB in the past, we ought to focus more on how paleopathological research contributes to understanding the present and achieving these sustainable development goals.

An important aspect of these two infections is that they are today "social diseases", and were in the past. Using archaeological and historical data helps us to explore that social history. Today, they both affect the poorer and more vulnerable sections of society, and often those whose immune systems are already compromised, who live in crowded unsanitary conditions, who are not well-nourished, and who do not necessarily have access to a good education or healthcare. There is strong reason to believe that many of these risk factors were relevant in the past. For instance, TB had a romantic image and was linked to "genius" (poets, writers). Yet, it "slaughtered the poor by the million" (Dormandy, 1999:73), and "the more prosperous were lauded while poor victims were stigmatized" (Day, 2017:29). Hence, documenting leprosy and TB in the archaeological and historical records contributes to our understanding of how these diseases impacted people and populations, enables those affected to tell their stories through paleopathology and history, and allows us to explore how resilient (or not) people might have been.

Pathogenesis and Epidemiology

Both leprosy and TB are transmitted primarily via droplet spread from infected lungs, but a large percentage (90–95%) of adults today have innate (present at birth) immunity (van Crevel et al., 2002; Moraes et al., 2017). Leprosy may be contracted from nine-banded armadillos (Da Silva et al., 2018), particularly through consumption of their meat. *M. bovis* is the second most common cause of TB in humans, after *M. tuberculosis*. *M. bovis* can be contracted from a range of animal products, such as contaminated milk from infected animals (Wilson, 2021). There are also other potential "environmental" reservoirs for these organisms, such as water and soil (e.g., Martinez et al., 2019; Ploemacher et al., 2020), a point explored in the past pertaining to leprosy (Irgens et al., 1981; Chakrabarty & Dastidar, 1989).

The most recent epidemiological data for leprosy and TB derive from the World Health Organization (2020a, 2020b). The number of people with leprosy at the end of 2018 was 177,175 and the number of people newly registered with leprosy in 2019 was 202,185, revealing a slight decline from previous years. The reduction has been "gradual [and] uniform over the past 10 years, both globally and in the WHO regions" (2020c:419), but "Leprosy continues to cause more physical deformity than other infectious diseases" (ibid.:417), and stigma can lead to discrimination and late diagnosis. This reduction is in no small part due to available drug therapy (antibiotics) that has been free since 1995. Brazil, India, and Indonesia are the most affected regions of the world.

TB was the leading cause of death from a single infectious agent (ranking above HIV/AIDS) prior to the SARS-CoV-2 pandemic (WHO, 2020b:xiii). Around 10 million people had TB in 2019, and 1.2 million died who did not have HIV as a co-morbidity. South-East Asia, Africa, and the Western Pacific had the highest number of people who developed TB. The TB incidence rate is declining very slowly (like leprosy), in part because of antibiotic resistance that develops over the course of TB (and leprosy) treatment. This challenge is more serious for people with TB (e.g., see Munir et al., 2020). Inevitably, during COVID-19, services and facilities responsible for detecting, diagnosing, and treating people with both leprosy and TB were affected, showing the impact of pandemics on the management of other health problems (Mahato et al., 2020; Togun et al., 2020). Consequently, the long-term effect of this means that targets to eliminate leprosy and TB in the future will be affected.

Signs and Symptoms

The manner in which leprosy and TB affect the body, including the skeleton, is generally dependent on a person's immune system strength. This is especially so for leprosy, which has a broad immune spectrum (Ridley & Jopling, 1966) that stretches from high (tuberculoid leprosy) to low resistance (lepromatous leprosy), with several stages in between. If the causative bacteria of either infection enters the body, become active rather than latent, and are not treated with the requisite "multiple drug therapy" (MDT), both can spread throughout the body via the blood and lymphatic systems. The (visible) signs and experienced symptoms linked to leprosy (Roberts, 2020:91–93) and TB (Roberts & Buikstra, 2003:20) can vary in occurrence and severity between individuals. Infection can also progress at different rates. This will depend on intrinsic factors, such as the strength of a person's immune system, the person's age and biological sex, and extrinsic factors, such their social standing, their diet, the environment in which they live and work, and how they and their community conceptualize and manage these conditions. Extrinsic factors can change over time and may vary geographically and between cultures.

Leprosy is a disease of the skin, peripheral nerves, and other parts of the body, including the eyes, testes, kidneys, upper respiratory tract, lining of blood vessels, and skeleton (Jopling, 1982). It can have a long incubation period during which people harbor the bacteria but do not experience symptoms; on average this is five years, but much longer periods have been reported. Leprosy can affect the five senses (hearing, sight, smell, taste and touch), leading to impairment and disability. For example, people with leprosy can develop eye infection and ultimately become blind, and hearing can be compromised. Sensory nerve involvement can lead to a lack of sensation affecting the sense of touch and the individual's ability to detect cuts and other trauma; secondary infection can then lead to ulceration, particularly of the feet and hands. There also may be nasal congestion that damages the normal taste and smell mechanisms. The impact of leprosy on the senses is an area warranting historical and archaeological research (e.g. see general studies on the senses, *per se*, by Woolgar, 2006; Skeates, 2010). For example, loss of the senses was associated with madness, and in medieval England, a lack of any one sense indicated that the person was evil. Hence, alongside the direct physiological effects of the disease, the social or community response could have exacerbated or worsened the person's lived experience.

TB can affect the lungs and gastrointestinal tract, but also the central nervous system, lymph nodes, kidneys, genitals, and skeleton (Reddy & Ellner, 2021). If a person's immunity is strong, then the TB bacteria are destroyed; if not, then the infection becomes latent in the body – known as primary TB (Daley, 2021). Later in life, the TB lesion can reactivate if the person's immune system is compromised or the person becomes infected with a different pathogen (Lucas, 2008). For instance, TB is the most common presenting illness among people living with HIV and is the major cause of HIV-related deaths globally (Mandimik & Friedland, 2021:267).

Evidence for Leprosy and TB from Paleopathology

Most paleopathologists study skeletons because there are relatively few preserved bodies in the archaeological record. However, leprosy has been identified in the bones of one mummy from El Bigha, northern Sudan, dated to around 500 AD (Møller-Christensen & Hughes, 1966), and TB has been noted in a number of mummies (e.g., Zimmerman, 1979:five-year-old child from Egypt with spinal TB, adhesion of the lungs to the chest wall, and fresh blood in the trachea and lungs; dated 1000BC–500AD). Detecting the presence of these infections in the past is challenging. First, people who died with leprosy and TB may have had latent/subclinical infection, leaving their skeletons unaffected. Further, only a minority of people who do not receive treatment will develop bone changes (Jaffe, 1972:TB; Paterson & Rad, 1961:leprosy). This means skeletal prevalence data grossly underestimate these diseases in the past. Research on the bone changes of both these infections in medicine and in bioarchaeology reveals specific and non-specific indicators of the diseases. However, it is not the place here to detail the bone changes of leprosy and TB, as there are many sources providing that information (e.g. Roberts & Buikstra, 2003:87–110; 2019:321–439, 2021; Roberts, 2020).

A range of methods is used to explore the presence/absence of bone changes associated with TB and leprosy, including macroscopic, radiological, histological, and biomolecular analyses (aDNA, mycolic acids, and proteins). Macroscopic analysis, while being the most common method used, presents a number of challenges. First, skeletons are often fragmented and poorly preserved, so it is important to know what bones are specifically affected by leprosy (facial – rhinomaxillary syndrome, and the hand and foot bones via nerve damage) and TB (spine – Pott's disease, hip, and knee joints). Second, TB can affect a number of other bones, creating non-specific alterations. For example, in TB, the long (hypertrophic pulmonary osteoarthropathy) and short bones (phalanges: dactylitis), endocranial surfaces (TB meningitis), and the pleura (calcification) can be affected. Similarly, gastrointestinal TB could affect the internal surfaces of the pelvic girdle bones. Third, in leprosy, the long and short bones can be affected (diffuse periosteal new bone formation, or a more focal reaction due to ulceration), and there could be a number of co-morbidities: osteopenia/osteoporosis, especially in males related to bioavailability of testosterone, upper (sinuses) and lower (ribs) respiratory tract disease, poor oral health (difficulty with oral hygiene), and trauma (impairments affecting normal mobility and sight). Fourth, we must always document the preservation of the bones of the skeleton and the bones that are affected when we are looking for pathological changes; and fifth, careful differential diagnoses for these bone changes are essential to consider – specific and non-specific bone changes associated with either of these infections could be the result of a range of other diseases, for example those caused by non-TB mycobacteria (NTM) that can cause osteomyelitic bone changes in humans. Although their pathogenesis is unclear and bone changes are generally non-specific (Bi et al., 2015), NTM should be considered in mycobacterial differential diagnoses (Roberts & Buikstra, 2019:331).

Early evidence for TB has been noted in Egypt, Israel, Germany, Hungary, Italy, Jordan, and Poland, dating as early as 9,000 years ago (if all the evidence is accepted). Most published evidence for TB, however, comes from late and post-medieval periods in Europe – 12th–19th centuries – when the transmission of TB (and leprosy) was facilitated by high urban population densities. Later, evidence has been found in Asia and the Pacific Islands. However, new data from China is almost 6,000 years old (Okazaki et al., 2019). In the Americas, evidence for TB is more recent compared to Europe (Roberts & Buikstra, 2021); the earliest accepted evidence is in the Americas (South America - 700 AD, Chile), with suggestive evidence occurring as early as 400 AD in Mesoamerica (González Miranda and Torres Sanders, 2014). In what is today the continental United States and Canada, TB has been confidently detected as early as 900 AD. The skeletal evidence for leprosy holds a similar picture to TB, with sparse evidence noted in Africa and Asia, and northern Europe yielding the most evidence, again dating to the 12th–16th centuries (Roberts, 2020:191–280). However, pre-conquest evidence for leprosy is absent in the Americas, suggesting that this infection was introduced during conquest and colonialism during the 16th century AD (Ruiz et al., 2020).

The majority of skeletons with bone changes of leprosy and TB have been excavated from funerary contexts that are considered "normal" for the time and place. This is notwithstanding that special hospitals were opened for people with leprosy in ancient Eurasia, and sanatoria in much more recent centuries. Evidence to date indicates that rarely were people with leprosy and TB buried in a different manner from those without leprosy and TB. This is particularly true for leprosy and with instances of people being given special high-status rites (e.g., a bed burial at Edix Hill, Anglo-Saxon England: Duhig, 1998). A few leprosy hospital cemeteries, particularly in England and Denmark, have revealed large numbers of skeletons with leprosy (e.g., Magilton et al., 2008). However, beyond leprosaria, there are many more archaeological sites that have revealed the overall extent of the evidence of leprous skeletons, suggesting people with the infection were accepted within their communities, contrary to assumptions of stigma and segregation promulgated in historical texts (Roberts, 2020:280; Filipek et al., 2021a).

Recent Developments in the Study of Mycobacteria

Documented Clinical and Statistical Approaches

Improving the diagnosis of leprosy and TB in skeletons using available methods and criteria is important, as reliance on biomolecular analysis for diagnosis presents many challenges and requires destruction of bone. Work on non-specific bone changes may hold value, particularly from skeletons from documented collections. Although these collections have inherent biases, and ethical concerns relating to how they were assembled (Henderson & Alves-Cardoso, 2018), we present two examples to illustrate their value in TB diagnosis. In their study of adult skeletons from the Coimbra Collection, Portugal, Santos and Roberts (2006) found vertebral end rib lesions more commonly in the central part of the rib cage in people who died of TB, with peritoneal TB linked to rib lesions of the lower rib cage. In another study, Spekker et al. (2020) considered skeletons from the Robert J Terry Collection, Smithsonian Institution, USA and focused on endocranial granular impressions in individuals who died from TB. Their study showed that granular impressions were more common in individuals who died of this infection compared to those who did not. The lesion location and distribution were described as similar to tubercles in tuberculous meningitis. They concluded that these lesions can be used for diagnosing this condition in paleopathology. Hence, careful use of documented collections can serve paleopathology well.

Probabilistic statistical approaches can also aid paleopathological diagnosis. For example, Boldsen (2001) and Dangvard Pedersen et al. (2019) have developed a lesion-specific probabilistic statistical approach for estimating the frequency of leprosy and TB in archaeological skeletons. This approach measures "*sensitivity* (the likelihood that a person has a disease given a certain skeletal indicator) and *specificity* (the likelihood that a person does not have a certain disease in the absence of said indicator)" (Kelmelis et al., 2020:154). For both infections, specific skeletal lesions were found to be variously associated with these infections, some of which are considered "classic" (e.g., alveolar process change in leprosy), some non-specific (e.g., rib lesions in TB), and some that would normally not be considered for a diagnosis (e.g., lytic changes to the acetabular fossa for TB). In their study of skeletons from 13 urban and rural medieval Danish cemeteries, Kelmelis et al. (2020) explored whether urbanization was relevant for the transmission/spread of leprosy/TB. They found that leprosy frequency was lower than TB (Kelmelis et al., 2020), attributed to the segregation of individuals displaying signs of the disease during life (thus reducing the risk to the wider population). Further, they found that TB was related to "urban growth facilitating economic exchanges between rural and urban communities, particularly through frequent contact with livestock and dairy consumption" (ibid.:176).

Clinical information is an essential tool for diagnosis. For example, with ethical approval, studying TB sanatorium medical and social records can furnish us with information on bone TB. In a survey of almost 2,000 patient records from the early-mid 20th century Stannington Children's Sanatorium, Morpeth, Northumberland, England, 60% of the children had pulmonary TB, with a 12% frequency of bone TB (Bernard, 2003). This percentage is obviously greater than the 3–5% commonly cited for bone involvement in people with untreated TB. The second example concerns a study of medical files from the 20th century Rovisco Pais Hospital-Colony, Tocha, Portugal. Here, Matos (2009) developed the first diagnostic criteria for tuberculoid (high resistant) leprosy in archaeological skeletons: unilateral or bilateral hand and foot bone changes with no rhinomaxillary involvement.

In addition to understanding treatment after death, pathological lesions present on the skeletons of people with TB/leprosy can be used and interpreted within a clinically based "Bioarchaeology of Care" framework (Tilley & Cameron, 2014, and see Chapter 25, this volume) to assess whether individuals were provided with care during their lives. Tilley and Nystrom (2019) applied this methodology to the mummified remains of a boy with chronic Pott's disease from the Late Nasca Period (700 AD) in Peru. The long-term nature of the "Nasca Boy's" illness, and the likely significant personal and community investment needed to support him during his life, led authors to conclude that care for children (both healthy and infirm) was a commonplace behavior for this time and place. Snoddy et al. (2020) similarly analyzed the remains of a British settler buried in Otago (New Zealand) whose identity, period of invalidity, and cause of death were documented. This person died as a result of secondary pulmonary TB and, using a wealth of contextual data, Snoddy et al. (2020) concluded that he was cared for and supported financially and palliatively by both his family and an established social support network for the infirm. Roberts (2017) and Filipek et al. (2021b) also applied the "Bioarchaeology of Care" method to male individuals with skeletal evidence of advanced leprosy buried in leprosaria cemeteries in southern England (i.e., in Chichester and Winchester). Both were able to conclude that direct and indirect support was likely provided, demonstrating that these individuals needed personal and community based care to live with leprosy. What they could not ascertain, however, is whether this care was provided within the leprosarium nor how long each individual had spent there prior to their deaths. Although these previous studies have suggested hints of a "community of care", the "Bioarchaeology of Care" framework can be limited in its application because of a number of challenges: the incomplete nature of osteological data; variable expressions of skeletal pathologies depending on immune system strength; the osteological paradox; and not knowing what symptoms these people were experiencing over the course of their disease (see Roberts, 2022). While "each person with leprosy [and TB] today experiences [common and] different signs and symptoms, levels of 'disability', attitudes from their communities, types of care given (if any), progress of infection, and rate of recovery" cannot be definitively established (Roberts, 2017:120). The further use of the Bioarchaeology of Care to produce more nuanced studies is merited to enrich these concepts of care in the past. In particular, studying more human remains with detailed documentation, as per Snoddy et al. (2020), will produce more informative and reliable interpretations.

Synergistic Approaches

Respiratory Disease and Vitamin D Deficiencies

Since the 1980s, and increasingly in the 1990s and the 21st century, the identification of upper and lower respiratory disease indicators in skeletal remains has been a focus of research. This is particularly true for indicators of maxillary sinusitis and inflammatory rib lesions (e.g., Boocock et al., 1995; Lambert, 2002), and sometimes both (e.g. Davies-Barrett, 2018), but less work has focused on rhinosinusitis, mastoiditis, and middle ear disease. In some studies, an association of these conditions has been established for leprosy and TB (although correlation is not necessarily causation), along with the wider context of the impact of poor air quality on respiratory health. For example, Lee and Boylston (2008) describe rib lesions in skeletons from the leprosarium site of St Mary Magdalene, Chichester, some associated with bone changes of TB. Of course, sinusitis has been documented in skeletons with evidence of leprosy (Boocock et al., 1995). In more recent work on sinusitis, Davies-Barrett et al. (2021) examined almost 500 skeletons from the Nile Valley, Sudan and noted that there were changes consistent with leprosy and TB in Medieval cemeteries in the Fourth Cataract, thus showing that these two infections were present amongst the population, and people with them could have been predisposed to respiratory disease (Davies-Barrett, 2018). Interestingly, more sophisticated methods of analysis now enable us to detect soot within dental calculus and, hence, to know if an individual was regularly exposed to open fires, and hence potentially respiratory disease. Respiratory (and oral) disease pathogens have also been found in dental calculus (e.g., see Millard et al., 2020). There is much more potential in this area for exploring the bioarchaeology of leprosy and TB.

Studies exploring the association between mycobacterial infections and conditions such as vitamin D deficiency (a clinically recognized co-morbidity for respiratory problems; and see Chapter 19, this volume) are critical to our understanding of respiratory disease in the past. Roberts and Brickley (2019), for instance, discuss known synergies between infectious (leprosy and TB) and metabolic diseases (e.g., vitamin D). Although there is substantial clinical literature on this relationship, the link is not always clear (e.g., see Charoenngam & Holick, 2020). There are very few paleopathological studies that have specifically linked respiratory disease with vitamin D deficiency (including leprosy and TB), a deficiency that affects normal immune system function and increases susceptibility to infection (Aranow, 2011). Exceptions include Ives (2018), where bone lesions indicating active rickets and respiratory infection were found in a few 19th-century London children, and Boyd's (2020) analysis of sinusitis and rib lesion data from 601 adult skeletons from the Wellcome Osteological Database, Museum of London. In this latter study, two adult individuals displayed respiratory disease and residual rickets (evidence of rickets in childhood). Roberts et al. (2016), in their study of a post-medieval 12–14-year-old boy, also reported rib lesions and rickets, amongst many other health challenges. However, there are very few studies directly linking leprosy/TB with this deficiency in the paleopathological record.

Given that both leprosy and TB would have flourished in crowded urban environments in the past and that people in these contexts often experienced poor air quality, predisposing them to vitamin D deficiency due to the lack of exposure to UV light and the synthesis of the vitamin in the skin, we should expect to see an association of this deficiency with leprosy and TB (e.g., see Lai et al., 2013 on TB). This would be especially seen at higher latitudes where UV light exposure may be reduced at certain times of the year. We also know that exposure to sunlight was a treatment for TB in many sanatoria (Bernard, 2003), despite the limited research needed to improve understandings of the link between TB and D deficiency (Ralph et al., 2013). More research on the connection between mycobacterial diseases and upper and lower respiratory tract disease is critical. This effort will likely be facilitated by the development of the Respiratory Disease Network (https://twitter.com/bioarchresp), designed to bring together researchers investigating the risk factors and drivers for respiratory disease in past societies.

The Role of Zoonoses in Leprosy and TB

Critical aspects of leprosy and TB are their wide host ranges and propensity for zoonotic transmission. Although the number of archaeozoological studies of pathological animal remains has increased in recent years (see Thomas, 2019, for examples), their value in paleopathology requires more attention and emphasis. This is especially essential since the One Health approach is key to understanding health in humans and other animals: *One Health is a collaborative, multisectoral, and transdisciplinary approach – working at the local, regional, national, and global levels – with the goal of achieving optimal health outcomes recognizing the interconnection between people, animals, plants, and their shared environment* (https://www.cdc.gov/onehealth/index.html) (and see Chapter 33, this volume). Having knowledge about the ecology and host ranges of infectious diseases and their continuing evolution is paramount to understanding them in the past and in the present (Roche et al., 2018; Bonilla-Aldana et al., 2020). Leprosy can affect hosts such as red squirrels (Avanzi et al., 2016), nine-banded armadillos, and non-human primates (Honap et al., 2018), while TB flourishes in a range of wild and domesticated animals (Wilson, 2021). Focusing upon the specific ways people interacted with and contracted leprosy and TB from animals in the past will help us to understand interactions inherent to the transmission of the diseases today. We need only look at COVID-19 and potential jumps of a novel virus to humans from animal reservoirs to note the importance of researching these complex host/pathogen relationships in the past (Prince et al., 2021).

Biomolecular Approaches to Studying Mycobacteria in the Past

aDNA

Ancient DNA (aDNA) analysis and that of other biomolecules involving sampling of a range of body tissues, including bones, teeth, and the soft tissues for destructive analysis, has generated nuanced studies of ancient pathogens and their diversity and evolution (genus, species, and strains) (see Chapter 8, this volume). While initial work focused on detecting traces of the pathogens in individual skeletons/mummies, in recent years advances in methods have enabled the analysis of larger numbers of samples and the recovery of whole ancient MTBC and *M. leprae* genomes (e.g. Bos et al., 2014:TB; Schuenemann et al., 2018). The resulting data are complex, but informative. For example, ancient and modern DNA evidence of different strains of *M. leprae* and their geographic location have contributed significantly to understanding the interplay between human migration and the spread of leprosy (e.g., see summary by Roberts, 2020:284–291). In more recent research, Pfrengle et al. (2021) incorporated new data from ancient genomes of strains collected from European sites in the hitherto unstudied regions of Russia, Scotland, and Iberia. Diverse *M. leprae* lineages were found at leprosarium sites, suggesting that people with leprosy were travelling to leprosaria from distant places. In comparison, Fotakis et al. (2020) applied a multi-omic approach to confirm the presence of *M. leprae* in a female skeleton from Trondheim, Norway. While the skeleton itself displayed early-stage leprosy lesions that were not definitive, diagnosis was confirmed by the recovery of a low-coverage *M. leprae* genome and mycobacterial peptides (proteins). This study appears to be the first finding of *M. leprae* in dental calculus, demonstrating that dental calculus is not only a valuable source for detecting opportunistic pathogens of the oral microbiome, but also for detecting localized oral and rhinomaxillary infections. While only small amounts of calculus are needed for analysis, it is not necessarily the least destructive sampling approach. However, a wide range of ancient materials are recoverable from calculus that cannot be recovered from any other skeletal substrate, ranging from soot particles and dietary constituents to pollen and pathogens (Warinner et al., 2014). Therefore, projects employing dental calculus samples should avoid oversampling and maximize the potential of this unique substrate (Austin et al., 2019).

For TB, like leprosy, there have been many studies focusing on aDNA. There are, however, fewer Next-Generation Sequencing (NGS) studies of MTBC than M. leprae; over three times as many M. leprae genomes have been recovered. This may reflect the stochastic nature of MTBC DNA preservation in bone, the difficulty of distinguishing between the genetic sequences of MTBC and closely related mycobacteria, or its apparent absence from the dental pulp chamber at the time of death. This is because the majority of ancient pathogen screening projects involve teeth. The few recovered ancient MTBC genomes, however, indicate that TB had a different trajectory in Europe than leprosy. Whereas most *M. leprae* lineages were present in Medieval Europe (Pfrengle et al., 2021), MTBC strains detected from 4th-century England through 17th-century Sweden and 18th-century Hungary (Müller et al., 2014; Kay et al., 2015; Sabin et al., 2020) belong to the Euro-American Lineage 4. The contrast between high *M. leprae* genetic diversity and long-term MTBC genetic continuity raises intriguing questions about how the disease ecologies, transmission rates, and social impact of leprosy and TB facilitated such different trajectories for these organisms.

aDNA studies in the Americas have also uncovered another perplexing trajectory of the MTBC. In Peru, Bos et al (2014) explore the links between TB, humans, and other animals. The researchers found that the ancient MTBC strains of three individuals with skeletal changes of TB derived from three sites from the Chiribaya culture (750–1350 AD) were closely related to strains that affect seals and sea lions. They posit that the spread of TB to these ancient humans came from pinnipeds moving across the ocean prior to European human contact. To determine whether these were terminal zoonotic transmissions or if *M. pinnipedii* was adapted to human-human transmission, Vågene and colleagues (2022) sequenced two more MTBC genomes from pre-conquest sites in Colombia, more than 600 kilometers away from any coastline. They found that these in-land MTBC infections were also caused by *M. pinnipedii*, suggesting that pinniped-associated strains of MTBC were likely human-to-human transmissible. Clearly, humans, animals, and the environment are interlinked and more work in this area in relation to ancient leprosy/TB is needed (Mackenzie & Jeggo, 2019).

Evolutionary Histories from Genetic Studies

Our ability to document the evolution and history of both mycobacteria has benefited over the last 20 years from the fields of ancient and modern genetics. Both infectious pathogens were the first infectious diseases to be studied using aDNA analysis, starting in the early 1990s (see Roberts et al., 2022a, 2022b and references within). The original focus was on confirming diagnoses already established through paleopathological studies (e.g.,

Spigelman & Lemma, 1993; Rafi et al., 1994), but more nuanced analyses have been undertaken in recent years with the advent of NGS of the causative pathogens. Challenges and problems aside (see Chapter 8, this volume), these analyses have allowed us to study different species and strains of mycobacteria through time. In turn, this has provided data that inform us about how, when, and where the bacteria infected human populations.

For example, *M. leprae* and MTBC genomes recovered from radiocarbon dated skeletal remains serve as calibration points in their evolutionary trees, enabling estimates of lineage divergence times (Bos et al., 2014; Schuenemann et al., 2018). Prior to the use of aDNA, divergence rate estimates of leprosy- and TB-causing pathogens were either biased by using human migratory times as calibration priors or by comparing samples isolated from small temporal windows, e.g., low-diversity datasets (Wirth et al., 2008; Monot et al., 2009; Comas et al., 2013). This led to last common ancestor (LCA) estimates ranging from 20,000 to 3 million years ago. The rapid accumulation of modern and ancient mycobacterial genomes has helped overcome these biases. aDNA datasets provide snapshots of diversity through time, allowing independent calibration of their molecular clocks. The sequencing of modern genomes from historically under-sampled areas, such as sub-Saharan Africa and the Pacific Islands, expands the known genetic diversity within *M. leprae* and MTBC lineages. Evolutionary dating analyses of combined modern and aDNA datasets have consistently reported surprisingly young LCA estimates from ~6,000 kya for MTBC (Bos et al., 2014, Sabin et al., 2020) and ~4,000 kya for *M. leprae* (Schuenemann et al., 2018; Blevins et al., 2020). Molecular clock calibration using ancient pathogen genomes, however, is still affected by sampling bias. For example, ancient MTBC strains have only been recovered for two (*M. tuberculosis* Lineage 4 and *M. pinnipedii*) of many animal and human-associated clades. It is plausible that these LCA estimates will continue to shift as genomes from underrepresented lineages are recovered from these ancient pathogens, but the growing body of evidence that indicates their relatively recent emergence as human pathogens raises questions about how human behavior enabled the pathogens to get a foothold.

Although ancient MTBC and *M. leprae* genomes have provided valuable insights into the timing and diversification of these pathogens, aDNA data have yet to conclusively contribute to our understanding of their geographic or zoonotic origins. Modern genetic research on TB was sparse until the late 1990s (Roberts et al., 2022b). However, relatively early biomolecular analyses revealed that TB in humans did not evolve from animals, but rather MTBC genetic diversity in strains seen in animals today was underpinned by a human strain (Brosch et al., 2002).

Further accrual of modern MTBC genomes continues to show that sub-Saharan east and west Africa contain the greatest diversity and the most basal MTBC lineages, indicating the MTBC likely evolved in one of these regions (Ngabonziza et al., 2020; Coscolla et al., 2021). Unlike for the MTBC, the geographic origins of *M. leprae* remain unclear. The unexpectedly high genetic diversity of lineages across medieval Europe could indicate the pathogen evolved on the European continent. Today, however, basal lineages are found in China, Japan, and the Pacific Islands.

Isotope Analysis

Multi-isotope analysis (e.g., carbon, $\delta^{13}C$; nitrogen, $\delta^{15}N$; sulfur, $\delta^{34}S$; oxygen, $\delta^{18}O$; strontium, $^{87}Sr/^{86}Sr$) is another biomolecular method that can be applied to answer archaeological questions regarding health and disease in the past (see Chapter 7, this volume). For example, through documenting mobility histories of skeletons of individuals with TB from Italy and

England (Goude et al., 2020 and Quinn, 2017, respectively), and with leprosy from England (Inskip et al., 2015; Roffey et al., 2017; Filipek et al., 2021a, 2022), the impact of people's mobility on the transmission of the bacteria has been explored. More generally, these analyses can provide contextual information not only about mobility histories and disease transmission, but also diet, physiological stress, and environmental conditions. Alongside non-normative funerary practices, including exotic artifacts, it is clear that people were moving to new areas from distant places.

Several studies illustrate the value of viewing different multi-isotope ratios from people with mycobacterial infections in the past. For example, Linderholm & Kjellström (2011) compared the isotope ratios ($\delta^{13}C$, $\delta^{15}N$, and $\delta^{34}S$) of late medieval individuals with leprosy and TB with "healthy" members of the community in Sigtuna (Sweden). Their analyses showed no significant differences between the groups, indicating that people from both groups had similar diets and originated from similar environs (Linderholm & Kjellström, 2011). Similarly, in a study of skeletons from two late medieval Danish leprosaria and four contemporary non-leprosarium sites, carbon and nitrogen isotope analyses were used to view lifetime dietary data of patients, and the medieval Danish community as a whole. Results indicated that a terrestrial diet with some marine resource protein was eaten by leprosy patients and people from other medieval Danish sites. The mobility histories of individuals with leprosy from $\delta^{34}S$, $^{87}Sr/^{86}Sr$ further indicated that they were born and raised locally within the regions of the leprosaria (Brozou et al., 2021). Filipek et al. (2021a) studied ten adolescents from 10th to 11th century Norwich in Eastern England. Strontium and oxygen isotope ratios revealed that people with leprous bone changes had been buried alongside their local community. The data from these studies, again like Roberts (2020:127–175), challenged the notion of social exclusion for people with leprosy. In a related study, isotopic evaluation of a young adult male buried in the medieval leprosarium cemetery in Winchester indicated that he was not local to the area (Roffey et al., 2017). Buried alongside him was a scallop shell derived from the Galician coast of Spain, perhaps signifying a pious pilgrimage to the shrine of St James the Greater at Compostela (Yeoman, 2018). While the geographic origin of birth of this individual is unknown, it is likely that he travelled extensively, contracted leprosy sometime during his life and travels, and was buried in the leprosarium cemetery. Further multi-isotope analysis of this site by Filipek et al. (2022) indicated that this leprosarium was accommodating both local adolescent males and females, as well as people who were raised outside Britain and likely migrated with the disease.

Studies of individuals with TB using multi-isotope analyses have also gained attention. For instance, Goude et al. (2020) focused on prehistoric Italy and cave burials in Liguria. Here, they use carbon and nitrogen isotope values to explore evidence for breastfeeding, weaning, stress, and mobility in a number of individuals. Of particular relevance to TB, was one adolescent who had bone changes of the infection and evidence for growth disturbance. Through incremental dentine analysis of carbon and nitrogen isotope values, a sharp increase in $\delta^{15}N$ at the age of 11.5 years was noted, accelerating up to the age of 14 years; this was accompanied by a decline in $\delta^{13}C$, suggesting malnutrition. This was interpreted to be the result of TB triggering a catabolic state and leading to progressive wasting in the last two years of this person's short life. In a related study, carbon and nitrogen stable isotope analysis of ten adults with similar dietary intakes from Pica (Chile, AD 900–1400) found no significant differences in the bulk $\delta^{13}C$ serine, $\delta^{15}N$, or amino acid $\delta^{13}C$ values of tendon and rib collagen between individuals with and without bone changes due to TB. However, rib $\delta^{13}C$ serine (a non-essential amino acid involved in protein biosynthesis) of those with TB was significantly lower than the control group, possibly due to increased protein catabolism and amino acid recycling, and/or indicative of an altered serine metabolism induced by bacterial infection (Mora et al., 2021).

In a different study, the mobility of people dated to the Roman period in England with specific and/or non-specific bone changes of TB was explored. Quinn (2017) tested the hypothesis that people with TB buried in Roman-dated sites had been "on the move" at some point in their lives. Using multi-isotope analyses ($\delta^{13}C$, $\delta^{15}N$, $\delta^{18}O^{87}$, $Sr/^{86}Sr$), the aim was to establish if they spent childhoods near or far from their burial locations. Of the 21 adult individuals studied for dietary information, all except three people consumed a C3 terrestrial diet (similar to other data in the same or contemporary cemeteries). In terms of strontium and oxygen isotope analysis, 6 of the 21 were not born local to the area where they were buried. One challenge, however, is not knowing when these individuals contracted TB in their lives, although in the future performing multi-isotope analysis of younger individuals may be useful because contracting TB during childhood/adolescence may lead to reduced mobility. Children/adolescents with TB buried in a cemetery might also be a good indicator that TB was present in the wider community and not unique to a traveller who died and was buried at that location (see also Filipek et al., 2021a, 2022).

Applications of multi-isotope analysis to explore mobility histories of people with evidence of infections are promising for understanding the implications of mobility on transmission of infectious diseases in the past. This is germane to the world today, as we have seen with the spread of SARS-CoV-2 associated with travel (Nouvellet et al., 2021).

Future Directions and Final Thoughts

In concert with the study of paleopathological evidence, biomolecular analyses (aDNA and multi-isotopes), archaeological and anthropological contextual data, and historical documents, where available, synergistic approaches like some of those described here will contribute to a more nuanced picture of the complexities of mycobacterial infections in the past and their impact on the present. Leprosy and TB will deeply affect populations worldwide for many years to come as long as inequality and limited access to essential resources, including health care, work, a living wage, a healthy enviroment and adquate nutrition are allowed to continue. Ultimately, paleopathologists should strive to make clear that research into the past helps shape the future. Otherwise, what is the point of what we do?.

References

Aranow, C. (2011). Vitamin D and the immune system. *Journal of Investigative Medicine* 59(6):881–886. DOI: 10.231/JIM.0b013e31821b8755.

Austin, R. M., Sholts, S. B., Williams, L., Kistler, L. & Hofman, C. A. (2019). Opinion: to curate the molecular past, museums need a carefully considered set of best practices. *Proceedings of the National Academy of Sciences* 116(5):1471–1474. DOI: 10.1073/pnas.1822038116.

Avanzi, C., Del-Pozo, J., Benjak, A., Stevenson, K., Simpson, V. R., Busso, P., McLuckie, J., Loiseau, C., Lawton, C., ... & Meredith, A. L. (2016). Red squirrels in the British Isles are infected with leprosy bacilli. *Science* 354(6313):744–747. DOI: 10.1111/tbed.13423.

Bernard, M. -C. (2003) *Tuberculosis: A Demographic Analysis and Social Study of Admissions to a Children's Sanatorium (1936–1954) in Stannington, Northumberland. Health* (Unpublished doctoral dissertation). Durham University, England.

Bi, S., Hu, F. S., Yu, H. Y., Xu, K. J., Zheng, B. W., Ji, Z. K., Li, J. J., Deng, M., Hu, H. Y. & Sheng, J. F. (2015). Nontuberculous mycobacterial osteomyelitis. *Infectious Diseases* 47(10):673–685. DOI: 10.3109/23744235.2015.1040445.

Blevins, K. E., Crane, A. E., Lum, C., Furuta, K., Fox, K. & Stone, A. C. (2020). Evolutionary history of *Mycobacterium leprae* in the Pacific Islands. *Philosophical Transactions of the Royal Society B.* https://doi.org/10.1098/rstb.2019.0582.

Boldsen, J. (2001). Epidemiological approach to the paleopathological diagnosis of leprosy. *American Journal of Physical Anthropology* 115:380–387. https://doi.org/10.1002/ajpa.1094.

Bonilla-Aldana, D. K., Dhama, K. & Rodriguez-Morales, A. (2020). Revisiting the One Health approach in the context of COVID-19: a look into the ecology of this emerging disease. *Advances in Animal and Veterinary Sciences.* DOI: http://dx.doi.org/10.17582/journal.aavs/2020/8.3.234.237.

Boocock, P., Roberts, C. A. & Manchester, K. (1995). Prevalence of maxillary sinusitis in leprous individuals from a medieval leprosy hospital. *International Journal of Leprosy* 63(2):265–268. DOI: 10.1002/ajpa.1330980408.

Bos, K. I., Harkins, K. M., Herbig, A., Coscolla, M., Weber, N., Comas, I., t, S. A., Bryant, J. M., Harris, S. R., … & Krause, J. (2014). Pre-Columbian mycobacterial genomes reveal seals as a source of New World human tuberculosis. *Nature* 514:94–497. DOI: 10.1038/nature13591.

Boyd, D. (2020). Respiratory stress at the periphery of Industrial-era London: insight from parishes within and outside the city. In Betsinger, T. K. & DeWitte, S. (Eds.), *The Bioarchaeology of Urbanization – The Biological, Demographic, and Social Consequences of Living in Cities*, pp. 379–402. Switzerland: Springer Nature.

Brosch, R., Gordon, S. V., Marmiesse, M., Brodin, P., Buchrieser, C., Eiglmeier, K., Garnier, T., Gutierrez, C., Hewinson, G., … & Cole, S. T. (2002). A new evolutionary sequence for the *Mycobacterium tuberculosis* complex. *Proceedings of the National Academy of Science USA* 99(6):3684–3689. DOI: 10.1073/pnas.052548299.

Brozou, A., Fuller, B. T., Grimes, V., Lynnerup, N., Boldsen, J. L., Jørkov, M. L., Dangvard Pederson, D., Olsen, J. & Mannino, M. A. (2021). Leprosy in medieval Denmark: exploring life histories through a multi-tissue and multi-isotopic approach. *American Journal of Physical Anthropology.* https://doi.org/10.1002/ajpa.24339.

Chakrabarty, A. N. & Dastidar, S. G. (1989). Correlation between occurrence of leprosy and fossil fuels: role of fossil fuel bacteria in the origin and global epidemiology of leprosy. *Indian Journal of Experimental Biology* 27:483–496.

Charoenngam, N. & Holick, M. F. (2020). Immunologic effects of vitamin D on human health and disease. *Nutrients* 12. DOI: 10.3390/nu12072097.

Comas, I., Coscolla, M., Luo, T., Borrell, S., Holt, K. E., Kato-Maeda, M., Parkhill, J., Malla, B., Berg, S., … & Gagneux, S. (2013). Out-of-Africa migration and Neolithic coexpansion of *Mycobacterium tuberculosis* with modern humans. *Nature Genetics* 45(10):1176–1182. https://doi.org/10.1038/ng.2744.

Coscolla, M., Gagneux, S., Menardo, F., Loiseau, C., Ruiz-Rodriguez, P., Borrell, S., Darko Otchere, I., Asante-Poku, A., Asare, P., … & Brites, D. (2021). Phylogenomics of *Mycobacterium africanum* reveals a new lineage and a complex evolutionary history. *Microbial Genomics.* https://doi.org/10.1099/mgen.0.000477.

Dangvard Pedersen, D., Milner, G., Kolmos, H. & Boldsen, J. (2019). The association between skeletal lesions and tuberculosis diagnosis using a probabilistic approach. *International Journal of Paleopathology* 27:88–100. DOI: 10.1016/j.ijpp.2019.01.001.

Daley, C. L. (2021). Extrapulmonary tuberculosis. In Friedman, L. N., Dedicoat, M. & Davies, P. D. O. (Eds.), *Clinical Tuberculosis* (6th ed.), pp. 249–265. Boca Raton, FL: CRC Press.

Da Silva, M. B., Portela, J. M., Li, W., Jackson, M., Gonzalez, M., Hidalgo, A. S., Belisle, J. T., Bouth, R. C., Gobbo, A. R., … & Spencer, J. S. (2018). Evidence of zoonotic leprosy in Pará, Brazilian Amazon, and risks associated with human contact or consumption of armadillos. *PloS Neglected Tropical Diseases* 12(6):e0006532. DOI: 10.1371/journal.pntd.0006532.

Davies-Barrett, A. (2018). *Respiratory Disease in the Middle Nile Valley: A Bioarchaeological Analysis of the Impact of Environmental and Sociocultural Change from the Neolithic to Medieval Periods* (Unpublished doctoral dissertation). Durham University, England.

Davies-Barrett, A., Roberts, C. A. & Antoine, D. (2021). Time to be nosy: evaluating the impact of environmental and sociocultural changes on maxillary sinusitis in the Middle Nile Valley (Neolithic to Medieval periods). *International Journal of Paleopathology* 34:182–196. DOI: 10.1016/j.ijpp.2021.07.004.

Day, C. (2017). *Consumptive Chic. A History of Beauty, Fashion, and Disease.* London: Bloomsbury Academic.

Dormandy, T. (1999). *The White Death. A History of Tuberculosis*. London: Hambledon.

Duhig, C. (1998). The human skeletal material. In Malin, T. & Hines, J. (Eds.), *The Anglo-Saxon Cemetery at Edix Hill (Barrington A) Cambridgeshire*, pp. 154–199. Council for British Archaeology Research Report 112. York: Council for British Archaeology.

Fine, P. E. M. (1984). Leprosy and tuberculosis – an epidemiological comparison. *Tubercle* 65:137–153. DOI: 10.1016/0041-3879(84)90067-9.

Filipek, K. L., Roberts, C. A., Gowland, R., Montgomery, J. & Evans, J. (2021a). Illness and inclusion: mobility histories of adolescents with leprosy from Anglo-Scandinavian Norwich (eastern England). *International Journal of Osteoarchaeology*. DOI: https://doi.org/10.1002/oa.3029.

Filipek, K. L., Roberts, C. A., Gowland, R. & Tucker, K. (2021b). Alloparenting adolescents: evaluating the biological and social impacts of leprosy on young people in Early-Late Medieval England (9th – 12th centuries AD) through cross-disciplinary models of care. In Kendall, E. J. & Kendall, R. (Eds.), *The Family in the Past Perspective*, pp. 37–50. London: Routledge.

Filipek, K. L., Roberts, C. A., Montgomery, J., Gowland, R., Moore, J., Tucker, K. & Evans, J. (2022). Creating communities of care: sex estimation and mobility histories of adolescents buried in the cemetery of St. Mary Magdalen Leprosarium (Winchester, England). *American Journal of Biological Anthropology*. Early View.

Fotakis, A. K., Denham, S. D., Mackie, M., Orbegozo, M. I., Mylopotamitaki, D., Gopalakrishnan, S., Sicheritz-Pontén, T., Olsen, J. V., Cappellini, E., … & Vågene, A. J. (2020). Multi-omic detection of *Mycobacterium leprae* in archaeological human dental calculus. *Philosophical Transactions of the Royal Society B* 375:20190584. http://dx.doi.org/10.1098/rstb.2019.0584.

González Miranda, L. A. & Torres Sanders, L. (2014). Personajes con tuberculosis del eriod Clásico teotihuacano. *Arqueología* 49:52–70.

Goude, G., Dori, I., Sparacello, V. S., Starnini, E. & Varalli, A. (2020) Multi-proxy stable isotope analyses of dentine microsections reveal diachronic changes in life history adaptations, mobility, and tuberculosis-induced wasting in prehistoric Liguria (Finale Ligure, Italy, northwestern Mediterranean). *International Journal of Paleopathology* 28:99–111. DOI: 10.1016/j.ijpp.2019.12.007.

Henderson, C. Y. & Alves-Cardoso, F. (2018). *Identified Skeletal Collections: The Testing Ground of Anthropology?* Oxford: Archaeopress.

Honap, T. P., Pfister, L. -A., Housman, G., Mills, S., Tarara, R. P., Suzuki, K., Cuozzo, F. P., Sauther, M. L., Rosenberg, M. S. & Stone, A. C. (2018). *Mycobacterium leprae* genomes from naturally infected nonhuman primates. *PloS Neglected Tropical Diseases* 12(1):e0006190. https://doi.org/10.1371/journal.pntd.0006190.

Inskip, S. A., Taylor, G. M., Zakrzewski, S. R., Mays, S. A., Pike, A. W. G., Llewellyn, G., Williams, C. M., Lee, OY. -C., Wu, H. H. T., … & Stewart, G. R. (2015). Osteological, biomolecular and geochemical examination of an Early Anglo-Saxon case of lepromatous leprosy. *PloS ONE* 10(5):e0124282. https://journals.plos.org/plosone/article?id=10.1371/journal.pone.0124282.

Irgens, L. M., Kazda, J., Müller, K. & Eide, G. E. (1981). Conditions relevant to the occurrence of acid-fast bacilli in sphagnum vegetation. *Acta Pathologica Microbiologica Scandinavica. Section B Microbiology* 89:41–47. DOI: 10.1111/j.1699-0463.1981.tb00150_89b.x.

Ives, R. (2018). Rare paleopathological insights into vitamin D deficiency rickets, co-occurring illnesses, and documented cause of death in mid-19th century London, UK. *International Journal of Paleopathology* 23:76–87. DOI: 10.1016/j.ijpp.2017.11.004.

Jaffe, H. L. (1972). *Metabolic, Degenerative and Inflammatory Diseases of Bones and Joints*, Philadelphia, PA: Lea and Febiger.

Jopling, W. H. (1982). Clinical aspects of leprosy. *Tubercle* 63:295–305. https://doi.org/10.1016/S0041-3879(82)80019-6.

Kay, G. L., Sergeant, M. J., Zhou, Z., Chan, J. Z. M., Millard, A., Quick, J., Szikossy, I., Pap, I., Spigelman, M., … & Pallen, M. J. (2015). Eighteenth-century genomes show that mixed infections were common at time of peak tuberculosis in Europe. *Nature Communications* 6:1–9. https://doi.org/10.1038/ncomms7717.

Kelmelis, K., Kristensen, V. R. L., Alexandersen, M. & Dangvard Pedersen, D. (2020). Markets and mycobacteria – a comprehensive analysis of the influence of urbanization on leprosy and tuberculosis prevalence in Denmark (AD 1200–1536). In Betsinger, T. K. & DeWitte, S. (Eds.), *The Bioarchaeology of Urbanization – The Biological, Demographic, and Social Consequences of Living in Cities*, pp. 147–182. Switzerland: Springer Nature.

Lai, P. C., Low, C. T., Tse, W. S., Tsui, C. K., Lee, H. & Hui, P. C. (2013). Risk of tuberculosis in high-rise and high-density dwellings: an exploratory spatial analysis. *Environmental Pollution* 183:40–45. DOI: 10.1016/j.envpol.2012.11.025.

Lambert, P. (2002). Rib lesions in a prehistoric Puebloan sample from Southwestern Colorado. *American Journal of Physical Anthropology* 117:281–292. https://doi.org/10.1002/ajpa.10036.

Lee, F. & Boylston, A. (2008). Infection: tuberculosis and other infectious diseases. In Magilton, J. R., Lee, F. & Boylston, A. (Eds.), *"Lepers outside the Gate": Excavations at the Cemetery of the Hospital of St James and St Mary Magdalene, Chichester, 1986–87 and 1993*, pp. 218–228. Council for British Archaeology Research Report 158 and Chichester Excavations Vol. 10. York: Council for British Archaeology.

Linderholm, A., & Kjellstrom, A. (2011). Stable Isotope Analysis of a Medieval Skeletal Sample Indicative of Systemic Disease from Sigtuna, Sweden. *Journal of Archaeological Science* 38: 925–933.

Lucas, S. B. (2008). Infections. In Levison, D. A., Reid, R., Burt, A. D., Harrison, D. J. & Fleming, S. (Eds.), *Muir's Textbook of Pathology* (14th ed.), pp. 508–543. Totnes, Devon, England: Hodder Arnold.

Mackenzie, J. S. & Jeggo, M. (2019). The One Health approach—why is it so important? *Tropical Medicine and Infectious Disease* 4(2).10.3390/tropicalmed4020088.

Magilton, J. R., Lee, F. & Boylston, A. (2008). *"Lepers Outside the Gate": Excavations at the Cemetery of the Hospital of St James and St Mary Magdalene, Chichester, 1986–87 and 1993.* Council for British Archaeology Research Report 158 and Chichester Excavations Volume 10. York: Council for British Archaeology.

Mahato, S., Bhattarai, S. & Singh, S. (2020). Inequities towards leprosy-affected people: a challenge during COVID-19 pandemic. *PloS Neglected Tropical Diseases* 14(7):e0008537. https://doi.org/10.1371/journal.pntd.0008537.

Mandimik, C. & Friedland, G. (2021). Tuberculosis and human immunodeficiency virus coinfection. In Friedman, L. N., Dedicoat, M. & Davies, P. D. O. (Eds.), *Clinical Tuberculosis* (6th ed.), pp. 267–300. London: CRC Press.

Martinez, L., Verma, R., Croda, J., Horsburgh, C. R., Walter, K. S., Degner, N., Middelkoop, K., Koch, A., Hermans, S., ... & Andrews, J. R. (2019). Detection, survival and infectious potential of *Mycobacterium tuberculosis* in the environment: a review of the evidence and epidemiological implications. *European Respiratory Journal* 53(6). DOI: 10.1183/13993003.02302-2018.

Matos, V. M. J. (2009). *Odiagnóstico Retrospective da Lepra: Complimentaridade Clínica e Paleopatológica no Arquivo Médico do Hospital-Colónia Rovisco Pais (Século X. X.,Tocha, Portugal) e na Colecção de Esqueletos da Leprosaria Medieval de St Jørgen's (Odense, Dinamarca).* (Unpublished doctoral dissertation or master's thesis), Universidade de Coimbra, Faculdade de Ciências e Technologia, Coimbra.

Millard, A. R., Annis, R. G., Caffell, A. C., Dodd, L. L., Fischer, R., Gerrard, C. M. & Graves, C. P. (2020). Scottish soldiers from the Battle of Dunbar 1650: a prosopographical approach to a skeletal assemblage. *Plos One*. https://doi.org/10.1371/journal.pone.0243369.

Møller-Christensen, V. & Hughes, D. R. (1966). An early case of leprosy from Nubia. *Man* 62:177–179.

Monot, M., Honoré, N., Garnier, T., Zidane, N., Sherafi, D., Paniz-Mondolfi, A., Matsuoka, M., Taylor, G. M., Donoghue, H. D., ... & Cole, S. T. (2009). Comparative genomic and phylogeographic analysis of *Mycobacterium leprae*. *Nature Genetics* 41:1282–1289. DOI: 10.1038/ng.477.

Mora, A., Pacheco, A., Roberts, C.A., & Smith, C. (2021). Palaeopathology and amino acid δ^{13}C analysis: Investigating pre-Columbian individuals with tuberculosis at Pica 8, northern Chile (1050–500 BP). *Journal Archaeological Science* 129: doi.org/10.1016/j.jas.2021.105367.

Moraes, M. O., Silva, L. R. B. & Pinheiro, R. O. (8 October 2017, posting date). Innate immunology. In Scollard, D. M. & Gillis, T. P. (Eds.), *International Textbook of Leprosy*, Chapter 6.1. www.internationaltextbookofleprosy.org.

Müller, R., Roberts, C. A. & Brown, T. A. (2014). Genotyping of ancient *Mycobacterium tuberculosis* strains reveals historic genetic diversity. *Proceedings of the Royal Society B* 281:20133236. DOI: 10.1098/rspb.2013.3236.

Munir, A., Vedithi, S. C., Chaplin, A. K. & Blundell, T. L. (2020). Genomics, computational biology and drug discovery for Mycobacterial infections: fighting the emergence of resistance. *Frontiers of Genetics* 11:965.DOI: 10.3389/fgene.2020.00965.

Ngabonziza, J. C. S., Loiseau, C., Marceau, M., Jouet, A., Menardo, F., Tzfadia, O., Antoine, R., Niyigena, E. B., Mulders, W., ... & Supply, P. (2020). A sister lineage of the *Mycobacterium tuberculosis* complex discovered in the African Great Lakes region. *Nature Communications* 11(1):1–11. https://doi.org/10.1038/s41467-020-16626-6.

Nouvellet, P., Bhatia, S., Cori, A. et al. (2021). Reduction in mobility and COVID-19 transmission. *Nature Communications* 12. https://doi.org/10.1038/s41467-021-21358-2.

Okazaki, K., Takamuku, S., Yonemoto, S., Itahashi, Y., Gakuhari, T., Yoneda, M. & Chen, J. (2019) A paleopathological approach to early human adaptation for wet-rice agriculture: the first case of Neolithic spinal tuberculosis at the Yangtze River Delta of China. *International Journal of Paleopathology* 24:236–244. DOI: 10.1016/j.ijpp.2019.01.002.

Paterson, D. E. & Rad, M. (1961) Bone changes of leprosy: their incidence, progress, prevention and arrest. *International Journal of Leprosy and Other Mycobacterial Diseases* 29:393–422.

Pfrengle, S., Neukamm, J., Guelil, M., Keller, M., Molak, M., Avanzi, C. et al. (2021). *Mycobacterium leprae* diversity and population dynamics in medieval Europe from novel ancient genomes. *BMC Biology* 19:220. https://doi.org/10.1186/s12915-021-01120-2.

Pin, D., Guérin-Faublée, V., Brevasse, F., Dumitrescu, O., Flandrois, J. -P. & Lina, G. (2014). Mycobacterium species related to *M. leprae* and *M. lepromatosis* from cows with bovine nodular thelitis. *Emerging Infectious Diseases* 20:2111–2114. DOI: 10.3201/eid2012.140184.

Ploemacher, T., Faber, W. R., Menke, H., Rutten, V. & Pieters, T. (2020). Reservoirs and transmission routes of leprosy; a systematic review. *PloS Neglected Tropical Diseases* 14(4):1–27. DOI: 10.1371/journal.pntd.0008276.

Prince, T., Smith, S. L., Radford, A. D., Solomon, T., Hughes, G. L. & Petterson, E. I. (2021). SARS-CoV-2 Infections in animals: reservoirs for reverse zoonosis and models for study. *Viruses* 13(3):494. DOI: 10.3390/v13030494.

Quinn, K. (2017). *A Bioarchaeological Study of the Impact of Mobility on the Transmission of Tuberculosis in Roman Britain* (Unpublished doctoral dissertation or master's thesis). Durham University, England.

Rafi, A., Spigelman, M., Stanford, J., Lemma, E., Donoghue, H. & Zias, J. (1994). DNA of *Mycobacterium leprae* detected by PCR in ancient bone. *International Journal of Osteoarchaeology* 4:287–290.

Ralph, A. P., Lucas, R. M. & Norval, M. (2013). Vitamin D and solar ultraviolet radiation in the risk and treatment of tuberculosis. *The Lancet Infectious Diseases* 13:77–88. DOI: 10.1016/S1473-3099(12)70275-X.

Reddy, D. B. & Ellner, J. J. (2021). Pathogenesis of tuberculosis. In Friedman, L. N., Dedicoat, M. & Davies, P. D. O. (Eds.), *Clinical Tuberculosis* (6th ed.), pp. 51–76. Boca Raton, FL: CRC Press.

Ridley, D. S. & Jopling, W. H. (1966). Classification of leprosy according to immunity: a five-group system. *International Journal of Leprosy and Other Mycobacterial Diseases* 34:255–273.

Roberts, C. A. (2017). Applying the "Index of care" to a person who experienced leprosy in late Medieval Chichester, England. In Tilley, L. & Schrenk, A. A. (Eds,), *New Developments in the Bioarchaeology of Care*, pp. 101–124. Switzerland: Springer.

Roberts, C. A. (2020). *Leprosy. Past and Present*. Gainesville, FL: University of Florida Press.

Roberts, C. A. (2022). Conceptual approaches to the bioarchaeology of "community" care using knowledge from personal experiences of care giving (Nursing). In Tremblay, L. & Schrenk, A. (Eds.), *A Community of Care: Expanding Bioarchaeology of Care to Population Level Analyses*. Gainesville, FL: University of Florida Press.

Roberts, C. A. & Brickley, M. (2019). Infectious and metabolic diseases: a synergistic bioarchaeology. In Katzenberg, A. & Grauer, A. (Eds.), *Biological Anthropology of the Human Skeleton* (3rd ed.), pp. 415–446. Wiley-Blackwell.

Roberts, C. A. & Buikstra, J. E. (2003). *The Bioarchaeology of Tuberculosis: A Global View on a Re-Emerging Disease*. Gainesville, FL: University Press of Florida.

Roberts, C. A. & Buikstra, J. E. (2019). Bacterial infections. In Buikstra, J. E. (Ed.), *Ortner's Identification of Pathological Conditions in Human skeletal Remains*, pp. 321–439. Amsterdam, The Netherlands: Elsevier.

Roberts, C. A. & Buikstra, J. E. (2021). History of tuberculosis from the earliest times to the development of drugs. In Friedman, L. N., Dedicoat, M. & Davies, P. D. O. (Eds.), *Clinical Tuberculosis* (6th ed.), pp. 3–15. Boca Raton, FL: CRC Press.

Roberts, C. A., Caffell, A., Filipek-Ogden, K. L., Jakob, T. & Gowland, R. (2016). 'Til poison phosphorous brought them death': an occupationally-related disease in a post-medieval skeleton from Coach Lane, North Shields, north-east England. *International Journal of Paleopathology* 13:39–48. DOI: 10.1016/j.ijpp.2015.12.001.

Roberts, C. A., Davies, P. D. O., Blevins, K. E. & Stone, A. C. (2022a). Preventable and curable, but still a global problem: tuberculosis from an evolutionary perspective. In Plomp, K. A., Roberts, C. A., Bentley, G. R. & Elton, S. E. (Eds.), *Evolving Health: Palaeopathology and Evolutionary Medicine*. Oxford: Oxford University Press.

Roberts, C. A., Scollard, D. M. & Fava, V. (2022b). Leprosy is down but not yet out: new insights shed light on its origin and evolution. In Plomp, K. A., Roberts, C. A., Bentley, G. R. & Elton, S. E. (Eds.), *Evolving Health: Palaeopathology and Evolutionary Medicine*. Oxford: Oxford University Press.

Roche, B., Broutin, H. & Simard, F. (Eds.). (2018). *Ecology and Evolution of Infectious Diseases. Pathogen Control and Public Health Management in Low-Income Countries.* Oxford: Oxford University Press.

Roffey, S., Tucker, K., Filipek-Ogden, K., Montgomery, J., Cameron, J., O'Connell, T., Evans, J., Marter, P. & Taylor, G. M. (2017). Investigation of a Medieval pilgrim burial from the *Leprosarium* of St Mary Magdalen Winchester, UK. *PloS Neglected Tropical Diseases* 11(1):e0005186. https://journals.plos.org/plosntds/article?id=10.1371/journal. Pntd.0005186.

Ruiz, G. J., Serrano, S. C. & Guilliem, A. S. (2020). Sociedad Novohispana y enfermedad. Un caso de lepra en el complejo funerario colonial de Tlatelolco, México. *Revista Espanola de Antropologia Fisica* 41:28–42.

Sabin, S., Herbig, A, Vågene, A. J., Ahlstrom, T., Bozovic, G, Arcini, C., Kühnert, D. & Bos, K. I. (2020). A seventeenth-century *Mycobacterium tuberculosis* genome supports a Neolithic emergence of the *Mycobacterium tuberculosis* complex. *Genome Biology* 21(1):201. DOI: https://doi.org/10.1186/s13059-020-02112-1.

Santos, A. L. & Roberts, C. A. (2006). Anatomy of a serial killer: differential diagnosis of tuberculosis based on rib lesions of adult individuals from the Coimbra Identified Skeletal Collection, Portugal. *American Journal of Physical Anthropology* 130:38–49. DOI: 10.1002/ajpa.20160.

Schuenemann, V. J., Avanzi, C., Krause-Kyora, B., Seitz, A., Herbig, A., Inskip, S., Bonazzi, M., Reiter, E., Urban, C., ... & Krause, J. (2018). Ancient genomes reveal a high diversity of *Mycobacterium leprae* in medieval Europe. *PLOS Pathogens* 14(5):e1006997-17. https://doi.org/10.1371/journal.ppat.1006997.

Skeates, R. (2010). *An Archaeology of the Senses: Prehistoric Malta.* Oxford: Oxford University Press.

Snoddy, A. M., Buckley, H., King, C., Kinaston, R., Nowell, G., Gröcke, D., Duncan, W. & Petchey, P. (2020). 'Captain of all these men of death': an integrated case study of tuberculosis in nineteenth-century Otago, New Zealand. *Bioarchaeology International* 3(4):217–237. https://doi.org/10.5744/bi.2019.1014.

Spekker, O., Hunt, D. R., Paja, L., Molnár, E., Pálfi, G. & Schultz, M. (2020). Tracking down the White Plague. The skeletal evidence of tuberculous meningitis in the Robert J. Terry anatomical skeletal collection. *PLoS ONE* 15(3):e0230418: DOI: 10.1371/journal.pone.0230418.

Spigelman, M. & Lemma, E. (1993). The use of polymerase chain reaction to detect *Mycobacterium tuberculosis* in ancient skeletons, *International Journal of Osteoarchaeology* 3:137–143. https://doi.org/10.1002/oa.1390030211.

Thomas, R. (2019). Nonhuman animal paleopathology—are we so different? In Buikstra, J. E. (Ed.), *Ortner's Identification of Pathological Conditions in Human Skeletal Remains,* pp. 809–822. Amsterdam, The Netherlands: Elsevier.

Tilley, L. & Cameron, T. (2014). Introducing the Index of Care: a web-based application supporting archaeological research into health-related care. *International Journal of Paleopathology* 6:5–9. DOI: 10.1016/j.ijpp.2014.01.003.

Tilley, L. & Nystrom, K. (2019). A 'cold case' of care: Looking at old data from a new perspective in mummy research. International J Paleopathol. 2019 Jun;25:72–81. DOI: 10.1016/j.ijpp.2018.08.001. Epub 2018 Aug 16. PMID: 30120031.

Togun, T., Kampmann, B., Stoker, N. G.,& Lipman, M. (2020). Anticipating the impact of the COVID-19 pandemic on TBpatients and TB control programmes. *PLoS Neglected Tropical Diseases* 14(7):e0008537. https://doi.org/10.1371/journal.pntd.0008537.

Vågene, Å. J, Honap, T. P., Harkins, K. M., Rosenberg, M. S, Giffin, K., Cárdenas-Arroyo, F., Paloma Leguizamón, L., Arnett, J., Buikstra, J. E., ... & Bos, K. I. (2022). Geographically dispersed zoonotic tuberculosis in pre-contact South American human populations. *Nature Communications* 13(1195). https://doi.org/10.1038/s41467-022-28562-8.

van Crevel, R. Ottenhoff, T. H. & van der Meer, J. W. (2002). Innate immunity to *Mycobacterium tuberculosis. Clinical Microbiology Reviews* 15(2):294–309. https://doi.org/10.1128/CMR.15.2.294-309.2002.

Warinner, C., Rodrigues, J. F. M., Vyas, R., Traschel, C., Shved, N., Grossmann, J., Radini, A., Hancock, Y., Tito, R. Y., ... & Cappellini, E. (2014). Pathogens and host immunity in the ancient human oral cavity. *Nature Genetics* 46:336–344. https://doi.org/10.1038/ng.2906.

Wilson. C. (2021). Animal tuberculosis. In Friedman, L. N., Dedicoat, M. & Davies, P. D. O. (Eds.), *Clinical Tuberculosis* (6th ed.), pp. 415–435. Boca Raton, FL: CRC Press.

Wirth, T., Hildebrand, F., Allix-Béguec, C., Wölbeling, F., Kubica, T., Kremer, K., van Soolingen, D., Rüsch-Gerdes, S., Locht, C., ... & Niemann, S. (2008). Origin, spread and demography of the

Mycobacterium Tuberculosis Complex. *PLOS Pathogens* 4(9):e1000160-10. https://doi.org/10.1371/journal.ppat.1000160.

Woolgar, C. M. (2006). *The Senses in Late Medieval England*. New Haven, CT: Yale University Press.

World Health Organization. (2020a). Global Leprosy Update, 2018: global leprosy (Hansen disease) update, 2019: time to step-up prevention initiatives. *Weekly Epidemiological Record* 94(35–36):389–412.

World Health Organization. (2020b). *Global Tuberculosis Report*. Geneva, Switzerland: World Health Organization.

World Health Organization. (2020c). Global leprosy (Hansen disease) update, 2019: time to step-up prevention initiatives. *Weekly Epidemiological Record* 95:417–440.

Yeoman, P. (2018). An archaeology of pilgrimage. In Gerrard, C. & Gutiérrez, A (Eds.), *The Oxford Handbook of Later Medieval Archaeology in Britain*, pp. 641–657. Oxford: Oxford University Press.

Zimmerman, M. R. (1979). Pulmonary and osseous tuberculosis in an Egyptian mummy. *Bulletin of the New York Academy of Medicine* 55:604–608.

18
PALEOPATHOLOGY OF INFECTIOUS DISEASES

Olivier Dutour

The human species is the most infected of the animal kingdom. Infectious diseases are directly responsible for more than a quarter of the world's annual human mortality. About 1,500 microbial species, representing bacteria, fungi, helminths, viruses, and protozoa, can cause infectious diseases in humans (Woolhouse & Gowtage-Sequeria, 2005). This very large diversity of pathogenic microbes potentially harbored by a single species can be explained by three of our particularities: the exponential character of our demographic growth since the Neolithic period, the multiplication of our interfaces with other animal species (wildlife, companions, livestock, commensals) and our unique capacity to profoundly and durably transform our environment by influencing our planet's climate. Of the pathogens that can use humans as hosts, nearly 60% are of animal origin, having crossed the species barrier at various times in our history: 40% are zoonoses not adapted to human-to-human transmission, requiring repeated contamination from animal reservoirs, 35% are pathogens of animal origin adapted to human-to-human transmission and the others are ancestral human pathogens contemporary with the emergence of the *Homo sapiens* species (7%) or the genus *Homo* (18%) (Reperant & Osterhaus, 2013). Thus, two successive steps are necessary for the emergence of a human infection: species jump from animal to human and adaptation to inter-human spread (Lederberg et al., 1992). This phenomenon of emergence has always existed, but it has increased markedly since the end of the 20th and beginning of the 21st centuries (Morens et al., 2004). Aidan Cockburn, the founder of the Paleopathology Association, already noted in 1971 "The importance of infectious diseases in the control of populations demands that more attention be given to the study of available evidence of infections in early man" (Cockburn, 1971). As Victor Hugo, the French writer and poet noted that "the future is a closed door to which the past is the key". To open the door and understand the dynamics of human infections over time, it is crucial to turn to the sciences of the past and especially to paleopathology.

The Paleopathology of Infections, Challenges, and Perspectives

Very few infectious diseases leave traces that can be identified on the skeleton. It can be estimated that less than 10% of common infections (represented essentially by bacteria and fungi and exceptionally by viruses) affect the osteoarticular system on a regular or occasional basis. This means that more than 90% of infections are located outside the field of vision of paleopathologists in their current practice of skeletal examination. The study of infections in paleopathology is therefore subject to the general "iceberg principle", according to which the visible part of the studied object is only a tiny part of the reality, which remains hidden from the observer's eyes.

The digital revolution that began in the 1980s has led to major technological advances that have revolutionized both social and scientific practices. The knowledge of infectious diseases in the past has benefited from this progress, which has made it possible to distinguish between two epistemological periods: before the 1990s, when infectious disease in the past was primarily studied by medical historians focusing on ancient epidemics and paleopathologists working on skeletal and mummified remains; and after the 1990s, when rapid progress of molecular biology techniques (PCR, NGS) has invited new specialists, such as biologists, geneticists, and bioinformaticists, into the debate. Thus, knowledge of the history of human infections is now based on the study of three main data sources: old bones and mummified remains, historical texts and accounts (see Chapters 10 and 12, this volume), and ancient and modern biomolecules (see Chapter 8, this volume) (Dutour, 2016). Medical books, especially those dating from the second part of the 19th century – a period when medical knowledge became modern but therapy had not – are a more valuable source for paleopathologists than modern medical literature, as the natural expression of human infectious disease is strongly influenced by our modern preventive and curative arsenal.

Microbial paleogenomics is also revolutionizing our knowledge of past infections, having the unique capability, in addition to demonstrating the diagnosis, to provide a number of key information on infections in the past such as the origins and spread of past epidemics or the transmission and virulence of ancient pathogens (e.g., Andam et al., 2016; Duchêne et al., 2020). These cutting-edge methods from the field of microbial genetics, applied to archaeological material, can significantly contribute to overcoming the limitations of the iceberg principle by revealing past infections that have hitherto remained hidden from medical historians and paleopathologists. However, it is important that this emerging field of research, coined "paleomicrobiology" by Raoult and Drancourt (2008), does not become an autonomous scientific discipline outside of paleopathology, as it might due to the specialization needed in order to undertake complex molecular techniques and use of methods derived from bioinformatics. It is a challenge to not restrict paleopathological research to macroscopic skeletal analyses due to technical limits. There ought to be no conceptual limits to paleopathological research, thanks to the broad definition of the discipline offered by Marc Armand Ruffer: "the science of the diseases which can be demonstrated in human and animal remains from ancient times" (Ruffer, 1913) in spite of some molecular biologists suggesting that genetic biomolecular research be called "genetic paleopathology"(Knapp, 2011).

Thus, to get the most comprehensive perspective of the paleopathology of infections, it is essential to adopt multidisciplinary approaches, including microbial paleobiology which includes paleogenetics, paleogenomics, and paleoproteomics (Raoult & Drancourt, 2008; Hendy et al., 2016; Bos et al., 2019), research into host susceptibility to pathogens (Krause-Kyora et al., 2018), paleoparasitology, which studies the traces of ancient parasites (Appelt et al., 2016, and see Chapter 9, this volume), archaeoentomology, which studies the remains of insects that can be vectors of infections (Bain, 2004; Raoult et al., 2006), the history of medicine and diseases (Alter & Carmichael, 1996), as well as the history of art (Grmek & Gourevitch, 1998). This holistic approach appears to be the most promising way to reconstruct the past dynamics of human and animal infections (Dutour, 2008, 2016; Duchêne et al., 2020).

Since skeletal ramifications and the paleopathology of specific infectious diseases have been dealt with by many researchers (see, for example, Aufderhiede & Rodriguez-Martin, 1998; Buikstra, 2019), and Chapters 16 and 17, this volume), I will focus here on the paleopathology of non-specific skeletal infections.

The Paleopathology of Non-Specific Skeletal Infections

Specific and Non-Specific: A Matter of Three Infectious Modes

Clinical practice in infectious diseases distinguishes two types of infections: specific infections due to particular pathogens responsible for a clinically unique disease identifiable by characteristic pathological lesions and non-specific infections responsible for tissue lesions that may be caused by or associated with different pathogens. This distinction is important to recognize in paleopathological practice *Brucella* because some infections leave characteristic traces on the skeleton and can be identified specifically (tuberculosis, leprosy, brucellosis, and treponematosis, for example), while others can only be recognized as infectious in origin without being attributed to a particular pathogen. The specificity (or lack of specificity) of lesions is mainly conditioned by the mechanisms by which the pathogenic microbes cause damage to tissues of the infected organism. Tissue damage can be the result of a direct action of the pathogen or can be the indirect consequence of the body's immune reaction in response to the pathogen infection. Three fundamental patterns of tissue damage can be recognized: septic, granulomatous, and angiitic (Ragsdale & Lehmer, 2012) (see Table 18.1).

The direct action of pathogens on tissues is undertaken by toxins or by cytopathic effect. Toxins are either released by microorganisms and act directly on host cells (exotoxins) or are present in the structure of the pathogens (endotoxins) and will trigger secretion of cytokines by the contaminated phagocytes, which will cause a rapid local inflammatory response (stimulation of angiogenesis and cell death) and a systemic reaction (fever). These mechanisms will lead to the production of pus (made up of dead cells, mainly neutrophilic polymorphonuclears leukocytes and microbes proliferating in a liquid exudate of cellular and extracellular origin), which may stay suppurative or collect as abscesses. Localization of this process in bone tissue is initially rapidly destructive, and if death does not occur as a result of the infection, the repair processes will lead to significant remodeling of the bone with important bone production. This process corresponds to the **septic pattern** of host reaction to infection. It is mainly due to "pyogenic" bacteria, including cocci (staphylococci, streptococci, pneumococci, meningococci) and bacilli (*Haemophilus influenza* and more recently *Kingella kingae*). Hence, this pattern, triggered by a multitude of pathogens, is termed "non-specific infection" in paleopathology not because the pathogen is non-specific, but rather, because of the host's rather generalized response. It is commonly observed in paleopathology, mainly represented by the presence of osteomyelitis. Cytopathic effects on bone result from viral infections (smallpox, chickenpox, measles, poliomyelitis, influenza, hepatitis), damaging tissues of various organs, including affecting bone and joint tissues (as seen in variola virus infections) or having an indirect impact on the skeleton through consequences of neurological cytopathy (such as poliomyelitis paralysis). Importantly, these are two rare examples of viral infections that are potentially identifiable by paleopathologists on skeletal remains.

Indirect mechanisms related to host immune responses are also responsible for tissue damage. Some pathogens stimulate cell-mediated immunity, and after infection, microbes will be encircled by an aggregate of macrophages and lymphocytes, forming a slow-growing and

Table 18.1 Physiopathogeny of common specific and non-specific infection observed in skeletal paleopathology

Microbial pathogenic species	Mechanism	Pathogenicity	Immune reaction	Effect	Basic lesions	Infectious pattern	Skeletal lesions	Specificity of lesions
Staphylococcus aureus, Streptococcus pyogenes, Streptococcus pneumonia, Haemophilus influenzae, Kingella kingae (recent)	Direct	Toxins (endo- or exotoxins)	Polymorphonuclear	Exudative reaction, pus production	Abscess	Septic	Osteomyelitis, Osteoarthritis (Spondylodiscitis)	Non-specific
Mycobacterium tuberculosis complex	Indirect	Non-toxic but Invasive and persistent pathogen	Cell mediated, macrophages and histiocytes	Focal aggregates of immune cells encircling slow growing pathogens, central caseous necrosis	Granuloma	Granulomatous	Spondylodiscitis Osteoarthritis	Specific
Brucella melitensis, abortus & suis							Osteomyelitis	specific (pseudotuberculotic)
Histoplasma duboisi, Blastomyces dermatidis, Coccidioides sp., Actinomyces israeli							Osteomyelitis Osteoarthritis	
Mycobacterium leprae Mycobacterium lepromatosis				Target tissues: myelin envelope of peripheral nerves, nasal and oral mucosa			Acro-osteolysis Rhinomaxillary syndrome	Specific
Treponema pallidum pallidum, Treponema pallidum pertenue, Treponema pallidum endemicum		Production of mucopolysac-charidase degrading MPS of capillaries vessels	Immune complexes, lymphocytes	Vasculitis, infarction, aseptic necrosis	Gumma	Angiitic	Osteoperiostitis	specific

tissue-invasive rounded focal structure called granulomas. The mechanism of these lesions is the progressive development of space-occupying masses destroying the surrounding tissue in a tumor-like process. When it concerns bone tissue, this granulomatous mode involves both bone (osteitis) and joint (arthritis), frequently associated (osteoarthritis) and leading to slow destruction followed by a repair process, often fusing (joint ankylosis). This process is characterized as the ***granulomatous pattern***, examples of which include infection by *Mycobacteria* from the *Mycobacterium tuberculosis* complex, pathogenic species of the genus *Brucella*, responsible for brucellosis, or pathogenic fungi. In case of leprosy (*Mycobacterium leprae* and *lepromatosis*), specific skeletal lesions are the consequence of granulomatous infection of peripheral nerves and nasal-oral mucosa. For other pathogens, tissue damage results from the action of immune complexes, precipitated by the binding of foreign or host antigens and host antibodies. The accumulation of antibody-producing cells (lymphocytes) around blood vessels will be responsible for vascular inflammation (vasculitis) and thrombosis that can lead to focal and successive necrosis of tissues, evolving toward healing and known as gumma. On bone tissue, there are strong bilateral and symmetrical reactions of the periosteum and bone gumma of different stages (some active, others healed), responsible for a characteristic gummatous osteoperiostitis. This process is characterized as the ***angiitic pattern***, associated with infection by pathogenic treponemes (*Treponema pallidum ssp*), responsible for yaws, bejel, and syphilis.

Naming the Infectious Conditions of Bone and Joints

The suffix "itis", added to an organ name, means the existence of an inflammatory process at level of the cited organ. This terminology is colloquially used in clinical infectiology for naming infections: meningitis, hepatitis, appendicitis, osteomyelitis. However, in formal medical language, inflammation and infection are not synonymous (Signore, 2013). This confusion arises because the vast majority of infections are accompanied by inflammatory reactions, but not all inflammation is of infectious origin. For instance, "arthritis" means joint inflammation that can be either septic or aseptic (reactive or rheumatoid, for instance). Therefore, formally speaking, the nature of inflammation, if infectious, should be mentioned after each medical word using the "itis" suffix: septic meningitis, viral hepatitis, infectious appendicitis, septic osteomyelitis. In this chapter, in which we only deal with infections, we do not systematically use this specification, but it should be kept in mind by the reader.

The three components of bone (periosteum, cortical bone, medullary space), and synovial joints, can be infected independently, this is named "periostitis", "osteitis", "myelitis" and "arthritis", respectively. The infectious process can involve several structures, whereby "osteomyelitis", "osteoperiostitis" and "osteoarthritis" can be recognized. Some particular locations have specific terms. When the infection reaches the spine, the most common term is "spondylodiscitis", which describes infections affecting both vertebrae and discs, since a single infection of the vertebral body or the intervertebral disc is not usually encountered. Another specific term is used in instances of osteoarthritis of sacroiliac joint: "sacroiliitis".

Natural History and Paleopathology of Non-Specific Skeletal Infection

The contamination of bone and joints by pyogenic pathogens can result from

i   direct inoculation (wound, open fracture, penetrating agent) resulting from accidental or voluntary trauma or from therapeutic action;

ii "neighborhood" contamination from a close infectious focus;
iii hematogenous diffusion of germs from a portal of entry (cutaneous or mucous) located at a distance from the bone tissue.

The prime causative pathogen associated with contamination of bone and joints is *Staphylococcus aureus*, identified by Louis Pasteur in 1880 as a major pathogen responsible for bone and joint infections, followed by *Streptococcus pyogenes*, *Streptococcus pneumoniae*, *Haemophilus influenzae*, and *Escherichia coli*. However, since the routine introduction of molecular screening techniques in clinical infectiology, the new dominant pathogen recognized as being responsible for more than half of the osteoarticular infections occurring in children in Europe is now *Kingella kingae* (Samara et al., 2019). This is a slow-growing Gram-negative bacillus identified in the 1960s, named in the 1970s, and recognized as pathogenic in the 1990s. It is difficult to know if this bacterium is a true emerging pathogen or whether its identification is new and, hence, represents a pathogen hidden in the submerged part of the "iceberg" of clinical bacteriology, simply because it is not easily cultivable. The promising key to answering this question is through paleomicrobiological research, but very little work has been conducted on the frequency, etiology, and evolution of ancient osteomyelitis. Paleogenomic and paleoproteomic research, however, was conducted on a case of osteomyelitis observed on a 17th-century Italian skeleton (attributed to the famous painter Caravaggio): the identified pathogen was *Staphylococcus aureus* (Drancourt et al., 2018).

Paleopathologists observe non-specific skeletal infections in three main forms: osteomyelitis, spondylodiscitis, and septic arthritis. Periosteal reactions are regularly associated with these conditions, but when observed alone, their attribution to an infectious process must be interpreted cautiously, taking into account the multiplicity of etiologies, including, in the youngest subjects, the physiological hyperactivity of a periosteum during a growth spurt.

Osteomyelitis

The most common form of this condition is hematogenous osteomyelitis. Its annual incidence ranges from 13 to 74 per 100000 children, varying by populations and occurring more frequently in an acute form than in subacute form (Riise et al., 2008). Male predominance is classically noted (70% of boys, according to Lannelongue in 1879) but today's sex ratio appears more balanced (Riise et al., 2008; Labbé et al., 2010). Osteomyelitis affects mostly children and adolescents, more rarely infants and young adults (Lannelongue, 1879; Trueta, 1959; Labbé et al., 2010). It appears that older teenagers and young adults were proportionally more affected at the end of the 19th than today (see Figure 18.1).

Infection mainly involves the long bones and follows the adage "near the knee and far from the elbow"; that is to say, the proximal part of the tibia, distal femur, proximal humerus, and distal radius are common locations, while flat and short bones are less commonly affected. In more than 90% of case of infection affecting gone, a single bone is involved. Infection of several bones is the result of severe forms with multi-visceral infections occurring in younger subjects (Labbé et al., 2010). The lower limb is more frequently involved than the upper limb, with comparable ratios noted before the antibiotic era (80% lower limb versus 15% upper limb [Lannelongue, 1879]) and today (70% versus 20% [Labbé et al, 2010]) (see Table 18.2). The femur was the most affected bone in the clinical series studied by Lannelongue (1879), but in the larger modern series studied by Labbé et al. (2010), it is the tibia. This difference may result from difference in sample size or from a secular trend of unknown origin.

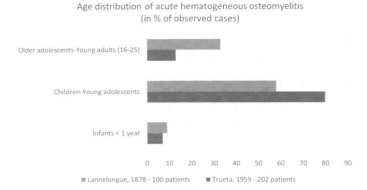

Figure 18.1 Comparison of age distribution of acute osteomyelitis at the end of the 19th century (Lannelongue, 1879) and at the mid-20th century (Trueta, 1959). Age categories of children – young adolescents (2–15 years old) are the most exposed. Older adolescents and young adults were proportionately more affected during the pre-antibiotic era than at present.

Table 18.2 Comparison of percentage skeletal distribution of hematogenous osteomyelitis on two clinical series observed in 1879 and in 2010

Bone involved	Labbé et al., 2010		Lannelongue, 1879		
	%	n	%	n	
Tibia	32.3	**70**	34.2	**80**	Lower limb
Femur	25.8		47.0		
Fibula	7.2		6.0		
Patella	1.1				
Tarsal bone	1.1				
Metatarsal-phalanges	2.3				
Ilium	5.7		1.15		
Humerus	1.4	**20**	7.0	**15**	Upper limb
Radius	5.3		3.5		
Ulna	3.0				
Metacarpal-phalanges	1.1				
Clavicle-scapula	0.5		1.15		
Ribs	2.7				
Mandible	0.5				
	450 patients		100 patients		
	[3 months–15 yrs]		[5 months–22 yrs]		

Due to age-related patterns of the growth plate and vascular anatomy of the long bones, the development of hematogenous osteomyelitis varies: in infancy, epiphyseal and articular infections are common and multiple bones can be affected; in childhood, the localization is metaphyseal with subperiosteal abscesses, the epiphyses and joints are generally preserved from infection; in adulthood, the epiphyses and joints are more commonly involved and infection of spine, flat and short tubular bones is more frequent (Resnick & Niwayama, 1995).

The classic pathophysiological mechanism of osteomyelitis begins as an initial focal infection of the metaphysis near the growth plate, which arrives by hematogenous route and stagnates in the anastomotic vascular network of the metaphyseal region, causing thrombosis and edema. The infection diffuses through the relatively thin cortical bone at this level and collects under the periosteum, detaching the membrane from the subperiosteal cortical bone and becoming a subperiosteal abscess, which may be voluminous. The production of a new layer of bone by the periosteum at a distance from the cortical bone creates an involucrum. This pattern, described by Trueta (1959), has been adopted by many authors (Resnick & Niwayama, 1995).

However, an alternative pathophysiological model has been more recently developed by Labbé and colleagues (2010) based on a retrospective study of 450 cases of acute osteomyelitis observed over a 20-year period between 1985 and 2004. According to their observations, ultrasound and CT imaging indicates that in most the cases a subperiosteal abscess occurs in the early phase if infection, whereas metaphyseal changes are only observed by imaging when the involucrum develops, corresponding to an advanced stage of the infection. Moreover, blunt force trauma preceding the clinical onset of infection by a few days was found in 63% of cases and is likely an underestimate of the true occurrence. They propose that Trueta's model is valid when subacute osteomyelitis occurs in childhood and intraosseous abscesses, known as "Brodie's" abscesses, form, but that most often, the initial process of acute osteomyelitis is linked to a direct trauma of the limb. They assert that the direct trauma produces edema or a subperiosteal hematoma, which will serve as a stopping point and culture medium for germs arriving through the blood stream to the rich vascular system of the periosteum. Consequently, Labbé and colleagues propose to change the term "acute osteomyelitis" to "acute osteoperiostitis". Interestingly, this "new" notion of initial subperiosteal abscess and of a blunt trauma preceding the first clinical signs by a few days was precisely described more than a century earlier by Lannelongue in 1879. Moreover, the term "acute osteoperiostitis" was already used as a synonym for osteomyelitis in the 19th century to designate the formation process of subperiosteal abscess. Therefore, during this period, two clinical expressions were recognized by surgeons: subperiosteal abscess, a severe condition which could be cured by rapid evacuation of the abscess after opening the periosteum; and osteomyelitis, a lethal condition occurring in the absence of rapid amputation (Lannelongue, 1879). This etiopathogenic debate is of interest today for their suggested therapeutic strategies and may assist paleopathologists seeking to understand historic period medical decisions and outcomes, however in most instances, when osteomyelitis is diagnosed in the archaeological record, it appears as an advanced form in which the medullary, cortical and periosteal compartments are involved.

Whatever the starting point of the infection, metaphyseal or osteoperiosteal, the diffusion of the infection will produce the same effects on tubular bones:

- in the metaphysis, the pus infiltrates the trabecular bone generating cavities, more or less circumscribed;
- the epiphysis is usually protected from infection by the growth plate in children but not in infants and adults. However, a purulent metaphyseal invasion under strong pressure may detach the epiphysis causing septic epiphysiolysis;
- the medullary canal fills with pus, which can drain outwards through an orifice called a cloaca (see Figure 18.2a);

- the infected cortical bone, deprived of vascularization, may become necrotic in the form of a sequestrum of variable size, sometimes consisting of a large part of the diaphysis, the ends of which are very irregular;
- the development of a subperiosteal abscess leads to a detachment of the periosteum, the production of new layers of bone constitutes the involucrum, which can be massive and opened by one or more cloacae, allowing the discharge of pus (skin opening);
- the extension of the infection to the whole diaphysis is referred to as pandiaphysitis.

Without effective treatment, this acute phase can result in rapid death within days or weeks or can become subacute evolving over several months. Mortality from acute or subacute osteomyelitis was probably very high in the pre-antibiotic era and has been estimated to be at least 20% (Roberts, 2019). During the years 1876 to 1878, of the 24 children that Lannelongue received at his hospital with a diagnosis of osteomyelitis, 12 died in his service, constituting a mortality rate of 50%. These historical documents are of interest to the paleopathologist, as deaths at hospital were followed by autopsies and indicate that skeletal changes are already visible two to three weeks after the first clinical signs appear. Thus, we can argue that acute osteomyelitis may be actually belong in the "visible part of the iceberg" and escape the osteological paradox, which warns that fatal acute diseases can produce "healthy" appearing skeletons because death occurs before bone tissue reacts (Wood et al., 1992).

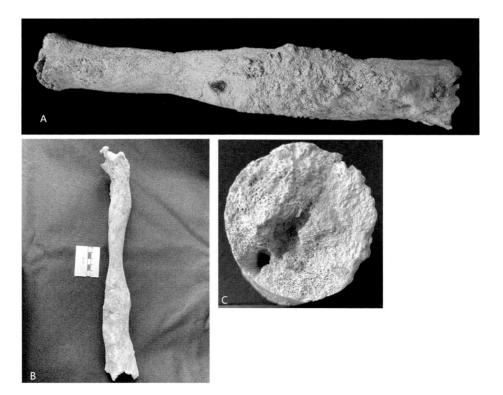

Figure 18.2 Paleopathological cases of chronic osteomyelitis: (a) Right tibia, showing the involucrum and the cloacal opening; (b) Diaphysis of femur displaying bifocal osteomyelitis; (c) Complete sclerosis of the medullar canal characteristic of Garré's sclerosing osteomyelitis.

In instances of survival without treatment, the infection becomes chronic, alternating between healing and recurrence, lasting several years, and with definitive healing being far less frequent. Two particular clinical forms are compatible with prolonged survival: the presence of a single central metaphyseal cavity surrounded by sclerosis, known as a Brodie's abscess (Brodie, 1832); and the development of a massive sclerosing reaction, both periosteal and endosteal, which induces a significant cortical thickening and completely obstructs the medullary canal (see Figure 18.2b), which is known as Garré's sclerosing osteomyelitis (Garré, 1893). In these two forms, there are no sequestrae or cloacae. For paleopathologists, these sclerosing forms of osteomyelitis involving femur or tibia may be difficult to differentiate from the osteoperiostitis of treponematoses (Roberts, 2019), but one of the diagnostic criteria of treponemal skeletal lesions is bilaterality and symmetry.

There is a paradox between the great frequency of osteomyelitis in historical periods, described in many contemporary medical records, and the relative scarcity of paleopathological references devoted to this subject for archaeological populations (noted by Lewis [2018] and Roberts [2019]). This does not mean that osteomyelitis was rare in osteoarchaeological populations. On the contrary, it may have been quite common. By studying large archaeological collections composed of hundreds of skeletons from late medieval and early modern periods, more than a dozen cases of chronic osteomyelitis were found (personal experience, unpublished, Figure 18.3). These numbers could be even more insightful if children's skeletons were examined for acute forms of osteomyelitis, which is responsible for quick death, but can be skeletally detectable even in early stages of infection.

Spondylodiscitis

Infection of vertebral bodies and intervertebral disks by pyogenic pathogens, known as vertebral or spinal osteomyelitis, is often included in chapters focusing on osteomyelitis because of its similar pathophysiology. However, its annual incidence is presently estimated at ~3 per 100000, which makes it an uncommon condition compared to osteomyelitis. It is more frequently found in females than in males, and more common in adults than in children (Resnick & Niwayama, 1995). The lumbar vertebrae are more frequently involved than the thoracic, which is more frequently involved than the cervical vertebrae.

The most frequent route of contamination is hematogenous, through the vascular system of vertebrae (nutrient arteries and Batson's venous system). The first phase of the infection is the development of a septic focus in the anterior part of the vertebral body, which will spread to the vertebral plate and the intervertebral disk, followed by the spread of the infection to the adjacent vertebra. In a further step, infection may spread through the anterior vertebral ligament and be responsible for paravertebral abscess (Resnick & Niwayama, 1995). Depending on the pathogen and host immunity, septic spondylodiscitis can be rapidly fatal, but as the vertebral and disk lesions appear within a few weeks, they can be detectable on archaeological specimens, constituting a theoretical counterexample to the osteological paradox. The most important challenge in paleopathology is to distinguish pyogenic spondylodiscitis from the first stages of tuberculous spondylodiscitis (Pott's disease). Pyogenic spondylodiscitis affects fewer vertebrae than Pott's disease and because it evolves more rapidly, may be more destructive, less sclerotic in appearance, and less likely to lead to vertebral fusion. Importantly, however, differential diagnosis is difficult in cases of vertebral collapse with bony bridging, which can be observed in vertebral osteomyelitis. It is hoped that through advances in paleomicrobiology and the identification of specific pathogens in individuals displaying pathological lesions that differential diagnosis can be improved.

Septic Arthritis

Infection at the site of joints can occur hematogenously, by contiguity (such as from osteomyelitis), or by direct inoculation. Single joints are most frequently affected (except when infection by specific germs such as gonococcus occurs, which is responsible for multi-joint infections). The knee is often affected regardless of age, and the hip is more often affected in children than in adults. Infection of the sacroiliac joint is observed at all ages (Resnick & Niwayama, 1995). The unique aspect of pyogenic infection of a joint is the development of joint fusion, which can occur following destruction of joint cartilage (Figure 18.3). This fusion may constitute a form of healing of the infection. In paleopathological practice, the distinction between septic arthritis and tuberculous osteoarthritis is often difficult (Roberts, 2019). Here again, advances in paleomicrobiology, which may isolate specific pathogens, might ultimately assist with differential diagnosis.

Periosteal Reactions/Periostitis

Periosteal reaction, appearing as new bone formation on the cortical surface of bones, is frequently observed in paleopathology. The lesions are sometimes mistakenly called periostitis, which suggests an infectious etiology. However, reactions of the periosteum can be related to or caused by many other pathological circumstances, such as trauma, metabolic conditions, and

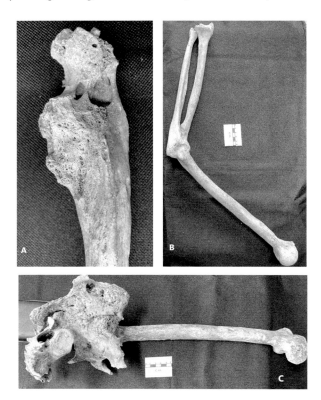

Figure 18.3 Three paleopathological examples of joint destruction and fusion due to infectious arthritis: (a) left ulna; (b) right humerus, radius, and ulna fused at elbow joint; (c) left femur fused to os coxae.

vascular diseases, tumors, and can also occur physiologically during growth spurts in childhood (Rittemard et al., 2019). Therefore, although the presence of periosteal reactions can be interpreted as indicators of "non-specific infection"; that is, infection by unknown pathogens (Weston, 2012), it is misleading (and perhaps outright false) to assert unequivocally that their presence indicates systemic pathogenic infection. Systematic and rigorous differential diagnosis is essential to undertake, especially since the causes of periosteal changes are particularly complex. An argument can be made that only in instances where periosteal reaction is clearly associated with osteomyelitic or osteoarthritic changes that the lesions can be called periostitis.

Pyogenic Bacteria, The Poor Relatives of Paleomicrobiology

The paleopathological understanding of infections has benefited from progress in molecular biology, allowing the identification of numerous pathogens (bacterial, viral, mycotic, and parasitic) and serving as the source of a considerable knowledge about human infection in the past (e.g., Raoult et al., 2006; Raoult & Drancourt, 2008; Appelt et al., 2016; Duggan et al., 2016; Bos et al., 2019; Duchêne et al., 2020). There is, however, a marked imbalance, with some pathogens serving as the source of inquiry much more often than others. As an example, in a recent synthesis on the past, present, and future of ancient bacterial DNA by Arning & Wilson (2020), only the "bacterial trio" of *Yersinia pestis* (69 genomic sequences), *Mycobacterium leprae* (27), and *Mycobacterium tuberculosis* (17) capture the attention of the scientists in the catalog of bacterial paleogenomes. No future is mentioned for the exploration of aDNA of pyogenic bacteria. This is regrettable, as knowledge of the evolution of human pyogenic bacteria remains *terra incognita*. *Staphylococcus aureus*, discovered in 1880 by Louis Pasteur from a clinical sample provided by Odilon Lannelongue from one of his young osteomyelitic patients, certainly deserves greater exploration of its evolutionary past, especially as the pathogen develops greater and greater antibiotic resistance in our modern world.

Conclusions

To conclude, infections (whether of known or unknown etiology) were and still are frequent and severe; killing vast proportions of affected children in the past and leaving survivors profoundly impacted. These infections remain a public health problem today. Considering that the pathophysiology, especially for acute osteomyelitis, has been the subject discussion for 150 years, and that a new pyogenic bacterium (*Kingella kingae*) other than *Staphylococcus aureus* has been recently discovered, the issue of "non-specific" infections should warrant keen attention from paleopathologists and other members of the scientific community. This is a great step forward as we seek to understand health and disease in the past, present, and future.

References

Alter, G. & Carmichael, A. (1996). Studying causes of death in the past: problems and models. *Historical Methods: A Journal of Quantitative and Interdisciplinary History* 29(2):44–48. https://doi.org/10.1080/01615440.1996.10112728.

Andam, C. P., Worby, C. J., Chang, Q. & Campana, M. G. (2016). Microbial genomics of ancient plagues and outbreaks. *Trends in Microbiology* 24(12):978–990. https://doi.org/10.1016/j.tim.2016.08.004.

Appelt, S., Drancourt, M. & Le Bailly, M. (2016). Human coprolites as a source for paleomicrobiology. *Microbiology Spectrum* 4(4). https://doi.org/10.1128/microbiolspec.PoH-0002-2014.

Arning, N. & Wilson, D. J. (2020). The past, present and future of ancient bacterial DNA. *Microbial Genomics* 6(7). https://doi.org/10.1099/mgen.0.000384.

Aufderheide, A. C. & Rodriguez-Martin, C. (1998). *The Cambridge Encyclopedia of Human Paleopathology.* Cambridge: Cambridge University Press.

Bain, A. (2004). Irritating Intimates: the archaeoentomology of lice, fleas, and bedbugs. *Northeast Historical Archaeology* 33(1):81–90. https://doi.org/10.22191/neha/vol33/iss1/8.

Bos, K. I., Kühnert, D., Herbig, A., Esquivel-Gomez, L. R., Andrades Valtueña, A., Barquera, R., … & Krause, J. (2019). Paleomicrobiology: diagnosis and evolution of ancient pathogens. *Annual Review of Microbiology* 73(1):639–666. https://doi.org/10.1146/annurev-micro-090817-062436.

Brodie, B. C. (1832). An account of some cases of chronic abscess of the tibia. *Medico-Chirurigical Transactions* 17:239–249. https://doi.org/10.1177/095952873201700111.

Buikstra, J. E. (2019). *Ortner's Identification of Pathological Conditions in Human Skeletal Remains.* Amsterdam, The Netherlands: Elsevier.

Cockburn, T. A. (1971). Infectious diseases in ancient populations. *Current Anthropology* 12(1):45–62. https://doi.org/10.1086/201168.

Drancourt, M., Barbieri, R., Cilli, E., Gruppioni, G., Bazaj, A., Cornaglia, G. & Raoult, D. (2018). Did Caravaggio die of *Staphylococcus aureus* sepsis? *The Lancet Infectious Diseases* 18(11):178. https://doi.org/10.1016/S1473-3099(18)30571-1.

Duchêne, S., Ho, S. Y. W., Carmichael, A. G., Holmes, E. C. & Poinar, H. (2020). The recovery, interpretation and use of ancient pathogen genomes. *Current Biology* 30(19):R1215–R1231. https://doi.org/10.1016/j.cub.2020.08.081.

Duggan, A. T., Perdomo, M. F., Piombino-Mascali, D., Marciniak, S., Poinar, D., Emery, M. V., Buchmann, J. P., Duchêne, S., Jankauskas, R. & Humphreys, M. (2016). 17th century variola virus reveals the recent history of smallpox. *Current Biology* 26(24):3407–3412.

Dutour, O. (2008). Archaeology of human pathogens: palaeopathological appraisal of palaeoepidemiology. In Raoult, D. & Drancourt, M. (Eds.), *Paleomicrobiology*, pp. 125–144. Springer Berlin Heidelberg. https://doi.org/10.1007/978-3-540-75855-6_8.

Dutour, O. (2016). Paleopathology of human infections: old bones, antique books, ancient and modern molecules. In Drancourt, M. & Raoult, D. (Éds.), *Paleomicrobiology of Humans*, pp. 93–106. ASM Press. https://doi.org/10.1128/9781555819170.ch10.

Garré, C. (1893). *Uber Besondere Formen Und Folgezustande Der Akuten Infekfionsen Osteomyelitis* 10:241–298.

Grmek, M., Drazen & Gourevitch, D. (1998). *Les Maladies dans l'Art Antique.* Fayard.

Hendy, J., Collins, M., Teoh, K. Y., Ashford, D. A., Thomas-Oates, J., Donoghue, H. D., Pap, I., Minnikin, D. E., Spigelman, M. & Buckley, M. (2016). The challenge of identifying tuberculosis proteins in archaeological tissues. *Journal of Archaeological Science* 66:146–153. https://doi.org/10.1016/j.jas.2016.01.003.

Knapp, M. (2011). The next generation of genetic investigations into the Black Death. *Proceedings of the National Academy of Sciences* 108(38):15669–15670. https://doi.org/10.1073/pnas.1112574108.

Krause-Kyora, B., Nutsua, M., Boehme, L., Pierini, F., Pedersen, D. D., Kornell, S. -C., … & Nebel, A. (2018). Ancient DNA study reveals HLA susceptibility locus for leprosy in medieval Europeans. *Nature Communications* 9(1):1569. https://doi.org/10.1038/s41467-018-03857-x.

Labbé, J. -L., Peres, O., Leclair, O., Goulon, R., Scemama, P., Jourdel, F., Menager, C., Duparc, B. & Lacassin, F. (2010). Acute osteomyelitis in children: the pathogenesis revisited? *Orthopaedics & Traumatology: Surgery & Research* 96(3):268–275. https://doi.org/10.1016/j.otsr.2009.12.012.

Lannelongue, O. M. (1879). *De l'Ostéomyélite Aiguë Pendant la Croissance.* Asselin & Cie; Bibliothèque nationale de France. https://gallica.bnf.fr/ark:/12148/bpt6k61090059.

Lederberg, J., Shope, R. E. & Oaks, S. (1992). *Emerging Infections—Microbial Threats to Health in the United States.* Washington, DC: National Academies Press.

Lewis, M. (2018). *Paleopathology of Children: Identification of Pathological Conditions in the Human Skeletal Remains of Non-Adults.* Academic Press.

Morens, D. M., Folkers, G. K. & Fauci, A. S. (2004). The challenge of emerging and re-emerging infectious diseases. *Nature* 430(6996):242–249. https://doi.org/10.1038/nature02759.

Ragsdale, B. D. & Lehmer, L. M. (2012). A knowledge of bone at the cellular (histological) level is essential to paleopathology. In Grauer, A. L. (Ed.), *A Companion to Paleopathology*, pp. 225–249. Wiley-Blackwell. https://doi.org/10.1002/9781444345940.ch13.

Raoult, D. & Drancourt, M. (Éds.). (2008). *Paleomicrobiology: Past Human Infections*. Berlin; Heideiberg: Springer Verlag.

Raoult, D., Dutour, O., Houhamdi, L., Jankauskas, R., Fournier, P. -E., Ardagna, Y., Drancourt, M., Signoli, M., La, V. D. & Macia, Y. (2006). Evidence for louse-transmitted diseases in soldiers of Napoleon's Grand Army in Vilnius. *The Journal of Infectious Diseases* 193(1):112–120.

Reperant, L. A. & Osterhaus, A. (2013). The human-animal interface. *Microbiology Spectrum* 1(1):1–15. https://doi.org/10.1128/microbiolspec.OH-0013-2012.

Resnick, D. & Niwayama, G. (1995). Osteomyelitis, septic arthritis and soft tissue infection. In D. Resnick & G. Niwayama (Éds.), *Diagnosis of Bone and Joint Disorders*, pp. 2525–2618. Saunders.

Riise, Ø. R., Kirkhus, E., Handeland, K. S., Flatø, B., Reiseter, T., Cvancarova, M., Nakstad, B. & Wathne, K.-O. (2008). Childhood osteomyelitis-incidence and differentiation from other acute onset musculoskeletal features in a population-based study. *BMC Pediatrics* 8(1):45. https://doi.org/10.1186/1471-2431-8-45.

Rittemard, C., Colombo, A., Desbarats, P., Dutailly, B., Dutour, O. & Coqueugniot, H. (2019). The periosteum dilemma in bioarcheology: normal growth or pathological condition? – 3D discriminating microscopic approach. *Journal of Archaeological Science: Reports* 24:236–243. https://doi.org/10.1016/j.jasrep.2018.12.012.

Roberts, C. A. (2019). Infectious disease. In Buikstra, J. (Ed.), *Ortner's Identification of Pathological Conditions in Human Skeletal Remains*, pp. 285–319. Elsevier. https://doi.org/10.1016/B978-0-12-809738-0.00010-7.

Ruffer, M. A. (1913). On pathological lesions found in Coptic bodies (400–500 AD). *Journal of Pathology and Bacteriology* 18:149–162.

Samara, E., Spyropoulou, V., Tabard-Fougère, A., Merlini, L., Valaikaite, R., Dhouib, A., Manzano, S., Juchler, C., Dayer, R. & Ceroni, D. (2019). *Kingella kingae* and osteoarticular infections. *Pediatrics* 144(6):e20191509. https://doi.org/10.1542/peds.2019-1509.

Signore, A. (2013). About inflammation and infection. *EJNMMI Research* 3(1):8. https://doi.org/10.1186/2191-219X-3-8.

Trueta, J. (1959). The three types of acute haematogenous osteomyelitis: a clinical and vascular study. *Journal of Bone and Joint Surgery* 41B(4):671–680.

Weston, D. A. (2012). Nonspecific infection in paleopathology: interpreting periosteal reactions. In Grauer, A. L. (Ed.), *A Companion to Paleopathology*, pp. 492–512. Wiley-Blackwell. https://doi.org/10.1002/9781444345940.ch27.

Wood, J. W., Milner, G. R., Harpending, H. C. & Weiss, K. M. (1992). The osteological paradox: problems of inferring prehistoric health from skeletal samples. *Current Anthropology* 33(4):343–370. https://doi.org/10.1086/204084.

Woolhouse, M. E. J. & Gowtage-Sequeria, S. (2005). Host range and emerging and reemerging pathogens. *Emerging Infectious Diseases* 11(12):1842–1847. https://doi.org/10.3201/eid1112.050997.

19
METABOLIC AND ENDOCRINE DISEASES

Megan B. Brickley and Brianne Morgan

Introduction

Metabolic and endocrine diseases are globally recognized as a major public health priority related to acute and chronic health consequences. Although within the group there are many exceptionally rare conditions, most readers will know somebody who has experienced one or more of these diseases and there is a strong possibility that you or someone you know is currently affected. Metabolic conditions such as anemias, vitamin D deficiency, and age-related bone loss and diabetes make up the majority of non-transmissible conditions experienced by 21st-century populations. With close links to immune response, and associated morbidity and mortality, the metabolic and endocrine diseases play a significant role in the lives and deaths in communities today and in the past.

Disorders of the endocrine and metabolic systems are frequently considered together due to close physiological links. Endocrine glands play an active role in the production and delivery of hormones and are critical to the processing of vitamins, minerals, and micro-nutrients, often with direct effects on the pathophysiology of bone and closely linked cells and tissues. The metabolic bone diseases are frequently classified as those that cause alterations in "normal bone formation, resorption, or mineralization, or a combination of these; in most conditions, these alterations are systemic" (Brickley & Mays, 2019:531), with many linked to nutrition and nutritional factors (e.g., New & Bonjour, 2003; Weaver & Heaney, 2013).

A number of metabolic and endocrine diseases have played a central role in paleopathological investigations. These include scurvy (vitamin C deficiency), rickets and osteomalacia (primarily vitamin D deficiency), and acquired anemias, where bioavailability of micro-nutrients such as iron, folate, and vitamin B_{12} are critical. The presence of osteoporosis has also been a focus of attention, as acquisition of peak bone mass (PBM) and bone maintenance are closely tied to dietary variables and, in the case of females, endocrine factors in hormonal changes. Secondary hyperparathyroidism exemplifies the complex association between the metabolic and endocrine diseases, while others, such as type 2 diabetes (T2D), present clear challenges for paleopathologists, so will be included in this chapter as we explore historical perspectives and current approaches.

Historical Perspectives and Current Approaches

The importance of understanding pathophysiology at the cellular level and an appreciation of hormonal involvement in disease processes have contributed to metabolic bone diseases assuming a central place in recent paleopathological investigation (see Grauer, 2019). However, sporadic paleopathological reporting of scurvy and rickets has occurred since the mid-19th century (Mays, 2014; Mays & Brickley, 2018). Pathological aspects of osteoporosis were also recognized centuries ago, with the clear association of bone loss with age made possible with the development of x-rays in 1895. Other epidemiological and pathophysiological aspects of the condition have been recognized in the last 70 years (Curate, 2014; Agarwal, 2018; Brickley et al., 2020:157; van Spelde et al., 2021), and the first studies within paleopathology date back 50 years (e.g., van Gerven et al., 1969). Understanding diabetes is also relatively new, and although possible references to symptoms of diabetes are present in the Ebres and Hearst papyri from ancient Egypt (1530 and 1479 BCE, respectively), a possible case has only recently been suggested in an archaeological individual (Dupras et al. 2010).

Scurvy

Scurvy, caused by severe deficiency of vitamin C, impairs collagen formation and reduces differentiation of osteoblasts (Aghajanian et al., 2015). This results in decreased bone formation and hemorrhaging of blood vessels. Clinically, scurvy is diagnosed using detailed questions on dietary history of the patient and evaluation of skin and oral conditions, such as petechiae (spots on the skin) and gum swelling/bleeding. Symptoms, such as tiredness, lethargy, leg pain, and refusal to walk (Ceglie et al., 2019), also help modern clinicians diagnose the disease. However, the use of radiography to diagnose scurvy played a more important role prior to the modern widespread use of blood tests and patient surveys. Hence, while there are limited descriptions of bone lesions that might be helpful to paleopathologists working directly with skeletal remains, early radiographs and autopsy reports linking vitamin C deficiency with hemorrhagic disorders can be useful.

Ortner and colleagues sought to explore these links through identifying biological mechanisms of vitamin C deficiency that could lead to recognizable bone changes. Over a period of 15 years, Ortner led a team that established a series of 13 commonly occurring lesions (see Table 19.1) (Ortner & Ericksen, 1997; Brown & Ortner, 2011). These lesions arise as a response to hemorrhage and consist of porosity of the original cortical surface of bone and newly formed bone beneath the periosteum. Both lesion types occur in active scurvy cases and are more readily observed in those undergoing rapid growth (Brickley et al., 2020:51). Paleopathologists have also identified what have been termed "mixed lesions", where new bone forms at the same sites where the porosity of the original cortex is present (Brickley & Mays, 2019).

While additional lesions likely linked to scurvy, such as new bone formation in the pterygoid fossae, have been noted (e.g., Snoddy et al., 2018), Ortner's criteria have provided a clear basis for investigation of scurvy from diverse contexts including Greece (1200–1300 CE) (Bourbou, 2014), the Pacific islands (1080–980 BCE) (Buckley et al., 2014), Predynastic Egypt (3800–3600 BCE) (Pitre et al., 2016), and sites from Peru (spanning 200–1470 CE) (Klaus, 2017). Historical texts in Europe, from the time of Hippocrates (460–370 BCE), describe probable cases of scurvy. Economic growth fueled wars and voyages of exploration from the Renaissance (15th century CE) to the early 18th century, producing numerous descriptions of scurvy in adults serving in the military or on ships (and recognition of the need for fruits, such as limes, to ward off the condition) (French, 1993). Assessment of archaeological material, however, demonstrates that skeletal lesions are much more clearly observed in rapidly growing individuals. In infants, scurvy reflects aspects of maternal health and specific practices used in feeding and weaning (Mays, 2014; Snoddy et al., 2017).

Studying the presence of vitamin C deficiency in the past can shed light on aspects of human life that extend beyond diet. For instance, the effects of military conquest on dietary factors were explored for individuals in the settlement of Oxford following the Norman conquest of England (1066 CE) (Craig-Atkins et al., 2020). Dietary information derived from paleopathology, serial stable isotopes, residue analysis, archaeobotanical, and zooarchaeological and contemporary documentary sources, revealed agricultural intensification and widespread adoption of practices used by elites. Evidence of scurvy was found in an individual with isotopic evidence suggesting limited early access to protein, dietary fluctuations, and/or physiological stress (Craig-Atkins et al., 2020). The use of multiple sources of evidence alongside conditions such as scurvy enabled a more nuanced understanding of political change and potential food insecurity at the community level. Importantly, scurvy often reflects food choices in the context of environmental availability and cultural determinants. Individuals and/or communities can often exercise some control over the acquisition,

Table 19.1 Typical sites for hemorrhagic lesions in scurvy

Lesion location – all arise due to hemorrhagic phenomena	Notes
Cranial	
1 Sphenoid, external surface, greater wing	Generally bilateral and symmetric
2 Zygomatic bone, medial surface/posterio-medial surface of maxillary zygomatic process.	
3 Posterior surface of maxilla	
4 Coronoid process of mandible, medial surface	
5 Inferior surface, palatine processes of maxillae	
6 Maxillary and/or mandibular alveolar bone	
7 Orbital walls	Superior wall most often affected. Alterations may show left/right asymmetry
8 Cranial vault	Ectocranial surface more often affected than endocranial
9 Infraorbital foramen of maxilla	
10 Foramen rotundum of sphenoid bone	
Post-cranial	
1 Long bones (porosity – primarily growing individuals, PNBF – primarily mature individuals)	Porosity especially seen on metaphyses, but rarely extends beyond 5–10 mm of the growth plate. Differentiate from growth-related cut-back zone porosity
2 Scapulae, supra- and infra-spinous fossae	
3 Ilia, medial surface	

Notes. PNBF = sub-periosteal new bone formation. Porosity is the most common lesion, but PNBF can occur at all sites with potential for 'mixed' lesions. All lesions are more common during growth. After Brickley and Mays (2019: Table 15.1)

processing, cooking, and storage of food. Hence, human behavior, along with environment, can serve as important determinants of disease.

Rickets and Osteomalacia

Vitamin D is obtained via two mechanisms: synthesis following exposure of the skin to sunlight (UVB) and ingestion. Few foods naturally contain this nutrient, so in the absence of modern fortified foods, sunlight is the main source of vitamin D (Jones, 2018). Often considered a hormone, vitamin D facilitates absorption from the gut and maintenance of optimal levels in the bloodstream, of both calcium and phosphate; all three are required for normal formation and maintenance of the skeleton. Disruption of the tightly linked triad of vitamin D, calcium, and phosphate leads to impaired mineralization of tissues and potentially development of skeletal diseases, rickets, and osteomalacia (Holick, 2010; Jones & Prosser, 2011; Rice et al., 2015). Vitamin D deficiency is a product of biophysical variables, such as geographic latitude, skin pigmentation, and bioavailability of vitamin D in food sources, as well as cultural variables such as behaviors and actions that may place an individual or population at risk (Brickley et al., 2014:48). Rickets develops in those still growing; impaired bone mineralization results in development of porous lesions and, with time, loss of the structural integrity of bone and bowing. A suite of 16 macroscopic lesions observed consistently in growing individuals from disparate contexts are now widely accepted as being indicative of rickets (see Table 19.2). Remnants of bone deformities may persist and have been referred to as *healed rickets* in growing individuals and *residual rickets* in adults. In adults, *osteomalacia* develops. Severe long-standing disruption of bone mineralization results in accumulation of osteoid, the unmineralized framework of bone, and resultant bone deformity, or more commonly pathological fractures referred to as pseudofractures. The presence/absence of mineralization defects of bones and teeth can indicate different disease stages during growth and later life.

Cases of rickets and osteomalacia have now been identified from past communities from a diverse range of contexts. Urban centers associated with the Industrial Revolution in Northern Europe and North America marked the high point in occurrence of vitamin D deficiency due to generally low levels of UVB in northern latitudes and workers' limited access to sunlight (e.g., Watts & Valme, 2018), but humans, and our ancestors, have likely always had the propensity to develop rickets and osteomalacia in situations where access to UVB was below levels required for adequate synthesis of vitamin D. For instance, a large-scale study of Roman period communities from Western Europe found rickets was linked to latitude, with higher levels in the north where UVB is more limited (Mays et al., 2018). Bioarchaeological data demonstrated that although some settlements had high population density and multi-storey housing, most people lived in low-density settlements with access to open space and sunlight (Lockau et al. 2019). Interestingly, rickets has been recorded at sites where cutaneous synthesis of vitamin D would have been possible all year, but strong social patterns of sun avoidance were practiced (e.g., Littleton, 1998). Examples of osteomalacia in adults are found less frequently than in childhood rickets in modern clinical studies and in paleopathological investigations. Osteomalacia has been reported from various contexts where both dietary sources of vitamin D and UVB access were limited. Osteomalacic individuals were identified at an early psychiatric hospital in Bloemendaal, North Holland, where bedrest was used for some patients, and at southern sites, such as the Roman city of Ostia, Italy, where the lived environment limited access to sunlight (van der Merwe et al., 2018; Lockau et al., 2019). Clearly, social and cultural contexts are important determinants of access to UVB (see Theoretical Approaches, below).

Table 19.2 Key lesions of impaired mineralization: Rickets and Osteomalacia

Lesion location and characteristics	Biological mechanism	Active/healed/residual
Macroscopic lesions – primarily found during growth		
1 Cranial vault porosity	Impaired mineralization.	A
2 Orbital roof porosity	Impaired mineralization.	A
3 Cranial vault thickening.	Mineralization of osteoid accumulated during impaired mineralization.	H
4 Deformed mandibular ramus	Deformation of weakened bone.	A, H + R
5 Rib bending deformity	Deformation of weakened bone.	A, H + R
6 Costochondral rib flaring	Deformation of weakened bone, and mineralization of osteoid accumulated during impaired mineralization.	A, H
7 Costochondral rib porosity	Impaired mineralization.	A
8 Ilium concavity	Deformation of weakened bone.	A, H
9 Bending deformity – upper limb long-bones	Deformation of weakened bone.	A, H + R
10 Bending deformity – lower limb long-bones	Deformation of weakened bone.	A, H + R
11 Long-bone metaphyseal flaring/cupping of ends	Deformation of weakened bone, and mineralization of osteoid accumulated during impaired mineralization.	A, H
12 Long-bone general thickening	Mineralization of osteoid accumulated during impaired mineralization.	H
13 Long-bone cortical (especially metaphyseal) porosity	Impaired mineralization at sites of rapid growth.	A
14 Superior flattening femoral metaphysis	Deformation of weakened bone.	A, H + R
15 Coxa vara (downward deformation with reduction of femoral neck angle)	Deformation of weakened bone.	A, H + R
16 Porosis/roughening on bone underlying growth plates	Impaired mineralization at sites of rapid growth.	A
Macroscopic lesions – Primarily found once growth complete		
1 Pathological fractures (pseudofractures)	Accumulations of osteoid and poorly mineralized bone.	A
Microscopic lesions		
1 Interglobular dentin. Permanent lesion	Impaired mineralization dentin.	A, H + R
2 Mineralization defects in bone (term osteomalacia often used). Transitory lesion	Impaired mineralization bone.	A

Notes: A = denotes disease active at time of death; feature generally transitory, being removed by remodeling in healed cases. R = may remain as residual lesions once growth has ceased. H = healed/healing disease. Sources drawn from Brickley et al. (2020) and Welsh et al. (2020).

Dietary factors play a limited role in past cases of vitamin D deficiency, but there has been discussion of dietary adaptations in groups living at latitudes where adequate cutaneous synthesis is only possible for part of the year (Chaplin & Jablonski, 2013). Early inhabitants are suggested to have established an "adaptive complex" in the Mesolithic and Neolithic, with both development of skin with low pigmentation levels (maximizing UVB absorption) and consumption of a diet rich in fish such as cod (cod liver oil is a rich source of vitamin D). Levels of deficiency may have increased slightly with adoption of farming at 5,000 years BCE, but foodstuffs such as black pudding, made from cow's blood, contained reasonable levels of vitamin D. From the 18th century, urbanization and industrialization occurred alongside profound dietary shifts for poorer members of society, many of whom relied heavily on potatoes. Dietary sources of vitamin D and UVB exposure were greatly reduced. Chaplin and Jablonski (2013) suggest these shifts underlie poor population-level health in Scotland today, with high levels of cardiovascular and autoimmune disease reported. Longer-term evolutionary aspects of vitamin D synthesis have also been considered with changes in levels of skin pigmentation, to boost absorption of UVB, and potential positive selection for ductal branching in the mammary glands increasing transfer of nutrients such as vitamin D (Hlusko et al., 2018; Jablonski & Chaplin, 2018). Understanding long-term patterns of vitamin D deficiency has clear implications for tackling public health issues, as the role vitamin D in immune response and other health consequences become clear (e.g., Khammissa et al., 2018; Owa & Owa, 2020).

Anemia

Anemia is one of the most widespread conditions experienced by humans today (Pasricha et al., 2013) and would likely have been common in the past. There are two categories of anemia: acquired anemia, which stems from environmental and behavioral conditions during the lifetime of the individual, and inherited anemias, which are linked to the presence of genes and gene expression. The term anemia is used to describe the physiological state of insufficient oxygen availability to meet the body's need. Red blood cells (RBCs) play a key role in the oxygenation of cells and tissues. Hence, disruption to the production, maintenance, and function of these cells are critical factors leading to anemia. Nutritional problems are a leading cause of acquired anemia. Although a balanced diet with key nutrients is important, availability of nutrients required for formation of sufficient normal RBCs can be disrupted for various reasons (Alzaheb & Al-Amer, 2017). Today, iron-deficiency anemia (IDA) is the most diagnosed form, but there are many cases where multiple factors play a role in disease development (DeLoughery, 2017). The prospect of acquired anemias providing insight into health and disease in past communities has led the condition being extensively investigated for close to a century (e.g., Williams, 1929; El Najjar et al., 1976).

Associating bone lesions with the presence of anemia is complicated. Bone lesions are not considered in clinical diagnosis of anemia, so as with scurvy, paleopathologists working directly with bone need to consider the underlying biological mechanisms of lesion formation before associating bone change with a diagnosis of anemia. For instance, researchers have used the presence of porous lesions as an indicator of anemia. However, porosity needs to have developed due to marrow hyperplasia (expansion) – a response by the body to produce more RBCs in order to increase oxygen transport to tissues. Acquired anemias are less likely to produce marked skeletal changes than those of genetic origin (e.g., see Lewis, 2012). Microscopic or micro-CT examination may allow evaluation of underlying mechanisms involved in lesion formation (see Table 19.3).

Table 19.3 Lesions in anemia

Lesion location	Notes
Cranial/mandibular	
Orbital roof: signs of marrow hyperplasia	Thinning of trabecular elements and cortical bone (initial changes). Perforation of original cortical surface produces porous lesions[a]
	Mixed lesions can arise in areas with marrow and PNBF
Cranial vault: signs of marrow hyperplasia	As above
	Porosity due to anemia will not develop at sites that lack RBC-producing marrow or muscle attachment sites
Post-cranial	
Vertebrae: signs of marrow hyperplasia	[a]Perforation of original cortical surface in vertebral bodies
Ribs: signs of marrow hyperplasia	Expansion in size can occur
	[a]Perforation of original cortical surface found (Thal)
Long bones: signs of marrow hyperplasia	[a]Perforation of original cortical surface
Long bones: necrosis of the femoral or humeral head	Found in SCA

Microscopic/micro-CT assessment is required to assess internal structural changes in the absence of post-depositional breakage.
[a]Anemia can only be inferred if the surface porosity is associated with marrow hyperplasia identified via enlarged marrow spaces. Notes: PNBF = sub-periosteal new bone formation, (Thal) = thalassemia, SCA= sickle cell anemia. Adapted from Brickley et al. 2020 Table 9-3.

It is also clear that the age at which increased RBC production occurs will play a key role in the presence and pattern of skeletal lesions (see Gurevitch et al., 2007; Guillerman, 2013; Chan et al., 2016; and summary in Brickley, 2018). Demand for RBCs is especially high during periods of rapid growth (infancy – early childhood) and with increased nutritional demands for women during pregnancy. Today anemia is common in these demographic groups (World Health Organization, 2001; Miller, 2016:179). Since anemia increases susceptibility to further health problems, it is often viewed as a marker for poor health and nutrition (World Health Organization, 2004). Used as an indicator of micro-nutrient deficiency, anemia has considerable potential to facilitate a deeper understanding of life in past communities. Women and children play a critical role as human capital in shaping social well-being, contributing to political and economic development, and providing community stability (World Health Organization, 2016; Richter et al., 2017). These constituents are often acutely affected by social changes but are usually poorly represented in historical texts. Integrating consideration of age of occurrence of lesions demonstrably caused by anemia into paleopathological research would facilitate understanding women and children in past communities.

Hyperparathyroidism

Over-production of thyroid hormone, hypothyroidism (either primary or secondary), is an endocrine disorder often considered alongside metabolic bone diseases due to the direct effect this hormone has on metabolism and bone health. Primary hyperparathyroidism is often caused by development of a benign tumor (adenoma) or hyperplasia (Masi, 2019). Secondary hyperparathyroidism will normally develop in the presence of long-standing vitamin D deficiency (Creo et al., 2017; Charoenngam et al., 2019). Vitamin D facilitates absorption of calcium and phosphate from the gut, maintaining healthy levels in circulation. Low levels of vitamin D, and other conditions that result in low serum calcium levels (hypocalcemia) and absorption, prompt the release of thyroid and resorption of bone, freeing minerals stored in the skeleton (Uday & Högler, 2017). Hence, this condition typifies the complex association between metabolic and endocrine disorders.

Micro-structural indicators of secondary hyperparathyroidism, such as linear resorptive tunneling of cortical bone, can be observed via radiography or microscopy, and characteristic lesions resulting from marked osteoclastic activity can develop (see Zink et al., 2005). Evidence of secondary hyperparathyroidism has been observed via microscopic examination of archaeological individuals with rickets (Mays et al., 2007), but lesions will develop in any condition with marked bone resorption. Consideration of cases, alongside biological, environmental, and social factors will enable fuller paleopathological contributions to research.

Low Bone Levels and Osteoporosis

Osteoporosis is a qualitative pathological state measured by increased fracture risk due to failure to acquire and/or subsequent bone loss. Most cases of osteoporosis involve bone loss in older individuals, but when linked to disease, injury, or immobility, the condition can be either localized or systemic. In current communities with good nutrition and healthcare, the primary cause of bone loss leading to fragility fractures occurs with hormonal change in females at the menopause. The propensity of bones to fracture is dependent on PBM attained, the rate of subsequent loss, and the quality of bone at the micro-structural level. PBM is achieved in the late teens or early twenties (Forwood, 2013). Nutritional status and activity levels during key periods of childhood and adolescent growth play a critical role in ensuring individuals attain their genetic potential for PBM (Weaver et al., 2016), but maternal health and early fetal development also contribute to accrual of bone and fracture risk (Harvey et al., 2014; see Chapter 28, this volume).

The amount of bone present in an individual has been evaluated in paleopathology using measures of bone mineral density (BMD), and bone quality – primarily structural aspects such as cortical thickness via radiogrammetry (Curate, 2014; Brickley & Mays, 2019). Developments in diagnostic approaches have permitted consideration of micro-structural aspects of bone quality, such as porosity, and overall structural integrity of bone (Johannesdottir et al., 2014; Cole et al., 2019). Micro-porosity cannot be observed in examination of skeletal material or standard computed tomography (CT) radiography. Rather, histomorphometric assessment is required either using micro-CT or microscopic evaluation. BMD is now accessible from CT scans with developments in quantitative CT (QCT), and assessment of structural integrity is achievable with peripheral QCT (pQCT) (Brickley et al., 2020:147).

Fragility fractures are the outcome of osteoporosis but, as one of the commonest findings in paleopathology, fractures should be assessed alongside bone mass and/or quantity to establish osteoporosis as an underlying cause. While individual cases can have strong circumstantial evidence that a fracture is linked to osteoporosis, to ensure maximum information is obtained from population-level studies, quantification is required. A useful dataset is provided for both fractures and bone quantity/quality from individuals that died in the Medieval farming community of Wharram Percy, England (summarized in Mays, 2007).

It has long been known that data from past communities could assist in understanding the high levels of osteoporosis and associated fractures in current groups, and recent paleopathological investigations are yielding useful information. Extensive work undertaken by Beauchesne and Agarwal (2017) at the Roman site of Velia, Italy, for example, showed that although overall patterns of loss were similar to those in current populations, there were important differences. Just two fragility fractures were identified, and a measure of trabecular bone micro-architecture was the only significant difference found between males and females that died at older ages. Results revealed the complexity of bone acquisition, maintenance, and loss; higher activity levels appear to play a critical role in bone maintenance (Beauchesne & Agarwal, 2017). The importance of activity levels for bone health in women from past groups was also illustrated by Macintosh and colleagues (Macintosh et al., 2017). Rigorous activity involving the upper limb was an important aspect of life during the first 5,500 years of farming in Central Europe, giving women in these communities comparable upper limb strength to modern athletes (Macintosh et al., 2017). At present, radiogrammetry provides a simple technique that allows direct comparison between recent and paleopathological data, but as techniques such as pQCT are developed (Stride et al., 2013) more detailed appraisals are likely forthcoming.

Diabetes (Type 2)

Diabetes mellitus (DM) is a group of metabolic diseases that result in high blood glucose levels (hyperglycemia) (Expert Committee on the Diagnosis and Classification of Diabetes Mellitus, 2003). T2D is the most common form in present day and was likely also present in past communities (Centers for Disease Control, 2011; Brickley et al., 2020:236–238). Individuals with T2D often produce insulin, but either insufficient amounts or they become resistant to its actions, so blood glucose is poorly regulated. It can be many years before complications such as kidney disease, nerve damage, and increased propensity to fractures develops arising from consistent hyperglycemia. It has been estimated that approximately 27% of those with T2D in the USA today do not realize that they have the condition (Centers for Disease Control, 2011). Treatments now used to manage T2D range from changes in diet and exercise, to oral medications and, in some cases, insulin injections.

The metabolic syndrome (MetS), a group of conditions linked to the risk of developing T2D and/or cardiovascular disease, is frequently discussed alongside T2D. Consensus on diagnosis of MetS is lacking. Measures of obesity, blood pressure, and assessment of blood chemistry for indicators such as glucose, cholesterol, and lipid levels are evaluated in making a diagnosis. It is argued that marked, long-standing cases of MetS produce disturbances of bone mineralization due to accumulation of advanced glycation end products (AGEs) (Rubin, 2016) and that skeletal pathology can develop as a secondary response to complications of T2D (Beeve et al., 2019; Brickley et al., 2020:237–238; Lauri et al., 2020). Peripheral nerve damage (neuropathy), ulceration, and infection of soft tissues arising from poor blood supply and neuropathy will, with time, lead to neuropathic joint disease, with secondary consequences for bone. For those working in paleopathology, the lack of primary lesions of T2D is a concern, as all secondary lesions are etiologically non-specific.

To date, the most convincing suggested case of T2D is that in an older adult male from Dayr al-Barsha, Egypt (2055–1650 BCE) (Dupras et al., 2010). Using evidence of lesions from across the skeleton that may be secondary to complications of T2D, including possible metatarsophalangeal amputation and contextual information, the presence of T2D was suggested. More recently, difficulties were highlighted during assessment of skeletal lesions in

38 individuals with documented DM (compared to 30 controls) in a contemporary skeletal collection from Milan, Italy (Biehler-Gomez et al., 2019). While the type of DM was not considered, no skeletal lesions were identified that could be used as a basis for diagnosis. Amputations of the lower leg were present in two individuals diagnosed with DM, and vascular calcifications were present in 21% (8/38) (Biehler-Gomez et al., 2019). No lesions, such as Charcot's joints, were found which, while still etiologically non-specific (Beck, 1959), are more clearly an indicator of peripheral nerve damage.

In the absence of clear diagnostic lesions, paleopathologists have considered data linked to conditions such as gout, which may have links to MetS (e.g., Buckley & Buikstra, 2019). Data on gout and long-term dietary factors were studied in Pacific Islanders as a means of recognizing the presence of MetS (Buckley & Buikstra, 2019). Theoretical approaches have also considered evolutionary aspects of the wide spectrum of susceptibility of conditions within MetS, both within and between communities (e.g., Gurven et al., 2016; Wells, 2017). Clearer understanding of links between MetS conditions, biochemical indicators, and diet, such as fiber and micro-nutrient intake, has received less attention, may facilitate development of more effective approaches to individual and community disease burden today and a better understanding of aspects of past lifestyle and disease development. Today, those with limited access to resources experience some of the highest levels of MetS, and although there are genetic components, levels of deprivation are clearly key (e.g., Kolb & Martin, 2017). In past groups, however, it is likely to have been those with greater access to resources who were at greater risk of developing these conditions. Most people would have consumed minimally processed foods that were unlikely to exceed their caloric requirements. Energy expenditure for the average person was higher than today; walking will have been the primary means of travel, and pre-mechanized daily tasks would have been energy intensive.

Recognizing and Interpreting Metabolic and Endocrine Disease in the Past

Work on metabolic and endocrine diseases has highlighted some core issues in paleopathology. Recent consideration of the ways in which disease is manifested prior to completion of growth and development has underlined the need to evaluate physiological mechanisms of lesion formation. Consideration of lived experiences of past communities, including the social and biological complexities of life, has highlighted the importance of adopting biocultural and bioarchaeological approaches when examining disease in the past. Similarly, recognizing the impact of both the co-occurrence of diseases and co-morbidity provides a greater understanding of variables contributing to disease and individual's and population's responses to it (Schattmann et al., 2016; Brickley et al., 2020:227–229). Paleopathologists can contribute to conversations about the complexity of human disease and offer diagnostic frameworks and theoretical approaches to support interpretations (Grauer, 2018; Mays, 2018, 2020; and see Chapter 3, this volume).

The Issue of Porotic Lesions

At the most basic level, whether on a macro and/or micro scale, porotic lesions develop in all the metabolic and endocrine diseases. The seemingly simple question of "what caused porotic lesions?" lies at the heart of what paleopathologists aim to do – reconstruct aspects of health, disease, and life histories at both the individual and wider community level. Lesions visible to those working directly with bone frequently have no clinical diagnostic correlate and, superficially, porotic lesions can have a similar appearance despite different mechanisms precipitating development (Brickley et al., 2020:35–38). To aid evaluation of porous lesions, consideration will be given to the basic mechanisms that underlie the development of this common group of lesions.

In essence, ante mortem porous lesions develop due to four basic biological mechanisms, illustrated in a generic post-cranial bone in Figure 19.1 (Brickley et al., 2020: Figures 3–6 show equivalent lesions in the orbit). Hence, it is critically important when diagnosing these lesions to consider other cranial lesions alongside porotic lesions, as well as lesions across the rest of the skeleton, and to evaluate when during the life course the condition/s occurred.

Porotic lesions of the roof of the orbit and cranial vault are amongst the most recorded pathological conditions on human skeletal remains, with those in the orbital roof referred to as cribra orbitalia and the term porotic hyperostosis applied to porous lesions of the cranial vault. One of the first researchers to evaluate porous lesions in paleopathology, Larry Angel, worked on collections in which thalassemia, a heritable condition initiating hemolytic anemia, was likely to have been present (Angel, 1966). Later, researchers considered whether acquired anemias, such as IDA, might also produce porous cranial lesions (e.g., see Stuart-Macadam, 1992) and whether porotic lesions of the orbital roof and cranial vault are etiologically linked (e.g.,

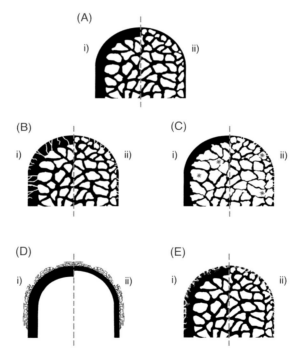

Figure 19.1 Generic bone with varying cortical thicknesses illustrating basic principles underlying lesion formation occurring in the four basic biological mechanisms that results in porotic lesions. Thick (i) and thin (ii) cortical bone are shown for each. Cortical thickness is a key determinant of lesion appearance and morphology. Idealized versions of the lesions caused by each mechanism are shown, but preservation, taphonomic variables, and presence of multiple conditions can all affect their appearance. (a) Normal bone. (b) Porosity due to a vascular inflammatory response. (c) Porosity due to marrow hyperplasia. Star = enlarged spaces in bone occupied by marrow. (d) Porosity due to deposition of porous sub-periosteal new bone (formed as a response in many conditions/circumstances). (e) Porosity due to impaired mineralization.

Suby 2014; Rivera & Lahr, 2017). The widespread occurrence of IDA in modern populations was noted by paleopathologists and with time a persistent assumption emerged that porous lesions of the orbits and cranial vault were synonymous with IDA.

To explore this deterministic association, Wapler et al. (2004) evaluated whether porous lesions in the orbital roof were linked to anemia using direct sectioning of crania to check for marrow expansion. After all, a physiological response to low oxygen levels ought to be increased production of RBCs in bone marrow. However, they found that other disease processes and post-depositional damage likely were responsible for some lesions. Regardless, the common association between the presence of cribra orbitalia and porotic hyperostosis and IDA prevailed, rendering this conflation of description with diagnosis a true hindrance to the understanding of health and disease in the past (see discussion in Mays, 2012; Grauer, 2019:514–515).

However, the identification of underlying biological mechanisms will not always lead to a clear understanding of health and disease in the past. This is particularly true for conditions where there is insufficient oxygen available to meet the body's need (anemia) prompting production of additional RBCs. Parsing out the multiple potential interacting causes in acquired cases of anemia may be impossible in paleopathology. Although development of anemia due to dietary inadequacies can occur, marrow hyperplasia occurs as a response to multiple other conditions, including infection, and the various acquired anemias all produce similar lesions. Various potential health correlates with porotic cranial lesions, caused by bone resorption due to marrow expansion (hyperplasia), were identified in a retrospective study using clinical CT data and aspects of medical history from modern individuals (O'Donnell et al., 2020). Links were found between those with porotic lesions and respiratory infections, and three potential mechanisms were discussed for marrow hyperplasia and perforation of the cortical bone. Obtaining data on nutritional status was not possible in this retrospective study, but some individuals had diseases of the digestive system (O'Donnell et al., 2020). The key take-home message is that factors that contribute to the development of anemia are complex (see Grauer, 2019:517), and further investigation of the causes of marrow hyperplasia, beyond acquired nutritional anemia, is necessary. Although nutritional status is clearly critical, this is not always directly linked to diet; multiple factors beyond dietary quality contribute to the need to produce more RBCs. Clinical cases with more than one condition acting simultaneously to produce anemia are common. Lesion expression will depend at least in part on the age at which the condition developed, with contributions from intensity of the condition, interactions with other factors affecting health, and the period over which these processes operated prior to the death. Consideration of the context and all available information, including human agency, are critical for both a basic diagnosis and interpretation of porotic lesions.

Porotic bone lesions don't arise simply as a response to the presence of anemia; they can arise due to an inflammatory response. In scurvy, hemorrhage causes inflammation, and a feedback mechanism is initiated that exacerbates both the hemorrhagic and inflammatory response. Formation of porous lesions that are characteristically <1 mm diameter and fully penetrate the outer cortex of bone occurs as a response to these processes (Brown & Ortner, 2011). In cases of inflammation following traumatic injury in the absence of scurvy, the feedback mechanism will not be initiated, and porosity is less likely to penetrate the bone cortex (see Figure 19.1b:i). Porosity can also develop following resorption of bone in response to marrow hyperplasia. As with lesions due to inflammation, thickness of the cortical bone will be a key factor in development of porosity. In cases of marrow hyperplasia, where change originates with expansion of marrow, there will always be changes that are invisible during macroscopic examination of bones (see Figure 19.1c:i). Only red marrow, or mixed marrow with a substantial component of red, has the propensity to expand in response to an increased demand for oxygen. Variation in the distribution of marrow type with age, and timing of increased demand for oxygen delivery, will thus play a role in skeletal distribution of lesions (see Brickley, 2018). Furthermore, the remodeling rates of specific bones and the amount of time an individual lived after the period of increased oxygen demand can also be factors in lesion distribution. Porous lesions and evidence of marrow hyperplasia can persist in bones with slower remodeling rates long past the episode of increased oxygen demand (e.g., cranial bones).

Sub-periosteal new bone formation can also have a porous appearance (see Figure 19.1d). New bone forms in many conditions/circumstances, and the appearance of these bone lesions differs depending on variables such as the level of the stimulus, physiological factors of skeletal location, time since initiation of formation, and individual biological factors, such as age and health. A porous appearance will also arise in growing individuals when mineralization is impaired (see Figure 19.1e); in past communities, this will likely be found in growing individuals with marked vitamin D deficiency. Although mineralization is also impaired in those whose growth has ceased, lower levels of bone turnover mean porosity will remain at the micro-structural level; appearance can be linked to disease severity and/or stage (see Table 19.2), so understanding the basic distinctions in causative mechanisms offers a way forward.

Multiple processes causing porous bone lesions can occur simultaneously as part of complex biological reactions to disease. The development of what have been termed 'mixed lesions' has recently been discussed for scurvy where inflammatory responses to hemorrhage can, in long-standing cases, include both porotic lesions of cortical bone and new bone formation (Brickley & Mays, 2019). Mixed lesions are also found in anemia, where sub-periosteal proliferation of marrow initiates inflammation, creating new bone in the vicinity of the porotic lesions through which marrow passed (Brickley et al., 2020:214). The presence of more than one disease could also initiate the development of mixed lesions and as discussed below bioarchaeologists and clinicians have begun to actively consider co-occurrence and co-morbidity.

Re-evaluation of photographs taken in 2002 from the St. Martin's project revealed cases with mixed lesions and potential co-occurrence. Figure 19.2 shows the orbit of a child with active rickets diagnosed from post-cranial lesions (Mays et al., 2006). Without re-examination of the skeleton, a diagnosis beyond active rickets cannot be made. New bone formed across the orbital roof of SMB217 is irregular (Figure 19.2: contoured line), likely

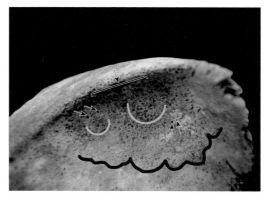

Figure 19.2 Porotic lesions of the orbit Individual SMB217 (1.3 years), St. Martin's UK. Active rickets was diagnosed from post-cranial lesions (Mays et al., 2006), but porotic lesions of the orbits indicate other metabolic diseases were also present. Notes: Impaired mineralization of bone formed during growth (contoured line), porosity of the original cortical surface (arrows and bracket), sub-periosteal new bone formation (PNBF; semi-circles).

due to impaired mineralization (vitamin D deficiency). The morphology of porotic new bone formed toward the orbital margin is however beyond that expected from impaired mineralization, another pathological process was likely also operating. Porotic lesions of the cortical surface are not typical of those caused by impaired mineralization (arrows and bracket). Mixed lesions are present, cortical porosity is situated beneath new bone formation (semi-circles). Cortical surface porosity could result from an inflammatory response to hemorrhage or thinning and perforation of the cortex due to marrow hyperplasia. Visualization of the underlying cortical bone and trabecular microstructure would be needed to differentiate between these two causes. Both processes could have occurred simultaneously. "Mixed lesions" develop in both scurvy and anemia; porotic new bone could be linked to either of these conditions or one of the multiple other conditions that initiate PNBF.

Although not seen in Figure 19.2, vitamin D deficiency can also create porotic lesions in the orbit and cranial bones. In a large-scale study of vitamin D deficiency in Roman Europe (Brickley et al., 2018), skeletal remains of individuals still undergoing growth were evaluated (n = 1119). Assessment of cranial and post-cranial remains individuals still undergoing growth showed that while vitamin D deficiency certainly caused many of the porous cranial lesions, other conditions likely contributed to lesion development – including anemia (Brickley et al., 2018). Grauer highlights the importance of considering context and required use of theoretical frameworks to get beyond "they were poor and had IDA" (Grauer, 2018). The underlying mechanisms driving lesions formation will be linked to a mix of biological and socio-cultural variables operating at the individual and community level. When considered alongside contextual data using theoretical frameworks, the presence of etiologically unknown porotic lesions can provide valuable data as signs of physiological stress (Watts, 2013; Geber, 2014; and see Chapter 22, this volume). Although more time consuming, recording detailed information on underlying etiology and disease stage in concert with robust theoretical approaches has considerable rewards in terms of understanding social cultural and environmental factors operating (e.g., Schattmann et al., 2016).

Co-Occurrence and Co-Morbidity

Until recently, most paleopathological studies of metabolic bone diseases focused on single conditions with singular etiologies. With the co-occurrence of metabolic and endocrine diseases, and consequences for physical impairment, quality of life, morbidity, and mortality, capturing the attention of medical clinicians (e.g., Bharati et al., 2018), it is evident that individuals with metabolic and endocrine diseases often have multiple dietary deficiencies (e.g., Haimi & Lerner, 2014; Tchaou et al., 2016) leading to etiologically complex conditions. When deficiencies are marked, metabolic diseases develop as either isolated or co-occurring diseases (e.g., see Ceglie et al., 2019) contributing to other associated risk factors or linked to underlying biological factors that influence the presence and manifestation of other diseases (Follis et al., 1940; Brickley et al., 2020:227–229). Many individuals who become the focus of paleopathological study will have experienced a number of diseases or conditions along their life course and these can influence the future development of metabolic and endocrine conditions. Distinct additional disease is referred to as co-morbidity.

When considering co-occurrence, researchers need to understand the underlying biological mechanisms contributing to lesions throughout the life course. Brickley and colleagues (2020) suggest consideration of whether each condition is active, healed, or re-current alongside the fact that the presence of one condition may modify the skeletal expression of a second disease. Co-occurrence should only be considered when a 'thorough differential diagnosis suggests that lesions indicative of more than one condition with potential for co-occurrence are present, or it is clear that one disease on its own cannot account for the gamut of lesions seen in a skeleton' (Brickley et al., 2020:230). Recognition that sequence and presence of co- and re-current disease episodes influence lesion development will facilitate a clearer understanding of the dynamics operating in past groups. The first paper that explicitly considered co-occurrence of metabolic bone disease in a skeletal population focused on rickets and scurvy in a 16th–18th century (CE) French collection and offered information on maternal deficiency and infant feeding practices (Schattmann et al., 2016). Further studies that have considered co-occurrence have focused on the interaction of vitamin D deficiency with various metabolic/infectious diseases (Ives, 2018) and metabolic disease clustering within a commingled sample (Perry & Edwards, 2021).

The investigation of health conditions within adults buried at an archaeological site in Northern Sudan by Wapler and colleagues (2004) illustrates how understanding underlying mechanisms of disease is essential to the recognition of co-occurrence of disease. While their primary aim was to evaluate evidence for physiological processes and to determine if porotic lesions recorded were caused by anemia, this team demonstrated that it was possible to determine cases where anemia co-occurred with other conditions such as inflammation. Importantly, they concluded that anemia was likely a chronic condition persisting throughout the life of some individuals. Evidence of age-related bone loss was also present in some individuals (Wapler et al., 2004).

Diagnosis of disease, and co-occurrence, requires consideration of multiple lines of evidence from across the skeleton (see Brickley et al., 2020:9 and Box 10–11). In isolation, orbital porosity in Figure 19.2 could be used as an indicator of "stress". At the most basic level, nutritional problems will have played a role in lesions formed – though care is required as, discussed in the text, not all issues are due to diet. Fuller information on the individual from conception to death could however be obtained with currently available approaches (Brickley et al., 2020). Understanding disease load, interactions between health conditions, and the interaction between disease and life histories will lead to a more nuanced understanding of past communities. The contribution that full integration of co-occurrence data can make in future studies is clear.

Theoretical Approaches

Systemic review of lesions and the biological mechanisms of formation is a key step in disease diagnosis and can feed into more nuanced consideration of past communities (see Figure 19.3). Humans do not exist in closed, simplistic systems. Hence, theoretical frameworks that go beyond reductionist or processual approaches, where deterministic links are assumed, are essential if we are to understand health and disease in past communities (Grauer, 2012:5–6). Clear health disparities experienced by those with limited access to resources are seen in many current groups (e.g., Braveman & Barclay, 2009), but health outcomes are complex. There are instances where access to more resources results in worse health outcomes (Giuffra et al., 2015; Roberts & Brickley, 2018:430).

Experiences that contribute to individual health status operate in open systems, so equifinality operates. Equifinality is the theory that an end point (in the context of paleopathology, a disease) can arise from multiple starting points and follow multiple pathways. For instance, Brickley et al. (2020:122) found that there were multiple context-dependent actions and behaviors that result in restricted access to sunlight (effective UVB) and, hence, rickets. Rickets arises in individuals with and without access to resources and/or of high or low socio-economic status. In some circumstances, individuals with inadequate housing and diet developed rickets,

Metabolic and Endocrine Diseases

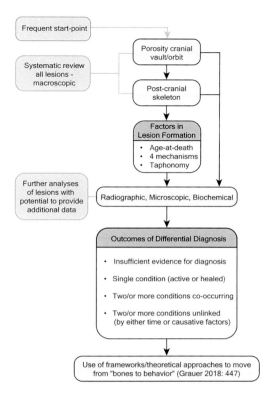

Figure 19.3 Systemic evaluation and interpretation of porotic lesions.

but in other contexts, regardless of housing and diet, individuals with access to resources chose to limit use of outdoor space and skin exposure to sunlight. In other examples, Brickley and colleagues found that biological factors such as skin pigmentation along with biophysical and social variables such as latitude, access to resources, and social standing were linked with the presence of rickets. Similarly, there can also be equifinality in the development of other metabolic and endocrine diseases such as osteoporosis. Multiple factors influence both the starting point of bone loss, PBM acquired during growth and development, and the ongoing trajectory of bone maintenance and subsequent loss. Disease is often multifactorial.

Final Comments

Metabolic and endocrine diseases play a key role in health outcomes, and paleopathology offers unique insights. The Neolithic Revolution and introduction of agriculture, and more recently the Industrial Revolution, have resulted in profound changes in the lifeways of significant sections of the world's population. The mismatch between evolved physiology and modern environments is recognized to have profound effects on health outcomes for contemporary groups (Carrera-Bastos et al., 2011; Jablonski & Chaplin, 2018). Changes in conditions in the MetS and T2D have received limited attention in paleopathology, but recognition of the difficulties involved, and the importance of issues facing modern populations, highlights the value of finding ways to investigate the past occurrence of these conditions. Contributions have been made to the understanding of long-term trends for both vitamin D deficiency and patterns of bone acquisition, loss, and associated fragility fractures in humans and other primates (Brickley et al., 2020:127; Ruff et al., 2020). Ongoing work puts paleopathology in a good position to provide a deeper appreciation of past health, disease, and life histories at both the individual and wider community levels, together with longer-term perspectives on current health debates.

References

Agarwal, S. C. (2018). Understanding bone aging, loss, and osteoporosis in the past. In Katzenberg, M. A. & Grauer, A. L. (Eds.), *Biological Anthropology of the Human Skeleton* (3rd ed.), pp. 385–414. Hoboken: John Wiley & Sons, Inc. https://doi.org/10.1002/9781119151647.ch11.

Aghajanian, P., Hall, S., Wongworawat, M. D. & Mohan, S. (2015). The roles and mechanisms of actions of vitamin C in bone: new developments. *Journal of Bone and Mineral Research* 30(11): 1945–1955. https://doi.org/10.1002/jbmr.2709.

Alzaheb, R. A. & Al-Amer, O. (2017). The prevalence of iron deficiency anemia and its associated risk factors among a sample of female university students in Tabuk, Saudi Arabia. *Clinical Medicine Insights: Women's Health* 10:1–8. https://doi.org/10.1177/1179562X17745088.

Angel, J. L. (1966). Porotic hyperostosis, anemias, malarias, and marshes in the prehistoric eastern Mediterranean. *Science* 153(3737):760–763. https://doi.org/10.1126/science.153.3737.760.

Beauchesne, P. & Agarwal, S. C. (2017). A multi-method assessment of bone maintenance and loss in an Imperial Roman population: implications for future studies of age-related bone loss in the past. *American Journal of Physical Anthropology* 164(1):41–61. https://doi.org/10.1002/ajpa.23256.

Beck, R. E. (1959). Roentgenographic findings in the complications of diabetes mellitus. *The American Journal of Roentgenology, Radium Therapy, and Nuclear Medicine* 82:887–896.

Beeve, A. T., Brazill, J. M. & Scheller, E. L. (2019). Peripheral neuropathy as a component of skeletal disease in diabetes. *Current Osteoporosis Reports* 17(5):256–269. https://doi.org/10.1007/s11914-019-00528-8.

Bharati, H. P., Kavthekar, S. O., Kavthekar, S. S. & Kurane, A. B. (2018). Prevalence of micronutrient deficiencies clinically in rural school going children. *International Journal of Contemporary Pediatrics* 5:234–238.
https://doi.org/10.18203/2349-3291.ijcp20175591.

Biehler-Gomez, L., Castoldi, E., Baldini, E., Cappella, A. & Cattaneo, C. (2019). Diabetic bone lesions: a study on 38 known modern skeletons and the implications for forensic scenarios. *International Journal of Legal Medicine* 133(4):1225–1239. https://doi.org/10.1007/s00414-018-1870-0.

Bourbou, C. (2014). Evidence of childhood scurvy in a Middle Byzantine Greek population from Crete, Greece (11th–12th centuries AD). *International Journal of Paleopathology* 5:86–94. https://doi.org/10.1016/j.ijpp.2013.12.002.

Braveman, P. & Barclay, C. (2009). Health disparities beginning in childhood: a life-course perspective. *Pediatrics* 124(Suppl. 3):S163–S175. https://doi.org/10.1542/peds.2009-1100D.

Brickley, M. B. (2018). Cribra orbitalia and porotic hyperostosis: a biological approach to diagnosis. *American Journal of Physical Anthropology* 167(4):896–902. https://doi.org/10.1002/ajpa.23701.

Brickley, M.B. Mays, S. George, M. & Prowse, T.L. (2018). Analysis and interpretation of patterning in the occurrence of skeletal lesions used as indicators of vitamin D deficiency in subadult and adult skeletal remains. *International Journal of Paleopathology* 23:43-53. https: doi: 10.1016/j.ijpp.2018.01.001.

Brickley, M. B., Ives, R. & Mays, S. (2020). *The Bioarchaeology of Metabolic Bone Disease* (2nd ed.). San Diego, CA: Academic Press.

Brickley, M. B. & Mays, S. (2019). Metabolic disease. In Buikstra, J. E. (Ed.), *Ortner's Identification of Pathological Conditions in Human Skeletal Remains* (3rd ed.), pp. 531–566. New York: Elsevier.

Brickley, M. B., Moffat, T. & Watamaniuk, L. (2014). Biocultural perspectives of vitamin D deficiency in the past. *Journal of Anthropological Archaeology* 36:48–59. https://doi.org/10.1016/j.jaa.2014.08.002.

Brown, M. & Ortner, D. J. (2011). Childhood scurvy in a medieval burial from Mačvanska Mitrovica, Serbia. *International Journal of Osteoarchaeology* 21(2):197–207. https://doi.org/10.1002/oa.1124.

Buckley, H. R. & Buikstra, J. E. (2019). Stone agers in the fast lane? How bioarchaeologists can address the paleo diet myth. In Buikstra, J. E. (Ed.), *Bioarchaeologists Speak Out: Deep Time Perspectives on Contemporary Issues*, pp. 161–180. Cham: Springer.

Buckley, H. R., Kinaston, R., Halcrow, S. E., Foster, A., Spriggs, M. & Bedford, S. (2014). Scurvy in a tropical paradise? Evaluating the possibility of infant and adult vitamin C deficiency in the Lapita skeletal sample of Teouma, Vanuatu, Pacific Islands. *International Journal of Paleopathology* 5:72–85. https://doi.org/10.1016/j.ijpp.2014.03.001.

Carrera-Bastos, P., Fontes-Villalba, M., O'Keefe, J. H., Lindeberg, S. & Cordain, L. (2011). The western diet and lifestyle and diseases of civilization. *Research Reports in Clinical Cardiology* 2:15–35. https://doi.org/10.2147/RRCC.S16919.

Ceglie, G., Macchiarulo, G., Marchili, M. R., Marchesi, A., Aufiero, L. R., Di Camillo, C. & Villani, A. (2019). Scurvy: still a threat in the well-fed first world? *Archives of Disease in Childhood* 104(4):381–383. http://dx.doi.org/10.1136/archdischild-2018-315496.

Centers for Disease Control and Prevention. (2011). National diabetes fact sheet: national estimates and general information on diabetes and prediabetes in the United States, 2011. *Atlanta, GA: US Department of Health and Human Services, Centers for Disease Control and Prevention* 201(1):2568–2569.

Chan, B. Y., Gill, K. G., Rebsamen, S. L. & Nguyen, J. C. (2016). MR imaging of pediatric bone marrow. *Radiographics* 36(6):1911–1930. https://doi.org/10.1148/rg.2016160056.

Chaplin, G. & Jablonski, N. G. (2013). The human environment and the vitamin D compromise: Scotland as a case study in human biocultural adaptation and disease susceptibility. *Human Biology* 85(4):529–552. https://doi.org/10.3378/027.085.0402.

Charoenngam, N., Shirvani, A. & Holick, M. F. (2019). Vitamin D for skeletal and non-skeletal health: what we should know. *Journal of Clinical Orthopaedics and Trauma* 10(6):1082–1093. https://doi.org/10.1016/j.jcot.2019.07.004.

Cole, M. E., Stout, S. D. & Agnew, A. M. (2019). Image processing techniques for extracting complex three-dimensional cortical pore networks from high-resolution micro-computed tomography (micro-CT) images of the human femoral neck and rib. *American Journal of Physical Anthropology* 168(S68):46.

Craig-Atkins, E., Jervis, B., Cramp, L., Hammann, S., Nederbragt, A. J., Nicholson, E., Taylor, A. E., Whelton, H. & Madgwick, R. (2020). The dietary impact of the Norman Conquest: a multiproxy archaeological investigation of Oxford, UK. *PloS One* 15(7):e0235005. https://doi.org/10.1371/journal.pone.0235005.

Creo, A. L., Thacher, T. D., Pettifor, J. M., Strand, M. A. & Fischer, P. R. (2017). Nutritional rickets around the world: an update. *Paediatrics and International Child Health* 37(2):84–98. https://doi.org/10.1080/20469047.2016.1248170.

Curate, F. (2014). Osteoporosis and paleopathology: a review. *Journal of Anthropological Sciences, Rivista di Antropologia: JASS* 92:119–146. https://doi.org/10.4436/jass.92003.

DeLoughery, T. G. (2017). Iron deficiency anemia. *Medical Clinics of North America* 101(2):319–332. https://doi.org/10.1016/j.mcna.2016.09.004.

Dupras, T. L., Williams, L. J., Willems, H. & Peeters, C. (2010). Pathological skeletal remains from ancient Egypt: the earliest case of diabetes mellitus? *Practical Diabetes International* 27(8):358–363. https://doi.org/10.1002/pdi.1523.

El-Najjar, M. Y., Ryan, D. J., Turner, C. G. & Lozoff, B. (1976). The etiology of porotic hyperostosis among the prehistoric and historic Anasazi Indians of Southwestern United States. *American Journal of Physical Anthropology* 44(3):477–487. https://doi.org/10.1002/ajpa.1330440311.

Expert Committee on the Diagnosis and Classification of Diabetes Mellitus. (2003). Report of the expert committee on the diagnosis and classification of diabetes mellitus. *Diabetes Care* 26(Suppl. 1):s5–s20. https://doi.org/10.2337/diacare.26.2007.S5.

Follis, R. H., Jackson, D. A. & Park, E. A. (1940). The problem of the association of rickets and scurvy. *American Journal of Diseases of Children* 60:745–747.

Forwood, M. R. (2013). Growing a healthy skeleton: the importance of mechanical loading. In Rosen, C. (Ed.), *Primer on the Metabolic Bone Diseases and Disorders of Mineral Metabolism*, pp. 149–155. Chichester: Wiley-Blackwell.

French, R. K. (1993). Scurvy. In Kiple, K. F. (Ed.), *The Cambridge World History of Human Disease*, pp. 1000–1005. Cambridge: Cambridge University Press.

Geber, J. (2014). Skeletal manifestations of stress in child victims of the Great Irish Famine (1845–1852): prevalence of enamel hypoplasia, Harris lines, and growth retardation. *American Journal of Physical Anthropology* 155(1):149–161. https://doi.org/10.1002/ajpa.22567.

Grauer, A. L. (2012). Introduction: the scope of paleopathology. In Grauer, A. L. (Ed.), *A Companion to Paleopathology*, pp. 1–14. Chichester: Wiley-Blackwell.

Grauer, A. L. (2018). Paleopathology: from bones to social behavior. In Katzenberg, A. & Grauer, A. (Eds.), *Biological Anthropology of the Human Skeleton* (3rd ed.), pp. 447–465. New Jersey: Wiley.

Grauer, A. L. (2019). Circulatory, reticuloendothelial, and hemopoietic disorders. In Buikstra, J. E. (Ed.), *Ortner's Identification of Pathological Conditions in Human Skeletal Remains*, (3rd ed.), pp. 491–529. London: Academic Press.

Guillerman, R. P. (2013). Marrow: red, yellow and bad. *Pediatric Radiology* 43(1):181–192. https://doi.org/10.1007/s00247-012-2582-0.

Gurevitch, O., Slavin, S. & Feldman, A. G. (2007). Conversion of red bone marrow into yellow–cause and mechanisms. *Medical Hypotheses* 69(3):531–536. https://doi.org/10.1016/j.mehy.2007.01.052.

Gurven, M. D., Trumble, B. C., Stieglitz, J., Blackwell, A. D., Michalik, D. E., Finch, C. E. & Kaplan, H. S. (2016). Cardiovascular disease and type 2 diabetes in evolutionary perspective: a critical role for helminths?. *Evolution, Medicine, and Public Health* 2016(1):338–357. https://doi.org/10.1093/emph/eow028.

Haimi, M. & Lerner, A. (2014). Nutritional deficiencies in the pediatric age group in a multicultural developed country, Israel. *World Journal of Clinical Cases: WJCC* 2(5):120. https://doi.org/10.12998/wjcc.v2.i5.120.

Harvey, N., Dennison, E. & Cooper, C. (2014). Osteoporosis: a life course approach. *Journal of Bone and Mineral Research* 29(9):1917–1925. https://doi.org/10.1002/jbmr.2286.

Hlusko, L. J., Carlson, J. P., Chaplin, G., Elias, S. A., Hoffecker, J. F., Huffman, M., …& Scott, G. R. (2018). Environmental selection during the last ice age on the mother-to-infant transmission of vitamin D and fatty acids through breast milk. *Proceedings of the National Academy of Sciences* 115(19):E4426–E4432. https://doi.org/10.1073/pnas.1711788115.

Holick, M. F. (2010). Vitamin D and health: evolution, biologic functions, and recommended dietary intakes for vitamin D. In Holick, M. F. (Ed.), *Vitamin D* (2nd ed.), pp. 3–33). New York: Springer Humana Press.

Ives, R. 2018. Rare paleopathological insights into vitamin D deficiency rickets, co-occurring illnesses, and documented cause of death in mid-19th century London, UK. *International Journal of Paleopathology* 23:76–87. https://doi.org/10.1016/j.ijpp.2017.11.004.

Jablonski, N. G. & Chaplin, G. (2018). The roles of vitamin D and cutaneous vitamin D production in human evolution and health. *International Journal of Paleopathology* 23:54–59. https://doi.org/10.1016/j.ijpp.2018.01.005.

Johannesdottir, F., Turmezei, T. & Poole, K. E. (2014). Cortical bone assessed with clinical computed tomography at the proximal femur. *Journal of Bone and Mineral Research* 29(4):771–783. https://doi.org/10.1002/jbmr.2199.

Jones, G. (2018). The discovery and synthesis of the nutritional factor vitamin D. *International Journal of Paleopathology* 23:96–99. https://doi.org/10.1016/j.ijpp.2018.01.002.

Jones, G. & Prosser, D. (2011). The activating enzymes of vitamin D metabolism (25- and 1α-hydroxylases). In Feldman, D. & Pike, J. A. (Eds.), *Vitamin D*, (3rd ed.), pp. 23–42. San Diego, CA: Academic Press.

Khammissa, R. A. G., Fourie, J., Motswaledi, M. H., Ballyram, R., Lemmer, J. & Feller, L. (2018). The biological activities of vitamin D and its receptor in relation to calcium and bone homeostasis, cancer, immune and cardiovascular systems, skin biology, and oral health. *BioMed Research International* 2018:1–9. https://doi.org/10.1155/2018/9276380.

Klaus, H. D. (2017). Paleopathological rigor and differential diagnosis: case studies involving terminology, description and diagnostic frameworks for scurvy in skeletal remains. *International Journal of Paleopathology* 19:96–110. https://doi.org/10.1016/j.ijpp.2015.10.002.

Kolb, H. & Martin, S. (2017). Environmental/lifestyle factors in the pathogenesis and prevention of type 2 diabetes. *BMC Medicine* 15(1):131. https://doi.org/10.1186/s12916-017-0901-x.

Lauri, C., Leone, A., Cavallini, M., Signore, A., Giurato, L. & Uccioli, L. (2020). Diabetic foot infections: the diagnostic challenges. *Journal of Clinical Medicine* 9(6):1779. https://doi.org/10.3390/jcm9061779.

Lewis, M. E. (2012). Thalassaemia: its diagnosis and interpretation in past skeletal populations. *International Journal of Osteoarchaeology* 22(6):685–693. https://doi.org/10.1002/oa.1229.

Littleton, J. (1998). A Middle Eastern paradox: rickets in skeletons from Bahrain. *Journal of Paleopathology* 10(1):13–30.

Lockau, L., Atkinson, S., Mays, S., Prowse, T., George, M., Sperduti, A., Bondioli, L., Wood, C., Ledger, M. & Brickley, M. B. (2019). Vitamin D deficiency and the ancient city: skeletal evidence across the life course from the Roman period site of Isola Sacra, Italy. *Journal of Anthropological Archaeology* 55:101069. https://doi.org/10.1016/j.jaa.2019.101069.

Macintosh, A. A., Pinhasi, R. & Stock, J. T. (2017). Prehistoric women's manual labor exceeded that of athletes through the first 5500 years of farming in Central Europe. *Science Advances* 3(11):eaao3893. https://doi.org/10.1126/sciadv.aao3893.

Masi, L. (2019). Primary hyperparathyroidism. *Frontiers of Hormone Research* 51:1–12. https://doi.org/10.1159/000491034.

Mays, S. (2007). The human remains. In Mays, S., Harding, C. & Heighway, C. (Eds.), *The Churchyard. Wharram: A Study of Settlement in the Yorkshire Wolds*, pp. 77–192; 337–397. York: York University Press.

Mays, S. (2012). The relationship between paleopathology and the clinical sciences. In Grauer, A. L. (Ed.), *A Companion to Paleopathology*, pp. 285–309. Chichester: Wiley-Blackwell.

Mays, S. (2014). The palaeopathology of scurvy in Europe. *International Journal of Paleopathology* 5:55–62. https://doi.org/10.1016/j.ijpp.2013.09.001.

Mays, S. (2018). How should we diagnose disease in paleopathology? Some epistemological considerations. *International Journal of Paleopathology* 20:12–19. https://doi.org/10.1016/j.ijpp.2017.10.006.

Mays, S. (2020). A dual process model for paleopathological diagnosis. *International Journal of Paleopathology* 31:89–96. https://doi.org/10.1016/j.ijpp.2020.10.001.

Mays, S. & Brickley, M. B. (2018). Vitamin D deficiency in bioarchaeology and beyond: the study of rickets and osteomalacia in the past. *International Journal of Paleopathology* 23:1. https://doi.org/10.1016/j.ijpp.2018.05.004.

Mays, S., Brickley, M. B. & Ives, R. (2006). Skeletal manifestations of rickets in infants and young children in a historic population from England. *American Journal of Physical Anthropology* 129(3):362–374. https://doi.org/10.1002/ajpa.20292.

Mays, S., Brickley, M. B. & Ives, R. (2007). Skeletal evidence for hyperparathyroidism in a 19th century child with rickets. *International Journal of Osteoarchaeology* 17(1):73–81. https://doi.org/10.1002/oa.854.

Mays, S., Prowse, T., George, M. & Brickley, M. B. (2018). Latitude, urbanisation, age and sex as risk factors for vitamin D deficiency disease in the Roman Empire. *American Journal of Physical Anthropology* 167(3):484–496. https://doi.org/10.1002/ajpa.23646.

Miller, E. M. (2016). The reproductive ecology of iron in women. *American Journal of Physical Anthropology* 159:S172–S195. https://doi.org/10.1002/ajpa.22907.

New, S. & Bonjour, J. P. (Eds.). (2003). *Nutritional Aspects of Bone Health*. Cambridge: Royal Society of Chemistry Publication.

O'Donnell, L., Hill, E. C., Anderson, A. S. A & Edgar, H. J. (2020). Cribra orbitalia and porotic hyperostosis are associated with respiratory infections in a contemporary mortality sample from New Mexico. *American Journal of Physical Anthropology* 173(4):721–733. https://doi.org/10.1002/ajpa.24131.

Ortner, D. J. & Ericksen, M. F. (1997). Bone changes in the human skull probably resulting from scurvy in infancy and childhood. *International Journal of Osteoarchaeology* 7(3):212–220. https://doi.org/10.1002/(SICI)1099-1212(199705)7:3<212::AID-OA346>3.0.CO;2-5.

Owa, O. T. & Owa, A. B. (2020). Vitamin D deficiency among children: more of a mountain than a molehill. *Pediatric Oncall Journal* 17(4):105–108. https://doi.org/10.7199/ped.oncall.2020.43.

Pasricha, S. R., Drakesmith, H., Black, J., Hipgrave, D. & Biggs, B. A. (2013). Control of iron deficiency anemia in low-and middle-income countries. *Blood* 121(14):2607–2617. https://doi.org/10.1182/blood2012-09-453522.

Perry, M.A. & Edwards, E. (2021). Differential diagnosis of metabolic disease in a commingled sample from 19th century Hisban, Jordan. *International Journal of Paleopathology* 33:220–233. https://doi.org/10.1016/j.ijpp.2021.05.003.

Pitre, M. C., Stark, R. J. & Gatto, M. C. (2016). First probable case of scurvy in ancient Egypt at Nag el-Qarmila, Aswan. *International Journal of Paleopathology* 13:11–19. https://doi.org/10.1016/j.ijpp.2015.12.003.

Rice, S. A., Carpenter, M., Fityan, A., Vearncombe, L. M., Ardern-Jones, M., Jackson, A. A., Cooper, C., Baird, J. & Healy, E. (2015). Limited exposure to ambient ultraviolet radiation and 25-hydroxyvitamin D levels: a systematic review. *British Journal of Dermatology* 172(3):652–661. https://doi.org/10.1111/bjd.13575.

Richter, L. M., Daelmans, B., Lombardi, J., Heymann, J., Boo, F. L., Behrman, J. R., ... & Darmstadt, G. L. (2017). Investing in the foundation of sustainable development: pathways to scale up for early childhood development. *The Lancet* 389(10064):103–118. https://doi.org/10.1016/S0140-6736(16)31698-1.

Rivera, F. & Mirazón Lahr, M. (2017). New evidence suggesting a dissociated etiology for cribra orbitalia and porotic hyperostosis. *American Journal of Physical Anthropology* 164(1):76–96. https://doi.org/10.1002/ajpa.23258.

Roberts, C. A. & Brickley, M. B. (2018). Infectious and metabolic diseases: a synergistic relationship. In Katzenberg, A. & Grauer, A. L (Eds.), *Biological Anthropology of the Human Skeleton* (3rd ed.), pp. 415–446. New Jersey: Wiley. https://doi.org/10.1002/9781119151647.ch12.

Rubin, M. (2016). Biomarkers of diabetic bone disease. In Lecka-Czernik, B. & Fowlkes, J. (Eds.), *Diabetic Bone Disease*, pp. 113–124. Heidelberg: Springer International. https://doi.org/10.1007/978-3-319-16402-1_6.

Ruff, C. B., Junno, J. A., Eckardt, W., Gilardi, K., Mudakikwa, A. & McFarlin, S. C. (2020). Skeletal ageing in Virunga mountain gorillas. *Philosophical Transactions of the Royal Society B* 375(1811):20190606. https://doi.org/10.1098/rstb.2019.0606.

Schattmann, A., Bertrand, B., Vatteoni, S. & Brickley, M. B. (2016). Approaches to co-occurrence: scurvy and rickets in infants and young children of 16th – 18th century Douai, France. *International Journal of Paleopathology* 12:63–75. https://doi.org/10.1016/j.ijpp.2015.12.002.

Snoddy, A. M. E., Buckley, H. R., Elliott, G. E., Standen, V. G., Arriaza, B. T. & Halcrow, S. E. (2018). Macroscopic features of scurvy in human skeletal remains: a literature synthesis and diagnostic guide. *American Journal of Physical Anthropology* 167(4):876–895. https://doi.org/10.1002/ajpa.23699.

Snoddy, A. M. E., Halcrow, S. E., Buckley, H. R., Standen, V. G. & Arriaza, B. T. (2017). Scurvy at the agricultural transition in the Atacama desert (ca 3600–3200 BP): nutritional stress at the maternal-foetal interface? *International Journal of Paleopathology* 18:108–120. https://doi.org/10.1016/j.ijpp.2017.05.011.

Stride, P. J., Patel, N. & Kingston, D. (2013). The history of osteoporosis: why do Egyptian mummies have porotic bones? *The Journal of the Royal College of Physicians of Edinburgh* 43(3):254. https://doi.org/10.4997/JRCPE.2013.314.

Stuart-Macadam, P. (1992). Porotic hyperostosis: a new perspective. *American Journal of Physical Anthropology* 87(1):39–47. https://doi.org/10.1002/ajpa.1330870105.

Suby, J. A. (2014). Porotic hyperostosis and cribra orbitalia in human remains from southern Patagonia. *Anthropological Science* 122:69–79. https://doi.org/10.1537/ase.140430.

Tchaou, M., Sanogo, S., Sonhaye, L., Amadou, A., Kolou, B., Rivoal, E., Sidibe, S. & N'Dakena, K. (2016). Late radiographic findings of infantile scurvy in northern Mali, a region facing a humanitarian and security crisis. *Hong Kong Journal of Radiology* 19:e10-e13. https://doi.org/10.12809/hkjr165303.

Uday, S. & Högler, W. (2017). Nutritional rickets and osteomalacia in the twenty-first century: revised concepts, public health, and prevention strategies. *Current Osteoporosis Reports* 15(4):293–302. https://doi.org/10.1007/s11914-017-0383-y.

van der Merwe, A. E., Veselka, B., Van Veen, H. A., Van Rijn, R. R., Colman, K. L. & de Boer, H. H. (2018). Four possible cases of osteomalacia: the value of a multidisciplinary diagnostic approach. *International Journal of Paleopathology* 23:15–25. https://doi.org/10.1016/j.ijpp.2018.03.004.

van Gerven, D. P., Armelagos, G. J. & Bartley, M. H. (1969). Roentgenographic and direct measurement of femoral cortical involution in a prehistoric Mississippian population. *American Journal of Physical Anthropology* 31(1):23–38. https://doi.org/10.1002/ajpa.1330310105.

van Spelde, A. M., Schroeder, H., Kjellström, A. & Lidén, K. (2021). Approaches to osteoporosis in paleopathology: how did methodology shape bone loss research? *International Journal of Paleopathology* 33:245–257. https://doi.org/10.1016/j.ijpp.2021.05.001.

Wapler, U., Crubézy, E. & Schultz, M. (2004). Is cribra orbitalia synonymous with anemia? Analysis and interpretation of cranial pathology in Sudan. *American Journal of Physical Anthropology* 123(4):333–339. https://doi.org/10.1002/ajpa.10321.

Watts, R. (2013). Childhood development and adult longevity in an archaeological population from Barton-upon-Humber, Lincolnshire, England. *International Journal of Paleopathology* 3(2):95–104. https://doi.org/10.1016/j.ijpp.2013.05.001.

Watts, R. & Valme, S. R. (2018). Osteological evidence for juvenile vitamin D deficiency in a 19th century suburban population from Surrey, England. *International Journal of Paleopathology* 23. https://doi.org/60-68. 10.1016/j.ijpp.2018.01.007.

Weaver, C. M., Gordon, C. M., Janz, K. F., Kalkwarf, H. J., Lappe, J. M., Lewis, R., O'Karma, T., Wallace, C. & Zemel, B. S. (2016). The National Osteoporosis Foundation's position statement on peak bone mass development and lifestyle factors: a systematic review and implementation recommendations. *Osteoporosis International* 27(4):1281–1386. https://doi.org/10.1007/s00198-015-3440-3.

Weaver, C. M. & Heaney R. P. (2013). Nutrition and osteoporosis. In Rosen, C. J. (Ed.), *Primer on the Metabolic Bone Diseases and Disorders of Mineral Metabolism* (8th ed.), pp. 361–366. Chichester: Wiley-Blackwell.

Wells, J. C. (2017). Body composition and susceptibility to type 2 diabetes: an evolutionary perspective. *European Journal of Clinical Nutrition* 71(7):881–889. https://doi.org/10.1038/ejcn.2017.31.

Welsh, H., Nelson, A. J., van der Merwe, A. E., de Boer, H. H. & Brickley, M. B. (2020). An investigation of micro-CT analysis of bone as a new diagnostic method for paleopathological cases of osteomalacia. *International Journal of Paleopathology* 31:23–33. https://doi.org/10.1016/j.ijpp.2020.08.004.

Williams, H. U. (1929). Human paleopathology-with some original observations on symmetrical osteoporosis of the skull. *Archives of Pathology* 7(5):839–902.

World Health Organization. (2001). *Iron Deficiency Anaemia: Assessment, Prevention, and Control - A Guide for Program Managers*. Geneva, Switzerland: World Health Organization (WHO/NHD/01.3).

World Health Organization. (2004). *WHO Scientific Group on the Assessment of Osteoporosis at Primary Health Care Level: Summary Meeting Report*. May 5–7, 2004, Brussels, Belgium. Geneva, Switzerland: World Health Organization.

World Health Organization. (2016). *The Global Strategy for Women's, Children's, and Adolescents' Health (2016–2030)*. Geneva, Switzerland: World Health Organization.

Zink, A. R., Panzer, S., Fesq-Martin, M., Burger-Heinrich, E., Wahl, J. & Nerlich, A. G. (2005). Evidence for a 7000-year-old case of primary hyperparathyroidism. *JAMA* 293(1):36–42. https://doi.org/10.1001/jama.293.1.40-c.

20
DENTAL DISEASE

Jaime Ullinger and Tisa Loewen

Introduction

In many burial environments, teeth preserve better than bone. And, despite their small size, they are a densely packed record of our lives. Various questions that interest biological anthropologists (including bioarchaeologists) can be addressed by examining dental paleopathology, including what food were people eating and did this vary in terms of age or status? Were some people ill or otherwise biologically stressed during childhood, and how did this affect their likelihood to make it to adulthood? What daily activities did people engage in? How does forced migration affect food choice and the oral microbiome? And, like other pathological indicators, dental disease can bear witness to the impacts of urbanization, starvation, climate change, warfare, and other social changes in the past. When combined with other paleopathological indicators, demographic analyses, and techniques such as stable isotope analysis, dental disease can provide a wealth of information about past behavior and social change (Gagnon, 2020). This chapter will review a variety of dental disease indicators and how they have been used in paleopathological and bioanthropological studies.

While teeth preserve well due to the structure of enamel, they are still prone to diagenetic effects, particularly those related to stable isotopes and trace elements (Kendall et al., 2018). Dental enamel is roughly 97% mineral by weight and 93% mineral by volume (Elliott et al., 1998), making it the hardest substance in the human body. Dentin has an inorganic/organic ratio that is more similar to human bone, and while dentin can repair itself, dental enamel cannot. This means that enamel preserves a record of diet and health across an individual's lifetime, preserving insults that occur even in childhood. However, it also means that once the enamel has worn away, it is gone – as is any information about the individual for which it could have borne witness.

What do we mean by dental disease? Some disease indicators are manifestations of normal processes that exceed a particular threshold, while other conditions generally considered with dental pathology are not direct analyses of disease expressions, but instead assessments of evidence left on or in dentition due to a complex etiology of genetics and environmental factors during development and/or use of the teeth. A helpful way to think about these changes might be to define the purpose of looking at dental disease and then examine indicators that assist in the analysis of classical disease. Therefore, we explore dental manifestations that are clinically pathological, as well as other physiological, chemical, and developmental indicators of pathogenesis, which provide us with an understanding of how past health, wellness, and other factors affected people's quality of life and longevity.

Such a proposal presents enormous complications, such as the complex nature of recognizing signs of health and/or disease in the past, along with methodological concerns, which further exacerbate interpretations. These complications are discussed in detail in Part I: Applications, Methods, and Techniques in Paleopathology in this book. And techniques for identifying and recording many of these conditions can be found in Hillson (2019). Instead, here we focus not on the *how*, but on the *why* of dental pathology. We discuss dental analyses as integral to contextualizing bioarchaeological and paleopathological work by exploring what the teeth can tell us. In addition to macroscopic disease, and developmental and physiological changes, we also discuss some microscale analyses that provide a wealth of knowledge both across a person's life and during their final days.

Many pathological indicators in the dentition can be examined macroscopically and non-invasively, making their study cost effective across a relatively large sample. The identification of carious lesions and antemortem tooth loss (AMTL), for example, does not require much technology and can be learned quickly. This can be applied to complete skeletons, as well as to commingled, fragmentary assemblages where teeth are often found loose (i.e., not situated within their sockets in the bone). Reporting condition by tooth type ensures comparable frequencies among different sites (Bentley & Perry, 2008; Albashaireh & Al-Shorman, 2010; Ullinger et al., 2015), although overall tooth counts can be used, as well. These rates can then be compared to any dataset where data were reported by tooth type (or tooth count). Reporting by tooth type can account for the fact that postmortem tooth loss occurs more frequently with anterior teeth, which may lead to an overestimation of tooth count frequencies for conditions seen more commonly in the posterior teeth (and similarly an underestimation of conditions in anterior teeth).

Microscopic analyses are increasingly useful (and possible) in dental analyses. However, newer approaches (such as aDNA analysis from dental calculus) may require an immense amount of labor and skill, as well as sampling of the material on the teeth. Other techniques employed in dental paleopathology, such as histological sampling, are destructive to the tooth itself. Photography and casting of the tooth should be done before any destructive analysis occurs, to provide a permanent representation of the complete tooth. The casts, images, and any sample taken should remain with the original collection. Aris (2020) encourages micro-CT use, when possible, but notes that some data are not captured through these images, and that the expense of micro-CT renders it inaccessible to many students and early career researchers. Recent studies demonstrate that oral pathologies can be identified using 3D digital microscopy (3D DM) and cone beam computed tomography (CBCT), which are in some cases less expensive and easier to use than scanning electron microscope (SEM) or microCT (Lozano et al., 2022).

Dental disease is widely prevalent around the globe today, with roughly 3.5 billion people affected, making the oral cavity one of the most expensive parts of the body to treat medically (James et al., 2018). Inequality plays a role in who is likely to experience dental disease (Petersen, 2004), and poor oral health is directly related to a higher risk of death (Adolph et al., 2017). Much of the dental disease experienced around the world today is associated with consumption of highly processed foods that contain sugars, tobacco use, and lack of access to health care (Jin et al., 2016). Some of these factors may play a role in the oral health of past populations, while others may not. An oft-repeated broad pattern that has emerged over time is that our early ancestors had relatively little dental disease [with a few significant exceptions, such as the Middle Pleistocene cranium from Broken Hill in Zambia (Lacy, 2014b)], that it increased significantly with the advent of agriculture, and then increased further with urbanization. However, Lacy (2014a) asserts that dental health was not great for Upper Paleolithic peoples, who had significant tooth loss and periodontal disease. And, while our early ancestors may not have had the same rates of infection, dental caries was still present, illustrating that we share a long history with all of the dental diseases that afflict us today (Humphrey et al., 2014).

Dental Caries

Dental caries (colloquially referred to as "cavities") is a common infectious disease that destroys dental enamel (Selwitz et al., 2007) and is seen in over 2.5 million people globally today (James et al., 2018) (Figure 20.1). Dental caries is the result of localized enamel demineralization due to acidic byproducts secreted by a polymicrobial biofilm. Experimentation suggests that *Streptococcus mutans*, often cited as the primary driver of caries, does not operate independently in this action, but is facilitated by other bacteria in the oral microbiome, which aid in the creation of a localized region of lower pH and enamel demineralization that, if not reversed, leads to cavitation (Kim et al., 2020) (Figure 20.1a). The human oral cavity houses approximately 700–1000 different species of microbes (Chen et al., 2020), and there is an argument that the microorganisms involved in dental caries should be identified as pathobionts and not as "infectious" pathogens (Simón-Soro & Mira, 2015) because they inhabit healthy mouths but tend not to trigger a pathogenic process in the absence of dietary sugars (Lamont et al., 2018). Much ink has been spilled on the etiology of dental caries, and while it has been associated primarily with carbohydrate consumption, there are numerous other contributors to this multifactorial disease, including salivatory functions and fluoride (Selwitz et al., 2007: Figure 3; Pitts et al., 2017). While dental caries may involve alternating periods of more and less activity, the disease is generally age-progressive, and any comparisons made must consider age groups (Hillson, 2019). When comparing samples with differential preservation, or when commingled with a lot of loose teeth, care must also be taken to make comparisons between similar tooth types, as occlusal lesions are more likely to appear on the posterior teeth, which have larger, more complex crown surfaces. Discussion of caries often includes site of initiation (i.e., occlusal, buccal, lingual, mesial, distal), and

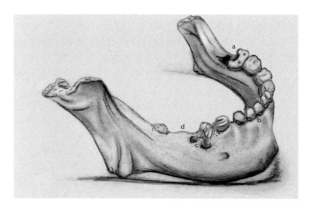

Figure 20.1 Illustration of (a) dental caries, (b) dental calculus, (c) periapical lesions, and (d) AMTL. Illustration by Rachel Heil.

lesions on the crown may be discussed separately from those on the root surface, or at the cemento-enamel junction (CEJ).

Dental caries has been used to estimate past subsistence strategies, with lower caries rates indicating foraging groups and higher rates suggesting an agricultural population (e.g., Turner, 1979; Larsen, 2006). However, a recent meta-analysis suggests that variation within the same subsistence strategy may be greater than variation between strategies (Marklein et al., 2019). For example, a high prevalence of dental caries – similar to rates found today – was noted in Pleistocene hunter-gatherers from Morocco (Humphrey, et al., 2014). Over 50% of all teeth from the site had at least one carious lesion, which may be related to the processing of carbohydrate-rich wild plants, such as acorn and pine nuts. Similarly, the consumption of tropical fruits may explain relatively high rates of caries among foragers at Lapa do Santo, an Early Holocene site in Brazil (Da-Gloria et al., 2017). Conversely, Tayles and colleagues (2000) found a decrease in caries rates after the intensification of rice agriculture in Thailand. Several researchers have cautioned that while caries is often discussed as having a complex, multifactorial etiology, it is then often associated with carbohydrate consumption almost exclusively (Tayles et al., 2009; Marklein et al., 2019).

There has been significant discussion around the difference in caries rate between bioarchaeological individuals estimated to be male or female, and disease prevalence due to sexual division of labor and differential access to food types (Temple, 2015). Studies have also reported higher rates of caries in women, particularly after the advent of agriculture, due to physiological life-history changes (Lukacs, 2008). Varying weight has been placed on the influence of hormonal changes and reproduction (Lukacs & Largaespada, 2006) and gendered difference in food choice (Larsen, 2018). However, many of these studies use biological sex estimation as a proxy for gender, and rarely incorporate a discussion of the interaction among sex, gender, age, status, and disease indicators (Zuckerman & Crandall, 2019). Several recent studies have found a great deal of variability when looking at sex estimation, age, and other factors associated with caries, such as AMTL, periodontal disease, bone mineral density, and survivorship, suggesting that hormonal differences between sexes sometimes seem to be a main causal agent, and sometimes do not (Kubehl & Temple, 2020; Mountain et al., 2021).

Calculus

Dental calculus, or mineralized plaque, can occur on both the supragingival and subgingival surfaces of teeth and lead to gingival loss and periodontal disease (Figure 20.1b). Supragingival calculus can adhere to enamel, dentin, and cementum, while subgingival calculus adheres to cementum only (White, 1997). There are a few other differences between these types of calculus, including their inorganic makeup and microstructures (Lieverse, 1999). Both supragingival and subgingival calculus have complex etiologies with a variety of factors influencing their formation, including the alkalinity of the oral environment, presence of microorganisms, and the composition of saliva and gingival crevice fluid (Lieverse, 1999; Warinner et al., 2015). Initial formation of the plaque biofilm occurs as microbes (primarily from the viridans group streptococci and *Actinomyces* species) adhere to a thin film on the tooth formed by salivary proteins (Warinner et al., 2015). As the plaque mineralizes, it becomes dental calculus.

A complex relationship exists between dental calculus and diet, particularly in the amount of protein and mineral consumption, which affect oral pH and mineralization. Therefore, the multifactorial origin of calculus means that macroscopic observation in paleopathological and bioarchaeological studies has often been recorded, but not used as a diagnostic element when reconstructing diet (Lieverse, 1999). In addition, the likelihood that calculus can detach from the teeth during life or postmortem could bias results (Radini et al., 2017).

However, recent work with dental calculus focuses on its potential to reveal information about diet from a microscopic perspective and the microbiome. As calculus forms, dietary microfossils (pollen, phytoliths) and environmental substances can become trapped within the mineral matrix, along with bacterial cells from the oral cavity (Warinner et al., 2015). The ability to sample and analyze these remains has opened up a new avenue for research.

Plant foods in the diet have been reconstructed by examination of microscopic remains trapped in calculus, such as starch grains and phytoliths (Tao et al., 2020; Zanina et al., 2021). Dental calculus samples can inform bioarchaeologists about other significant questions such as trade and daily activity (Radini et al., 2017). Blatt and colleagues (2011) found evidence of cotton fibers trapped in dental calculus from four individuals from a Late Woodland site in Ohio. These fibers appeared most closely related to those from the Southwest U.S., and when considered with other material culture from the site, suggest the community was involved in long-distance trade with communities from the western Gulf of Mexico. It also suggests that cotton fibers may have been processed or anchored in the mouth, by some community members (Blatt et al., 2011). Another study not only identified the presence of grain and grasses by observing microfossils but also used gas-chromatography mass-spectrometry to reveal wine derivatives, mushrooms, and medicinal plants in calculus from a medieval Italian group. These results, particularly the presence of non-local tea alkaloids, beyond establishing dietary and medicinal practices, also suggested trade with the Near East (Gismondi et al., 2018).

Evidence of nicotine alkaloids in dental calculus from pre-contact individuals at sites in central California suggested tobacco use that could be tied to specific individuals (Eerkens et al., 2018). This may allow bioarchaeologists to test hypotheses about who would have used tobacco, and if tobacco was being smoked or chewed (depending on what teeth the alkaloids were associated with). Identification of chemical indicators associated with medicinal plants may provide new information on how ancient peoples treated particular conditions, which can be incorporated with other pathological indicators noted in the skeleton to offer a more complete biocultural understanding of health and disease in the community (Gismondi et al., 2018).

One promising avenue of future research is to analyze genomic sequences found within the calculus matrix, although some caution that there are still many limitations to identifying dietary organisms via genetic evidence from calculus (Mann et al., 2020). The identification of specific proteins may also provide direct evidence for consumption of particular foods in the past. Warinner and colleagues (2014) identified the presence of b-lactoglobulin (BLG), a milk whey protein, in dental calculus from ancient and historic Europe, southwest Asia, and Norse Greenland, providing direct evidence of dairy consumption. Further, they were able to separate sequences consistent with cattle, sheep, and goats. This offers the ability to not only reconstruct diet but also examine recent natural selection of lactase persistence in humans. Another study found proteomic evidence of dairy, cereal grains, legumes, and other plant crops in 100 archaeological samples from Iron Age to post-medieval England, and noted that while the technique may be used to describe a group's diet in general, comparisons among individuals cannot yet be made (Hendy et al., 2018).

Researchers have also used dental calculus samples to analyze oral microbiota genomes. Eisenhofer and colleagues (2020), looking at individuals from the Japanese Jomon (ca. 2400–3000BP) and Edo (ca. 400-150BP) time periods, found that oral microbiome composition did not change much between the two despite a shift from foraging to farming. They note that this is consistent with other findings that show stability in oral microbiota over great swathes of time, unlike the gut microbiome. A study underway of the oral microbiome among 20 generations of African Americans in the U.S. may elucidate changes in foodways and disease from the 17th to early 20th centuries, providing insight into the transition from African to African-American identities and outcomes of marginalization (Jackson et al., 2016). Another study was able to identify a *Mycobacterium leprae* genome in a dental calculus sample from a 16th-century Norwegian, along with mycobacterial peptides, confirming that the person was likely infected with leprosy, despite a lack of definitive evidence in the skeleton (Fotakis et al., 2020). In addition, tuberculosis DNA was sequenced from calculus from several individuals in the Smithsonian's Huntington Collection (Young, 2017).

Periodontal Disease

As with other oral diseases, the etiology of periodontitis is multifactorial and complex. Similar to dental caries, polymicrobial communities occur regularly in the human oral cavity, but the presence of inflammation can lead to dysbiosis (microbial imbalance), and ultimately, periodontitis (Lamont et al., 2018). The microbes involved include *Porphyromonas gingivalis*, *Tannerella forsythia*, *Treponema denticola* ("red complex" species), and *Aggregatibacter actinomycetemcomitans* (Jin et al., 2016). Effectively, plaque on the teeth mineralizes into dental calculus, as mentioned in the previous section, leading to gingivitis, which is the inflammation of the gum tissue around the tooth. Chronic gum inflammation can lead to a hypersensitive reaction of the immune response, damaging the tissues of the periodontium, and causing separation of the gum from the tooth (Page & Schroeder, 1976). These pockets then can lead to deep, chronic infections, known as periodontitis. Periodontitis can lead to exfoliation of the tooth, which must be considered when assessing AMTL. Its complexity and the fact that periodontal disease is episodic, with sporadic progression and recession, may be why periodontal disease is often not incorporated into diet reconstruction (Page & Schroeder, 1976; Bonsall, 2014; Tuggle & Watson, 2019).

Nevertheless, macroscopically, periodontal disease can be assessed on archaeological skeletal material (Whiting et al., 2019). Many studies that incorporate periodontal disease into bioarchaeological analysis discuss possible sex-based differences (Šlaus, 2000; Delgado-Darias et al., 2006; DeWitte, 2012; Bonsall, 2014). These efforts are influenced by clinical studies, which suggest there may be hormonally related microbial sexual dimorphism and gendered social-cultural differences in oral health care (Ioannidou, 2017). Tuggle and Watson (2019) found that females living in the prehistoric American Southwest exhibited greater tooth and alveolar bone loss, as well as more significant wear and alveolar crest depth. The difference was greatest when comparing males and females aged between 30 and 50 years, suggesting that changes in estrogen, associated with reproductivity across the female life course, may play a role. On the other hand, at Neolithic Jomon sites, sex differences were attributed to potentially different levels of both food competition and gendered divisions of labor (Saso & Kondo, 2019).

Recent genomic analyses of the oral microbiome have contributed to a new understanding of human-bacterial coevolution. Bravo-Lopez and colleagues (2020) identified aDNA from *Tannerella forsythia* in individuals from Pre-Hispanic and Colonial Mexico. They found that some strains of the bacteria dated to the earliest arrival of humans in the Americas and those other strains were introduced during the colonial period. Genomic analysis of the oral microbiome of males and females in the Edo period from Japan indicated the absence of red complex bacteria in individuals with periodontal disease but did identify the archaeon

Methanobrevibacter oralis (Eisenhofer et al., 2020). Females were found to have greater abundance of this microbe, which is associated with periodontitis (Horz & Conrads, 2011). The greater abundance of *Methanobrevibacter oralis* was of particular interest, as the women with periodontal disease also practiced Ohagaru, or staining of the teeth with a black paste, which was believed to prevent oral disease (Eisenhofer et al., 2020).

Apical Periodontal Lesions

Small cavities in the alveolar bone have often erroneously been identified as dental abscesses when they are more likely to be benign granulomas or cysts (Dias & Tayles, 1997). These bony hollows can form when the pulp cavity becomes infected following heavy wear, dental caries, and/or trauma, which produces an inflammatory response in the periapical tissues (Dias & Tayles, 1997) (Figure 20.1c). There are various stages of the inflammation response, including a possibly infective state [see Figure 2 of Dias and Tayles (1997) for a useful pathogenesis model]. Dias and colleagues (2007:626) suggest that periapical lesions smaller than 3mm should be identified as periapical granulomas, while those larger than 3mm should be referred to as apical periodontal cysts. A lesion with an asymmetrical margin, roughened wall, and drainage sinus would be identified as an abscess (Rufino et al., 2017). Alternatively, Nelson (2020) suggests referring to any bony cavity as a "periapical void" to reduce confusion, particularly when diagnosis is unknown, and Pilloud and Fancher (2019) suggest "periapical lesion" or "anatomical lesion," arguing that the identification of a granuloma, cyst, or abscess necessitates soft tissue examination.

Kieser and colleagues (2001) reported relatively high rates of periapical lesions in precontact Māori. They found that 18% of teeth examined had lesions and that males had more lesions than females. Most of the periapical lesions were associated with heavily worn teeth, suggesting that inflammation and pulp exposure resulted from grit in the diet that caused excessive wear. Dental caries and heavy wear can both contribute to the development of periapical lesions, as seen in the Romano-British Poundbury sample where many individuals had periapical activity linked with both caries and wear (Raitapuro-Murray et al., 2014).

Dental Wear and Chipping

Dental wear is a normal physiological phenomenon where teeth are worn down during occlusion throughout life. Dental wear may take several forms including attrition (tooth-on-tooth wear), abrasion (wear from foreign substances in the mouth, such as food, phytoliths, or sand), erosion/corrosion (chemical destruction of enamel), and abfraction (loss of tooth structure at the CEJ caused by occlusal biomechanical loads) or other trauma (Kaidonis, 2008; Sarode & Sarode, 2013; Burnett, 2020; Crane et al., 2020) (Figure 20.2). Dental wear patterning has been associated with diet and food processing, occupation or habitual behaviors, and as the result of traumatic mechanical loads. Wear that is inconsistent with the patterns expected from the normal mechanical forces of mastication are described as aberrant or the result of a whole suite of idiosyncratic behaviors that may not be related to pathology but socio-cultural practices (Stojanowski et al, 2015; Burnett and Irish, 2017; Crane et al., 2020). While many masticatory and habitual patterns should not be identified as disease processes, alteration and damage to dental enamel and dentin that reach the pulp cavity can lead to significant dental disease (Pilloud & Fancher, 2019). Therefore, dental wear's value for paleopathology is in providing additional context to other dental diseases and dietary indicators, keeping in mind that it is age-progressive (Bartlett & Dugmore, 2008; Kaidonis, 2008).

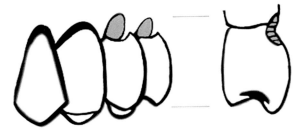

Figure 20.2 Illustration of abfraction. Illustration by Tisa Loewen.

Mastication and Alimentary Use

Abrasion due to mastication is not typically considered pathological unless dentin or the pulp cavity are exposed, in which case exposure of tooth nerves can cause dentin sensitivity (DS) or hypersensitivity (DH) and pain, impacting quality of life. Clinical research on DS/DH describes the etiology, in which wear-produced exposure of nerves is irritated by hydrodynamic movement through dentinal tubules of foreign substances; a process that predominantly results from erosion, a more recent concern due to modern diets (West et al., 2013) (Figure 20.3). This suggests that the experience of pain in an individual with worn teeth may vary depending on the nature of the wear. Chemical alteration of the teeth can occur due to frequent consumption of acidic foods and beverages, as well as frequent vomiting and reflux. Archaeological cases are not common but have been reported. A three-year-old child from the Pedra do Cachorro site in Brazil, dating to roughly 1470 BP, had evidence of corrosion on their maxillary incisors. Oliveira and colleagues (2020) suggest that the child may have had chronic episodes of vomiting and/or reflux due to a gastric disorder. There were few indicators of generalized stress, except that the child's skeleton aged much younger than the dentition.

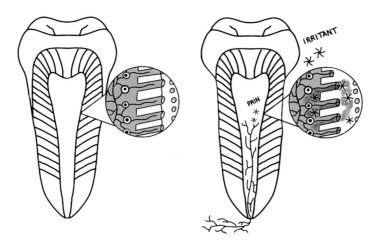

Figure 20.3 Illustration of irritation of dentinal tubules that can lead to dental sensitivity and dental hypersensitivity. Illustration by Tisa Loewen.

Teeth as Tools and Occupational Indicators (Non-Alimentary)

While patterned dental wear may indicate the relative hardness of foods in the diet, it can also indicate activity. Comparing rates of wear between anterior and posterior teeth, Albaishareh and Al-Shorman (2010) suggested that Byzantine inhabitants at Sa'ad may have been using their teeth to grasp materials for leather processing and/or basket making. In another study of individuals from Neolithic Sweden, Molnar (2008) found that females and males had similar rates of typical dental wear, chipping, and periapical lesions, but differed in atypical patterns. These differences suggested that most people in the group were using their teeth as tools, but that there may have been gendered differences in labor and extramasticatory tooth use. Molnar (2011) provides a helpful overview of identifying the characteristics associated with using teeth as tools. The standard tools for scoring dental macrowear may obscure our ability to identify non-masticatory wear, therefore Crane and colleagues (2020) provide a model for consideration of dental wear and its implications on social embodiment and a community of practice.

Trauma

Traumatic dental injury (TDI) alterations to tooth surfaces may be sudden, in the case of facial injury, or slow, such as with bruxism (grinding of the teeth). TDI may be an injurious lesion manifest in the dentition that is also indicative of pathologies elsewhere in the body, such as psychosocial stress. Foley (2020) notes that there are no pathognomonic indicators of bruxism, but that heavy wear combined with other indicators (such as mandibular and maxillary exostoses, degenerative joint disease of the temporomandibular joint, or hypercementosis) may aid bioarchaeologists in the identification of bruxing behavior in individuals. Bruxism was suggested as the cause for heavy dental wear in a young adult from the Roman-era site of Oğlanqala in Azerbaijan, where this individual may have been affiliated with the Roman army and may have experienced bruxism as a response to psychological stress (Nugent, 2013). Psychological stress is also implicated in heavy wear that may have been caused by bruxism among Nubians at Tombos living under Egyptian colonialism (Buzon & Bombak, 2010). Worne (2017) also considers bruxism as a cause of heavy dental wear on an individual that may have had cerebral palsy in 19th-century Kentucky.

Chipping of teeth is another form of damage that can be due to traumatic injury or long-term use such as with abfraction, where a large wedge-shaped crack results from microfractures at the CEJ due to indirect mechanical loading on the teeth (Sarode & Sarode, 2013). Chipping of the crown has been used as evidence extensively in paleoanthropology. Distribution of chipping in Neandertals led to an interpretation of gendered divisions of labor (Estalrrich & Rosas, 2015). It was also identified as occurring frequently in *Homo naledi* fossils compared to other hominins, suggesting a unique dietary etiology (Towle et al., 2017). Microwear pits and scratches also provide a wealth of information related to diet, health, and development and are commonly used in paleoanthropology (Ungar & Berger, 2018) as well as bioarchaeology (Scott & Halcrow, 2017; Schmidt et al., 2019).

Antemortem Tooth Loss (AMTL)

AMTL refers to the loss of a tooth before death that may be due to wear, caries, trauma, periodontal disease, and/or intentional ablation. It can be distinguished from postmortem dental loss by the presence of remodeled alveolar bone, and ultimately, the absence of a tooth socket (Figure 20.1d). It may be impossible to identify which particular event led to AMTL although it may be inferred if other individuals have excessive dental wear, or a high incidence of caries. Congenital absence of a tooth typically leaves no space for a socket, while AMTL results in a gap where the tooth was housed, with remodeled bone. Mesial drift of remaining distal teeth may narrow this space over time. AMTL may be particularly useful for reconstructing dental health in fragmentary, commingled burial contexts, particularly in cremations, where teeth may not have been preserved well (Ullinger et al., 2015). While loose teeth necessitate tooth count analyses, AMTL can often still be examined by individual count and considered with age and sex if some of the cranium is still present.

Intentional ablation (the purposeful removal of teeth) is a form of dental modification that may reflect the embodiment of a social identity (Smith-Guzmán et al., 2020) or act as a medicinal practice (Bolhofner, 2017). Ablation is considered to be a biosocial marker when the evulsion of highly visible teeth (such as healthy anterior teeth) co-occurs with a persistent pattern of prevalence across a group (De Groote & Humphrey, 2016). The oldest example of ablation in the archaeological record thus far is of a maxilla belonging to a 35–40-year-old male from the Early Epipaleolithic Levantine site of Ohalo II H2 (approx. 22,500 cal BP) that exhibited the antemortem loss of the right maxillary central incisor (Willman & Lacy, 2020). Taken to its extreme, ablation can result in edentulism (the complete lack of dentition). While edentulism can be the result of natural causes, such as aging or disease process, ablative edentulism can have its own cultural and ritual purposes.

Enamel Defects

Enamel hypoplastic defects may form as a result of over 100 different conditions as a tooth develops; referring to their cause as childhood "stress" glosses over their complex etiology (Edinborough & Rando, 2020). Hypoplastic defects can appear in a number of different ways (e.g., as pits, striations, or grooves). The most commonly examined defects are linear enamel hypoplasias (LEH), which manifest as horizontal depressions that circle the crown, following the perikymata (Cares Henriquez & Oxenham, 2020). LEH are enamel defects due to growth disruption during ontology and have been used to indicate biocultural transitions, such as employing a life-history approach to examine LEH and the ecological impact of health and subsistence on development in Neolithic Liguria (Italy) (Orellana-González et al., 2020). While they are nonspecific in nature, they are often combined with other pathological markers by bioarchaeologists to make inferences about conditions that have multiple effects on the human skeleton. For example, they have been used in conjunction with other pathological indicators to identify starvation (Simpson, 2020). Enamel defects, therefore, do not necessarily indicate oral health, but systemic health (Pilloud & Fancher, 2019). Because enamel does not remodel, LEH represent childhood growth disruption regardless of an individual's age.

There are a variety of ways to examine LEH, which can make comparison complicated across sites (Cares Henriquez & Oxenham, 2020). Researchers, therefore, should be very explicit in their description of technique and method when reporting on LEH. An additional consideration when comparing LEH frequencies is the composition of the sample. A recent study found that there may be an intergenerational, familial risk in the development of LEH, and that the condition may be over-represented if a sample is composed of relatively closely related individuals (Lawrence et al., 2021). Towle and Irish (2020) offer a similar note of caution when examining LEH; researchers should be recording all forms of defects, contextualizing dental morphology, and considering genetic conditions.

Biological distance studies that use data derived from living populations with known familial relationships are useful in understanding the etiologies of pathologies like LEH because they are able to account for variance in both genetic and environmental contributions without the uncertainty posed by the osteological paradox. For example, while increased LEH from one generation to the next might suggest stress, it could also be indicative of greater survivorship in an archaeological population. But if analyses can be made from dentition of individuals who were still alive at the time of recording (from radiographs or casts), coupled with information on genealogy, they can demonstrate when predisposition to a disease is kin-structured. Therefore, differences in "frailty" can be assessed more specifically and show whether gene flow is influenced by variance in the shared environment. These insights then inform our interpretations of past populations that are contextualized by location, time, or other pathologies.

Developmental Variation

There are a wide variety of developmental variants that can occur in the dentition, including (among others) (1) more teeth than expected (supernumerary teeth); (2) fewer teeth than expected (agenesis); (3) teeth exchanging position (transposition); (4) migration of dental buds during development (ectopic teeth); (5) teeth that are significantly smaller than others; and (6) impaction. While variants such as these are not uncommon when considered together, specific types may only be found in one or a few individuals from any given site or sample. Therefore, they are not often reported, and when they are, may be included as a descriptive note within a larger volume on osteology, or presented as a case study (e.g., Lieverse et al., 2014; Phillips et al., 2021).

Transposition and agenesis have been used to contextualize biological relatedness. For example, relatively high frequencies of maxillary canine-first premolar transposition among Early Period Channel Islands inhabitants may suggest high rates of endogamy that later decline in the Middle and Late Period, as evidenced by lower rates of transposition (Sholts et al., 2010). Decreasing rates of agenesis between the Late Antique and Early Medieval periods in Croatia were interpreted as evidence for arrival of new groups of people in the later period, while decreasing rates of dental crowding were related to heavier wear with more abrasive diets in those later groups (Vodanović et al., 2012). Edgar and colleagues (2016) combined several developmental variants, along with other rare dental non-metric traits, to examine population formation in prehistoric Mexico and the American Southwest. Their analysis found that examination of these rare traits reinforced the same patterns seen with more common dental morphological traits.

Reconstruction of Past Lives

By combining various dental pathological indicators with each other, along with other lines of evidence (stable isotope analysis, mortuary analysis, and theory), paleopathologists and bioarchaeologists can interpret social and cultural factors beyond dental disease through a biocultural lens. One of the most common bioarchaeological reconstructions using dental indicators is diet. Questions about foodways may examine different subsistence practices over time, across contemporaneous groups, or among genders. Alfonso-Durruty and colleagues (2019) used both stable isotope analysis and dental pathologies to explore diet in Chilean coastal and inland communities. For one of the coastal groups, AMTL was likely the result of strong wear, and not caries, as evidenced by low rates of carious lesions, but also by relatively high $\delta^{15}N$ values, indicative of a reliance on marine resources that required more chewing than other foods. Inland groups had higher levels of AMTL and caries, suggesting greater consumption of terrestrial foods. The examination of dental disease and stable isotope analysis, along with archaeological and ethnographic information, led to the conclusion that groups in the Arica culture had two identities – one coastal and reliant on marine resources; the other inland and dependent on agricultural foods (Alfonso-Durruty et al., 2019).

Cheung and colleagues (2019) also combined stable isotope and dental caries data from 77 different sites in a meta-analysis of northern China. They found enrichment in $\delta^{13}C$ values from 9000–4500 BP, corresponding to the domestication and increasing use of millet across northern China, with some sites retaining a mixed rice/millet economy. Dental caries rates were variable before 4500 BP and may reflect reliance on a variety of wild foods, which were more or less cariogenic. Eventually, C_3 plants increase in popularity after 4500 BP, as rates of carious lesions increase, suggesting that people relied more heavily on these crops in the later time period. Furthermore, these changes, which seem to revolve around 4500–3500 BP, are linked to a global shift in aridity, concurrent with increasing population size.

Fabra and González (2019) combined stable isotope analysis, dental wear, and dental caries rates to infer that people in central Argentina from 4000–300BP practiced agriculture, but collected wild foods – and wild fruits, in particular – for a relatively large component of their diet. This was further linked to the practice of wild food collection used by later Indigenous peoples to create a cohesive community identity in response to the colonial Spanish system. Other studies have shown that diet changed more significantly, particularly for females, under Spanish colonialism in South America than it did under Incan imperialism (Gagnon, 2020). In Mali, dental disease increased significantly from the pre-Dogon (7th–14th century AD) to the Dogon period (17th–19th century AD), with caries, AMTL, and abscesses doubling in frequency while dental wear and periodontitis did not change (Dlamini et al., 2019). This was accompanied by a concomitant decrease in $\delta^{13}C$ values, indicating increasing consumption of C_3 foods, such as rice, and that preparation techniques may have affected the cariogenicity of this food.

As noted in the section on dental caries, there has been significant discussion around the etiology of sex differences and dental caries. One possible solution identified by Gagnon and Wiesen (2013) was to compare a variety of dental pathological indicators with fertility rates. Looking at individuals dating to a period of agricultural intensification and population centralization before the formation of the Moche State, they concluded that increased sex differences in dental disease without corresponding changes in fertility pointed to behavior as a primary driver for these disparities. They also analyzed dental calculus samples, finding evidence of maize starch in more teeth from females than males in later periods. Ultimately, the discussion surrounding sex differences and dental caries highlights the importance of contextualizing bioarchaeological data with a life-course approach, among other theoretical considerations.

Dental pathological indicators have also been used to assess "health" among and within different social groups [for a discussion of the use of the word "health" as used in bioarchaeology, see Reitsema and McIlvaine (2015)]. Betsinger and DeWitte (2021) examine a number of different studies on the comparison of dental health and diet between urban and rural contemporary groups. They found no consistent pattern, with various rural groups exhibiting both worse and better dental health than their urban counterparts. Similarly, Zejdlik and colleagues (2019) found that patterns of dental disease varied, even when examining individuals from the same time period and general location (medieval Romania), highlighting that context is important. They also refer to Pilloud and Fancher's (2019) call for standardizing data collection, as well as consideration of what conditions should be included when discussing "oral health." A study of individuals buried in vaults beneath the 19th-century Spring Street Presbyterian Church in New York City found high rates of caries and AMTL, even when comparing the group to their contemporaries (Hosek et al., 2020). Hosek and colleagues (2020) argue that relatively few examinations of dental disease have incorporated social aspects of oral health and dental care. They link the ideals of 19th-century nationalism and citizenry with oral health, illustrating the complex biocultural nature of paleopathology and ways in which embodiment theory can explain unexpected biological phenomena.

Dental pathological analysis can offer insight into the effects of marginalization. At the First African Baptist Church in Philadelphia, researchers discovered that while free African-American individuals buried there experienced better overall health than enslaved individuals, they still suffered from periodic undernutrition and infectious disease; 92.5% of deciduous teeth (from 21 non-adults) had enamel defects, as did all 50 adults (Rankin-Hill, 2016). This corroborated earlier work by Blakey and colleagues (1994) that found that enslaved males in the plantation south all had hypoplastic defects, and that 70% of females did, as well. Therefore, individuals in the "free" north experienced similar stress and infectious disease to those enslaved in the south (Blakey, 2001). Similarly, de la Cova (2014) found that African Americans experienced more nutritional stress and infectious disease than Euro-Americans in the 19th–20th centuries, although rates of caries and AMTL were higher among the Euro-Americans.

While hypoplastic defects have been used to infer childhood stress in adults, less attention has been paid to non-adults and oral disease in deciduous dentition. In non-adults, periodontal disease, periapical lesions, calculus, and AMTL are rare (Rohnbogner & Lewis, 2016; Alfonso-Durruty et al., 2019). But dental caries (which is often only recorded in permanent dentition) can elucidate meaningful differences between children and adults from the same community, highlighting differences in diet related to age and weaning (Halcrow et al., 2013; Hosek et al., 2020). Microwear of deciduous dentition may also be able to reveal timing, as well as the kinds of foods introduced during weaning (Scott & Halcrow, 2017).

Closing Comments

It is important that in the study of dental pathology, anthropologists engage with clinical research. Previous authors have written on or exemplified the need for communication between clinical and anthropological/evolutionary studies, highlighting application of knowledge across the disciplines (Kaidonis, 2008; Kaidonis et al., 2012; Reitsema & McIlvaine, 2015; Whiting et al., 2019; Ungar, 2020; Boyd et al., 2021). The most obvious examples involve comparisons of developmental evolutionary mismatches with post-industrial life that result in modern pathology (Corruccini, 1984). However, assumptions about pain, quality of life, genetics, environment, evolution, and plasticity in the past can be tempered by insights from modern dental research. For example, pulp calcification, which is fairly common in modern dentition, has been demonstrated to increase during life (Goga et al., 2008). The pulp chamber's physiological response to aging and use can have a pathological presentation (pulp stones), has a genetic component, and has an effect on sensory response (Goga et al., 2008). They may also be of interest to forensic odontologists and bioarchaeologists as pulp stones or pulp calcifications, sometimes called denticles, can survive in the archaeological record, and show on radiographs, CT scans, and histological sections (Nicklisch et al., 2021). Additionally, pulp stones are associated with trauma, diet, cardiovascular disease, and renal calcifications, among other systemic diseases (Goga et al., 2008; Nicklisch et al.,

2021). Calcific metamorphosis (CM), a deposition of hard tissue in the pulp cavity, can also lead to necrosis of the tooth or result in either complete or partial obliteration of root canals following trauma (Amir et al., 2001). These clinical insights challenge the ways we, as anthropologists, think about pain and wellness, environmental influence, and evolutionary response mechanisms.

Anthropologists are increasingly incorporating new techniques and theoretical approaches into their analyses. Both proteomics and genomics have revolutionized our ability to understand diet and disease from dental calculus. The inclusion of skeletal data, dental data, stable isotope analyses, along with archaeological and historical evidence has provided richer, more contextualized understandings of past lives. The integration of theoretical approaches with dental anthropology, such as life-course analysis and the theory of embodiment, has led to a stronger biocultural discussion of lived experiences in the past.

References

Adolph, M., Darnaud, C., Thomas, F., Pannier, B., Danchin, N., Batty, G. D. & Bouchard, P. (2017). Oral health in relation to all-cause mortality. *Scientific Reports* 7:44604.

Albashaireh, Z. S. M. & Al-Shorman, A. A. (2010). The frequency and distribution of dental caries and tooth wear in a Byzantine population of Sa'ad, Jordan. *International Journal of Osteoarchaeology* 20:205–213.

Alfonso-Durruty, M. P., Gayo, E. M., Standen, V., Castro, V., Latorre, C., Santoro, C. M. & Valenzuela, D. (2019). Dietary diversity in the Atacama desert during the Late intermediate period of northern Chile. *Quaternary Science Reviews* 214:54–67.

Amir, F. A., Gutmann, J. L. & Witherspoon, D. E. (2001). Calcific metamorphosis. *Quintessence International* 32(6):447–455.

Aris, C. (2020). The Histological Paradox. *Papers from the Institute of Archaeology* 29(1):1–16.

Bartlett, D. & Dugmore, C. (2008). Pathological or physiological erosion—is there a relationship to age? *Clinical Oral Investigations* 12(1):27–31.

Bentley, G. R. & Perry, V. J. (2008) Dental analyses of the Bab edh-Dhra' human remains. In Ortner, D. J. & Frohlich, B. (Eds.), *The EBI Tombs and Burials of Bâb edh Dhrâ, Jordan*, pp. 281–296. Lanham, MD: AltaMira Press.

Betsinger, T. K. & DeWitte, S. N. 2021. Toward a bioarchaeology of urbanization. *Yearbook of Physical Anthropology* 175(S72):79–118.

Blakey, M. L. (2001). Bioarchaeology of the African diaspora in the Americas. *Annual Review of Anthropology* 30:387–422.

Blakey, M. L., Leslie, T. E. & Reidy, J. P. (1994). Frequency and chronological distribution of dental enamel hypoplasia in enslaved African Americans. *American Journal of Physical Anthropology* 95:371–384.

Blatt, S. H., Redmond, B. G., Cassman, V. & Sciulli, P. W. (2011). Dirty teeth and ancient trade. *International Journal of Osteoarchaeology* 21:669–678.

Bolhofner, K. L. (2017). Identity marker or medicinal treatment? In Burnett, S. E. & Irish, J. D. *A World View of Bioculturally Modified Teeth*, pp. 48–61. Gainesville: University Press of Florida.

Bonsall, L. (2014). A comparison of female and male oral health in skeletal populations from late Roman Britain. *Archives of Oral Biology* 59(12):1279–1300.

Boyd, K., Saccomanno, S., Lewis, C. J., Paskay, L. C., Quinzi, V. & Marzo, G. (2021). Culture, industrialisation and the shrinking human face: why is it important?. *European Journal of Paediatric Dentistry* 22(1–2021):80–82.

Bravo-Lopez, M., Villa-Islas, V., Rocha Arriaga, C., Villaseñor-Altamirano, A. B., Guzmán-Solís, A., … Ávila-Arcos, M. C. (2020). Paleogenomic insights into the red complex bacteria *Tannerella forsythia* in Pre-Hispanic and Colonial individuals from Mexico. *Philosophical Transactions of the Royal Society B: Biological Sciences* 375(1812):20190580.

Burnett, S. E. (2020). Crown wear: identification and categorization. In Irish, J. D. & Scott, G. R. (Eds.), *A Companion to Dental Anthropology*, pp. 415–432. Chichester: John Wiley & Sons.

Burnett, S. E., & Irish, J. D. (Eds.). (2017). *A World View of Bioculturally Modified Teeth*. Gainesville, FL: University Press of Florida.

Buzon, M. R. & Bombak, A. (2010). Dental disease in the Nile Valley during the New Kingdom. *International Journal of Osteoarchaeology* 20:371–387.

Cares Henriquez, A. & Oxenham, M. (2020). A new comprehensive quantitative approach for the objective identification and analysis of linear enamel hypoplasia (LEH) in worn archaeological dental assemblages. *Journal of Archaeological Science* 113:105064.

Chen, X., Daliri, E. B. -M., Kim, N., Kim, J. -R., Yoo, D. & Oh, D, -H. (2020). Microbial etiology and prevention of dental caries: exploiting natural products to inhibit cariogenic biofilms. *Pathogens* 9(7):569–584.

Cheung, C., Zhang, H., Hepburn, J. C., Yang, D. Y., & Richards, M. P. (2019). Stable isotope and dental caries data reveal abrupt changes in subsistence economy in ancient China in response to global climate change. *PLOSONE* 14(7):1–27.

Corruccini, R. S. (1984). An epidemiologic transition in dental occlusion in world populations. *American Journal of Orthodontic* 86(5):419–426.

Crane, A., Watson, J. T. & Haas, R. (2020). The effects of aberrant tooth wear on occlusal relationships. In Schmidt, C. W. & Watson, J. T. (Eds.), *Dental Wear in Evolutionary and Biocultural Contexts*, pp. 99–121. London: Academic Press.

Da-Gloria, P., Oliveira, R. E. & Neves, W. A. (2017). Dental caries at Lapa do Santo, central-eastern Brazil. *Anais da Academia Brasileira de Ciências* 89(1):307–316.

De Groote, I. & Humphrey, L. (2016). Characterizing evulsion in the Later Stone Age Maghreb. *Quaternary International* 413:50–61.

de la Cova, C. (2014). The biological effects of urbanization and in-migration on 19th-century-born African Americans and Euro-Americans of low socioeconomic status. In Zuckerman, M. K. (Ed.), *Modern Environments and Human Health*, pp. 243–264. New York: John Wiley & Sons.

Delgado-Darias, T., Velasco-Vázquez, J., Arnay-de-la-Rosa, M., Martín-Rodríguez, E. & González-Reimers, E. (2006). Calculus, periodontal disease and tooth decay among the prehispanic population from Gran Canaria. *Journal of Archaeological Science* 33(5):663–670.

DeWitte, S. N. (2012). Sex differences in periodontal disease in catastrophic and attritional assemblages from medieval London. *American Journal of Physical Anthropology* 149(3):405–416.

Dias, G. & Tayles, N. (1997) 'Abscess cavity' – a misnomer. *International Journal of Osteoarchaeology* 7:548–554.

Dias, G., Prasad, K., & Santos, A. L. (2007). Pathogenesis of apical periodontal cysts. *International Journal of Osteoarchaeology* 17:619–626.

Dlamini, N., Sealy, J. & Mayor, A. (2019). Diet variability among pre-Dogon and early Dogon populations (Mali) from stable isotopes and dental diseases. *American Journal of Physical Anthropology* 169:287–301.

Edgar, H. J. H., Willermet, C., Ragsdale, C. S., O'Donnell, A. & Daneshvari, S. (2016). Frequencies of rare incisor variations reflect factors influencing precontact population relationships in Mexico and the American Southwest. *International Journal of Osteoarchaeology* 26(6):987–1000.

Edinborough, M. & Rando, C. (2020). Stressed out. *Journal of Archaeological Science* 121:105197.

Eerkens, J. W., Tushingham, S., Brownstein, K. J., Garibay, R., Perez, K., Murga, E., Kaijankoski, P., Rosenthal, J. S. & Gang, D. R. (2018). Dental calculus as a source of ancient alkaloids. *Journal of Archaeological Science: Reports* 18:509–515.

Eisenhofer, R., Kanzawa-Kiriyama, H., Shinoda, K. & Weyrich, L. S. (2020). Investigating the demographic history of Japan using ancient oral microbiota. *Philosophical Transactions B* 375:20190578.

Elliott, J. C., Wong, F. S. L., Anderson, G. R. D. & Dowker, S. E. P. (1998). Determination of mineral concentration in dental enamel from x-ray attenuation measurements. *Connective Tissue Research* 38:1–4.

Estalrrich, A. & Rosas, A. (2015). Division of labor by sex and age in Neandertals: an approach through the study of activity-related dental wear. *Journal of Human Evolution* 80:51–63.

Fabra, M. & González, C. V. (2019). Oral health and diet in populations of central Argentina during the Late Holocene: bioarchaeological and isotopic evidence. *Latin American Antiquity* 30(4):1–18.

Foley, A. J. (2020) The daily grind. *Journal of Archaeological Science* 117:105117.

Fotakis, A. K., Denham, S. D., Mackie, M., Orbegozo, M. I., Mylopotamitaki, D., Gopalakrishnan, S., …Vågene, Å. (2020). Multi-omic detection of *Mycobacterium leprae* in archaeological human dental calculus. *Philosophical Transactions of the Royal Society B* 375:20190584.

Gagnon, C. M. (2020). Exploring oral paleopathology in the Central Andes. *International Journal of Paleopathology* 29:24–34.

Gagnon, C. M. & Wiesen, C. (2013). Using general estimating equations to analyze oral health in the Moche Valley of Perú. *International Journal of Osteoarchaeology* 23:557–572.

Gismondi, A., D'Agostino, A., Canuti, L., Di Marco, G., Martínez-Labarga, C., Angle, M., Rickards, O., & Canini, A. (2018). Dental calculus reveals diet habits and medicinal plant use in the Early Medieval Italian population of Colonna. *Journal of Archaeological Science: Reports* 20:556–564.

Goga, R., Chandler, N. P. & Oginni, A. O. (2008). Pulp stones. *International Endodontic Journal* 41(6):457–468.

Halcrow, S. E., Harris, N. J., Tayles, N., Ikehara-Quebral, R. & Pietrusewsky, M. (2013). From the mouths of babes. *American Journal of Physical Anthropology* 150:409–429.

Hendy, J., Warinner, C., Bouwman, A., Collins, M. J., Fiddyment, S., Fischer, R., ... & Speller, C. F. (2018). Proteomic evidence of dietary sources in ancient dental calculus. *Proceedings of the Royal Society B* 285:20180977.

Hillson, S. (2019). Dental pathology. In Katzenberg, M. A. & Grauer, A. L. (Eds.) *Biological Anthropology of the Human Skeleton* (3rd ed.), pp. 293–333. New York: John Wiley & Sons.

Horz, H. -P. & Conrads, G. (2011). Methanogenic *Archaea* and oral infections. *Journal of Oral Microbiology* 3:5940.

Hosek, L., Warner-Smith, A. L. & Watson, C. C. (2020). The body politic and the citizen's mouth. *Historical Archaeology* 54:138–159.

Humphrey, L. T., De Groote, I., Morales, J., Barton, N., Collcutt, S., Ramsey, C. B. & Bouzouggar, A. (2014). Earliest evidence for caries and exploitation of starchy plant foods in Pleistocene hunter-gatherers from Morocco. *PNAS* 111(3):954–959.

Iaonnidou, E. (2017). The sex and gender intersection in chronic periodontitis. *Frontiers in Public Health* 5:189.

Jackson, F. L. C., Jackson, l., Cross, C. & Clarke, C. (2016). What could you do with 400 years of biological history on African Americans? Evaluating the potential scientific benefit of systematic studies of dental and skeletal materials on African Americans from the 17th through 20th centuries. *American Journal of Human Biology* 28 (4):510–513.

James, S. L., Abate, D., Abate, K. H., Abay, S. M., Abbafati, C., Abbasi, N., ...& Murray, C. J. L. (2018). Global, regional, and national incidence, prevalence, and years lived with disability for 354 diseases and injuries for 195 countries and territories, 1990–2017. *The Lance* 392(10159):1789–1858.

Jin, L. J., Lamster, I. B., Greenspan, J. S., Pitts, N. B., Scully, C. & Warnakulasuriya, S. (2016). Global burden of oral diseases. *Oral Diseases* 22(7):609–619.

Kaidonis, J. A. (2008). Tooth wear. *Clinical Oral Investigations* 12(Suppl 1):21–26.

Kaidonis, J. A., Ranjitkar, S., Lekkas, D. & Townsend, G. C. (2012). An anthropological perspective: another dimension to modern dental wear concepts. *International Journal of Dentistry* 2012:741405.

Kendall, C, Høier Eriksen, A. M., Kontopoulos, I., Collins, M. J. & Turner-Walker, G. (2018). Diagenesis of archaeological bone and tooth. *Palaeogeography, Palaeoclimatology, Palaeoecology* 491(1):21–37.

Kieser, J. A., Kelsen, A., Love, R., Herbison, P. G. P. & Dennison, K. J. (2001). Periapical lesions and dental wear in the early Maori. *International Journal of Osteoarchaeology* 11:290–297.

Kim, D., Barraza, J. P., Arthur, R. A., Hara, A., Lewis, K., Liu, Y., Scisci, E. L., Hajishengallis, E., Whitely, M. & Koo, H. (2020). Spatial mapping of polymicrobial communities reveals a precise biogeography associated with human dental caries. *PNAS* 117(22):12375–12386.

Kubehl, K. & Temple, D. H. (2020). Reproductive life histories influence cariogenesis. *American Journal of Physical Anthropology* 172(3):376–385.

Lacy, S. A. (2014a). *Oral Health and its Implications in Late Pleistocene Western Eurasian Humans*. Ph.D. dissertation. St. Louis: Washington University in St. Louis.

Lacy, S. A. (2014b). The oral pathological conditions of the Broken Hill (Kabwe) 1 cranium. *International Journal of Paleopathology* 7:57–63.

Lamont, R. J., Koo, H. & Hajishengallis, G. (2018). The oral microbiota. *Nature Reviews: Microbiology* 16(12):745–759.

Larsen, C. S. (2006). The agricultural revolution as environmental catastrophe. *Quaternary International* 150(1):12–20.

Larsen, C. S. (2018). The bioarchaeology of health crisis. *Annual Review of Anthropology* 47:295–313.

Lawrence, J., Stojanowski, C. M., Paul, K. S., Seidel, A. C. & Guatelli-Steinberg, D. (2021). Heterogeneous frailty and the expression of linear enamel hypoplasia in a genealogical population. *American Journal of Physical Anthropology* 176(4):638–651.

Lieverse, A. R. (1999). Diet and the aetiology of dental calculus. *International Journal of Osteoarchaeology* 9:219–232.

Lieverse, A. R., Pratt, I. V., Schulting, R. J., Cooper, D. M. L., Bazaliiskii, V. I. & Weber, A. W. (2014). Point taken. *International Journal of Paleopathology* 6:53–59.

Lozano, M., Gamarra, B., Hernando, R. & Ceperuelo, D. (2022). Microscopic and virtual approaches to oral pathology *Annals of Anatomy-Anatomischer Anzeiger* 239:151827.

Lukacs, J. R. (2008). Fertility and agriculture accentuate sex differences in dental caries rates. *Current Anthropology* 49(5):901–914.

Lukacs, J. R. & Largaespada, L. L. (2006). Explaining sex differences in dental caries prevalence. *American Journal of Human Biology* 18:540–555.

Mann, A. E., Yates, J. A. F., Fagernäs, Z., Austin, R. M., Nelson, E. A. & Hofman, C. A. (2020). Do I have something in my teeth? the trouble with genetic analyses of diet from archaeological dental calculus *Quaternary International*. DOI: 10.1016/j.quaint.2020.11.019

Marklein, K. M., Torres-Rouff, C., King, L. M. & Hubbe, M. (2019). The precarious state of subsistence. *Current Anthropology* 60(3):341–368.

Molnar, P. (2008). Dental wear and oral pathology: possible evidence and consequences of habitual use of teeth in a Swedish Neolithic sample. *American Journal of Physical Anthropology* 136:423–431.

Molnar, P. (2011). Extramasticatory dental wear reflecting habitual behavior and health in past populations. *Clinical Oral Investigations* 15:681–689.

Mountain, R. V., Wilson, J. A., McPherson, C. B., Blew, R. M. & Watson, J. T. (2021). Sex differences in age-related bone loss and antemortem tooth loss in East-Central Arizona (AD 1200–1450). *International Journal of Osteoarchaeology* 31(5):716–726.

Nelson, G. (2020). A host of other dental diseases and disorders. In Irish, J. D. & Scott, G. R. (Eds.), *A Companion to Dental Anthropology*, pp.575–638. Chichester: John Wiley & Sons.

Nicklisch, N., Schierz, O., Enzmann, F., Knipper, C., Held, P., Vach, W., … & Alt, K. W. (2021). Dental pulp calcifications in prehistoric and historical skeletal remains. *Annals of Anatomy-Anatomischer Anzeiger* 235:151675.

Nugent, S. (2013). *Death on the Imperial Frontier: An Ostebiography of Roman Burial from Oğlanqala, Azerbaijan*. M.A. Thesis. Columbus, OH: The Ohio State University.

Oliveira, R. E., Solari, A., Silva, S. F. S. M., Martin, G., Soares, C. B. & Strauss, A. (2020). Dental corrosion in preindustrial societies. *Dental Anthropology* 33(2):3–16.

Orellana-González, E., Sparacello, V. S., Bocaege, E., Varalli, A., Moggi-Cecchi, J. & Dori, I. (2020). Insights on patterns of developmental disturbances from the analysis of linear enamel hypoplasia in a Neolithic sample from Liguria (northwestern Italy). *International Journal of Paleopathology* 28:123–136.

Page, R. C. & Schroeder, H. E. (1976). Pathogenesis of inflammatory periodontal disease. *Laboratory Investigation* 34(3):235–249.

Petersen, P. E. (2004). Challenges to improvement of oral health in the 21st century. *International Dental Journal* 54(6):329–343.

Phillips, E. L. W., Irish, J. D. & Antoine, D. (2021). Ancient anomalies. *International Journal of Osteoarchaeology* 31(3):456–461.

Pilloud, M. & Fancher, J. 2019. Outlining a definition of oral health within the study of human skeletal remains. *Dental Anthropology* 32(02):3–11.

Pitts, N. B., Zero, D. T., Marsh, P. D., Ekstrand, K., Weintraub, J. A., Ramos-Gomez, F., Tagami, J., Twetman, S., Tsakos, G. & Ismail, A. (2017). Dental caries. *Nature Reviews Dental Primers* 3(17030):1–16.

Radini, A., Nikita, E., Buckley, S., Copeland, L. & Hardy, K. (2017). Beyond food: the multiple pathways for inclusion of materials into ancient dental calculus. *American Journal of Physical Anthropology* 162:71–83.

Raitapuro-Murray, T., Molleson, T. I. & Hughes, F. J. (2014). The prevalence of periodontal disease in a Romano-British population c. 200–400 AD. *British Dental Journal* 217(8):459–466.

Rankin-Hill, L. M. (2016). Identifying the First African Baptist Church: searching for historically invisible people. In Zuckerman, M. K. & Martin, D. L. (Eds.), *New Directions in Bioculural Anthropology*, pp.133–156. New York: John Wiley & Sons.

Reitsema, L. J. & McIlvaine, B. K. (2015). Reconciling "stress" and "health" in physical anthropology. *American Journal of Physical Anthropology* 155(2):181–185.

Rohnbogner, A. & Lewis, M. (2016). Dental caries as a measure of diet, health, and difference in non-adults from urban and rural Roman Britain. *Dental Anthropology* 29(01):16–31.

Rufino, A. I., Ferreira, M. T. & Wasterlain, S. N. (2017). Periapical lesions in intentionally modified teeth in a skeletal sample of enslaved Africans (Lagos, Portugal). *International Journal of Osteoarchaeology* 27:288–297.

Sarode, G. S. & Sarode, S. C. (2013). Abfraction. *Journal of Oral and Maxillofacial Pathology* 17(2):222–227.

Saso, A. & Kondo, O. (2019). Periodontal disease in the Neolithic Jomon. *Anthropological Science* 127(1):13–25.

Schmidt, C. W., Remy, A., Van Sessen, R., Willman, J., Krueger, K., Scott, R., … & Herrmann, N. (2019). Dental microwear texture analysis of *Homo sapiens sapiens*. *American Journal of Physical Anthropology* 169(2):207–226.

Scott, R. M. & Halcrow, S. E. (2017). Investigating weaning using dental microwear analysis. *Journal of Archaeological Science: Reports* 11:1–11.

Selwitz, R. H., Ismail, A. I. & Pitts, N. B. (2007). Dental caries. *The Lancet* 369(9555):51–59.

Sholts, S. B., Clement, A. F. & Wärmländer, S. K. T. S. (2010) Brief communication: additional cases of maxillary canine-first premolar transition in several prehistoric skeletal assemblages from the Santa Barbara Channel Islands of California. *American Journal of Physical Anthropology* 143:155–160.

Simón-Sora, A. & Mira, A. (2015). Solving the etiology of dental caries. *Trends in Microbiology* 23(2):76–82.

Simpson, R. (2020). New and emerging prospects for the paleopathological study of starvation. *Pathways* 1:66–83.

Šlaus, M. (2000). Biocultural analysis of sex differences in mortality profiles and stress levels in the late Medieval population from Nova Rača, Croatia. *American Journal of Physical Anthropology* 111:193–209.

Smith-Guzmán, N. E., Rivera-Sandoval, J., Knipper, C. & Sánchez Arias, G. A., (2020). Intentional dental modification in Panamá. *Journal of Anthropological Archaeology* 60:101226.

Stojanowski, C. M., Johnson, K. M., Paul, K. S. & Carver, C. L. (2015). Indicators of idiosyncratic behavior in the dentition. In Irish, J. D. & Scott, G. R. (Eds.), *A Companion to Dental Anthropology*, pp. 377–395. Chichester: John Wiley & Sons.

Tao, D., Zhang, G., Zhou, Y. & Zhao, H. (2020). Investigating wheat consumption based on multiple evidence. *International Journal of Osteoarchaeology* 30(5):594–606.

Tayles, N., Domett, K. & Halcrow, S. (2009). Can dental caries be interpreted as evidence of farming? The Asian experience. In Koppe, T., Meyer, G. & Alt, K. W. (Eds.), *Comparative Dental Morphology*, pp.162–166. Basel: Karger.

Tayles, N., Domett, K. & Nelsen, K. (2000). Agriculture and dental caries? The case of prehistoric Southeast Asia. *World Archaeology* 32(1):68–83.

Temple, D. H. (2015). Caries. In Irish, J. D., & Scott, G. R. (Eds.), *A Companion to Dental Anthropology*, pp.433–449. Chichester: John Wiley & Sons.

Towle, I. & Irish, J. D. (2020). Recording and interpreting enamel hypoplasia in samples from archaeological and palaeoanthropological contexts. *Journal of Archaeological Science* 114:105077.

Towle, I., Irish, J. D. & De Groote, I. (2017). Behavioral inferences from the high levels of dental chipping in *Homo naledi*. *American Journal of Physical Anthropology* 164:184–192.

Tuggle, A. & Watson, J. T. (2019). Periodontal health and the lifecourse approach in bioarchaeology. *Dental Anthropology* 32(2):12–21.

Turner, C. G. II. (1979). Dental anthropological indicators of agriculture among the Jomon people of central Japan. *American Journal of Physical Anthropology* 51:619–636.

Ullinger, J., Sheridan, S. G. & Guatelli-Steinberg, D. (2015). Fruits of their labour. *International Journal of Osteoarchaeology* 25:753–764.

Ungar, P. (2020). Why we have so many problems with our teeth. *Scientific American* 322(4):44–49.

Ungar, P. S. & Berger, L. R. (2018). Brief communication: Dental microwear and diet of *Homo naledi*. *American Journal of Physical Anthropology* 166(1):228–235.

Vodanović, M., Galić, I., Strujić, M., Peroš, K., Šlaus, M. & Brkić, H. (2012). Orthodontic anomalies and malocclusions in Late Antique and Early Mediaeval period in Croatia. *Archives of Oral Biology* 57(4):401–412.

Warinner, C., Speller, C. & Collins, M. J. (2015). A new era in palaeomicrobiology. *Philosophical Transactions of the Royal Society B* 370:20130376.

Warinner, C., Hendy, J., Speller, C., Cappellini, E., Fischer, R., Trachsel, C., … & Collins, M. J. (2014). Direct evidence of milk consumption from ancient human dental calculus. *Scientific Reports* 4:7104.

West, N. X., Lussi, A., Seong, J. & Hellwig, E. (2013). Dentin hypersensitivity. *Clinical Oral Investigations* 17(1):9–19.

White, D. J. (1997). Dental calculus. *European Journal of Oral Sciences* 105(5):508–522.

Whiting, R., Antoine, D. & Hillson, S. (2019). Periodontal disease and 'oral health' in the past. *Dental Anthropology* 32(2):30–50.

Willman, J. C. & Lacy, S. A. (2020). Oral pathological conditions of an Early Epipaleolithic human from Southwest Asia. *International Journal of Paleopathology* 30:68–76.

Worne, H. (2017). Bioarchaeological analysis of disability and caregiving from a nineteenth-century institution in central Kentucky. *Bioarchaeology International* 1(3–4):116–130.

Young, S. (2017). *Please Forget to Floss: Developing an Assay for Identifying Tuberculosis in Dental Calculus from the Smithsonian's Huntington Collection (1893–1921)*. Syracuse University Honors Program Capstone Projects 1006. Syracuse, NY: Syracuse University.

Zanina, O. G., Tur, S. S., Svyatko, S. V., Soenov, V. I. & Borodovskiy, A. P. (2021) Plant food in the diet of the Early Iron Age pastoralists of Altai *Journal of Archaeological Science: Reports* 35:1–14.

Zejdlik, K., Bethard, J. D., Nyárádi, Z. & Gonciar, A. (2019). The Medieval Transylvanian oral condition. *Dental Anthropology* 32(02):77–88.

Zuckerman, M. K. & Crandall, J. (2019). Reconsidering sex and gender in relation to health and disease in bioarchaeology. *Journal of Anthropological Archaeology* 54:161–171.

PART III

Theoretical Approaches and New Directions

21
ETHICAL CONSIDERATIONS FOR PALEOPATHOLOGY

Carlina de la Cova

Introduction

Biological anthropology, or physical anthropology, has evolved in the generations since its initial founding. Methodological and theoretical advancements in the discipline have resulted in a plethora of new knowledge about the past. This is also true with respect to its subdiscipline of paleopathology. Unfortunately, this knowledge was acquired, especially when these fields were in their nascent stages, by, according to today's standards, unethical or dubious means that targeted marginalized groups and "exoticized" others. In recent years, scholars have begun to wrestle with this past and decolonize the discipline in a manner that addresses the social violence and resonating harm done to these groups and their descendants. Despite the positive nature of these intentions, biological anthropology and its associated subdisciplines, including paleopathology, continue to struggle with questionable ethical practices. The lack of consistent ethical guidelines across the broader discipline is also problematic (Fluehr-Lobban, 2006; Zuckerman et al., 2014). Furthermore, these past misdeeds cannot be erased by shifts in attitudes or even discipline names (e.g., changing the term "physical" anthropology to "biological" anthropology). Regardless of how noble our intentions are, these actions do not change past behaviors and violence perpetrated by our anthropological founding fathers, which continue to resonate into the present. Name changes and calls to decolonize the discipline may make us, as scholars and academics, feel better but it means little to the communities we have harmed for generations and will continue to harm unless we seriously question how, or even if, we have the right to engage with the dead, ancestors, and descendant communities. If we fail to grapple with these underlying and chronic issues then calls for diversity and decolonization will become empty, performative gestures tantamount to placing a band-aid on a purulent, gangrenous wound that has been festering for decades. While a shift in name, such as the American Association of Physical Anthropologists (AAPA) renaming itself the American Association of Biological Anthropologists (AABA), is a cosmetic reflection of how the discipline desires to embrace a new biological anthropology, name changes, as we have seen in the world of corporatized social media, do not modify the processes of behavior associated with an organization. Substantive actions are required for a field that continues to struggle with its past, with diversity, and embracing diverse perspectives.

There are deeper issues that scholars and ambassadors for a new inclusive bioarchaeology and paleopathology should focus on to make concrete, effective changes. The discipline must vocally address and come to terms with its troublesome origins and past, which is painfully enmeshed with grave-robbing, scientific racism, eugenics, preying on the marginalized other, and dehumanization. It must clearly demonstrate, on a unified front, how it has attempted to make amends for past violations and how it will proceed ethically in a manner that is inclusive and values input from descendant communities and communities of care. Furthermore, it must hold scholars who engage in unethical practices accountable, including those that harm the dead and, by proxy, their descendants. To date, the discipline has not done the latter, but it must if it wishes to heal the wounds created by both past and modern scholars. Ultimately, the purpose of this chapter is to discuss and provide suggestions for best ethical practices in bioarchaeology and paleopathology in a manner that will encourage scholars to be ethically conscious about their work and research agendas. This work also serves as a starting point for students, scholars, and the public to better understand the complicated ethical issues that the discipline must disentangle if it wishes to proceed in a manner that is inclusive of all perspectives and includes meaningful descendant community engagement.

The perspectives shared in this chapter will shed light on the problematic issues that plague the discipline and illustrate how we, as scholars in a new and emerging bioarchaeology and paleopathology, have ethical obligations that extend beyond our own research agendas to the broader public. As paleopathologists, our research certainly matters and resonates into the present, especially in the current contexts of social movements, health disparities, and pandemics. We are also in a unique position to use our paleopathological knowledge for the greater good as a tool for social justice. However, to do this, we need to pause and turn our high-powered microscopic lenses back on ourselves and our discipline to re-evaluate its history and our own research practices. For decades we have skirted around deep ethical issues, which is problematic, as we are a discipline that engages with and studies the dead, and for many of us, their descendant communities. Current social and political movements that seek justice for both the living and their deceased ancestors are unfolding before our eyes. In the public sphere, perceptions of our discipline are not favorable, particularly among Black and Brown communities. It is time for us to heed the calls for humanistic change. It will be challenging, as we currently have neither the answers nor the tools for navigation, but we must start the process and develop these tools, skill sets, and policies. If not, the public (particularly marginalized groups) will continue to perceive us as grave-robbers, non-consensual experimenters, and night doctors who violate the postmortem rights of their dead and continue to harm the living.

I suspect what follows in this chapter may make some uncomfortable. I firmly believe that the discipline needs to change, but I also have immense respect for my colleagues, especially those that have mentored me over the years. Therefore, I want to stress that the perspectives presented in this chapter come from my positionality as a scholar of color. Ultimately, I view the history of bioarchaeology and paleopathology and its current practices through this lens. This means my perspectives and experiences in the discipline will be influenced and biased by my positionality as a person of color and by someone raised in culture where the dead play active roles in the lives of the living. However, I wish to stress that the spaces provided by paleopathology have been more welcoming to me than those in the broader discipline of biological anthropology. My hope is that this chapter will provide a starting point for us to do better and to be better scholars, anthropologists, and advocates for the public. As space is limited, very little time will be spent reviewing literature and a discussion will ensue about ethical practices moving forward.

Moving Toward an Ethical Paleopathology and Bioarchaeology

In the past three decades an increasing number of publications, including both edited volumes and articles, have focused on ethics in the broader discipline of biological anthropology and its subdisciplines of bioarchaeology and forensic anthropology (Walker, 2000; Larsen & Walker, 2005; Turner, 2005; Alfonso & Powell, 2007; Lambert, 2012; Passalacqua et al., 2014; DeWitte, 2015; Lambert and Walker, 2018; Passalacqua & Pilloud, 2018; Turner et al., 2018; Squires et al., 2020, 2022; Williams & Ross, 2022). The discipline is also in a state of change as it begins to wrestle with ethics and integrate more theoretical approaches to better understand past individuals' and groups' experiences. This state of flux makes it more malleable and adaptive to change. However, in many ways, our discipline lags behind others, especially in the broader field of anthropology.

The lag is likely due to the fact, as discussed by Larsen and Walker (2005) and reiterated by Zuckerman et al. (2014), that it is only within recent decades that bioarchaeologists have been forced to consider the ethical implications of their work, in part due to the legislative passing of the Native American Graves Protection and Repatriation Act (NAGPRA) (Martin et al., 2013; also see: https://www.nps.gov/subjects/nagpra/index.htm), the growing public awareness of human rights violations, the rise of anti-racism activism, especially in the context of the African Burial Ground (LaRoche & Blakey, 1997; Mack & Blakey, 2004; Blakey, 2010), the painfully recent MOVE debacle (see All Things Considered, 2021; Kassutto, 2021; Levenson, 2021; and The Tucker Law Group, 2021 for information), and the national loss of African American graves through land redevelopment (Dunnavant et al., 2021). Turner et al. (2018:942) also point out that the "formal consideration of ethical norms by professional societies is often triggered by societal events or by allegation of misconduct by practitioners". They illustrate that the AAPA (now the AABA) was spurred to "publish a series of position statements, and eventually establish its own Code of Ethics in 2003" (see https://physanth.org/documents/3/ethics.pdf) by sociopolitical events including Kennewick Man or the Ancient One (McManamon, 2004; Kaestle & Smith, 2005; Owsley & Jantz, 2014), the publication of *The Bell Curve* (Herrnstein and Murray, 1994; Marks, 2005), the removal of teaching the theory of evolution in K-12 curricula, and the creation of the Human Genome Diversity Project (Greely, 1998; Cavalli-Sforza, 2005; Turner et al. 2018:942–943). Prior to the AABA developing its original Code of Ethics, biological anthropologists utilized guidelines from related organizations. In the midst of the above political issues and prior to formulating its ethical guidelines, the AAPA published a statement on the Biological Aspects of Race (see https://physanth.org/about/position-statements/aapa-statement-race-and-racism-2019/; AAPA, 1996:569) signaling to the public and to the membership that there was no place in the discipline for older concepts of "race", especially those that historically have been "used to support racist doctrines" or "foster institutional discrimination". During this same year, in 1996, at the business meeting of the association, it was pointed out that the organization lacked a code of ethics (Turner et al., 2018). This pushed the AAPA to form an ad-hoc committee on ethics and eventually compose a Code of Ethics, which became part of AAPA documentation in 2003 (Turner et al., 2018).

We are currently experiencing renewed calls for ethical reform within anthropology. This push for reformation is once again tied to social events, including the rise of anti-racism movements, calls for an African American Graves Protection and Repatriation Act (Dunnavant et al., 2021), the distressing MOVE events, and increasing demands to decolonize the discipline. Only after the occurrence of these events and the rise in popularity of these movements have anthropological organizations revisited their now outdated ethical guidelines. This is especially true in biological anthropology, where guidelines regarding human remains, or deceased individuals/ancestors, have not been re-evaluated since 2003.

The MOVE issue was especially heartbreaking for me as a scholar of color. In April of 2021, it was revealed by the press that the remains of two child victims associated with the 1985 Philadelphia police bombing of the Black liberation community MOVE were unethically retained by the Penn Museum and being utilized in an online forensics course without consent of their living descendants. The University of Pennsylvania and the Penn Museum retained a law firm to independently examine the issue (The Tucker Law Group, 2021). Their investigation found that the forensic anthropologists involved did not violate professional, ethical, or legal standards; however, their actions demonstrated "poor judgment" and "insensitivity" (The Tucker Law Group, 2021:75). They further stated that "none of the statements of condemnation issued by several…organizations when this controversy arose identified the specific ethical standards of their associations that were violated" and how they might apply to the conduct of the anthropologists involved (The Tucker Law Group, 2021:75). This case and this statement reveal the problematic, outdated ethical issues associated with the discipline. However, more heartbreaking for me as a person of color was reading the comments as the story broke on different news and social media outlets. The sentiments that biological anthropologists were experimenters and were being compared to J. Marion Sims (the mid-19th-century surgeon, known as the "father of gynecology" who practiced techniques on enslaved women without consent or anesthesia), night doctors (18th through 19th-century medical practitioners who dissected and practiced techniques on the remains of African American individuals whose bodies were robbed from graves and/or sold by slave owners), and Nazis, were deeply upsetting. Many in my academic generation had worked to improve ethical approaches in the discipline, but because of old, problematic thought processes and murky legalities that allow for the retention of elements of individuals by forensic anthropologists, our work in the public eye was destroyed. Even more disappointing, especially for scholars of color, was the silence of our flagship association, the AABA, immediately following the reporting of the MOVE fiasco.

This event illustrated to me and other scholars the problematic nature and vagaries of our ethical guidelines. There has been little grappling with the disposition and treatment of deceased individuals beyond the phrase: treat them "with dignity and respect". Everyone agrees that all ancestors should be treated with dignity and respect, but exactly what does this mean? And from whose perspective? How one culture, or even subgroup of a society, defines dignity and respect may differ from another. Certainly, what scientists term "dignity" and "respect" may very well differ from how a community defines dignity and respect. This fact is made evident in our ethical codes that emphasize how "human remains" should be "preserved for future generations" and research on these remains "should be communicated to appropriate groups" (Larsen and Walker, 2005:116). What does this mean? Who are "appropriate groups"? What if descendant communities, either genetic or self-described communities of practice/care, do not wish this? These are very real issues we must begin to address. In the process of doing this, we must be conscious of the history of structural violence in the discipline (including paleopathology), which preyed, and in some respects continues to prey, on the marginalized, the poor, the mentally ill, and the othered.

To start the process of healing and new ethical thinking, we must engage with the history of the discipline. From its origins in scientific racism, to its role in the creation of racial and criminal typologies and eugenics, we must acknowledge that our mother discipline, biological anthropology, was founded on the concept of white superiority. Even 64 years after Samuel Morton's *Crania Americana* and 65 years following the publication of Nott and Glidden's

Types of Mankind, Aleš Hrdlička (1919:18) explicitly stated in the first volume of the *American Journal of Physical Anthropology*:

> The paramount scientific object of Physical Anthropology is the gradual completion, in collaboration with the anatomist, the physiologist, and the chemist, of the study of the normal white man living under ordinary conditions. And our knowledge must not extend to the averages or mean conditions alone, but to the complete range of normal variation of every important feature of the human body, and to the laws governing their correlation. Such knowledge of the white race is eventually indispensable for anthropological comparisons. The goal, however, is still very distant, notwithstanding the results already accomplished. It is necessary to renew and to extend the investigations to every feature, every organ, every function of the white man, until these are known in every detail. The facility and value of all comparative work will increase in direct proportion to the degree of consummation of efforts in this direction. The choice of the white man for the standard is only a matter of most direct concern and convenience; the yellow-brown or the black man would serve equally well, if not better, were we of his blood and were he as readily available.

The discipline would stagnate along these lines for decades, focusing on basic typological categories tied to racialized categories (Caspari, 2003; Marks, 2017; Turner et al. 2018). World War II may have been the first ethical wake-up call in the discipline, when the realization that its methods were being used by Nazi Germany to bolster the belief of the "Aryan Race" and to justify the Final Solution, which resulted in the genocide of millions. Knowledge about unethical Nazi experimentation and sterilization horrified the West, resulting in the passage of the Nuremburg Code in 1947, which established a set of research ethics for experimentation and human subjects that emphasized informed consent, preventing harm in the form of physical and mental suffering, and advocated experimentation for the good of society (Washington, 2006). After World War II, the discipline experienced shifts in its focus, slowly stepping away from racialized approaches to formulating and adopting broader evolutionary approaches. However, we cannot sweep the discipline's past under the rug. Our first goal should be to wrestle with it and decolonize it. In this context, decolonizing bioarchaeology and paleopathology means addressing its unsavory history, taking definitive measures to include perspectives of scholars who come from marginalized and oppressed groups, deconstructing colonial stereotypes, and allowing descendant communities to have active roles in the creation, production, and control of knowledge about their ancestors (Harrison, 1997; Martin et al., 2013; Robertson, 2018; Lans, 2021; Buikstra et al., 2022).

Wrestling With and Decolonizing the Past

The first step toward embracing best ethical practices and decolonizing our field is wrestling with its past. Broadly speaking, biological anthropology and by default bioarchaeology and paleopathology have a complicated past, which has contributed to the (un)ethical issues it struggles with today. I firmly believe this convoluted past can be traced to the Enlightenment Period (1685–1815), which emphasized that reason, rationality, and science could be employed to understand the world and improve humanity. The rise of anthropology as a discipline is strongly linked to this era (Harris, 2001). This is especially true of biological anthropology, as the first racial classification schemes emerged as part of the Enlightenment era. Scientists, including François Bernier, Carolus Linnaeus, Georges-Louis Leclerc, and

Johann Friedrich Blumenbach, eager to understand the physical differences among the new and different groups who were being encountered globally, attempted to classify people into races based on their physical characteristics and geographic locations. However, it was natural theologist and father of modern taxonomy, Carolus Linnaeus, who planted the seeds for scientific racism in his 10th edition of *Systema Naturae*, when he altered his four varieties of humans (*Europaeus albus*, *Americanus rubescens*, *Asiaticus fuscus*, and *Africanus niger*) to include behavioral traits. Now for the first time in history "races" were associated with intellectual qualities and behaviors, with Europeans being the wisest of all humanity. These assertions would persist, inspiring the American School of Ethnology in the 19th century and the Eugenics movement in the 20th century.

Other Enlightenment scientists attempted to classify the human race. Leclerc, who believed that racial variation was linked to environment and cultural beliefs, labeled six "varieties" of humankind (Polar Negro, Tartar, American, Australian, Asiatic, and European). Johann Friedrich Blumenbach, a German anatomist, considered the father of physical anthropology, used craniometrics to separate humans into five races: Caucasian, Mongolian, Malayan, Ethiopian, and American. In the process of creating this classification scheme, Blumenbach managed to acquire 240 skulls from colleagues, by means considered unethical today (Böker, 2018). Blumenbach, like many of his anatomy colleagues (discussed in greater detail below), normalized the process of collecting disembodied parts of people, particularly skulls, for scientific inquiry without consent.

Thus, by default, early biological anthropology and paleopathology (as discussed below) was the "bastard child" of anatomy and medicine, particularly Enlightenment-period medicine (Shapiro, 1959). This era ushered in changes in public perceptions about the dead and medical perceptions about anatomy and disease processes. In Western society, prior to the Enlightenment, the living actively engaged with the dead, whether it was through visiting charnel houses, catacombs, or other areas where the remains of ancestors were visible and tangible (Koudounaris, 2011). The dead were an active part of life, always present and available for comfort and consultation. This changed during the Enlightenment as beliefs about decomposition transformed the dead into unhygienic objects to be hidden from view via burial (Jenner, 2005). Ultimately, on a social level, burying the dead and hiding our ancestors from view culturally reinforced the separation of the living from the dead.

During the Enlightenment Period, the fields of anatomy and medicine also flourished. Increasing emphasis was placed on observation, dissection, demonstration, and the application of the scientific method to comprehend physiology, disease, pathology, and body functions (Porter, 1998; Moore, 2007; Mitchell, 2012). Hypothesis testing replaced antiquated concepts of humoral balances. Dissection became the paramount way to obtain anatomical knowledge of the human form. This shift toward anatomization coincided with clinical treatment of the living and marginalization of the dead. The collecting of human remains became normalized, including the amassment of disembodied parts of people for curation in anatomical cabinets. Anatomists and physicians began to prepare and collect isolated anatomical "specimens" from decedents whose bodies were either robbed from graves or whose social status rendered them powerless to consent. The bodies and body parts of these decedents were competitively collected as dehumanized objects to be prized, valued for their otherness (whether it be cultural affiliation or pathological disease), traded, and displayed in private anatomical cabinets or museums. In many instances, scholars competed with each other to have the largest collection of deceased humans; a practice that continued in early 20th-century America as anthropology's founding fathers, Franz Boas and Aleš Hrdlička, engaged in "skull wars" by non-consensually robbing remains of marginalized and BIPOC individuals to include in their museum collections (Thomas, 2000).

In addition to the dehumanization and objectification of the dead, the emergence of racial classification schemes during the Enlightenment paved the way for scientific racism in the decades that followed. The largest stain on the discipline that continues to have ethical ramifications is anthropology's unsavory ties to the origins of scientific racism, criminal anthropology, and eugenics. In recent years, scholars have discussed this history and the practices of early physical anthropologists (Thomas, 2000; Fabian, 2010; DeWitte, 2015; Redman, 2016). This past continues to resonate in the present as the discipline struggles not only with diversity issues that extend beyond the color line but also with public perceptions.

Guideline I: Challenging Our Past by Engaging With It and Deconstructing It

First, we cannot, as scholars of this discipline, ignore or erase the past misdeeds (or sins) committed by our academic forefathers, upon whose shoulders we sometimes stand. We also cannot alter the history of the field. However, we can atone for the wrongs committed by engaging with the unsavory past of our discipline. This is critical for moving forward. The eras of the past must be addressed with respect to their temporal contexts in which colonial attitudes of superiority, scientific racism, eugenics, and systemic racism were normalized as a part of white Western society. We must proactively speak to these issues in our teaching, research, and public engagement in a manner that clearly conveys that we do not support the biologically deterministic and discriminatory beliefs of past physical anthropologists. We must openly discuss the context of the time period in which these men existed, actively engage with it, address it, teach about it, and *clearly articulate and demonstrate* how we are moving the discipline forward in a way that embraces a new ethically based paleopathology (Blakey, 1998; Blakey, 2008; Martin et al., 2013). This will require changing how we engage with the dead and how we educate the next generation of bioarchaeologists and paleopathologists. However, in order to embrace an ethical and new bioarchaeology and paleopathology, it is *critical* that we discuss, teach, and address this past in a manner that makes it clear to both our students and the public that we are not like our forefathers.

Guideline II: Acknowledging That We Are the Bastard Child of Enlightenment Medicine and Need to Break Free of Our Enlightenment Chains

For generations, we have been comfortable with ideals inherited from the Enlightenment, chiefly the separation of an individual's identity from their physical corpus. This cultural disconnect between the living and the dead in the West continues into the present day. It is reflected in our social construction of the dead and the persons that we study in our discipline. Bioarchaeologists, paleopathologists, and forensic anthropologists often strip persons, groups, or individuals of their identities. Individuals or groups are referred to as "specimens", "populations", "skeletal material", "bones", "corpses", or simply "dead bodies". They are no longer considered people with names or lived experiences. This disconnect has seeped into bioarchaeology and paleopathology, where studies of the body, including the skeleton, exist "between two…conflicting and continually developing, traditions within the discipline" (Sofaer, 2006:1). One is scientifically based, examining the human body metrically and/or assessing age at death, estimating sex, evaluating diet and biodistance, and evidence of pathology (Sofaer, 2006). While human variation is acknowledged in the use of osteologically based methods at the scientific level, individuals lose their identity, becoming objectified as "skeletal remains" and are reduced to the scientific results generated from their skeletal bodies. Sofaer (2006:xiii) acknowledges that these methods are "necessarily fixed, universal and transhistorical in order that the body may be subjected to scientific analysis and comparisons between bodies made" (Sofaer, 2006:xiii). However, not only are one's mortal remains objectified but their identity is also denied, or silenced; they become the embodiment of the pathologies, anomalies, and metric traits observed within them. Thus, an individual's identity ceases to exist and a new identity, predicated on their biology, is formed so that they can be compared to other nameless and identity-less bodies.

According to Soafer (2006:xiii), the other disciplinary tradition, based in social theory, views the "body as a social construction that is contextually and historically produced". However, human remains are rarely addressed, and the focus is more on agency, sociocultural construction, and culturally defined identity. These two very different approaches affect bioarchaeological and paleopathological analyses, as skeletal remains are often separated from their sociocultural, environmental, and historical contexts and reduced to pathological frequencies and case studies. We must break free of our Enlightenment chains and stop separating the identity and social body of an individual from their physical corpus. Both are intimately intertwined; one's social identity and social self, as well as perception of one's social self within society, strongly influences one's cultural interactions in both life and death. To be ethical in a discipline that deals solely with the dead requires embracing a humanistic approach and actively acknowledging that we study individuals. As interpreters of the past, we must do better by abandoning these debasing descriptions that continue to perpetuate the structural violence started by our academic fathers.

How do we move forward ethically? As bioarchaeologists and paleopathologists that regularly interact with the dead, we have a responsibility to treat those we study, as well as their descendant communities, with care and respect. The first step in this process means breaking out of our entrenched thought processes. The individuals that we study are not specimens, materials, or disembodied disease processes. They were actual, living people. The structurally violent Enlightenment-era practice continues today when we sever the social and cultural identity of an individual from their corpus. Thus, to be ethical means reconciling the social with the biological. This requires envisioning the remains of individuals not as separate, disembodied "elements", "specimens", materials, or even samples, but as actual persons with lived experiences. When we remember those close to us who have died, we recollect their lives via rich nuanced memories entrenched in sociocultural identity. Don't those we study deserve the same respect? Death can't eradicate one's humanity.

Guideline III: Restoring the Social and the Biological through Multidimensional Analyses

Many scholars in the discipline have begun to move away, or completely abandon, one-dimensional analyses that simply report paleopathological descriptions, disease frequencies, metrics (this includes forensics), anomalies, and DNA presence (Agarwal & Glencross, 2011; Martin et al., 2013; Watkins & Muller, 2015; Mant & Holland, 2016; de la Cova, 2017, 2019, 2020a, 2020b; Blakey, 2020). To be better ethically based paleopathologists, we need to step away from old descriptive approaches and address broader societal issues at the individual and group level. This does not mean that case studies do not have a place in paleopathology. They most certainly do. However, we need to embrace a new bioarchaeology and paleopathology that strives "to transcend the skeletal body into the realm of lived experience and to make a significant contribution to our understanding of social processes and life in the past"

(Agarwal and Glencross, 2011:3). Key to this is the integration of cross-disciplinary methodologies and theoretical approaches that employ biological, social, behavioral, and ecological research (Blakey, 2008; Agarwal and Glencross, 2011; Cheverko et. al., 2020; de la Cova, 2020b, 2022; DeWitte and Yaussy, 2020; Mant et al., 2021; Buikstra, 2022). Readers will note that many chapters in this volume directly employ these approaches and bring to light innovative and critical ways in which paleopathology enriches our understanding of peoples of the past, not simply the diseases from which they may have suffered. These methods force us to think beyond mortal remains and material culture to identity, lived experience, and the true relationship between biology, social experience, and environmental influences. Adopting humanistic approaches provide us with holistic, multidimensional views of the past that tie directly to historical social injustices of the past and, importantly, to modern day social inequalities (de la Cova, 2019, 2020b, 2022; Blakey, 2020; Lans, 2021; Mant et al., 2021).

Guideline IV: Remember Your Privilege and Positionality

As scholars, we are viewed by the public as elites and specialists. This places us in a position of privilege and power. We have the privilege of a higher education, an opportunity that not all can attain due to economic and other sociocultural constraints. Education provides status, allowing us to generate knowledge. The acquisition and production of knowledge is powerful; it can result in good deeds, elicit change, and inform public policy. However, with knowledge and power comes great responsibility. Our words can be manipulated by the press and public to fit political and social agendas, or can be sensationalized for financial gain (Snoddy et al., 2020). Hence, while our words and work can do good, they can also generate mistrust and cause harm, especially to and within descendant communities.

It is also essential that we critically evaluate and be reflexive about our own biases and our own positionality as we seek to understand the past (Blakey, 1998; Muller, 2020; Watkins, 2020; Buikstra et al., 2022). Critical questions to address include:

- What biases do we have as Western-trained scientists?
- What biases are we bringing to our research that may impact how we collect, analyze, and interpret our data?
- How does our cultural background, our position, and how we interact with society, including how we perceive ourselves and how we feel we are perceived, impact how we position ourselves within the framework of our research, data analyses, and interpretation?

Furthermore, we must ask ourselves if we even have the right to collect, study, and create knowledge among the groups we currently are or may be interested in studying. This is a critical question that many of us are uncomfortable grappling with, but it must be addressed. For years we have assumed that because deceased ancestors and individuals have been obtained in a legal manner, or that we have received permissions at the governmental-level to study certain groups, that this is acceptable. This thinking is ethically problematic. For example, as a scholar who has worked with documented anatomical collections (that is, collections that include the name and often other aspects of the decedant's life) for most of my career, I have recently asked myself whether our discipline has the right to perform research on these individuals as the persons in the Hamann-Todd Human Osteological Collection (comprising 3,100 persons that died in Cleveland, Ohio, between 1893 and 1938), the Robert J. Terry Anatomical Human Skeletal Collection (composed of individuals that died in Missouri from

1910 to 1967), and the William Montague Cobb Collection (which includes persons that died in Washington, D.C. between 1932 and 1969) were non-consensually anatomized and amassed in a dehumanizing manner (de la Cova, 2019, 2020a, 2020b). Although the bodies of the individuals included in these series were obtained in abidance of the law, this does not address ethical considerations of the practice. In other words, just because these persons were legally dissected and curated, it does not make it ethical, or right, that we use their bodies in the pursuit of scientific inquiry. These individuals did not consent to these decisions or actions. They were stripped of the power to advocate or chose their postmortem treatment by virtue of their socioeconomic means, their ancestry, and/or legal status. Thus, the structural violence they experienced in life continued long after their death (Muller et al., 2017; de la Cova, 2012, 2017, 2019, 2020a, 2020b).

Therefore, it is time for us to take a pause in our work to truly evaluate our ethics. This means, as Guideline V will address below, that we need to engage with descendant communities to determine if our work is (a) welcome and (b) contributes to the narratives of the lives of those we study, as well as their descendants. We must stop framing the "good" we do simply around our personal research agendas. Our research should focus on the communities with whom we scientifically engage and should seek to improve lives through the exploration of relationships between health, culture, biology, and environment in both the past and present.

Guideline V: What We Do Matters! We Must Clearly Communicate With the Public and Descendant Communities

If we truly intend to be ethical in our practices, we must communicate clearly not only to the public but also with descendant communities in regard to our research methods and intentions. We must stop relying on "disciplinary-speak" that limits our audience to those extremely familiar with our field. We must convey our work in a manner that is cross-disciplinary and comprehensible to the general public. This is critical if we want our work to assist in the transformation of public policy and benefit descendant and marginalized communities. Openness and clarity with the public about what we do can combat the negative connotations associated with our discipline, especially when scholars violate ethical norms.

We must also *engage* with descendant communities. Descendent groups may be defined genetically or socially as communities of care/practice. Communities of care/practice do not need to be genetically related, but have an emotional, personal, broader ancestry-based, or geographic tie to the ancestors under study. Hence, the researcher must determine what constitutes a descendant community and ensure that it is broad and inclusive and within the context of a project. Once defined, the investigator must commit to initiating and continuing conversations with descendants in order to formulate questions and to determine what responsible and joint actions should be taken regarding the care, treatment, and/or reburial of the ancestors. Descendants must be welcomed in the scientific processes of planning, collecting information, and analyzing and interpreting data if we are to move beyond the singular production of knowledge by settlers, colonizers, and those socially, culturally, and politically imbued with power.

Thomas and Krupa (2021:349–353) discuss, in detail, important ethical questions for bioarchaeologists that paleopathologists should also consider. They assert that, first, determine whether answering your research question truly requires working with human remains. Then ask:

1   What are the wishes of the deceased?
2   What are the wishes of the descendant community/communities?
3   What are the wishes of the local community?
4   What are the wishes of relevant cultural and religious groups?
5   What were the wishes of people who lived during that time period in the region?
6   Deep time should not alter our decisions regarding what is ethical.

Engagement with descendant communities is critical and is rapidly changing bioarchaeological practices. Paleopathology is not exempt from this change. Scholars are now required to address the ethics of their research when submitting to academic journals and applying for grants. Furthermore, they are being queried about how their research engages with and impacts descendant communities. Increasing calls to decolonize the discipline has also resulted in many scholars advocating for cross-disciplinary approaches that integrate theory, while others question whether or not we have the right to study and retain the remains of marginalized others without having conversations with descendants (Robertson, 2018; Lans, 2020; Thomas & Krupa, 2021; Squires et al. 2022; Williams & Ross, 2022).

Hence, the next question is "What is engagement?"; it is not simply informing groups about what you intend to do or sharing your scientific conclusions. Rather, it requires intensive communication and collaboration between researchers and descendant communities. A superb example of engagement was demonstrated by researchers involved in the New York African Burial Ground project (NYABGP): the first ethically engaged bioarchaeology project that employed informed consent and was committed to scientific study alongside the respect for human rights (Blakey, 1998, 2008, 2010; 2020). Blakey utilized a clientage model of public engagement that acknowledged the subjectivity of science and operated on the platform of informed consent, which required all research to be based on the wishes of the self-identified and associated African American descendant community (Blakey, 2008, 2020; Williams & Ross, 2022). According to Blakey (2008:21), two types of clientage emerged from the NYABGP,

> …the descendant community most affected by our research (the ethical client) and the GSA that funds the research (the business client). While both clients have rights that should be protected, the ethical requirements of the field privilege the voices of descendants. Descendants have the right to refuse research entirely and the researcher's obligation is to share what is known about the potential value of bioarchaeological studies.

Hence, in this project, a research design draft was presented to the descendant community to "elicit comment, criticism, and new ideas and questions to which the descendant community was most interested in having answers" (Blakey, 2008:21). This resulted in a stronger research design with more engaging questions that would not have come from researchers alone. Blakey indicates, "A sense of community empowerment, in contrast to the preexisting sense of desecration, was fostered by our collaboration".

I, too, wrestle with these issues in my own work. As mentioned previously, I have worked extensively with the individuals whose remains make up the Hamann-Todd, Terry, and Cobb anatomical collections. While individuals were legally anatomized, it does not make their current disposition ethically sound, in my opinion, as none of the individuals consented to their inclusion in the collections. What, then, are the next ethical steps to take? I have tried my best to do right by these individuals and atone for what happened to them by publishing their stories and struggles, including how their societal marginalization affected both their lived and postmortem experiences (de la Cova, 2019, 2020a, 2020b). They were stripped of their identities; their lives were made to "disappear" through structural violence and social apathy. My goal has been to restore their identities, reconcile their social and biological lives, and to offer immortality so future scholars will not forget who they were, what they suffered, and how their experiences still resonate in present-day marginalized groups. I am also committed to illustrating how factors that created health disparities in the past persist today.

This process has been extraordinarily difficult. I feel, however, that this is the proper approach, but as a female scholar of color, I am also conflicted. Where are the descendants to whom I should reach out for inclusion and guidance? How do I engage a broader community? My goals and intentions have been honest and clear. I have been resolute in my commitment to understand and communicate past injustices, including the biological impact that social movements and marginalization had and continue to have on the poor, the institutionalized, and people of color. Will this lead to change? It must.

Guideline VI: Stop the Perpetual Cycle of Structural Violence

All of the guidelines above address some form of structural violence. If we continue to neglect the identities of the individuals we study and not take a multifaceted approached to reunite their social and biological identities then we are continuing the cycle of structural violence, or what I term **structural apathy.** Refusing to acknowledge the humanity and identities of those we study, denying descendant input, and assuming we have the right to study the dead for the sake of science without adopting a humanistic approach are the very embodiment of structural apathy in our discipline. Structural apathy is more insidious than structural violence, as it is invisible to society and causes harm that spans generations. While we may have been benevolently ignorant of our role in structural apathy, we can no longer partake or perpetuate in it.

It is also critical that we acknowledge, as part of our positionality, that our definition of science and what we deem as ethically appropriate are defined by culture and Westernized values. Thus, science is inherently ethnocentric since it is derived from and confined by Western cultural constructs (see Blakey, 1998). This extends to how we view, construct, interact, define, and study the dead. We must deconstruct our concepts of Western science, particularly those of us who work within other cultures and belief systems. Adhering to Western values and definitions outside of Western cultural contexts is yet another form of structural apathy from which we must break free.

Lastly, our ethical guidelines are outdated and legally murky, especially regarding forensic protocols. While human subject legislation in America may view the individuals we study as specimens because they are not living persons, this does not mean that we must abide by and perpetuate these notions. Furthermore, just because legislation and law enforcement may allow forensic practitioners to retain elements of individuals for over 30 years, with or without permission of close living relatives, this does not mean it is ethical. Legality and ethics are two separate concepts that we all struggle with, depending on the context of our respective situations. Regardless, I assert that both forensic and archaeological individuals should not be used in teaching or research without explicit informed consent from immediate family or permission is obtained from descendant communities.

Perhaps the final point to address is accountability. We must, as a discipline, start holding colleagues accountable for unethical practices. To date, this has not been done. This will be a long conversation within the discipline, but it is time for that conversation to occur. My fear is that if we do not hold individuals accountable for unethical practices, we will continue to be viewed negatively in eyes of the public and BIPOC communities.

Guideline VII: Ethical "Bias" and Fluidity

It is essential that we are aware of our own ethical biases. While ethics are a set of principles guiding us to act morally, we must remember that all ethical systems are culturally based. What I believe is ethical, in a relational manner, is tied to my perceptions and experiences in the world, which in turn is tied to my cultural (and subcultural) beliefs as an American trained scholar (of color). Therefore, there may be times when scholars, researchers, students, and the public are unaware that they are perpetuating or engaging in unethical or inappropriate practices in the eyes of others who do not share their lived experiences. Their decisions and actions are based on naiveté, benevolent ignorance, unconscious bias, or, perhaps, shifting and fluid concepts and definitions of ethical behavior. To avoid these culturally entrenched biases, we must be cognizant of how Western training, culture, and perspectives influence our actions and decisions and how, subsequently, this influences our interactions with the dead. Ethics, and what defines best ethical practices, is culturally constructed and temporally labile. This means that what is considered appropriate ethical behavior by a society will always be in flux as cultural beliefs change through time, which in turn shifts ethical belief systems. Thus, ethics cannot remain static or in a state of stasis. Ethics will change as cultural ethos redefines what is and is not appropriate.

Conclusion

Biological anthropologists, and in turn paleopathologists, are situated to address the relationship between biology, health, environment, identity, and the social conditions of past and current populations. Bones and the diseases, disorders, or forms of biological stress they reflect provide critical insights into social, cultural, and political forces that impact health. The knowledge we acquire transcends understandings of the past by allowing us to connect past injustices and disparities to current inequalities. Our findings have the potential to help combat social marginalization, allow us to better understand epidemiological patterns of disease and nutritional stress, and reveal the biological impact of racism. Thus, bioarchaeology can contribute to a broader and deeply contextual dialogue on social justice.

However, to do this, we must uncomfortably move out of the shadow of our past into an ethical future. As anthropologists, our work extends beyond the "samples" we study. We have a responsibility to the public and to the communities with whom we work. If we are doing research solely to advance our careers or to gain knowledge for knowledge's sake alone then it may be time to re-evaluate what it means to be an anthropologist. As we move into a new era, gathering paleopathological and paleoepidemiological data simply to comply with a research agenda despite potential ethical issues is problematic. This is self-serving and perpetuates ethnocentric colonial approaches that enhance the power within which our academic forefathers operated and flourished. It also continues the cycle of structural apathy. The time has come for us to break this cycle.

This chapter has laid out ethical guidelines, which I hope instigates important discussions about why and how we must move forward with a more ethically-based paleopathology that benefits descendants of the individuals we study and humanity as a whole. As scientists we have a responsibility to the public to improve the human condition. We have an obligation, as a discipline, to change the world for the better.

References

AAPA. (1996). AAPA statement on biological aspects of race. *American Journal of Physical Anthropology*, 101(4), 569–570. https://doi.org/10.1002/ajpa.1331010408.

Agarwal, S. C. & Glencross, B. A. (2011). *Social Bioarchaeology*. John Wiley & Sons.

Alfonso, M. P. & Powell, L. (2007). Ethics of flesh and bone, or ethics in the practice of paleopathology, osteology and bioarchaeology. In Cassman, V., Odegaard, N. & Powell, J. (Eds.), *Human Remains: Guide for Museums and Academic Institutions*, pp. 5–19. Alta Mira Press.

All Things Considered. (2021, April 27). Penn museum apologizes for 'unethical possession of human remains'. National Public Radio. Last accessed May 2022 at: https://www.npr.org/2021/04/27/988972736/penn-museum-apologizes-for-unethical-possession-of-human-remains.

Blakey, M. L. (1998) Beyond European enlightenment: toward a critical and humanistic human biology. In Goodman, A. H. & Leatherman, T. L. (Eds.), *Building a New Biocultural Synthesis: Political-Economic Perspectives on Human Biology*, pp. 379–405. University of Michigan Press.

Blakey, M. L. (2008). An ethical epistemology of publicly engaged biocultural research. In Haau, J., Fawcett, C. & Matsunaga, J. M. (Eds.), *Evaluating Multiple Narratives: Beyond Nationalist, Colonialist, Imperialist Archaeologies*, pp. 17–28. Springer.

Blakey, M. L. (2010). African burial ground project: paradigm for cooperation? *Museum International* 62(1&2):61–68.

Blakey, M. L. (2020) Archaeology under the blinding light of race. *Current Anthropology* 61(S22):S183–S197. https://doi.org/10.1086/710357.

Böker, W. (2018) Blumenbach's collection of human skulls. In Rupke, N. G. & Lauer (Eds.), *Johann Friedrich Blumenbach: Race and Natural History*, pp. 1750–1850. Routledge. 10.4324/9781315184777.

Buikstra, J. E., DeWitte, S. N., Agarwal, S. C., Baker, B. J., Bartelink, E. J., Berger, E., & Zakrzewski, S. R. (2022). Twenty-first century bioarchaeology: taking stock and moving forward. *Yearbook of Biological Anthropology* Early View:1–61. https://doi.org/10.1002/ajpa.24494.

Caspari, R. (2003). From types to populations: a century of race, physical anthropology, and the American Anthropological Association. *American Anthropologist* 105(1):65–76.

Cavalli-Sforza, L. L. (2005). The human genome diversity project: past, present and future. *Nature Reviews Genetics* 6(4):333–340.

Cheverko, C. M., Prince-Buitenhuys, J. M. & Hubbe, M. (2020). *Theoretical Approaches in Bioarchaeology*. Routledge.

de la Cova, C. (2012) Patterns of trauma and violence in 19th-century-born African American and Euro-American females. *International Journal of Paleopathology* 2(2–3):61–68.

de la Cova, C. (2017). Fractured lives: structural violence, trauma, and recidivism in urban and institutionalized 19th-century-born African Americans and Euro-Americans. In Tegemeyer, C. & Martin, D. (Eds.), *Broken Bones, Broken Bodies: Bioarchaeological and Forensic Approaches for Accumulative Trauma and Violence*, pp. 153–180. Lexington Press.

de la Cova, C. (2019). Marginalized bodies and the construction of the Robert J. Terry anatomical skeletal collection: a promised land lost. In Mant, M. & Holland, A. J. (Eds.), *Bioarchaeology of Marginalized People*, pp. 133–155. Elsevier Academic Press. https://doi.org/10.1016/C2017-0-02300-5.

de la Cova, C. (2020a). Processing the destitute and deviant dead: inequality, dissection, politics, and the structurally violent legalization of social marginalization in American anatomical collections. In Osterholtz, A. J. (Ed.), *The Poetics of Processing: Memory Formation, Identity, and the h]Handling of the Dead*, pp. 212–234. University Press of Colorado.

de la Cova, C. (2020b). Making silenced voices speak: restoring neglected and ignored identities in anatomical collections. In Cheverko, C. M., Prince-Buitenhuys, J. M. & Hubbe, M. (Eds.), *Theoretical Approaches in Bioarchaeology*, pp. 150–169. Routledge.

de la Cova, C. M. (2022). Ethical issues and considerations for ethically engaging with the Robert J. Terry, Hamann-Todd, and William Montague Cobb anatomical collections. *American Journal of Biological Anthropology* 177(S73): 42.

DeWitte, S. N. (2015) Bioarchaeology and the ethics of research using human skeletal remains, *History Compass* 13:10–19. DOI: 10.1111/hic3.12213.

DeWitte, S. & Yaussy, S. (2020). Bioarchaeological applications of intersectionality. In Cheverko, C. M., Prince-Buitenhuys, J. R. & Hubbe, M. (Eds.), *Theoretical Approaches in Bioarchaeology*, pp. 45–58. Routledge.

Dunnavant, J., Justinvil, D. & Colwell, C. (2021). Craft an African American Graves Protection and Repatriation Act. *Nature* 593:337–340. https://doi.org/10.1038/d41586-021-01320-4.

Fabian, A. (2010). *The Skull Collectors: Race, Science, and America's Unburied Dead*. University of Chicago Press.

Fluehr-Lobban, C. (2006). *Race and Racism: An Introduction*. Rowman & Littlefield.

Greely, H. T. (1998). Legal, ethical, and social issues in human genome research. *Annual Review of Anthropology* 27:473–502. https://doi.org/10.1146/annurev.anthro.27.1.473.

Harris, M. (2001). *The Rise of Anthropological Theory: A History of Theories of Culture*. AltaMira Press.

Harrison, F. (1997) *Decolonizing Anthropology: Moving Further Toward an Anthropology for Liberation* (2nd ed.). American Anthropological Association and Association of Black Anthropologists.

Herrnstein, R. J. & Murray, C. A. (1994). *The Bell Curve: Intelligence and Class Structure in American Life*. Free Press.

Hrdlička, A. (1919). Physical anthropology: its scope and aims: its history and present status in America. *American Journal of Physical Anthropology* 1(2):133–182.

Jenner, M. (2005). Death, decomposition and dechristianisation? Public health and church burial in Eighteenth-Century England. *The English Historical Review* 120(487):615–632. http://www.jstor.org/stable/3489409.

Kaestle, F. & Smith, D. G. (2005). Working with ancient DNA: NAGPRA, Kennewick Man, and other ancient peoples. In Turner, T. R. (Ed.), *Biological Anthropology and Ethics: From Repatriation to Genetic Identity*, pp. 241–262. SUNY Press.

Kassutto, M. (2021, April 21). Remains of children killed in MOVE bombing sat in a box at Penn Museum for decades. Last Accessed May 2022 at: https://billypenn.com/2021/04/21/move-bombing-penn-museum-bones-remains-princeton-africa/.

Koudounaris, P. (2011). *Empire of Death: A Cultural History of Ossuaries and Charnel Houses*. Thames & Hudson.

Lambert, P. M. (2012). Ethics and issues in the use of human skeletal remains in paleopathology. In Grauer, A. L. (Ed.), *Companion to Paleopathology*, pp. 17–33. Wiley-Blackwell.

Lambert, P. M. & Walker, P. L. (2018). Bioarchaeological ethics: perspectives on the use and value of human remains in scientific research. In Katzenberg, M. A. & Grauer, A. L. (Eds.), *Biological Anthropology of the Human Skeleton* (3rd ed.), pp. 1–42. Wiley-Blackwell. DOI: https://doi.org/10.1002/9781119151647.ch1.

Lans, A. M. (2021). Decolonize this collection: integrating black feminism and art to re-examine human skeletal remains in museums. *Feminist Anthropology* 2(1):130–142.

LaRoche, C. J. & Blakey, M. L. (1997). Seizing intellectual power: the dialogue at the New York African Burial Ground. *Historical Archaeology* 31(3):84–106.

Larsen, C. S. & Walker, P. L. (2005). The ethics of bioarchaeology. In Turner, T. R. (Ed.). *Biological Anthropology and Ethics: from Repatriation to Genetic Identity*, pp. 11–119. SUNY Press.

Levenson, M. (2021, May 15). Discovery of bones from MOVE bombing jolts Philadelphia once again. *New York Times*. Last Accessed May 2022 at: https://www.nytimes.com/2021/05/15/us/philadelphia-move-bombing-cremation.html.

Mack, M. E. & Blakey, M. L. (2004). The New York African Burial Ground Project: past biases, current dilemmas, and future research opportunities. *Historical Archaeology* 38(1):10–17. http://www.jstor.org/stable/25617128.

Mant, M. & Holland, A. (2016). *Beyond the Bones: Engaging with Disparate Data Sets*. Academic Press.

Mant, M., de la Cova, C., & Brickley, M. B. (2021). Intersectionality and trauma analysis in bioarchaeology. *American Journal of Physical Anthropology* 74: 583–594. DOI: https://doi.org/10.1002/ajpa.24226

Marks, J. (2005). Anthropology and the bell curve. In Besteman, C. & Gusterson, H. (Eds.), *Why America's Top Pundits Are Wrong: Anthropologists Talk Back*, pp. 206–228. University of California Press. https://doi.org/10.1525/9780520938489-011.

Marks, J. (2017). *Is Science Racist?* John Wiley & Sons.

Martin, D. L., Harrod, R. P. & Pérez, V. R. (2013). *Bioarchaeology: An Integrated Approach to Working with Human Remains*. Springer New York.

McManamon, F. P. (2004). *Kennewick Man*. National Park Service, U.S. Department of the Interior. Last accessed May 2022 at: https://www.nps.gov/archeology/kennewick/index.htm.

Mitchell, P. (2012). *Anatomical Dissection in Enlightenment England and Beyond: Autopsy, Pathology and Display* (1st ed.). Routledge. https://doi.org/10.4324/9781315566962.

Moore, W. (2007). *The Knife Man: Blood, Body Snatching, and the Birth of Modern Surgery*. Crown.

Muller, J. L. (2020). Reflecting on a more inclusive historical bioarchaeology. *Historical Archaeology* 54:202–211. DOI: https://doi.org/10.1007/s41636-019-00222-7.

Muller, J., Pearlstein, K. & de la Cova, C. (2017). Dissection and documented skeletal collections: embodiments of legalized inequality. In Nystrom, K. (Ed.), *The Bioarchaeology of Dissection and Autopsy in the United States*, pp. 185–201. Springer.

Owsley, D. W. & Jantz, R. L. (2014). *Kennewick Man: The Scientific Investigation of an Ancient American skeleton*. Texas A&M University Press.

Passalacqua, N. V. & Pilloud, M. A. (2018). *Ethics and Professionalism in Forensic Anthropology*. Academic Press.

Passalacqua, N. V., Pilloud, M. A. & Gruters, G. A. (2014). Professionalism: ethics and scholarship in forensic science. *Journal of Forensic Sciences* 59:573–575.

Porter, R. (1998). *The Greatest Benefit to Mankind: A Medical History of Humanity*. W. W. Norton.

Redman, S. J. (2016). *Bone Rooms*. Harvard University Press.

Robertson, H. (2018). Decolonizing bioarchaeology: an autoethnographic reflection. *New Proposals: Journal of Marxism and Interdisciplinary Inquiry* 9(2):19–33.

Shapiro, H. L. (1959). The History and development of physical anthropology. *American Anthropologist* 61(3):371–379. http://www.jstor.org/stable/667203.

Snoddy, A. M. E., Beaumont, J., Buckley, H. R., Colombo, A., Halcrow, S. E., Kinaston, R. L & Vlok, M. (2020). Sensationalism and speaking to the public: scientific rigour and interdisciplinary collaborations in Palaeopathology. *International Journal of Paleopathology* 28:88–91. https://doi.org/10.1016/j.ijpp.2020.01.003.

Sofaer, J. R. (2006). *The Body as Material Culture: A Theoretical Osteoarchaeology*. Cambridge University Press.

Squires, K., Errickson, D. & Márquez-Grant, N. (2020). *Ethical Approaches to Human Remains: A Global Challenge in Bioarchaeology and Forensic Anthropology*. Springer Nature.

Squires, K., Roberts, C. A. & Márquez-Grant, N. (2022). Ethical considerations and publishing in human bioarcheology. *American Journal of Biological Anthropology* 177(4):615–619. https://doi.org/10.1002/ajpa.24467.

The Tucker Law Group. (2021). The Odyssey of the MOVE Remains: Report of the Independent Investigation Into the Demonstrative Display of MOVE Remains at the Penn Museum and Princeton University, August 20, 2021.

Thomas, D. H. (2000). *Skull Wars: Kennewick Man, Archaeology, and the Battle for Native American Identity*. Basic Books.

Thomas, J. & Krupa, K. L. (2021). Bioarchaeological ethics and considerations for the deceased. *Human Rights Quarterly* 43(234):4–354. DOI: 10.1353/hrq.2021.0022.

Turner, T. R. (2005). *Biological Anthropology and Ethics: From Repatriation to Genetic Identity*. SUNY Press.

Turner, T. R., Wagner, J. K. & Cabana, G. S. (2018). Ethics in biological anthropology. *American Journal of Physical Anthropology* 165(4): 939–951. https://doi.org/10.1002/ajpa.23367.

Walker, P. L. (2000). Bioarchaeological ethics: a historical perspective on the value of human remains. In Katzenberg, M. A. & Saunders, S. R. (Eds.), *Biological Anthropology of the Human Skeleton*. pp. 3–39. Wiley-Liss.

Washington, H. A. (2006). *Medical Apartheid: the Dark History of Medical Experimentation on Black Americans from Colonial Times to the Present*. Doubleday.

Watkins, R. J. (2020). An alter(ed)native perspective on historical bioarchaeology. *Historical Archaeology* 54:17–33. https://doi.org/10.1007/s41636-019-00224-5.

Watkins, R. & Muller, J. (2015), Repositioning the Cobb human archive: the merger of a skeletal collection and its texts. *American Journal of Human Biology* 27(1):41–50. https://doi.org/10.1002/ajhb.22650.

Williams, S. E. & Ross, A. H. (2022). Ethical dilemmas in skeletal collection utilization: implications of the Black Lives Matter movement on the anatomical and anthropological sciences. *Anatomical Record* 305(4):860–868. https://doi.org/10.1002/ar.24839.

Zuckerman, M., Kamnikar, K. & Mathena, S. (2014). Recovering the 'body politic': a relational ethics of meaning for bioarchaeology. *Cambridge Archaeological Journal* 24(3):513–522. DOI: 10.1017/S0959774314000766.

22
SYNTHESIZING STRESS IN PALEOPATHOLOGICAL PERSPECTIVE

Theory, Method, Application

Daniel H. Temple and Haagen D. Klaus

The vertebrate skeletal system embodies a legacy of nearly half a billion years of evolution (Hall, 2015). Skeletal tissue was once seen as a simple biological construct, providing mostly a rigid body structure and a calcium reservoir. Current perspectives reveal the skeleton to host previously unknown and functionally profound interactions with the brain and peripheral nervous systems, immune function, gut health, inflammation, and more (Crespo, 2021; Guder et al., 2020). Vertebrate skeletal tissue interacts with, and can be disrupted by, external stressors and commonality in this experience is demonstrated in the physiological pathways that operate in response to stress across vertebrate taxa (Crespi & Denver, 2005; Thayer et al., 2018). This body of research suggests that changes in skeletal phenotypes attributable to stress illustrate physiological responses that reflect deep homologies among vertebrata and that the shared characters of skeletal tissue provide an important opportunity to document these experiences in the human past. This begins with the observation and recording of abnormal states of tissue loss or formation. Proper theorization and contextualization of stress-related lesions is then foundational for the development of more rigorous, scientific, and insightful approaches in paleopathology – especially regarding accurate and perceptive interpretations of what skeletal pathological conditions represent.

This chapter explores the physiological, theoretical, and methodological study of stress in paleopathology and helps develop models introduced by previous research (Huss-Ashmore et al., 1982; Goodman et al., 1988; Temple & Goodman, 2014; Temple & Edes, 2022) within paleopathological contexts. These works established a series of skeletal indicators of stress (Figure 22.1) and theoretical models for interpretation. This chapter has five sections, and each sequentially builds upon the previous section. The work opens with an overview of the conceptualization of "stress" in human biology. The second section discusses the basic physiological "nuts and bolts" of stress response mechanisms on the organismal level. This is followed by an overview of how stress translates into observable skeletal phenotypes and pathological conditions. The fourth section proposes a working model of systemic stress for paleopathology and bioarchaeology. The chapter closes with thoughts on future directions for the paleopathological study of systemic stress and skeletal disease.

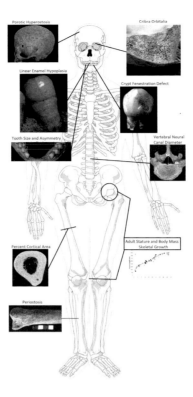

Figure 22.1 Commonly used phenotypic alterations associated with stress experience in paleopathology. Photos: DHT and HDK.

Stress in Human Biology

Stress, Homeostasis, and Allostasis

Stress is traditionally defined as a *disruption of physiological homeostasis caused by an external agent* (Huss-Ashmore et al., 1982; Goodman et al., 1988). The concept of homeostasis was derived from the term *interior milieu*, which referenced the capacity to maintain physiological stability despite unpredictable environmental conditions (Bernard, 1865). This concept was later modified through experimental studies that clarified relatively constant physiological states that shifted in response to environment (Cannon, 1915, 1932). By 1936, many of these ideas saw further development in the extensive and highly impactful body of work of Hans Selye (Jackson, 2014). Selye (1936) reported that a variety of disruptions to physiological homeostasis prompted a common response associated with the actions of the hypothalamic–pituitary–adrenal (HPA) axis. This response occurs according to a triphasic process reflecting alarm, resistance, and exhaustion (Selye, 1936).

The first phase, alarm, engages the HPA axis and stimulates secretion of adrenaline and cortisol. This is followed by the second phase, resistance, in which elevated glucose levels and increased blood pressure persist as the body attempts a return to homeostasis. Should stress fail to abate, a third phase, exhaustion, will emerge where morbidity and mortality risk elevates. This work had three primary arguments that formed the basis of stress research for the past century (Selye, 1946): first, physiological disruption is undergirded by the tripartite response and is found across vertebrates. Second, this response is demonstrative of adaptation energy – which elicits survival in response to stress but may reduce the capacity for survival at later stages. Finally, the general adaptation syndrome was defined as the sum of all bodily reactions to non-specific stress events that produces a kind of "wear and tear" over the lifetime.

Later studies emphasized the cumulative impacts of ecological and cultural conditions of stress on general health against contexts such as drastic transformation and inequality (Cassel & Tyroler, 1961; Toffler, 1970). However, the bigger argument associated with the general adaptation syndrome posited that cumulative adversity promoted greater risk of morbidity and mortality across the lifespan (Selye, 1946). Contemporary approaches to the study of stress argue that organisms experience near-daily fluctuations away from homeostasis across organ systems and have dubbed these fluctuations allostasis (Sterling, 2012). Allostatic states end when stressors are removed, though these states may be repeatedly entered or exist as continuous states if organisms fail to achieve homeostasis. Allostatic load defines the cumulative impact of allostasis across the life course which may increase risk of morbidity and mortality (McEwen & Stellar, 1993; McEwen & Wingfield, 2003). Cortisol is one of the primary hormones contributing to allostatic load (Sapolsky, 1998). However, allostatic load is now measured using more than five dozen biomarkers, and relationships with morbidity and mortality are well established (Edes & Crews, 2017).

In addition, theoretical advancements in the study of stress emphasize a life history perspective. These ideas are best represented in the theoretical perspectives surrounding the concept of allostasis and allostatic load as well as the Developmental Origins of Health and Disease (DOHaD). DOHaD is a quasi-academic discipline that references relationships between the conditions of early life (ranging from fetal to infancy and childhood) and relationships with morbidity and mortality at later ages (Barker & Osmond, 1986; Barker et al., 1989; and see Chapter 28, this volume). These studies contributed to the development of the thrifty phenotype hypothesis which predicts that individuals survive neonatal stress through energy sparing but are at a greater risk of metabolic disease at later stages of life (Bateson et al., 2004). Further theoretical development integrated these findings within life history theory (LHT). Using the role of cortisol in the stress response as an example, it is demonstrated that the HPA axis promotes short-term survival for the individual, with long-term consequences in terms of reduced investment in growth, maintenance, and reproduction (Worthman & Kuzara, 2005).

Physiological Mechanisms of Stress

The first component of a stress response involves perception of an acute or chronic stressor, whether it is a conscious or unconscious function of the central nervous system. The first act is undertaken by the HPA axis, which releases corticotropic-releasing hormone (CRH) from the hypothalamus into the anterior pituitary to release adrenocorticotropic-releasing hormone (ACTH) from the anterior pituitary into systemic circulation (Charmandari et al., 2005). ACTH subsequently triggers release of mineralocorticoids and glucocorticoids into systemic circulation from the adrenal cortices to regulate blood plasma volume, electrolyte balance, and blood pressure (Everly & Lating, 2013).

While the HPA axis is active, the hypothalamus engages the sympathetic-adrenal-medullary (SAM) axis to secrete catecholamines from the adrenal medulla to increased blood pressure and heart rate, release free fatty acids, and decreased blood flow to currently nonessential tissues (e.g., skin, gastrointestinal, and kidneys), further readying an organism for confrontation with the stressor through either fight or flight (Everly & Lating, 2013). Catecholamines also enhance emotional memory formation allowing future anticipatory responses to stressors (McEwen, 2004; Korte et al., 2005). The posterior pituitary, thyroid, and somatotropic axes are activated during stress responses. The posterior pituitary stimulates release of vasopressin/antidiuretic hormone (ADH) to further modulate blood pressure (Everly & Lating, 2013), while the hypothalamus drives the anterior pituitary to release thyroid-stimulating hormone (TSH) elevating basal metabolic rate (Seaward, 2006). The anterior pituitary also releases somatotropic hormone (human growth hormone) for tasks that remain uncertain.

Testosterone, oxytocin, and prolactin play roles in stress responses as well (Everly & Lating, 2013). While acute stress may increase testosterone production, chronic stress lowers it (Kalantaridou et al., 2010) to potentially inhibit reproduction (Charmandari et al., 2005). Luteinizing hormones are similarly downregulated by glucocorticoids, reducing sexual receptivity (Carter, 2002). Androgens reduce oxytocin production in response to stressors and negatively influence maternal behavior, pair bonding, aggression behavior, and fear responses and reducing sympathetic nervous system activity to lower fear responses. Beyond neuroendocrine and sex hormone activity, stress responses also involve release of albumin (Murata et al., 2004), C-reactive protein (Hostinar et al., 2015), dehydroepiandrosterone-sulfate (Buford & Willoughby, 2008), inflammatory cytokines interleukin-6 (IL6) and tumor necrosis factor-α (TNF-α) (Hostinar et al., 2015), luteinizing hormone (Kalantaridou et al., 2010), oxytocin (Taylor et al., 2000), prolactin (Lennartsson & Jonsdottir, 2011), and lipids and lipoproteins (Steptoe & Brydon, 2005) that represent activity occurring far beyond the boundaries of just the HPA axis and secretion of cortisol.

Translations of Stress in the Skeleton

Infection and Disease

Infection is not equivalent to disease. Variations of pathogenicity, transmission mechanism, and host response are mediating factors. Therefore, the inabilities of the body to defend against, mitigate, or otherwise eliminate chronic and lower mortality infectious process has long been interpreted as a broad reflection of a systemically stressed physiology and immune response. In settings where high mortality processes are at play (e.g., bubonic plague, see Chapter 31, this volume), differential patterns of survivorship are more reflective of stressed physiologies. There is also natural underlying heterogeneity of human immune responses to the same stressors, including our inflammatory phenotypes (Crespo, 2020).

Skeletal diseases tend to be a manifestation of stress that has opened the door to some downstream disease state. That is, many skeletal lesions are symptoms of stress, and often not the cause of it. Yet, this can be more complicated, since when a disease state is entered, it can produce feedback relationships exacerbating extant states of physiological stress. Examples of this include the process of hematogenous dissemination of bacteria from an osteomyelitic focus or the spread of tuberculosis across multiple tissue types and sites where the progression of disease contributes to its spread and then intensifies that stress.

Specific infectious diseases such as tuberculosis, leprosy (see Chapter 17,, this volume), syphilis (Baker, this volume), osteomyelitis, and other disorders (see Chapter 18, this volume) have long been in the paleopathological spotlight as reflections of biological stress. Perhaps the most commonly observed form of chronic abnormal bone disease in archaeological skeletons is periostosis. Periostosis is most commonly observed on the tibiae and represents a non-specific, formative response to an infectious condition. However, differential diagnoses of unilateral periosteal lesions are suggestive of isolated events (traumatic impact to the shin). Especially when conditions such as hypertrophic (pulmonary) osteoarthropathy, melorheostosis, fluorosis, and other conditions can be reasonably ruled out, bilateral periosteal manifestations are indicative of a systemic process most commonly linked to infectious organisms in the *Staphylococcus* or *Streptococcus* genera (Roberts, 2019).

Infection-related periostosis likely manifests in the wake of systemic infection following an inflammatory response that activates the periosteal membrane – the thin, fibrous connective tissue that tightly adheres to bone surfaces. The innermost layer of the periosteum is the cambium, and it possesses an osteogenic capacity (Ito et al., 2001). The cambium can be perturbed by a variety of stressors, such as infection, trauma, and venous stasis. In response, fibroblasts differentiate into osteogenic precursor cells and, eventually, mature osteoblasts to produce new, reactive pathological bone (Resnick, 2002). Persistent infection promotes a sustained inflammatory response where mononuclear leukocytes, neutrophils, and fibroblasts migrate to an infection site and, among other effects, produce pus. Subsequent accumulation of interstitial pressure between the bone and periosteal membrane can compress, stretch, and tear capillaries. Extravagated blood produces hematomas, and hematomas in the periosteal envelope are organized into reactive new bone (Ragsdale & Lehmer, 2011).

Not all bones are equal in their osteogenic potential, and even a single bone varies in osteogenic potential by anatomical region (Gallay et al., 1994). However, the tibia may be particularly sensitive to chronic infection. It is the least vascularized area of the entire body, has less intervening soft tissue between it and the outside environment, is slow to mount an immune response, and its diaphysial periosteum possesses an elevated osteogenic potential (Gallay et al., 1994). Moreover, the prevalence abnormal tibial reactions frequently increase in settings of elevated stress, population density, increasing sedentism, socioeconomic marginalization, and other negative biocultural changes such that the presence of the bilateral periostosis has been widely used to make baseline inferences about ancient health, biological stress, immunocompetence, and community-level stress buffering systems (Larsen, 2015).

Nutrient Deficiencies

Cribra orbitalia and porotic hyperostosis are morphological syndromes that arise as downstream products secondary to chronic anemias and in response to a functional need to increase the surface area of hematopoietic marrow. Anemia can be a result of blood loss, impaired erythropoiesis (red blood cell [RBC] production), parasitism, hemolysis (RBC destruction), and other factors (Walker et al., 2009; Kumar et al., 2020). Under any of these conditions, chronic anemia may generate a state of delinquent oxygen transport and hypoxia. To compensate, the kidneys secrete the hormone erythropoietin (Stockmann & Fandrey, 2006) elevating RBC production and accelerating cellular maturation.

Sustained erythropoietin production stimulates hematopoietic marrow hypertrophy (Stockman & Fandrey, 2006). Associated lesions are observed in the form of abnormal porosity of the superior orbits (cribra orbitalia) and cranial vault surface (porotic hyperostosis). In the human skeleton, red marrow resides in multiple sites, and importantly, it changes in distribution throughout the life course (Brickley, 2018). RBC production first begins in the yolk sack, then moves to the spleen, liver, and eventually, fetal bone marrow. In preadults, marrow spaces in the mandible, cranial vault, and long bones take over the work, and in the adult skeleton, erythropoiesis shifts mostly to trabecular spaces of the vertebrae, sternum, and ribs (Hoffbrand & Lewis, 1981; Brickley, 2018). Under conditions of chronic anemia, nearly all expressions of marrow hypertrophy are contained in the long bones without eliciting macroscopic changes (exceptions include genetic anemias such as thalassemia major or sickle cell disease) (Ortner, 2003). Yet, the cranium possesses a much thinner lamellar bone surface and expansion of the diploë is directional – outward and away from the brain. The resulting pressure exerted from within the diploë upon the outer table activates osteoclasts to remove bone so that the porous morphology of expanding marrow space becomes visible. Diverse clinical and anatomical studies demonstrate that porotic hyperostosis reflects chronic anemia (see citations in Walker et al. 2009; also, Ortner, 2003). In skeletal remains, abnormal orbital and vault porosity reflects childhood metabolic disruption, particularly since red hematopoietic marrow in the diploë converts to fatty yellow marrow beginning around age ten years (Brickley, 2018; Lewis, 2018). Active lesions are observed most frequently in the remains of preadults, but due to the lack of functional demand for cranial remodeling, the "scars" of childhood anemia in the form of inactive porotic features may persist for decades in the adult cranium.

The etiology of porotic hyperostosis was historically attributed to iron deficiency anemia (Stuart-Macadam, 1992). Today, it is clear that a far more intricate range of conditions is likely. Walker et al. (2009) contend that chronically deficient iron status actually inhibits erythropoiesis and that hemolytic anemias, vitamin B_9 and B_{12} anemias, and megaloblastic anemias are most likely the root causes of porotic hyperostosis. Nevertheless, iron deficiency anemia remains a plausible etiology for porous cranial lesions as a chronic lack of iron bioavailability may also produce ineffective erythropoiesis and result in a comparable morphological syndrome (Oxenham & Cavill, 2010). Other work points to parasitic and diarrheal diseases (Kent, 1986) and malarial infection (Smith-Guzmán, 2015), though lesions related to scurvy may be varyingly distinguished from marrow hypertrophy by both histological (Wapler et al., 2004) and macroscopic (Klaus, 2017) methods.

Another area of debate involves whether or not vault lesions share a common pathogenesis with orbital lesions. While some have reasoned that orbital lesions represent a chronologically earlier expression of anemia, more recent work proposes that vault and orbital lesions represent different *types* of anemia. Cribra orbitalia is also linked to marrow hypoplasia (caused by chronic diseases, aplastic/endocrine anemias, and renal failure), while vault lesions are generated by marrow hyperplasia (megaloblastic and hemolytic anemias) (Rivera & Mirazón Lahr, 2017).

Vitamin C and D deficiencies, once neglected stress markers, have garnered major attention over the last two decades (Ortner & Mays, 1998; Ortner, 2003; Brickley & Ives, 2008; Crandall & Klaus, 2014b; Lewis, 2018; Snoddy et al., 2018, and see Chapter 19, this volume). All human beings are susceptible to vitamin C deficiency, owing to a common mutation of the gene that produces l-gluno-γ-lactone oxidase, which is the final enzyme needed to synthesize ascorbic acid, or vitamin C (Nishikimi & Udenfriend, 1977). Obtaining at least 10 mg/day of dietary vitamin C is required. If sufficient quantities are not ingested, substandard Type I collagen formation promotes the production of defective osteoid, fragile blood vessels prone to rupture, and periosteal membranes with a propensity to tear. Hemorrhage is thus a hallmark of scurvy. Outside the circulatory system, the body treats blood as an inflammatory substance. Bleeding adjacent to bone surfaces stimulates incursion of osteoclasts into existing cortical bone that creates channels for newly formed capillaries usually less than 1 mm in diameter (Ortner et al., 1999), which are pathways for removal of hemorrhagic blood. Should hemorrhage elevate the periosteum, hematomas are progressively organized into abnormal hypertrophic bone (Ragsdale and Lehmer, 2012).

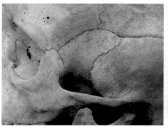 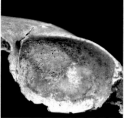 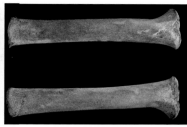

Figure 22.2 Scurvy is an increasingly scrutinized indicator of preadult biological stress in paleopathology. A chronic insufficiency of vitamin C leads to production of subperiosteal hemorrhages and osseous responses to inflammation in multiple anatomic sites, such as abnormal porosity of the greater wing of the sphenoid bone (left; Chornancap South Platform Burial 2, Late pre-Hispanic period, Peru; CNS Burial U4AE-2, Colonial Period, Peru), abnormal formation of heterotrophic bone on the orbits (center), and abnormal new bone formation on limb bones (right; CNS Burial U3-91, Colonial Period, Peru). Photos: HDK.

Common skeletal sites associated with scurvy, particularly in preadults, include the orbits, ecto- and endocranial regions of the cranial vault, alveolar bone, the hard palate, and the posterior maxilla and mandible (Figure 22.2) (Ortner et al., 1999; Klaus, 2014b; Snoddy et al., 2018). Ortner et al. (1999) argued abnormal bilateral porosity of the greater wing of the sphenoid bone is virtually pathognomonic for scurvy. Endocranially, scurvy can produce epidural bleeding as arteries in the dura rupture and leak into surrounding tissue space which tears the dura, periosteum, and the bridging vessels between the arachnoid and dura layers (Lewis, 2004; Kumar et al., 2020). In the postcranial skeleton, movement of the muscles of the rotator cuff is implicated in the formation of porous lesions and new bone deposition in the supra- and infraspinatus fossa of the scapula. Osteochondral junctions of ribs and long bone metaphyses may fracture. New bone ≤ 1 cm thick may be deposited on affected regions of long bone diaphyses. The largest subperiosteal hematomas are observed on the weight-bearing long bones of the lower limb, especially in infants and children (Ortner, 2003:384). The ilium and the foramen rotundum of the sphenoid bone are also identified as potential sites of scorbutic inflammation (Geber & Murphy, 2012).

Developmental Defects of Enamel

Developmental defects of enamel are arguably the most widely studied indicator of stress in human remains (Hillson, 2014; Larsen, 2015; and see Chapter 20, this volume). Of the developmental defects of enamel, linear enamel hypoplasia (LEH) is most frequently incorporated into paleopathological research (Hillson, 2014; Larsen, 2015). LEH is produced when shortened enamel prisms are deposited by ameloblasts following acute or chronic stress events (Hillson & Bond, 1997). These defects are most commonly manifested as transverse grooves or furrows across the enamel surface – but also can appear as irregular pits or otherwise insufficient tooth enamel thickness. Physiological pathways associated with stress are likely related to defect formation. For example, cortisol dysregulates calcium absorption within ameloblasts, and this may disrupt enamel development by reducing energy transport and moving cellular mitochondria away from the enamel organ (Sasaki & Garrant, 1987; Seow et al., 1989). In this sense, LEH is linked to over 100 known particular causes from nutritional deprivation, weanling diarrhea, infection, febrile states, parasitism, and toxin exposure (Goodman & Rose, 1991; Suckling, 1989; Schultz et al., 1998), though direct links with LEH formation and stress have not been demonstrated (Hillson, 2014). Differential diagnosis can rule out hereditary and traumatic etiologies especially when multiple defects occur at comparable developmental stages on more than one tooth (Hillson, 2014).

LEH may be identified macroscopically or microscopically. LEH are macroscopically recorded as deficiencies in enamel thickness distributed along the longitudinal axis of the tooth. The prevalence of these defects has been compared to characterize stress experiences during adaptive transitions (reviewed by Larsen, 2015). Relationships between LEH and mortality risk have been found, but these are culturally and ecologically contingent (Cook & Buikstra, 1979; DeWitte & Wood, 2008; Amoroso et al., 2014; Wilson, 2014). Because enamel is formed chronologically, the relative location of LEH on teeth is used to estimate and compare age-at-defect formation between skeletal samples (Goodman and Rose, 1991). Striae of Retzius angulation and non-linear growth of enamel do, however, create problems in objective identification of LEH and estimation of age-at-defect formation (Hillson & Bond, 1997; Reid & Dean, 2000; Guatelli-Steinberg et al., 2012; Hassett, 2012).

Microscopic studies provide an objective approach to the identification of LEH and estimations of age-at-defect formation. Incremental microstructures outcrop onto the enamel surface as perikymata (Nanci, 2007), and histological studies demonstrate a modal periodicity for these structures at around 7–8 days (Reid et al., 1998; Reid & Ferrell, 2006; Nanci, 2007). These structures may be studied using high-resolution replicas of the enamel surface and an engineer's measuring microscope (Hillson, 1992; King et al., 2002). LEH are identified based on enlarged perikymata (Figure 22.3) (Hillson and Bond, 1997; King et al., 2002). Enlarged perikymata are defined using standard deviations from surrounding microstructures or residuals of observed and predicted perikymata size (Bocaege et al., 2010; Hassett, 2012). Age-at-defect formation may be estimated using perikymata counts and estimates of cuspal enamel formation and crown initiation times (Reid et al., 1998; King et al., 2002). Studies have also used counts of perikymata in the occlusal wall of LEH to estimate stress episode duration (Guatelli-Steinberg et al., 2004).

Thin sections of enamel allow for the visualization of long period (striae of Retzius) and short period (cross-striations) striae in enamel when viewed under transmitted or polarized light microscopy (Figure 22.4). Accentuated striae of Retzius appear with darkened coloration and are frequently associated with abnormal enamel prisms (Rose et al., 1978). Accentuated striae are frequently matched with LEH and found in association with medical records documenting stress events in non-human primates (Hillson and Bond, 1997; Schwartz et al., 2006). Timing of these events may be estimated using measurements between the neonatal line and accentuated striae that are reliant on daily secretion rate (Mahoney, 2008) or compared between sections of teeth that overlap in formation time (Antoine et al., 2009).

Crypt fenestration enamel defects (CFEDs) are developmental defects of enamel characterized by the presence of an oval or roughly circular area of deficient, thinned, or missing enamel in the form of a flattened or concave pit, generally located on the midlabial surface of the tooth crown (Skinner & Hung, 1986). Bioarchaeological studies find that CFED frequencies increase in samples with archaeologically and bioarchaeologically documented evidence for dietary insufficiency, climatic deterioration, and skeletal growth disruption (Lukacs et al., 2001; Stojanowski & Carver, 2011), and interactions with mortality and colonialism are reported (Thomas et al., 2019).

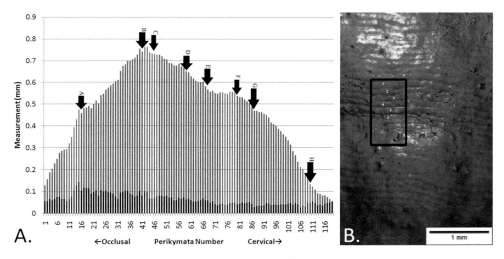

Figure 22.3 Enamel surface and perikymata spacing profile of a right mandibular second incisor for individual 194 from the Takasago site, Hokkaido, Japan. Black bars indicate measurements of perikymata spacing, while gray bars indicate the distance between the optical lens and the focal point (enamel depth). Matched LEH defects are identified by letters and arrows. LEH defect E is pictured in Figure 22.2. Photos: DHT.

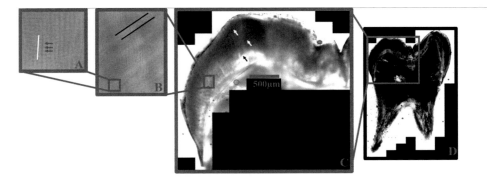

Figure 22.4 Enamel cross-striations each representing approximately one day of growth. These images were captured within long period striae from a first deciduous molar of a preadult recovered from the Charterhouse Warren site, United Kingdom.

Growth Disruption

While it is important to recognize the diverse hormones associated with stress experiences (Edes & Crews, 2017; Temple & Edes, 2022), cortisol is a master regulator derived from the activation of the HPA-axis that is deeply involved in growth suppression. Cortisol dysregulates skeletal growth by suppressing growth hormone pulsations and expression in the growth plate as well as osteoblast differentiation in the periosteal mesenchyme (Chyun et al., 1984; Martinelli & Moirera, 1994). Cortisol also inhibits pulsations of gonadotropin hormones during puberty, which may suppress the adolescent growth spurt (Seeman et al., 2001; Oakley et al., 2009). Experimental work further implicates vasoconstriction and limited nutrient delivery to the growth plate in skeletal growth disruption (Riesenfeld, 1973). This process reflects trade-offs in energetic allocation that reduce investments in growth to maintain essential tissue function. A truly substantial body of scholarship has linked poor growth to reduced bioavailability of nutrients reflecting infection, food insecurity and poor nutrition, and poor living conditions – especially in contexts of socioeconomic inequality (Bogin, 2020). Stress can either delay the timing of developmental events or slow rates of growth rates, but may also return to its original trajectory by increasing the rate or duration of growth following stress events (Stinson, 2012). This is frequently recorded in association with changing nutritional environments but may also reflect a deeper degree of canalization in body size.

Comparisons of long bone length relative to age is commonly performed in paleopathological research with the general expectation that negative deviations from the line of best fit reflects growth disruption (Cook, 1984; Lovejoy et al., 1990). Long bone length can be compared as a percentage of achieved growth or estimates of velocity (Lovejoy et al., 1990; Klaus & Tam, 2009). Polynomial models fit to growth data using methods such as forward selection provide a useful method that can extrapolate growth curves into adolescence (Schillaci et al., 2011; Ruff et al., 2013; Temple et al., 2014). Comparisons of preadult growth to standards derived from living populations help identify if mortality in these samples approximate growth in living individuals (Saunders & Hoppa, 1993; Schillaci et al., 2011; Stull et al., 2021). Negative residuals in growth may be compared across age categories to explore lived experiences such as ontologies of personhood or weaning schedules (Schillaci et al., 2011; Temple et al., 2014). Deficiencies of cortical bone mass also capture a record of stress as general measures of cortical area or percentages of cortical area (Mays et al., 2009; Robbins Schug & Goldman, 2014; Van Gerven et al., 1985). Several studies do, however, point out that cortical area is responsive to biomechanical loading and may not capture growth disruptions observed in diaphyeal lengths (Ruff et al., 2013; Robbins et al., 2014; Temple et al., 2014).

Terminal adult stature represents the culmination of growth across ontogeny. Stature is typically estimated using regression equations derived from long bones that approximate adult height (Sciulli et al., 1990; Raxter et al., 2006), though growth of the lower limbs are most consistently impacted by stress (Bogin et al., 2002). Therefore, paleopathological research also incorporates singular skeletal elements (i.e., femur or tibia) or leg length (i.e., femur + tibia) as proxies for stature (DeWitte & Hughes-Morey, 2012; Hughes-Morey, 2016). Frequentist comparisons of mean stature are a common way that stress is explored in paleopathological research (reviewed in Larsen, 2015). However, relationships between reduced stature and mortality may demonstrate changes in selective mortality, particularly in relation to epidemic disease (DeWitte & Hughes-Morey, 2012; Hughes-Morey, 2016). Catch-up growth may obscure relationships between stature and other indicators of early life stress (Stinson, 2012). Insights from human biology, however, indicate that growth faltering sustained during the first intense phase of human growth (birth-two years) has the most appreciable impact on adult height (Floyd & Littleton, 2006).

Another promising method involves the study of vertebral neural canal (VNC) diameters. Transverse diameter appears to reach adult size no later than four years of age suggesting that this measurement is a useful indicator of early life stress (Clark et al., 1986; Newman & Gowland, 2015; Watts, 2015). Anterior-posterior diameter achieves adult dimensions in early adolescence suggesting that this measurement is a more cumulative measure of stress experience (Clark et al., 1986). VNC growth tracks with the development of the hypothalamus and lymphatic system, and disruptions to growth during this time may reflect deeper systemic challenges (Clark et al., 1986). Numerous studies have demonstrated relationships between VNC stunting and mortality, though the relationships are complex and appear to result from both early life and cumulative stress experiences (Clark et al., 1986; LoPresto, 2020; Watts, 2015).

Disruption to growth may also manifest in tooth size. Heritability in tooth size is estimated as high as 90% (Townsend & Brown, 1978) suggesting that these measurements express high levels of genetic variance. However, tooth size may reflect stressors associated with poor maternal health, low birth weight, chronic disease, congenital disease, and nutritional deprivation (Garn et al., 1979). Several studies point to non-evolutionary reductions of tooth size associated with the transition from foraging to farming (Larsen, 1981) and relationships between reduced adult tooth size and age-at-death are reported in non-polar teeth (Stojanowski et al., 2007).

Developmental stability references the capacity for structures to grow and develop along genetically canalized pathways (Waddington, 1957), and this produces similarity in size between right and left antimeres in bilaterally symmetrical organisms (Van Valen, 1962). Random deviations from bilateral symmetry are indicators of developmental instability and are termed fluctuating asymmetry acknowledging the non-directional distribution of these measurements (Van Valen, 1962). Studies of fluctuating asymmetry compare stress experience using measurements of antimeric teeth, craniofacial elements, and epiphyseal fusion (Albert & Greene, 1999; DeLeon, 2007; Barrett et al., 2012; Sciulli, 2002; Weisensee, 2013). Relationships between fluctuating asymmetry and age-at-death are used to understand mortality risk and developmental stability (Weisensee, 2013).

Additional measures of stress have been explored over the years, and while worth mentioning, efficacy remains unclear. Cranial base height was proposed (Angel, 1982), but lacks a clear causative mechanism. The adult pelvic girdle appears as a far more likely skeletal structure to be affected by a confluence of weight, gravity, and nutritional stress (Brickley and Ives, 2008) to include pelvic flattening and alterations of pelvic outlet and greater sciatic notch geometry (Walker, 2005). Harris lines have also been incorporated into paleopathological studies of stress, though experimental work now suggests that these features may be produced during periods of accelerated growth (Alfonso-Durruty, 2011).

Modeling Stress in Paleopathology

In general, paleopathology has recently adopted a lifespan framework to indicators of stress and disease based on four distinct yet overlapping bodies of method and theory: skeletal pathophysiology, allostasis and allostatic load, life course theory, and evolutionary life history (Temple & Edes, 2022). Skeletal pathophysiology identifies the molecular and physiological signaling mechanisms associated with skeletal and dental indicators of stress (Gosman, 2011; Klaus, 2014a). Careful description and identification of stress mechanisms that alter skeletal phenotypes is imperative as allostatic load models have identified a multitude of biomarkers associated with this process (see Edes & Crews, 2017). For example, Klaus (2014a) argues that osteogenic signaling factors are triggered as downstream responses to inflammatory stress events, and this challenges assertions that periostosis does *not* reflect stress due to the general osteoclastogenic response of cortisol. Stress hormones such as parathyroid hormone act as signaling factors for bone morphogenic proteins, while other osteogenic transcription factors are independently expressed in response to inflammation. In another example, deeper understanding of the underlying skeletal pathophysiology responsible for cribra orbitalia has helped identify the systemic conditions responsible for these lesions (Schultz, 2001;

Wapler et al., 2004). Pushing further, studies of isotopes and proteins culled from dentin have identified increases in barium in relation to weight-loss and heat shock protein (HSP-70) originating from buffering mechanisms that prevent denaturation of odontoblasts (Austin et al., 2016). Finally, cortisol has recently been identified in archaeological enamel and dentin, suggesting that stress experiences that originate through HPA pathways may be studied in the deep past (Quade et al., 2021).

Studies of allostasis and allostatic load emphasize the use of multiple biomarkers related to stress (e.g., Edes and Crews, 2017), and multiple stress indicators have been used to calculate a skeletal frailty index (SFI) (Marklein et al., 2016). The goal was to compare the SFI between skeletal samples or model SFI relative to mortality risk, though little relationship between these indices and mortality were found (Marklein et al., 2016). While the use of multiple indicators of stress is valuable and may at some point act as a measure for allostatic load, the research design and assumptions of these works require attention. Many stress indicators included in this work originate from diverse developmental and physiological pathways, and altered phenotypes may reflect experiences that are unrelated to mortality. Future models that incorporate multiple measures of stress into studies of stress in human skeletal remains may work to ensure that the approach reflects data collected from similar developmental and physiological pathways.

Life course and evolutionary life history models both incorporate epidemiological methods and emphasize plasticity as a key factor in phenotypic alteration (Temple & Goodman, 2014; Gowland, 2015; Agarwal, 2016; Temple, 2019; and see Chapter 28, this volume). Life course perspectives explore questions related to the developmental trajectory of individuals, which include mortality, formation of lesions at later ages, social context, or general patterns of growth (Gowland, 2015; Agarwal, 2016). In addition, life course studies include intra-generational experiences through modeling stress experiences reflecting maternal health and well-being in relation to offspring (Gowland, 2015). Evolutionary life history is interested in physiological constraints associated with surviving stress at earlier ages and, therefore, explores factors such as mortality risk, growth disruption, and infectious disease at future stages of the lifespan (Temple, 2014, 2019). A recent adjunct to evolutionary life history models includes sensitive developmental windows framework (McPherson, 2021). These studies test the hypothesis that relationships with morbidity and mortality at later stages of development are closely associated with physiological disruption at developmentally sensitive ages (Temple, 2014; McPherson, 2021). The use of epidemiological models integrated with evolutionary and social theory surrounding the life course and life history has produced important models for exploration in the paleopathological analysis of stress. The models view a mutually constitutive relationship between early life experiences and outcomes at later stages of development, while focusing on the contextual or experiential inequalities that may foster or inhibit these reciprocal interactions (i.e., Ingold & Pallson, 2013).

Taken as a whole, modeling stress in human skeletal remains requires careful understanding of the pathophysiological principles governing the formation of altered skeletal phenotypes. These principles help reveal the underlying physiological pathways that produce skeletal and dental indicators of stress and the ages at which these phenotypes may develop. This knowledge may be built upon by indices of skeletal frailty, life course, and evolutionary life history models of stress. It is important to emphasize that none of these approaches represent a "best-fit" model, but that all approaches should begin with a careful understanding of skeletal pathophysiology as this helps identify the mechanisms associated with skeletal indicators of stress.

The Future

The study of stress in paleopathological perspective will benefit from approaches that orient this research in cultural, temporal, systemic, and developmental context. For example, high-resolution studies of individual life history rely on radiocarbon dating of human skeletal remains, incremental microstructures of enamel to identify stress, and incremental sectioning of teeth to reveal diet (Zvelebil & Weber, 2013). Other research has used incremental sections of enamel to identify diet and stress events associated with the weaning process, exposure to toxins, and climatic challenges (Dirks et al., 2010; Smith et al., 2018). Pathological expressions of stress never exist in a vacuum, and the study of hyperinflammatory responses helps further demonstrate this integrative pathway. For instance, a growing body of bioarchaeological and experimental evidence suggests that periodontal disease and periostosis may be linked by a common axis involving heightened systemic inflammation (DeWitte & Bekvalac, 2011). These and other findings make a case for exploring the degrees to which the field of osteoimmunology can contribute unique perspectives to studies of stress and disease (Crespo et al., 2017; Tsukasaki & Takayanagi, 2019).

Finally, human biology links colonial histories, marginalization, and racism to physiological adversity in early life environments, at later stages of the lifespan, and across generations (Gravlee, 2009; Kuzawa & Sweet, 2009; Thayer et al., 2017). Much of this violence is historically and epigenetically documented suggesting that studies of stress in the past have much to offer. While the impacts of colonialism, racism, and marginalization have been documented by bioarchaeological research (Blakey et al., 1994; Rankin-Hill, 1997; Murphy & Klaus, 2012; de la Cova, 2014), few studies have incorporated life course or evolutionary life history perspectives into addressing these questions (Daniels-Hill, 2021). Paleopathological studies of systemic stress that emphasize life history combined with theoretical paradigms that give voice to marginalized experience will help illustrate the deeply embodied history of these social challenges (Watkins, 2020; Daniels-Hill, 2021). The future of stress research in paleopathological context portends great transformative potential through both methodological innovation and theoretical paradigms that are socially relevant.

Acknowledgments

We thank Anne Grauer for the invitation to participate in this edited volume and expressing near-limitless patience as we strove toward completion of the chapter. Conversations with Clark Larsen, Jane Buikstra, Jim Gosman, and Laurie Reitsema were highly influential as we formulated the ideas that form the basis for this work.

References

Agarwal, S. C. (2016). Bone morphologies and histories: life course approaches in bioarchaeology. *American Journal of Physical Anthropology* 159(S61):130–149.

Albert, A. M., & Greene, D. L. (1999). Bilateral asymmetry in skeletal growth and maturation as an indicator of environmental stress. *American Journal of Physical Anthropology* 110(3):341–349.

Alfonso-Durruty, M. P. (2011). Experimental assessment of nutrition and bone growth's velocity effects on Harris lines formation. *American Journal of Physical Anthropology* 145(2):169–180.

Amoroso, A., Garcia, S. J. & Cardoso, H. F. V. (2014). Age at death and linear enamel hypoplasias: testing the effects of childhood stress and adult socioeconomic circumstances in premature mortality. *American Journal of Human Biology* 26(4):461–468.

Angel, J. L. (1982). A new measure of growth efficiency: skull base height. *American Journal of Physical Anthropology* 58(3):297–305.

Antoine, D., Hillson, S. & Dean, M. C. (2009). The developmental clock of dental enamel: a test for the periodicity of prism cross-striations in modern humans and an evaluation of the most likely sources of error in histological studies of this kind. *Journal of Anatomy* 214(1):45–55.

Austin, C., Smith, T. M., Farahani, R. M. Z., Hinde, K., Carter, E. A., Lee, J., … & Arora, M. (2016). Uncovering system-specific stress signatures in primate teeth with multimodal imaging. *Scientific Reports* 6(1):18802.

Barker, D. J. & Osmond, C. (1986). Infant mortality, childhood nutrition, and ischaemic heart disease in England and Wales. *Lancet* 1(8489):1077–1081.

Barker, D. J. P., Osmond, C., Winter, P. D., Margetts, B. & Simmonds, S. J. (1989). Weight in infancy and death from ischaemic heart disease. *The Lancet* 334(8663):577–580.

Barrett, C. K., Guatelli-Steinberg, D. & Sciulli, P. W. (2012). Revisiting dental fluctuating asymmetry in Neandertals and modern humans. *American Journal of Physical Anthropology* 149(2):193–204.

Bateson, P., Barker, D., Clutton-Brock, T., Deb, D., D'Udine, B., Foley, R. A., … & Sultan, S. E. (2004). Developmental plasticity and human health. *Nature* 430(6998):419–421.

Bernard, C. (1865). *Introduction á le´Étude de la Médicine Expérimentale*. Paris: J.-B. Balliere.

Blakey, M. L., Leslie, T. E. & Reidy, J. P. (1994). Frequency and chronological distribution of dental enamel hypoplasia in enslaved African Americans: a test of the weaning hypothesis. *American Journal of Physical Anthropology* 95(4):371–383.

Bocaege, E., Humphrey, L. T. & Hillson, S. (2010). Technical note: a new three-dimensional technique for high resolution quantitative recording of perikymata. *American Journal of Physical Anthropology* 141(3):498–503.

Bogin, B. (2020). *Patterns of Human Growth* (3rd ed.). Cambridge University Press.

Bogin, B., Smith, P., Orden, A. B., Varela Silva, M. I. & Loucky, J. (2002). Rapid change in height and body proportions of Maya American children. *American Journal of Human Biology* 14(6):753–761.

Brickley, M. B. (2018). Cribra orbitalia and porotic hyperostosis: a biological approach to diagnosis. *American Journal of Physical Anthropology* 167(4):896–902.

Brickley, M. B. & Ives, R. (2008). *The Bioarchaeology of Metabolic Bone Disease*. Academic Press.

Buford, T. W. & Willoughby, D. S. (2008). Impact of DHEA(S) and cortisol on immune function in aging: a brief review. *Applied Physiology, Nutrition, and Metabolism* 33(3):429–433.

Cannon, W. (1915). *Bodily Changes in Pain, Hunger, Fear, and Rage: An Account of Recent Researches into the Function of Emotional Excitement*. D Appleton and Company.

Cannon, W. (1932). *The Wisdom of the Body*. W.W. Norton and Company.

Carter, S. (2002). Hormonal influences on human sexual behavior. In Becker, J. (Ed.), *Behavioral Endocrinology* (2nd ed.), pp. 205–222. Cambridge, MA: MIT Press.

Cassel, J. & Tyroler, H. A. (1961). Epidemiological studies of culture change. *Archives of Environmental Health: An International Journal* 3(1):25–33.

Charmandari, E., Tsigos, C. & Chrousos, G. (2005). Endocrinology of the stress response. *Annual Review of Physiology* 67:259–284.

Chyun, Y.S., Kream, B.E., & Raisz, L. (1984). Cortisol decreases bone formation by inhibiting periosteal cell proliferation. *Endocrinology* 114:477–480.

Clark, G. A., Hall, N. R., Armelagos, G. J., Borkan, G. A., Panjabi, M. M. & Wetzel, F. T. (1986). Poor growth prior to early childhood: decreased health and life-span in the adult. *American Journal of Physical Anthropology* 70(2):145–160.

Cook, D. C. (1984). Subsistence and health in the Lower Illinois Valley: osteological evidence. In Cohen, M. N. & Armelagos, G. J. (Eds.), *Paleopathology at the Origins of Agriculture*, pp. 235–269. London: Academic Press.

Cook, D. C. & Buikstra, J. E. (1979). Health and differential survival in prehistoric populations: prenatal dental defects. *American Journal of Physical Anthropology* 51(4):649–664.

Crandall, J. J. & Klaus, H. D. (2014). Advancements, challenges, and prospects in the paleopathology of scurvy: current perspectives on vitamin C deficiency in human skeletal remains. *International Journal of Paleopathology* 5:1–8.

Crespi, E. J., & Denver, R. J. (2005). Ancient origins of human developmental plasticity. *American Journal of Human Biology* 17(1):44–54.

Crespo, F. A., Klaes, C. K., Switala, A. E., & DeWitte, S. N. (2017). Do leprosy and tuberculosis generate a systemic inflammatory shift? Setting the ground for a new dialogue between experimental immunology and bioarchaeology. *American Journal of Physical Anthropology* 162(1):143–156.

Crespo, F. K. (2021). Reconstructing immune competence in skeletal samples: a theoretical and methodological approach. In Cheverko, C. M., Prince-Buitenhuys, J. R. & Hubbe, M. (Eds.), *Theoretical Approaches in Bioarchaeology*, pp. 76–77. Abingdon: Routledge.

Daniels-Hill, L. (2021). *The Souls of Embodiment: Early Life Stress, Inequality, and Racism in 20th Century Black and White Americans*. Fairfax, Virginia: George Mason University.

de la Cova, C. (2014). The biological effects of urbanization and in-migration on 19th-century-born African Americans and European Americans of low socioeconomic status: an anthropological and historical approach. In Zuckerman, M. K. (Ed.), *Are Modern Environments Bad for Health? Revisiting the Second Epidemiological Transition*, pp. 243–364. Chichester: Wiley-Blackwell.

DeLeon, V. B. (2007). Fluctuating asymmetry and stress in a medieval Nubian population. *American Journal of Physical Anthropology* 132(4):520–534.

DeWitte, S. N. & Bekvalac, J. (2011). The association between periodontal disease and periosteal lesions in the St. Mary Graces cemetery, London, England A.D. 1350–1538. *American Journal of Physical Anthropology* 146(4):609–618.

DeWitte, S. N. & Hughes-Morey, G. (2012). Stature and frailty during the Black Death: the effect of stature on risks of epidemic mortality in London, A.D. 1348–1350. *Journal of Archaeological Science* 39(5):1412–1419.

DeWitte, S. N. & Wood, J. W. (2008). Selectivity of Black Death mortality with respect to preexisting health. *Proceedings of the National Academy of Sciences* 105(5):1436–1441.

Dirks, W., Humphrey, L. T., Dean, M. C. & Jeffries, T. E. (2010). The relationship of accentuated lines in enamel to weaning stress in juvenile baboons (Papio hamadryas anubis). *Folia Primatol (Basel)* 81(4):207–223.

Edes, A. N. & Crews, D. E. (2017). Allostatic load and biological anthropology. *American Journal of Physical Anthropology* 162(S63):e23146.

Everly, G. S. & Lating, J. M. (2013). The anatomy and physiology of the human stress response. In Everly, G. S. & Lating, J. M. (Eds.), *A Clinical Guide to the Treatment of the Human Stress Response*, pp. 17–51. New York: Springer.

Floyd, B. & Littleton, J. (2006). Linear enamel hypoplasia and growth in an Australian Aboriginal community: not so small, but not so healthy either. *Annals of Human Biology* 33(4):424–443.

Gallay, S. H., Miura, Y., Commisso, C. N., Fitzsimmons, J. S. & O'Driscoll, S. W. (1994). Relationship of donor site to chondrogenic potential of periosteum in vitro. *Journal of Orthopaedic Research* 12(4):515–525.

Garn, S. M., Osborne, R. H. & McCabe, K. D. (1979). The effect of prenatal factors on crown dimensions. *American Journal of Physical Anthropology* 51(4):665–677.

Geber, J. & Murphy, E. (2012). Scurvy in the Great Irish Famine: evidence of vitamin C deficiency from a mid-19th century skeletal population. *American Journal of Physical Anthropology* 148(4):512–524.

Goodman, A. H., Brooke Thomas, R., Swedlund, A. C. & Armelagos, G. J. (1988). Biocultural perspectives on stress in prehistoric, historical, and contemporary population research. *American Journal of Physical Anthropology* 31(S9):169–202.

Goodman, A. H. & Rose, J. C. (1991). Dental enamel hypoplasias as indicators of nutritional status. In Kelley, M. A. & Larsen, C. S. (Eds.), *Advances in Dental Anthropology*, pp. 279–294. New York: Wiley-Liss.

Gosman, J. H. (2011). The molecular biological approach in paleopathology. In Gauer, A. L. (Ed.), *A Companion to Paleopathology*, pp. 76–96. Chichester: Wiley-Blackwell.

Gowland, R. L. (2015). Entangled lives: implications of the developmental origins of health and disease hypothesis for bioarchaeology and the life course. *American Journal of Physical Anthropology* 158(4):530–540.

Gravlee, C. C. (2009). How race becomes biology: embodiment of social inequality. *American Journal of Physical Anthropology* 139(1):47–57.

Guatelli-Steinberg, D., Ferrell, R. J. & Spence, J. (2012). Linear enamel hypoplasia as an indicator of physiological stress in great apes: reviewing the evidence in light of enamel growth variation. *American Journal of Physical Anthropology* 148(2):191–204.

Guatelli-Steinberg, D., Larsen, C. S. & Hutchinson, D. L. (2004). Prevalence and the duration of linear enamel hypoplasia: a comparative study of Neandertals and Inuit foragers. *Journal of Human Evolution* 47(1):65–84.

Guder, C., Gravius, S., Burger, C., Wirtz, D. C. & Schildberg, F. A. (2020). Osteoimmunology: a current update of the interplay between bone and the immune system [Review]. *Frontiers in Immunology* 11(58). https://doi.org/10.3389/fimmu.2020.00058

Hall, B. K. (2015). *Bones and Cartilage: Developmental and Evolutionary Skeletal Biology*. Elsevier.

Hassett, B. R. (2012). Evaluating sources of variation in the identification of linear hypoplastic defects of enamel: a new quantified method. *Journal of Archaeological Science* 39(2):560–565.

Hillson, S. W. (1992). Impression and replica methods for studying hypoplasia and perikymata on human tooth crown surfaces from archaeological sites. *International Journal of Osteoarchaeology* 2(1):65–78.

Hillson, S. W. (2014). *Tooth Development in Human Evolution and Bioarchaeology*. Cambridge University Press.

Hillson, S. W. & Bond, S. (1997). Relationship of enamel hypoplasia to the pattern of tooth crown growth: a discussion. *American Journal of Physical Anthropology* 104(1):89–103.

Hoffbrand, A. V. & Lewis, S. M. (1981). *Postgraduate Haematology*. Butterworth Ltd.

Hostinar, C. E., Lachman, M. E., Mroczek, D. K., Seeman, T. E. & Miller, G. E. (2015). Additive contributions of childhood adversity and recent stressors to inflammation at midlife: findings from the MIDUS study. *Developmental Psychology* 51(11):1630–1644.

Hughes-Morey, G. (2016). Interpreting adult stature in industrial London. *American Journal of Physical Anthropology* 159(1):126–134.

Huss-Ashmore, R., Goodman, A. H. & Armelagos, G. J. (1982). Nutritional inference from paleopathology. *Advances in Archaeological Method and Theory* 5:395–474.

Ingold, T. & Pallson, G. (2013). *Biosocial Becomings: Integrating Biological and Social Anthropology*. Cambridge, UK: Cambridge University Press.

Ito, Y., Fitzsimmons, J. S., Sanyal, A., Mello, M. A., Mukherjee, N. & O'Driscoll, S. W. (2001). Localization of chondrocyte precursors in periosteum. *Osteoarthritis Cartilage* 9(3):215–223.

Jackson, M. (2014). Evaluating the role of Hans Selye in the modern history of stress. In Cantor, D. & Ramsden, E. (Eds.), *Stress, Shock, and Adaptation in the Twentieth Century*, pp. 21–48. Woodbrigdge, Suffolk, UK: Boydell & Brewer.

Kalantaridou, S. N., Zoumakis, E., Makrigiannakis, A., Lavasidis, L. G., Vrekoussis, T. & Chrousos, G. P. (2010). Corticotropin-releasing hormone, stress and human reproduction: an update. *Journal of Reproductive Immunology* 85(1):33–39.

Kent, S. (1986). Influence of sedentism and aggregation on porotic hyperostosis and anemia: a case study. *Man* 21:605–636.

King, T., Hillson, S. & Humphrey, L. T. (2002). A detailed study of enamel hypoplasia in a post-medieval adolescent of known age and sex. *Archives of Oral Biology* 47(1):29–39.

Klaus, H. D. (2014a). Frontiers in the bioarchaeology of stress and disease: cross-disciplinary perspectives from pathophysiology, human biology, and epidemiology. *American Journal of Physical Anthropology* 155(2):294–308.

Klaus, H. D. (2014b). Subadult scurvy in Andean South America: evidence of vitamin C deficiency in the late pre-Hispanic and Colonial Lambayeque Valley, Peru. *International Journal of Paleopathology* 5:34–45.

Klaus, H. D. (2017). Paleopathological rigor and differential diagnosis: case studies involving terminology, description, and diagnostic frameworks for scurvy in skeletal remains. *International Journal of Paleopathology* 19:96–110.

Klaus, H. D. & Tam, M. E. (2009). Contact in the Andes: bioarchaeology of systemic stress in colonial Mórrope, Peru. *American Journal of Physical Anthropology* 138(3):356–368.

Korte, S. M., Koolhaas, J. M., Wingfield, J. C. & McEwen, B. S. (2005). The Darwinian concept of stress: benefits of allostasis and costs of allostatic load and the trade-offs in health and disease. *Neuroscience and Biobehavior Reviews* 29(1):3–38.

Kumar, V., Abbas, A. & Aster, J. (2020). *Robbins and Coltran Pathologic Basis for Disease* (Vol. 10). London: Elsevier.

Kuzawa, C. W. & Sweet, E. (2009). Epigenetics and the embodiment of race: developmental origins of US racial disparities in cardiovascular health. *American Journal of Human Biology* 21(1):2–15.

Larsen, C. S. (1981). Skeletal and dental adaptations to the shift to agriculture on the Georgia coast. *Current Anthropology* 22(4):422–423.

Larsen, C. S. (2015). *Bioarchaeology: Interpreting Behavior from the Human Skeleton*. Cambridge: Cambridge University Press.

Lennartsson, A. K. & Jonsdottir, I. H. (2011). Prolactin in response to acute psychosocial stress in healthy men and women. *Psychoneuroendocrinology* 36(10):1530–1539.

Lewis, M. E. (2004). Endocranial lesions in non-adult skeletons: understanding their aetiology. *International Journal of Osteoarchaeology* 14(2):82–97.

Lewis, M. E. (2018). *The Paleopathology of Children: Identification of Pathological Conditions in the Human Skeletal Remains of Non-Adults.* London: Academic Press.

LoPresto, S. L. (2020). *Vertebral Neural Canal Growth and Developmental Stress: A Case Study from the American Southwest.* Master's thesis. George Mason University. Fairfax, Virginia

Lovejoy, C. O., Russell, K. F. & Harrison, M. L. (1990). Long bone growth velocity in the Libben population. *American Journal of Human Biology* 2(5):533–541.

Lukacs, J. R., Nelson, G. C. & Walimbe, S. R. (2001). Enamel hypoplasia and childhood stress in prehistory: new data from India and Southwest Asia. *Journal of Archaeological Science* 28(11):1159–1169.

Mahoney, P. (2008). Intraspecific variation in M1 enamel development in modern humans: implications for human evolution. *Journal of Human Evolution* 55(1):131–147.

Marklein, K. E., Leahy, R. E. & Crews, D. E. (2016). In sickness and in death: assessing frailty in human skeletal remains. *American Journal of Physical Anthropology* 161(2):208–225.

Martinelli, C.E. & Moira, A.C. (1994). Relationship between growth hormone and spontaneous cortisol secretion in children. *Clinical Endocrinology* 41:117–121.

Mays, S., Ives, R. & Brickley, M. (2009). The effects of socioeconomic status on endochondral and appositional bone growth, and acquisition of cortical bone in children from 19th century Birmingham, England. *American Journal of Physical Anthropology* 140(3):410–416.

McEwen, B. S. (2004). Protection and damage from acute and chronic stress: allostasis and allostatic overload and relevance to the pathophysiology of psychiatric disorders. *Annals of the New York Academy of Sciences* 1032:1–7.

McEwen, B. S. & Stellar, E. (1993). Stress and the individual. Mechanisms leading to disease. *Archives of Internal Medicine* 153(18):2093–2101.

McEwen, B. S., & Wingfield, J. C. (2003). The concept of allostasis in biology and biomedicine. *Hormones and Behavior* 43(1):2–15.

McPherson, C. B. (2021). Examining developmental plasticity in the skeletal system through a sensitive developmental windows framework. *American Journal of Physical Anthropology* 176(2):163–178.

Murata, H., Shimada, N., & Yoshioka, M. (2004). Current research on acute phase proteins in veterinary diagnosis: an overview. *The Veterinary Journal* 168(1):28–40.

Murphy, M. S. & Klaus, H. D. (2012). *Colonized Bodies: Worlds Transformed.* University Press of Florida.

Nanci, A. (2007). *Ten Cate's Oral Histology.* Mosby.

Newman, S. L. & Gowland, R. L. (2015). The use of non-adult vertebral dimensions as indicators of growth disruption and non-specific health stress in skeletal populations. *American Journal of Physical Anthropology* 158(1):155–164.

Nishikimi, M. & Udenfriend, S. (1977). Scurvy as an inborn error of ascorbic acid biosynthesis. *Trends in Biochemical Sciences* 2(5):111–113.

Oakley, A. E., Breen, K. M., Clarke, I. J., Karsch, F. J., Wagenmaker, E. R. & Tilbrook, A. J. (2009). Cortisol reduces gonadotropin-releasing hormone pulse frequency in follicular phase ewes: influence of ovarian steroids. *Endocrinology* 150(1):341–349.

Ortner, D. J. (2003). *Identification of Pathological Conditions in Human Skeletal Remains.* London: Elsevier.

Ortner, D. J., Kimmerle, E. H. & Diez, M. (1999). Probable evidence of scurvy in subadults from archeological sites in Peru. *American Journal of Physical Anthropology* 108(3):321–331.

Ortner, D. J. & Mays, S. (1998). Dry-bone manifestations of rickets in infancy and early childhood. *International Journal of Osteoarchaeology* 8(1):45–55.

Oxenham, M. F. & Cavill, I. (2010). Porotic hyperostosis and cribra orbitalia: the erythropoietic response to iron-deficiency anaemia. *Anthropological Science* 118(3):199–200.

Quade, L., Chazot, P. L. & Gowland, R. (2021). Desperately seeking stress: a pilot study of cortisol in archaeological tooth structures. *American Journal of Physical Anthropology* 174(3):532–541.

Ragsdale, B. D., & Lehmer, L. M. (2011). A knowledge of bone at the cellular (histological) level is essential to paleopathology. In Grauer. A. L. (Ed.), *A Companion to Paleopathology,* pp. 225–249. Wiley.

Rankin-Hill, L. M. (1997). *A Biohistory of 19th Century Afro-Americans: The Burial Remains of a Philadelphia Cemetery.* Koln, Germany: Berin and Garvey.

Raxter, M. H., Auerbach, B. M. & Ruff, C. B. (2006). Revision of the fully technique for estimating statures. *American Journal of Physical Anthropology* 130(3):374–384.

Reid, D. J., Beynon, A. D. & Ramirez Rozzi, F. V. (1998). Histological reconstruction of dental development in four individuals from a medieval site in Picardie, France. *Journal of Human Evolution* 35(4):463–477.

Reid, D. J. & Dean, M. C. (2000). Brief communication: the timing of linear hypoplasias on human anterior teeth. *American Journal of Physical Anthropology* 113(1):135–139.

Reid, D. J. & Ferrell, R. J. (2006). The relationship between number of striae of Retzius and their periodicity in imbricational enamel formation. *Journal of Human Evolution* 50(2):195–202.

Resnick, D. W. (2002). *Diagnosis of Bone and Joint Disorders*. Philadelphia: W.B. Saunders.

Riesenfeld, A. (1973). The effect of extreme temperatures and starvation on the body proportions of the rat. *American Journal of Physical Anthropology* 39(3):427–459.

Rivera, F. & Mirazón Lahr, M. (2017). New evidence suggesting a dissociated etiology for cribra orbitalia and porotic hyperostosis. *American Journal of Physical Anthropology* 164(1):76–96.

Roberts, C. A. (2019). Bacterial infections. In Buikstra, J. E. (Ed.), *Ortner's Identification of Pathological Conditions in Human Skeletal Remains*, pp. 321–439. London: Elsevier.

Robbins Schug, G., & Goldman H. (2014). Birth is but our death begun: a bioarchaeological assessment of skeletal emaciation in immature human skeletons in the context of environmental, social, and subsistence transition. *American Journal of Physical Anthropology* 155(2):243–259.

Rose, J. C., Armelagos, G. J. & Lallo, J. W. (1978). Histological enamel indicator of childhood stress in prehistoric skeletal samples. *American Journal of Physical Anthropology* 49(4):511–516.

Ruff, C. B., Garofalo, E. & Holmes, M. A. (2013). Interpreting skeletal growth in the past from a functional and physiological perspective. *American Journal of Physical Anthropology* 150(1):29–37.

Sapolsky, R. M. (1998). *Why Zebras Don't Get Ulcers*. New York" W.H. Freeman and Company.

Sasaki, T. & Garrant, P. R. (1987). Mitochondrial migration and Ca-ATPase modulation in secretory ameloblasts of fasted and calcium loaded rats. *American Journal of Anatomy* 179(2):116–130.

Saunders, S. R. & Hoppa, R. D. (1993). Growth deficit in survivors and non-survivors: biological mortality bias in subadult skeletal samples. *American Journal of Physical Anthropology* 36(S17):127–151.

Schillaci, M. A., Nikitovic, D., Akins, N. J., Tripp, L. & Palkovich, A. M. (2011). Infant and juvenile growth in ancestral Pueblo Indians. *American Journal of Physical Anthropology* 145(2):318–326.

Schug, G. R. & Goldman, H. M. (2014). Birth is but our death begun: a bioarchaeological assessment of skeletal emaciation in immature human skeletons in the context of environmental, social, and subsistence transition. *American Journal of Physical Anthropology* 155(2):243–259.

Schultz, M. (2001). Paleohistopathology of bone: a new approach to the study of ancient diseases. *American Journal of Physical Anthropology* 116(S33):106–147.

Schwartz, G. T., Reid, D. J., Dean, M. C. & Zihlman, A. L. (2006). A faithful record of stressful life events recorded in the dental developmental record of a juvenile gorilla. *International Journal of Primatology* 27(4):1201–1219.

Schultz, M., Carlie-Thiele, P., Schmidt-Schultz, T.H., Keirdof, H., Teegen, W.R. & Kreutz, K. (1998). Enamel hypoplasias in archaeological skeletal remains. In Alt, K.W., Rosing, F.W., Teschler-Nicola, M., (Eds.), *Dental Anthropology: Fundamentals, Limits, and Prospects*, pp. 293–311. Berlin: Springer-Verlag.

Sciulli, P. W. (2002). Dental asymmetry in a Late Archaic and Late Prehistoric skeletal sample of the Ohio Valley Area. *Dental Anthropology* 16:33–44.

Sciulli, P. W., Schneider, K. N. & Mahaney, M. C. (1990). Stature estimation in prehistoric Native Americans of Ohio. *American Journal of Physical Anthropology* 83(3):275–280.

Seeman, T. E., Singer, B., Wilkinson, C. W. & McEwen, B. (2001). Gender differences in age-related changes in HPA axis reactivity. *Psychoneuroendocrinology* 26(3):225–240.

Selye, H. (1936). A syndrome produced by diverse nocuous agents. *Nature* 138(3479):32–32.

Selye, H. (1946). The general adaptation syndrome and diseases of adaptation. *The Journal of Clinical Endocrinology & Metabolism* 6(2):117–230.

Seaward, B.L. (2006). *Managing Stress: Principles and Strategies for Health and Well-Being*, (5th Ed). Boston, MA: Jones and Barlett Publishers.

Seow, W. K., Masel, J. P., Weir, C. & Tudehope, D. I. (1989). Mineral deficiency in the pathogenesis of enamel hypoplasia in prematurely born, very low birthweight children. *Pediatric Dentistry* 11(4):297–302.

Skinner, M. F. & Hung, J. T. W. (1986). Localized enamel hypoplasia of the primary canine. *ASDC Journal of Dentistry for Children* 53(3):197–200.

Smith-Guzmán, N. E. (2015). The skeletal manifestation of malaria: an epidemiological approach using documented skeletal collections. *American Journal of Physical Anthropology* 158(4):624–635.

Smith, T. M., Austin, C., Green, D. R., Joannes-Boyau, R., Bailey, S., Dumitriu, D., … & Arora, M. (2018). Wintertime stress, nursing, and lead exposure in Neanderthal children. *Science Advances* 4(10):eaau9483.

Snoddy, A. M. E., Buckley, H. R., Elliott, G. E., Standen, V. G., Arriaza, B. T., & Halcrow, S. E. (2018). Macroscopic features of scurvy in human skeletal remains: a literature synthesis and diagnostic guide. *American Journal of Physical Anthropology* 167(4):876–895.

Steptoe, A. & Brydon, L. (2005). Associations between acute lipid stress responses and fasting lipid levels 3 years later. *Health Psychology Journal* 24(6):601–607.

Sterling, P. (2012). Allostasis: a model of predictive regulation. *Physiology & Behavior* 106(1):5–15.

Stinson, S. (2012). Growth variation: biological and cultural factors. In Stinson, S., Bogin, B. & O'Rourke, D. (Eds.), *Human Biology: An Evolutionary and Biocultural Perspective*, pp. 587–636. Chicester: Wiley-Blackwell.

Stockmann, C. & Fandrey, J. (2006). Hypoxia-induced erythropoietin production: a paradigm for oxygen-regulated gene expression. *Clinical and Experimental Pharmacology and Physiology* 33(10):968–979.

Stojanowski, C. M. & Carver, C. L. (2011). Inference of emergent cattle pastoralism in the southern Sahara desert based on localized hypoplasia of the primary canine. *International Journal of Paleopathology* 1(2):89–97.

Stojanowski, C. M., Larsen, C. S., Tung, T. A. & McEwan, B. G. (2007). Biological structure and health implications from tooth size at Mission San Luis de Apalachee. *American Journal of Physical Anthropology* 132(2):207–222.

Stuart-Macadam, P. (1992). Porotic hyperostosis: a new perspective. *American Journal of Physical Anthropology* 87(1):39–47.

Stull, K. E., Wolfe, C. A., Corron, L. K., Heim, K., Hulse, C. N. & Pilloud, M. A. (2021). A comparison of subadult skeletal and dental development based on living and deceased samples. *American Journal of Physical Anthropology* 175(1):36–58.

Suckling, G. W. (1989). Developmental defects of enamel - Historical and present-day perspectives of their pathogenesis. *Advances in Dental Research* 3(2):87–94.

Taylor, S. E., Klein, L. C., Lewis, B. P., Gruenewald, T. L., Gurung, R. A. & Updegraff, J. A. (2000). Biobehavioral responses to stress in females: tend-and-befriend, not fight-or-flight. *Psychology Review* 107(3):411–429.

Temple, D. H. (2014). Plasticity and constraint in response to early-life stressors among Late/Final Jomon period foragers from Japan: evidence for life history trade-offs from incremental microstructures of enamel. *American Journal of Physical Anthropology* 155(4):537–545.

Temple, D. H. (2019). Bioarchaeological evidence for adaptive plasticity and constraint: Exploring life-history trade-offs in the human past. *Evolutionary Anthropology: Issues, News, and Reviews* 28(1):34–46.

Temple, D. H., Bazaliiskii, V. I., Goriunova, O. I. & Weber, A. W. (2014). Skeletal growth in early and Late Neolithic foragers from the Cis-Baikal region of Eastern Siberia. *American Journal of Physical Anthropology* 153(3):377–386.

Temple, D. H. & Edes, A. N. (2022). Stress in bioarchaeology, epidemiology, and evolutionary medicine: an integrated conceptual model of shared history from the descriptive to the developmental In Plomp, K., Roberts, C. A., Elton, S. & Bentley, G. (Eds.), *Evolving Health: Palaeopathology and Evolutionary Medicine*. Oxford:Oxford University Press.

Temple, D. H. & Goodman, A. H. (2014). Bioarcheology has a "health" problem: conceptualizing "stress" and "health" in bioarcheological research. *American Journal of Physical Anthropology* 155(2):186–191.

Thayer, Z. M., Blair, I. V., Buchwald, D. S. & Manson, S. M. (2017). Racial discrimination associated with higher diastolic blood pressure in a sample of American Indian adults. *American Journal of Physical Anthropology* 163(1):122–128.

Thayer, Z. M., Wilson, M. A., Kim, A. W. & Jaeggi, A. V. (2018). Impact of prenatal stress on offspring glucocorticoid levels: a phylogenetic meta-analysis across 14 vertebrate species. *Scientific Reports* 8(1):4942.

Thomas, J. A., Temple, D. H. & Klaus, H. D. (2019). Crypt fenestration enamel defects and early life stress: contextual explorations of growth and mortality in Colonial Peru. *American Journal of Physical Anthropology* 168(3):582–594.

Toffler, A. (1970). *Future Shock*. New York: Random House.

Townsend, G. C. & Brown, T. (1978). Heritability of permanent tooth size. *American Journal of Physical Anthropology* 49(4):497–504.

Tsukasaki, M. & Takayanagi, H. (2019). Osteoimmunology: evolving concepts in bone-immune interactions in health and disease. *Nature Reviews Immunology* 19(10):626–642.

Van Gerven, D. P., Hummert, J. R. & Burr, D. B. (1985). Cortical bone maintenance and geometry of the tibia in prehistoric children from Nubia's Batn el Hajar. *American Journal of Physical Anthropology* 66(3):275–280.

Van Valen, L. (1962). A study of fluctuating asymmetry. *Evolution* 16(2):125–142.

Waddington, C. H. (1957). *The Strategy of Genes*. Stuttgart, Germany: MacMillan.

Walker, P. L. (2005). Greater sciatic notch morphology: sex, age, and population differences. *American Journal of Physical Anthropology* 127(4):385–391.

Walker, P. L., Bathurst, R. R., Richman, R., Gjerdrum, T. & Andrushko, V. A. (2009). The causes of porotic hyperostosis and cribra orbitalia: a reappraisal of the iron-deficiency-anemia hypothesis. *American Journal of Physical Anthropology* 139(2):109–125.

Wapler, U., Crubézy, E. & Schultz, M. (2004). Is cribra orbitalia synonymous with anemia? Analysis and interpretation of cranial pathology in Sudan. *American Journal of Physical Anthropology* 123(4):333–339.

Watkins, R. J. (2020). An alter(ed)native perspective on historical bioarchaeology. *Historical Archaeology* 54(1):17–33.

Watts, R. (2015). The long-term impact of developmental stress: evidence from later medieval and post-medieval London (AD1117–1853). *American Journal of Physical Anthropology* 158(4):569–580.

Weisensee, K. E. (2013). Assessing the relationship between fluctuating asymmetry and cause of death in skeletal remains: a test of the developmental origins of health and disease hypothesis. *American Journal of Human Biology* 25(3):411–417.

Wilson, J. J. (2014). Paradox and promise: research on the role of recent advances in paleodemography and paleoepidemiology to the study of "health" in Precolumbian societies. *American Journal of Physical Anthropology* 155(2):268–280.

Worthman, C. M. & Kuzara, J. (2005). Life history and the early origins of health differentials. *American Journal of Human Biology* 17(1):95–112.

Zvelebil, M. & Weber, A. W. (2013). Human bioarchaeology: group identity and individual life histories – Introduction. *Journal of Anthropological Archaeology* 32(3):275–279.

23
THEORETICAL APPROACHES TO THE PALEOPATHOLOGY OF INFANTS, CHILDREN, AND ADOLESCENTS

Structural Violence as a Holistic Interpretive Tool in Paleopathology

Siân E. Halcrow and Gwen Robbins Schug

Introduction

Research on infants and children is central to a holistic understanding of the human condition (Gottlieb, 2000; Baxter, 2005; Lewis, 2006, 2017; Lillehammer, 2015; Nowell & Kurki, 2020). For paleopathologists and bioarchaeologists, including infant and children's skeletons in our research has the potential to yield meaningful insights into historical and socio-cultural variation in concepts of identity, personhood, the life course, social age, social structure, violence, and disease across the lifespan (e.g., Thompson et al., 2014; Geber, 2016; Martin & Tegtmeyer, 2017; Beauchesne & Agarwal, 2018; Ellis, 2020; Gowland & Halcrow, 2020). Paleopathological focus on immature remains increasingly contributes to understanding the etiology, pathogenesis, progression, and differential diagnoses of specific pathological conditions in infants and children – infectious, developmental, nutritional and congenital conditions, and traumatic injuries – in a manner that cannot always be accomplished through clinical or experimental work in contemporary populations (e.g., Lewis, 2006, 2014, 2017). Due to these theoretical and methodological advances, the past ten years have witnessed a burgeoning interest in using paleopathology of infants and children to develop a more comprehensive archaeology of the human experience across the life course (Halcrow & Tayles, 2008; Robbins Schug, 2011; Halcrow et al., 2017; Snoddy et al., 2017; see Mays et al., 2017; & Halcrow & Ward, 2017 for a review).

Historically, anthropological research on children was focused on their provision, protection, and limited participation across cultural contexts, following a paradigm outlined by the United Nations Convention on the Rights of the Child (1989). In the 21st century, our discipline turned away from the static view of children as objects of care or benchmarks for development; increasingly children are recognized as actors embedded within wider social structures, working, providing care, and enacting violence and social change (see review in Korbin, 2003; Bluebond-Lagner & Korbin, 2007). Analogously, paleopathologists were once primarily interested in skeletal manifestations of disease in childhood and measuring visible disruptions to homeostasis in children as a proxy for the "health" of past populations or to examine the adaptive value of larger social and environmental systems (Goodman & Armelagos, 1989; Larsen, 2002). Now, however, many biocultural stress markers are recognized to have a complex relationship with "health" in past populations (Reitsema & McIlvaine, 2014; Temple & Goodman, 2014). Combined with the recent acknowledgment in paleopathology and bioarchaeology of the particular vulnerabilities, interconnectedness, and agency of children and childhood, a more sophisticated appreciation of social theory around these themes has developed (e.g., Halcrow & Tayles, 2008; Gowland, 2015; Beauchesne & Agarwal, 2018). Childhood is increasingly understood to be a social life stage and an experience, one that is entangled with many other aspects of identity and enmeshed in relationships with other individuals (mothers, caregivers, family members, community members, and others) and societal structures (Gowland, 2020; Halcrow, 2020; Halcrow et al., 2020; Robbins Schug, 2020; Kendall & Kendall, 2021).

Our goal in this chapter is to explore the multivocality of infancy and childhood in paleopathology through the lens of structural violence and to examine the tension between vulnerability and agency in different socio-cultural contexts through time (Gottlieb, 2000; Korbin, 2003; Baxter, 2005; Montgomery, 2008; Lancy, 2012; Gowland, 2020). In this chapter, we highlight relevant examples from the paleopathological literature, beginning with a brief description of the framework of structural violence, specifically as it pertains to the experience of past childhood pathology. We review some of the work that has been conducted on traumatic injuries at the nexus of power and sacrifice, explore debates about applying the concept of structural violence to evidence for past violence, and how this framework can reconcile relativism with human rights. Next, we briefly examine the recent focus in paleopathology on the maternal-fetal nexus as a contributor to infant health and lifelong experience (see Chapter 28, this volume, for a more detailed discussion on the Developmental Origins of Health and Disease (DOHaD) hypothesis; Gowland, 2015; Han et al., 2017; Gowland & Halcrow, 2020) and how this approach can be extended using the structural violence framework. Finally, we highlight research on the varied and adaptive nature of family relationships and structures and how these support systems may be constrained and/ or provide resilience in the face of structural violence (Hodson & Gowland, 2020; Filipek et al., 2021; Kendall & Kendall, 2021). Although the body of work we explore touches on these themes, there has not been a comprehensive research program to explore these issues in the paleopathology of children and thus there is much additional work to be done.

Structural Violence

Structural violence is a framework developed in peace and conflict studies that describes how social structures (social relations, economy, laws, etc.) and institutions impinge, impair, or harm individuals or groups (Galtung, 1969). The term describes a state of "unrecognizable, socially recognized violence" that is both visible and hidden, as it is deeply interwoven into the fabric of a society (Bourdieu, 1977:191–192; Scheper-Hughes, 1996; Bourgois, 2001, see also Chapters 21, 26 and 27, this volume). Structural violence operates through unequal access to resources, including health and safety, and is arguably the leading cause of human suffering, mortality, and disability today (Farmer, 1997, 2004; Farmer et al., 2006; Larchanché, 2012). The application of the concept of structural violence, specifically to health and pathology, falls under the rubric of "social suffering", or the way that political, economic, and institutional systems of power are complicit in the oppression of certain individuals and communities, including through illness, violence, and death (Kleinman et al., 1997). Paul Farmer, for example, uses this framework to demonstrate the extreme human suffering caused by colonialism-induced landlessness and poverty, the racist and sexist beliefs that exacerbate the consequences of starvation and endemic disease, and the global inequities that create and maintain the "texture of dire affliction" that is life for these communities (Farmer, 1997:263).

Since structural violence was initially defined, the theoretical framework has become a guiding explanatory principle for sociologists and medical anthropologists investigating socially induced inequality in the experience of symbolic and physical violence, famine and starvation, and disease and ill-health, more generally (Leatherman & Goodman, 2011; Bright, 2020). Because social structure is universal for humans, and the power dynamics of institutional inequality have been shown to have a potentially severe impact on human health and suffering (Kleinman et al., 1997), a consideration of structural violence is a particularly useful biocultural approach in bioarchaeology and paleopathology (Grauer & Buikstra, 2019). Indeed, bioarchaeological research on structural violence described below has elucidated how human remains can inform us about social relations of power and control in the past.

Structural violence has been an important framework in paleopathology and bioarchaeology since Carlina de la Cova articulated how gender, race, and class formed the basis for structural and physical violence to be enacted against certain bodies (de la Cova, 2008, 2011, 2012, 2020). A structural violence framework has been applied to historic communities (Tremblay & Reedy, 2020), and to other documented historical skeletal collections (Lans, 2020; Watkins, 2012, 2015, 2018a, 2018b), which are primarily derived from marginalized communities who have not given informed consent, and sometimes no consent (Dunnavant et al., 2021). Over the past decade structural violence is starting to be employed in bioarchaeological and paleopathological research on infants and children in a variety of cultural and social contexts, both historic and more ancient (Martin et al., 2010; Klaus, 2012; Martin & Harrod, 2012; Robbins Schug et al., 2012; Stone, 2012; Nystrom, 2014, 2017; Geber, 2015; Ellis, 2020; Nystrom & Robbins Schug, 2020; Sheridan & Gregoricka, 2020; Filipek et al., 2021). Some of this work is directly focused on children's experience of identity performance (Torres-Rouff, 2020), warfare (Tegtmeyer & Martin, 2017), or environmental marginalization (Harrod & Martin, 2014), although the framework of structural violence is not always explicitly articulated (Barrett, 2014).

Although some scholars have suggested that structural violence may only be relevant to hierarchical societies (Klaus, 2012), this question deserves further attention. Indeed, conflict has always been a feature of human communities and the othering process that can lead to greater risk of violence is not limited to complex societies. In addition, archaeologists have broadened our understanding of conflict to include physical and everyday violence within the rubric of structural or institutional violence (Gonzáles-Ruibal & Moshenska, 2014). Anthropological research has repeatedly confirmed that infants and children (along with women) are most often the targets of structural violence cross-culturally and that they are at greatest risk of social suffering (Scheper-Hughes, 1996; Farmer, 1997; Panter-Brick et al., 2011). Infants and children are disproportionately affected by the risk of deprivation, violence, and disease within populations and are, therefore, particularly sensitive barometers of environmental and social deprivation, which is seen to increase during times of social unrest and conflict (Panter-Brick et al., 2011). Their experiences are also important lines of evidence for inferring the impacts of social structure and institutionalized violence, as well as personal struggles and resistance. Despite the importance of theorizing structural violence in the context of infant and child paleopathology, there is a dearth of literature on the topic.

There are special concerns when applying the structural violence framework to children's remains. There can be an uncomfortable tension when anthropologists describe violence as perpetrated in the context of structural inequality because the framework does not inherently include a recognition of human agency for all actors or a recognition of resilience (Galtung, 1969). This tension may be felt most keenly in the application of ideas about social suffering in children, for whom social structure is but one of many potential constraints on agency and for whom the concept of complicity may run into additional ethical dilemmas (i.e., age of consent or responsibility, victim blaming, and the like) when larger social forces promote and sustain violence and children are potentially violent actors (Scheper-Hughes, 1987; Scheper-Hughes & Sargent, 1998; Korbin, 2003). Childhood is relational; parents, families, older children, and adults have particular roles to play in the perception of children and childhood – children's identity, agency, and resilience – and in shaping the health and nutritional outcomes for infants and children (Kendall & Kendall, 2021). Although vulnerabilities and limitations apply to infants, social bioarchaeologists have described children as competent agents, working within the constraints of social structure (Barrett 2014; Ellis 2020; Thompson et al., 2014) and as people who experience suffering in conditions of disease (Lewis, 2006), deprivation (Robbins Schug & Goldman, 2014), poverty (Geber, 2015), violence (Robbins Schug et al., 2012), and war (Tegtmeyer & Martin, 2017).

The following sections review some major themes in infant and child paleopathology, which lend themselves to an exploration of structural violence, including violent injuries; patterns of mortality, stress, and disease; social life course; and structures of childcare, family, and resilience.

Violent Injuries in Infant and Children's Remains

Structural violence is often at the root of behavioral violence against children (Lee, 2019), and children's suffering in general (Kleinman et al., 1997). Behavioral violence has a long legacy in human communities (Hrdy, 1999; Fry, 2006; Sala et al., 2015) and past forms of institutionally-sanctioned violence – including infanticide, massacres, captivity, torture, and sexual violence – pose unique interpretive challenges for bioarchaeologists (Geller, 2011; Kuckleman et al., 2017; Osterholtz & Martin, 2017; Tegtmeyer & Martin, 2017). Anthropologists recognize the concept of cultural relativism – that some collective practices of a given society may be traditionally sanctioned while other societies deem these same practices to be "detrimental" – but anthropologists also acknowledge there is a certain point where relativism "falls short" in the translation of pain, fear, and bodily harm (see Korbin, 2003). This chapter acknowledges the fact that women and children have been the targets of behavioral violence, and we review a couple of examples of how paleopathologists use skeletal evidence to demonstrate manipulation and control of individuals, to obtain or maintain power, terrorize, and/or demoralize the whole.

Women and children's bodies are prominently featured in anthropological studies of warfare and the organized use of violence in the American Southwest, Mesoamerica, and the Andes (Scherer & Verano, 2014; Tung et al., 2016; Toyne, 2018). Importantly, detailed interpretation is possible in this region because of the rich iconographic, epigraphic, and archaeological record, which provides deep contextualization for the human remains (e.g., Scherer & Verano, 2014). Women and children were frequent targets of direct violent action that falls under the rubric of violence as a means of social control or to gain power: massacres of entire families or communities based on their identity; the taking of captives for trophies, slavery, torture, or sacrifice; and ritual practices of body manipulation, intended to subordinate, annihilate, or remake society once the conflict event reached a conclusion (Martin & Harrod, 2020; Osterholtz, 2020). Osterholtz and Martin (2017) for example, describe disarticulated assemblages in the American Southwest whose demographic profiles suggest the massacre of entire families or clans and for whom the extensive level of processing indicated a repetitious, ritualized performance of restoration through the dehumanization and annihilation of entire groups and their identity. In this case, perimortem injuries in children's remains resemble the pattern of injuries found in adult men and women, which may suggest their agency as combatants (Toyne & Narvaez-Vargas, 2014; Osterholtz & Martin, 2017). Whether the people involved in this communal violence were seeking "power to" (capability) or "power over", physical and social control were the invisible forces driving the behavior (Foucault, 1980; Arnold & Hastorf, 2008:23), and its institutionalization makes structural violence a relevant construct for understanding the reverberations of these behaviors in the community.

Infant and child sacrifice also played a role in Mesoamerican and Andean ceremonies distinct from war-related violence (Hooton, 1940; Beck & Sievert, 2005; Gaither et al., 2008; Klaus et al., 2010; Tung & Knudson, 2010; Andrushko et al., 2011; Geller, 2011; Balderas, 2014; Crandall & Thompson, 2014; Bentley & Klaus, 2016; Klaus & Shimada, 2016; Klaus & Toyne, 2016). Among many pre-Columbian people, it has been argued that childhood death was "intimately tied to sacrifice" and age identity, and the practice of sacrifice was used to sanctify, rather than violate an individual's personhood (Geller, 2011:79). Crandall and Thompson (2014) took a social approach to arguing for infant and child sacrifice at a cave site of La Cueva de los Muertos Chiquitos (AD 660-1430), Durango, Mexico, addressing questions about cultural variation in ideology surrounding the human life course, liminality, and disease. Many Meso- and North American Ancestral communities believed that children had not attained full personhood prior to adolescence; thus, Mesoamerican infants and children were often conceptualized as a precious yet precarious resource (Joyce, 2000; Hamann, 2006; Geller, 2011). Based on the age structure of the infant burials, the high frequency of pathological conditions related to metabolic disturbances from micronutrient deficiencies, ethnographic analogy, and the extraordinary elaboration found in the grave goods of the sickest individuals, Crandall and Thompson (2014) argued that the infants and children interred at La Cueva de los Muertos Chiquitos represented sacrificial victims. This example is interesting because their argument was constructed despite having no evidence for traumatic injuries. At a time of high infant mortality, it is argued that these liminal beings were more fluid in their existence and identity, more proximal to the dead, and most suitable as sacrificial offerings. The authors discuss how it is unclear whether these individuals were chosen from the local community or whether they were captured in raiding activities of nearby marginalized communities. In either case, this Ancestral Tepehuán assemblage expresses how the community's perceptions of infancy and disease ideology structured their choice of offerings and how childhood experiences can be shaped by religious and political systems of power. Structural violence may be applied in circumstances of child sacrifice (*cf.* Geller, 2011), such as in the case of Aztec ceremonies, where the intent was certainly political and religious performance, devotions to imperial power, as well as gifts to Tlaloc (Aztec water god) and other deities.

Beyond Physical Violence: The Social Life Course Approach to Structural Violence in Infants and Children's Remains

Structural violence leads to varied and cumulative health effects that span the life course and that can extend across generations (Lupu & Peisakhin, 2017). This section reviews the effects that structural violence can have on subadult health, starting *in-utero*, through a lens of the social life course approach, and how paleopathologists can assess the relationships between political, economic, and institutional power, which shape illness and mortality across social life stages.

Social life course theory developed from within sociology and assesses how factors including chronological age, social identity, relationships, life events, and agency shape people's lives across the life course within specific social and historical contexts (Hutchison, 2011). For example, social beliefs around consumption of some foods during pregnancy and different life stages may have beneficial or detrimental effects on the health of mothers and their unborn, infants, and children (Vallianatos et al., 2006). Another example of social beliefs around consumption is the finding of children being fed different foods based on their gender, as has been identified in the bioarchaeological record (Miller et al., 2020).

Life course approaches in paleopathology address socio-cultural phenomena related to identity (i.e., age, gender, disability, socio-economic status, community membership) across the life course (Agarwal, 2016; Beauchesne & Agarwal, 2018; Inglis & Halcrow, 2018; Cheverko, 2020). Combined with the structural violence perspective, this approach is informative about the effects of health across the life course as it considers multiple aspects of identity and the wider social and political determinants of these impacts. The life course approach considers social structure and institutions and has an explicit focus on embodied historical forces, so therefore easily lends itself to work on structural violence, e.g., social age and gender are central factors for how people are treated within a social healthcare system, and how this may change over the life course.

The investigation of childhood as a socio-cultural phenomenon in paleopathology will necessarily begin with an investigation of the corporeal body that is embodied with social and environmental experiences (Sofaer, 2006). Studies of paleopathology that use the life course approach acknowledge the cumulative effect of environmental circumstances and identity across one's life. Adult bodies represent a palimpsest of experiences, insults, and healing from the start of life through to older age, whereas infants and children provide a thinner slice of experience. However, it is at the start of the life course that people are particularly susceptible to illness, malnutrition, and infection as when developing physically and immunologically (Lewis, 2006, 2017). This social life course research shows how plasticity across an individual's lifespan, and also across generations, is integral to understanding the influence of growth, disease, stress, diet, activity, and aging on the skeleton (Agarwal, 2016; Cheverko, 2020).

The nature of bone development in fetuses, infants, and children means that they are more susceptible to some pathological bone lesions and indicators of physiological stress and growth disturbance compared with adults (Lewis, 2006, 2019). In ways that have only become visible in the past few decades for paleopathologists, the *in-utero* period is an extremely sensitive time for both mother and baby, where both are more susceptible to infection and malnutrition (Robbins Schug & Blevins, 2016; Snoddy et al., 2017; Halcrow, 2020), and these insults *in-utero* can have lifelong repercussions on health (see Chapter 28, this volume). This challenges the notion of individual life courses, as Gowland (2015: 530) articulates, "Individual life courses can no longer be regarded as discrete, bounded, life histories, with clearly defined beginning and end points. If socioeconomic circumstances can have intergenerational effects, including disease susceptibility and growth stunting, then individual biographies should be viewed as nested or "embedded" within the lives of others."

Recent work on the development of methods for the examination of the timing of adolescence in the past, interpreted in relation to "health" and disease (e.g., Shapland & Lewis,

2013; Lewis et al., 2016a, 2016b) is central to extending our understanding of the subadult life course. Further work comparing growth and maturation status for age (e.g., vertebral canal size) with the timing of stress markers (e.g., linear enamel hypoplasia), may elucidate how early life stress has implications for growth in adolescence. In some cases, the investigation of adolescent health could contribute to our understanding of social age; for example, elucidating the life experiences of those who, although not yet biologically mature, may be taking on the adult roles of labor and subsistence in the community and becoming mothers themselves.

Social changes with the development of the Industrialization Era led to extreme structural violence experienced by the vulnerable working-class children in these communities. For example, in England during this period, children from the working class were sent to work for 10–15 hours a day from as young as six years old. There is bioarchaeological and historical evidence for the severe health consequences this had on the young in the form of growth stunting, and infectious and nutritional diseases (Gowland et al., 2018; Hodson & Gowland, 2020). Paleopathological work on the victims of the Great Irish Famine from the Kilkenny workhouse illustrates the deleterious effects that structural violence, occurring as the result of institutionalization and legislation, had on quality of life, and in particular the dire effects at the start of life (Geber, 2015, 2016). In this case, the poor and destitute, with nowhere else to go during the time of famine, were forced to reside and work within this institution. The inhabitants experienced inhumane working and living conditions and the very young were forcibly removed from their parents, which contributed to the devastating effects of severe illness and suffering. The victims of the Kilkenny workhouse, of which there were more than 1,000, were buried in a mass grave with evidence for a very high infant and child mortality rate, and extensive disease and starvation in this age cohort (Geber, 2015, 2016). This analysis considers the intersections of poverty, social status, gender, age, and disability, and the harrowing effects this had on the institutionalized population at this time.

Despite the potential of structural violence as a heuristic tool for understanding infant and child paleopathology and lived experiences, there is a dearth of literature outside of assessing physical violence in this age group. The effects of structural violence across the life course could possibly be assessed using isotopic evidence of dietary change over the life course in comparison with age-specific pathological profiles within a skeletal population (Knudson et al., 2012; Miller et al., 2018; Halcrow et al., 2022 and see Chapter 7, this volume). One challenge in the assessment of the social life course in infant and child paleopathology is that biological sex is often unknown without the application of aDNA techniques. However, methodological development in peptide analyses of dental enamel, which is very minimally destructive, is proving effective in sex determination (Stewart et al., 2017; Gowland et al., 2021). For example, recent bioarchaeological work in Industrial Era England and Europe has shown that girls are more affected by growth stunting compared with boys across low, middle, and high socio-economic status communities as a result of structural violence related to food preference (Reedy, 2020). Reedy (2020) argues that although boys may have worked in more strenuous situations outside of the home, there was preferential treatment for boys who received more nutritious food compared with girls (Humphries, 2013). Of course, biological sex is a poor proxy for gender identity and there is an entire avenue of investigation there that has only recently been recognized.

Structural Violence and the Pregnant Body

The exploration of fetal remains and the maternal-fetal nexus (Halcrow et al., 2017; Lewis 2017; Gowland & Halcrow 2020), and therefore the DOHaD hypothesis (Amoroso et al.,

2014; Amoroso & Garcia, 2018; and see Chapter 28, this volume), is becoming acknowledged as a sensitive barometer of health-related stress because of the biological constraints imposed through high energy expenditure during pregnancy and breastfeeding, coupled with increased vulnerability to illness during pregnancy.

Over the past few years, there has been a stimulation of paleopathological work assessing *in-utero* and early infancy stress as a proxy for maternal physiological stress (Beaumont et al., 2015; Snoddy et al., 2017; King et al., 2018; Lewis, 2019; Ellis, 2020; Hodson & Gowland, 2020; Adams et al., 2021). Avenues to assess maternal-fetal deprivation include the analyses of fetal bone growth stunting (e.g., Robbins Schug & Goldman, 2014; Hodson & Gowland, 2020) and deciduous dental enamel defects (Adams et al., 2021). Although fetal remains can tell their own stories of deprivation and disease (Robbins Schug, 2011; Robbins Schug & Goldman, 2014), they can also give cues to the maternal state (Robbins Schug & Blevins, 2016; Snoddy et al., 2017) due to the fundamental interactions between two deeply interdependent individuals (Gowland, 2020).

When structural inequalities inhibit appropriate antenatal care, biological constraints on the pregnant body and fetus are often exacerbated. Today, with the medicalization of the maternal body and the childbirth process, we see evidence for structural violence toward vulnerable pregnant and birthing people (Neely et al., 2020). Inadequacies of antenatal and postnatal support and care can also result in poorer perinatal outcomes. For example, it has been found that preventable maternal and infant deaths are significantly higher in some populations related to inequalities related to race, gender, and poverty (e.g., Gamlin & Holmes, 2018). Similarly, there is historical evidence for structural violence in maternal care and birth where poor and/or unmarried pregnant people received inferior medical care compared with those who were wealthy enough to pay for a private doctor to attend their birth (McIntosh, 2012).

The impact of structural violence on antenatal health and care and the nexus with perinatal outcomes can be considered in interpretations of the study of infant and child paleopathology. An example that demonstrates the usefulness of this approach is growth, mortality, and morbidity research in the resource-poor setting in post-Medieval London (Hodson & Gowland, 2020). Hodson and Gowland (2020) assessed the bone growth of perinates and older infants from several archaeological sites and found significant growth disruption in long bones and bone pathology indicating deprivation of mothers and their babies *in-utero* in these poor, working-class communities as the result of unequal access to resources. Their findings are interpreted by the historic evidence for maternal deprivation and lack of access to appropriate medical care and resources post-birth (Hodson & Gowland, 2020). Recent historical research has used the framework of structural violence to explain how maternal bodies at this time were marginalized and institutionalized which created health inequalities and an allostatic load (Mathena-Allen & Zukerman, 2020). Unfortunately, even if these babies who were deprived *in-utero* lived past the perinatal period, they likely experienced further negative health effects upon their already compromised state. Most working-class parents in these communities were forced back into long hours of work for very low wages when their babies were very young. The limited social and government support and insufficient access to medical care meant that parents often had to leave their infants with other very young family members, often young children themselves.

Structural violence has a strong interrelationship with the medicalization of the maternal body. The use of invasive medical interventions during birth such as forceps and cesarean sections has been shown to have a negative effect on physical and mental health of mother and baby (Peters et al., 2018). As noted, the structural violence framework is also a useful lens to consider the treatment of vulnerable people's bodies after death historically. This seems particularly pertinent for the treatment of the maternal and fetal body and the history of retention of fetal and infant remains from mothers who were socially deprived and disadvantaged, e.g., there is evidence that infants held in some anatomy legacy collections are babies from unwed mothers who lacked resources and social support (Clarke, 2012; Muller & Butler, 2018; Southorn, 2019).

The nature of maternal and infant care has been thoroughly theorized from the evolutionary anthropological context (Halcrow et al., 2020). The exploration of the intersection between structural violence and maternal-fetal outcome in paleopathology can be further illuminated through a consideration of care for a birthing mother from an evolutionary biology perspective (Halcrow et al., 2020). For example, Abrams and Rutherford (2011) have explored postpartum hemorrhage (PPH) in humans from an evolutionary biology perspective and argue that the maternal body can be subjected to structural violence through the loss of traditional practices in birth care. Humans have developed vulnerability to PPH from changes in placental invasiveness and vascular changes to counteract gravitational effects of bipedalism. They argue that the cross-cultural occurrence of indigenous traditional childbirth attendants' actions (Lefèber & Voorhoeve, 1998) mimics World Health Organization recommendations on cord traction and uterine massage to induce placental birth illustrating the deep evolutionary past of placental vulnerability (Abrams & Rutherford, 2011).

Childcare, Family, and Resilience in the Face of Structural Violence

Care can be defined as "the provision of what is necessary in order to maintain another person's state of health and welfare" (Powell et al., 2016:1). The definition can be expanded to include aspects of emotion in the provision of care: "A feeling of affection and responsibility combined with actions that provide responsibility for an individual's personal needs or well-being, in a face-to-face relationship. Caregiving includes physical care, such as bathing or feeding a person, as well as emotional care, such as tender touch, supportive talk, empathy, and affection." (Cancian and Oliker, 1999:2).

Structural violence has major impacts on emotional and physical care and the disruption for care for the mother, infant, and child today (Scheper-Hughes, 1992; McIntosh, 2012; Gamlin & Holmes, 2018), and in the past (Geber, 2015, 2016; Halcrow, 2020; Halcrow et. al., 2020; Filipek et al., 2021). Recently, models to investigate infant and childcare in paleopathology have been presented that consider cultural and social aspects of infant feeding and weaning, social organization, family structure and size, the disease environment, and the archaeology of emotion, including grief around the loss of an infant (Murphy, 2011; Geber, 2015; Halcrow, 2020; Halcrow et al., 2020; Hodson & Gowland, 2020; Robbins Schug, 2020; Supernant et al., 2020; Filipek et al., 2021). These models (Halcrow, 2020; Halcrow et al., 2020) could be extended to focus on structural violence through a consideration of social structures and individual identity, including gender, race, and socio-economic status, which mediate inequity in care.

There is a tendency to assume that because infant and child mortality and morbidity in the past were often high, that parents withheld emotional attachment toward their young, and/or were neglectful (Ariès, 1962:39; Shorter, 1975: 200; Schepher-Hughes, 1992; Cannon & Cook, 2015). However, recent archaeological and bioarchaeological work has challenged these interpretations in the context of many archaeological settings, where intense grief of parents toward the death of infants in the past has been illustrated (Carroll, 2011; Murphy, 2011; Gowland, 2020).

Research that incorporates paleopathological data and theoretical approaches to disability, emotion, and childhood in the past can help in our interpretation of infant and childhood experiences of health and care in the past, and social responses to their deaths. For example, Robbins Schug (2017) in her examination of two child crania from the site of Harappa identified that the individuals suffered plagiocephaly and were likely twins based on genetic and developmental processes. She argues that aspects of personhood, emotion, and behavior can be inferred from these individuals' remains since physical care was required throughout their infancy and the unusual mortuary ritual after their death may represent a personal connection, or social value (Robbins Schug, 2020b).

There is growing acknowledgment within anthropology of the considerable resilience and adaptability of family structures that can work to combat structural violence, highlighting the efforts that parents made to secure the welfare of their children in the face of considerable inequality, including marginalization and stigma (e.g., Powell et al., 2016; Filipek et al., 2021; Kendall & Kendall, 2021). We do, however, recognize that many social factors including oppressive institutions, colonialism, and slavery were structured to undermine family structures (e.g., the forcible removal of Indigenous children from their families and schooling in colonial institutions, as occurred in the United States, Canada, Australia, New Zealand Aotearoa, etc.). Furthermore, family structures themselves can contribute to oppression of women and children (Montesanti & Thurston, 2015).

Kendall and Kendall (2021) consider family structure and colonial oppression in the representation of parenting in 19th century Fens, a wetland region in Eastern England. They assess the portrayal of parenting and the impact of colonial powers on the family and childhood health and wellbeing. "Othering" of the inhabitants was (and continues to be) a significant issue for Fenlanders, with those in power (colonists) creating a culture of fear and condemnation toward these communities. The Fenlanders were known by groups outside of this region to be haunted by demons, an area rife with "ague", and were characterized by maternal neglect and indifference toward their children. However, Kendall and Kendall (2021) present an alternate model that decolonizes the discourse of childcare in the 19th century Fens. They present evidence that shows the valued position of children and their care, and consider the childcare provisions that women made when they worked outside of the home (Kendall & Kendall, 2021).

Filipek et al. (2021) assessed constructions of care for adolescents suffering from leprosy in Saxo-Norman period England using evidence for medical care and treatment, social age and institutionalization from historiographical sources, and pathology from the skeletons. They interrogate the assumptions that medieval leprosy hospitals represented neglect and confinement with minimal care. Filipek et al. (2021) argue that although there is evidence for a complex level of care at the group level for these young patients, there was significant structural inequality for families seeking this care for their young.

Although structural violence is known to disproportionately affect some segments in society (i.e., infants, children, and mothers), we acknowledge that the framework presented here is also relevant to the study of adults in the past. Furthermore, it is important that we study both the survivors and non-survivors to gain a more holistic perspective of human experience of disease, and an understanding of the human experience over the entire life course. A consideration of both the survivors and non-survivors can also help to test important interpretive issues in paleopathology such as the "osteological paradox", including the formation of skeletal lesions and the relationship with survivorship (DeWitte & Stojanowski, 2015; and see Chapter 31, this volume).

Conclusion

Infant and child paleopathology has developed significantly, both methodologically and theoretically, over the past two decades to contribute to a more holistic understanding of the past. This chapter reviewed the potential uses of a structural violence framework as a heuristic tool for interpreting evidence of infant and childhood paleopathology in the past and the importance of the exploration of the maternal-infant nexus. Women, infants, and children are particularly informative about social suffering, institutionalized violence, struggle, and resistance because they are disproportionately affected by the risk of deprivation, violence, and disease within populations. Furthermore, biological fragility during *in-utero* development and early postnatal life exacerbates the impact of structural violence and health deficits during this time. Recent social bioarchaeological work has illustrated the resilient and adaptive nature of family and social structures of maternal, infant, and childcare that can offset some of these deleterious effects of structural violence toward the pregnant body and infants and children.

References

Abrams, E. T. & Rutherford, J. N. (2011). Framing postpartum hemorrhage as a consequence of human placental biology: an evolutionary and comparative perspective. *American Anthropologist* 113(3):417–430. https://doi.org/10.1111/j.1548-1433.2011.01351.x

Adams, A. B., Halcrow, S. E., King, C. L., Miller, M. J., Vlok, M., Millard, A. R., … & Oxenham, M. F. (2021). We're all in this together: accessing the maternal-infant relationship in prehistoric Vietnam. In Kendall, E. J. & Kendall, R. (Eds.), *The Family in Past Perspective: An Interdisciplinary Exploration of Familial Relationships Through Time*, pp. 191–221. Abingdon: Routledge.

Agarwal, S. C. (2016). Bone morphologies and histories: life course approaches in bioarchaeology. *American Journal of Physical Anthropology* 159(S61):130–149. https://doi.org/10.1002/ajpa.22905

Amoroso, A. & Garcia, S. J. (2018). Can early-life growth disruptions predict longevity? Testing the association between vertebral neural canal (VNC) size and age-at-death. *International Journal of Paleopathology* 22:8–17. https://doi.org/10.1016/j.ijpp.2018.03.007

Amoroso, A., Garcia, S. J. & Cardoso, H. F. V. (2014). Age at death and linear enamel hypoplasias: testing the effects of childhood stress and adult socioeconomic circumstances in premature mortality. *American Journal of Human Biology* 26(4):461–468. https://doi.org/10.1002/ajhb.22547

Andrushko, V. A., Buzon, M. R., Gibaja, A. M., McEwan, G. F., Simonetti, A. & Creaser, R. A. (2011). Investigating a child sacrifice event from the Inca heartland. *Journal of Archaeological Science* 38(2):323–333. https://doi.org/10.1016/j.jas.2010.09.009

Ariès, P. (1962). *Centuries of Childhood.* New Jersey: Cape.

Arnold, D. Y. & Hastorf, C. A. (2008). *Heads of State: Icons, Power, and Politics in the Ancient and Modern Andes.* Abingdon: Routledge.

Barrett, A. (2014). Childhood, colonialism, and nation-building. In Thompson, J. L., Alfonso-Durruty, M. P. & Crandall, J. J. (Eds.), *Tracing Childhood: Bioarchaeological Investigations of Early Lives in Antiquity*, pp. 159–182. Gainesville: University Press of Florida.

Baxter, J. E. (2005). *The Archaeology of Childhood Children, Gender and Material Culture.* Lanham, MD: AltaMira.

Beauchesne, P. & Agarwal, S. C. (2018). *Children and Childhood in Bioarchaeology.* Gainesville: University Press of Florida.

Beaumont, J., Montgomery, J., Buckberry, J. & Jay, M. (2015). Infant mortality and isotopic complexity: new approaches to stress, maternal health, and weaning. *American Journal of Physical Anthropology* 157(3):441–457. https://doi.org/10.1002/ajpa.22736

Beck, L. A. & Sievert, A. K. (2005). Mortuary pathways leading to the cenote at Chichén Itzá. In Rakita, G. M., Buikstra, J. E., Beck, L. A. & Williams, S. R. (Eds.), *Interacting with the Dead: Perspectives on Mortuary Archaeology for the New Millennium*, pp. 290–304. Gainesville: University Press of Florida.

Bentley, S. & Klaus, H. D. (2016). Reconsidering retainers: identity, death and sacrifice in high-status funerary contexts on the North Coast of Peru. In Klaus, H. D. & Toyne, J. M. (Eds.), *Ritual Violence in the Ancient Andes*, pp. 266–290. Austin: University of Texas Press.

Bluebond-Langner, M. & Korbin, J. E. (2007). Challenges and opportunities in the anthropology of childhoods: an introduction to children, childhoods, and childhood studies. *American Anthropologist* 109(2):241–246. https://doi.org/10.1525/aa.2007.109.2.241

Bourdieu, P. (1977). *Outline of a Theory of Practice*. Cambridge University Press.

Bourgois, P. (2001). The power of violence in war and peace: post-cold War lessons from El Salvador. *Ethnography* 2(1):5–34. https://doi.org/10.1177/14661380122230803

Bright, L. N. (2020). Structural violence: epistemological considerations for bioarchaeology. In Cheverko, C. M., Prince-Buitenhuys, J. R. & Hubbe, M. (Eds.), *Theoretical Approaches in Bioarchaeology*, pp. 131–149. Abingdon: Routledge.

Cancian, F. M. & Oliker, S. J. (1999). *Gender and Care*. Altamira.

Cannon, A. & Cook, K. (2015). Infant death and the archaeology of grief. *Cambridge Archaeological Journal* 25(2):399–416. https://doi.org/10.1017/S0959774315000049

Carroll, M. (2011). Infant death and burial in Roman Italy. *Journal of Roman Archaeology* 24:99–120. https://doi.org/10.1017/S1047759400003329

Chávez Balderas, X. (2014). Sacrifice at the Templo Mayor of Tenochtitlan and its role in regard to warfare. In Scherer, A. K. & Verano, J. W. (Eds.), *Embattled Bodies, Embattled Places: War in Pre-Columbian Mesoamerica and the Andes*, pp. 173–199. Washington, DC: Dumbarton Oaks.

Cheverko, C. M. (2020). Life course approaches and life history theory. In Cheverko, C. M., Prince-Buitenhuys, J. R. & Hubbe, M. (Eds.), *Theoretical Approaches in Bioarchaeology*, pp. 59–74. Abingdon: Routledge.

Clarke, A. (2012). *Born to a Changing World: Childbirth in Nineteenth-Century New Zealand*. Wellington, New Zealand: Bridget Williams Books.

Crandall, J. J. & Thompson, J. L. (2014). Beyond victims: exploring the identity of sacrificed infants and children at La Cueva de Los Muertos Chiquitos, Durango, Mexico (AD 571–1168). In Thompson, J. L., Alfonso-Durruty, M. P. & Crandall, J. J. (Eds.), *Tracing Childhood: Bioarchaeological Investigations of Early Lives in Antiquity*, pp. 36–57. Gainesville: University Press of Florida.

de la Cova, C. (2008). *Silent Voices of the Destitute: An Analysis of African American and Euro-American Health During the Nineteenth Century*. Doctoral thesis, Indiana University. Bloomington, Indiana. ProQuest Dissertations & Theses Global.

de la Cova, C. (2011). Race, health, and disease in 19th-century-born males. *American Journal of Physical Anthropology* 144(4):526–537. https://doi.org/10.1002/ajpa.21434

de la Cova, C. (2012). Patterns of trauma and violence in 19th-century-born African American and Euro-American females. *International Journal of Paleopathology* 2(2–3):61–68. https://doi.org/10.1016/j.ijpp.2012.09.009

de la Cova, C. (2020). Making silenced voices speak: Restoring neglected and ignored identities in anatomical collections. In Cheverko, C. M., Prince-Buitenhuys, J. R. & Hubbe, M. (Eds.), *Theoretical Approaches in Bioarchaeology*, pp. 150–169. Abingdon: Routledge.

DeWitte, S. N. & Stojanowski, C. M. (2015). The osteological paradox 20 years later: past perspectives, future directions. *Journal of Archaeological Research* 23(4):397–450. https://doi.org/10.1007/s10814-015-9084-1

Dunnavant, J., Justinvil, D. & Colwell, C. (2021, May 19). Craft an African American graves protection and repatriation act. *Nature* 593:337–340. https://www.nature.com/articles/d41586-021-01320-4

Ellis, M. A. B. (2020). Still life: a bioarchaeological portrait of perinatal remains buried at the Spring Street Presbyterian Church. *Historical Archaeology* 54(1):184–201. https://doi.org/10.1007/s41636-019-00216-5

Farmer, P. (1997). Ethnography, social analysis, and the prevention of sexually transmitted HIV infection. In Inhorn, M. C. & Brown, P. J. (Eds.), *The Anthropology of Infectious Disease: International Health Perspectives*, pp. 413–438. Philadelphia: Gordon and Breach.

Farmer, P. (2004). An anthropology of structural violence. *Current Anthropology* 45(3):305–325. https://doi.org/10.1086/382250

Farmer, P. E., Nizeye, B., Stulac, S. & Keshavjee, S. (2006). Structural violence and clinical medicine. *PLoS Med* 3(10):e449. https://doi.org/10.1371/journal.pmed.0030449

Filipek, K. L., Roberts, C., Gowland, R. L. & Tucker, K. (2021). Alloparenting adolescents: Evaluating the social and biological impacts of leprosy on young people in Saxo-Norman England (9th to 12th centuries AD) through cross-disciplinary models of care. In Kendall, E. J. & Kendall, R. (Eds.), *The Family in Past Perspective: An Interdisciplinary Exploration of Familial Relationships Through Time*, pp. 30–57. Abingdon: Routledge.

Foucault, M. (1980). *Power/Knowledge*. New York: Pantheon.
Fry, D. P. (2006). *The Human Potential for Peace: An Anthropological Challenge to Assumptions About War and Violence*. Oxford: Oxford University Press.
Gaither, C., Kent, J., Sánchez, V. V. & Tham, T. R. (2008). Mortuary practices and human sacrifice in the middle Chao Valley of Peru: their interpretation in the context of Andean mortuary patterning. *Latin American Antiquity* 19(2):107–121. https://doi.org/10.1017/S1045663500007744
Galtung, J. (1969). Violence, peace, and peace research. *Journal of Peace Research* 6(3):167–191.
Gamlin, J. & Holmes, S. (2018). Preventable perinatal deaths in indigenous Wixárika communities: an ethnographic study of pregnancy, childbirth and structural violence. *BMC Pregnancy and Childbirth* 18(1):243. https://doi.org/10.1186/s12884-018-1870-6
Geber, J. (2015). *Victims of Ireland's Great Famine: The Bioarchaeology of Mass Burials at Kilkenny Union Workhouse*. Gainesville: University Press of Florida.
Geber, J. (2016). 'Children in a ragged state': seeking a biocultural narrative of a workhouse childhood in Ireland during the Great Famine (1845–1852). *Childhood in the Past* 9(2):120–138. https://doi.org/10.1080/17585716.2016.1205344
Geller, P. L. (2011). The sacrifices we make of and for our children: making sense of pre-Columbian Maya practices. In Baadsgaard, A., Boutin, A. T. & Buikstra, J. E. (Eds.), *Breathing New Life into the Evidence of Death: Contemporary Approaches to Mortuary Analysis*, pp.79–106. Santa Fe, NM: School for Advanced Research Press.
González-Ruibal, A. & Moshenska, G. (2014). *Ethics and the Archaeology of Violence* (Vol. 2). New York: Springer International Publishing.
Goodman, A. H. & Armelagos, G. J. (1989). Infant and childhood morbidity and mortality risks in archaeological populations. *World Archaeology* 21(2):225–243. https://doi.org/10.1080/00438243.1989.9980103
Gottlieb, A. (2000). Where have all the babies gone? Toward an anthropology of infants (and their caretakers). *Anthropological Quarterly* 73(3):121–132.
Gowland, R. L. (2015). Entangled lives: Implications of the developmental origins of health and disease hypothesis for bioarchaeology and the life course. *American Journal of Physical Anthropology* 158(4):530–540. https://doi.org/10.1002/ajpa.22820
Gowland, R. L. (2020). Ruptured: reproductive loss, bodily boundaries, time and the life course in archaeology. In Gowland, R. & Halcrow, S. E. (Eds.), *The Mother-Infant Nexus in Anthropology; Small Beginnings, Significant Outcomes,* pp. 257–274. New York: Springer International Publishing.
Gowland, R. L., Caffell, A. C., Newman, S., Levene, A. & Holst, M. (2018). Broken childhoods: rural and urban non-adult health during the industrial revolution in Northern England (eighteenth-nineteenth centuries). *Bioarchaeology International* 2(1):44–62. https://doi.org/10.5744/bi.2018.1015
Gowland, R. L. & Halcrow, S. E. (Eds.) (2020). *The Mother-Infant Nexus in Anthropology: Small Beginnings, Significant Outcomes*. New York: Springer International Publishing. https://doi.org/10.1007/978-3-030-27393-4
Gowland, R. L., Stewart, N. A., Crowder, K. D., Hodson, C., Shaw, H., Gron, K. J. & Montgomery, J. (2021). Sex estimation of teeth at different developmental stages using dimorphic enamel peptide analysis. *American Journal of Physical Anthropology* 174(4):859–869. https://doi.org/10.1002/ajpa.24231
Grauer, A. L. & Buikstra, J. E. (2019). Themes in paleopathology. In Buikstra, J. E. (Ed.), *Ortner's Identification of Pathological Conditions in Human Skeletal Remains* (3rd ed), pp. 21–33. London: Academic Press.
Halcrow, S. E. (2020). Infants in the bioarchaeological past: who cares? In Gowland, R. & Halcrow, S. E. (Eds.), *The Mother-Infant Nexus in Anthropology: Small Beginnings, Significant Outcomes*, pp.19–38. New York: Springer International Publishing. https://doi.org/10.1007/978-3-030-27393-4_2
Halcrow, S. E., Miller, M. J., Pechenkina, K., Dong, Y. & Fan, W. (2022). The bioarchaeology of infant feeding. In Han, S. & Tomori, C. (Eds.), *The Routledge Handbook of Anthropology and Reproduction,* pp. 541–558. Abingdon: Routledge.
Halcrow, S. E. & Tayles, N. (2008). The bioarchaeological investigation of childhood and social age: problems and prospects. *Journal of Archaeological Method and Theory* 15(2):190–215. https://doi.org/10.1007/s10816-008-9052-x
Halcrow, S. E., Tayles, N. & Elliott, G. E. (2017). The bioarchaeology of fetuses. In Han, S., Betsinger, T. K. & Scott, A. B. (Eds.), *The Anthropology of the Fetus: Biology, Culture, and Society* (1st ed), pp. 83–111. Oxford, New York: Berghahn Books.

Halcrow, S. E. & Ward, S. M. (2017). Bioarchaeology of childhood. In Montgomery, H. (Ed.), *Oxford Bibliographies in Childhood Studies*. Oxford: Oxford University Press. https://www.oxfordbibliographies.com/view/document/obo-9780199791231/obo-9780199791231-0178.xml. DOI: 10.1093/OBO/9780199791231-0178

Halcrow, S. E., Warren, R., Kushnick, G. & Nowell, A. (2020). Care of infants in the past: bridging evolutionary anthropological and bioarchaeological approaches. *Evolutionary Human Sciences* 2:e47. https://doi.org/10.1017/ehs.2020.46

Hamann, B. E. (2006). Child martyrs and murderous children: age and agency in sixteenth-century transatlantic religious conflicts. In Ardren, T. & Hutson, S. (Eds.), *The Social Experience of Childhood in Ancient Mesoamerica*, pp. 203–231. Boulder: University of Colorado Press.

Han, S., Betsinger, T. K. & Scott, A. B. (Eds.). *The Anthropology of the Fetus: Biology, Culture, and Society*. Oxford, New York: Berghahn Books.

Harrod, R. P. & Martin, D. (2014). *Bioarchaeology and Environmental Change and Violence*. New York: Springer.

Hodson, C. M. & Gowland, R. (2020). Like mother, like child: investigating perinatal and maternal health stress in post-medieval London. In Gowland, R. & Halcrow, S. (Eds.), *The Mother-Infant Nexus in Anthropology: Small Beginnings, Significant Outcomes*, pp. 39–64. New York: Springer International Publishing. https://doi.org/10.1007/978-3-030-27393-4_3

Hooton, E. A. (1940). Skeletons from the *cenote* of sacrifice at chichén Itzá. In Hay, C. L., Linton, R., Lothrop, S. K. & Vaillant, G. C. (Eds.), *The Maya and Their Neighbors: Essays on Middle American Anthropology and Archaeology*, pp. 272–280. Norwalk, CT: Appleton Century.

Hrdy, S. B. (1999). *Mother Nature: A History of Mothers, Infants, and Natural Selection*. New York: Pantheon.

Hutchison, E. D. (2011). Life course theory. In Levesque, R. J. R. (Ed.), *Encyclopedia of Adolescence*, pp. 2141–2150. New York: Springer International Publishing.

Humphries, J. (2013). The lure of aggregates and the pitfalls of the patriarchal perspective: a critique of the high wage economy interpretation of the British industrial revolution. *Economic History Review* 66(3): 693–714.

Inglis, R. M. & Halcrow, S. E. (2018). The bioarchaeology of childhood: theoretical development in the field. In Beauchesne, P. & Agarwal, S. (Eds.), *Children and Childhood in Bioarchaeology*, pp.33–60. Gainesville: University Press of Florida.

Joyce, R. A. (2000). *Gender and Power in Prehispanic Mesoamerica*. Austin: University of Texas Press.

Kendall, E. J. & Kendall, R. (Eds.) (2021). *The Family in Past Perspective: An Interdisciplinary Exploration of Familial Relationships Through Time*. Abingdon: Routledge.

King, C. L., Halcrow, S. E., Millard, A. R., Gröcke, D. R., Standen, V. G., Portilla, M. & Arriaza, B. T. (2018). Let's talk about stress, baby! Infant-feeding practices and stress in the ancient Atacama desert, Northern Chile. *American Journal of Physical Anthropology* 166(1):139–155. https://doi.org/10.1002/ajpa.23411

Klaus, H. D. (2012). The bioarchaeology of structural violence: a theoretical model and a case study. In Martin, D. L., Harrod, R. P. & Perez, V. R. (Eds.), *The Bioarchaeology of Violence*, pp. 29–62. Gainesville: University Press of Florida.

Klaus, H. D., Centurión, J. & Curo, M. (2010). Bioarchaeology of human sacrifice: violence, identity and the evolution of ritual killing at Cerro Cerrillos, Peru. *Antiquity* 84(326):1102–1122. https://doi.org/10.1017/S0003598X00067119

Klaus, H. D. & Shimada, I. (2016). Bodies and blood: Middle Sicán human sacrifice in the Lambayeque valley complex (AD 900–1100). In Klaus, H. D. & Toyne, J. M. (Eds.), *Ritual Violence in the Ancient Andes: Reconstructing Sacrifice on the North Coast of Peru*, pp.120–149. Austin: University of Texas Press.

Klaus, H. D. & Toyne, J. M. (2016). *Ritual Violence in the Ancient Andes: Reconstructing Sacrifice on the North Coast of Peru*. Austin: University of Texas Press.

Kleinman, A., Das, V. & Lock, M. M. (1997). *Social Suffering*. Oakland: University of California Press.

Knudson, K. J., Pestle, W. J., Torres-Rouff, C. & Pimentel, G. (2012). Assessing the life history of an Andean traveller through biogeochemistry: stable and radiogenic isotope analyses of archaeological human remains from Northern Chile. *International Journal of Osteoarchaeology* 22(4):435–451. https://doi.org/10.1002/oa.1217

Korbin, J. E. (2003). Children, childhoods, and violence. *Annual Review of Anthropology* 32(1):431–446. https://doi.org/10.1146/annurev.anthro.32.061002.093345

Kuckleman, K. A. (2017). Cranial trauma and victimization among ancestral pueblo farmers of the Northern San Juan region. In Martin, D. L. & Tegtmeyer, C. E. (Eds.), *Broken Bones, Broken Bodies: Bioarchaeological and Forensic Approaches for Accumulative Trauma and Violence*, pp. 43–60. Lanham, MD: Lexington Books.

Lans, A. M. (2020). Embodied discrimination and "mutilated historicity": archiving Black women's bodies in the Huntington Collection. In Tremblay, L. A. & Reedy, S. (Eds.), The Bioarchaeology of Structural Violence, pp. 31–52. Bioarchaeology and Social Theory. Cham: Springer. https://doi.org/10.1007/978-3-030-46440-0_3

Lancy, D. (2012). Unmasking children's agency. *AnthropoChildren* 1(2). https://digitalcommons.usu.edu/sswa_facpubs/277/

Larchanché, S. (2012). Intangible obstacles: health implications of stigmatization, structural violence, and fear among undocumented immigrants in France. *Social Science and Medicine* 74(6):858–863. https://doi.org/10.1016/j.socscimed.2011.08.016

Larsen, C. S. (2002). Bioarchaeology: the lives and lifestyles of past people. *Journal of Archaeological Research* 10(2):119–166.

Leatherman, T. & Goodman, A. H. (2011). Critical biocultural approaches in medical anthropology. In Singer, M. & Erickson, P. I. (Eds.), *A Companion to Medical Anthropology*, pp. 29–48. Chichester: Wiley-Blackwell.

Lee, B. X. (2019). *Violence: An Interdisciplinary Approach to Causes, Consequences and Cures*. New York: Wiley.

Lefeber, Y. & Voorhoeve, H. W. A. (1998). *Indigenous Customs in Childbirth and Child Care*. Assen, Drenthe, The Netherlands: Van Gorcum and Company.

Lewis, M. E. (2006). *The Bioarchaeology of Children: Perspectives from Biological and Forensic Anthropology*. Cambridge: Cambridge University Press.

Lewis, M. E. (2014). Sticks and Stones: exploring the nature and significance of child trauma in the past. In Knüsel, C. & Smith, M. (Eds.), *The Routledge Handbook of the Bioarchaeology of Human Conflict*, pp. 39–63. Abingdon: Routledge.

Lewis, M. E. (2017). *Paleopathology of Children: Identification of Pathological Conditions in the Human Skeletal Remains of Non-Adults*. London: Academic Press.

Lewis, M. E. (2019). Fetal paleopathology: an impossible discipline? In Han, S., Betsinger, T. K. & Scott, A. B. (Eds.), *The Anthropology of the Fetus: Biology, Culture, and Society*, pp. 112–131. Oxford, New York: Berghahn Books. https://doi.org/10.2307/j.ctvw04h7z.11

Lewis, M., Shapland, F. & Watts, R. (2016a). On the threshold of adulthood: a new approach for the use of maturation indicators to assess puberty in adolescents from medieval England. *American Journal of Human Biology* 28(1):48–56. https://doi.org/10.1002/ajhb.22761

Lewis, M. E., Shapland, F. & Watts, R. (2016b). The influence of chronic conditions and the environment on pubertal development: an example from medieval England. *International Journal of Paleopathology* 12:1–10. https://doi.org/10.1016/j.ijpp.2015.10.004

Lillehammer, G. (2015). 25 years with the 'child' and the archaeology of childhood. *Childhood in the Past* 8(2):78–86. https://doi.org/10.1179/1758571615Z.00000000030

Lupu, N. & Peisakhin, L. (2017). The legacy of political violence across generations. *American Journal of Political Science* 61(4):836–851. https://doi.org/10.1111/ajps.12327

Martin, D. L. & Harrod, R. P. (2012). *The Bioarchaeology of Violence*. University Press of Florida.

Martin, D. L. & Harrod, R. P. (2020). Gendered violence in small-scale societies in the past. In O'Toole, L. L., Schiffman, J. R. & Sullivan, R. (Eds.), *Gender Violence: Interdisciplinary Perspectives* (3rd ed), pp. 13–24. New York: New York University Press.

Martin, D. L., Harrod, R. P. & Fields, M. (2010). Beaten down and worked to the bone: bioarchaeological investigations of women and violence in the ancient Southwest. *Landscapes of Violence* 1(1):3.

Mathena-Allen, S. & Zuckerman, M. K. (2020). Embodying industrialization: inequality, structural violence, disease, and stress in working-class and poor British women. In Tremblay, L. A. & Reedy, S. (Eds.), *The Bioarchaeology of Structural Violence*, pp. 53–79. New York: Springer International Publishing.

Mays, S., Gowland, R., Halcrow, S. E. & Murphy, E. (2017). Child bioarchaeology: perspectives on the past 10 years. *Childhood in the Past* 10(1):38–56. https://doi.org/10.1080/17585716.2017.1301066

McIntosh, T. (2012). *A Social History of Maternity and Childbirth: Key Themes in Maternity Care*. Abingdon: Routledge.

Miller, M. J., Agarwal, S. C. & Langebaek, C. H. (2018). Dietary histories: tracing food consumption practices from childhood through adulthood using stable isotope analysis. In Beauchesne, P. &

Agarwal, S. (Eds.), *Children and Childhood in Bioarchaeology*, pp. 262–293. Gainesville: University Press of Florida.

Miller, Melanie, J., Dong, Y., Pechenkina, K., Fan, W. & Halcrow, S. E. (2020). Raising girls and boys in early China: stable isotope data reveal sex differences in weaning and childhood diets during the eastern Zhou era. *American Journal of Physical Anthropology* 172(4):567–585. https://doi.org/10.1002/ajpa.24033

Montesanti, S. R. & Thurston, W. E. (2015). Mapping the role of structural and interpersonal violence in the lives of women: implications for public health interventions and policy. *BMC Women's Health* 15(1):100. https://doi.org/10.1186/s12905-015-0256-4

Montgomery, H. (2008). *An Introduction to Childhood: Anthropological Perspectives on Children's Lives*. Chicester: Wiley-Blackwell.

Muller, J. L. & Butler, M. S. (2018). At the intersections of race, poverty, gender, and science: a museum mortuary for twentieth century fetuses and infants. In Stone, P. K. (Ed.), *Bioarchaeological Analyses and Bodies: New Ways of Knowing Anatomical and Archaeological Skeletal Collections*, pp. 71–86. New York: Springer International Publishing.

Murphy, E. M. (2011). Children's burial grounds in Ireland (Cilliní) and parental emotions toward infant death. *International Journal of Historical Archaeology* 15(3):409-428. https://doi.org/10.1007/s10761-011-0148-8

Neely, E., Raven, B., Dixon, L., Bartle, C. & Timu-Parata, C. (2020). "Ashamed, silent and stuck in a system"—Applying a structural violence lens to midwives' stories on social disadvantage in pregnancy. *International Journal of Environmental Research and Public Health* 17(24):9355. https://doi.org/10.3390/ijerph17249355

Nowell, A. & Kurki, H. (2020). Moving beyond the obstetrical dilemma hypothesis: birth, weaning and infant care in the plio–pleistocene. In Gowland, R. & Halcrow, S. (Eds.), *The Mother-Infant Nexus in Anthropology: Small Beginnings, Significant Outcomes*, pp.173–192. New York: Springer International Publishing. https://doi.org/10.1007/978-3-030-27393-4_10

Nystrom, K. C. (2014). The bioarchaeology of structural violence and dissection in the 19th-century United States. *American Anthropologist* 116(4):765–779. https://doi.org/10.1111/aman.12151

Nystrom, K. C. (2017). *The Bioarchaeology of Dissection and Autopsy in the United States*. New York: Springer International Publishing.

Nystrom, K. & Robbins Schug, G. (2020). A bioarchaeology of social inequality and environmental change. In Robbins Schug, G. (Ed.), *The Routledge Handbook of the Bioarchaeology of Climate and Environmental Change*, pp. 159–188. Abingdon: Routledge.

Osterholtz, A. (2020). Pain as power: Torture as a mechanism for social control. In. Sheridan, S. G & Gregoricka, L. A. (Eds.), *Purposeful Pain: The Bioarchaeology of Intentional Suffering*, pp. 215–231. New York: Springer International Publishing.

Osterholtz, A. J. & Martin, D. L. (2017). The poetics of annihilation: on the presence of women and children at massacre sites in the ancient southwest. In Martin, D. L. & Tegtmeyer, C. (Eds.), *Bioarchaeology of Women and Children in Times of War*, pp. 111–128. New York: Springer International Publishing.

Panter-Brick, C., Goodman, A., Tol, W. & Eggerman, M. (2011). Mental health and childhood adversities: a longitudinal study in Kabul, Afghanistan. *Journal of the American Academy of Child & Adolescent Psychiatry* 50(4):349–363. https://doi.org/10.1016/j.jaac.2010.12.001

Peters, L. L., Thornton, C., de Jonge, A., Khashan, A., Tracy, M., Downe, S., Feijen-de Jong, E. I. & Dahlen, H. G. (2018). The effect of medical and operative birth interventions on child health outcome in the first 28 days and up to 5 years of age: a linked data population-based cohort study. *Birth: Issues in Perinatal Care* 45:347–357. https://doi.org/10.1111/birt.12348

Powell, L., Southwell-Wright, W. & Gowland, R. (2016). *Care in the Past: Archaeological and interdisciplinary perspectives*. Oxford: Oxbow Books.

Reedy, S. (2020). Patriarchy in industrial era Europe: skeletal evidence of male preference during growth. In Tremblay, L. A. & Reedy, S. (Eds.), *The Bioarchaeology of Structural Violence: A Theoretical Framework for Industrial Era Inequality*, pp. 81–108. New York: Springer International Publishing. https://doi.org/10.1007/978-3-030-46440-0_5

Reitsema, L. J. & McIlvaine, B. K. (2014). Reconciling "stress" and "health" in physical anthropology: what can bioarchaeologists learn from the other subdisciplines? *American Journal of Physical Anthropology* 155(2):181–185. https://doi.org/10.1002/ajpa.22596

Robbins Schug, G. (2011). *Bioarchaeology and Climate Change: A View from South Asian Prehistory*. Gainesville: University Press of Florida.

Robbins Schug, G. (2017). A hierarchy of values: the bioarchaeology of complexity, order, health, and hierarchy at Harappa. In Klaus, H. D., Harvey, A. R. & Cohen, M. N. (Eds.), *Bones of Complexity: Osteological Indicators of Emergent Heterarchy and Hierarchy*, pp. 263–298. Gainesville: University Press of Florida.

Robbins Schug, G. (2020a). *The Routledge Handbook of the Bioarchaeology of Climate and Environmental Change*. Abingdon: Routledge.

Robbins Schug, G. (2020b). Touching the surface: biological, behavioural, and emotional aspects of plagiocephaly at Harappa. In Gowland, R. & Halcrow, S. E. (Eds.), *The Mother-Infant Nexus in Anthropology: Small Beginnings, Significant Outcomes*, pp. 235–274. New York: Springer International Publishing. https://doi.org/10.1007/978-3-030-27393-4_13

Robbins Schug, G. & Blevins, K. E. (2016). The center cannot hold: a bioarchaeological perspective on environmental crisis in the second millennium BCE, South Asia. In Robbins Schug, G. & Walimbe, S. R. (Eds.), *A Companion to South Asia in the Past*, pp. 255–273. New York: John Wiley and Sons.

Robbins Schug, G. & Goldman, H. M. (2014). Birth is but our death begun: a bioarchaeological assessment of skeletal emaciation in immature human skeletons in the context of environmental, social, and subsistence transition. *American Journal of Physical Anthropology* 155(2):243–259. https://doi.org/10.1002/ajpa.22536

Robbins Schug, G., Gray, K., Mushrif-Tripathy, V. & Sankhyan, A. R. (2012). A peaceful realm? Trauma and social differentiation at Harappa. *International Journal of Paleopathology* 2(2–3):136–147. https://doi.org/10.1016/j.ijpp.2012.09.012

Sala, N., Arsuaga, J. L., Pantoja-Pérez, A., Pablos, A., Martínez, I., Quam, R. M., Gómez-Olivencia, A., Bermúdez de Castro, J. M. & Carbonell, E. (2015). Lethal interpersonal violence in the middle pleistocene. *PloS One* 10(5):e0126589. https://doi.org/10.1371/journal.pone.0126589

Sargent, C. & Scheper-Hughes, N. (1998). *Small Wars: The Cultural Politics of Childhood*. Oakland: University of California Press.

Scheper-Hughes, N. (1987). *Child Survival: Anthropological Perspectives on the Treatment and Maltreatment of Children* (Vol. 11). Berlin: Springer Science & Business Media.

Scheper-Hughes, N. (1992). *Death Without Weeping: The Violence of Everyday Life in Brazil*. Oakland: University of California Press.

Scheper-Hughes, N. (1996). Maternal thinking and the politics of war. *Peace Review* 8(3):353–358.

Scherer, A. K. & Verano, J. W. (2014). *Embattled Bodies, Embattled Places: War in Pre-Columbian Mesoamerica and the Andes*. Washington, DC: Dumbarton Oaks Research Library and Collection.

Shapland, F. & Lewis, M. E. (2013). Brief communication: a proposed osteological method for the estimation of pubertal stage in human skeletal remains. *American Journal of Physical Anthropology* 151(2):302–310. https://doi.org/10.1002/ajpa.22268

Sheridan, S. G. & Gregoricka, L. A. (2020). A bioarchaeology of purposeful pain. In Sheridan, S. G. & Gregoricka, L. A. (Eds.), *Purposeful Pain: The Bioarchaeology of Intentional Suffering*, pp. 1–17. New York: Springer International Publishing.

Shorter, E. (1975). *The Making of the Modern Family*. Honley, UK: Collins.

Snoddy, A. M. E., Halcrow, S. E., Buckley, H. R., Standen, V. G. & Arriaza, B. T. (2017). Scurvy at the agricultural transition in the Atacama desert (ca 3600–3200 BP): nutritional stress at the maternal-foetal interface? *International Journal of Paleopathology* 18:108–120. https://doi.org/10.1016/j.ijpp.2017.05.011

Sofaer, J. R. (2006). *The Body as Material Culture: A Theoretical Osteoarchaeology* (Vol. 4). Cambridge: Cambridge University Press.

Southorn, M. J. (2019). *Forgotten Children: The Foetal and Infant Skeletal Remains of the W.D. Trotter Anatomy Museum*. Unpublished Honours thesis. University of Otago, New Zealand.

Stewart, N. A., Gerlach, R. F., Gowland, R. L., Gron, K. J. & Montgomery, J. (2017). Sex determination of human remains from peptides in tooth enamel. *Proceedings of the National Academy of Sciences* 114(52):13649–13654. https://doi.org/10.1073/pnas.1714926115

Stone, P. K. (2012). Binding women: ethnology, skeletal deformations, and violence against women. *International Journal of Paleopathology* 2(2–3):53–60. https://doi.org/10.1016/j.ijpp.2012.09.008

Supernant, K., Baxter, J. E., Lyons, N. & Atalay, S. (2020). *Archaeologies of the Heart*. New York: Springer International Publishing.

Tegtmeyer, C. E. & Martin, D. L. (2017). The bioarchaeology of women, children, and other vulnerable groups in times of war. In Martin, D. L. & Tegtmeyer, C. (Eds.), *Bioarchaeology of Women and*

Children in Times of War: Case Studies from the Americas, pp. 1–14. New York: Springer International Publishing.

Temple, D. H. & Goodman, A. H. (2014). Bioarcheology has a "health" problem: conceptualizing "stress" and "health" in bioarcheological research. *American Journal of Physical Anthropology* 155(2):186–191. https://doi.org/10.1002/ajpa.22602

Thompson, J. L., Alfonso-Durruty, M. P. & Crandall, J. J. (2014). *Tracing Childhood: Bioarchaeological Investigations of Early Lives in Antiquity.* Gainesville: University Press of Florida.

Torres-Rouff, C. (2020). Binding, wrapping, constricting, and constraining the head: a consideration of cranial vault modification and the pain of infants. In Sheridan, S. G. & Gregoricka, L. A. (Eds.), *Purposeful Pain: The Bioarchaeology of Intentional Suffering,* pp. 233–252. New York: Springer International Publishing.

Toyne, J. M. (2018). A childhood of violence: a bioarchaeological comparison of mass death assemblages from ancient Peru. In Beauchesne, P. & Agarwal, S. (Eds.), *Children and Childhood in Bioarchaeology,* pp. 171–204. Gainesville: University Press of Florida. https://doi.org/10.2307/j.ctvx0794d.12

Toyne, J. M. & Narváez-Vargas, A. (2014). The fall of Kuelap: bioarchaeological analysis of death and destruction on the eastern slopes of the Andes. In Scherer, A. K. & Verano, J. W. (Eds.), *Embattled Bodies, Embattled Places: War in Pre-Columbian Mesoamerica and the Andes,* pp. 341–364. Cambridge, MA: Harvard University Press.

Tremblay, L. A. & Reedy, S. (Eds.) (2020). *The Bioarchaeology of Structural Violence: A Theoretical Framework for Industrial Era Inequality.* New York: Springer International Publishing.

Tung, T. A. & Knudson, K. J. (2010). Childhood lost: abductions, sacrifice, and trophy heads of children in the Wari empire of the ancient Andes. *Latin American Antiquity* 21(1):44–66.

Tung, T. A., Miller, M., DeSantis, L., Sharp, E. A. & Kelly, J. (2016). Patterns of violence and diet among children during a time of imperial decline and climate change in the ancient Peruvian Andes. In VanDerwarker, A. & Wilson, G. D. (Eds.), *The Archaeology of Food and Warfare: Food Insecurity in Prehistory,* pp. 193–228. New York: Springer International Publishing. https://doi.org/10.1007/978-3-319-18506-4_10

United Nations Commission for Human Rights, (1989). *Convention on the Rights of the Child.* United Nations Human Rights Office of the High Commissioner. https://www.ohchr.org/en/professionalinterest/pages/crc.aspx

Vallianatos, H., Brennand, E. A., Raine, K., Stephen, Q., Petawabano, B., Dannenbaum, D. & Willows, N. D. (2006). Beliefs and practices of first nation women about weight gain during pregnancy and lactation: implications for women's health. *Canadian Journal of Nursing Research* 38(1):102–119.

Watkins, R. J. (2012). Variation in health and socioeconomic status within the W. Montague Cobb skeletal collection: degenerative joint disease, trauma and cause of death. *International Journal of Osteoarchaeology* 22(1):22–44. https://doi.org/10.1002/oa.1178

Watkins, R. J. (2018a). Anatomical collections as the anthropological other: Some considerations. In Stone, P. K (Ed.), *Bioarchaeological Analyses and Bodies: New Ways of Knowing Anatomical and Archaeological Skeletal Collections,* pp. 27–47. New York: Springer International Publishing.

Watkins, R. J. (2018b). The fate of anatomical collections in the US: bioanthropological investigations of structural violence. In Henderson, C. Y. & Cardoso, F. A. (Eds.), *Identified Skeletal Collections: The Testing Ground of Anthropology?,* pp. 169–18. Archaeopress.

Watkins, R. & Muller, J. (2015). Repositioning the Cobb human archive: the merger of a skeletal collection and its texts. *American Journal of Human Biology* 27(1):41–50. https://doi.org/10.1002/ajhb.22650

24
ISSUES OF GENDER, IDENTITY, AND AGENCY IN PALEOPATHOLOGY

Pamela K. Stone and Adam Netzer Zimmer

Introduction

Thirty years ago, Conkey and Gero published their groundbreaking work *Engendering Archaeology* (1991), which was one of the earliest calls to action to move archaeological research away from a static binary. They challenged anthropologists to recognize the broad spectrum of human identity, to look beyond assumptions of contemporary sex/gender roles, and to see the body as a reflection of the lived experiences of that time and space in which the individual lived. Since Conkey and Gero's groundbreaking work, many have expanded and explored the complexities of gender, identity, and agency in the past. For the paleopathologist, this is evidenced in Buikstra's (2019) recently revised edition of *Ortner's Identification of Pathological Conditions in Human Remains*. This updated version reimagines Ortner's seminal text, foregrounding advancements "in the vibrant field of paleopathology in the 21st Century" (xvi-preface). Buikstra's revisions present the complex ways that paleopathology is beginning to embrace and intertwine empirical data with theoretical analyses to offer more nuanced interpretations.

However, there continue to be gaps in the ways in which this engagement is understood. These gaps result in narrow and often inconsistent interpretations, which reproduce static, and often antiquated ideas of human experience. In particular, these reproduced ideas see the past as a reflection only of 19th-century binary, heteronormative, White, cisgender perspectives (Zuckerman et al., 2016; Stone, 2020a). By continuing to reproduce and build on old and biased models instead of interrogating them, paleopathological studies miss the opportunity to read the past and see the agency of people whose lives are being narrated. Today more than ever, older models need to be reworked, challenged, and in some cases disrupted.

As Conkey and Gero (1991) established, the broadening of our analysis to consider a wider, and yet more inclusive understanding of people calls for self-reflexivity. This process of self-reflexivity has been central in recent years to the growth of knowledge in the related field of bioarchaeology, but paleopathology seems to be slower to take up these calls. Perhaps, as Buikstra (2019) suggests, this has to do with paleopathology's closer alignment with medicine. This idea may not be surprising, given that "hard" sciences have traditionally rebuffed accusations of human bias in data collection and have neglected to consider humanistic impacts that may result in different outcomes of analyses. Regardless, in this chapter, we aim to show how such re-examinations can better inform our interpretations of skeletal disease and trauma and, in the end, produce better and more nuanced interpretations of paleopathological data that provides a wider spectrum of identities and agency in the past and the present.

Our goal is to offer ways that theoretical models can expand paleopathology's understanding of gender, identity, and agency in the past. To do this, we explore how traditional paleopathological studies aim to unpack but not interrogate data by way of sex and gender, and race, while also considering what we mean when we evoke the concept of agency in our analyses. We then briefly define four complex theoretical frameworks that we see as integral to paleopathological analyses: sex and gender theory, structural violence theory, embodiment theory, and queer theory. Through examples and then two vignettes, we illuminate how the *status quo* in paleopathological analysis can be reframed, illustrating how more nuanced paleoanthropological analysis can be used to expand understandings of gender, identity, and human agency in the past.

Gender, Identity, and Agency

Gender and Sex in Paleopathology

Before we begin to unpack sex and gender's roles in paleopathological analyses, we must first define what we mean by these terms. Many researchers, the authors included, often use these terms without explicitly acknowledging how we are defining them. Here we offer how sex and gender are complex concepts, ones that are biologically and culturally constructed, that may not be understood universally, cross-culturally, or even through time. While we do not precisely define these terms, we instead acknowledge that sex and gender require us to read them in their cultural contexts, else we miss their complexity and potentially misunderstand people's roles and positions in the past.

Often when the term "sex" is used it suggests that we are referring only to the biological elements that differentiate male and female physiology, namely the primary and secondary sexual characteristics that lead to an individual being assigned the sex of "male" or "female" at birth. Because of this, "sex" is often thought of as more easily defined, but this reinforces the historical concept of a biological binary of male versus female (Fausto-Sterling, 2000). However, we know that even in the biological sense, sex does not belong to a simple binary (Ainsworth, 2015; Astorino, 2019). Instead, sex can be thought of as an individual's combined expression of many different polymorphic biological characteristics. Most individuals will have traits that fall more or less into one column or the other and it is this combination, and our cultural understanding of what said combination codes for, that determines sex.

As you can see in Table 24.1, there are various biological characteristics that are presumed to belong to either females or males. Biological researchers assume uncritically that most individuals will have the prescribed combination of external genitalia, gonads, chromosomal makeup, and hormonal levels seen in the "female" or "male" columns. All these traits, though, can exist polymorphically instead of bimorphically (Astorino, 2019), with many humans exhibiting any combination of traits from either column, often without even knowing it (Ainsworth, 2015; Davis, 2015). Nor do these traits individually parse neatly into bimorphic categories. For example, when does a large clitoris pass the threshold for definition as a penis? Similarly, should a female with naturally occurring high levels of testosterone, which match levels more often seen in males, be excluded from that very category of femalehood?

Table 24.1 Common biological characteristics used in defining a bimorphic model of sex in humans

Polymorphic sex characteristic	Assumed "female" trait	Assumed "male" trait	Example of other possible expressions★
External genitalia	Vulva, clitoris	Penis, scrotum, descended testicles	Fused labia resembling a scrotum
Gonads	Paired ovaries	Paired testes	Combination of ovarian and testicular tissue (ovotestis)
Chromosomal pairing	XX	XY	Extra sex chromosome (e.g., 47, XXY)
Hormonal expression	Higher estrogen	Higher testosterone	Congenital adrenal hypoplasia (CAH)

★Such examples are not comprehensive of all the possible polymorphic variations of the described characteristic and merely reflect one possible polymorphism.

Such questions are not simply rhetorical exercises – these definitions of sex are currently being debated and have real-world implications (see Block, 2021).

With this in mind, *what exactly* are we assessing when we include skeletal sex in our paleopathological studies? To be frank, we do not know. Yet, identification of sex (alongside age and stature estimation) is one of the primary analytical tools used by all paleopathologists in studies of past populations. These skeletal markers of sex are predicated on the assumption that there are two clear categories of bodies: "female" and "male"; in which "female" refers to people of "all genders whose anatomy is assigned to be female, and the same gender inclusivity applies to "male'" (Dunsworth, 2020:108). In paleopathology, sex determination continues to be considered a biological fact, making its use in skeletal analysis seem a simple way to begin to understand differences; male versus female.

Our goal here is not to dispute that there are the skeletal markers of sex, which almost certainly reflect physiological responses to the sex hormones, estrogen, and testosterone, all of which are related to the reproductive systems of an individual, and result in structural differences of the pelvis (see Dunsworth, 2020). We instead want to bring forward the implicit biases that come with sex; biases that impact how the skeletal transcript is read, how the past is narrated, and how these ideas serve to reproduce binary understandings and, until recently, are rarely questioned. As such we need to remind ourselves that, in our analyses, we should not assume that skeletal markers of sex hormones tell us anything more than something about the physical structures an individual lived with, and perhaps little about their identity and roles in their society.

In much of the paleopathological research, "sex" determination results in descriptions of lived experiences that tend to conflate and subsequently ascribe sex with gender identity and roles. But defining gender is just as an elusive a concept as sex and may be even harder to define. Understanding "gender" requires one to understand individual and cultural definitions and associations that relate to aspects of identity, behavior, and an individual's relationship to society (Delphy, 1993; Gottlieb, 2002; Butler, 2011; Oakley, 2016). But in paleopathology, the use of "gender", and more specifically "gender roles", reveals subtle (and not so subtle) assumptions of what it means to be "male" or "female" without interrogating the implicit biases of these interpretations. As such it is important for us to recognize "…that neither [sex or gender] divide into uniform, discrete, or binary categories" (Dunsworth, 2020:108).

The roots of these narrow categories of sex and gender, commonly used in paleopathology research, stem from the history of scientific inquiry. Historically, the traits ascribed to the terms, "male" and "female" or "man" and "woman", are reflections of the Victorian period's scripting of sex and gender in cultural and societal expectations. These categories are what we would now call gender-normative definitions of male and female, and they rely on the idea that an individual's assigned sex directly aligns with their gender identity, and therefore their biologically predicted cultural performance of identity (Stone & Sanders, 2020). At the same time that these sex/gender norms were developing, so too were allopathic medicine and anthropology. White male scientists worked to understand human variations and differences, while simultaneously perpetuating the way in which sex and gender, and race (discussed in more detail below) were being defined and used to frame expectations of "males" and "females". Their definitions directly reflected the era they were forged within.

Victorian definitions of sex and gender were fixed, binary, and biologically deterministic. "Sex" differentiated the biologically visible elements of male and female physiology. "Gender" was used to define aspects of identity, behavior, and social expectations, but was also tied directly to sex as all were seen as biologically determined. The notion that sex and gender were fixed served to enforce male/man as superior in all areas. This, in turn, gave males greater agency. They were the competitors while female/woman were deemed as purely reproductive vessels and passive participants in community (Schiebinger, 1987; Martin, 2001; Warsh, 2019; Dunsworth, 2020; Stone & Sanders, 2020). Any deviation from these set categories suggested biological inferiority. Today we see the complexity of both sex and gender as encompassing a mosaic of identities, biological variations, and human experiences, but our work in paleopathology continues to neglect the more complex ways expressions of gender, identity, and agency may have been experienced in other cultures and timeframes.

The distinction between "male" and female" in paleopathology needs to consider the wide range of anatomical, chromosomal and hormonal variations in human sex identity, while also understanding that "sex" and "gender" are far more complex than simply identifying someone as a girl or a boy, a man or a woman. Our interpretations need to be framed in lived, cultural, and political contexts. Like Conkey and Gero's (1990) work, it has been 30 years since Judith Butler's (1990) influential text *Gender Trouble* in which they interrogated the conventional distinctions between sex and gender. Yet these concepts continue to be "troubled" by the fact that sex does not exist before or without gender (Stone & Sanders, 2020). The performativity of gender now plays an important role in the fields of queer and transgender studies, opening up key questions about the nature of sex and gender in contemporary culture as well as in (pre)history. For paleopathology, this means we must be careful in our assessments and recognize that skeletal morphological characteristics associated with sex (i.e., the capacity to bear children) do not tell us about the lived experience of the individual (gender). They only allow us an opportunity to consider that an individual *may* have played a reproductive role in the community and yet could have been a warrior or a laborer, as well.

We must also emphasize that the majority of paleopathological analyses focused on sex rely on a specific binary model of ascertaining *skeletal sex*. That is, we code for traits of the (most often pelvic) skeletal elements that are most commonly seen in individuals of one sex or another (Astorino, 2019). But again, we are assessing *skeletal* sex and skeletal sex only, not behavior or experiences. Neither are we necessarily assessing biological sex in its other manifestations. This recognition of sex itself existing outside of an all-or-nothing binary is the first step in our "data first, interpretation second" call.

Race in Paleopathology

A discussion about gender and agency in paleopathology would be incomplete if race were not critically addressed. In addition to sex, stature, and age, osteologists are often asked to conduct ancestry estimation as a part of a standard biological profile. Ancestry estimation, which for years has been short-handed as "assessing race", has a harmful and dangerous history within biological anthropology (Armelagos & Van Gerven, 2003; Watkins, 2012, 2018; Blakey, 2020; DiGangi & Bethard, 2021; and see Chapter 21, this volume). From the founding of the discipline, craniometric traits have been used by White researchers to construct biological arguments for racial hierarchy and have consistently placed White males at the top (DiGangi & Bethard, 2021). DiGangi and Bethard (2021) have called for an end to skeletal ancestry assessment by arguing that its continued use in any context only serves to uphold White supremacy. We echo these arguments and wish to expand upon them to argue for why race *as a social construct that nonetheless has biological consequences* must be included as a key marker in paleopathological research.

Again, we must begin with defining our terms. Race, like the other categorical factors discussed in this chapter, is a complicated phenomenon whose purview goes beyond a singular, agreed-upon definition. It goes beyond our abilities to even begin to disentangle the various definitions within this chapter, but we refer readers to the American Association of Biological Anthropology's statement on race as one suitable resource to start with (see Fuentes et al., 2019).

While there *are* phenotypic differences that are observable in humans, perhaps most notably in skin color, these differences are not discrete and assignable to any particular "race" or genetic or geographical cluster.

"Instead, the Western concept of race must be understood as a classification system that emerged from, and in support of, European colonialism, oppression, and discrimination. It thus does not have its roots in biological reality, but in policies of discrimination" (Fuentes et al., 2019:400). However, the fact that race is not a discrete genetic phenomenon does not negate its impact on many groups. "While typological races are not valid descriptors of clinal human biological variation, they are both socially powerful and potentially biologically impactful, particularly in terms of structuring human interactions and negatively affecting the biological wellbeing and health outcomes of people who experience racism, discrimination, and stress due to structural inequities perpetuated by a fixed notion of race" (Tallman et al., 2021:1–2).

Scholars like Wynter (2003) and Weheliye (2014) have even argued that racialization's original purpose was not to divide groups of our species into a hierarchy of *human* categories but instead define groups as human, subhuman, or even nonhuman, with people of African descent placed into that lowest category of nonhuman. It is important to note here that biological anthropology has been long intertwined with the biocentricity of the racialization process, that is, a focus on defining and codifying racial categories according to "measurable" phenotypic traits (Watkins, 2018; DiGangi & Bethard, 2020).

We must also re-emphasize in this discussion that race, as the term is used in most biological research, is a socially defined phenomenon. By this, we mean those racial categories that readers in the continental United States are familiar with (i.e., White, Black, Asian, Latino) are culturally specific and not fixed categories that are necessarily legible elsewhere across other geographic or temporal spaces. To underscore this, we direct readers to Gravlee et al.'s (2005) seminal work on race-correlated health inequalities in Puerto Rico. In this study, the researchers tested the association between blood pressure and "race" by assessing if phenotypic skin pigmentation (as measured by reflectance spectrophotometry) or culturally specific *color*, as determined by a multitude of phenotypic and social factors, correlated with blood pressure levels. The researchers found that *color* was indeed a determining factor in blood pressure, while skin pigmentation was not. By using a cultural model of race that is particular to Puerto Rico, one that includes categories like *trigueño*, *negro*, and *blanco*, Gravlee et al. (2005) were able to demonstrate the biological impacts of social categorization of race that is not a one-to-one correlate of genetic phenotypes.

But regardless of how well-acquainted researchers are with the biological falsity of race, individuals (both living and deceased) are still often relegated to their "racial category", regardless of how it is defined. Yet it is well documented that "race" can be seen as a dialectical relationship by which sociocultural, political, legal, and economic forces work to form and solidify racial categories and are then reformed by the very categories created (Omi & Winant, 2014). As Gravlee et al.'s (2005) research in Puerto Rico demonstrates, the existence of a socially defined race exacerbates differential health outcomes. Unfortunately, this is often misinterpreted to mean that these disparities are an in-born trait ascribable to biological race rather than caused by sociocultural factors impacting each socially defined racial category differently. The nature of this relationship and its misinterpretation creates an almost "common sense" aspect of race, one that has real implications for each racial category it helps define, simultaneously creating even more disparities between those categories.

Our emphasis here on race, in a chapter mainly focused on sex and gender, is necessary because the scientific delineation of racial categories has always been intertwined with sex and gender. In particular, we draw readers' attention to the intersection of race and gender in skeletal studies when specifically discussing pelvic morphology. Markowitz (2017) deftly demonstrates that studies of pelvic dimorphism were never truly binary in defining "male" versus "female" because race has been a controlling factor since the emergence of formalized sexological research. We can see this with an 1886 quote from famed sexologist Richard von Krafft-Ebing, "The secondary sexual characteristics differentiate the two sexes; they present the specific male and female types. The higher the anthropological development of the race, the stronger these contrasts between man and woman, and vice versa" (Krafft-Ebing, 1886/1939:42). Markowitz traces such anthropological research into pelvic dimorphism over time showing that, even into the late 1950s, anthropological studies of the pelvis sought to show race-specific differences in the degree of sexual dimorphism. We highlight this work because it demonstrates that even "objective" attempts to discern sexual dimorphism in skeletal samples cannot be separated from a history of overt racialization attempts. Nor is "sex" separable from a history of racist tropes of, in particular, Black women's gender.

With this in mind, how can we include race in paleopathology without continuing to reify racial categories? In short, we cannot. But given the very real biological impact that racial disparity has, we also cannot ignore it. White researchers have shied away from critically engaging with race unless it somehow benefits them materially; this is a concept Derek Bell (1995) has deemed "interest convergence". Ignoring *socially determined* race completely as a factor in skeletal studies would create a false narrative that it has no physiological effects, which we know not to be true (e.g., de la Cova, 2011, 2014; Watkins, 2012). Therefore, we advocate for an intersectional analysis of skeletal health as advocated by Mant et al. (2021:2): "Intersectionality extends biocultural understandings of past lives by engaging with multiple axes of identity, stress, and inequality when they can be ascertained and recognizes these 'distinctive dynamics at their multi- dimensional interface' […] we should avoid projecting contemporary ideals of identity, such as age, sex, and status, into the past or assume they were salient in a society so distant in time and space from our own".

Such an intersectional approach recognizes that factors influencing the skeletal health of one gender or another in the past are entirely inseparable from other social categories into which that individual fits. For example, de la Cova (2012) found while examining remains in the Terry Skeletal Collection that fracture patterning in 19th-century-born females was almost entirely race dependent; higher rates of cranial, nasal, and hand phalanx trauma were found in African American females, whereas hip and radial fractures were more common in Euro-American females. By closely examining the historical framework in which these populations existed, de la Cova (2012) demonstrated that eliding these racial groups into one would obscure the particular forms of interpersonal, institutional, and structural violence enacted specifically against women of color in 19th-century Cincinnati. de la Cova did not "assess race" from craniometric traits, thereby perpetuating the idea that race is skeletally coded by genetics, but rather used documentary evidence to show that the social race that individuals in the Terry Collection belonged to had a biological impact on their health. Of course, as Mant et al. (2021) cautioned, intersectional interpretations like this are not always easy, especially when dealing with prehistoric skeletal collections. However, by including other lines of evidence (material culture, stable isotope analysis, etc.), a more nuanced understanding of intersecting identities' effects on skeletal health in the past, even in the ancient past, may be enacted.

Agency in Paleopathology

Before we could address how agency is framed in paleopathological analyses, we needed to unpack sex, gender, and race and explore the cultural biases that shape and frame our interpretations. Doing this allows us a window into how interpretations of agency have been impacted and influenced by the ways in which we "see" sex, gender, and race today, which informs how we then "see" agency, and in how narratives of people in the past are then crafted.

While the concept of agency in anthropology is invoked frequently, it is often left undefined (Smith, 2013). In addition, when you explore the idea of a definition of "agency" in anthropology you quickly learn that there are multiple ways the concept of agency is deployed (Ahern, 1999; Frank, 2006; Smith, 2013; and many others). While it is not in the scope of this chapter to explore all the ways in which "agency" can be defined, we offer below a brief example from the ancient American Southwest of new ways to see female agency by locating the body through its individual, social, and political experiences (Scheper-Hughes & Locke, 1987; Ahern, 1999), which offers a useful heuristic tool for how paleopathology should read skeletal markers of illness, trauma, nutrition, care, and life experiences.

Unpacking and understanding agency through the analysis of human remains requires us to read the mortuary context and position of a body juxtaposed with pathological analyses. New interpretations of individual bodies from burials found at the La Plata site (c.1000–1300AD) in northern New Mexico offer an excellent example of how agency can be redefined. Martin et al. (1995), Martin (1997), and Stone (2012) offer reinterpretations of the burials and bodies from La Plata, revealing new ways to consider patterns of traumatic injuries, chronic ill-health, and stress by sex, by age, and by mortuary context. The mortuary contexts and pathological analysis revealed that the females were found without grave goods and in a haphazard manner – not your "normal" flexed burial. Each had multiple cranial traumas and most postcranial trauma was consistent with defensive injuries (Martin et al., 1995). In contrast, only a few males presented with traumatic head injuries (each only a single incidence) and postcranial trauma. Burial position was only reported for one male, and while he was without grave goods, he was buried in the "normal" flexed position (Martin et al.,

1995). Further, Martin and colleagues (1995) discuss the biological variability in epigenetic traits and stature, noting that the females found with the differential burial context may not be from the local Puebloan community in which they died.

As both Stone (2012) and Martin (1997) have noted, a new interpretation of these burials and paleopathological data from La Plata suggests that local females might have been dominant over the non-local females, resulting in sanctioned disciplinary actions toward the non-local females, which manifests in the form of hitting someone in the head (of which there is biological evidence of). This suggests that injuries associated with interpersonal encounters may be the result of women–women as opposed to the originally assumed male-on-female conflict. This new way of seeing the burials and pathologies places women at the center of violent acts, and makes them active participants in the ways in which early Puebloan communities may have functioned, enforcing the structural systems of power within the domestic spheres. It is well documented that domestic spheres in Puebloan communities are female-centered spaces (Lowell, 1991; Mobly-Tanka, 1997; Fowels, 2005). Combined, the higher incidences of trauma and chronic ill-health suggest something about how the stressors of displacement and captivity support a different picture of social controls and interpersonal relationships of power and resistance between females, not between males and females. These data require us to reframe assumptions of who perpetrates violence and how this might reflect established norms and other modes of control that are often invisible but have a lasting impact on the lived experiences of individuals. Expanding our rethinking of how we understand human experiences and agency in the past, it is the addition of theoretical modeling that adds dimension to the stories we can tell.

Theoretical Modeling

Theoretical modeling moves our analyses of past populations away from reductionist examinations and pushes the researcher to interrogate the ways in which ideological and structural systems in the past may have regulated expressions and practices of human social systems (Giffney, 2008). The integration of theoretical frameworks with paleoanthropological data allows us to begin to more fully consider individuals' experiences and roles within their own specific temporal and cultural contexts. But, as we will see, when we consider biological data alongside social theorizing, it allows us to more fully understand the ways in which people participated within their communities in all aspects of life (Geller, 2016).

Sex and Gender Theory

Emanating out of feminist approaches, sex and gender theory offers a lens from which to view the biophysical body and the cultural contexts of life and death. While this has permeated bioarchaeology to a greater degree, sex and gender theory in paleopathology itself has not had a long history. While conceptually complicated, sex and gender theory is not about "adding" sex or gender but about disentangling our current cultural frameworks of sex/gender roles. By asking what the data reveal before we add sex/gender, more nuanced and complex understandings of people in the past can be gleaned.

As we have noted, paleopathology is still largely dominated by prevailing masculine paradigms and assumptions of social roles as dictated by "sex/gender" and not ability. For example, when we consider our own cultural assumptions about reproductive females, in which we see the parturient or childrearing female as weak, fragile, helpless, and at risk for early death, we have just perpetuated the idea of biologically constructed social roles and gender identity established in the Victorian era (Stone & Sanders, 2020). This "truth" about females, constructed in the 1800s, was supported by the cultural practices of corset use and tight-lacing, as well as a series of other expectations that ultimately resulted in increases in ill-health and high rates of maternal mortality for reproductive-aged Victorian women (e.g., Stone, 2016, 2020a). Consider now that paleoanthropological and archaeological demographic analyses, in which the data often demonstrates high mortality for reproductive-aged pre-contact females, rely on these early assessments of reproductive-aged women as biological facts. This has meant that these data are interpreted through a filter in which the concept of "the biologically weak female" is a biological fact: thus, all females who die during their reproductive years do so as a result of pregnancy-related complications (Martin et al., 1991; Lovejoy et al., 1977). Stone (2016) has argued that studies such as these rely only on age-at-death as the indicator of "maternal mortality" without considering other factors that may have resulted in early death. These studies offer little to support or refute the notion that complications in parturition resulted in the death of the individual. Instead, they reproduce an unsubstantiated assumption that reproductive-aged females are weak and fragile, and this has remained mostly unchallenged as biological fact. However, this "fact" is a cultural narrative that permeates anthropological (and medical) dialogues.

The last ten years have seen new scholarship that questions these types of biologically deterministic frameworks and offer new perspectives for considering bodies before assuming social roles (e.g., Agarwal & Glencross, 2011; Rakita, 2014; Geller, 2016). These biological anthropologists have not shied away from pushing back on the value-laden (androcentric and heterosexual) models rooted in historical and political contexts but bring to light the ways in which the early "sexual sciences" were rooted in typological approaches seated in biological deterministic frameworks. In addition, Dunsworth and colleagues (2012) and Dunsworth (2020) continue to offer new physiological frameworks in which to consider human experiences related to growth and development and reproduction. Dunsworth et al. (2012) strongly support the concept of biological limits for in-uterine growth for fetal brains, such that when the caloric needs of brain growth exceed what the mother can provide around nine months of gestation, it leads to the initiation of labor and birth. Expanding on this, Dunsworth (2020) explores the roles of hormones and sexual organs in sexual dimorphism. Combined, this research serves to counter long-held beliefs that evolution failed the female pelvis, making it flawed, instead suggesting that we don't know enough about the complex physiological processes that result in sexual dimorphism, to determine that one body is flawed and another is normal. Work such as this offers us new entry points in which to consider how the evolutionary and physiological forces that result in skeletal dimorphism are far more complex than a simple sex-differentiated process aimed at sexual selection and reveals that long-held ideas of male and female need further investigations.

Structural Violence

Structural violence, first defined by Galtung (1969), is used as a framework to examine how human actions can and should be examined. Galtung brought forward the idea that violence is perpetrated in both visible and invisible ways: visibly through physical, direct, manifestations; broken bones, depression fracture, etc.; and invisibly through indirect forces of violence stemming from behaviors, attitudes, and conditions in society. While the indirect forces are harder to see and unpack (e.g., long-term chronic stress, body modifications, nutritional stressors), they reflect how the social structures or institutions harm people who do not comply. "Seeing" the invisible, indirect forces that harm people requires a deeper understanding of the cultural and social arena of lived experiences of the individual within the social and political expectations of the larger community to inform paleopathological analyses.

Paleopathology's tendency to only focus on direct, physical responses to violence seen on bone is evidenced in the sorting of pathologies into clear categories: disease and trauma. But these categories may miss markers of structural violence or may be misread when we fail to consider the larger social forces that may impact people within a community. Understanding what structural violence looks like in temporally different cultural spaces requires us to define what we mean by violence. It then requires us to consider how a body is implicated in the performance of violence. Building on Galtung's work, Whitehead (2004) reminds us that we need to understand the complexity of violence and that it is framed in different ways in different cultural and temporal contexts. So as our inquiries evolve, we need to more fully explore the intersectional and intertwined "…emotional meanings of violence in conjunction with the social positioning of the participants" (Whitehead, 2004:71), and how this produces the actors: aggressors, victims, and witnesses. In addition to the actors, we need to understand the underlying cultural experiences and expectations. This brings us back to Galtung's (2002) root forces (behaviors, attitudes, conditions), which shape how the actions of the individual or the social group respond to the threat of, or actual occurrence of, direct violence which reinforce the systems of power.

As an example, Stone (2020b) explores the ways in which footbinding reflects intergenerational (mothers to daughters) compliance with social expectations, by hobbling females for their lifetime. Binding feet results in life-long chronic stress, poor bone health, and disability, while simultaneously resulting in females being seen as compliant with the social and political scripts they are meant to follow (Cummings et al., 1997; Munk & Poon, 1996; Zhang et al., 2014; Gu et al., 2015). Here, the systems of power positioned women whose feet were bound as socially acceptable, beautiful, marriageable, while "an unbound foot reflected socioeconomic and ethnic minority status, and in some cases, unbound feet could lead to punishments imparted on the parents" (Stone, 2020b:41). This cultural practice is clearly a form of structural violence, but the direct consequences (low bone density and increases in hip fractures from lack of stability) are often overlooked or attributable to issues of aging or even assumed to be the product of multiparous experiences of females who present with these stress markers in paleopathological analyses. Yet, footbinding and its consequences can be used to decipher the values of family, community, and the state, while also defining the individual within each of these arenas. Expanding the analyses requires the paleopathologist to understand something about the culture, its history, and the larger contexts of the practice to understand the bodily consequences of having a bound foot, or not.

Identifying structural violence may also require paleopathologists to look outside the skeleton itself and instead examine associated data in order to identify subtler violence. Zimmer (2017, 2018) examined skeletal remains from the Huntington Anatomical Collection (1893–1921) from New York City that were acquired from medical school anatomical dissections. Despite the fragmentary nature of the skeletal material, the associated documentation, which showed the last known address of each individual in the collection, suggested a particular pattern of "definitional violence" (Miller, 1994), wherein Black residents of New York were defined by the physicians who collected their bodies as "appropriate" subjects for dissection regardless of income level, occupation, or location within the city. The documentary data suggested that a decedents' race was the main determining factor in whether or not someone was selected for dissection. Black New Yorkers were automatically perceived as "appropriate research subjects" purely based on their being Black, whereas White decedents were protected by their very Whiteness. In other words, physicians saw Blackness itself as co-constitutive with "cadaver subject", whereas a decedents' Whiteness required additional factors of poverty, joblessness, *and* residence within the city far from other wealthy Whites in order to be taken. In just looking at the skeletal material itself, researchers might fall into the trap of believing that all individuals selected for dissection belonged to a catch-all category of "the unclaimed poor" regardless of race. By expanding the included data sets, a much more nuanced story of how White physicians were implicated in anti-Black structural violence is revealed. This also allows us to see how specific social definitions of race, rather than some biological definition of race, is embodied within a skeletal population.

Embodiment Theory

Embodiment theory, as formulated by anthropologist Csordas (1990), offers a framework to consider how our bodies are both objects of, and subjects in, our expressions of self through the lens of cultural expectations and adherence to and deviance from social norms. In Csordas' (1990: 5) words, studying embodiment "begins from the methodological postulate that the body is not an object to be studied in relation to culture, but is to be considered as the subject of culture, or in other words as the existential ground of culture". As we consider sex and gender, and structural violence in paleopathology, we need to weave in embodiment theory to uncover how the body reflects lived experiences in life as the individual performed social expectations; and in death as the body reveals the consequences of structural systems in the ways in which they were intentionally (or not intentionally) buried.

For many paleopathological studies the body is central to analysis, but the addition of embodiment theory requires us to consider the larger constellation of the social and political lived experiences of the individuals we are examining. This means we need to consider the body as a transcript not only of direct experiences but also of indirect ones. The historical social subjects we examine, and the pathologies and traumas we can read from the skeletal body, need to be understood through a broader, intersectional lens that is informed by the cultural and environmental landscape. Employing embodiment theory, we can locate the body as simultaneously a subject and object that is quantifiable and qualitative and as a reflection of the individual, the social, and the political (Scheper-Hughes & Locke, 1987; Ahern, 1999; Mascia-Lees, 2011).

An example of embodiment can be seen in the *castrati*, a group of individuals based predominantly in Italy who underwent orchiectomies before puberty in order to preserve an upper-register, child-like voice. They were considered some of the most elite of the upper-class citizens of Italian society through much of the 17th, 18th, and 19th centuries (Rosselli, 1988; Clapton, 2008), with some living even into the 20th century, like Alessandro Moreschi who performed with the Sistine Chapel choir until 1913 (Clapton, 2008).

Pre-pubertal castration in the *castrati* would have resulted in unique skeletal changes, like continued growth of long bones, delayed onset or lack of epiphyseal fusion, barrel-shaped chests, and reduced cortical bone density (Peschel & Peschel, 1987). Prior pathological and physiological studies on the *castrati* have attempted to lump them together with eunuchs of other cultures, such as the Skotpzy religious sect of imperial Russia or eunuch guards of the Ming royal palace (Wilson & Roehrborn, 1999; Scholz, 2001). The justification behind such groupings is that all males who have been subject to castration will exhibit similar physiological responses to a lack of testosterone within their bodies. However, Zanatta et al. (2016) examined the remains of *castrato* Gaspare Pacchierotti (1740–1821) and found that he not only exhibited bone growth anomalies consistent with primary hypogonadism but also osteophytic growth on the ribs at respiratory muscle insertion sites. This suggests extremely high amounts of lung activity, as one would expect from an individual whose very body was shaped to be a professional singer. Furthermore, gender-oriented studies of the operatic characters, costumes, and musical pieces created for *castrati* show us that, due to the physiological changes manifested in their bodies, they occupied a unique niche in Italy's gender axis at the time, lying somewhere between male and female in the Baroque-era vertical axis of gender (Freitas, 2001).

The *castrati* reveal that in any cultural context, an individual is both shaped by and performs within a system of understandings composed of individual, social, and political ideologies within that particular society. In paleoanthropology, the body becomes a site to read how the cultural systems in place at the time are revealed through burial, material culture, and the skeleton. Embodiment and structural violence theory serve to inform our inquiries and shape how we engage with reading lived experiences in the past. Further examination of the intersections of ideology and embodiment in temporal and environmental landscapes need to be considered and contextualized through the fabric of the social world the individual lived within.

Queer/Queering Theory

Paleoanthropology, as a part of Western science, is embedded within a heteronormative and androcentric culture. Therefore, most researchers will bring biases developed from this culture with them to their interpretations. Without reflexivity, this means that interpretations can often say more about the culture of the researcher themselves than it does about the cultural context of the people being examined. In turn, this reinforces a heterosexual-only version of the past. This does not mean that the goals of queer inquiry are solely to find material evidence of non-binary experiences (often cast as sexual deviance/deviants), but that any/all normative paradigms need to be critiqued and any presuppositions which characterize traditional binary interpretations should be called into question. If the majority of archaeologists bring heteronormative biases with them to research, then queer archaeologists who do not live their day-to-day lives following binary structures can potentially bring fundamentally different understandings of the past to their own research (Voss, 2009). Queer theory enables this by offering a tripartite model of disciplinary reflection: (1) ask who is given disciplinary authority; (2) expose the disciplinary "rules" which those voices of authority have established to keep their own voices dominant; and (3) illuminate how those rules shape our interpretations of the past (Dowson, 2000; Zimmer, 2021).

As such, queer theory may be more readily understood in the context of examining socio-sexual aspects of lives in the past than it is in skeletal differential diagnosis (Geller, 2016). However, we argue that this deconstructive queer theory is actually necessary when discussing manifestations of skeletal health and disease in the past. As Mant et al. (2021) have recently discussed, paleopathologists need to do a better job in untangling the health effects of individuals' intersecting identities on their skeletal health. Queer theory offers a mechanism to do this by explicitly centering both subjects and researchers who are typically rejected as outliers. The inclusion of those subjects/researchers typically classified as queer (in the sense of non-normative) serves to broaden the interpretations of the past that are possible.

One example that highlights a queered approach to disease studies readily applicable to paleopathology is Nagington's (2015) assessment of aging in HIV-positive gay men in England. Nagington discusses how HIV infection (particularly in gay men) has been studied as a disease of both medical and social deficiencies. It is associated with a host of co-morbidities and, despite the introduction of highly active antiretroviral therapy (HAART), the "near-normal" life of HIV-positive people can often be seven to ten years less than their HIV-negative counterparts. Similarly, aging HIV-positive gay men are often the last of their early-life social groups (Owen & Catalan, 2012), thereby eliminating the potential ameliorating effects of community support later in life. Yet, Nagington (2015) synthesizes a queered approach to studying aging in HIV-positive gay men and proposes that this population offers a radically different sense of both temporality and kinship that we argue could be useful to other paleopathological studies. For many HIV-positive men, the uncertainty of a potential "future" might be resisted by rejecting heteronormative ideas of time based on socially sanctioned reproductive markers (e.g., having biological children) and instead by focusing purely on "a kind of nirvana where one just exists in a purely queer moment with no care for the future, the passage of time and certainly not the reproduction of heteronormative social structures" (Nagington, 2015:12). Kinship ties, too, can be constructed outside of traditionally Western frameworks of biological family units, instead focusing on ones' ties to others who are HIV-positive, both in the past and future. This demonstrates how a viral infection itself can become a part of identity (de)construction and might therefore have analogues in the paleopathological past, including how disease itself can drive identity.

New Approaches to Studying the Body in the Past

The body is a site of complex interactions between social and political expectations and controls, in both the lived experiences as well as in who is telling the story. In paleopathology, understanding pathological lesions on the skeleton as reflections of illness and violence is just the first step. Paleopathological analyses need to be considered within the temporal and cultural practices of the time to fully understand the sociopolitical meaning of the lived experiences of the individual(s) being examined. While we unpack the story written on bones, we also need to recognize our own biases, as well as how the foundations of paleopathology are deeply linked to and informed by the history of science and medicine. These foundations are framed by the gaze of the 19th century White male scientists whose implicit biases constructed the concept of a "normal" body, as well as the consequences of deviance from their prescribed archetype, through racist and sexist lenses (Blake, 1994; Reischer & Koo, 2004). The quest to understand human difference was fueled by the Bible, imperialism, economics, and a desire to elevate White humans, especially males, as superior and apart from everyone else; the result was that certain bodies became valued over others.

While we may think that today our ideas of a "normal body" have moved beyond the 19th-century platform of White supremacist masculine superiority, they have not. The "normal body" is still the White male body, as this is still the backdrop to how all bodies are measured today. It is critical for us to disrupt these biases, implicit or overt, and to engage in new models and ways to think that do not reinforce White, cis-gendered male frameworks and gazes. Disrupting these constructs of a "normal body" allows for new ways to see the past. This is especially important in paleoanthropological studies as people in the past may not fit cultural assumptions framed in how we "see" male and female today.

Exploring new theoretical frameworks and perspectives that can inform how the bodies we examine in paleopathology can be reimagined may seem daunting. But it is important for our analyses to expand and evolve. Here we offer two paleopathological "case studies", which we have reframed as *vignettes* in an attempt to show how to destabilize paleopathology's reliance solely on differential diagnosis and classifications by intertwining empirical data with theoretical analyses. In each case the incorporation of theory leads to reframing the way the data is read, resulting in more complex understandings of gender, identity, and agency in paleopathological interpretations of the past.

Who are We Studying? Biases in Comparative Skeletal Collections

I also do not feel comfortable claiming to "speak for the dead," and instead acknowledge the post-mortem careers of the women I study and collaborate with.

(Lans, 2021: 134)

When conducting paleopathological studies of the skeletal body, we rely on a set of standards as a baseline. Perhaps the most commonly cited is *Standards for Data Collection from Human Skeletal Remains* (Buikstra & Ubelaker, 1994). In this publication, the editors did the essential job of compiling the most agreed-upon methodologies for skeletal analysis, including the assessment of skeletal sex. One of the most well-known methodologies for skeletal sex assessment outlined in our standards is the Phenice method of examining architectural features of the subpubic region of the pubis. Per its definition as a standard, this method of sex assessment is interpreted to be applicable to most all skeletal analyses with populations across both time and geographic region. In the original publication, Phenice (1969) discusses that the method was developed and tested on 275 individuals in the Robert J. Terry Skeletal Collection. However, as researchers who study anatomical skeletal collections have pointed out, the use of such individuals, who were often collected for dissections and then retained as skeletal samples afterward, as a pan-demographic representative sample is fraught at best (Muller et al., 2017; Nystrom, 2018; Lans, 2018, 2020; Zimmer, 2018, 2021). Those remains came from persons who were often most subjected to external factors of racism, classism, and other forms of structural violence (Muller et al., 2017). The Terry Collection itself, upon which the Phenice method was developed, represents a very particular swath of St. Louis, Missouri's most marginalized residents, most especially African-Americans (de la Cova, 2019).

In order for a standard methodology to be sound, the data from whence it sprung must also be sound. In assessing a related anatomical skeletal collection, the George S. Huntington Skeletal Collection, Lans (2020, 2021) discusses how the Black women whose bodies now reside as research specimens in the anatomical collection were subject to specific intersecting forces of racism and sexism in life that undoubtedly impacted the skeletal manifestations which are left to be read by osteologists. By utilizing a Black feminist lens to reconsider these women as individuals subject to "catchment" rather than as an aggregate "Black woman population", Lans interrogates their use as data points for standards at all. And, as stated earlier, Zimmer (2018) also demonstrated that differing criteria were used when selecting White versus Black persons for dissections in the Huntington Collection. What this suggests is that those individuals upon whom our standards are based are not truly "standard" at all but are a particular slice of the human population and perhaps methodologies developed on their bodies are not as standard and broadly applicable as they are portrayed.

Furthermore, Lans (2018) argues that the collections themselves may shine just as much light on those doing the collecting as they do the individuals collected. The catchment of remains amassed by Huntington is now known by his name, officially deemed the George S. Huntington Anatomical Collection. In other words, individuals within that collection were, at some point, transformed from individual actors into segments of Huntington's own legacy. Lans flips this orientation on its head, seeing Huntington himself as a person constructed through his acts of dissection. The man we think of as the physician George S. Huntington is inseparable from the remains of other lives that he rendered and cataloged. In this sense, we can see that the act of collection, the collection itself, and the person-as-collector are all part of one entity. In recognizing this, one gathered data point from one skeletal feature from one skeletal element from one deceased individual can never truly be just that: one anonymized data point. Even those collections which are used as anonymized standards have a unique history all their own.

This is not to say that skeletal standards should never be used for sex assessment. In fact, they become more important than ever when we use them to truly examine the basis of the data themselves *before our interpretations of those data can begin*. However, this can only happen when we step back and keep the consideration of where our standards came from when we begin data collection. In doing so, we can use these methods to create a more nuanced understanding of the complex cultural forces working on the skeletal body.

Sex and Agency: Is There Really an Obstetrical Dilemma?

Childbirth is an intimate and complex transaction whose topic is physiological and whose language is cultural.

(Jordan, 1993: 3)

The concept of the "obstetrical dilemma" (OD) assumes that the evolutionary structural changes associated with bipedalism and encephalization resulted in a fetal head at odds with the smaller, bipedal pelvis, making hominin childbirth difficult, dangerous, and often deadly (Turner, 1885; Caldwell & Moloy, 1933; Krogman, 1951; and others). The construction of the OD from human evolutionary studies is a tale of compromise told within the adaptive paradigm of paleoanthropology. The story begins with male pelvic morphology, which is used to illustrate the pure unfettered adaptation to bipedal locomotion, the "normal" bipedal pelvis". Conversely, the functional morphology of the female pelvis is interpreted as a compromise between the structural requirements of bipedal locomotion and those of childbirth, thus deviant from the "normal"; making it a pathological condition (Krogman, 1951). This evolutionary explanation, of competing demands of bipedalism and childbirth, is said to leave humans with what Washburn coined as the "obstetrical dilemma" (1960). Paleopathology continues to reinforce this concept as fact by drawing attention to the increase in maternal mortality for White women from the late 19th to the mid-20th century (Schultz, 1949; Krogman, 1951; Washburn, 1960; Rosenberg, 1992; Rosenberg & Trevathan, 1995; Wittman & Wall, 2007; Franciscus, 2009; Trevathan, 2011; Grabowski, 2013). This historic increase in maternal mortality is then juxtaposed with demographic analyses of ancient remains where there are often more reproductive-aged females represented in our skeletal samples. But rarely do we interrogate this idea; in fact, we have embraced the idea of an obstetrical dilemma, holding Krogman's (1951:56) explanation published in *Scientific American* as truth: "…there can be no doubt that many of the obstetrical problems of Mrs. H. Sapiens are due to the combination of a narrower pelvis and a bigger head in the species". The pathological female pelvis as a "fact" of evolution has secured childbirth as the single killer of reproductive age females across time and space. However, if we examine more closely the concept of the OD, especially prior to the 19th century, we find little to any evidence of its persistence. So, what if the OD is a cultural construction and in fact there is no OD?

As noted, within archaeological and paleopathological research demographic analyses suggest that reproductive-aged females are more likely to present in skeletal and cemetery samples, but there is often little tying these deaths directly to childbirth; yet these deaths are almost always read as the product of an OD. Prehistorically and historically, there is actually little direct physical data to support the western pathologized picture of risky birth. The few paleopathological studies that have employed direct clinical pelvic metric analyses on prehistoric skeletal samples (Arriaza et al., 1988; Sibley et al., 1992; Tague, 1994; Stone, 2016) all reveal dimensions of the pelvis that fall within or very close to the current "normal" size standards set by obstetricians over the last two centuries (Cunningham et al., 2010). These data counter many assumptions of reproductive complications of the pelvis. These data strongly suggest that birth took a very similar path biologically in the ancient world. So maybe something about cultural contexts puts females at risk for early death, as pregnancy and childbirth most likely add an additional strain on females, but may not be why they died.

Historically, when birth is considered outside of the western medical culture another picture develops. For example, G. J. Englemann (1882), an obstetrician and gynecologist, presented his ethnological study of birth in non-western cultures, offering strong testimony about the lack of obstructed or dangerous labors for non-Whites (or in his words "the other races") in contrast to the "civilized" or evolved White-female: "[Childbirth] seems to be an equally easy process among all people who live in a near natural state" (8). In contrast, "[t]he nearer civilization' is approached, the more trying does the ordeal of childbirth become" (9).

Consider the experiences of midwife Martha Ballard, who practiced on the frontiers of Maine from 1785 to 1812. Midwife Ballard was well-educated and kept a diary that provided the records of her daily life and of all the births she attended during the 50 years she practiced midwifery. Of the 800 births she records, she did not lose a single mother or child to childbirth death (Thatcher-Urlich, 1991; Stone, 2016). While texts and diaries from midwives and doctors have the potential to reveal much, they are few and far between, but clinical and social frameworks of pregnancy and birth can also be examined in the historic context through other forms of documentation.

Data from preindustrial Europe reveals that death in childbirth was not as common an issue before medicine's interventions. For example, in Great Britain, the Royal Medical Society reported on childbirth deaths between 1752 and 1781. In 1781 there were four maternal deaths out of 1,897 deliveries (0.21%) and from 1752 to 1784 only 229 females died in childbirth, out of 19,786 deliveries (1.15%) (Shelton, 2010, 47). French statistics reported even lower death rates in Paris, where from January 1740 to January 1742 of the 3,743 women who gave birth, five died, and 29 children were still-born (Shelton, 2010:47). In France, the majority of births were home births, as those who died were noted as being "taken directly from their homes to the churchyard" (Shelton, 2010:47). These statistics change dramatically as more females deliver in controlled clinical spaces, known as lying-in hospitals. With lying-in births, there is an alarming increase in rates of infections, puerperal fevers, hemorrhage, and subsequent childbed deaths. Clearly, the 19th century was a very risky time to give birth, but prior to this, it may not have been so risky (Loudon, 2000; De Costa, 2002; Hallett, 2005).

What is it about the persistence of an evolutionary OD, and why does it continue to be taught in medical and anthropological introductory texts? This 20th-century "fact" of life has become entrenched in biomedical obstetrics, anthropology, and in the eyes of the public: females are held captive by their difficult and dangerous reproductive situations. Why are we not questioning the cultural and medical systems that resulted in dramatic increase in maternal mortality? Is there an obstetrical dilemma, or is this a narrative set to the implicit bias of the scientists reading the data?

Disentangling the OD from the historic frameworks that established it as a fact of evolution requires us to consider the 18th- and 19th-century cultural constructions of race, sex roles and gender expectations, and the constructs of agency in male/female, strong/weak, normal/deviant, which were woven together with scientific and medical language serving to reinforce the idea of risky childbirth as biologically set. Through the lens of structural violence, as well as embodiment theory, we can begin to see this dominant White, Euro-American, biomedical, cultural narrative has become embedded in how we read female bodies and their agency within society. Of further concern is that we may be missing larger issues of structural violence that place females at risk for higher rates of morbidity and mortality that are often exacerbated by pregnancy and birth, but not caused by them. MacDonald (2013) notes that maternal mortality has been shown to be a sensitive indicator of inequality and social development. Is paleopathology falling into this same trap, where females are no more than their reproductive capacities, and supporting the biologically fragile reproductive female who is the product and prisoner of the obstetric dilemma, without agency.

Conclusion

Though brief, our reflections here seek to show how paleopathology's continued reliance on a clinical "objective" analysis of the skeleton ignoring the implicit biases of these reductionist methodologies, has the potential to misread or reproduce problematic or biased understandings of the lived experience in the past. Our examples are aimed at showing how new readings that weave together social theory to complicate gender, identity, and agency in the past, lead to new and more nuanced understandings of human experiences. Further, we have shown how engaging with questions of gender, identity, and agency within theoretical frameworks requires us to break these antiquated models of analysis. However, these theoretical frameworks we offer here are just one component of more nuanced and inclusive analyses of the past. As we consider more inclusive ways to think about paleopathology, we emphasize Watkins and Muller's (2015) call for "a critical and humanistic orientation toward human biological study" (2015:41). This call hinges upon two key ideas. The first is that Science, a human-invented methodology toward investigating the world, is not an objective practice. The second is that, in order for research on the human condition to be relevant, researchers themselves must make themselves knowledgeable and competent with those social justice issues which impact said human condition. With this orientation in mind, paleopathological study has several potential venues to explore as it becomes a more humanistic endeavor.

For example, in the course of writing this chapter, literature searches related to the topics revealed only two paleopathology papers that explicitly incorporate the concept of "intersectionality" into the title (see DeWitte & Yaussey, 2020; Mant et al., 2021). That is not to say that paleopathological researchers, especially women of color, have not been conducting such studies, but it seems clear that such work has often been pushed aside or relegated as less serious than more clinically oriented studies. As discussed previously in this chapter, intersectional analyses of health in the past can be extremely difficult, but the outcomes of such effort reveal to us closely nuanced understandings of how individuals' multifaceted identities impacted their health. It is therefore our responsibility to recognize that human experiences transcend the traditional boundaries of race, gender, and social hierarchies of modern times, and to see the past through a modern lens is to miss the mosaic of human experiences. Acknowledging, and then disrupting the biases that have infiltrated how we understand, and how we narrate the stories the data offers, can only result in expanding the ways in which paleopathology considers gender, identity, and agency.

References

Ahern, L. M. (1999). Agency. *Journal of Linguistic Anthropology* 9(1/2):12–15. https://doi.org/10.1525/jlin.1999.9.1-2.12.

Ainsworth, C. (2015). Sex redefined. *Nature* 518(7539):288– 291. https://doi.org/10.1038/518288a.

Agarwal, S. C. & Glencross, B. A. (2011). Building a social bioarchaeology. In Agarwal, S. C. & Glencross, B. A. (Eds.), *Social Bioarchaeology*, pp. 1–11. New York:Wiley.

Armelagos, G. J. & Gerven, D. P.V. (2003). A century of skeletal biology and paleopathology: contrasts, contradictions, and conflicts. *American Anthropologist* 105(1):53–64. https://doi.org/10.1525/aa.2003.105.1.53.

Astorino, C. M. (2019). Beyond dimorphism: sexual polymorphism and research bias in biological anthropology. *American Anthropologist* 121(2):489–490. https://doi.org/10.1111/aman.13224.

Arriaza, B., Allison, M. & Gerszten, E. (1988). Maternal mortality in pre-Columbian Indians of Arica, Chile. *American Journal of Physical Anthropology* 77(1):35–41. https://doi.org/10.1002/ajpa.1330770107.

Bell, D. A. (1995). Who's afraid of critical race theory? *University of Illinois Law Review* 4:893–910.

Blake, C. F. (1994). Foot-binding in neo-Confucian China and the appropriation of female labor. *Signs* 19(3):676–712. https://doi.org/10.1086/494917.

Blakey, M. L. (2020). Archaeology under the blinding light of race. *Current Anthropology* 61(S22):S183–S197. https://doi.org/10.1086/710357.

Block, M. (2021, July 28). Olympic runner Caster Semenya wants to compete, not defend her womanhood. National Public Radio. https://www.npr.org/sections/tokyo-olympics-live-updates/2021/07/28/1021503989/women-runners-testosterone-olympics.

Buikstra, J. E. (Ed.). (2019). *Ortner's Identification of Pathological Conditions in Human Skeletal Remains* (3rd ed.). London: Academic Press.

Buikstra, J. E. & Ubelaker, D. H. (1994). *Standards for Data Collection from Human Skeletal Remains*. Research Series 44, Arkansas Archaeological Survey, Fayetteville.

Butler, J. (1990). *Gender Trouble: Feminism and the Subversion of Identity*. Abingdon: Routledge.

Butler, J. (2011). *Bodies That Matter: On the Discursive Limits of Sex*. Abingdon: Routledge.

Caldwell, W. E. & Moloy, H. C. (1933). Anatomical variations in the female pelvis and their effect in labor with a suggested classification. *American Journal of Obstetrics and Gynecology* 26(4):479–505. https://doi.org/10.1016/S0002-9378(33)90194-5.

Clapton, N. (2008). *Moreschi: The Last Castrato*. Haus Publishing.

Cummings, S. R., Ling, X. & Stone, K. (1997). Consequences of foot binding among older women in Beijing, China. *American Journal of Public Heath* 87(10):1677–1679. https://doi.org/10.2105/AJPH.87.10.1677.

Cunningham, F. G., Leveno, K. J., Bloom, S. L., Hauth, J. C., Gilstrap, L. C. & Wenstrom, K. D. (Eds.). (1997). *Williams Obstetrics* (20th ed.). Stamford, CT: Appleton & Lange.

Conkey, M. W. & Gero, J. M. (1991). *Engendering Archaeology Women and Prehistory*. Wiley-Blackwell.

Csordas, T. J. (1990). Embodiment as a paradigm for anthropology. *Ethos* 18(1):5–47. https://doi.org/10.1525/eth.1990.18.1.02a00010.

Davis, G. (2015). *Contesting Intersex: The Dubious Diagnosis*. New York: NYU Press.

De Costa, C. M. (2002). "The contagiousness of childbed fever": a short history of puerperal sepsis and its treatment. *Medical Journal of Australia* 177(11):668–671.

de la Cova, C. (2011). Race, health, and disease in 19th-century-born males. *American Journal of Physical Anthropology* 144(4):526–537. https://doi.org/10.1002/ajpa.21434.

de la Cova, C. (2012). Patterns of trauma and violence in 19th-century-born African American and Euro-American females. *International Journal of Paleopathology* 2(2–3):61–68. https://doi.org/10.1016/j.ijpp.2012.09.009.

de la Cova, C. (2014). The biological effects of urbanization and in-migration on 19th-century-born African Americans and Euro-Americans of low socioeconomic status: an anthropological and historical approach. In Zuckerman, M. K. (Ed.), *Modern Environments and Human Health: Revisiting the Second Epidemiological Transition*, pp. 243–264. Hoboken: Wiley Blackwell. https://doi.org/10.1002/9781118504338.ch13.

de la Cova, C. (2019). Marginalized bodies and the construction of the Robert J. Terry anatomical skeletal collection: a promised land lost. In Mant, M. L & Holland, A. J. (Eds.), *Bioarchaeology of Marginalized People*, pp. 133–155. London: Academic Press. https://doi.org/10.1016/B978-0-12-815224-9.00007-5.

Delphy, C. (1993, January). Rethinking sex and gender. In *Women's Studies International Forum* (Vol. 16, No. 1), pp. 1–9. Oxford: Pergamon. https://doi.org/10.1016/0277-5395(93)90076-L.

DeWitte, S. N. & Yaussy, S. L. (2020). Bioarchaeological applications of intersectionality. In Cheverko, C. M., Prince-Buitenhuys, J. R. & Hubbe, M. (Eds.), *Theoretical Approaches in Bioarchaeology*, pp. 45–58. Abingdon: Routledge.

DiGangi, E. A. & Bethard, J. D. (2021). Uncloaking a lost cause: decolonizing ancestry estimation in the United States. *American Journal of Physical Anthropology* 175(2):422–436. https://doi.org/10.1002/ajpa.24212.

Dowson, T. A. (2000). Why queer archaeology? An introduction. *World Archaeology* 32(2):161–165. https://doi.org/10.1080/00438240050131144.

Dunsworth, H. M. (2020). Expanding the evolutionary explanations for sex differences in the human skeleton. *Evolutionary Anthropology: Issues, News, and Reviews* 29(3):108–116. https://doi.org/10.1002/evan.21834.

Dunsworth, H. M., Warrener, A. G., Deacon, T., Ellison, P. T. & Pontzer, H. (2012). Metabolic hypothesis for human altriciality. *Proceedings of the National Academy of Sciences* 109(38):15212–15216. https://doi.org/10.1073/pnas.1205282109.

Englemann, G. (1882). *Labor Among Primitive Peoples*, London: Chambers & Co.

Fausto-Sterling, A. (2000). *Sexing the Body: Gender Politics and the Construction of Sexuality*. New York: Basic Books.

Fowles, Severin M. (2005). Our father (our mother): gender, praxis, and marginalization in Pueblo religion. In Hegmon, M. & Eiselt, S. (Eds.), *Engaged Anthropology*, pp. 27–51. Ann Arbor: University of Michigan Press.

Franciscus, R. G. (2009). When did the modern human pattern of childbirth arise? New insights from an old Neandertal pelvis. *Proceedings of the National Academy of Sciences* 106(23):9125–9126. https://doi.org/10.1073/pnas.0903384106.

Frank, K. (2006). Agency. *Anthropological Theory* 6(3):281–302. https://doi.org/10.1177/1463499606066889.

Freitas, R. (2001). *Portrait of a Castrato: Politics, Patronage, and Music in the Life of Atto Melani*. Cambridge: Cambridge University Press.

Fuentes, A., Ackermann, R. R., Athreya, S., Bolnick, D. A., Lasisi, T., Lee, S. H., McLean, S. A. & Nelson, R. G. (2019). AAPA statement on race and racism. *American Journal of Physical Anthropology* 169:400–402. https://doi.org/10.1002/ajpa.23882.

Galtung, J. (1969). Violence, Peace, and Peace Research. *Journal of Peace Research* 6(3):167–191. https://doi.org/10.1177/002234336900600301.

Galtung, J. (2002). Violence, war, and their impact: on visible and invisible effects of violence. Polylog. http://them.polylog.org/5/fgj-en.htm.

Geller, P. L. (2016). *The Bioarchaeology of Socio-Sexual Lives*. New York: Springer.

Giffney, N. (2008). Queer apocal(o)ptic/ism: the death drive and the human. In Hird, M. J. & Giggney, N. (Eds.), *Queering the Non/Human*, pp. 55–78. Milton Park, UK: Taylor & Francis.

Gottlieb, A. (2002). Interpreting gender and sexuality: approaches from cultural anthropology. In MacClancy, J. & Bennett, G. (Eds.), *Exotic No more: Anthropology on the Front Lines*, pp.167–189. Chicago University of Chicago Press.

Grabowski, M. W. (2013). Hominin obstetrics and the evolution of constraints. *Evolutionary Biology* 40:1–19. https://doi.org/10.1007/s11692-012-9174-7.

Gravlee, C. C., Dressler, W. W. & Bernard, H. R. (2005). Skin color, social classification, and blood pressure in southeastern Puerto Rico. *American Journal of Public Health* 95(12):2191–2197. https://doi.org/10.2105/AJPH.2005.065615.

Gu, Y., Mei, Q., Fernandez, J., Li, J., Ren, X. & Feng, N. (2015). Foot loading characteristics of Chinese bound feet women: a comparative analysis. *PloS One* 10(4):p.e0121695. https://doi.org/10.1371/journal.pone.0121695.

Hallett, C. (2005). The attempt to understand puerperal fever in the eighteenth and early nineteenth centuries: the influence of inflammation theory. *Medical History* 49:1–28. https://doi.org/10.1017/S0025727300000119.

Jordan, B. (1993). *Birth in Four Cultures. A Crosscultural Investigation of Childbirth in Yucatan, Holland, Sweden and the United States*. Prospect Heights: Waveland Press.

Krafft-Ebing, R. (1939). *Psychopathia Sexualis*. (12th ed.). William Heinemann (Medical Books) Ltd. (Original work published 1886).

Krogman, W. M. (1951). The scars of human evolution. *Scientific American* 185(6):54–57.
Lans, A. (2018). "Whatever was once associated with him, continues to bear his stamp": articulating and dissecting George S. Huntington and his anatomical collection. In *Bioarchaeological analyses and bodies*, pp. 11–26. Cham: Springer. https://doi.org/10.1007/978-3-030-46440-0_3.
Lans, A. M. (2020). Embodied discrimination and "mutilated historicity": archiving Black women's bodies in the Huntington collection. In Trembly, L. A. & Reedy, S. (Eds.), *The Bioarchaeology of Structural Violence*, pp. 31–52. Cham: Springer.
Lans, A. M. (2021). Decolonize this collection: integrating black feminism and art to re-examine human skeletal remains in museums. *Feminist Anthropology* 2(1):130–142. https://doi.org/10.1002/fea2.12027.
Loudon, I. (2000). *The Tragedy of Childbed Fever*. New York: Oxford University Press.
Lovejoy, C. O., Meindl, R. S., Pryzbeck, T. R., Barton, T. S., Heiple, K. & Knotting, D. (1977). Paleodemography of the Libben Site, Ottawa County Ohio. *Science* 198:291–293.
Lowell, J. C., (1991). Reflections of sex roles in the archaeological record: insights from Hopi and Zuni ethnographic data. In Walde, D. & Willows, N. D. (Eds.), *The Archaeology of Gender Proceedings of the 22nd Chacomool Conference*, pp. 452–461. Calgary: The Archaeological Association of the University of Calgary.
MacDonald, M. E. (2013). The biopolitics of maternal mortality: anthropological observations from the Women Deliver Conference in Kuala. *Somatosphere*. http://somatosphere.net/2013/the-biopolitics-of-maternal-mortality-anthropological-observations-from-the-women-deliver-conference-in-kuala-lumpur.html/.
Mant, M., de la Cova, C. & Brickley, M. B. (2021) Intersectionality and trauma analysis in bioarchaeology. *American Journal of Physical Anthropology* 174(4):583–594. https://doi.org/10.1002/ajpa.24226.
Markowitz, S. (2017). Pelvic politics: sexual dimorphism and racial difference. *Signs* 26(2):386–414. https://doi.org/10.1086/495598.
Martin, D. L. (1997). Violence against women in the La Plata River Valley (A.D. 1000–1300). In Martin, D. L. & Frayer, D. W. (Eds.), *Troubled Times: Violence and Warfare in the Past*, pp. 45–76. Philadelphia: Gordon and Breach Publishers.
Martin, D. L., Akins, N. J., Goodman, A. H. & Swedlund, A. H., (1995*). Harmony and Discord: Bioarchaeology of the La Plata Valley Santa Fe, New Mexico*. Albuquerque: Museum of New Mexico Press.
Martin, D. L, Goodman, A. H., Armelagos, G. J. & Magennis, A. L. (1991). *Black Mesa Anasazi Health: Reconstructing Life from Patterns of Death and Disease*. Center for Archaeological Investigations: Southern Illinois University at Carbondale. Occasional Article No. 14.Martin, E. (2001). *The Woman in the Body: A Cultural Analysis of Reproduction*. New York: Beacon Press.
Mascia-Lees, F. E. (2011). *A Companion to the Anthropology of the Body and Embodiment*. Hoboken, NJ: Wiley-Blackwell.
Miller, D. L. (1994). Definitional violence and Plains Indian life: ongoing challenges to survival. In Taylor, W. B. & Pease, F. (Eds.), *Violence, Resistance, and Survival in the Americas: Native Americans and the Legacy of Conquest*, pp. 226–248. Washington: Smithsonian Institution.
Mobley-Tanaka, Jeanette L. (1997). Gender and ritual space during the Pithouse to Pueblo transition: subterranean mealing rooms in the North American Southwest. *American Antiquity* 62(3):437–448. https://doi.org/10.2307/282164.
Muller, J. L., Pearlstein, K. E. & de la Cova, C. (2017). Dissection and documented skeletal collections: embodiments of legalized inequality. In Nystrom, K. (Ed.), *The Bioarchaeology of Dissection and Autopsy in the United States*, pp. 185–201. Springer, Cham. https://doi.org/10.1007/978-3-319-26836-1_9.
Munk, P. L. & Poon, P. Y. (1996). Bound feet in an elderly Chinese woman. *American Journal of Roentgenology* 167(5):1216–1216. https://doi.org/10.2214/ajr.167.5.8911183.
Nagington, M. (2015). The utility of queer theory in reconceptualising ageing in HIV-positive gay men. *Aporia* 7(4):6–17. https://doi.org/10.18192/aporia.v7i4.2801.
Nystrom, K. C. (2018). Conclusion: challenging the narrative. In Stone, P. (Ed.), *Bioarchaeological Analyses and Bodies*, pp. 231–242. Cham: Springer. https://doi.org//10.1007/978-3-319-71114-0_12.
Oakley, A. (2016). *Sex, Gender and Society*. Abingdon: Routledge.
Omi, M. & Winant, H. (2014). *Racial Formation in the United States*. Abingdon: Routledge.
Owen, G. & Catalan, J. (2012). 'We never expected this to happen': narratives of ageing with HIV among gay men living in London, UK. *Culture, Health & Sexuality* 14:59–72. https://doi.org/10.1080/13691058.2011.621449.

Peschel, E. R. & Peschel, R. E. (1987). Medical insights into the castrati in opera. *American Scientist* 75(6):578–583.

Phenice, T. W. (1969). A newly developed visual method of sexing the os pubis. *American Journal of Physical Anthropology* 30(2):297–301. https://doi.org/10.1002/ajpa.1330300214.

Rakita, G. F. (2014). Bioarchaeology as a process: an examination of bioarchaeological tribes in the USA. In O'Donnabhain, B. & Lozada, M. C. (Eds.), *Archaeological Human Remains*, pp. 213–234. New York: Springer International Publishing. https://doi.org/10.1007/978-3-319-06370-6_16.

Reischer, E. & Koo, K. S. (2004). The body beautiful: symbolism and agency in the social world. *Annual Review of Anthropology* 33:297–317. https://doi.org/10.1146/annurev.anthro.33.070203.143754.

Rosenberg, K. R. (1992). The evolution of modern human childbirth. *American Journal of Physical Anthropology* 35(S15):89–124. https://doi.org/10.1002/ajpa.1330350605.

Rosenberg, K. & Trevathan, W. (1995). Bipedalism and human birth: the obstetrical dilemma revisited. *Evolutionary Anthropology: Issues, News, and Reviews* 4(5):161–168. https://doi.org/10.1002/evan.1360040506.

Rosselli, J. (1988). The castrati as a professional group and a social phenomenon, 1550-1850. *Acta Musicologica* 60(Fasc. 2):143–179.

Scheper-Hughes, N. & Lock, M. M. (1987). The mindful body: a prolegomenon to future work in medical anthropology. *Medical Anthropology Quarterly* 1(1):6–41. https://doi.org/10.1525/maq.1987.1.1.02a00020.

Schiebinger, L. (1987). *Skeletons in the Closet: The First Illustrations of the Female Skeleton in Eighteenth-Century Anatomy*. Oakland: University of California Press.

Scholz, P. O. (2001). *Eunuchs and Castrati: A Cultural History*. Princeton, NJ: Markus Wiener Publishers.

Schultz, A. H. (1949). Sex differences in the pelves of primates. *American Journal of Physical Anthropology* 7(3):401–424.

Shelton, D. C. (2010). The emperor's new clothes. *Journal of the Royal Society of Medicine* 103:46–50. https://doi.org/10.1258/jrsm.2009.090295.

Sibley, L. M., Armelagos, G. J. & Van Gerven, D. P. (1992). Obstetric dimensions of the true pelvis in a medieval population from Sudanese Nubia. *American Journal of Physical Anthropology*, 89(4):421–430.

Smith, E. A. (2013). Agency and adaptation: new directions in evolutionary anthropology. *Annual Review of Anthropology* 42:103–120. https://doi.org/10.1146/annurev-anthro-092412-155447.

Stone, P. K. (2012) Binding women: ethnology, skeletal deformations, and violence against women. *International Journal of Paleopathology* 2(2–3):53–60. https://doi.org/10.1016/j.ijpp.2012.09.008.

Stone, P. K. (2016). Biocultural perspectives on maternal mortality and obstetrical death from the past to the present. *American Journal of Physical Anthropology* 159(S61):150–171. https://doi.org/10.1002/ajpa.22906.

Stone, P. K. (2020a). Bound to please: the shaping of female beauty, gender theory, structural violence, and bioarchaeological investigations. In Sheridan, S. & Gregoricka, L. (Eds.), *Purposeful Pain: The Bioarchaeology of Intentional Suffering*, pp. 39–62. Cham: Springer. https://doi.org/10.1007/978-3-030-32181-9_3.

Stone, P. K. (2020b). Female beauty, bodies, binding, and the bioarchaeology of structural violence in the industrial era through the lens of critical white feminism. In Trembly, L. A & Reedy, S. (Eds.), *The Bioarchaeology of Structural Violence*, pp. 13–30. Cham: Springer. https://doi.org/10.1007/978-3-030-46440-0_2.

Stone, P. K. & Sanders, L. S. (2020). *Bodies and Lives in Victorian England: Science, Sexuality, and the Affliction of Being Female*. Abingdon: Routledge.

Tague, R. G. (1994). Maternal mortality or prolonged growth: age at death and pelvic size in three prehistoric Amerindian populations. *American Journal of Physical Anthropology* 95:27–40. https://doi.org/10.1002/ajpa.1330950103.

Tallman, S., Parr, N. & Winburn, A. (2021). Assumed differences; unquestioned typologies: the oversimplification of race and ancestry in forensic anthropology. *Forensic Anthropology* 4(4):73–96. https://doi.org/10.5744/fa.2020.0046.

Trevathan, W. R. (2011). *Human Birth: An Evolutionary Perspective* (2nd ed.). Hawthorne, NY: Aldine de Gruyter.

Turner, W. (1885). The index of the pelvic brim as a basis of classification. *Journal of Anatomy and Physiology* 20(1):125–143.

Urlich, L. T. (1991). *A Midwife's Tale: The Life of Martha Ballard, Based on Her Diary, 1785–1812*. New York: Vintage Books.

Voss, B. L. (2009). Looking for gender, finding sexuality: a queer politic of archaeology, fifteen years later. *Que(e)Rying Archaeology: Proceedings of the 37th Annual Chacmool Archaeological Conference*, pp. 29–39.

Warsh, C. K. (2019). Chapter Five: Future childbirth: doctors and babies. In Warsh, C. K. (Ed.), *Prescribed Norms: Women and Health in Canada and the United States Since 1800*, pp.153–171. Toronto: University of Toronto Press.

Washburn, S. L. (1960). The tools of human evolution. *Scientific American* 203(3):63–75.

Watkins, R. J. (2012). Variation in health and socioeconomic status within the W. Montague Cobb skeletal collection: degenerative joint disease, trauma and cause of death. *International Journal of Osteoarchaeology* 22(1):22–44. https://doi.org/10.1002/oa.1178.

Watkins, R. J. (2018). Anatomical collections as the anthropological other: some considerations. In Stone, P. K. (Ed.), *Bioarchaeological Analyses and Bodies*, pp. 27–47. Cham: Springer. https://doi.org/10.1007/978-3-319-71114-0_3.

Watkins, R. J. & Muller, J. L. (2015). Repositioning the Cobb human archive: the merger of a skeletal collection and its texts. *American Journal of Human Biology* 27(1):41–50. https://doi.org/10.1002/ajhb.22650.

Weheliye, A. G. (2014). *Habeas Viscus: Racializing Assemblages, Biopolitics, and Black Feminist Theories of the Human*. Durham, NC: Duke University Press.

Whitehead, Neil L. (2004). On the poetics of violence. In Whitehead, N. L. (Ed.), *Violence*, pp. 55–77. Santa Fe: School of American Research. http://www.loc.gov/catdir/toc/ecip0420/2004017171.html

Wilson, J. D. & Roehrborn, C. (1999). Long-term consequences of castration in men: lessons from the Skoptzy and the eunuchs of the Chinese and Ottoman courts. *The Journal of Clinical Endocrinology & Metabolism* 84(12):4324–4331. https://doi.org/10.1210/jcem.84.12.6206.

Wittman, A. B. & Wall, L. L. (2007). The evolutionary origins of obstructed labor: bipedalism, encephalization, and the human obstetric dilemma. *Obstetrical & Gynecological Survey* 62(11):739–748. https://doi.org/10.1097/01.ogx.0000286584.04310.5c.

Wynter, S. (2003). Unsettling the coloniality of being/power/truth/freedom: towards the human, after man, its overrepresentation—An argument. *CR: The New Centennial Review* 3(3):257–337.

Zanatta, A., Zampieri, F., Scattolin, G. & Bonati, M. R. (2016). Occupational markers and pathology of the castrato singer Gaspare Pacchierotti (1740–1821). *Scientific Reports* 6(1):1–9. https://doi.org/10.1038/srep28463.

Zhang, Y., Li, F. L., Shen, W. W., Li, J. S., Ren, X. J. & Gu, Y. D. (2014). Characteristics of the skeletal system of bound foot: a case study. *Journal of Biomimetics, Biomaterials and Tissue Engineering*. http://dx.doi.org/10.4172/1662-100X.1000120.

Zimmer, A. N. (2017). Unpacking the definitional violence of skeletal collections in the United States (Abstract). *Paper presented at the annual meeting of the American Anthropological Association*, Washington, DC.

Zimmer, A. N. (2018). More than the sum total of their parts: restoring identity by recombining a skeletal collection with its texts. In Stone, P. K. (Ed.), *Bioarchaeological Analyses and Bodies*, pp. 49–69. Cham: Springer. https://doi.org/10.1007/978-3-319-71114-0_4.

Zimmer, A. N. (unpublished paper). *Queer Theory & Identified Skeletal Collections*. Keynote talk presented at the annual meeting of the British Association of Biological Anthropology & Osteoarchaeology, Middlesbrough, England.

Zuckerman, M. K., Harper, K. N. & Armelagos, G. J. (2016). Adapt or die: three case studies in which the failure to adopt advances from other fields has compromised paleopathology. *International Journal of Osteoarchaeology* 26(3):375–383. https://doi.org/10.1002/oa.2426.

25
DISABILITY AND CARE IN THE BIOARCHAEOLOGICAL RECORD

Meeting the Challenges of Being Human

Lorna Tilley

Introduction

[A]pproaches to reconstructing disability in the past are currently underutilized by bioarchaeologists … [B]ioarchaeology would benefit… from an increased awareness of the implications of disease, impairment and disability in our interpretations.

(Knudson and Stojanowski, 2008:409)

Disease and injury are constants of human existence. There is now an increasing body of bioarchaeological research suggesting that caregiving in response to disability arising from disease or injury is an equally well-established feature of human history. Knudson and Stojanowskis' (2008:409) observation has proven prescient: the last decade has seen an exponential growth of publications on "disability" and on "disability and care", opening up new, and more nuanced, ways of looking at the past. Focusing on disability has required bioarchaeologists to think through what disability may have signified in the period under scrutiny – both to the person identified as experiencing this state and to the community in which it was experienced: how, by whom, under what conditions, and with reference to what expectations was an individual's "disability" determined? Health-related caregiving occurs through personal interactions which can be intimate, complicated, physically exhausting, and emotionally rewarding yet emotionally demanding for everyone involved; the care given is a product of values, beliefs, traditions, access to resources, knowledge, and skills, and it is shaped within a social, economic, and physical environment (Bates & Linder-Pelz, 1990; Pol & Thomas, 2001; Raphael et al., 2019; Weiss & Copelton, 2020). A focus on care allows insights into the people, practices and priorities of the community in which it occurred.

Identification of both disability and care in the bioarchaeological record is based on indicators in human remains suggesting an individual survived with, or following, a pathology which – for a period of time – compromised their ability to operate independently and/or participate appropriately within their lifeways setting (disability), and to counteract which they received a level of support from others (care). The premise is straightforward, but the reality more complex. This chapter concentrates on the *what*, *how*, and *why* of applied bio-archaeological research into disability and care. Part 1 discusses issues central to identifying and interpreting evidence for disability and care in the archaeological record; Part 2 examines how research into past disability and care is undertaken in practice; and Part 3 addresses why understanding past disability and care is relevant for modern times.

The 'What' of Research into Past Disability and Care: Definitions, Debates, Principles, and Problems

Disagreement over Definitions of "Disability" …

> It is important, therefore, to appreciate… the case… for viewing disablement as a universal human phenomenon.
>
> *(Bickenbach et al., 1999:1179)*

Modern estimates suggest that at any one time over 15% of the population is experiencing disability and, furthermore, that almost everyone will experience at least one temporary or permanent activity-limiting disability at some stage of life (Bickenbach et al., 1999; WHO, 2011; AIHW, 2020). It is unlikely this situation was any different in the past; in what seems more than mere coincidence, Ortner (2003:112) reports that "[i]n typical archaeological human skeletal samples about 15 per cent of burials will show evidence of significant disease". Experience of disability is integral to the experience of being human; disability is "part of the human condition" (WHO, 2011:7) and, as such, an important focus for archaeological research.

Dictionary definitions of "disability" are deceptively straightforward, casting disability simply as "a physical, mental, cognitive, or developmental condition that impairs, interferes with, or limits a person's ability to engage in certain tasks or actions or participate in typical daily activities and interactions" (Merriam-Webster, 2022). In practice, the meaning of this term is often fiercely contested, depending upon the way 'disability' is conceptualized – and there are multiple and sometimes diametrically opposed models of disability in play (Bickenbach, 2019). At one end of the spectrum, the 'medical model' depicts disability as a biological or "medical health" problem to be remedied, with the individual as the primary focus of intervention (Areheart, 2008). At the other end, critical disability studies theory situates disability as a sociopolitical construction, arguing that it is society that needs fixing, not the individual: "[disability is] not fundamentally a question of medicine or health… rather it is a question of politics and power" (Devlin & Pothier, 2006:2; Goodley et al., 2019). The interactionalist conception of disability lies between these extremes, rejecting the medical model for its failure to acknowledge that experience of disability involves far more than pathology impact and rejecting the social model for not only "fail[ing] to capture the complexity of disabled people's lives" (Shakespeare, 2008:11) but also disempowering those experiencing disability by denying the very real medical impacts of disease (Shakespeare, 2008, 2013; Vehmas, 2008). The interactional model, which now forms the basis for most policy and research in the area of disability, acknowledges disease or injury as a precondition for the existence of disability but establishes *actual* "disability" as the outcome of interactions between biological, psychological, and social factors (Bickenbach, 1999, 2019; Shakespeare, 2008, 2013).

An agreed understanding of what disability comprises is key to enabling its identification in the archaeological record. Perhaps predictably, there is a history of debate surrounding the use of this term in our discipline. Thirty years ago, on the back of the emergent Disability Studies movement, Dettwyler (1991) argued that disability cannot be identified in the archaeological record because it is, above all, a *social* phenomenon. Conflating care (a behavior) with compassion (a motivation), she critiqued attempts to identify either care or compassion on the basis of archaeological evidence, asserting there can be no justification for "drawing conclusions either about the quality of life for disabled individuals in the past or about the motives or attitudes of the rest of the community from skeletal evidence of physical impairment" (Dettwyler, 1991:375). Although recently comprehensively critiqued, this widely cited article played a major role in discouraging (bio)archaeological research into disability and care for at least 20 years (Tilley, 2015a:43–48; Doat, 2017), reflecting sensitivities around the question of what constitutes disability rather than quality of argument. In 1999, a dedicated issue of the *Archaeological Review from Cambridge* sought to stimulate interest in research on disablement and, more particularly, the development of an archaeological model of disability (Cross, 1999; Metzler, 1999; Roberts, 1999). Again, the pressure to frame disability in the archaeological past within the (then) dominant social model (Shakespeare, 1999; Southwell-Wright, 2013: 61–78) resulted in little of practical relevance to a discipline which, regardless of its reliance on interpretation, has the notion of materiality at its core. A few unrelated papers canvassed the possibility of an 'archaeology of disability' in the years following (e.g., Roberts, 2000; Battles, 2009), but it is only in the last decade that interest in exploring the topic of disability has flourished (e.g., Byrnes & Muller, 2017).

In 2011, the article which first introduced the bioarchaeology of care approach argued for adoption of the World Health Organization (WHO) definition (Tilley & Oxenham, 2011; Tilley, 2015:69–71), which (following the interactional model) positions disability as "... an umbrella term, covering impairments, activity limitations, and participation restrictions. An impairment is a problem in body function or structure; an activity limitation is a difficulty encountered by an individual in executing a task or action; while a participation restriction is a problem experienced by an individual in involvement in life situations. Thus disability is a complex phenomenon, reflecting an interaction between features of a person's body and features of the society in which he or she lives" (WHO, 2011).

This "biopsychosocial" definition of disability provides a conceptual framework within which experience of disability can be operationalized (WHO, 1997, 2011; Bickenbach et al., 1999) and is embodied in the WHO International Classification of Functioning, Disability and Health (ICF) (Bickenbach et al., 1999; WHO, 2003; Bickenbach, 2019), the global standard for describing and measuring the effects of disease on life experience (Bickenbach et al., 1999; Bickenbach, 2019). The ICF describes and assesses the nature and physiological implications of pathology, but focuses on the impact of these on an individual's capacity to meet the demands (and desires) of their individual lifeways context. In effect, this translates the concept of 'disability' into 'ability to function' (Bickenbach, 2019).

It is this focus on "ability to function" which makes the WHO definition of disability so apposite for bioarchaeological research. Bioarchaeology can never retrieve the multi-faceted whole of an individual's experience of disability. However, if there is skeletal or preserved soft tissue evidence for an individual having experienced, for a period, a pathology typically posing "a problem in body function or structure" (WHO, 2011), then assessment of the likely clinical implications of this condition can be examined in relation to cultural, social, economic and physical environments and associated lifeways expectations which may have challenged the person's ability to function. Pragmatically, operationalizing pathology impact in terms of "ability to function" and analyzing the result in the context of what is known of past lifeways allows an appreciation of disability experiences (however superficial) that is the most objective, and sometimes the *only*, option available to bioarchaeologists.

... But (By and Large) Embracing The Concept of 'Care'

> We suggest care is a fundamental social dynamic, connecting caregivers from early to contemporary times. Caregivers can be viewed as a shared global community, transcending community and time.
>
> *(Hale & Jaye, 2018:120)*

If we can characterize 'disablement as a universal phenomenon' (Bickenbach et al., 1999:1179), then history and personal experience allow us to characterize caregiving as a human behavior of equal universality (Hale & Jaye, 2018). As Carter (1997:1) puts it: "[t]here are only four kinds of people in the world: those who have been caregivers, those who are currently caregivers, those who will be caregivers, and those who will need caregivers". The ubiquity of caregiving behavior, and what this behavior may reveal about the individual and their wider world, renders health-related care a compelling topic for bioarchaeological research.

In sharp contrast to the continuing debate around the meaning of "disability", most bioarchaeologists seem willing to accept a working definition of "health-related care" as an action or process intended to help address needs and limitations arising from disease or injury. There also appears a general in-principle acceptance that provision of care may be inferred from evidence in human remains that indicates an individual lived, for a period of time, with a pathology likely compromising their ability to function independently in one or more domains. There is less agreement about how severe such impacts must have been before care was needed: should pathology be completely incapacitating, or is it sufficient that the individual was likely excluded from certain – even if not all – activities in particular areas of life? But one thing that paleopathologists and bioarchaeologists agree on is that the circumstances under which care is considered necessary and/or appropriate, and the form and/or content of this care, may vary significantly between and within different cultures and during different time periods. Caregiving may indeed be a "fundamental social dynamic" (Hale & Jaye, 2018:120), but it is one which relies on context for its production and for our subsequent interpretation (see e.g., Tilley, 2015a:66–71, 79–84; Powell et al., 2016; Tilley & Schrenk, 2017).

Until recently, little thought had been given to care as a potential topic for bioarchaeological research. When Knudson and Stojanowski presented their vision for "new directions in bioarchaeology" in 2008, "disability" was highlighted, but "care" was not on their radar. Yet there were several reports prior to this – some dating back half a century – in which the likely practice of caregiving in response to disease, injury, and disability had been noted. These studies chronicled health challenges ranging from traumatic injury (e.g., Solecki, 1971; Lovejoy & Heiple, 1981; Trinkaus & Zimmerman, 1982; Orschiedt et al., 2003; Buquet-Marcon et al., 2007), through activity and/or life-limiting congenital conditions (e.g., Frayer et al., 1987; Dickel & Doran, 1989; Webb & Thorne, 1995; DiGangi et al., 2009), to (variously) acute, chronic, infectious, systemic, and degenerative diseases (Suzuki et al., 1984; Formicola et al., 1987; Walker & Shipton, 1996; Hawkey, 1998; Luna et al., 2008), with cases sourced from all continents and extending from Homo erectus to Early Modern times. Unfortunately, the primary aim in all these studies was description and diagnosis of pathology; identification of possible care provision was usually relegated to brief mention in a concluding paragraph. Studies rarely attempted consideration of what such care practice may have entailed, or more than anodyne generalization about what caregiving might imply about the society in which it occurred (Tilley, 2015:13–29).

With publication of the first bioarchaeology of care case study in 2011 (Tilley & Oxenham, 2011), identification of caregiving moved from being the by-product of research to its focus. Defining health-related care as the delivery of assistance to those experiencing short-, medium-, or long-term disability, the bioarchaeology of care methodology conceptualizes the behavior of caregiving as a continuum extending from "direct support", referring to the more labor-intensive forms of caregiving required when an individual is mostly or wholly reliant on others, to "accommodation of difference", comprising adoption of strategies making it easier for an individual to take their place in the community when challenges to function render "normal" participation difficult or impossible. These forms of care are not mutually exclusive; most people requiring "direct support" will almost certainly require "accommodation", and levels of care required will typically vary over time as well. Importantly, the continuum of care concept means that disease experience suggested by skeletal evidence need not have resulted in complete incapacitation, nor have been lifelong and/or ultimately fatal, in order to qualify for bioarchaeology of care analysis.

Ten years on, bioarchaeologists have already produced an impressive number of studies exploring different aspects and implications of health-related caregiving. A valuable paper by Stodder and Byrnes (2019) lays out the relationship between "traditional" paleopathology and the "new kids on the block" bioarchaeologies of disability and care, and is recommended for readers interested in untangling where (and how) research into care fits within our discipline. A rich body of theory underpinning bioarchaeological research into health-related care is also emerging. Some fundamental questions are being asked: for example, how is bioarchaeological evidence suggesting receipt of care by early Homo to be reconciled with the tenets of evolutionary "selection of the fittest"? What enabling role might health-related care itself have played in human evolution? Can archaeological evidence suggesting individual and community willingness to undertake (often onerous) costs of care be explained by purely biologically based mechanisms of "reciprocal altruism" – and how do we balance the claims of social learning and the notion of agency with those of biological determinism? Can evidence which allows the inference of caregiving in the archaeological record also be read as revealing the presence of compassion? (For detailed discussion see Fàbrega, 1999; Spikins et al., 2010, 2019; Tilley, 2015a:95–119; Doat, 2016, 2017; Thorne, 2016; Millela, 2017.)

Principles: The Obvious, The Not-So-Obvious, and the Ethical

Establishing context is both the most important and the most obvious principle to be observed in bioarchaeological research into disability and care. While some basic symptoms of particular pathologies will be biologically determined and, as such, common across individuals, concepts of "health" and "disease" are understood very differently across time and culture. Form, content, and meaning of disability experience, along with caregiving response, will be, to a very large extent, determined by context (e.g., Scheper-Hughes & Lock, 1987; Martin & Horowitz, 2003; Levin & Browner, 2005). As Zuckerman et al. (2014) assert, contextualizing skeletal evidence of lived experience (the authors look specifically at inscribed signatures of power, oppression, and privilege) means bioarchaeology can recover stories which may be "otherwise obscured or invisible in the historical or archaeological record" (2014:514).

Dettwyler's (1991) critique of the archaeological inference of care and compassion rests, in part, on assessing the subject's state on the basis of culturally *in*appropriate practices and expectations. For example, Romito 2, a male aged 17–20 years at time of death, lived with a rare and potentially disabling form of disproportionate dwarfism in a mobile, hunter-gatherer community operating in the mountainous Calabrian terrain around 11 000 years ago. Frayer et al.'s (1987, 1988) analyses of Romito 2's remains determined that Romito 2 faced obstacles to meeting economic and environmental challenges which required ongoing community support for his survival (Frayer et al., 1987, 1988). Critiquing this conclusion, Dettwyler (1991:381) compared Romito 2's situation to that of a man with the same condition who was able to function independently as an office-based draftsman in 20th-century USA, and with the situation of !Kung children, who traverse the flat Kalahari desert with no special concession made for similar stature. There is obviously no equivalence in these comparisons, and by using such examples to support an argument that we need to look at how people with particular diseases function in *today's* society rather than "assume" experience of disability in the past, Dettwyler (1991) illustrates why the principle of contextualization is paramount.

The second obvious principle in researching past questions of disability and care is that this must be approached as a quintessentially transdisciplinary endeavor. Teasing out the complexity inherent in understanding disability and care calls for the integration of theories and methodologies from across all fields of archaeology and bioanthropology, as well as from non-archaeological disciplines such as medicine and clinical practice, social and medical anthropology, ethnography and sociology, psychology, history of medicine and disability studies. Conlogue et al. (2017) provide a compelling example of a cross-disciplinary approach. Their paper, focusing on the remains of a mature male from late 18th century London manifesting severe skeletal anomalies, results from a collaboration between specialists in bioarchaeology, history, medicine, medical imaging, forensics and orthopedics – a combination producing an historically and socially contextualized analysis of disease impact on functioning which is exceptionally rich in background and meticulous in detail.

Not as immediately obvious – but no less important – is the principle placing agency at the center of research into past disability and care. Care is not a default response. The act of caregiving, typically consisting of a sequence of actions over a period of time (however brief this period may be), always embodies intent: although the decision to care, the aims of care and the features of care often change over the caregiving process, each element of the care provided is the result of choices made and options rejected – whether consciously or not. Evidence for care provision can be deconstructed in terms of "agency" and "context" operating in a recursive relationship. Agency is shaped by the lifeways context in which the caregivers are operating, and in turn, context will be shaped by the care given and the outcomes of this care (Tilley, 2015:130–137).

Those experiencing disability requiring care also exercise agency. In fact, these material remnants of life we study can be perceived as representing both actor and artifact: *actor*, because these remains represent a once living person who met the challenges of disability and who survived; *artifact*, because – in cases of severe pathology at least – the disease indicators supporting inference of disability exist, in part, by virtue of the care which enabled survival. Care recipients are not passive. Their negotiation of, contribution to, and cooperation with care are integral to its design and outcomes (e.g., Lupton, 1997; Nusselder et al., 2005; Lussier & Richard, 2008; Kim, 2010).

The final principle considered here is the one which demands that bioarchaeological research into disability and care meet the ethical responsibilities incumbent on *all* archaeological research involving human remains: to respect, protect and preserve the integrity of the individuals under examination, recognizing that their remains "serve as essential portals to the past" (Grauer, 2018:908).

Research into disability seeks access to experiences and behaviors which, in a living individual, are always personal, often powerful, and sometimes deeply private. While the human remains at the center of study no longer retain sentient existence, the research process itself endows them with *social* existence (Tarlow, 2000). The potential for misrepresentation is ever-present. Chamoun (2020) notes that study subjects are often the ancestors of colonized peoples and/or come from the ranks of the disadvantaged, and asks whether attempts to (re)construct personal stories of disability and care are not a form of appropriation which "demonstrates an esoteric custodianship of bodies, a (post)colonial privilege many bioarchaeologists enact ... performed on bodies which literally cannot speak back" (Chamoun, 2020:38; see Chapter 22, this volume, for further discussion on ethics and the use of human remains in research).

From different perspectives, Doat (2014; 2017) maintains the human species is defined by interdependence, suggesting that disability and care research can overturn misconceptions of human development as the "survival of the fittest": in fact, survival demanded cooperation between, and care for, the strong, the weak, the healthy and the sick. Doat (2017) argues that there is an ethical imperative to provide a balanced representation of our early ancestors, noting that disability and caregiving are often written out of historical records and at stake is a more accurate understanding of human evolution. Mennear (2017), meanwhile, calls on bioarchaeologists to recognize that questions of disability and care have an immediate relevance for many people. Because the primary rationale of archaeology is engendering greater understanding of the present through discoveries about the past, bioarchaeologists have an ethical responsibility both to pursue this research and to encourage public engagement in this process.

Problems: Obstacles and Limitations (and Possible Responses to Some of These)

When working with skeletal remains, reliance on osteological and/or dental indicators to identify disease is a continuing constraint in bioarchaeological research on disability and care. Relatively few pathologies (other than bone fracture, periodontal disease, and degenerative joint conditions) consistently register in bone, and even those with this potential usually do so only 10–20% of the time (Ortner, 2009:328). In many diseases frequency of bone involvement may be lower – for example, diagnostic markers are found in only 1–5% of cases of leprosy, syphilis, and tuberculosis (Ortner, 2003:112–115). Skeletal involvement usually occurs with advanced disease, meaning those who recovered or died before bone was implicated cannot be identified as experiencing pathology (Wood et al., 1992; Ortner 2009), much less requiring care. In the absence of a distinctive pattern of disease response diagnosis may be impossible, ruling out consideration of comorbidities; the ability to identify disease is further compromised when remains are incomplete or poorly preserved (Ortner 2003; Waldron 2009). Soft tissue preservation may provide superior opportunities for diagnosis of certain pathologies and for charting impacts of pathology over time, and recent studies involving mummified subjects reveal this as a promising area for future investigation (Nystrom & Tilley, 2019).

Another unavoidable problem is that every individual responds to disease symptoms, even symptoms of the *same* disease, differently, reflecting individual biology, psychology, and personal life experience (see Roush, 2017; Roberts, 2017) and meaning that there can be no presumption of an invariable relationship between pathology and its consequences. Moreover, conceptions of disability also differ, and a pathology considered incapacitating in one setting may not be so in another. See, for example, Scheer and Groce (1988) in relation to "normalization" of deafness, Knusel (1999) and Anand (2017) on cultural differences in perceptions of individuals with microcephaly; and Tarlow (2000) and Anand (2017) on infertility experienced as disabling in cultures in which family size defines social and economic status.

Finally, archaeology rarely provides a representative sample of a population. If we cannot obtain an accurate picture of disease prevalence, then it is clearly impossible to estimate the need for care at a population level with any precision, although with "about 15 per cent" of human remains in archaeological samples "show[ing] evidence of serious disease" (Ortner, 2003:112), we can be confident such need existed. In fact, there is evidence for human experience of systemic infection, trauma, and congenital disease from Middle Palaeolithic times onwards (e.g., Cohen & Armelagos, 1984; Berger & Trinkaus 1995; Steckel & Rose, 2002; Cohen & Crane-Kramer, 2003; Roberts & Manchester, 2005; Larsen, 2018; Spikins et al., 2018).

The obstacles outlined dictate that conclusions regarding the need for health-related care, and for the provision of care in response to this need, must err on the side of caution. Nonetheless, human biology dictates a level of uniformity in physical expressions of, and physiological reactions to, specific pathology across time and culture. In other words, some conditions will generate requirements for forms of treatment which are so essential that, if they are not met, the individual will most likely not survive – or be unlikely to survive for the length of time necessary to produce skeletal or soft tissue indicators meeting the criteria for inclusion in bioarchaeology of disability and care analyses. Kleinman (1980) observes that, in relation to ethnomedical studies, "the problem…is not that [these studies] impose an alien category on indigenous materials, *but rather that they fail to apprehend a profound cross-cultural similarity in clinical interest and practice*" (Kleinman 1980:83, italics added). Drawing directly from the work of the nursing theorist Virginia Henderson (Henderson, 1964, 1966), the bioarchaeology of care approach nominates ten "constants of care" (Table 25.1) for use in developing a model of caregiving practice based on evidence for likely need for care in human remains.

Table 25.1 'Constants of care'[a,b]

1	Provision of food and water (may include special diet, assistance with eating/drinking).	6	Monitoring health status (to allow timely response to physiological needs, and to avoid health crises – see [7], [8], and [9] in particular).
2	Maintaining body temperature within normal range (may include protection from elements – provision of shade/shelter)	7	Maintaining personal hygiene/protection of integument cleanliness is essential for skin integrity and preventing and treating infection.
3	Facilitation of rest and sleep (may include postural adjustment, provision of pain relief)	8	Physical manipulation (turning, lifting, stretching and massage essential maintain/improve body system and organ function in cases of immobility, and see [9])
4	Ensuring physical safety (may include protection from self-harm, domestic and wider environmental [e.g. human, animal, reptile] hazards – may require regular monitoring [see 6])	9	Maintaining physiological functioning (involves timely response to metabolic, respiratory, gastrointestinal, circulatory, urinary, etc. dysfunction – includes physical manipulation, temperature control, diet, and hydration)
5	Maintaining/assisting mobility (integral to management of/recovery from disease as immobility can be fatal – see also [8])	10	Specific intervention(s)/technologies (includes invasive/non-invasive surgery e.g. orthopaedic, trepanation, amputation; control of hemorrhage; pharmaceuticals; practical aids e.g., prosthetics, walking aids)

[a]Table 25.1 borrows from, and adapts, Henderson's (1964) components of nursing practice.
[b]For a more detailed discussion, see Tilley 2015:79–83.

In any given case, aspects of care may be unknowable – particularly when caregiving corresponds to "accommodation". Without direct evidence it will likely be impossible to establish spiritual, psychological, or emotional care provision (although this may be suggested by context). However, from the earliest medical texts onwards, it is clear that spiritual care, at least, was often an inseparable element of caregiving, and historic and ethnographic evidence attests to spiritual and psychological needs being recognized as of equal (if not greater) importance than physical ones (e.g., Lewis, 1975; Scheper-Hughes & Lock, 1987; Wesp, 2017; Gilchrist, 2020:71–109).

The 'How': Retrieving Disability and Care from the Archaeological Record

The Bioarchaeology of Care Approach: Theory, Practice, and Feedback

The bioarchaeology of care approach provides a framework for case study-based research into disability and care that offers a systematic, theorized process for identifying, ordering, analyzing, and interpreting evidence and which encourages rigour and transparency. Starting with evidence from human remains displaying lived experience of potentially activity-limiting pathology, the methodology divides analysis into four incremental stages (see Table 25.2 and Figure 25.1, which illustrates the application of the methodology). The associated Index of Care (www.indexofcare.com) (Tilley & Cameron, 2014, 2021) is an open-access instrument designed to assist researchers work through a bioarchaeology of care case study.

Feedback from researchers using the bioarchaeology of care approach has been generally positive, and the methodology has been widely adopted and creatively extended in ways unimagined when first developed. However, the uncertainties of retrospective diagnosis and heterogeneity in disease response have led to some researchers expressing reservations arising from practical constraints in accurately identifying disability impact. This is an understandable concern and only addressed by conservatism at every step in analysis (emphasized throughout the methodology and built into the Index of Care algorithm). Other researchers have expressed concern at the amount of interpretation called for in Stages 3 and 4 of the methodology. The further a case study progresses, the more analysis relies on inference from evidence rather than on material evidence itself, and interpretation of inference is, to put it bluntly, speculation. The immediate response is that while Stages 3 and 4 unarguably call for a degree of speculation, it is speculation based on a firm foundation of evidence and reason, and the methodology calls for all inferences and assumptions to be explicitly identified. An equally valid response is that this level of interpretation takes archaeology beyond simple description and into a more sophisticated and much more meaningful engagement with the past (Campanaro 2021). Thorpe (2016), for instance, situates interpretation as a moral duty: "[p]aleoanthropological analysis following the [bioarchaeology of care] model cannot continue to treat interpretation of the consequences of impairment as an optional extra. … [By integrating interpretation into analysis] [p]aleoanthropologists could thereby contribute fully to some of the most significant debates about the origins and development of human society` (Thorpe, 2016:125). Ultimately, of course, researchers alone will decide how far they are comfortable in interpreting their data. Table 25.3 contains synopses of a very small selection of studies illustrating the scope and flexibility of the bioarchaeology of care approach – and the wealth of the information it is capable of generating.

Table 25.2 The four stages of the bioarchaeology of care

Stage 1: Describe, diagnose, document	**Stage 1** begins with evidence in human remains suggesting life with, or following, serious pathology: pathology lesions and diagnoses are documented, and sociodemographic characteristics, physical remains, mortuary treatment, and contemporary cultural, social, economic and physical environments described. It produces a baseline osteobiography (a 'social identity' expanded over the course of analysis), establishes lifeways context, and is the foundation for analysis and interpretation in Stages 2–4.
Stage 2: Assess disability[a] and need for care	**Stage 2** comprises three parts. i. **Clinical Impacts** uses modern medical sources to identify clinical signs and symptoms associated with pathology described in Stage 1 and factors in complications/comorbidities unlikely to register in remains. ii. **Functional Implications** considers likely effects on performance of (a) 'essential (or basic) activities of daily living' (e.g., hygiene maintenance, self-feeding, control of body position – Katz et al., 1970); if independent performance of any 'essential' task is impossible, the subject will depend on care as "direct support" for survival; and (b) 'instrumental activities of daily living' (everyday economic, social, cultural and domestic activities typical of the subject's sociodemographic – Chong, 1995; WHO, 2003). These latter are context-dependent [Stage 1], usually not essential for physical survival but important for group inclusion and quality of life; inability to perform activities may require care as 'accommodation'. iii. **Assessment** asks whether, *on the balance of probabilities*, the individual required care provision in either activity category. If "<u>Yes</u>", the study continues to Stage 3. If "<u>No</u>", the study ends here.
Stage 3: Construct a model of care[b]	**Stage 3** produces a model of likely care in response to impact on essential and instrumental activities of daily living [Stage 2] within the constraints of lifeways context and individual osteobiography [Stage 1]. Some components of care as "*direct support*" may be confidently deduced from known clinical and functional impacts of a particular pathology (see Table 25.1). Inferring care as "*accommodation*" involves reviewing likely difficulties in performing instrumental activities of daily living and identifying possible adjustments made to expectations and practices to enable management of these. Likely duration of care, changes to care over time, identity and number of caregivers, and direct and indirect costs of care are also considered. Dependent on context, it may be possible to infer interventions by "formal" healers, use of medicines, spiritual, and/or psychological care.
Stage 4: Interpret implications of care	**Stage 4** unpacks and interprets the model of care developed over Stages 1–3. Behaviors in both provision and receipt of care constitute expressions of agency; Stage 4 explores what constituent elements of the care model - singly and in combination - indicate about contemporary social relations, practices and organization in the community in which care is given and about individual identity. A generic 'decision pathway' extending from the decision to provide care, through design, implementation, revision, and withdrawal of care, to mortuary treatment ("care after death"[c]) considers what the choices adopted at each step suggest about the community. Generic questions around personal experiences of disability and care prompt researchers to consider the unique lived experience of the individual.

[a]The methodology adopts the WHO (2011) definition of "disability" as a state (temporary or longer-term) arising from an impairment in body function or structure and associated with activity limitations and/or participation restrictions.

[b]"Care" is used as an inclusive term for behaviors along a continuum extending from hands-on, often time-consuming "direct support" (e.g. nursing, hygiene maintenance, physical therapy, provisioning) to "accommodation of difference" (e.g., strategies to facilitate participation in lifeways activities).

[c]Mortuary treatment is included on the decision pathway because in some circumstances it may reflect on treatment during life – see Figure 25.1.

Man Bac Burial 9

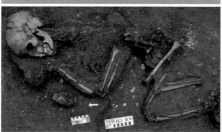

1. **DESCRIBE** ~4000 BP; male; ~20-25 yrs., North Vietnam. ~75% complete. C1-T3 fused, extreme bone atrophy, fused sacroiliac joint, no evidence trauma or infection. Pathology: quadriplegia (acquired ~12-14yrs, complication congenital Klippel-Feil Syndrome). Mortuary: cemetery, flexed N-S (standard supine E-W), 2 pots. Lifeways: small group, sedentary, hunter-gatherer (fishing), estuarine environment.

2. **ASSESS NEED FOR CARE** *Clinical*: Certain - upper (partial) and lower (complete) body paralysis; torticollis; osteoporosis. Probable - depressed immune system; cardiovascular, gastrointestinal, and respiratory dysfunction; kidney failure; pressure sores. Possible - pain; depression.
Functional: Immobile - incapable of all *'Essential activities of daily living'* and of all physically demanding *'Instrumental activities of daily living'*. Lived ~10 yrs with quadriplegia.
Care Needed? YES

3. **MODEL OF CARE** *Direct support:* all *'constants of care'* - continuing and intensive nursing, including regular monitoring of health status, hygiene (waste removal, bathing, protect integument), feeding (special diet?), maintain hydration and temperature regulation, massage and positioning (encourage organ function, prevent pressure sores).
Accommodation: likely included efforts to enable participation in social activities (important for psychological wellbeing).

4. **INTERPRET** *Community*: long-term survival and absence of infection/fracture reflect skilled, labour-intensive care; community cooperation and flexibility in managing 'costs' of, and organising around, care; non-fatalist philosophy - 'cure' impossible but care given (suggesting value placed on lives of all group members); 'deviant' burial - burial in community cemetery indicates inclusion, but positioning acknowledges and respects difference?
Individual: survival reflects strong will to live; ability to adapt; social engagement; strong self-esteem.

The Nasca Boy

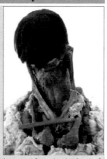

1. **DESCRIBE** ~700AD; male; 8yrs; Nasca ,Peru. Well-preserved mummy. Pathology: histological / radiographic evidence for tuberculosis; Pott's disease (TB of spine), onset ~2+yrs, progressing to paraplegia ~6-7yrs; Miliary TB at 8yrs, death in days/ weeks. Mortuary: pit tomb; textile-wrapped 'mummy bundle' - body sits on adobe stool used in life for transport (unique arrangement); grave goods standard for child except for *atypical* set of panpipes. Lifeways: small farming settlement; likely kin-based; harsh climate, stressful political environment, declining population health. **N.B.** *Very little known about status / treatment of children in Nasca culture.*

2. **ASSESS NEED FOR CARE** *Clinical:* Pott's disease: fever, weight loss, delayed growth, back and/or chest pain, respiratory / general immune system dysfunction. Neurological impacts (eventual immobility) potential to compromise all organ systems. Miliary TB - blood-borne infection overwhelms all body systems.
Functional: delays in motor / social skills development, unable to participate in most 'normal' childhood activities (e.g. play, domestic tasks); paralysis results in problems with most *'Essential activities of daily living'*.
Care Needed? YES

3. **MODEL OF CARE** *Accommodation:* modifying expectations; strategies facilitating inclusion (e.g. stool); time-consuming reassurance, encouragement and general comforting (way beyond normal 'child care', requirements ,overlaps with 'nursing' below).
Direct support: with disease progression all 'constants of care': full-time nursing, health monitoring, hygiene management, special diet / feeding, pain and fever relief, massage and repositioning.

4. **INTERPRET** *Community*: survival to 8yrs in harsh lifeways reflects commitment to care despite economic and emotional costs; primary carers likely immediate family, but enabled by group support. Unique mortuary inclusions: stool may e.g. reflect cosmology (needed for passage to, or use in, the afterlife?) or mark identity; panpipes may have shamanic significance or reflect love of music. Care in life *and* death indicate *this* child was highly valued; extrapolation suggests Nasca children *in general* valued as individuals with distinct personalities and needs, filling existing knowledge gap.
Individual: persistence of caregiving, burial treatment suggest capable of inspiring affection and respect.

[a]Tilley and Oxenham (2011), [b]Tilley and Nystrom (2019).

Figure 25.1 Examples of BoC application – Man Bac Burial 9[a] and the Nasca Boy[b]. Photographs © Lorna Tilley.

Table 25.3 Summaries of selected bioarchaeology of care case studies

Date Location	Case study synopsis
60–45000BP *Dordogne, France*	**Tilley (2015)** describes two Neanderthal adult males, La Chapelle-aux-Saints 1 and La Ferrassie 1, who both experienced progressively debilitating pathologies requiring care firstly as "accommodation" and later as "direct support". Assessment of Neanderthal cognitive potential has typically relied on extrapolation from anatomically modern human morphology and/or inference from tool manufacture, economic activity, and mortuary treatment. Analysis of likely care provided to these individuals offers new insights into Neanderthal social organization and contributes to an increased appreciation of Neanderthal cognition and behavior.
6610–6200BP *North-eastern Brazil*	**Solari et al. (2020)** analyze the remains of a ~9-month-old infant displaying evidence of severe disease in the weeks/months before death and afforded uniquely rich and complex burial rites. They conclude length of survival indicates a level of care exceeding normal infant nurturing practice, and that mortuary treatment suggests caregiving continued after death. The first bioarchaeology of care case to address the challenge of differentiating between altricial care and *health*-related care for young children, this study extends the methodology's application.
2475–2334BC *Sweden*	**Tornberg and Jacobsson (2018)** (a bioarchaeology and rehabilitation medicine collaboration) present the case of an older male with evidence of healed cranial trauma, identifying likely immediate and longer-term cognitive, psychological, and behavioral sequelae; care received; and insights into contemporary social relations and organization. Northern European Neolithic and Bronze Age remains suggest high rates of survival following cranial trauma. Extrapolating from their study to the sociocultural implications of high frequency brain injury during this ~4000yr period, the authors conclude that care provision for those with such pathology was 'a necessity for survival and maintenance of a socially sustainable society' (2018:188).
2220–2000BC *United Arab Emirates*	**Schrenk and Martin (2017)** apply the Index of Care to remains of a young woman displaying evidence for lower limb paralysis for which there is no clear diagnosis – the most likely being cerebral palsy or polio, diseases with different trajectories over the life course. Uncertainty regarding diagnosis is common in paleopathology, and the authors address this by constructing parallel models of 'disability and care'; each based on the same physical indicators of pathology, but exploring likely differences in clinical experience, functional impacts and sociocultural traditions of caregiving.
2050–1000BC *Bahrain*	**Boutin (2016)** employs the Index of Care to identify likely functional impacts of, and caregiving required in response to, multiple bone deformities displayed in the remains of a young woman. The author applies her (then) recently developed Bioarchaeology of Personhood approach, producing a "fictive osteobiographical narrative" revolving around her subject's disability experience and treatment by family and wider community. The paper brings the past vividly to life, illustrating how bioarchaeology of care analysis can inform research which has something other than disability or care as its primary focus.
1000–1250AD *Highland Peru*	**Jolly and Kurin (2017)** use the study of a young male displaying cranial and postcranial fractures, evidence for impaired mobility, and several healed trepanations to explore healthcare response to injury resulting from culturally-sanctioned interpersonal violence. Focusing on the social organization required to manage brain injury treatment and outcomes, as well as on the impact of acquired brain injury on social identity, this is the first study examining the complex interplay between caregiving and violence. The authors conclude that study of 'healthcare and impairment … illuminates the ramifications of warfare and conflict for community decision-making' (2017:193).

Date Location	Case study synopsis
AD1000–1534AD Central Coast Peru	**Sutherland (2019)** employs computed tomography scanning in a "virtual" analysis of a mummy bundle containing remains of a middle-aged male with chronic osteomyelitis in his right tibia; human neonate remains attached to this bone were inserted in a secondary burial and grave goods included seeds with medicinal properties. Working systematically through the Index of Care, the author develops a detailed account of the man's treatment in his last years of life and after death, asking more sophisticated questions than previously attempted in this technology-dependent area of mummy studies.
1150–1300AD Arizona, USA	**Dongoske et al. (2015)** describe a young woman who lived for over a decade with systemic infection, scoliosis and premature degenerative bone disease resulting in progressively severe clinical and functional impacts, initially requiring "accommodation" and ultimately labor-intensive "direct support". Analyzing the implications of caregiving in relation to cultural context and social organization, and considering the possible significance of her rich funerary assemblage, the authors focus on the individual's social identity. The first study following publication of the bioarchaeology of care to address social identity, the paper remains an example of how to approach this question.
1888–1890AD West Virginia, USA	**Beckett and Conlogue (2019)** examine soft tissue evidence of chronic obstructive pulmonary disease in a mummified adult female inpatient of the Trans-Allegheny Lunatic Asylum, identifying fine detail of disease impacts and care required. Pathophysiological analyses enable description of disease processes at cellular, organ, and system levels, allowing use of modern tools in assessing likely effects on everyday functioning. While stopping short of Stage 4 interpretation, this transdisciplinary study is remarkable for its precision in reconstructing the experience and lifeways of the individual, and demonstrates the potential of pathophysiological analysis and the value of interdisciplinary collaboration.

Alternative Options for Addressing the 'How'

While the bioarchaeology of care is given prominence in this chapter, there are a number of different (and often complementary) approaches available to bioarchaeologists interested in past disability and care. As few examples are briefly discussed below.

Other Ways of Assessing Disease Impact

Young and Lemaire (2014, 2017) present a method for estimating functional severity of knee osteoarthritis in archaeological samples based on rating lesions in the knee joints of skeletal remains, using a scale developed from scans of modern knee osteoarthritis sufferers for whom clinical impacts are known. Although this methodology cannot allow for certainty at an individual level, a rating may give interpretive power to (or gain interpretive power from) a more complete subject osteobiography. Additionally, aggregation of knee osteoarthritis impact ratings for members of a particular community might add to understanding of a population's age and gender-associated health status and activity levels.

Emphatically differentiating between "impairment" and "disability", Byrnes (2017) proposes a method for quantifying evidence of trauma-initiated orthopaedic "impairment" in human remains based on formulae contained in the American Medical Association *Guidance to the evaluation of permanent impairment* (Rondinelli et al., 2008). Criticizing the absence of standardized descriptions of impairment in bioarchaeological research, she claims her methodology permits not only calculation of the percentage impairment specific to the area affected but also conversion of this measure to a "whole person impairment" rating. However, the *Guidance's* goal in standardizing evaluation of impairment is to provide a baseline for determining access to compensation for injury and other disability entitlements in modern American populations; the translation of impairment rating into ability to function across daily living domains still has to be assessed individually and in context – as the *Guidance* makes clear (Rondinelli et al., 2008).

Stodder (2017) presents an elegant approach for estimating the cost burden of pathology evidenced in human remains based on Global Burden of Disease disability weightings (Murray & Lopez, 1996). "Disability weights" are internationally agreed values (ranked on a scale of 0 equals full health and 1 equals death) assigned to particular disease states and, where relevant, associated complications. Stodder (2017) uses these to generate individual morbidity scores (with potential for including likely comorbidities) and multiplies disease prevalence by corresponding disability weight to calculate "years lived with disability" – a proxy for "disease burden" – at a group level. She employs disability weights as indicators of generalized "cost" of specific pathologies to both the individual and their group, and this provides a basis for comparing disease burden over time, as well as between different demographic cohorts and different communities. Schrenk (2019) applies Stodder's (2017) methodology, together with the bioarchaeology of care approach, in analyzing remains spanning the Archaic Period (10,000–1,000BP) in Pre-Columbian Illinois with rewarding results.

Different Ways of Looking at Questions of Care

While most bioarchaeologists working on health-related care will refer to relevant ethnographic, ethnohistoric, and/or historic materials where these are available, a number of studies draw particularly heavily from such sources. Some have done so in conjunction with the bioarchaeology of care, using these sources to guide and ground identification and interpretation of caregiving; others rely almost entirely on these sources to frame their focus on past care practice.

The former category includes studies by Willett and Harrod (2017), Matczak and Kozlowski (2017), and Snoddy et al. (2020). Willett and Harrod (2017) use the Index of Care in the case of an adult woman from pre-Columbian south-west USA who experienced permanent mobility-limiting trauma. The authors' comprehensive (and convincing) discussion of their subject's probable social role and care received, including coverage of skills required in care provision and potential involvement of traditional healers, is only made possible by extensive reference to ethnographic and ethnohistoric accounts. Matczak and Kozlowski (2017) rely on ethnohistoric and historic sources to produce a vivid lifeways context informing detailed osteobiographies of two adult women from medieval Poland – one diagnosed with leprosy, the other with gigantism, and both with traumatic injury. The authors use the bioarchaeology of care framework to structure assessment of the functional implications of pathology and related health needs, and to assist consideration of interactions between social status; medical, magical, and religious treatments in common use; and likely care received. Snoddy et al.'s (2020) study of a middle-aged man from mid-19th-century New Zealand, for whom all basic biographical details (age at and cause of death, occupation, marital status, origins, migration pathway, even "Friendly Society" membership) are known, employs the empirical approaches of paleopathology, morphological analysis and isotope analyses, and the interpretive approaches of the bioarchaeology of care and the bioarchaeology of personhood (Boutin 2016) to "ground-truth" the historic evidence of the subject's life and death. The detail enabled by focusing on one man's experience of disease and care opens a pathway into the social institutions and practices of that time, while application of the bioarchaeology of personhood approach converts this experience into a unique narrative. In Snoddy et al.'s (2020) report, history and bioarchaeology operate in equal partnership to recover the recent past.

The work by Wesp (2017) and Krutak (2019) explores methods for looking at non-material elements of care provision. West (2019) uses historic and ethnohistoric sources documenting the emergence of Christian institutions in the early post-contact Americas to engage with one of the most problematic concerns for a bioarchaeology of care: how to give weight to the role of psychological, spiritual, and emotional caregiving. Describing pathologies evidenced in cemetery remains recovered from the first hospital established in Mexico for treating the indigenous population, she considers contemporary beliefs in the relationship between bodily and spiritual health, and the implications of these for developing a more rounded model of care practice. Krutak (2019) considers whether some of the tattoos occasionally observed on mummified remains can be interpreted in terms of health-related care (see also Nystrom & Piombino-Mascali, 2017; Zink et al., 2019). He presents archaeological, ethnographic, and historic evidence from Arctic populations for the use of tattoos to protect the bearer from physical and supernatural disease, arguing that the tattooed body can be read as a reflection of social and cultural forces and norms, and that "specific forms of curative tattooing offer interpretive models for the … bioarchaeological study of care through an ontological framework of analysis" (Krutak, 2019:99).

The growing interest in prospects for a population-level approach to past caregiving practice is another example of an alternative way of looking at care provision. Oxenham and Willis (2017) confront the vexed issue of distinguishing archaeologically between "normal" altricial care and specifically *health*-related care in infancy and early childhood. Situating their study in Neolithic South-East Asia, a period of elevated childhood morbidity and mortality, they apply the staged approach of the bioarchaeology of care to developing a "bioarchaeology of care for children". Extensive previous research into childhood disease type and frequency in this period provides the authors with a solid base for analyzing level of need for health-related care among children in this population and for addressing the likely identity of their caregivers. This paper provides an excellent model for analyzing experience in a particular demographic cohort. Filipek et al. (2021) combine evidence from history and bioarchaeology to evaluate the experience of leprosy in adolescents from Medieval England (9–12th century AD), including assessment of care needs using the Index of Care framework; likely alloparental (i.e., "other than parental") treatment provided within hospitals/leprosaria; familial motivations behind securing such care; and an overview of sociocultural perceptions of, and responses to, this disease and its sufferers. The authors also present an "Index of Effort", a guide for identifying direct and indirect costs likely incurred in obtaining medical care for children (Filipek et al., 2021:34) which might be easily adapted to other contexts and cohorts. At the opposite end of the demographic spectrum, Gowland (2017) considers the situation of the elderly, who are popularly assumed as likely to require special health-related care by virtue of age-associated functional decline. In this concept paper, the author discusses health, safety, disability and care in older age, highlighting the elderly's vulnerability to neglect and abuse, often from family members (usually their children and grandchildren) over whom they once held authority and upon whom they become reliant. Finally, a recent volume edited by Schrenk and Tremblay-Critcher (2022) presents a collection of case studies of care practice among specific populations ranging from hunter-gatherer communities in Archaic Period USA, through sub-adults in the Late Medieval/Early Modern period, to inmates of the 19th century Mississippi State Asylum. Of particular importance, many authors in this volume detail modifications to existing research methodologies and present new methodologies developed in the course of their work.

Sometimes evidence for specific treatments employed in response to pathology, such as use of medicines, changes to diet, or surgical intervention, offers a starting point for considering broader sociocultural and experiential aspects of care. For example, in the first study to address the application of a bioarchaeology of care approach to mummified remains, Nystrom & Piombino-Mascali (2017, and see Chapter 12, this volume) discuss the potential for identifying consumption of substances with medicinal properties (through microscopic and biochemical assays of intestinal contents, coprolites, hair, and soft tissue) and use this information as the basis for inferring details of care. They illustrate this with the study of an adult male from 18–19th century Sicily who suffered multiple myeloma and whose remains show evidence for ingestion of materials known for their use in medical treatments. Brown and Wilson (2019) use data from preserved hair (drug, stable light isotope, and aDNA analyses) in the bioarchaeology of care study of a mummified adult female with Chagas disease from pre-Columbian Chile, eliciting a meticulous and intimate account of her life with chronic illness; hair analysis allowed identification of dietary changes, increased physiological stress and consumption of coca (likely treatment for gastrointestinal symptoms) in the year before death. Using a similar approach, Verostick et al. (2019) combine stable isotope analysis of hair with coprolite analysis, reconstructing declining health, and identifying likely attempts at dietary therapy, in the final months of life of a mummified adult male diagnosed with megacolon and dating to the late Archaic Period, Texas.

Turning to surgery, Van Cant's (2018) bioarchaeology of care study of a young woman from late mediaeval Belgian who survived an above-the-knee amputation begins with detail of the procedure and its likely consequences, and flows into discussion of the specific social and historical context in which this procedure was negotiated and the associated after-care required. Phillips et al. (2021) analyze evidence for successful single foot amputation in the remains of two young women, separated in time by up to 300–400 years but from the same region of pre-Columbian Peru; they apply bioarchaeology of care analysis to explore the women's lived experiences and social identities. Giving equal weight to considering the likely medical, social and emotional care received by both women, the authors locate this care within an extraordinarily thorough account of cultural and cosmological influences possibly in play, using the evidence of the surgical procedure, which appears to illustrate continuity of medical knowledge and skills, to reflect upon cultural, social and political practice. Trepanation (removal of a portion of bone from the cranial vault, usually in response to health insult) is the most commonly observed surgery in the archaeological record, evidenced in most parts of the world and with the earliest known example dating to around 12,000 years (Arnott et al., 2003). Combining archaeological and ethnographic evidence, Kurin's (2016) comprehensive discussion of techniques of, motivations for, and care required following, trepanation practices in the pre-modern Andean region is required reading. Dastugue (1980) best summarizes the far-reaching implications of this surgical procedure, relating how evidence for trepanation in Mesolithic Taforalt (Morocco) led him "[t]o consider the mental development and the social behaviour of that poor population of snail eaters. Achievement of such a technique involves skilled hands and observing and reasoning gifts that are generally considered as the essential part of the "scientific genius". Besides, performing such an operation requires between patient and operator, the existence of bonds of mutual trust indicating an already elaborate social organization" (Dastugue, 1980:4).

In recent years, many bioarchaeologists have argued for explicit adoption of a "life course" approach to examining past experience of disease and care (Agarwal, 2016; Boutin, 2016; Gowland, 2017; Zuckerman et al., 2019; and see Chapter 29, this volume), and Hawkey (1998), in a still-unequalled reconstruction of the progressively disabling impacts of degenerative disease (juvenile-onset chronic arthritis in a man aged around 40 years at death), illustrates its descriptive power. Most recently, Cormier and Buikstra (2021) have published a framework for applying a life course approach to disability and care in archaeological cases of rare disease (i.e. complex, usually congenital, chronically debilitating, or life-threatening diseases affecting fewer than one in 2000 people [www.raredisease.org.uk 2021]). The authors demonstrate the framework's potential in an analysis of the remains of an adult woman, born into a Middle Woodland community (Illinois, USA) with achondroplasia and Leroy-Weill dyschondrosteosis, who presents a clinical profile suggesting increasingly severe physical limitations over time. Cormier and Buikstra (2021) explicitly link their work to current research and policy development in the area of rare diseases, taking on board concerns of modern disease communities with the dual aim of better understanding disease impacts in the past and "raising awareness and advancing contemporary perspectives on impairment and disability" in the present (2021:196). The second aim is directly relevant to considerations raised in the following – and final – part of this chapter.

The 'Why'? Relevance of Past Disability and Care Research for Modern Times

> The problem with archaeology…is that it has not sufficiently embraced the enormous potentialities provided to create new pasts, new knowledges and new truths and to use the differences of the past to challenge and restructure the black side of modernity: domination, exploitation, repression, alienation, violence.
>
> *(Tilley, 1990:129)*

Both bioarchaeologists and members of the general public have when into past disability and care. It is easy to explain this reaction among the former. A focus on disability and care presents unparalleled opportunities for diving into some of the finer detail of personal lives, interpersonal dynamics, and collective values and behaviors in the past. This focus adds nuance to our view of history; it can introduce unanticipated complexities, fill gaps in our knowledge, and sometimes overturn long-held assumptions. Simply put, it is a rewarding field of study.

Understanding why there is such widespread interest among the latter when this research makes it into the public domain is more complicated (see Chapter 32 for further discussion on paleopathology in the public eye). It seems counterintuitive that, in a rapidly changing, high pressure, and increasingly transactional world, research into disability experience and caregiving practice among the long dead is perceived as relevant to life today. Yet it *is*, and on occasion has given rise to wide-ranging, even impassioned, discussion. In 2012, for example, the New York Times published a story about Man Bac Burial 9 (Gorman, 2012). It was picked up by global print and electronic media, reproduced in countless special-interest newsletters and blogs, and inspired innumerable comments (Tilley, 2015:294–297). As featured archaeologist, I received a flood of emails from people with no formal archaeology background but with sophisticated questions about the practicalities and implications of my research; without exception, correspondence was supportive and constructive. Colleagues teaching and publishing in this area have told me of similarly positive responses to their work.

On the question of public interest, it is undeniable that archaeology holds a fascination for the public. Archaeology allows us to place ourselves in a wider perspective; to think about our origins, to understand who we are and how we have become who we are. As Cross (1999:8), writing about prospects for an "archaeology of disability", explains: "[a]rchaeology…serves the function once served by origin myths – the creation and explanation of identity".

When research focuses on disability and care, archaeology is operating on a "human scale" (Hodder, 2000:31). The subject is immediately accessible because there is nothing "exceptional" about either state. Most of us, at some stage, will experience disability requiring care, and most of us, at some stage, will be called on to provide care. Almost everyone has a stake in this research. The possibilities for creative public engagement are tantalizing, and active and inclusive outreach at all stages of disability and care research is not only an ethical imperative for bioarchaeology (Mennear, 2017) but is critical for best practice, as this engagement adds great value to our work. At a time when some archaeologists are attempting, with mixed success, to elucidate the relevance of our discipline for addressing current challenges such as climate change, environmental management, and unprecedented urbanization (Sabloff, 2008; Boivin & Crowther, 2021; Smith, 2021), there is no doubt about the political and social relevance of the bioarchaeologies of disability and care. Holding a mirror to current practice in an increasingly neoliberal world, Fitzpatrick points out that "…Developing an archaeology of care helps to reveal that care of others was regularly practised, and that not everyone ascribed to narrow definitions of worth that unfortunately are still perpetuated today; that your potential for labour did not equate to your value as a person, that you [did not have] to prove that you were worthy of care and support.… Sick and disabled people existed and were given care in the past – so what's the excuse of those in power in the present?" (Fitzpatrick, 2021:1)

This relevance can support conversations on critically important subjects in our communities, which are often too difficult to broach or are simply overlooked. For example, "discomfort" is reportedly felt by as many as one in five people when they are talking to, or about, those with a disability (Kearnan, 2021). This "discomfort" is typically a response born of ignorance, but has the potential to manifest in passive discriminatory, and actively cruel, behaviors: it is poisonous for perpetrators and victims alike, as well as for society in general – as the Australian Royal Commission into Violence, Abuse, Neglect and Exploitation of People with Disability (2020) is currently bearing witness to. Croucher (2021; Buster et al., 2018), in collaboration with colleagues from end-of-life medicine, nursing, and psychology, has used her research in mortuary archaeology in workshops for palliative care workers and others "to open dialogues around death and bereavement, and to challenge the concept of "right" or "normal" ways to grieve or deal with death" (Croucher, 2021:2). Her work could provide a model for challenging concepts of disability. Initially, it may be easier for people to talk about experiences of, and responses to, disability in the archaeological past before dealing with their own beliefs and behaviors in the present; as Shakespeare (199:99) suggests, "[situated at] the crossover between the sciences and the humanities … archaeology has the capacity to revisit and problematize issues of the human body in time and to connect the physical to the sociocultural".

The widespread undervaluing of informal caregivers (those providing care in non-institutional capacities) is another example of an issue to which bioarchaeological research can contribute. The work performed by informal caregivers is essential (without it, state health systems would collapse) and can be unrelenting, taking a massive toll on carers (Buckner & Yeandle, 2015; Deloitte Access Economics, 2020), yet it often goes unappreciated and unrecognized. Evidence of the unbroken chain of health-related caregiving extending from the most distant past to the present, and the reliance of human survival on this earliest of behaviors (e.g., Doat, 2016; 2017), can help to (re)establish the recognition that carers deserve. "*Care, The Great Human Tradition*" (McKenzie, 2018) was a pilot project bringing together archaeologists, historians, anthropologists, carer advocates, caregivers, and artists to develop strategies for elevating awareness of the role of carers and their need for support in public and political agendas. Participant feedback on archaeological contributions, provided to me in September 2019 during the concluding events associated with this project, demonstrated that the deep history of caregiving and caregivers can serve as an affirmation of caregiver identity and provide carers with ammunition in the struggle to achieve greater visibility and respect.

It is possible to envisage research into past experience of disability and care informing debate around contemporary concerns in many ways, and the existing level of public interest in this research suggests that research contributions will find a receptive audience. The quote by Christopher Tilley, which opens this section, credits archaeology with 'enormous potentialities … to challenge and restructure the dark side of modernity' (Tilley, 1990:129). If true, the bioarchaeologies of disability and care have an exciting part to play in this process.

Acknowledgement

I would like to thank (although this word is inadequate) Anne Grauer for the patience, kindness, perseverance, generosity, encouragement, and understanding she has shown me during the writing of this chapter. I'm sure that when Anne invited me to contribute to this volume she had no inkling of what she had let herself in for; while content, errors, and views expressed are all my own, in every other way this paper is as much hers as mine.

References

Agarwal, S. C. (2016). Bone morphologies and histories: life course approaches in bioarchaeology. *American Journal of Physical Anthropology* 159:130–149.

Anand, S. (2017). Historiography of disablement and the South Asian context: the case of Shah Daula's Chuhas. In Byrnes. J. F. & Muller, J. L. (Eds.), *Bioarchaeology of Impairment and Disability*, pp. 57–74. Switzerland: Springer.

Areheart, B. A. (2008). When disability isn't just right: the entrenchment of the medical model of disability and the goldilocks dilemma. *Indiana Law Journal* 83:181–232.

Arnott, R., Finger, S. & Smith, C. (Eds.) (2003). *Trepanation*. United Kingdom: Taylor & Francis.

Australian Institute of Health and Welfare (AIHW), (2020). *People with Disability in Australia 2020*. Canberra: AIHW.

Australian Royal Commission into Violence, Abuse, Neglect and Exploitation of People with Disability, (2020). *Interim Reports*. Accessed 2 February2022 https://disability.royalcommission.gov.au/policy-and-research

Bapty, I. & Yates, T. (2014). *Archaeology After Structuralism: Post-Structuralism and the Practice of Archaeology*. London: Routledge.

Bates, E. & Linder-Pelz, S. (1990). *Health Care Issues* (2nd ed.). Sydney: Allen and Unwin.

Battles, H. T. (2009). Long bone bilateral asymmetry. *The Canadian Student Journal of Anthropology* 21:1–5.

Beckett, R. G. & Conlogue, G. J. (2019). The importance of pathophysiology to the understanding of functional limitations in the bioarchaeology of care approach. *International Journal of Paleopathology* 25:118–128.

Berger, T. D. & Trinkaus, E. (1995). Patterns of trauma among the Neandertals. *Journal of Archaeological Science* 22:841–852.

Bickenbach, J. E. (2019). The ICF and its relationship to disability studies. In Watson, N. & Vehmas, S. (Eds.), *Routledge Handbook of Disability Studies*, pp. 55–71. London: Routledge.

Bickenbach, J. E., Chatterji, S., Badley, E. M. & Üstün, T. B. (1999). Models of disablement, universalism and the international classification of impairments, disabilities and handicaps. *Social Science & Medicine* 48(9):1173–1187.

Boivin, N. & Crowther, A. (2021). Mobilizing the past to shape a better Anthropocene. *Nature Ecology & Evolution* 5(3): 273–284.

Boutin, A. T. (2016). Exploring the social construction of disability: an application of the bioarchaeology of personhood model to a pathological skeleton from ancient Bahrain. *International Journal of Paleopathology* 12:17–28.

Brown, E. L. & Wilson, A. S. (2019). Using evidence from hair and other soft tissues to infer the need for and receipt of health-related care provision. *International Journal of Paleopathology* 25:91–98.

Buckner, L. & Yeandle, S. (2015). *Valuing Carers 2015. The Rising Value of Carers' Support*. United Kingdom: Carers UK.

Buquet-Marcon, C., Charlier, P. & Samzun, A. (2007). The oldest amputation on a Neolithic skeleton in France. *Nature Precedings*. Accessed January 12, 2011 http://precedings.nature.com/documents/1278/version/1/html

Büster, L. S., Croucher, K. T., Dayes, J. E., Green, L. I. & Faull, C. (2018). From plastered skulls to palliative care: what the past can teach us about dealing with death. *AP: Online Journal in Public Archaeology* 3:249–276.

Byrnes, J. F. (2017). Injuries, impairment, and intersecting identities: the poor in Buffalo, NY 1851–1913. In Byrnes, J. F. & Muller, J. L. (Eds.), *Bioarchaeology of Impairment and Disability,* pp. 201–222. Switzerland: Springer.

Byrnes, J. F. & Muller, J. L. (Eds.) (2017). *Bioarchaeology of Impairment and Disability*. Switzerland: Springer.

Campanaro, D. M. (2021). Inference to the best explanation (ibe) and archaeology: old tool, new model. *European Journal of Archaeology* 24(3):412–432.

Carter, R. (1997). Address by the former first lady of the USA on 13 February 1997 in her role as chair of last acts, a coalition of organisations campaigning for better end-of-life palliative care. Accessed 20 February 2019 http://gos.sbc.edu/c/carter.html

Chamoun, T. J. (2020). Caring differently: some reflections. *Historical Archaeology* 54(1):34–51.

Chong, D. K. H. (1995). Measurement of instrumental activities of daily living in stroke. *Stroke* 26:1119–1122.

Cohen, M. N. & Armelagos, G. J. (Eds.) (1984). *Paleopathology at the Origins of Agriculture*. Orlando, FL: Academic Press.

Cohen, M. N. & Crane-Kramer, G. (2003). The state and future of paleoepidemiology. In Greenblatt, C. L. & Spigelman, M. (Eds.), *Emerging Pathogens: The Archaeology, Ecology, and Evolution of Infectious Disease*, pp. 79–91. Nueva York: Oxford University Press.

Conlogue, G., Viner, M., Beckett, R., Bekvalac, J., Gonzalez, R., Sharkey, M., Kramer, K. & Koverman, B. (2017). A post-mortem evaluation of the degree of mobility in an individual with severe kyphoscoliosis using direct digital radiography (Dr) and multi-detector computed tomography (Mdct). In Tilley, L. & Schrenk, A. (Eds.), *New Developments in the Bioarchaeology of Care*, pp. 1553–173. Switzerland: Springer.

Cormier, A. A. & Buikstra, J. E. (2021). Thundering hoofbeats and dazzling zebras: a model integrating current rare disease perspectives in paleopathology. *International Journal of Paleopathology* 33:196–208.

Cross, M. (1999). Accessing the inaccessible: disability and archaeology. *Archaeological Review from Cambridge* 15:7–30.

Croucher, K. (2021). Scales of relevance and the importance of ambiguity. *Antiquity* 95(382):1081–1084.

Dastugue, J. (1980). Possibilities, limits and prospects in paleopathology of the human skeleton. *Journal of Human Evolution* 9:3–8.

Deloitte Access Economics *The Value of Informal Care in* 2020. Australia: Carers Australia. Accessed 20 February 2022 https://www.carersaustralia.com.au/wp-content/uploads/2020/07/FINAL-Value-of-Informal-Care-22-May_2020_No-CIC.pdf

Dettwyler, K. A. (1991). Can paleopathology provide evidence for "compassion"? *American Journal of Physical Anthropology* 84(4):375–384.

Devlin, R. & Pothier, D. (2006). Introduction: Toward a critical theory of dis-citizenship. In Pothier, D. & Devlin, R. (Eds.), *Critical Disability Theory: Essays in Philosophy, Politics, Policy and the Law*, pp. 1–22. Vancouver: University of British Columbia Press.

Dickel, D. N. & Doran, G. H. (1989). Severe neural tube defect syndrome from the early Archaic of Florida. *American Journal of Physical Anthropology* 80:325–334.

DiGangi, E. A., Bethard, J. D. & Sullivan, L. P. (2009). Differential diagnosis of cartilaginous dysplasia and probable Osgood–Schlatter's disease in a Mississippian individual from East Tennessee. *International Journal of Osteoarchaeology* 20:424–442.

Doat, D. (2014). Evolution and human uniqueness: Prehistory, disability and the unexpected anthropology of Charles Darwin. In Bolt, D. (Ed.), *Changing Social Attitudes: Disability, Culture, Education*, pp. 15–25. London: Routledge.

Doat, D. (2016). Setting the scene for an evolutionary approach to care in prehistory: a historical and philosophical journey. In Powell, L., Southwell-Wright, W. & Gowland, R. (Eds.), *Care in the Past: Archaeological and Interdisciplinary Perspectives*, pp. 131–148. Oxford: Oxbow Books.

Doat, D. (2017). What ethical considerations should inform bioarchaeology of care analysis?. In Tilley, L. & Schrenk, A. (Eds.), *New Developments in the Bioarchaeology of Care*, pp. 319–342. Switzerland: Springer.

Dongoske, K. E., Cox, E. S. & Rogge, A. E. (2015). Bioarchaeology of care: a Hohokam example. *Kiva* 80(3–4):304–323.

Fábrega, H. (1999). *Evolution of sickness and healing*. Berkeley: University of California Press.

Filipek, K. L., Roberts, C., Gowland, R. L. & Tucker, K. (2021). Alloparenting adolescents: evaluating the social and biological impacts of leprosy on young people in Saxo-Norman England (9th to 12th centuries AD) through cross-disciplinary models of care. In Kendall, E. J. & Kendall, R. (Eds.), *The Family in Past Perspective*, pp. 30–57. London: Routledge.

Fitzpatrick, A. (2021) The radical potential of making an archaeology of care visible. Accessed 10 January 2022 https://animalarchaeology.com/tag/disability-justice/

Formicola, V., Milanesi, Q. & Scarsini, C. (1987). Evidence of spinal tuberculosis at the beginning of the fourth millennium BC from Arene Candide cave (Liguria, Italy). *American Journal of Physical Anthropology* 72:1–6.

Frayer, D. W., Horton, W. A., Macchiarelli, R. & Mussi, M. (1987). Dwarfism in an adolescent from the Italian late upper palaeolithic. *Nature* 330(6143):60–62.

Frayer, D. W., Macchiarelli, R. & Mussi, M. (1988). A case of chondrodystrophic dwarfism in the Italian late upper paleolithic. *American Journal of Physical Anthropology* 75(4):549–565.

Gilchrist, R. (2020). *Sacred Heritage: Monastic Archaeology, Identities, Beliefs*. Cambridge: Cambridge University Press.

Goodley, D., Lawthom, R., Liddiard, K. & Runswick-Cole, K. (2019). Provocations for critical disability studies. *Disability & Society* 34(6):972–997.

Gorman, J. (2012). Ancient Bones That Tell a Story of Compassion. *New York Times*, 17 December 2012. Accessed 12 November 2021 http://www.nytimes.com/2012/12/18/science/ancient-bones-that-tell-a-story-of-compassion. html?_r=1&

Gowland, R. (2017). Growing old: biographies of disability and care in later life. In Tilley, L. & Schrenk, A. (Eds.), *New Developments in the Bioarchaeology of Care*, pp. 237–251. Switzerland: Springer.

Grauer, A. L. (2018). A century of paleopathology. *American Journal of Physical Anthropology* 165(4):904–914.

Greenblatt, C. & Spigelman, M. (2003). *Emerging Pathogens: The Archaeology, Ecology, and Evolution of Infectious Disease*, pp. 79–91. Oxford: Oxford University Press.

Hale, B. & Jaye, C. (2018). Revealing cosmopolitanism through an examination of informal elder care in seventeenth-eighteenth century England and nineteenth century colonial north America. *Sites: A Journal of Social Anthropology and Cultural Studies* 15(2):120–143.

Hawkey, D. E. (1998). Disability, compassion and the skeletal record: using musculoskeletal stress markers (MSM) to construct an osteobiography from early New Mexico. *International Journal of Osteoarchaeology* 8(5):326–340.

Henderson, V. (1964). The nature of nursing. *The American Journal of Nursing* 64:62–68.

Henderson, V. (1966). *The Nature of Nursing: A Definition and its Implications for Practice, Research, and Education*. New York: Macmillan.

Hodder, I. (2000). Agency and individuals in long-term processes. In Dobres, M. A. & Robb J. E. (Eds.), *Agency in Archaeology*, pp. 21–33. London: Routledge.

Jolly, S. & Kurin, D. (2017). Surviving trepanation: approaching the relationship of violence and the care of "war wounds" through a case study from prehistoric Peru. In Tilley, L. & Schrenk, A. (Eds.), *New Developments in the Bioarchaeology of Care*, pp. 175–195. Switzerland: Springer.

Katz, S., Downs, T. D., Cash, H. R. & Grotz, R. C. (1970). Progress in development of the index of ADL. *The Gerontologist* 10:20–30.

Kearnan, J. (2021). Paralympians say many still don't know how to talk about disability. *ABC News*. Accessed 5 October 2021 https://www.abc.net.au/news/2021-09-04/more-education-needed-for-disability-terminology-use/100424224

Kim, H. S. (2010). *The Nature of Theoretical Thinking in Nursing* (3rd ed.). New York: Springer.

Kleinman, A. (1980). *Patients and Healers in the Context of Culture: An Exploration of the Borderland between Anthropology, Medicine, and Psychiatry*. California: University of California Press.

Knudson, K. J. & Stojanowski, C. M. (2008). New directions in bioarchaeology: recent contributions to the study of human social identities. *Journal of Archaeological Research* 16(4):397–432.

Knüsel, C. (1999). Orthopaedic disability: some hard evidence. *Archaeological Review from Cambridge* 15:31–53.

Krutak, L. (2019). Therapeutic tattooing in the Arctic: ethnographic, archaeological, and ontological frameworks of analysis. *International Journal of Paleopathology* 25:99–109.

Kurin, D. S. (2016). *The Bioarchaeology of Societal Collapse and Regeneration in Ancient Peru*. Switzerland: Springer.

Levin, B. W. & Browner, C. H. (2005). The social production of health: critical contributions from evolutionary, biological, and cultural anthropology. *Social Science and Medicine* 61:745–750.

Lovejoy, C. O. & Heiple, K. G. (1981). The analysis of fractures in skeletal populations with an example from the Libben site, Ottawa County, Ohio. *American Journal of Physical Anthropology* 55:529–541.

Luna, L. H., Aranda, C. M., Bosio, L. A. & Beron, M. A. (2008). A case of multiple metastasis in Late Holocene hunter-gatherers from the Argentine Pampean region. *International Journal of Osteoarchaeology* 18:492–506.

Lupton, D. (1997). Consumerism, reflexivity and the medical encounter. *Social Science and Medicine* 45:373–381.

Lussier, M. & Richard, C. (2008). Because one shoe doesn't fit all: a repertoire of doctor-patient relationships. *Canadian Family Physician* 54:1089–1092.

Martin, D. L. & Horowitz, S. (2003). Anthropology and alternative medicine: orthopaedics and the other. *Techniques in Orthopaedics* 18:130–138.

Matczak, M. D. & Kozłowski, T. (2017). Dealing with difference: using the osteobiographies of a woman with leprosy and a woman with gigantism from medieval Poland to identify practices of care. In Tilley, L. & Schrenk, A. (Eds.), *New Developments in the Bioarchaeology of Care*, pp. 125–151. Switzerland: Springer.

Mennear, D. J. (2017). Highlighting the importance of the past: public engagement and bioarchaeology of care research. In Tilley, L. & Schrenk, A. (Eds.), *New Developments in the Bioarchaeology of Care*, pp. 343–364. Switzerland: Springer.

Merriam-Webster, (2022). https://www.merriam-webster.com/dictionary/disability

Metzler, I. (1999). The palaeopathology of disability in the middle ages. *Archaeological Review from Cambridge* 1:56–67.

Milella, M. (2017). Subadult mortality among hunter-gatherers: implications for the reconstruction of care during prehistory. In Tilley, L. & Schrenk, A. (Eds.), *New Developments in the Bioarchaeology of Care*, pp. 289–300. Switzerland: Springer.

Nusselder, W. J., Looman, C. W. & Mackenbach, J. P. (2005). Nondisease factors affected trajectories of disability in a prospective study. *Journal of Clinical Epidemiology* 58:484–494.

Nystrom, K. C. & Tilley, L. (2019). Mummy studies and the bioarchaeology of care. *International Journal of Paleopathology* 25:64–71.

Nystrom, K. & Piombino-Mascali, D. (2017). Mummy studies and the soft tissue evidence of care. In Tilley, L. & Schrenk, A. (Eds.), *New Developments in the Bioarchaeology of Care*, pp. 199–218. Switzerland: Springer.

Orschiedt, J., Häuber, A., Haidle, M. N., Alt, K. W. & Buitrago-Téllez, C. H. (2003). Survival of a multiple skull trauma: the case of an early Neolithic individual from the LBK enclosure at Herxheim (Southwest Germany). *International Journal of Osteoarchaeology* 13:375–383.

Ortner, D. J. (2003). *Identification of Pathological Conditions in Human Skeletal Remains* (2nd ed.). New York: Elsevier.
Oxenham, M. & Willis, A. (2017). Towards a bioarchaeology of care of children. In Tilley, L. & Schrenk, A. (Eds.), *New Developments in the Bioarchaeology of Care*, pp. 219–236. Switzerland: Springer.
Phillips, M., Cruz, V., Martin, E., Smith, D., Elias, B., Villalta, J. & Toyne, J. M. (2021). Two (Missing) left feet: caring for foot amputees in late pre-Hispanic Túcume, Lambayeque, Peru. *Bioarchaeology International*, 5(1–2):1–20.
Pol, L. G. & Thomas, R. K. (2001). *The Demography of Health and Health Care* (2nd ed.). Switzerland: Springer Science and Business Media.
Powell, L., Southwell-Wright, W. & Gowland, R. (Eds.) (2016). *Care in the Past: Archaeological and Interdisciplinary Perspectives*. Oxford: Oxbow Books.
Raphael, D., Bryant, T. & Rioux, M. (Eds.) (2019). *Staying Alive: Critical Perspectives on Health, Illness, and Health Care*. Ontario: Canadian Scholars.
Roberts, C. (2017). Applying the 'index of care' to a person who experienced leprosy in late medieval Chichester, England. In Tilley, L. & Schrenk, A. (Eds.), *New Developments in the Bioarchaeology of Care*, pp. 101–124. Switzerland: Springer.
Roberts, C. A. (1999). Disability in the skeletal record: assumptions, problems and some examples. *Archaeological Review from Cambridge* 15:79–97.
Roberts, C. A. & Manchester, K. (2005). *The Archaeology of Disease* (3rd ed.). New York: Cornell University Press.
Rondinelli, R. D., Genovese, E., Katz, R. T., Mayer, T. G., Mueller, K., Ranavaya, M. & Brigham, C. R. (2008). *AMA Guides to the Evaluation of Permanent Impairment*. New York: American Medical Association.
Roush, S. E. (2017). Consideration of disability from the perspective of the medical model. In Byrnes, J. F. & Muller, J. L. (Eds.), *Bioarchaeology of Impairment and Disability*, pp. 39–55. Switzerland: Springer.
Sabloff, J.A. (2008) *Archaeology Matters: Action Archaeology in the Modern World*. New York: Routledge.
Scheer, J. & Groce, N. (1988). Impairment as a human constant: cross-cultural and historical perspectives on variation. *Journal of Social Issues* 44:23–37.
Scheper-Hughes, N. & Lock, M. M. (1987). The mindful body: a prolegomenon to future work in medical anthropology. *Medical Anthropology Quarterly* 1:6–41.
Schrenk, A. A. (2019). *A Community of Care: Patterns of Pathology and Trauma with a Focus on the Bioarchaeology of Care at Carrier Mills, IL (10,000–1000 BP)* (Doctoral dissertation, University of Nevada, Las Vegas).
Schrenk, A. A. & Martin, D. L. (2017). Applying the index of care to the case study of a bronze age teenager who lived with paralysis: moving from speculation to strong inference. In Byrnes, J. F. & Muller, J. L. (Eds.), *Bioarchaeology of Impairment and Disability*, pp. 47–64. Switzerland: Springer.
Schrenk, A. & Tremblay-Critcher, L. (2022). *Bioarchaeology of Care through Population-Level Analyses*. Florida: University of Florida Press.
Shakespeare, T. (1999). Commentary: observations on disability and archaeology. *Archaeological Review from Cambridge* 15:99–101.
Shakespeare, T. (2008). Debating disability. *Journal of Medical Ethics* 34:11–14.
Shakespeare, T. (2013). *Disability Rights and Wrongs Revisited*. London: Routledge.
Shuttleworth, R. & Meekosha, H. (2017). Accommodating critical disability studies in bioarchaeology. In Byrnes, J. F. & Muller, J. L. (Eds.), *Bioarchaeology of Impairment and Disability*, pp. 19–38. Switzerland: Springer.
Smith, M. E. (2021). Why archaeology's relevance to global challenges has not been recognised. *Antiquity* 95(382):1061–1069.
Snoddy, A. M., Buckley, H., King, C., Kinaston, R., Nowell, G., Gröcke, D., … & Petchey, P. (2020). 'Captain of all these men of death': an integrated case study of tuberculosis in nineteenth-century Otago, New Zealand. *Bioarchaeology International* 3(4):217–237.
Solari, A., da Silva, S. F., Pessis, A. M., Martin, G. & Guidon, N. (2020). Applying the bioarchaeology of care model to a severely diseased infant from the middle Holocene, north-eastern Brazil: a step further into research on past health-related caregiving. *International Journal of Osteoarchaeology* 30(4):482–491.
Solecki, R. S. (1971). *Shanidar: The First Flower People*. New York: Alfred A. Knopf.

Southwell-Wright, W. (2013). Past perspectives: what can archaeology offer disability studies? In Wappett, M. & Arndt, K. (Eds.), *Emerging Perspectives on Disability Studies,* pp. 67–95. New York: Palgrave Macmillan.

Spikins, P. A., Rutherford, H. E. & Needham, A. P. (2010). From homininity to humanity: compassion from the earliest archaics to modern humans. *Time and Mind* 3:303–325.

Spikins, P., Needham, A., Tilley, L. & Hitchens, G. (2018). Calculated or caring? Neanderthal healthcare in social context. *World Archaeology* 50(3):384–403.

Steckel, R. H. & Rose, J. C. (Eds.) (2002a). *The Backbone of History: Health and Nutrition in the Western Hemisphere.* Cambridge: Cambridge University Press.

Stodder, A. L. (2017). Quantifying impairment and disability in bioarchaeological assemblages. In Byrnes, J. F. & Muller, J. L. (Eds.), *Bioarchaeology of Impairment and Disability,* pp. 183–200. Switzerland: Springer.

Stodder, Ann L. W. & Jennifer F. Byrnes. (Re)Discovering Paleopathology. In Willermet, C. & Lee, S. H. (Eds.), *Evaluating Evidence in Biological Anthropology: The Strange and the Familiar,* pp. 103–117. Cambridge: Cambridge University Press.

Sutherland, M. L. (2019). Use of computed tomography scanning in a 'virtual' bioarchaeology of care analysis of a central coast Peruvian mummy bundle. *International Journal of Paleopathology* 25:129–138.

Suzuki, T., Mineyama, I. & Mitsuhashi, K. (1984). Paleopathological study of an adult skeleton of Jomon period from Irie shell mound, Hokkaido. *Journal of the Anthropological Society of Nippon* 92:87–104.

Tarlow, S. (2000). Emotion in archaeology. *Current Anthropology* 41(5):713–746.

Thorpe, N. (2016). The Palaeolithic compassion debate–alternative projections of modern-day disability into the distant past. In Powell, L., Southwell-Wright, W. & Gowland, R. (Eds.), *Care in the Past: Archaeological and Interdisciplinary Perspectives,* pp 114–130. Oxford: Oxbow Books.

Tilley, C. (1990). On modernity and archaeological discourse. In Bapty, I. & Yates T. (Eds.), *Archaeology After Structuralism: Post-Structuralism and the Practice of Archaeology,* pp. 128–152. London: Routledge.

Tilley, L. (2015). *Theory and Practice in the Bioarchaeology of Care.* Switzerland: Springer.

Tilley, L. & Cameron, T. (2014). Introducing the index of care: a web-based application supporting archaeological research into health-related care. *International Journal of Paleopathology* 6:5–9.

Tilley, L., & Cameron, T. (2021). A user's guide to the index of care: navigating the open-access cloud application supporting bioarchaeology of care research. In Kacki, S., Réveillas, H. & Knusel, C. (Eds.), *Rencontre Autour du Corps Malade: Prise en Charge et Traitement Funéraire des Individus Souffrants à Travers les Siècles,* pp. 267–276. Actes de la 10e Rencontre du Gaaf, 23–25 mai 2018, Groupe d'anthropologie et d'archéologie funéraire, Bordeaux. Reugny: Gaaf, 2021.

Tilley, L. & Nystrom, K. (2019). A 'cold case' of care: looking at old data from a new perspective in mummy research. *International Journal of Paleopathology* 25:72–81.

Tilley, L. & Oxenham, M. F. (2011). Survival against the odds: modeling the social implications of care provision to seriously disabled individuals. *International Journal of Paleopathology* 1(1):35–42.

Tilley, L. & Schrenk, A. (Eds.) (2017). *New Developments in the Bioarchaeology of Care.* Switzerland: Springer.

Tornberg, A. & Jacobsson, L. (2018). Care and consequences of traumatic brain injury in Neolithic Sweden: a case study of ante mortem skull trauma and brain injury addressed through the bioarchaeology of care. *International Journal of Osteoarchaeology* 28(2):188–198.

Trinkaus, E. & Zimmerman, M. R. (1982). Trauma among the Shanidar Neandertals. *American Journal of Physical Anthropology* 57:61–76.

Van Cant, M. (2018). Surviving amputations: a case of a late-medieval femoral amputation in the rural community of Moorsel (Belgium). In Turner, W. J. & Lee, C. (Eds.), *Trauma in Medieval Society,* pp. 180–214. Leiden: Brill.

Vehmas, S. (2008). Philosophy and science: the axes of evil in disability studies? *Journal of Medical Ethic* 34:21–23.

Verostick, K. A., Teixeira-Santos, I., Bryant Jr, V. M. & Reinhard, K. J. (2019). The Skiles mummy: care of a debilitated hunter-gatherer evidenced by coprolite studies and stable isotopic analysis of hair. *International Journal of Paleopathology* 25:82–90.

Waldron, T. (2009). *Palaeopathology.* Cambridge: Cambridge University Press.

Walker, A. & Shipman, P. (1996). *The Wisdom of Bones.* London: Weidenfeld and Nicolson.

Webb, S. G., & Thorne, A. G. (1985). A congenital meningocoele in prehistoric Australia. *American Journal of Physical Anthropology* 68:525–533.

Weiss, G. L. & Copelton, D. A. (2020). *The Sociology of Health, Healing, and Illness*. London: Routledge.

Wesp, J. K. (2017). Caring for bodies or simply saving souls: the emergence of institutional care in Spanish Colonial America. In Tilley, L. & Schrenk, A. (Eds.), *New Developments in the Bioarchaeology of Care*, pp. 253–276. Switzerland: Springer.

Willett, A. Y. & Harrod, R. P. (2017). Cared for or outcasts: a case for continuous care in the Precontact US Southwest. In Tilley, L. & Schrenk, A. (Eds.), *New Developments in the Bioarchaeology of Care*, pp. 65–84. Switzerland: Springer.

Wood, J. W., Milner, G. R., Harpending, H. C. & Weiss, K. M. (1992). The osteological paradox: problems of inferring prehistoric health from skeletal samples. *Current Anthropology* 33:343–370.

World Health Organization, (1997). *The International Classification of Impairments, Activities and Participation (ICIDH-Beta 2)*. Switzerland: World Health Organization.

World Health Organization, (2003). *International Classification of Functioning, Disability and Health (Version 2.1)*. Switzerland: World Health Organization.

World Health Organization, (2011). *World Report on Disability*. Switzerland: World Health Organization.

Young, J. L. & Lemaire, E. D. (2014). Linking bone changes in the distal femur to functional deficits. *International Journal of Osteoarchaeology* 24(6):709–721.

Young, J. L. & Lemaire, E. D. (2017). Using population health constructs to explore impairment and disability in knee osteoarthritis. In Byrnes, J. F. & Muller, J. L. (Eds.), *Bioarchaeology of Impairment and Disability*, pp. 159–182. Switzerland: Springer.

Zink, A., Samadelli, M., Gostner, P. & Piombino-Mascali, D. (2019). Possible evidence for care and treatment in the Tyrolean Iceman. *International Journal of Paleopathology* 25:110–117.

Zuckerman, M. K., Kamnikar, K. R. & Mathena, S. A. (2014). Recovering the 'body politic': a relational ethics of meaning for bioarchaeology. *Cambridge Archaeological Journal* 24(3):513–522.

Zuckerman, M. K., Kamnikar, K. R., Osterholtz, A. J., Herrmann, N. P. & Franklin, J. D. (2019). Applying the index of care to the Mississippian period: a case study of treponematosis, physical impairment, and probable health-related caregiving from the Holliston Mills site, TN. *International Journal of Osteoarchaeology* 29(5):843–853.

26
DEFINING THE MARGINS, EMBODYING THE CONSEQUENCES

Madeleine Mant and Lauren September Poeta

Introduction

Paleopathological engagement with questions of marginalization and social disenfranchisement reveals the multidisciplinary nature of paleopathological inquiry itself. The goal of this chapter is to highlight the demonstrated strengths of paleopathology in engaging with the concept of marginalization while emphasizing potential future research directions. The chapter opens with a discussion of the multidisciplinary integration of a definition of marginalization and how structural violence has been operationalized in paleopathological research. Next, it explores how paleopathologists have investigated marginalization in skeletal and archival datasets. Finally, it examines the role of the researcher in paleopathological inquiry and closes with a call to action for paleopathologists to consider their role in social justice.

Defining marginalization has interested practitioners beyond paleopathology; disciplines such as social and feminist theory, health geography, epidemiology, nursing, and medical anthropology, to name a few, have grappled with the concept. Holland and Mant wrestled with defining the concept in their introduction to *Bioarchaeology of Marginalized People*, defining it as "a social process, whereby members perceived to be part of a specific group are treated differently than others in a society" (Mant & Holland, 2019a:1), concluding that it is "both a process and a product, an embodied force, that is the result of a nexus of political, social, economic, and environmental factors" (2019b:266). The physical and/or social peripheralization of people, the creation of an in-group and an out-group, the "othering" of certain individuals (Douglas, 1966; Chand et al., 2017; Weheliye, 2014; Hall & Carlson, 2016; Baah et al., 2018) – these themes echo through the literature, as scholars seek to define the edges of the "positions of ambiguity" populated by the marginalized (Lynam & Cowley, 2007:141).

Marginalization in paleopathological and bioarchaeological datasets might appear in varied ways, including (1) marginalization as a process of peripheralization; (2) marginalization as a loss of identity; (3) marginalization: positivity through difference; and (4) marginalization as a divorce from context or a process of forgetting (Mant & Holland, 2019a). These themes represent the effects of this powerful process both during life and after death, as the health of peripheralized individuals may be examined from osteological or mummified remains. The persistence of human remains in the present allows both for the uncovering and amplifying of the narratives of vulnerable individuals in the past and for a critical consideration of the role of the researcher in committing potential harm. The history of the amassment of anatomical and osteological research collections in particular reveals how biological anthropology, and paleopathology as an extension, has benefited from the collection of the bodies of the marginalized without their consent (Watkins, 2018; de la Cova, 2019, 2020, and see Chapter 21 volume).

Being marginalized may have many effects, including differential environmental exposures, stigma and scapegoating, and disparate access to resources. The uneven distribution of resources is key to Galtung's (1969:171) coining of the term *structural violence*, in which "the power to decide over the distribution of resources is unevenly distributed." These inequities, woven directly and silently into the fabric of a group, may result in both "bodily harm" and "psychological violence" (Galtung, 1969:177). Medical anthropologist Paul Farmer and colleagues applied this term to questions of clinical and public health, noting that "structural violence remains a high-ranking cause of premature death and disability" (Farmer, 2004; Farmer et al., 2006:1690). Marginalization is described as "a meta-process from which persistent, severe health disparities emerge" (Hall & Carlson, 2016:206), as the biological world, its physical and mental effects, become literally incorporated into the body. Embodiment theory communicates that bodies are storytellers, revealing the effects of a person's social and physical environment, and sometimes telling tales that a person is otherwise unable or unwilling to share (Krieger, 2005). An individual's context and the social determinants of health to which they are exposed, including neighborhood conditions, working conditions, education achieved, income, socially ascribed race, and stress, may have direct or indirect effects upon health (Marmot, 2005; Gravlee, 2009; Palmer et al., 2019), the chronic and embodied effects of which may be visible to the paleopathologist in human remains (e.g., Ellis, 2019).

Marginalization in the Bones

Paleopathological interpretation of marginalization demands both careful examination and contextualization of skeletal remains. Environmental, sociocultural, and biological pressures may be exerted on the body, affecting the immune and cardiovascular systems and even the bones. The skeleton can literally tell a story from the inside out. The challenge to the researcher is to consider how the patterning of lesions – be they cancerous, traumatic, infectious, metabolic, non-specific, etc. – within and between bodies reveals, emphasizes, or potentially reframes the margins. Increasingly, paleopathologists have engaged with broader contextual evidence to query not only what health issues might be affecting human groups, but the "how" and the "why" (Grauer, 2012:4) of such evidence. In the past decades, there has been increasing engagement with the concept of identity plasticity and embodiment in paleopathology and bioarchaeology, highlighting the effects of age (Gowland, 2006; Halcrow & Tayles, 2008; Sofaer, 2011; and see Chapter 23, this volume); gender (Sofaer, 2006; Geller, 2008, 2016; Hollimon, 2017; Zuckerman, 2020, and see Chapter 24, this volume); ethnogenesis (Klaus & Chang, 2009; Hu, 2013); and personhood (Boutin, 2016) on the body. Examinations of how individuals fit into broader understandings of populations have focused upon the creation and expression of social identity (Knudson & Stojanowski, 2009, 2020; Stodder & Palkovich, 2012). The recognition and problematizing of varied identities encourage researchers to consider *how* and *why* an individual's skeleton might display evidence of certain lesions. How did their identities affect their access to care? The care received? Their cultural currency?

Structural Violence

de la Cova's (2008, 2011, 2012, and see Chapter 21, this volume) work, investigating skeletal health, disease, and trauma, was instrumental in introducing the concept of structural violence to paleopathology. Klaus (2012) also incorporated the concepts of embodiment and structural violence into examinations of skeletal health and biological stress, drawing upon Walker's (2001) definition of violence, wherein a "dominant group shows callous disregard for the safety and physical well-being of the people they have marginalized" (quoted in Klaus, 2012:32; 2014). Recently, Nelson (2021) examined anthropology's previous approach to violence in its broadest conceptualization, concluding that the discipline's history of knowledge production has been hampering our ability to engage with the diversified reality of violence, and thus resulting pathologies, past people faced and the true scope and embodiment of human experience relating to vulnerability, risk, and survival (see Chapter 27, this volume).

Chronic stress can lead to an overburdening of the neuroendocrine, autonomic, immune, and metabolic systems, resulting in disease (McEwen, 2017). These pathological responses can be understood through energetic trade-offs and life history theory. For example, individuals that report higher feelings of social connectivity tend to have better rates of survival (Holt-Lunstad et al., 2015) and lower levels of inflammation (Kiecolt-Glaser et al., 2010). In contrast, socially isolated individuals are likely to have higher rates of inflammation (Yang, et al., 2014; Eisenberger, et al., 2017), yielding increased risks for mortality (Proctor et al., 2015; Raffetti et al., 2017). Further, childhood trauma has been associated with adverse health risks such as cardiovascular disease, obesity, diabetes, cancer, and issues including substance abuse (Felitti et al., 1998; Hughes et al., 2017; Condon et al., 2019). The children of pregnant people who suffer trauma may have adverse health outcomes such as low birth weight and development issues during childhood (Madigan et al., 2017; Folger et al., 2018). Forensic work has focused upon indicators of stress in and the treatment of migrant bodies, investigating borders as political margins with biological consequences (e.g., Beatrice & Soler, 2016; Kovras & Robins, 2016). As Syme and Hagen (2019) declared, "mental health is biological health" – the complex interplay of identity, experience, and stress may affect the body in myriad ways and acknowledging this complexity is critical for biological anthropology and paleopathology in particular (see Chapter 22, this volume)).

Studies of structural violence using skeletal collections of historically confirmed marginalized groups, such as Chinese immigrants and laborers in the late-19th-century United States (Harrod et al., 2012; Harrod & Crandall, 2015) and enslaved individuals from varied geographical and temporal contexts, have provided insights concerning the health effects of violence, segregation, forced labor, and nutritional stress, which might result in traumatic injuries, degenerative joint disease, dental trauma and/or infection, infectious disease, and malnutrition (e.g., Corruccini et al., 1982; Rose, 1989; Blakely & Harrington, 1997; Rankin-Hill, 1997; Rathbun & Steckel, 2002; Blakey & Rankin-Hill, 2004; Lambert, 2006; Perry et al., 2009; Shuler, 2011; Cardoso et al., 2018; Ferreira et al., 2019). Dent (2017:7) investigates antebellum slavery in the United States, citing hypoplastic enamel defects, carious lesions, tuberculosis, cranial porosity, and the distribution of periosteal new bone as the "embodied consequences of marginalization." Musculoskeletal markers, Harris lines, and short stature, in addition to carbon and nitrogen isotopes, may provide further clues to unequal nutrition and labor burdens between groups in a population (Quinn & Beck, 2016). Context is critical to these investigations, however, as there is no "check-list" of health indicators that confirm an individual experienced captivity or enslavement; incorporation of multiple lines of data such as primary documents, funerary data, ethnography, and taphonomic context is necessary to understand the structural violence an individual may have endured (Handler & Lange, 2006; Pearson et al., 2012; Redfern, 2018, 2020; Fricke, 2019). Simply put, context is everything.

A multifactorial approach to paleopathological investigation is critical. de la Cova (2011), comparing skeletal health disparities between 19th-century African American and Euro-American men of low socioeconomic status (SES), discovered that the African Americans had significantly higher frequencies of tuberculosis and treponematoses (diseases that include pinta, yaws, bejel, and syphilis), though there were no significant differences when examining other signs of skeletal stress or undernutrition. DeWitte and colleagues (2016:242) explain that there is "hidden heterogeneity in frailty," emphasizing that the "relationship between health and SES in past populations…may be context-specific rather than universal." SES is an important predictor of mortality in living populations, but its effects in the skeleton are varied. Studies incorporating skeletal stress indicators, such as long bone length (Mays et al., 2009), dental enamel hypoplasia (Miszkiewicz, 2015), and dental caries (Mant & Roberts, 2015), found mixed results when considering the relationship of the stress indicator to social status. Stature may be used as a more sensitive indicator of environmental conditions; Ives and Humphrey (2017) found both male and female children suffered from growth faltering in a mid-19th-century London, UK urban poor cemetery, suggesting early weaning and impoverishment as likely causes.

Considering the hidden heterogeneity of frailty and its effects on skeletal groups that we excavate and evaluate (Wood et al. (1992), Garland et al. (2016) discuss how the lower prevalence of infant stress indicators from the Early to Late colonial periods of the Lambayeque Valley of Peru can be interpreted in multiple ways. These include changing epidemiological patterns and differential access to resources from possibly adapting to Spanish influences, but also the potential that longer, more survivable periods of stress in the Early Colonial period may have been replaced by shorter, but less survivable periods of stress in the Late Colonial period. Here, social, political, and environmental changes intersected to affect epidemiological patterns and the pathological record demonstrating how a demographic change in health patterns may not be transparent.

In some cases, the effects of structural violence may be visible in the skeleton as physical trauma. "Reading" trauma has interested paleopathologists (e.g., Martin, et al., 2012; Knüsel & Smith, 2014; Redfern, 2016) who incorporate material culture and mortuary patterning to better understand the circumstances that may have created or encouraged violent acts. Martin and colleagues (2010) use Ancestral Pueblo remains from La Plata Valley to ask whether patterns of violence might be revelatory of gender and status identity within a group. Studies of intimate partner violence (Redfern, 2017) and injury recidivists (Mant, 2019) integrate clinical, forensic, and bioarchaeological datasets, noting the limitations inherent in skeletal datasets when studying antemortem fractures. Still, Martin and Osterholtz emphasize that studying "trauma on human remains from the past is a form of bioarchaeological 'witnessing' of violent events" (2016:472). While trauma might appear unambiguously in the skeletal remains, the context surrounding a fracture is more difficult to access. An accidental fall or a fall due to a push might leave the same evidence in the bones. Additionally, while what we interpret to be an act of violence may appear mechanically similar, a particular act may have different cultural value or significance than what has been traditionally associated with the definition of "violence" (Koziol, 2017). For example, a skull fracture could be the sign of ritualized violence or an indicator of interpersonal violence.

The embodiment of biological and social stresses from urbanization, and particularly industrialization, is an area of increased focus in paleopathology and bioarchaeology, evidenced by the publication of *The Bioarchaeology of Urbanization* (Betsinger & DeWitte, 2020), *Manufactured Bodies: The Impact of Industrialisation on London Health* (Western & Bekvalac, 2020), and several chapters in *The Bioarchaeology of Structural Violence* (Tremblay & Reedy, 2020). Paleopathological lesions (e.g., hypoplastic dental defects, dental caries, osteoarthritis, metabolic disorders such as scurvy and rickets, infectious diseases such as syphilis and tuberculosis), when taken together, may provide an indication of allostatic load (Mathena-Allen & Zuckerman, 2020). Examining the body for multifactorial signs of stress can provide insights about marginalized individuals, such as women and children for whom historical contextual information might be more difficult to access (Grauer, 2003).

Marginalized Bones

Autopsy and Dissection

The effects of marginalization may be noted *in bone*, as well as *to bone*. For instance, there has been increasing attention paid in paleopathology to the roles of dissection and autopsy in acting out structural violence upon bodies of the dead. Waldron and Rogers described these skeletal alterations as medical interventions, or "iatrogenic paleopathology" (1988), without distinguishing clearly between autopsy and dissection. More recent work has sought to clarify the difference, noting that, depending upon the temporal context, an autopsy may have been undertaken to clarify the cause of an individual's death, while a dissection may have had a basis in medical education, or may have been done to "hurt" the body or demonstrate power (Crossland, 2009; Nystrom, 2017).

Autopsies tend to be less invasive, generally involving a craniotomy (resulting in saw marks around the cranium) and removal of the anterior thoracic wall (indicated by transection of the ribs) (Geller, 1983). Cases suggestive of amateur surgical practice might show repeated false-starts and bone chipping (Novak, 2017). The challenge in paleopathology is distinguishing between evidence of antemortem surgical procedures (for trauma or chronic infectious diseases, e.g., amputations), postmortem autopsies, postmortem dissection, and postmortem experimentation (Owsley, 1995). Bioarchaeological evidence suggesting dissection might include the presence of duplicated skeletal elements, considerable fragmentation, transected elements, saw marks, material culture such as pins (for preparation of the bones in anatomical teaching), and "cuts that clearly would have been of no therapeutic value" (Western, 2012:30; Fowler & Powers, 2012; Nystrom, 2017). In cases of isolated remains, these distinctions provide even greater challenges (Walker, 2001), though the incorporation of historical research provides important context for future work (Dittmar & Mitchell, 2015; Flies et al., 2017).

Incorporating biocultural and social context is critical, not only to distinguish what type of intervention has taken place, but also why and to whom. In the United States, the bodies of poor individuals, almshouse inmates, prisoners, immigrants, and racialized minorities – particularly Black individuals – were historically targeted as sources for anatomical collections (Humphrey, 1973; Halperin, 2007). The edited collection *The Bioarchaeology of Dissection and Autopsy in the United States* (Nystrom, 2017) covers over 300 years of American history and characterizes dissection as a form of structural violence against the marginalized, noting its historical connection as a crime deterrent and association with social transgressions. Evidence of dissection and autopsy in marginalized groups has been found in sites as varied as American medical colleges (e.g., Blakely & Harrington, 1997; Hodge, 2013), 18th-century English hospital refuse (Boston & Webb, 2012; Chamberlain, 2012; Chaplin, 2012; Kausmally, 2012), poor farms (Richards et al., 2017), and burial sites including enslaved individuals such as the New York African Burial Ground (Perry et al., 2009). These varied contexts illuminate the importance of incorporating biocultural context to skeletal remains.

Multiple Lines of Data

Investigating institutional records, such as those of hospitals or poorhouses, can provide alternative means of accessing marginalized experiences. Mitchell (2011; and see Chapter 10, this volume) emphasizes the value in utilizing historical records to examine health and disease, outlining the paired biological-social diagnosis inherent in examining historical sources; biological being the diagnosis reflecting modern understandings of a disease and the social how individuals living in the past were likely to have understood it. Historic hospital records have been used to access the health and disease experience of individuals marginalized due to remote geography, peripatetic occupation, or SES (Mant, 2020a, b, c), where possible drawing together skeletal and historical sources (Mant, 2016, 2019) to emphasize the possibilities and limitations inherent in both lines of data. Nineteenth-century United States poorhouses, such as the Erie County Poorhouse (Nystrom et al., 2017; Muller et al., 2020), the Dunning Poorhouse (Grauer et al., 2017), and St. Lawrence County Poorhouse (Mant et al., 2019), offer embodied datasets of individuals pushed to the margins within their societies. Asylum skeletal samples can reveal the embodied inequities of 19th-century ideas of "labor therapy" (Phillips, 2003) in groups such as the mentally ill who may remain otherwise invisible (Phillips, 2015).

Burial practices, particularly those that appear nonnormative, have been harnessed as evidence of deviance, which could potentially reflect marginalization during life. Groups such as "criminals, women who died during childbirth, unbaptised infants, people with disabilities, and supposed revenants" (Murphy, 2008:xii) have been previously singled out as potential marginalized groups. Chapters in *The Odd, the Unusual, and the Strange: Bioarchaeological Explorations of Atypical Burials* (Betsinger et al., 2020) challenge the concept of a typical/atypical burial binary, exploring the spectrum of mortuary practices in a range of past societies. Lorna Tilley's (2015; Tilley & Schrenk, 2017) explorations of disability and care provision in the past reject the simplistic assumption that those with disabilities are automatically candidates for marginalization and exclusion (see Chapter 25, this volume). For example, in Peru, Mackey and Nelson (2020) report an elderly female (G T11) with cerebral palsy at Farfán, who has elliptical femoral heads and acetabulae which led to chronic flexion of the hips. Wear facets of the knees and ankles suggest chronic contracture of her lower limbs as well. While chronically flexed in life, her burial included the intentional dislocation of joints for burial in an extended position. Because adults and older nonadults are typically buried in flexed positions in this time period (Late Horizon, 1472–1532 AD) and only the youngest nonadults are buried in extended positions (Jijon y Caamaño, 1949), this is a significant aspect of her mortuary identity. Her grave offerings were also among the richest at Farfán, containing ceramic vessels, animal remains, rings, and two retainer burials – additional individuals that were sacrificed and buried with the main individual. Since G T11 lived to an old age with considerable status, it is evident the community was able and willing to adapt to her needs and abilities for her to thrive (Poeta & Nelson, 2021). Ethnohistoric accounts of Incan census categories further contextualize individuals with a disability, females referred to as

Unquq k'umu, as socially accepted, loved, and highly respected (Poma de Ayala, 1615; Poeta & Nelson, 2021). An individual with such serious pathology and nonnormative burial traits could have been socially marginalized, but this is clearly not the case when incorporating multiple lines of contextual evidence. Evidence of apotropaic burial practices such as prone burials, decapitation, stakes through the heart, and sickles across the throat (e.g., Gregoricka et al., 2014; Alterauge et al., 2020) have also been interpreted within a biocultural context, questioning whether the burial evidence suggests an individual being set apart during life, or whether the practice relates only to their corpse.

Robbins Schug (2016:1) investigated evidence of leprosy in South Asia, demonstrating that while stigma toward those suffering from leprosy today is rampant, "ignominy to the point of exclusion" only appears after the first millennium BCE. Stigma and resulting marginalization are cultural and contextual. Interestingly, Zuckerman's (2017) study of postmedieval cemeteries containing individuals with syphilis did not find evidence of segregated burial practices for the infected, despite evidence of community exclusion of those with the disease during life. She noted that mortuary groups should not be directly equated with "an actual lived, dynamic, and interacting community in the past" (2017:98). Understanding the status of an individual in life is important to consider in investigations of their apparent status in death. As the saying goes, the dead do not bury themselves.

Persistence into the Present

There is an uneven distribution of power in the researcher/research subject relationship in paleopathology. The skeletal remains of past individuals persist in the present with the researcher allowed the privilege to learn from and speak to the experience of the dead. The skeletons of marginalized, disenfranchised, or otherwise vulnerable individuals might best tell the stories of individuals whose lives might be invisible in written or archeological materials; without context, however, harm can be done to these individuals in the search to "deriv[e] *meaning from* and creat[e] *meaning for* human remains" (Zuckerman et al., 2014:514, original emphasis). A researcher may actively do harm if they do not consider their own positionality. Stone (2020), examining the structural violence of corsetry on female bodies in the Victorian era through critical white feminism, emphasizes the importance of looking beyond what we might "expect" to see in skeletal samples. She notes that while researchers have used the "white female body as the universal transcript," these "normal" bodies reflect only a small group of individuals (2020:28). To privilege a tight-laced, white, middle-class body as "normal" is to relegate all other bodies to a "deviant" category. Defining what is "normal" and "deviant" is an extension of our understandings of the world; further, researchers should not project the present into the past by assuming that identities had the same meanings in the past as they may today (Boutin, 2017).

This power differential should make researchers uneasy, as we consider how the "disinterred skeleton is the currency of the bioarchaeologist" (Dougherty & Sullivan, 2017:230). The theme of bodies as currency echoes throughout the literature concerning the amassment of biological anthropological reference collections. American collections, such as the George S. Huntington Anatomical Collection, Robert J. Terry Anatomical Collection, Hamann-Todd Osteological Collection, and William Montague Cobb Human Skeletal Collection, include the unclaimed dead from public hospitals, mental institutions, charity clinics, city morgues, almshouses, workhouses, and prisons (Watkins & Muller, 2015; Muller et al., 2017; Watkins, 2018; de la Cova, 2019, 2020, and see Chapter 21, this volume). The Samuel George Morton Cranial Collection, curated at the University of Pennsylvania, is composed of more than 1,300 crania, including those of enslaved people (Wolff Mitchell, 2021). While biological anthropological standards were built on these bones (de la Cova, 2022) and these bodies are the foundation of countless thesis projects, the exploitive history of their creation is often sidestepped.

While it is true that analyses of these remains, including contextual, biocultural analysis can "give voice to the impacts of impoverishment, marginalization, and institutionalization on individual lives and biologies" (Muller et al., 2017:199), a lack of contextualization may continue to harm these individuals, whose consent to be studied is doubly lacking, both because they are dead and because the circumstances of their death, in many cases, did not provide them with an opportunity to consent. For instance, in April 2021, it was reported that the remains of two children killed in the 1985 bombing of the MOVE headquarters in Philadelphia, Pennsylvania, had been stored and studied at two American universities without their families' knowledge or consent (McGreevy, 2021), resulting in intense media scrutiny and an independent investigative report (Tucker Law Group, 2021). It is important to remember that many marginalized communities and individuals maintain deep sociocultural relationships with their Ancestors and the dead – relationships that may or may not differ from those holding positions of power and privilege. Recent calls for the passing of an African American Graves Protection and Repatriation Act, modeled upon the Native American Graves Protection and Repatriation Act (Dunnavant et al., 2021), insist upon the immediate voluntary cataloguing of existing osteological collections in museums and universities as a means of addressing our science's long history of racism and subsequent marginalization.

Similarly, in the case of Indigenous Ancestral remains, Indigenous-led partnerships are crucial to ensuring research is respectful, culturally sensitive, and works for the needs and actual desires of descendant communities. Recent repatriation efforts have brought global attention to the fact that Indigenous Ancestors from around the world are still held in Euro-American institutions with extractive colonial histories (e.g., Shariatmadari, 2019; Hicks, 2020; Wambu, 2020). These colonial endeavors objectified Ancestral remains and lacked the documentation for repatriations to be handled effectively in contemporary institutions. Of course, national, cultural, and individual factors must be considered for each repatriation, as Indigenous Peoples refers to an exceptionally heterogenous grouping of Peoples globally. Respectful collaborations driven by descendant groups (e.g., Clark et al., 2019; chapters in Meloche et al., 2020; Nash & Colwell, 2020; Supernant et al., 2020; Wadsworth et al., 2021) can ensure that further harm is not done to either the Ancestors or their descendant communities.

It is an uncomfortable truth that the dead are vulnerable. Bones may be damaged during excavation or research, whether accidentally or due to destructive testing; collection managers understand that "taphonomy…does not stop at the doors of a curating institution" (Redfern & Bekvalac, 2017:378). Further, the individuals upon whose remains osteological education is conducted may not have consented to their inclusion in such a collection. Both authors clearly recollect being informed that the osteological learning collections we were training on as undergraduate students were primarily comprised of the remains of unclaimed individuals from Southeast Asia. This is not an uncommon reality for many North American university osteological collections and anatomy education laboratories (Habicht et al., 2018), a painful fact highlighted powerfully by Michelle Rodrigues (2021) and Sabrina Agarwal (2022). Reflecting on this knowledge now and taking stock of our own positionality emphasizes how much power we have previously unthinkingly wielded during our educations and continue to wield as researchers. This process of unlearning and re-examining the bioethics of education, the power of white privilege, and research using human remains is a lifelong process (e.g., Pérez, 2019; Warren & Kleisath, 2019; Beliso-De Jesús & Pierre, 2020).

Squires and colleagues (2022:3) outline the necessity of including an ethics statement in all publications centered upon archaeological human remains, emphasizing that skeletal remains "are not only a resource for teaching, research publication, and ultimately career development, but they represent once living individuals that deserve to be treated with dignity and respect."

While acknowledging the vulnerability of the marginalized individuals we may study, Klaus expounds that "we must be on guard against portraying recipients of structural violence as passive victims. While the agency of subordinate groups is often constrained, marginalized people should be expected to exercise as much agency as possible" (2012:37). We respect this agency by seeking to amplify their stories as comprehensively as possible, providing translational opportunities to seek social justice through paleopathological research. Importantly, the most respectful path forward may be "taking a pause" (Watkins, 2022) in examining skeletal collections known to include marginalized people.

Present and Future Directions

Incorporating themes from epidemiological, medical anthropological, and feminist theory has enriched the conversation about how adverse contexts and life stresses may affect the body. Life history theory and embodiment have become linked, leading researchers to examine how exposures to environmental influences and stresses in utero and during postnatal growth and development affect both short- and long-term health (Barker, 2012; Charles et al., 2016). The Developmental Origins of Health and Disease (DOHaD) hypothesis emphasizes that taking a life course and interdisciplinary approach to considering topics such as poverty, nutrition, education, and sanitation will have effects on the health of multiple generations (Mandy & Nyirenda, 2018; and see Chapter 28, this volume). Bioarchaeologists have only just begun to consider the effects of epigenetics and intergenerational health stresses upon skeletal manifestations of disease (e.g., Klaus, 2014; Gowland, 2015b), noting the difficulties in untangling the many threads. The medical anthropological concept of syndemics, wherein social, economic, and environmental conditions affect the interaction of two or more diseases present in a population, potentially leading to exacerbated disease effects and poor health outcomes (Singer & Clair, 2003), can be revealing when considering the health of those pushed to the margins of society, particularly for skeletal samples with associated historical context.

Whitney Battle-Baptiste (2011), Maria Franklin (2001), and Aja Lans (2021) call for the integration of Black feminist thought into archaeological studies of inequality and identified skeletal collections in museums, noting that conceptions of race, class, and gender must be problematized to understand "neglected histories" (Battle-Baptiste, 2011:30). Finally, intersectionality, the concept outlined by Kimberlé Crenshaw (1989, 1991) to examine the multiply-burdened position of Black women in the United States, has important lessons for studies of marginalization and health. The overlapping and intersecting axes of a person's social identity create and influence societal inequalities and discrimination, which may affect their health outcomes (Veenstra, 2011; Sen & Iyer, 2012). While intersectional approaches have certainly been taken in bioarchaeological and paleopathological studies, it is only recently that the term has been used and foregrounded explicitly (Byrnes, 2017; Torres-Rouff & Knudson, 2017; Yaussy, 2019; Mant et al., 2021). Further integration of paradigms emphasizing the interrelation of individuals' multifaceted identities and contexts upon their health will aid in both identifying margins in particular groups and their potential embodied effects. After all, a skeleton is not simply a snapshot of an individual at the end of their life, but the result of accumulated and intersecting identities and experiences throughout their life course.

Individuals may move within and between identities, fortunes, statuses, environments, and relationships during their lives that affect their access to resources and therefore their health. Gowland (2017a) employs a life course analysis to examine the cumulative identity of aging and how it may intersect with disability in older individuals, noting bioarchaeological examples suggestive of elder abuse (Gowland, 2015a, 2017b). Grauer (2018) highlights a young woman from the mid-19th-century Dunning Poorhouse Cemetery whose dentition displays evidence of gold foil restorative dentistry. Mant observed similar expensive dental work in an older adult individual of unknown sex (FAO90 1716) from the St. Bride's lower churchyard cemetery in London, UK, curated at the Museum of London Centre for Human Bioarchaeology. Despite poor overall skeletal completeness, the presence of a gold filling in this individual's right maxillary first molar provides a clue to their shifting SES throughout their life course. While both bodies were interred in cemeteries for individuals of lower SES in their respective societies, their teeth reveal the "fluid and subjective" relationship individuals may negotiate with poverty and status through their lives (Levene, 2006:ix).

Lessons from DOHaD and intersectionality – that an individual's many identities may overlap and exacerbate inequalities while potentially having effects on multiple generations – are fruitful ground for paleopathological analysis of marginalization. The concept of the hidden heterogeneity of risk, that individuals in the past were not equally likely to be exposed to, contract, or die from various diseases, forms part of the osteological paradox (Wood et al., 1992) and can be used to think through issues of frailty (DeWitte & Hughes-Morey, 2012; Yaussy, 2019) and cases where geographical marginalization appeared to benefit a group (Martin, 2019). Appreciating the potential intersections of varied identities encourages researchers to consider such complexity and how these intersections might have interacted to create or entrench a marginalized identity. Recognizing the complexity of sex and gender to health (Agarwal, 2017; Lukacs, 2017; Wesp, 2017), the presence of nonbinary genders (Weismantel, 2013; Hollimon, 2017; Moen, 2019), and the effects of sexuality (Voss, 2008; Voss & Casella, 2011; Geller, 2016) and how these varied identities may become embodied represents the continued unbinding of sex from gender in osteological analyses (Grauer & Stuart-Macadam, 1998). Tremblay and Reedy (2020) emphasize the importance of communicating with medical anthropologists and cultural anthropologists as we investigate the embodied evidence of past lives. While wholesale projecting of modern understandings of identity must be avoided (Boutin, 2017), integrated interdisciplinary scholarship will ensure that researchers asking similar questions and pursuing similar goals are communicating with one another. Further, it is critical to acknowledge and resist the "marginalization of scholarship produced by people on [the] margins" and the biases of Western knowledge production more broadly (Wynter, 1994; McKittrick, 2015; Athreya, 2019; Watkins, 2020:2). Championing the concept of "slow scholarship," better incorporating non-English language research, and increasing accessibility to peer-reviewed journals to all researchers are immediate steps that can be taken. With archaeological investigations occurring globally, it is also crucial that we respect, acknowledge, and cite the paleopathological work conducted outside our own circles. The centering of varied voices in paleopathological research enriches our understanding of the past.

Conclusion

Paleopathologists are trained to recognize the sometimes glaring, sometimes understated clues to the lived experience recorded in the skeleton. As researchers, we learn to recognize the subtle curve of healed childhood rickets in adult long bones, eye the pathway of a hairline fracture, and read timelines from the seeming chaos of freshly laid down woven bone. These observations, ensuring they are accurate and consistent, can provide insight into lived lives. It is the integration of context, however, that can shed light on marginalization in past groups.

Following Scheper-Hughes and Lock (1987), the body is individually experienced, social, and political. It can also be emotional, vulnerable, intimate, private, public, remembered, and forgotten. As researchers, our work is a product of our own context and our own experience in navigating the world. It is our responsibility to seek a deeper understanding of the context in which past individuals lived. We owe it to the individuals whose remains we have the privilege of studying to consider their complexities and sit with our discomfort in how much we do not know and may never know. Some aspects of an individual's identity may be mutable, others may not. Some aspects of one's identity may be unimaginable to some researchers, underlining the necessity of collaborating with researchers with diverse experiences and identities. Life experiences may be clearly "written in the bones," while others may remain invisible, even to a microscopic histopathological view.

Research is political. The powerful position of the researcher in reference to their research subject(s) must be acknowledged. Paleopathologists, through international collaborations with colleagues of varied backgrounds and experiences, are ideally positioned to use our research as a platform for social justice, particularly when analyzing the skeletal remains of individuals who negotiated marginalization during life. The Paleopathology Association's motto, *mortui viventes docent* (the dead teach the living), is predicated upon the understanding that the living are ready to learn from the dead, no matter how uncomfortable may be the truths that their bones reveal.

References

Agarwal, S. C. (2017). Understanding sex- and gender-related patterns of bone loss and health in the past: a case study from the Neolithic community of Çatalhöyük. In Agarwal, S. C. & Wesp, J. K. (Eds.), *Exploring Sex and Gender in Bioarchaeology*, pp. 165–188. Albuquerque: University of New Mexico Press.

Agarwal, S. C. (2022). The legacy and disposability of brown bodies: the bioethics of skeletal anatomy collections from India. *American Journal of Biological Anthropology* 177(S73):2.

Alterauge, A., Meier, T., Jungklaus, B., Milella, M, & Lösch, S. (2020). Between belief and fear – reinterpreting prone burials during the Middle Ages and early modern period in German-speaking Europe. *PloS One* 15(8):e0238439. https://doi.org/10.1371/journal.pone.0238439.

Athreya, S. (2019). "But you're not a *real* minority": the marginalization of Asian voices in paleoanthropology. *American Anthropologist* 121:472–474. https://doi.org/10.1111/aman.13216.

Baah, F. O., Teitelman, A. M. & Riegel, B. (2018). Marginalization: conceptualizing patient vulnerabilities in the framework of social determinants of health—an integrative review. *Nursing Inquiry* 26(1):e12268. https://doi.org/10.1111/nin.12268.

Barker, D. J. P. (2012). Developmental origins of chronic disease. *Public Health* 126(3):185–189.

Battle-Baptiste, W. (2011). *Black Feminist Archaeology*. Oakland, CA: Left Coast Press.

Beatrice, J. S. & Soler, A. (2016). Skeletal indicators of stress: a component of the biocultural profile of undocumented migrants in Southern Arizona. *Journal of Forensic Sciences* 61(5):1164–1172. https://doi.org/10.1111/1556-4029.13131.

Beliso-De Jesús, A. M. & Pierre, J. (2020). Special section: anthropology of white supremacy. *American Anthropologist* 122(1):65–75. https://doi.org/10.1111/aman.13351.

Betsinger, T. K., & DeWitte, S. N. (2020). *The Bioarchaeology of Urbanization*. New York: Springer. https://doi.org/10.1007/978-3-030-53417-2.

Betsinger, T. K., Scott, A. B. & Tsaliki, A. (2020). *The Odd, the Unusual, and the Strange: Bioarchaeological Explorations of Atypical Burials*. Gainesville: University of Florida Press. https://doi.org/10.5744/florida/9781683401032.001.0001.

Blakey, M. & Rankin-Hill, L. M. (2004). *The New York African Burial Ground Skeletal Biology Final Report, Vol. 1 the United States General Services Administration, Northeast and Caribbean Region: The African Burial Ground Project*. Washington, DC: Howard University.

Blakely, T. D. & Harrington, S. (1997). *Bones in the Basement: Postmortem Racism in Nineteenth-Century Medical Training*. Washington, DC: Smithsonian Institution Press.

Boston, C. & Webb, H. (2012). Early medical training and treatment in Oxford: a consideration of the archaeological and historical evidence. In Mitchell, P. D. (Ed.), *Anatomical Dissection in Enlightenment England and Beyond: Autopsy, Pathology and Display*, pp. 43–68. Aldershot, UK: Ashgate. https://doi.org/10.4324/9781315566962.

Boutin, A. (2016). Exploring the social construction of disability: an application of the bioarchaeology of personhood model to a pathological skeleton from ancient Bahrain. *International Journal of Paleopathology* 12:17–28. https://doi.org/ 10.1016/j.ijpp.2015.10.005.

Boutin, A. (2017). Reply to C. Torres-Rouff and K. J. Knudson. *Current Anthropology* 58(3):399–400. https://doi.org/10.1086/692026.

Byrnes, J. F. (2017). Injuries, impairment, and intersecting identities: the poor in Buffalo, NY 1851–1913. In Byrnes, J. F. & Muller, J. L. (Eds.), *Bioarchaeology of Impairment and Disability*, pp. 201–222. New York: Springer. https://doi.org/10.1007/978-3-319-56949-9.

Cardoso, H. F. V., Spake, L., Wasterlain, S. N. & Ferreira, M. T. (2018). The impact of social experiences of physical and structural violence on the growth of African enslaved children recovered from Lagos, Portugal (15th–17th centuries). *American Journal of Physical Anthropology* 168(1):209–221. https://doi.org/10.1002/ajpa.23741.

Chamberlain, A. T. (2012). Morbid osteology: Evidence for autopsies, dissection and surgical training from the Newcastle infirmary burial ground (1753–1845). In Mitchell, P. D. (Ed.), *Anatomical Dissection in Enlightenment England and Beyond: Autopsy, Pathology and Display*, pp. 11–22. Aldershot, UK: Ashgate. https://doi.org/10.4324/9781315566962.

Chand, R., Nel, E. & Pelc, S. (2017). *Societies, Social Inequalities, and Marginalization*. New York: Springer. https://doi.org/10.1007/978-3-319-50998-3.

Chaplin, S. (2012). Dissection and display in eighteenth-century London. In Mitchell, P. D. (Ed.), *Anatomical Dissection in Enlightenment England and Beyond: Autopsy, Pathology and Display*, pp. 95–114. Aldershot, UK: Ashgate. https://doi.org/10.4324/9781315566962.

Charles, M. -A., Delpierre, C., & Bréant, B. (2016). Le concept des origines développementales de la santé – Évolution sur trois décennies. *Médecine/Sciences (Paris)* 32(1):15–20. https://doi.org/10.1051/medsci/20163201004.

Clark, T., Betts, M., Coupland, G., Cybulski, J. S., Paul, J., Froesch, P., Feschuk, S., Joe, R. & Williams, G. (2019). Looking into the eyes of the ancient chiefs of shíshálh: the osteology and facial reconstructions of a 4000-year-old high-status family. In Mant, M. & Holland, A. J. (Eds.), *Bioarchaeology of Marginalized People*, pp. 53–67. Cambridge, MA: Elsevier Academic Press. https://doi.org/10.1016/C2017-0-02300-5.

Condon, E. M., Holland, M. L., Slade, A., Redeker, N. S., Mayes, L. C. & Sadler, L. (2019). Maternal adverse childhood experiences, family strengths, and chronic stress in children. *Nursing Research* 68(3):189–199. https://doi.org/10.1097/NNR.0000000000000349.

Corruccini, R. S., Handler, J. S., Mutaw, R. J., & Lange, F. W. (1982). The osteology of a slave burial population from Barbados, West Indies. *American Journal of Physical Anthropology* 159:443–459. https://doi.org/10.1002/ajpa.1330590414.

Crenshaw, K. (1989). Demarginalizing the intersection of race and sex: a Black feminist critique of antidiscrimination doctrine, feminist theory and antiracist politics. *University of Chicago Legal Forum* 1, Article 8, pp. 139–167.

Crenshaw, K. (1991). Mapping the margins: intersectionality, identity politics, and violence against women of color. *Stanford Law Review* 43(6):1241–1299. https://doi.org/10.2307/1229039.

Crossland, Z. (2009). Acts of estrangement: the post-mortem making of self and other. *Archaeological Dialogues* 16(1):101–125. https://doi.org/10.1017/S1380203809002827.

de la Cova, C. (2008). *Silent Voices of the Destitute: An Analysis of African American and Euro-American Health During the Nineteenth Century*. Unpublished doctoral dissertation. Bloomington: Indiana University.

de la Cova, C. (2011). Race, health, and disease in 19th-century-born males. *American Journal of Physical Anthropology* 144:526–537. https://doi.org/10.1002/ajpa.21434.

de la Cova, C. (2012). Trauma patterns in 19th-century-born African American and Euro-American females. *International Journal of Paleopathology* 2(2–3):61–68.

de la Cova, C. (2019). Marginalized bodies and the construction of the Robert J. Terry anatomical skeletal collection: a promised land lost. In Mant, M. & Holland, A. J. (Eds.), *Bioarchaeology of Marginalized People*, pp. 133–155. Cambridge, MA: Elsevier Academic Press. https://doi.org/10.1016/C2017-0-02300-5.

de la Cova, C. (2020). Processing the destitute and deviant dead: inequality, dissection, politics, and the structurally violent legalization of social marginalization in American anatomical collections. In Osterholtz, A. J. (Ed.), *The Poetics of Processing: Memory Formation, Identity, and the Handling of the Dead*, pp. 212–234. Boulder: University Press of Colorado.

de la Cova, C. M. (2022). *Ethical Issues and Considerations for Ethically Engaging with the Robert J. Terry, Hamann-Todd, and William Montague Cobb Anatomical Collections* [Abstract]. American Journal of Biological Anthropology 177(s73):42.

Dent, S. (2017). Individual differences in embodied marginalization: osteological and stable isotope analysis of antebellum enslaved individuals. *American Journal of Human Biology* 29(4):e23021. https://doi.org/10.1002/ajhb.23021.

DeWitte, S. N. & Hughes-Morey, G. (2012). Stature and frailty during the Black Death: the effect of stature on risks of epidemic mortality in London, A.D. 1348–1350. *Journal of Archaeological Science* 39:1412–1419. https://doi.org/10.1016/j.jas.2012.01.019.

DeWitte, S. N., Hughes-Morey, G., Bekvalac, J. & Karsten, J. (2016). Wealth, health and frailty in industrial-era London. *Annals of Human Biology* 43(3):241–254. https://doi.org/10.3109/03014460.2015.1020873.

Dittmar, J. M. & Mitchell, P. D. (2015). A new method for identifying and differentiating human dissection and autopsy in archaeological human skeletal remains. *Journal of Archaeology Science: Reports* 3:73–79. https://doi.org/10.1016/j.jasrep.2015.05.019.

Dougherty, S. P., & Sullivan, N. C. (2017). Autopsy, dissection, and anatomical exploration: the postmortem fate of the underclass and institutionalized in Old Milwaukee. In Nystrom, K. C. (Ed.), *The Bioarchaeology of Dissection and Autopsy in the United States*, pp. 205–235. New York: Springer. https://doi.org/10.1007/978-3-319-26836-1_10.

Douglas, M. (1966). *Purity and Danger*. Routledge.

Dunnavant, J., Justinvil, D., & Colwell, C. (2021). Craft an African American Graves Protection and Repatriation Act. *Nature* 593:337–340. https://doi.org/10.1038/d41586-021-01320-4.

Eisenberger, N. I., Moieni, M., Inagaki, T. K., Muscatell, K. A. & Irwin, M. R. (2017). In sickness and in health: the co-regulation of inflammation and social behavior. *Neuropsychopharmacology* 42:242–253. https://doi.org/10.1038/npp.2016.141.

Ellis, M. A. B. (2019). *The Children of Spring Street*. Springer. https://doi.org/10.1007/978-3-319-92687-2.

Farmer, P. E. (2004). Anthropology of structural violence. *Current Anthropology* 45(3):305–325. https://doi.org/10.1086/382250.

Farmer, P. E., Nizeye, B., Stulac, S. & Keshavjee, S. (2006). Structural violence and clinical medicine, *PloS Medicine* 3(10):e449. https://doi.org/10.1371/journal.pmed.0030449.

Felitti, V. J., Anda, R. F., Nordenberg, D., Williamson, D. F., Spitz, A. M., Edwards, V. & Marks, J. S. (1998). Relationship of childhood abuse and household dysfunction to many of the leading causes of death in adults: the Adverse Childhood Experiences (ACE) study. *American Journal of Preventive Medicine* 14:245–258. https://doi.org/10.1016/s0749-3797(98)00017-8.

Ferreira, M. T., Coelho, C., Cunha, E. & Wasterlain, S. N. (2019). Evidences of trauma in adult African enslaved individuals from Valle de Gafaria, Lagos, Portugal (15th–17th centuries). *Journal of Forensic and Legal Medicine* 65:68–75. https://doi.org/10.1016/j.jflm.2019.05.005.

Flies, M. J., Winther, S. D. & Lynnerup, N. (2017). Skeletal material from the cemetery of the 19th-century Copenhagen hospital for the poor: autopsies, surgical training, and anatomical specimens. *International Journal of Osteoarchaeology* 27(6):1012–1021. https://doi.org/10.1002/oa.2612.

Folger, A. T., Eismann, E. A., Stephenson, N. B., Shapiro, R. A., Macaluso, M., Brownrigg, M. E. & Gillespie, R. J. (2018). Parental adverse childhood experiences and offspring development at 2 years of age. *Pediatrics* 141:e20172826. https://doi.org/10.1542/peds.2017-2826.

Fowler, L., & Powers, N. (2012). *Doctors, Dissection and Resurrection Men: Excavations in the 19th-century Burial Ground of the London Hospital, 2006. MOLA Monograph 62*. Museum of London Archaeology.

Franklin, M. (2001). A Black feminist-inspired archaeology? *Journal of Social Archaeology* 1(1):108–125. https://doi.org/10.1177/146960530100100108.

Fricke, F. J. (2019). *The Lifeways of Enslaved People in Curacao, St Eustatius, and St Maarten/St Martin: A Thematic Analysis of Archaeological, Osteological, and Oral Historical Data.* Unpublished doctoral dissertation. University of Kent.

Galtung, J. (1969). Violence, peace, and peace research. *Journal of Peace Research* 6(3):167–191. https://doi.org/10.1177/002234336900600301.

Garland, C. J., Turner, B. L., & Klaus, H. D. (2016). Biocultural consequences of Spanish contact in the Lambayeque Valley region of Northern Peru: internal enamel micro-defects as indicators of early life stress. *International Journal of Osteoarchaeology* 26(6):947–958. https://doi.org/10.1002/oa.2505.

Geller, P. (2008). Conceiving sex: fomenting a feminist bioarchaeology. *Journal of Social Archaeology* 8(1):113–138. https://doi.org/10.1177/1469605307086080.

Geller, P. (2016). *The Bioarchaeology of Socio-Sexual Lives: Queering Common Sense About Sex, Gender, and Sexuality.* New York: Springer. https://doi.org/10.1007/978-3-319-40995-5.

Geller, S. (1983). Autopsy. *Scientific American* 248(3):124–137. https://doi.org/10.1038/scientificamerican0383-124.

Gowland, R. (2006). Embodied identities in Roman Britain: a bioarchaeological approach. *Britannia* 48:177–194. https://doi.org/10.1017/S0068113X17000125.

Gowland, R. (2015a). Elder abuse: evaluating the potentials and problems of diagnosis in the archaeological record. *International Journal of Osteoarchaeology* 26(3):514–523. https://doi.org/10.1002/oa.2442.

Gowland, R. (2015b). Entangled lives: implications of the developmental origins of health and disease hypothesis for bioarchaeology and the life course. *American Journal of Physical Anthropology* 158:530–540. https://doi.org/10.1002/ajpa.22820.

Gowland, R. (2017a). Growing old: biographies of disability and care in later life. In Tilley, L. & Schrenk, A. A. (Eds.), *New Developments in the Bioarchaeology of Care*, pp. 237–251. New York: Springer. https://doi.org/10.1007/978-3-319-39901-0.

Gowland, R. (2017b). That "tattered coat upon a stick" the ageing body: elder marginalization and abuse in Roman Britain. In Powell, L. A., Southwell-Wright, W. & Gowland, R. L. (Eds.), *Care in the Past: Interdisciplinary Perspectives*, pp. 71–90. Oxford: Oxbow Books.

Grauer, A. L. (2003). Where were the women? In Herring, D. A. & Swedlund, A. C. (Eds.), *Human Biologists in the Archives*, pp. 266–288. Cambridge: Cambridge University Press. https://doi.org/10.1017/cbo9780511542534.013.

Grauer, A. L. (2012). Introduction: the scope of paleopathology. In Grauer, A. L. (Ed.), *A Companion to Paleopathology*, pp. 1–14. Chichester: Wiley-Blackwell.

Grauer, A. L. (2018). Paleopathology: from bones to social behavior. In Katenberg, M. A. & Grauer, A. L. (Eds.), *Biological Anthropology of the Human Skeleton* (3rd ed.), pp. 447–465. New York: John Wiley & Sons, Inc. https://doi.org/10.1002/9781119151647.

Grauer, A. L., Lathrop, V. & Timoteo, T. (2017). Exploring evidence of nineteenth century dissection in the Dunning Poorhouse cemetery. In Nystrom, K. C. (Ed.), *The Bioarchaeology of Dissection and Autopsy in the United States*, pp. 301–313. New York: Springer. https://doi.org/10.1007/978-3-319-26836-1_14.

Grauer, A. L. & Stuart-Macadam, P. (1998). *Sex and Gender in Paleopathological Perspective.* Cambridge: Cambridge University Press.

Gravlee, C. C. (2009). How race becomes biology: embodiment of social inequality. *American Journal of Physical Anthropology* 139:47–57. https://doi.org/10.1002/ajpa.20983.

Gregoricka, L. A., Betsinger, T. K., Scott, A. B. & Polcyn, M. (2014). Apotropaic practices and the undead: a biogeochemical assessment of deviant burials in Post-Medieval Poland. *PloS One* 9(11):e113564. https://doi.org/10.1371/journal.pone.0113564.

Habicht, J. L., Kiessling, C., & Winkelmann, A. (2018). Bodies for anatomy education in medical schools: an overview of the sources of cadavers worldwide. *Academic Medicine* 93(9):1293–1300. https://doi.org/10.1097/ACM.0000000000002227.

Halcrow, S. E. & Tayles, N. (2008). The bioarchaeologist investigation of childhood and social age: problems and prospects. *Journal of Archaeological Method and Theory* 15:190–215. https://doi.org/10.1007/s10816-008-9052-x.

Hall, J. M. & Carlson, K. (2016). Marginalization: a revisitation with integration of scholarship on globalization, intersectionality, privilege, microaggressions, and implicit biases. *Advances in Nursing Science* 39(3):200–215. https://doi.org/10.1097/ANS.0000000000000123.

Halperin, E. C. (2007). The poor, the Black, and the marginalized as the source of cadavers in United States anatomical education. *Clinical Anatomy* 20:489–495. https://doi.org/10.1002/ca.20445.

Handler, J. S. & Lange, F. W. (2006). On interpreting slave status from archaeological remains. *African Diaspora Archaeology Newsletter* 9(2):Article 11. https://scholarworks.umass.edu/adan/vol9/iss2/11.

Harrod, R. P. & Crandall, J. J. (2015). Rails built of the ancestors' bones: the bioarchaeology of the overseas Chinese experience. *Historical Archaeology* 49(1):148–161. https://doi.org/10.1007/bf03376965.

Harrod, R. P., Thompson, J. L., & Martin, D. L. (2012). Hard labor and hostile encounters: what human remains reveal about institutional violence and Chinese immigrants living in Carlin, Nevada (1885–1923). *Historical Archaeology* 46(4):85–111. https://doi.org/10.1007/bf03376880.

Hicks, D. (2020). *The Brutish Museums: The Benin Bronzes, Colonial Violence and Cultural Restitution.* London: Pluto Press.

Hodge, C. J. (2013). Non-bodies of knowledge: anatomized remains from the Holden Chapel collection, Harvard University. *Journal of Social Archaeology* 13(1):122–149. https://doi.org/10.1177/1469605312465692.

Hollimon, S. (2017). Bioarchaeological approaches to nonbinary genders: case studies from Native North America. In: Agarwal, S. C. & Wesp, J. K. (Eds.), *Exploring Sex and Gender in Bioarchaeology*, pp. 51–69. Albuquerque: University of New Mexico Press.

Holt-Lunstad, J., Smith, T. B., Baker, M., Harris, T. & Stephenson, D. (2015). Loneliness and social isolation as risk factors for mortality: a meta-analytic review. *Perspectives on Psychological Science* 10:227–237. https://doi.org/10.1177/1745691614568352.

Hu, D. (2013). Approaches to the archaeology of ethnogenesis: past and emergent perspectives. *Journal of Archaeological Research* 21(4):371–402. https://doi.org/10.1007/s10814-013-9066-0.

Hughes, K., Bellis, M. A., Hardcastle, K. A., Sethi, D., Butchart, A., Mikton, C. & Jones, L., Dunne, M. P. (2017). The effect of multiple adverse childhood experiences on health: a systematic review and meta-analysis. *Lancet Public Health* 2(8):e356–66. https://doi.org/10.1016/S2468-2667(17)30118-4.

Humphrey, D. C. (1973). Dissection and discrimination: the social origins of cadavers in America, 1760–1915. *Bulletin of the New York Academy of Medicine* 49(9):819–827.

Ives, R., & Humphrey, L. (2017). Patterns of long bone growth in a mid-19th century documented sample of the urban poor from Bethnal Green, London, UK. *American Journal of Physical Anthropology* 163(1):173–186. https://doi.org/10.1002/ajpa.23198.

Jijon y Caamaño, J. (1949). *Maranga: Contribución al Conocimiento de Los Aborígenes del Valle del Rimac, Perú.* La Prensa Catolica.

Kausmally, T. (2012). William Hewson and the Craven St Anatomy School. In Mitchell, P. D. (Ed.), *Anatomical Dissection in Enlightenment England and Beyond: Autopsy, Pathology and Display*, pp. 69–76. Aldershot, UK: Ashgate. https://doi.org/10.4324/9781315566962.

Kiecolt-Glaser, J. K., Gouin, J. P. & Hantsoo, L. (2010). Close relationships, inflammation, and health. *Neuroscience and Biobehavioral Reviews* 35:33–38. https://doi.org/10.1016/j.neubiorev.2009.09.003.

Klaus, H. (2012). The bioarchaeology of structural violence: a theoretical model and a case study. In Martin, D. L., Harrod, R. P. & Pérez, V. R. (Eds.), *The Bioarchaeology of Violence*, pp. 29–62. Gainesville: University Press of Florida.

Klaus, H. (2014). Frontiers in the bioarchaeology of stress and disease: cross-disciplinary perspectives from pathophysiology, human biology, and epidemiology. *American Journal of Physical Anthropology* 155:294–308. https://doi.org/10.1002/ajpa.22574.

Klaus, H. D. & Tam Chang, M. E. (2009). Surviving contact: biological transformation, burial, and ethnogenesis in the colonial Lambayeque Valley, North Coast of Peru. In Knudson, K. J. & Stojanowski, C. M. (Eds.), *Bioarchaeology and Identity in the Americas*, pp. 126–152. Gainesville: University Press of Florida. https://doi.org/10.5744/florida/9780813036786.001.0001.

Kovras, I. & Robins, S. (2016). Death as the border: managing missing migrants and unidentified bodies at the EU's Mediterranean frontier. *Political Geography* 55:40–49. https://doi.org/10.1016/j.polgeo.2016.05.003.

Knudson, K. J. & Stojanowski, C. M. (2009). *Bioarchaeology and Identity in the Americas.* Gainesville: University Press of Florida. https://doi.org/10.5744/florida/9780813036786.001.0001.

Knudson, K. J. & Stojanowski, C. M. (2020). *Bioarchaeology and Identity Revisited.* Gainesville: University Press of Florida. https://doi.org/10.2307/j.ctv1198zkk.Knüsel, C. J. & Smith, M. J. (Eds.) (2014). *The Routledge Handbook of the Bioarchaeology of Human Conflict*. Abingdon: Routledge. https://doi.org/10.4324/9781315883366.

Koziol, K. M. (2017). Shattered mirrors: Gender, age, and Westernized interpretations of war (and violence) in the past. In Martin, D. B. & Tegtmeyer, C. (Eds.), *Bioarchaeology of Women and Children in Times of War: Case Studies from the Americas*, pp. 15–26. Berlin: Spring International Publishing. https://doi.org/10.1007/978-3-319-48396-2.

Krieger, N. (2005). Embodiment: a conceptual glossary for epidemiology. *Journal of Epidemiology and Community Health* 59(5), 350–355. https://doi.org/10.1136/jech.2004.024562.

Lambert, P. M. (2006). Infectious disease among enslaved African Americans at Eaton's Estate, Warren County, North Carolina, ca. 1830–1850. *Memórias do Instituto Oswaldo Cruz* 101(s2):107–117. https://doi.org/10.1590/S0074-02762006001000017.

Lans, A. M. (2021). Decolonize this collection: integrating Black feminism and art to re-examine human skeletal remains in museums. *Feminist Anthropology* 2:130–142. https://doi.org/10.1002/fea2.12027.

Levene, A. (2006). General introduction. In King, S., Nutt, T. & Tomkins, A. (Eds.), *Narratives of the Poor in Eighteenth-Century Britain* (Vol. 1), pp. vii–xix. London: Pickering & Chatto.

Lukacs, J. R. (2017). Bioarchaeology of oral health: sex and gender differences in dental disease. In Agarwal, S. C. & Wesp, J. K. (Eds.), *Exploring Sex and Gender in Bioarchaeology*, pp. 263–285. Albuquerque: University of New Mexico Press.

Lynam, M. J. & Cowley, S. (2007). Understanding marginalization as a social determinant of health. *Critical Public Health* 17(2):137–149. https://doi.org/10.1080/09581590601045907.

Mackey, C. J. & Nelson, A. J. (2020). Life, death, and burial practices during the Inca occupation of Farfán on Peru's North Coast. *Andean Past Special Publications*. 6. https://digitalcommons.library.umaine.edu/andean_past_special/6.

Madigan, S., Wade, M., Plamondon, A., Maguire, J. L. & Jenkins, J. M. (2017). Maternal adverse childhood experience and infant health: biomedical and psychosocial risks as intermediary mechanisms. *Journal of Pediatrics* 187:282–9e1. https://doi.org/10.1016/j.jpeds.2017.04.052.

Mandy, M. & Nyirenda, M. (2018). Developmental origins of health and disease: the relevance to developing nations. *International Health* 10(2):66–70. https://doi.org/10.1093/inthealth/ihy006.

Mant, M. (2016). 'Readmitted under urgent circumstance': uniting archives and bioarchaeology at the Royal London Hospital. In Mant, M & Holland, A. (Eds.), *Beyond the Bones: Engaging with Disparate Datasets*, pp. 37–59. San Diego: Elsevier Academic Press. https://doi.org/10.1016/c2015-0-04028-x.

Mant, M. (2019). Time after time: individuals with multiple fractures and injury recidivists in long eighteenth century (c. 1666–1837) London. *International Journal of Paleopathology* 24:7–18. https://doi.org/10.1016/j.ijpp.2018.08.003.

Mant, M. (2020a). Inpatients at the St. John's General Hospital: Morbidity in late 19th-century Newfoundland and Labrador. *Canadian Bulletin of Medical History* 37(2):360–394. https://doi.org/10.3138/cbmh.433-032020.

Mant, M. (2020b). For those in peril on and off the sea: Merchant marine bodies in 19th-century St. John's, Newfoundland. *International Journal of Maritime History* 32(1):23–44. https://doi.org/10.1177/0843871420904188.

Mant, M. (2020c). 'A little time woud compleat the Cure': Broken bones and fracture experiences of the working poor in London's general hospitals during the long eighteenth century. *Social History of Medicine* 33(2):438–462. https://doi.org/10.1093/shm/hky023.

Mant, M., de la Cova, C. & Brickley, M. (2021). Intersectionality and trauma analysis in bioarchaeology. *American Journal of Physical Anthropology* 174(4):583–594. https://doi.org/10.1002/ajpa.24226.

Mant, M., & Holland, A. J. (2019a). Introduction. In Mant, M. & Holland, A. J. (Eds.), *Bioarchaeology of Marginalized People*, pp. 1–9. Cambridge, MA: Elsevier Academic Press. https://doi.org/10.1016/C2017-0-02300-5.

Mant, M. & Holland, A. J. (2019b). Mapping marginalized pasts. In Mant, M. & Holland, A. J. (Eds.), *Bioarchaeology of Marginalized people*, pp. 261–267. Cambridge, MA: Elsevier Academic Press. https://doi.org/10.1016/C2017-0-02300-5.

Mant, M., Pitre, M., McCarthy, C. & Hale, A. (2019). Demographic reconstruction of health and disease at the St. Lawrence County Poorhouse, Canton, NY. *American Journal of Physical Anthropology* 168(S68):153.

Mant, M., & Roberts, C. (2015). Diet and dental caries in post-Medieval London. *International Journal of Historical Archaeology* 19:188–207. https://doi.org/10.1007/s10761-014-0286-x.

Marmot, M. (2005). Social determinants of health inequalities. *Lancet* 365:1099–1104. https://doi.org/10.1016/S0140-6736(05)71146-6.

Martin, D. L. (2019). Marginalized by choice – Kayenta Pueblo communities in the Southwest (AD 800–1500). In Mant, M. & Holland, A. J. (Eds.), *Bioarchaeology of Marginalized People*, pp. 115–132. Cambridge, MA: Elsevier Academic Press. https://doi.org/10.1016/C2017-0-02300-5.

Martin, D. L., Harrod, R. P. & Fields, M. (2010). Beaten down and worked to the bone: bioarchaeological investigations of women and violence in the Ancient Southwest. *Landscapes of Violence* 1(1):Article 3. https://scholarworks.umass.edu/lov/vol1/iss1/3.

Martin, D. L., Harrod, R. P. & Pérez, V. (2012). *The Bioarchaeology of Violence*. Gainesville: University of Florida Press. https://doi.org/10.5744/florida/9780813041506.001.0001.

Martin, D. L. & Osterholtz, A. J. (2016). Broken bodies and broken bones: biocultural approaches to ancient slavery and torture. In Zuckerman, M. K. & Martin, D. L. (Eds.), *New Directions in Biocultural Anthropology*, pp. 471–490. Chichester: Wiley Blackwell. https://doi.org/10.1002/9781118962954.ch23.

Mathena-Allen, S. & Zuckerman, M. K. (2020). Embodying industrialization: inequality, structural violence, disease, and stress in working-class and poor British women. In Tremblay, L. A. & Reedy, S. (Eds.), *The Bioarchaeology of Structural Violence*, pp. 53–79. New York: Springer.

Mays, S., Ives, R. & Brickley, M. (2009). The effects of socioeconomic status on endochondral and appositional bone growth, and acquisition of cortical bone in children from 19th century Birmingham, England. *American Journal of Physical Anthropology* 140:410–416. https://doi.org/10.1002/ajpa.21076.

McEwen, B. S. (2017). Neurobiological and systemic effects of chronic stress. *Chronic Stress* 1:1–11. https://doi.org/10.1177/2470547017692328.

McGreevy, N. (2021, April 26). Museum kept bones of Black children killed in 1985 police bombing in storage for decades. *Smithsonian News*. https://www.smithsonianmag.com/smart-news/outrage-over-penn-and-princetons-handling-move-bombing-victims-remains-180977583/.

McKittrick, K. (2015). Yours in the intellectual struggle: Sylvia Wynter and the realization of the living. In McKittrick, K. (Ed.), *Sylvia Wynter: On Human Being as Praxis*, pp. 1–8. Durham, NC: Duke University Press. https://doi.org/10.1215/9780822375852.

Meloche, C. H., Spake, L. & Nichols, K. L. (Eds.) (2020). *Working With and for Ancestors*. Abingdon: Routledge. https://doi.org/10.4324/9780367809317.

Miszkiewicz, J. (2015). Linear enamel hypoplasia and age-at-death at Medieval (11th – 16th centuries) St. Gregory's priory and cemetery, Canterbury, UK. *International Journal of Osteoarchaeology* 25:79–87. https://doi.org/10.1002/oa.2265.

Mitchell, P. (2011). Retrospective diagnosis and the use of historical texts for investigating disease in the past. *International Journal of Paleopathology* 1:81–88. https://doi.org/10.1016/j.ijpp.2011.04.002.

Moen, M. (2019). Gender and archaeology: where are we now? *Archaeologies* 15(2):206–226. https://doi.org/10.1007/s11759-019-09371-w.

Muller, J. L., Byrnes, J. F. & Ingleman, D. A. (2020). The Erie County Poorhouse (1828–1926) as a heterotopia: a bioarchaeological perspective. In Tremblay, L. A. & Reedy, S. (Eds.), *Bioarchaeology of Structural Violence: a Theoretical Framework for Industrial Era Inequality*, pp. 111–137. New York: Springer. https://doi-org.myaccess.library.utoronto.ca/10.1007/978-3-030-46440-0_6.

Muller, J. L., Pearlstein, K. E., & de la Cova, C. (2017). Dissection and documented skeletal collections: embodiments of legalized inequality. In Nystrom, K. C. (Ed.), *The Bioarchaeology of Dissection and Autopsy in the United States*, pp. 185–201. New York: Springer. https://doi.org/10.1007/978-3-319-26836-1_9.

Murphy, E. M. (2008). *Deviant Burial in the Archaeological Record*. Oxford: Oxbow Books.

Nash, S. E. & Colwell, C. (2020). NAGPRA at 30: the effects of repatriation. *Annual Review of Anthropology* 49:225–239. https://doi.org/10.1146/annurev-anthro-010220-075435.

Nelson, R. G. (2021). The sex in your violence: power and patriarchy in anthropological world building and every life. *Current Anthropology* 62(23):S92–S102. https://doi.org/10.1086/711605.

Novak, S. A. (2017). Partible persons or persons apart: postmortem interventions at the Spring Street Presbyterian Church, Manhattan. In Nystrom, K. C. (Ed.), *The Bioarchaeology of Dissection and Autopsy in the United States*, pp. 87–111. New York: Springer. https://doi.org/10.1007/978-3-319-26836-1_5.

Nystrom, K. C. (Ed.) (2017). *The Bioarchaeology of Dissection and Autopsy in the United States*. New York: Springer. https://doi.org/10.1007/978-3-319-26836-1.

Nystrom, K. C., Sirianni, J., Higgins, R., Perrelli, D. & Liber Raines, J. L. (2017). Structural inequality and postmortem examination at the Erie County Poorhouse. In. Nystrom, K.C (Ed.), *The Bioarchaeology of Dissection and Autopsy in the United States*, pp. 279–300. New York: Springer. https://doi.org/10.1007/978-3-319-26836-1_13.

Owsley, D. W. (1995). Contributions of bioarchaeological research to knowledge of nineteenth-century surgery. In Saunders, S. R. & Herring, A. (Eds.), *Grave Reflections: Portraying the Past Through Cemetery Studies*, pp. 120–151. Toronto: Canadian Scholars' Press.

Palmer, R. C., Ismond, D., Rodriquez, E. J. & Kaufman, J. S. (2019). Social determinants of health: future directions for health disparities research. *American Journal of Public Health* 109:S70–S71. https://doi.org/10.2105/AJPH.2019.304964.

Pearson, A., Jeffs, B., Witkin, A. & MacQuarrie, H. (2012). *Infernal Traffic: Excavation of a Liberated African Graveyard in Rupert's Valley, St Helena*. Cambridge: Cambridge University Press.

Pérez, V. R. (2019). "Until the brains ran out": White privilege, physical anthropology, and coopted narratives. *American Anthropologist* 121(2):470–472. https://doi.org/10.1111/aman.13215.

Perry, W. R., Howson, J., & Bianco, B. (2009). *The Archaeology of the New York African Burial Ground Part 2: Descriptions of Burials*. Washington, DC: Howard University.

Phillips, S. (2003). Worked to the bone: the biomechanical consequences of 'labor therapy' at a nineteenth century asylum. In Herring, D. A. & Swedlund, A. C. (Eds.), *Human Biologists in the Archives*, pp. 96–129. Cambridge: Cambridge University Press. https://doi.org/10.1017/CBO9780511542534.

Phillips, S. (2015). 'Just can't work em hard enough': a historical bioarchaeological study of the inmate experience at the Oneida County Asylum. In Knowles, T. & Trowbridge, S. (Eds.), *Insanity and the Lunatic Asylum in the Nineteenth Century*, pp. 85–100. Abingdon: Routledge. https://doi.org/10.4324/9781315654263.

Poeta, L. S. & Nelson, A. J. (2021, October 28). Age, disability, and status: a case study in the expression of mortuary identity in Pre-Columbian Peru [Poster]. Annual Meeting of the Canadian Association for Biological Anthropology, Hamilton, Ontario. https://doi.org/ 10.13140/RG.2.2.10932.99201.

Poma de Ayala, F. G. (1615). *El primer nueva corónica y buen gobierno*. http://www5.kb.dk/permalink/2006/poma/info/es/frontpage.htm

Proctor, M. J., McMillan, D. C., Horgan, P. G., Fletcher, C. D., Talwar, D. & Morrison, D. S. (2015). Systemic inflammation predicts all-cause mortality: a Glasgow Inflammation Outcome Study. *PLoS One* 10:e0116206. https://doi.org/10.1371/journal.pone.0116206.

Quinn, C. P. & Beck, J. (2016). Essential tensions: a framework for exploring inequality through mortuary archaeology and bioarchaeology. *Open Archaeology* 2(1):18–41. https://doi.org/10.1515/opar-2016-0002.

Raffetti, E., Donato, F., Casari, S., Castelnuovo, F., Sighinolfi, L., Bandera, A., … & Quiros-Roldan, E. (2017). Systemic inflammation-based scores and mortality for all causes in HIV-infected patients: a MASTER cohort study. *BMC Infectious Diseases* 17:193. https://doi.org/10.1186/s12879-017-2280-5.

Rankin-Hill, L. (1997). *A Biohistory of 19th Century Afro-Americans: The Burial Remains of Philadelphia Cemetery*. New York: Bergin and Garvey.

Rathbun, T. A. & Steckel, R. H. (2002). The health of slaves and free Blacks in the East. In Steckel, R. H. & Rose, J. C., *The Backbone of History: Health and Nutrition in the Western Hemisphere*, pp. 208–225. Cambridge: Cambridge University Press. https://doi.org/10.1017/cbo9780511549953.010.

Redfern, R. C. (2020). Iron Age 'predatory landscapes': a bioarchaeological and funerary exploration of captivity and enslavement in Britain. *Cambridge Archaeological Journal* 30(4):531–554. https://doi.org/10.1017/S0959774320000062.

Redfern, R. C. (2016). *Injury and Trauma in Bioarchaeology: Interpreting Violence in Past Lives*. Cambridge: Cambridge University Press. https://doi.org/10.1017/9780511978579.

Redfern, R. C. (2017). Identifying and interpreting domestic violence in archaeological human remains: a critical review of the evidence. *International Journal of Osteoarchaeology* 27(1):13–34. https://doi.org/10.1002/oa.2461.

Redfern, R. C. (2018). Blind to chains? The potential of bioarchaeology for identifying the enslaved of Roman Britain. *Britannia* 49:251–282. https://doi.org/10.1017/S0068113X18000119.

Redfern, R. C. & Bekvalac, J. J. (2017). Collection care and management of human remains. In Schotsmans, E. M. J., Márquez-Grant, N. & Forbes, S. L. (Eds.), *Taphonomy of Human Remains*, pp. 369–384. New York: Wiley. https://doi.org/10.1002/9781118953358.

Richards, P. B., Jones, C. R., Epstein, E. M., Richards, N. W., Drew, B. L. & Zych, T. J. (2017). "You couldn't identify your grandmother if she were in that party": the bioarchaeology of the postmortem investigation at the Milwaukee County Poor Farm cemetery. In Nystrom, K. C. (Ed.), *The Bioarchaeology of Dissection and Autopsy in the United States*, pp. 237–257. New York: Springer. https://doi.org/10.1007/978-3-319-26836-1_11.

Robbins Schug, G. (2016). Begotten of corruption? Bioarchaeology and "othering" of leprosy in South Asia. *International Journal of Paleopathology* 15:1–9. https://doi.org/10.1016/j.ijpp.2016.09.002.

Rodrigues, M. A. (2021, August 17). Haunted by my teaching skeleton. *SAPIENS.* https://www.sapiens.org/archaeology/where-do-teaching-skeletons-come-from/.

Rose, J. C. (1989). Biological consequences of segregation and economic deprivation: a post-slavery population from Southwest Arkansas. *Journal of Economic History* 49(2):351–360. https://doi.org/10.1017/S0022050700007981.

Scheper-Hughes, N. & Lock, M. M. (1987). The mindful body: a prolegomenon to future work in medical anthropology. *Medical Anthropology Quarterly* 1(1):6–41. https://doi.org/10.1525/maq.1987.1.1.02a00020.

Sen, G. & Iyer, A. (2012). Who gains, who loses and how: leveraging gender and class intersections to secure health entitlements. *Social Science & Medicine* 74:1802–1811. https://doi.org/10.1016/j.socscimed.2011.05.035.

Shariatmadari, D. (2019, April 23). 'They're not property': the people who want their ancestors back from British museums. *The Guardian: UK Edition.* https://www.theguardian.com/culture/2019/apr/23/theyre-not-property-the-people-who-want-their-ancestors-back-from-british-museums.

Shuler, K. A. (2011). Life and death on a Barbadian sugar plantation: historic and bioarchaeological view of infection and mortality at Newton Plantation. *International Journal of Osteoarchaeology* 21:66–81. https://doi.org/10.1002/oa.1108.

Singer, M. & Clair, S. (2003). Syndemics and public health: reconceptualizing disease in bio-social context. *Medical Anthropology Quarterly* 17(4):423–441. https://doi.org/10.1525/maq.2003.17.4.423.

Sofaer, J. (2006). *The Body as Material Culture: A Theoretical Osteoarchaeology.* Cambridge University Press. https://doi.org/10.1017/cbo9780511816666.

Sofaer, J. (2011). Toward a social bioarchaeology of age. In Agarwal, S. C. & Glencross, B. A. (Eds.), *Social Bioarchaeology,* pp. 285–311. Chichester: Wiley-Blackwell. https://doi.org/10.1002/9781444390537.

Squires, K., Roberts, C. A. & Márquez-Grant, N. (2022). Ethical considerations and publishing in human bioarchaeology. *American Journal of Biological Anthropology* 177(4):615–619. https://doi.org/10.1002/ajpa.24467.

Stodder, A. L. W. & Palkovich, A. M. (2012). *The Bioarchaeology of Individuals.* Gainesville: University Press of Florida. https://doi.org/10.5744/florida/9780813038070.001.0001.

Stone, P. (2020). Female beauty, bodies, binding, and the bioarchaeology of structural violence in the Industrial Era through the lens of critical white feminism. In Tremblay, L. A. & Reedy, S. (Eds.), *Bioarchaeology of Structural Violence: a Theoretical Framework for Industrial Era Inequality,* pp. 13–30. New York: Springer. https://doi.org/10.1007/978-3-030-46440-0_2.

Supernant, K., Baxter, J. E., Lyons, N. & Atalay, S. (2020). *Archaeologies of the Heart.* New York: Springer. https://doi.org/10.1007/978-3-030-36350-5.

Syme, K. L. & Hagen, E. H. (2019). Mental health is biological health: why tackling "diseases of the mind" is an imperative for biological anthropology in the 21st century. *American Journal of Physical Anthropology* 171(S70):87–117. https://doi.org/10.1002/ajpa.23965.

Tilley, L. (2015). *Theory and Practice in the Bioarchaeology of Care.* New York: Springer. https://doi.org/10.1007/978-3-319-18860-7.

Tilley, L. & Schrenk, A. A. (2017). *New Developments in the Bioarchaeology of Care.* New York: Springer. https://doi.org/10.1007/978-3-319-39901-0.

Torres-Rouff, C. & Knudson, K. J. (2017). Integrating identities: an innovative bioarchaeological and biogeochemical approach to analyzing the multiplicity of identities in the mortuary record. *Current Anthropology* 58(3):381–409. https://doi.org/10.1086/692026.

Tremblay, L. A. & Reedy, S. (2020). *The Bioarchaeology of Structural Violence.* New York: Springer. https://doi.org/10.1007/978-3-030-46440-0.

Tucker Law Group. (2021). The odyssey of the MOVE remains: report of the independent investigation into the demonstrative display of MOVE remains at the Penn Museum and Princeton University. https://www.penn.museum/documents/pressroom/MOVEInvestigationReport.pdf.

Veenstra, G. (2011). Race, gender, class, and sexual orientation: intersecting axes of inequality and self-rated health in Canada. *International Journal for Equity in Health* 10(3). https://doi.org/10.1186/1475-9276-10-3.

Voss, B. L. (2008). Sexuality studies in archaeology. *Annual Review of Anthropology* 37:317–336. https://doi.org/10.1146/annurev.anthro.37.081407.085238.

Voss, B. L. & Casella, E. C. (2011). *The Archaeology of Colonialism: Intimate Encounters and Sexual Effects.* Cambridge: Cambridge University Press.

Wadsworth, W. T. D., Supernant, K., Dersch, A. & the Chipewyan Prairie First Nation. (2021). Integrating remote sensing and Indigenous archaeology to locate unmarked graves: a case study from Northern Alberta, Canada. *Advances in Archaeological Practice* 9(3)1–13. https://doi.org/10.1017/aap.2021.9.

Waldron, T. & Rogers, J. (1988). Iatrogenic palaeopathology. *Journal of Paleopathology* 1(3):117–129.

Walker, P. L. (2001). A bioarchaeological perspective on the history of violence. *Annual Review of Anthropology* 30:573–596. https://doi.org/10.1146/annurev.anthro.30.1.573.

Wambu, O. (2020, Sept 2). Human remains held in Western museums must be returned to Africa. *New African Magazine.* https://newafricanmagazine.com/24029/.

Warren, J. & Kleisath, M. (2019). The roots of US anthropology's race problem: whiteness, ethnicity, and ethnography. *Equity & Excellence in Education* 52(1):55–67. https://doi.org/10.1080/10665684.2019.1632230.

Watkins, R. (2018). The fate of anatomical collections in the US: bioanthropological investigations of structural violence. In Henderson, C. Y. & Cardoso, F. A. (Eds.), *Identified Skeletal Collections: The Testing Grounds of Anthropology?*, pp. 169–185. Oxford.

Watkins, R. (2022). *Discussant* [podium presentation]. Ethics in the Curation and Use of Human Skeletal Remains. American Association of Biological Anthropologists, Denver, CO.

Watkins, R. J. (2020). "[This] system was not made for [you]:" a case for decolonial Scientia. *American Journal of Physical Anthropology* 175(2):350–362. https://doi.org/10.1002/ajpa.24199.

Watkins, R. & Muller, J. (2015). Repositioning the Cobb Human Archive: the merger of a skeletal collection and its texts. *American Journal of Human Biology* 27:41–50. https://doi.org/10.1002/ajhb.22650.

Weheliye, A. G. (2014). *Habeas Viscus.* Durham, NC: Duke University Press. https://doi.org/10.1515/9780822376491.

Weismantel, M. J. (2013). Towards a transgender archaeology: a queer rampage through history. In Stryker, S. & Aizura, A. Z. (Eds.), *The Transgender Studies Reader 2*, pp. 319–334. Abingdon: Routledge.

Wesp, J. K. (2017). Embodying sex/gender systems in bioarchaeological research. In Agarwal, S. C & Wesp, J. K. (Eds.), *Exploring Sex and Gender in Bioarchaeology*, pp. 99–126. Albuquerque: University of New Mexico Press.

Western, G. & Bekvalac, J. (2020). *Manufactured Bodies: The Impact of Industrialisation on London Health.* Oxford: Oxbow Books. https://doi.org/10.2307/j.ctv13gvh5j.

Western, A. G. (2012). A star of the first magnitude: osteological and historical evidence for the challenge of provincial medicine at the Worcester Royal Infirmary in the nineteenth century. In Mitchell, P. D. (Ed.), *Anatomical Dissection in Enlightenment England and Beyond: Autopsy, Pathology and Display*, pp. 23–41. Aldershot, UK: Ashgate. https://doi.org/10.4324/9781315566962.

Wolff Mitchell, P. (2021). Black Philadelphians in the Samuel George Morton anatomical collection. *Penn Arts & Sciences.* https://prss.sas.upenn.edu/penn-medicines-role/black-philadelphians-samuel-george-morton-cranial-collection.

Wood, J. W., Milner, G. R., Harpending, H. C. & Weiss, K. M. (1992). The osteological paradox: Problems of inferring prehistoric health from skeletal samples [and comments and reply]. *Current Anthropology* 33(4):343–370. https://doi.org/10.1086/204084.

Wynter, S. (1994). No humans involved: an open letter to my colleagues. *Forum N.H.I.: Knowledge for the 21st century* 1(1):42–73.

Yang, Y. C., Schorpp, K. & Harris, K. M. (2014). Social support, social strain and inflammation: evidence from a national longitudinal study of U.S. adults. *Social Science and Medicine* 107:124–35. https://doi.org/10.1016/j.socscimed.2014.02.013.

Yaussy, S. L. (2019). The intersections of industrialization: variation in skeletal indicators of frailty by age, sex, and socioeconomic status in 18th– and 19th-century England. *American Journal of Physical Anthropology* 170:116–130. https://doi.org/10.1002/ajpa.23881.

Zuckerman, M. K. (2017). The "poxed" and the "pure": a bioarchaeological investigation of community and marginalization relative to infection with acquired syphilis in post-medieval London. *Archaeological Papers of the American Anthropological Association* 28(1):91–103. https://doi.org/10.1111/apaa.12091.

Zuckerman, M. K. (2020). Gender in bioarchaeology. In Cheverko, C. M., Prince-Buitenhuys, J. R. & Hubbe, M. (Eds.), *Theoretical Approaches in Bioarchaeology*, pp. 28–44. Abingdon: Routledge. https://doi.org/10.4324/9780429262340-3.

Zuckerman, M. K., Kamnikar, K. R. & Mathena, S. A. (2014). Recovering the 'body politic': a relational ethics of meaning for bioarchaeology. *Cambridge Archaeological Journal* 24(3):513–522. https://doi.org/10.1017/S0959774314000766.

27
INTERPRETING TRAUMA AND SOCIAL VIOLENCE FROM SKELETAL REMAINS

Debra L. Martin, Aurora Marcela Pérez-Flórez, Claira Ralston and Ryan P. Harrod

Introduction

Violence is a fundamental part of human existence. Research into the causes, consequences, nature, and logic of violence in the past is complicated by the difficulty of interpreting the motivations and cultural explanations informing violent practices using only material culture. The nuanced, motivating factors behind violent behaviors can be explored further, however, using multidisciplinary approaches drawing on ethnographic work, historic and ethnohistorical accounts, forensic medicine, archaeological reconstructions, and most importantly, the bodies themselves.

Bodies are truth tellers. There is a physicality and corporeality to them that express a wealth of information from the individual body to the social body to the collective body politic (Scheper-Hughes & Lock, 1987; Sofaer, 2006; Geller, 2021). A body is both biologically and culturally produced and as such is a physical expression of accumulated biological (individual) responses to lived (cultural) experiences in the world. By extension, a person's skeleton contains their cumulative record of lived experiences and conditions; a process that commences when skeletal and dental tissues begin to form in utero and concludes only at death (Agarwal, 2016).

In forensic research, a range of scientific evidence is collected from not only the bones but the contexts within which they were found to identify details informing the likely cause of death of an individual. Attempting to ascertain the cause of death for bodies from the deep past is difficult because the skeletal evidence is less conclusive, and the context is often not possible to completely reconstruct (Martin, 2015; Tegtmeyer & Martin, 2017). However, as discussed by Byrnes and Gaddis (Chapter 13, this volume), the analysis of trauma on bones has seen an explosion of new multidisciplinary methods and techniques that provide increasingly more nuanced information about skeletal trauma and its manufacture.

Human-induced trauma to bones can be identified through differential diagnosis (Ortner, 2008; Redfern & Roberts, 2019) and careful consideration of the taphonomic processes that can mimic trauma. The next step in the analysis for those interested in social violence (defined below) is to offer a detailed reconstruction and interpretation of the circumstances that led to the individual becoming a victim of violence. Always challenging, interpretations of social violence from skeletal remains is key in providing data that informs us on the origin and evolution of violence in human groups and comprehending how and why violence is used by humans to solve a problem or produce an effect (see Martin & Harrod, 2016 for overview).

Violence has many definitions and causes but invariably includes some form of assault on individuals (Whitehead, 2004). While violence is often physical, it can also cause pain, suffering, and death through emotional and psychological pathways. The World Health Organization (2002) differentiates violence into three categories: self-directed violence, such as suicide; interpersonal violence, including homicides, assaults, and intimate partner violence; and collective violence such as political violence and warfare. While there are many laws, prohibitions, and cultural norms that aim to limit violence, it continues to operate on multiple complex levels in every society during every time period (Martin & Harrod, 2015).

Social violence refers to any type of violence that is culturally meaningful and is enacted and reproduced through the normalization of particular forms of violence and widespread cultural sanctions for the use of violence against specific groups or individuals (Harrod, 2018; Bright, 2020; Standish, 2020). Social violence is patterned or ritualized in terms of how it is manifested, and it is often motivated by political and social agendas that include the targeting of specific individuals and particular (usually marginalized) social groups. Social violence is distinguishable by its ubiquity and familiarity within cultural systems, and for its culturally specific motivations, meanings, historical use, and practices that have significant and historically contingent social impacts on individuals and communities.

Even in small-scale societies, power relations structure a range of violent behaviors within social systems, from gender relations to political alliances, captive-taking, and slavery, to the mechanisms of social control used to create and perpetuate deep inequalities within many societies (Redfern, 2020). The interpretation of violence from trauma and injury on human remains is particularly important for forensic anthropologists and bioarchaeologists who often work with the skeletal remains of people who died at the hands of others (Walker, 2001). Increasingly, researchers present new approaches and methodologies to make violence visible in the archaeological record, which challenge old notions about the nature and direction of violent practices, the relatedness of violence and inequality, and the way power structures how and why violence is used in human groups through time (Knüsel & Smith, 2014; Anderson & Martin, 2018; Harrod, 2018; Tremblay & Reedy, 2020; Mant et al., 2021).

Importantly, we must recognize that our perception and interpretation of violence in the past is shaped by our own social conditioning, cultural frameworks, and lived experiences. What is considered violence in one society may not be so in others. Furthermore, the culturally specific meaning of violence depends on the perspective from which one is observing it. Violence generally includes one or more aggressors or perpetrators, one or more victims, and usually several witnesses, bystanders, and survivors (Krohn-Hansen, 1994). Each of these participants perceives and interprets violent acts from their own, contextually contingent perspectives and frameworks, and can easily shift roles in the perpetration of the violent act depending on context and perspective. This perspective allows us to understand that violent behaviors overlap and, consequently, that a descriptive or superficial examination of trauma and violence is not revealing of the social impact of violent actions. Formulating careful interpretations of social violence is best carried out using multiple lines of evidence to account for the multiplicity of meanings given to violent behaviors. What is needed is the development of a broader appreciation that allows us to compare the evidence provided by our studies across different groups.

Age, sex, social identity and standing, place of birth, ancestry, and larger social, ideological, and political structures all must be simultaneously considered as one moves from trauma on bones to interpretations of social violence (Bright, 2020). We must also consider the patterning, severity, and type of trauma on bodies in the context of understanding the antemortem (before death), the perimortem (around the time of death), and the postmortem (after death) context. This includes the treatment and manipulation of bodies by the living, the mortuary context of bodies, the cultural and environmental context, and the historicity of violent events within the cultural system. The data obtained from skeletal remains and ethnohistorical evidence can be compared to ethnographic data (e.g., the Human Relations Area Files [HRAF]), ethnological research (e.g., Ember & Ember, 1997), and other resources demonstrating culturally specific forms of violence and their motivations to detect analogous patterns that can inform our interpretations of the skeletal data (Klaus, 2012; Geller, 2021). Therefore, going from trauma on bones to comprehending large-scale social and political motivations for using violence is not straight-forward and requires many and diverse datasets, but there are methods and approaches that help structure our analysis and guide interpretations.

Through the integration of biological and contextual data with social theory, bioarchaeologists have identified and interpreted a broad range of violent practices, including warfare, ritualized combat, hand to hand fighting, raids and ransacking, massacres, torture, executions, witchcraft, captive-taking, slavery, anthropophagy, intimate partner and child abuse, scalping, and human sacrifice (Martin & Harrod, 2016; Redfern, 2020). Distinguishing trauma due to social violence versus trauma from accidents and other causes is similarly challenging but possible by integrating all available skeletal and contextual information to identify socially significant patterns in the skeletal data (Redfern & Roberts, 2019). Integrating biological and contextual data within theoretical frameworks provides us different ways of thinking about the patterns we observe in skeletal remains. Case studies in edited volumes such as *The Bioarchaeology of Violence* (Martin et al., 2013) and *The Routledge Handbook of the Bioarchaeology of Human Conflict* (Smith, 2014), *The Bioarchaeology of Structural Violence. A Theoretical Framework for Industrial Era Inequality* (Tremblay & Reedy, 2020), offer great examples of theoretically informed empirical analyses that demonstrate how violence manifests in a wide variety of forms and expressions and is historically contingent and specific to time and place. In this chapter, we offer overviews of the various evidence for and interpretations of violence offered by bioarchaeological studies of the social role and cultural meaning of different manifestations of violence in ancient small-scale human groups.

Bones to Bodies to Behavior: The Value of Social Theory

The study of human skeletal remains is an evidence-based field of study, and the goal of many studies utilizing skeletal remains is to elucidate how people in the past lived and died within their societies, how populations changed over time, and how societies interacted within and between regions (Schrader & Torres-Rouff, 2020). Social theory provides a framework for clarifying the ways in which behavior and social processes are entwined and the motivations for certain behaviors over others. Identifying culturally specific patterns of behavior provides a way to move from the bone data to bodies that demonstrate agency and resistance and that are also broken by subordination and violence (Gowland & Kacki, 2020). From these violated bodies, we can reconstruct some of the more salient aspects of the culture that may provide insight into the motivation for violence and who, in any given society, benefits from violence. Social theories are frameworks that help focus the attention on particular facets of human social interactions, organization, and behaviors (Powers, 2010:5). Without social theories, studies are simply descriptions of the trauma found on bone (Klaus, 2012).

While osteological methods provide the raw data, social theory provides the framework from which to generate questions about human behavior that can be answered with those data. The development of the biocultural approach in bioarchaeology provided an integrative theoretical framework for the inclusion of data from the cultural and environmental context in the interpretation of patterns in the skeletal data (see Martin et al., 2013 for an in-depth review of the biocultural framework). What has developed from the biocultural approach is a body of scholarship that simultaneously examines the interactions between human biology, the natural and built environments, cultural innovations, adaptations and shortcomings, and changes in these relationships over time (Leatherman & Goodman, 2020). Researchers using this model have shown that violence is best understood as a form of social behavior (Martin et al., 2013; Martin & Harrod, 2015).

The importance of using social theory as a guiding framework to move from descriptive data to interpretations that have broader significance cannot be understated. It is the combination of standardized methods, robust empirical data, and social theory that takes bioarchaeology beyond simple descriptions of skeletal data. Geller (2021) provides an extensive overview of social theories used in bioarchaeology, many of which refer to forms of violence that underscore power relationships leading to inequality, subordination, and death. Therefore, it is the use of biological and contextual data integrated with social theory that permits bioarchaeological analyses to go beyond descriptions of violence to interpreting its social meaning (Klaus, 2012; Perez, 2012; Geller, 2021).

Is it Violence or Something Else?

Violence-related traumas are injuries sustained in the context of interpersonal conflict wherein participants generally use hands or other expedient weapons to inflict injury. Violence-related injuries are broadly classified into two categories: intragroup and intergroup violence. But how do we tell the difference between trauma sustained in violence-related contexts versus those received because of accidents or occupation-related hazards? As discussed by Byrnes and Gaddis (Chapter 13, this volume), the type, severity, number, timing, and location of fractures are important for distinguishing between violence-related and accidental trauma. Some types and locations of trauma are more diagnostic of violence-related injuries, and others more frequently reflect accidental injuries.

To help with ascertaining the cause and manner of traumatic skeletal injuries in the past, we (Harrod and Martin) have argued elsewhere that bioarchaeologists must incorporate two perspectives/approaches: ethnography and forensics (Harrod et al., 2012). Furthermore, Martin and Anderson (2014:5) state that "These integrated bioarchaeological–forensic approaches are useful in constructing the contexts in which violence takes place. Ultimately, both subdisciplines aim to reconstruct and explain complex human behavior and so can benefit from directly sharing case studies, methods of analysis, and theoretical approaches to interpretation." In both bioarchaeology and forensic anthropology studies, the further use of ethnographic research on the causes and context of trauma as well as archival resources can provide what Walker and colleagues call "ethnobioarchaeology" (Walker et al., 1998:389; Harrod, 2012; Harrod et al., 2012). The value of this approach is that we can observe injuries and the contexts in which they are received in extant small-scale societies who engage in different types of violence and compare the trends observed to potential analogous patterns in prehistoric skeletal remains.

In ancient populations, trauma to the skull – especially injuries located in the area between the Frankfort plane and the parallel line that passes through the skull at glabella (hat brim line) – are more susceptible to being classified as direct violence than trauma located in the postcranial (back of the head) region (Kremer et al., 2008; Guyomarc'h et al., 2010), which are usually associated with accidental etiologies (Lambert & Welker, 2019), however, this is not always the rule. For example, Harrod et al. (2012) used questionnaires and body diagrams to document and map the location of all nonlethal traumatic injuries sustained by the Turkana, an extant herding community in Kenya. The authors documented 38 individuals' age, sex, status, and other lifestyle variables with the questionnaire and used the body diagrams to map the locations of various traumatic injuries and the specific causes and contexts that resulted in those injuries. Studies by Harrod and colleagues (2012) and contemporary ethnographic studies of hunter-gatherer-forager societies like the Hadza in Tanzania (see Pollom et al., 2020) demonstrate how violence in small-scale societies is complex, nuanced, and patterned according to individual, sociocultural, ideological, and political factors. Therefore, bioarchaeological analyses are significant because they inform the models and theoretical frameworks bioarchaeologists use to interpret osteological and contextual information and test hypotheses about the social processes that created differential patterns of health, disease, and traumatic injury among past peoples.

Patterns in the location (e.g., cranial, appendicular), number, timing, and type of trauma on human skeletal remains are fundamental datasets from which violence and its meaning in the past is interpreted. Type, timing, and location of cranial traumata are particularly useful for interpreting the nature of their production, as well as the circumstances wherein they were acquired. As an early example, Walker (1989) demonstrated ways that cranial depression fractures can be diagnostic of violence-related activities and reveal information about the cultural context and motivation for particular types of violence. He analyzed the distribution of healed cranial depression fractures from 598 individuals from the Channel Islands of precontact southern California (AD 600–1400). Combining the osteological data with archaeological context and ethnohistoric documents, Walker ruled out warfare or raiding as an explanation for the comparatively equal distribution of cranial trauma observed between males and females exhibiting elite status mortuary contexts. Instead, he argued that the cranial trauma was likely produced by ritualized fighting between elite adult members of both sexes. Therefore, the patterning of trauma between individuals combined with cultural context informs us on whether the trauma was sustained in violent or occupation-related contexts and whether it is patterned according to age, sex, gender, or other biosocial categories.

Bioarchaeology's engagement with theoretical lenses in the interpretation of trauma and violence in the past reveals the inherent complex factors and circumstances exposing individuals to risk for injury and experiences with violence. For example, Mant et al. (2021) compare osteobiographical case studies of two unclaimed individuals from different geographical and temporal contexts and interpret them using the intersectional methodology outlined by de la Cova (2020). This four-step methodology incorporates all available anthropological, biological, historical, and sociopolitical datasets into the interpretation of observed traumatic injury on individual skeletal remains. The two individuals evaluated in this study lived during the 19th and 20th centuries, were of low socioeconomic status, died in public hospitals, and exhibited injury recidivism. They are represented by a white adult male (TC 361) from the Robert J. Terry skeletal anatomical collection with associated contextual information, and an old adult female (RLPO5 247) from the Royal London Hospital, Center for Human Bioarchaeology without any associated contextual information.

The osteological analysis of TC 361 revealed injury recidivism likely received in contexts of both interpersonal conflict and accidental trauma. The biographical and historical contextual analysis of this individual revealed a lifetime of personal tragedies and lifestyle choices that intersected and precipitated his eventual impoverishment, alcohol abuse and dependency, poor health outcomes (including poor bone health), risk for repeated traumatic injuries, and eventual death and unclaimed status. The osteological analysis of RLPO5 247 also revealed injury recidivism likely produced as the result of accidental trauma and reflected injury patterns typically experienced by older females.

Through their intersectional approach, Mant and coworkers (2021) demonstrated how the differences and intersections of these individuals' age, sex, gender, socioeconomic status, race, physical and mental health, and their life histories affected their osteological health, overall health outcomes, and resulted in their traumatic injury patterns, deaths, and unclaimed status (see also Chapter 26, this volume). In doing so, they show how the broken bones observed on the individuals' skeletons are a product of the intersection of the unique biological, histomorphological, sociocultural, environmental, and behavioral factors framing these individuals' lived experiences in the context of structural inequality. This study highlights the importance of theoretically informed trauma analyses and utility of osteobiographical approaches for identifying the presence and mechanisms of traumatic injury and inferring the unique biosocial factors that precipitate the physiological and sociocultural events that underwrite broken bones.

Therefore, bioarchaeological methods emphasizing skeletal data, mortuary context, and archaeological reconstruction provide a means to answer questions about patterns of violence going back thousands of years. Walker's (2001) summary of bioarchaeological approaches to violence suggest that the analysis of violence must not begin and end with the discovery of fractures or implements causing trauma but must integrate contextual data that distinguishes violence from accidental or occupational injuries and utilizes theoretical frameworks to ascertain the underlying motivations and cultural effects of violence.

Social Violence Between Groups in Small-Scale Societies

Paleopathologists and bioarchaeologists look to small-scale societies to understand the deep past and the origins and use of violence. By small-scale, we refer to early foraging, non-intensive horticulturalist/agriculturalist, and non-city state societies with small populations and (typically) no written records.

In small-scale societies, ritualized acts of violence are intertwined with ideology, socioeconomics, kinship, and masculinity (Martin, 2021). Abbink's (2000) study of the Suri in Ethiopia showed that violence can have many functions that benefit the larger community. He showed how ritualized acts of violence functioned as a "circuit breaker" for young males. While the Suri are traditionally considered to be a "violent" group, Abbink demonstrated that when placed within its broader cultural and historical context, violence among the Suri was a productive response to local and regional tensions and a pathway for males to obtain wives, cattle, and other resources necessary for a successful life.

In other small-scale societies, like the Yukpa (Halbmayer, 2001) and the Apache (Schröder, 2001), violence was just one of many culturally sanctioned, predictable, and managed social activities that facilitated group cohesion and built identity. In culturally sanctioned violence, there are often specific rules and regulations concerning the performance of raiding, warfare, ritualized fighting, and other violent practices (Martin, 2021). Therefore, in many small-scale societies, violence is an important part of socialization for young males and is seen as a positive and necessary social activity (Maringira, 2021).

In 2006, Fry examined evidence of lethal aggression in a large ethnographic sample, concluding that all complex and unequal societies of food gatherers participated in war, but most of the mobile foragers in the sample did not (Fry, 2006). Fry and Soderberg (2013) examined ethnographic data from mobile gatherer gang societies. Within these 21 populations, they extracted data on 148 lethal events, where 55% of these involved a victim and a murderer. Of the 148 events, 85% of them involved participants from the same society and instigations that included revenge killings and interpersonal disputes.

Thus, trauma to the body may bear witness to violence, but interpretation of that trauma is far more complex. Because pain, discomfort, disability, and death are not universally named nor experienced identically cross-culturally (Dominguez, 2015; Martin & Harrod, 2015), interpreting the meaning and motivations behind violent acts is challenging. Yet, there are aspects of violence between groups that can be interpreted. Some examples are presented here.

Warfare and Massacres

Intergroup violence (violence between two or more different groups) includes activities like warfare, massacres, raiding, feuding, and ambushes (Durrant, 2011). Massacres are often associated with warfare and raiding in small-scale societies, with convincing evidence for massacres occurring as early as 13,000 years ago (Erdal, 2012).

Massacres, defined by Alfsdotter et al. (2018:428) as "an act of intentional murder upon a mass of people who were not prepared for battle, with the killing being conducted by a group," have considerable time depth, variability in perpetration, and served contextually contingent social, political, and ideological purposes. Interpreting the social meaning behind massacres begins with identifying the victims (e.g., age, sex, ancestry) and their social and genetic relatedness to one another and other populations. The incorporation of paleogenomic analyses enhances researchers' abilities to identify genetic relationships between victims of massacres, providing insight into whether victims were genetically related to one another and/or to the perpetrators.

Evaluating the postmortem treatment of victims of violence has also been used to explore culturally specific meanings of violence. Alfsdotter (et al., 2018; 2019) and Alfsdotter and Kjellström (2020) discuss evidence of a massacre that took place within the Sandby borg ringfort (AD 400–550) on the island of Öland in modern southeast Sweden. Alfsdotter (2019:433) notes that the remains lack indicators offensive-related trauma, appear to have been killed with few (expedient) lethal blows, and show no evidence of mutilation or trophy taking. This suggests that the victims were taken by surprise and that the purpose of the attack was to kill. Alfsdotter and Kjellström (2020) also present a taphonomic analysis of the massacred individuals using a combination of techniques, including skeletal element preservation via zoning (Knüsel & Outram, 2004), weathering stages (Behrensmeyer, 1978), fracture analysis (Outram, 2002), and archaeothanatology, to determine the original depositional context of the massacred individuals. Also known as *anthropologie de terrain*, archaeothanatology is the in situ taphonomic analysis of a body that considers the postmortem manipulation and decomposition process of a corpse within mortuary contexts (Alfsdotter & Kjellström, 2020:267; Duday et al., 2009). Alfsdotter and Kjellström (2020) conclude that the spatial distribution, random positioning of the bodies, presence of rodent and carnivore gnawing, weathering, and the lack of evidence that the remains were manipulated from their primary depositional context by other humans suggest that the victims were left exposed and unburied. To understand how these remains were perceived by those who potentially witnessed the events and why these remains were left unburied, Alfsdotter (2019), Alfsdotter et al. (2018), and Alfsdotter and Kjellström (2020) frame the lack of burial as a deliberate and aggressive social tactic designed to manipulate the social and spatial memory of survivors and witnesses and to redraw the social and territorial landscape (Alfsdotter, 2019:438).

Novak et al. (2021) also offer deeply contextualized analyses of trauma. Here, the authors combine bioarchaeological analyses with genome-wide DNA analyses to extrapolate the relationships and identities of 38 out of the 41 victims of a 6,200-year-old massacre recovered from an Eneolithic (Copper Age) mass burial in Potočani, Croatia. The bioarchaeological analyses of the recovered individuals revealed that the group was represented by adult males and females and subadults from a wide range of age groups. At least 13 (6 subadults, 3 adult males, 4 adult females) individuals exhibit perimortem cranial trauma to the back and side of the head, which were inflicted by different weapons and likely by numerous attackers. The archaeological context suggests that the collective group were all interred during a single depositional event. A paleogenomic analyses revealed that the majority of the victims were not members of a closely related family group but likely represented a large farming community of several diverse lineages, were members of a homogenous population, and therefore unlikely to be immigrants to the region. Novak et al. (2021) conclude that the Potočani mass burial represents an indiscriminate massacre of an unrelated whole or part of a community and provides further evidence that large-scale massacres were a significant and important social process in pre-state societies.

Captives and Slaves

Violence against females and children from raiding, captivity, and enslavement, documented well in the context of the African slave trade in colonial America (Singleton, 1995; Blakey, 2001), was not uncommon in the past and has been documented in many early societies (see Brooks, 2002; Marshall, 2015; Cameron, 2016). Wilkinson and Van Wagenen (1993) identified evidence of precontact raiding and captives among groups ancestral to the modern Iroquois at Riviere aux Vase in Michigan (AD 1000–1300). When they mapped the location and number of nonlethal cranial trauma across age and sex categories, they found that three times more females than males exhibited healed cranial trauma. They also found that cranial trauma among males tended to concentrate on the forehead, whereas females experienced cranial trauma to all regions of the head (Wilkinson & Van Wagenen, 1993). Wilkinson (1997) used the combined cranial trauma data, ethnohistoric accounts, and archaeological context to argue that the cranial trauma data represents interpersonal violence targeted at young adult females and was perpetrated using blunt objects. Based on the ethnographic record for the region, he also argues that the violence perpetrated against these women reflects a well-established pattern of female captive-taking practices that included subduing and coercing women into submission, leading to acceptance of their captive status through nonlethal violence.

Based on similarities in the mortuary contexts of adult females with healed cranial trauma to adult females who did not have healed cranial trauma, Wilkinson (1997) posits that female captives who were integrated into their captive society were accorded similar status to non-captive female members of the group. Therefore, using multiple lines of evidence, Wilkinson (1997) shows how targeted nonlethal violence was used as a form of social control and how the victims of this violence survived and gained social mobility. By combining trauma and health data from burials, alongside mortuary and archaeological contexts and ethnohistoric resources, this case study demonstrates how violence is not only an expedient tool for social control but also a dialectical relationship between perpetrators, victims, and witnesses.

Social Violence within Groups in Small-Scale Societies

Interpersonal violence is defined as "violence between family members and intimates, and violence between acquaintances and strangers that is not intended to further the aims of any formally defined group or cause" (Waters et al., 2004). Although violence within a group can be between any member of the community (e.g., domestic abuse or child abuse), the motivations behind male-on-male interpersonal violence is arguably different. While it can vary, it is typically motivated by competition for females, status, prestige, and resources, or retaliation and revenge (Wrangham & Peterson, 1996; Gat, 2006). Using careful demographic and skeletal indicators of injury and trauma, violence against women and violence against children present some avenues of analysis that aid in exploring interpersonal violence.

Gendered Violence

Gendered violence has significant time depth and variable manifestations across time and space (Agarwal & Wesp, 2017; Zuckerman & Crandall, 2019; O'Toole et. al., 2020). In its variable ideations, manifestations, and applications, gendered violence is best described, for the purposes of this chapter, as the intentional exertion of control (e.g., physical, social, psychological) over the biological lives and functions of others through relational, organizational, and/or political structures predicated on their sex, gender identity, sexual orientation, ethnicity, and socioeconomic status within social systems (O'Toole et al., 2020:xiii). Before discussing how gendered violence is identified and interpreted in bioarchaeological analyses, we must define what we mean by the terms *sex* and *gender* as they relate to individual identity and lived experience and how these categories of identity are reconstructed in bioarchaeological investigations.

In bioarchaeology, sex is understood to be a biological category derived from the phenotypic expression of genetic information enabling sexual reproduction, with sex categories assigned based on the perception and interpretation of secondary sex traits, sex chromosomes, or gonads (Sofaer, 2012; Hollimon, 2017; Zuckerman & Crandall, 2019). Methodologically, the assignment of sex to skeletons is based on the assessment of morphological characteristics of the cranium and pelvis, overall size (long bone lengths), robusticity (Buikstra & Ubelaker, 1994), and metric characteristics of the postcranial skeleton (Spradley & Jantz, 2011).

Gender is understood to be a biosocial category distinct from, but related to, biological sex (Zuckerman & Crandall, 2019). It is assumed that the perception of sex-based differences (i.e. an individual's "maleness" or "femaleness") over an individual's life course plays a role in the assignment and socialization of individuals into particular gender roles and gender identities (Perry, 2004; Agarwal, 2017; Wesp, 2017). Gender is best described as a practice, rather than a static state, that is manifested in the performance of defined social roles, behaviors, and relationships (Hollimon, 2017; Wesp, 2017, and see Chapter 24, this volume).

While individual bodies are lived differently and distinctly and each individual's gendered experience is unique, there are broader trends of similarity that social institutions (e.g., gender systems) constrain into repetitive patterns of activity, behavior, and treatment that become incorporated into the bodies of those who perform them. It is these patterns that are the target for bioarchaeological analyses of gender (Joyce, 2017:5). The goal of bioarchaeological analyses of gender is not to simply describe sex-based differences in the past, but to interrogate the intersection of individual biology, environmental contexts, and social institutions in order to explore how social processes contribute to the production of differential experiences of disease, workload, trauma, and violence within and between individuals and groups. As a result, bioarchaeological analyses of gendered experiences are fundamentally comparative in that they involve a multi-scalar approach that integrates individual case studies (e.g., osteobiographies) and population-level analyses with archaeological and mortuary data and, whenever possible, ethnographic and ethnohistoric knowledge to capture the subtleties and culturally specific manifestations of gendered violence (O'Toole et al., 2020:1).

An example of this approach can be found in Redfern (2006). Here, the author discusses bioarchaeological evidence for female-perpetuated interpersonal violence in Iron Age Britain (c. 750BC-AD43). Fifty-one adult female individuals recovered from cemetery contexts at several different sites in Dorset England and were evaluated for the presence, patterning, and distribution of direct violence in the form of sharp force injuries, fractures, and injury recidivism. Redfern's (2006) research questions center around the paucity of studies addressing female relationships and engagement with violence in Iron Age Britain, despite the consistent references to it in Celtic literature and mythology. She found that there were no statistically significant differences between the number of males and females who exhibited observable fractures in the Dorset sample and that, based on the type and distribution of perimortem and antemortem injuries on crania and extremities, the majority of the injuries observed were delivered via interpersonal violence. Redfern (2006:9) interprets this to suggest that females may have been active participants in violence and/or were members of a group at risk for being victims of violence in Iron Age Britain. She then compared her data to that from several other national British Iron Age cemeteries, female burials from Aymyrlyg, an Iron Age cemetery in southern Siberia with archaeological evidence for female warriors, and to modern clinical datasets on domestic violence, warfare, and small-scale skirmishes. These comparative analyses collectively suggested that the fractures and sharp-force trauma patterns observed on the Dorset females are consistent with participation – as both perpetrators and victims – of interpersonal violence and that violence played a role in female lifeways in Iron Age Britain.

In bioarchaeology, the estimation of sex of skeletal remains is an important step in the construction of the biological profile at both the individual and population level and is used to generate empirical data that can be used in comparative frameworks for interrogating observed patterns of pathology, activity, and trauma. Specifically, for trauma analysis, like many other pathological bone lesions, the occurrence and consequence of a lesion in the musculoskeletal system will be different depending on the biological characteristics of the individual and the factors associated with their gender and lifestyle. Mainly, the changes associated with age have an impact on the morphology, size, and composition of bone. Age-related changes also have an impact on an individual's activity patterns and nutritional and occupational status, which influence the prevalence and nature of fracture patterns observed. These variations influence a bone's response to energy and the direction of external force, as well as an individual's ability to recover from injury. Therefore, an assessment of accumulated skeletal fractures throughout life provides opportunities to understand injury over time, and not as a singular and static event (Glencross, 2011).

Providing important methodological notes, however, Agarwal (2017), Geller (2017), and Sofaer (2012) have argued that the common method of dividing skeletal assemblages into distinct sex categories as the *first* step in bioarchaeological analyses automatically conflates biological sex and gender and could artificially position biological sex as the only critical variable structuring experience. To avoid this, these scholars recommend researchers analyze collected skeletal data with the estimated sex categories initially combined to assess whether observed patterns truly vary by sex (as opposed to other biosocial categories such as age or status) before examining within and between sexed patterns. By examining these patterns through the lens of gender, we can interpret the relative importance or insignificance of sex with respect to other aspects of social identity (i.e. age, social status, occupation) and begin to explore differential experiences of health, disease, and trauma in the past. Hence, it is through the contextualization and theoretical interpretation of observed patterns within and between social and biological categories that allow paleopathologists and bioarchaeologists to understand gender, gendered behaviors, and gendered violence in the past (Knudson & Stojanowski, 2008).

Violence Against Children

Child abuse, commonly referred to as child maltreatment today, involves the neglect and harm of children by adults responsible for their caretaking. In the US alone, the rate of abuse is staggering. In 2019, an estimated 656,000 children were victims of child abuse and neglect, rendering a victimization rate of 8.9 victims per 1,000 children in the national population (U.S. Department of Health and Human Services, 2019:20), a statistic that might have increased during the current pandemic (Kovler et al., 2021).

Tracking child abuse in modern society is difficult because it is often caregivers or trusted adults who are the perpetrators. According to Kleinman (1998:214), "A fall is also the most common event offered as an explanation for significant inflicted injury in childhood." In regard to head trauma related to falls, Brogdon (1998:302–303) asserts that falls from low heights, such as from baby chairs or tables, sofas, and beds rarely cause linear fractures and are usually not associated with intracranial damage. Fields such as radiology, medical pathology, and forensics, have helped to develop indicators of child abuse and means by which injuries can be differentiated from those arising from accidents.

Patterns of child abuse include several key features: (1) multiple injuries over the course of the lifetime of a young child; (2) fractures to the same bones of specific areas of the body; (3) and evidence of a fracture that does not heal because of repeated injury to the same location (Brogdon, 1998; Kleinman, 1998; Kleinman, 2015, see also Chapter 23, this volume for discussion on structural violence and children). Hence, recognizing the pattern of trauma is arguably the most important element to identifying child abuse. Evidence of healed injuries is key to the identification of child abuse. Therefore, it is important to understand how healing differs among children. According to Symes and colleagues (2012:358), osteogenic (bone-forming) activity in the periosteum and endosteum of bones is very high during infancy and childhood, which progressively decreases each year to a lower, more constant rate in young adulthood where it remains until old age. This means that children of different ages heal at different rates, which is important because very young children may appear to have a long history of trauma based on evidence of repeated injury on their bones, while the chronology of abuse may in fact be much shorter.

Violence as a Product of Inequalities

Medical anthropology has contributed a great deal to framing violence in ways that assist paleopathologists and bioarchaeologists (Klaus, 2012; Perez, 2012). Violence that is intricately part of the political, economic, or religious structures of a society is known as structural violence. Paul Farmer asserts that "Social factors including gender, ethnicity ("race"), and socioeconomic status may each play a role in rendering individuals and groups vulnerable to extreme human suffering…simultaneous consideration of various social "axes" is imperative in efforts to discern a political economy of brutality" (Farmer, 2003). Recipients (or victims) of culturally sanctioned violence are often those who do not have access to resources, decision-making, and capital. Structural violence can be viewed as a tactic that creates harm for some individuals based on social, political, or economic processes within the culture and can become institutionalized, repetitive, and ritualistic (Galtung, 1990).

An example of institutionalized violence can be found in Klaus (2012) (see also Chapter 22, this volume). Here, the author systematically collected data on trauma (healed and unhealed blunt and sharp force trauma) and general health (developmental dental defects and oral health, subadult growth, adult stature, anemia, infections, osteoarthritis, and age-at-death) to compare health profiles at the individual and population level within precolonial and postcolonial burials in Peru. Surprisingly, he did not find significant differences in direct violence in the form of trauma in either the precolonial or postcolonial groups. In the postcolonial group, however, he found that new rules and cultural pressures from colonizers were associated with statistically significant increases in nutritional problems, infections, and osteoarthritis in adults. Hard labor in the local gypsum mines, living in close quarters, eating contaminated food (all parts of a systematic structural system of violence) were the likely cause of increases in chronic health problems. Postcolonial children in the cemeteries did not show increased poor health compared to their precolonial counterparts. Klaus (2012) suggests that this may be because postcolonial children died younger and faster, not surviving long enough to accumulate indicators of stress on their bones.

Ritual, Performance, and Symbolism

Violence, in both interpersonal and collective contexts, in small-scale societies is often performative rather than being deviant, erratic, or episodic. It can, in fact, be deeply imbued with meaning to the participants that become ritualized. Ritualized violence plays many roles and has well-known effects, including reducing anxiety, boosting confidence, and communicating culturally specific meaning about the violence in that context (Whitehead, 2004). The following sections provide an example of the complex, performative, and ritualized nature of some acts of violence.

Head Hunting/Trophy Taking

Head hunting and trophy taking are common forms of ritual violence found worldwide in archaeological contexts (Chacon & Dye, 2007) and within ethnographic accounts that conceptualize these practices within cultural ideologies (Haddon, 1901; Hodson, 1909; Durham, 1923). Bioarchaeologists working in South America have demonstrated how the human head was a crucial aspect of social and political interaction (Forgey & Williams, 2005; Tung, 2008; Tung & Knudson, 2008; 2010). In Borneo, Okumura and Siew (2013) identified headhunting practices in a sample of 112 individuals represented by crania and/or mandibles. The sample was comprised of young adult males and females. Evidence of sharp force trauma was observed on more than half of the individuals, along with evidence of decapitation. Most of the skulls showed some evidence of burning and a significant number show evidence of drilled perforations (likely to put a string through). Osteological evidence and ethnographic data suggest that these skulls exemplify trophy taking, rather than being an example of ancestor veneration. Ethnographically, the authors found that acquiring trophy heads among the ethnic groups of Borneo was and is a significant behavior within their cultures.

Scalping

Similar to acquiring trophy heads, scalping has also been interpreted as a ritual act associated with interregional or interethnic violence. Scalping has been recorded in ethnohistoric accounts (Owsley & Berryman, 1975; Axtell & Sturtevant, 1980), representing a symbol of conquest and revenge and a spiritual token of the deceased's captured power. The behavior has also been noted in the bioarchaeological record (Neumann, 1940; Allen et al., 1985; Toyne, 2011; Baustian et al., 2012). For example, Toyne (2011) examined evidence of scalping (and healing) on skeletal remains excavated from Kuelap in the highlands of Peru. This precolonial site has been of particular interest to archaeologists due to its massive stone wall and its defensive architecture. There is also evidence of a stratified society with ceremonial elites living in the village. Skeletal remains were examined and cut mark morphology and pathological lesions were analyzed. A young adult female and older male showed evidence of scalping with early stage healing. This suggests that these individuals survived the event for at least a short time. It is possible that death resulted from infection to the exposed underlying bone. The adult male also showed evidence of cut marks with an inflammatory response to the outer table of the cranium. This individual appears to have survived the scalping for a longer period than the female.

The practice of scalping persisted after European contact in some areas of the Americas, often in the context of ritual or ceremonial behavior. For example, Dozier (1970) discusses the importance of symbolically consuming the scalps of fallen warriors in the Women's Scalp Association among the Pueblo people in the U.S. Southwest.

Anthropophagy

Anthropophagy, more colloquially known as cannibalism, is found in many cultures across time. Present in a wide variety of settings, its expression is highly varied. The long history of anthropophagy underscores that it is not a simple or easily understandable phenomenon, and that there are multiple cultural factors and practices motivating the practice of consuming human flesh. Anthropophagy is present in the archaeological record, both before European contact and after. Two of the most prominent archaeological examples are the highly processed remains found in the U.S. Southwest (Turner et al., 1999) and the infamous doomed expedition of the Donner Party in the Sierra Nevada mountain range (Dixon et al., 2010).

Jones et al. (2015) also provide an excellent bioarchaeological case-study examining the underlying motivations for anthropophagy in the Lau skeletal collection from prehistoric Fiji. Skeletal remains from midden and burial contexts were examined and compared. The authors examined sharp force trauma patterns. Almost all the individuals exhibited cut marks, and the patterning and distribution of the cut marks suggested dismemberment and muscle removal, particularly at the joints. Isotopic data indicated that the majority of the Lauan diet was plant based, with small amounts of meat protein consumed. The authors conclude that if anthropophagy occurred among these groups, it was likely non-nutritive and possibly nonviolent.

While motivations for the behavior traditionally include nutritional, ideological, and ritual factors, the authors present a complex view of anthropophagy as a form of violation as well as veneration.

Conclusion

The approaches discussed here provide nuanced and a deeper perspectives about the ways in which violence is integrated within cultural practices. We advocate for the development of research questions and strategies that will help identify the culturally specific characteristics of violence and that will examine how violence is embedded in other social processes such as subsistence activities, health status, gender roles, technologies, climate change, migration, inequality, power structures, and political-economic processes. Social violence carried out and perpetrated individually or in groups not only involves physical trauma, but it also reflects norms and motivating factors. Any interpretation of trauma must include deep and rich evaluations of mortuary and cultural contexts. In small-scale societies, violence (both lethal and nonlethal) is expressed in diverse and complex ways precisely because it is interlinked with and dependent upon ideologies associated with its purpose and meaning. Using fine-grained biocultural analyses, culture-specific patterns of violence can be better interpreted.

References

Abbink, J. (2000). Restoring the balance violence and culture among the Suri of Southern Ethiopia. In Abbink, J. & Aijmer, G. (Eds.), *Meanings of Violence*, pp. 77–100. Abingdon: Routledge.

Agarwal, S. C. (2016). Bone morphologies and histories: life course approaches in bioarchaeology. *American Journal of Physical Anthropology* 159:130–149. https://doi.org/10.1002/ajpa.22905.

Agarwal, S. C. (2017). Understanding sex-and gender-related patterns of bone loss and health in the past. In Agarwal, S. C. & Wesp, J. K. (Eds.) *Exploring Sex and Gender in Bioarchaeology*, pp. 165–188. University of New Mexico Press.

Alfsdotter, C. (2019). Social implications of unburied corpses from intergroup conflicts: postmortem agency following the Sandby borg massacre. *Cambridge Archaeological Journal* 29(3):427–442. https://doi.org/10.1017/S0959774319000039.

Alfsdotter, C. & Kjellström, A. (2020). A taphonomic interpretation of the postmortem fate of the victims following the massacre at Sandby Borg, Sweden. *Bioarchaeology International* 3(4):262–282. https://doi.org/10.5744/bi.2019.1016.

Alfsdotter, C., Papmehl-Dufay, L. & Victor, H. (2018). A moment frozen in time: evidence of a late fifth-century massacre at Sandby borg. *Antiquity* 92(362):421–436. https://doi.org/10.15184/aqy.2018.21.

Allen, W. H., Merbs, C. F. & Birkby, W. H. (1985). Evidence for prehistoric scalping at Nuvakwewtaqa (Chavez Pass) and Grasshopper Ruin, Arizona. In Merbs, C. F. & Miller, R. (Eds.), *Health and Disease in the Prehistoric Southwest*, pp. 23–41. Arizona State University Anthropological Research Papers No. 34.

Anderson, C. P. & Martin, D. L. (2018). *Massacres: Bioarchaeology and Forensic Anthropology Approaches*. University Press of Florida. https://muse.jhu.edu/book/62728.

Axtell, J. & Sturtevant, W. C. (1980). The unkindest cut, or who invented scalping. *The William and Mary Quarterly* 37(3):451–472. https://doi.org/10.2307/1923812.

Baustian, K. M., Harrod, R. P., Osterholtz, A. J. & Martin, D. L. (2012). Battered and abused: analysis of trauma at grasshopper pueblo (AD 1275–1400). *International Journal of Paleopathology* 2(2):102–111. https://doi.org/10.1016/j.ijpp.2012.09.006.

Behrensmeyer, A. K. (1978). Taphonomic and ecologic information from bone weathering. *Paleobiology* 4(2):150–162. https://doi.org/10.1017/S0094837300005820.

Blakey, M. L. (2001). Bioarchaeology of the African diaspora in the Americas: its origins and scope. *Annual Review of Anthropology* 30(1):387–422. https://doi.org/10.1146/annurev.anthro.30.1.387.

Bright, L. N. (2020). Structural violence: epistemological considerations for bioarchaeology. In Cheverko, C. M., Prince-Buitenhuys, J. R. & Hubbe, M. (Eds.), *Theoretical Approaches in Bioarchaeology*, pp. 131–149. Abingdon: Routledge.

Brogdon, B. G. (1998). The scope of forensic radiology. *Clinics in Laboratory Medicine* 18(2):203–240. https://doi.org/10.1016/S0272-2712(18)30169-0.

Brooks, J. F. (2002). *Captives and Cousins: Slavery, Kinship, and Community in the Southwest Borderlands*. Durham, NC: University of North Carolina Press.

Buikstra, J. E. & Ubelaker, D. H. (1994). *Standards for Data Collection from Human Skeletal Remains: Proceedings of a Seminar at the Field Museum of Natural History*. Arkansas Archeological Survey Research Series, No. 44, Fayetteville, AR.

Cameron, C. M. (2016). *Captives: How Stolen People Changed the World*. University of Nebraska Press.

Chacon, R. J. & Dye, D. H. (2007). Introduction to human trophy taking. In Chacon, R. J. & D. Dye, H. (Eds.), *The Taking and Displaying of Human Body Parts as Trophies by Amerindians*, pp. 5–31. New York: Springer US. https://doi.org/10.1007/978-0-387-48303-0_2.

de la Cova, C. (2020). Making silenced voices speak: restoring neglected and ignored identities in anatomical collections. In Cheverko, C. M., Prince-Buitenhuys, J. R. & Hubbe, M. (Eds.), *Theoretical Approaches in Bioarchaeology*, pp. 150–169. Abingdon: Routledge.

Dixon, K. J., Novak, S. A., Robbins, G., Schablitsky, J. M., Scott, G. R. & Tasa, G. L. (2010). Men, women, and children starving: archaeology of the Donner family camp. *American Antiquity* 75(3):627–656. https://doi.org/10.7183/0002-7316.75.3.627.

Dominguez, V. R. (2015). Violence: anthropologists engaging violence 1980–2012: introduction. *American Anthropologist*, Virtual Issue. https://experts.illinois.edu/en/publications/violence-anthropologists-engaging-violence-1980-2012-introduction.

Dozier, E. P. (1970). *The Pueblo Indians of North America*. New York: Holt, Reinhard, and Winston.

Duday, H., Cipriani, A. M. & Pearce, J. (2009). *The Archaeology of the Dead: Lectures in Archaeothanatology*. Oxford: Oxbow Books.

Durham, M. E. (1923). 11. Head-hunting in the Balkans. *Man* 23:19–21. https://doi.org/10.2307/2788856.

Durrant, R. (2011). Collective violence: an evolutionary perspective. *Aggression and Violent Behavior* 16(5):428–436. https://doi.org/10.1016/j.avb.2011.04.014.

Ember, C. R. & Ember, M. (1997). Violence in the ethnographic record: results of cross cultural research on war and aggression. In Martin, D. L. & Frayer, D. (Eds.), *Troubled Times: Osteological and Archaeological Evidence of Violence*, pp. 1–20. Philadelphia: Gordon and Breach.

Erdal, Ö. D. (2012). A possible massacre at early bronze age Titriş Höyük, Anatolia. *International Journal of Osteoarchaeology* 22(1):1–21. https://doi.org/10.1002/oa.1177.

Farmer, P. (2003). *Pathologies of Power: Health, Human Rights, and the New War on the Poor*. Oakland: University of California Press.

Forgey, K. & Williams, S. R. (2005). Were Nasca trophy heads war trophies or revered ancestors? In Rakita, G. F. M., Buikstra, J. E., Beck, L. A. & Williams, S. R. (Eds.), *Interacting With the Dead: Perspectives on Mortuary Archaeology for the New Millennium*, pp. 251–276. Gainesville: University Press of Florida.

Fry, D. (2006). *The Human Potential for Peace: An Anthropological Challenge to Assumptions about War and Violence*. Oxford: Oxford University Press.

Fry, D. P. & Soderberg, P. (2013). Lethal aggression in mobile forager bands and implications for the origins of war. *Science* 341:270–273.

Galtung, J. (1990). Cultural violence. *Journal of Peace Research* 27(3):291–305. https://doi.org/10.1177/0022343390027003005.

Gat, A. (2006). *War in Human Civilization*. Oxford: Oxford University Press.

Geller, Pamela (2017). *The Bioarchaeology of Socio-Sexual Lives: Queering Common Sense About Sex, Gender, and Sexuality*. New York: Springer International Publishing.

Geller, P. L. (2021). What is intersectionality? In Geller, P. L. (Ed.), *Theorizing Bioarchaeology*, pp. 61–86. New York: Springer International Publishing. https://doi.org/10.1007/978-3-030-70704-0_4.

Glencross, B. A. (2011). Skeletal injury across the life course: towards understanding social agency. In Agarwal, S. C. & Glencross, B. A. (Eds.), *Social Bioarchaeology*, pp. 390–409. London: Blackwell Publishing Ltd.

Gowland, R. & Kacki, S. (2020). Theoretical approaches to bioarchaeology: the view from across the pond. In Cheverko, C. M., Prince-Buitenhuys, J. R. & Hubbe, M. (Eds.), *Theoretical Approaches in Bioarchaeology*, pp. 170–183. Abingdon: Routledge.

Guyomarc'h, P., Campagna-Vaillancourt, M., Kremer, C. & Sauvageau, A. (2010). Discrimination of falls and blows in blunt head trauma: a multi-criteria approach. *Journal of Forensic Sciences* 55(2):423–427.

Haddon, A. C. (1901). *Head-hunters: Black, White, and Brown*. London: Methuen & Company.

Halbmayer, E. (2001). Socio-osmological contexts and forms of violence. In Schmidt, B. E. & Schröder, I. W. (Eds.), *Anthropology of Violence and Conflict*, pp. 49–75. Abingdon: Routledge.

Harrod, R. P. (2012). Ethnobioarchaeology. New Directions in Bioarchaeology, Special Forum. *The SAA Archaeological Record* 12(2):32–34.

Harrod, R. P. (2018). Subjugated in the San Juan Basin: identifying captives in the American Southwest. *KIVA: Journal of Southwestern Anthropology and History* 84(4):480–497.

Harrod, R. P., Liénard, P. & Martin, D. L. (2012). Deciphering violence: the potential of modern ethnography to aid in the interpretation of archaeological populations. In Martin, D. L., Harrod, R. P. & Pérez, V. (Eds.) *The Bioarchaeology of Violence*, pp. 63–80. Gainesville: University of Florida Press.

Hodson, T. C. (1909). Head-hunting among the hill tribes of Assam. *Folklore* 20(2):131–143. https://doi.org/10.1080/0015587X.1909.9719869.

Hollimon, S. E. (2017). Bioarchaeological approaches to non-binary genders: case studies from native North America. In Agarwal, S. C. & Wesp, J. K. (Eds.), *Exploring Sex and Gender in Bioarchaeology*, pp. 51–70. Albuquerque: University of New Mexico Press.

Jones, S., Walsh-Haney, H. & Quinn, R. (2015). Kana Tamata or feasts of men: an interdisciplinary approach for identifying cannibalism in prehistoric Fiji. *International Journal of Osteoarchaeology* 25(2):127–145. https://doi.org/10.1002/oa.2269.

Joyce, R. A. (2017). Sex, gender, and anthropology: moving bioarchaeology outside the subdiscipline. In Agarwal, S. C. & Wesp, J. K. (Eds.), *Exploring Sex and Gender in Bioarchaeology*, pp. 1–14. Albuquerque: University of New Mexico Press.

Klaus, H. D. (2012). The bioarchaeology of structural violence: a theoretical model and a case study. In Martin, D. L., Harrod, R. P. & Pérez, V. R. (Eds.), *The Bioarchaeology of Violence*, pp. 29–62. Gainesville: University Press of Florida.

Kleinman, P. K. (1998). Differential diagnosis III: accidental and obstetric trauma. In Kleinman, P. K. (Ed.). *Diagnostic Imaging of Child Abuse* (2nd ed.), pp. 214–224. London: Elsevier Health Sciences.

Kleinman, P. K. (2015). *Diagnostic Imaging of Child Abuse*. Cambridge: Cambridge University Press.

Knudson, K. J. & Stojanowski, C. M. (2008). New directions in bioarchaeology: recent contributions to the study of human social identities. *Journal of Archaeological Research* 16:397–432.

Knüsel, C. J. & Outram, A. K. (2004). Fragmentation: the zonation method applied to fragmented human remains from archaeological and forensic contexts. *Environmental Archaeology* 9(1):85–98. https://doi.org/10.1179/env.2004.9.1.85.

Knüsel, C. & Smith, M. J. (2014). The Osteology of Conflict: what does it all mean? In Knüsel, C. & Smith, M. J. (Eds.), *The Routledge Handbook of the Bioarchaeology of Human Conflict*, pp. 656–694. Abingdon: Routledge.

Kovler, M. L., Ziegfeld, S., Ryan, L. M., Goldstein, M. A., Gardner, R., Garcia, A. V. & Nasr, I. W. (2021). Increased proportion of physical child abuse injuries at a level I pediatric trauma center during the Covid-19 pandemic. *Child Abuse & Neglect* 116:104756. https://doi.org/10.1016/j.chiabu.2020.104756.

Kremer, C., Racette, S., Dionne, C. -A. & Sauvageau, A. (2008). Discrimination of falls and blows in blunt head trauma: systematic study of the hat brim line rule in relation to skull fractures. *Journal of Forensic Sciences* 53:716–719.

Krohn-Hansen, C. (1994). The anthropology of violent interaction. *Journal of Anthropological Research* 50(4):367–381. https://doi.org/10.1086/jar.50.4.3630559.

Lambert, P. M. & Welker, M. H. (2019). Revisiting traumatic injury risk and agricultural intensification: postcranial fracture frequency at Cerro Oreja in the Moche Valley of north coastal Peru. *American Journal of Physical Anthropology* 169(1):143–151.

Leatherman, T. & Goodman, A. (2020). Building on the biocultural syntheses: 20 years and still expanding. *American Journal of Human Biology* 32(4):e23360. https://doi.org/10.1002/ajhb.23360.

Mant, M., de la Cova, C. & Brickley, M. B. (2021). Intersectionality and trauma analysis in bioarchaeology. *American Journal of Physical Anthropology* 174(4):583–594. https://doi.org/10.1002/ajpa.24226.

Maringira, G. (2021). Soldiers, masculinities, and violence: war and politics. *Current Anthropology* 62(S23):S103–S111. https://doi.org/10.1086/711687.

Marshall, L. W. (2015). *The Archaeology of slavery: A Comparative Approach to Captivity and Coercion*. Southern Illinois University Press, Center for Archaeological Investigations, Occasional Paper No. 41.

Martin, D. L. (2015). Excavating for truths: forensic anthropology and bioarchaeology as ways of making meaning from skeletal evidence. In Crossland, Z. & Joyce, R. (Eds.), *Disturbing Bodies: A Relational Exploration of Forensic Archaeological Practice*, pp. 157–168. Santa Fe, NM: School of Advanced Research Press.

Martin, D. L. (2021). Violence and masculinity in small-scale societies. *Current Anthropology* 62(S23):S169-S181. https://doi.org/10.1086/711689.

Martin, D. L. & Anderson, C. P. (2014). Introduction. In Martin, D. L. & Anderson, C. P. (Eds.), *Massacres: Bioarchaeology and Forensic Anthropological Approaches*, pp. 1–11. Gainesville: University of Florida Press.

Martin, D. L. & Harrod, R. P. (2015). Bioarchaeological contributions to the study of violence. *American Journal of Physical Anthropology* 156(S59):116–145. https://doi.org/10.1002/ajpa.22662.

Martin, D. L. & Harrod, R. P. (2016). The bioarchaeology of pain and suffering: human adaptation and survival during troubled times. *Archaeological Papers of the American Anthropological Association* 27(1):161–174. https://doi.org/10.1111/apaa.12080.

Martin, D. L., Harrod, R. P. & Pérez, V. R. (2013). *Bioarchaeology: An Integrated Approach to Working with Human Remains*. New York: Springer.

Neumann, G. K. (1940). Evidence for the antiquity of scalping from central Illinois. *American Antiquity* 5(4):287–289. https://doi.org/10.2307/275199.

Novak, M., Olalde, I., Ringbauer, H., Rohland, N., Ahern, J., Balen, J., Janković, I., Potrebica, H., Pinhasi, R. & Reich, D. (2021). Genome-wide analysis of nearly all the victims of a 6200-year-old massacre. *PLOS ONE* 16(3):e0247332. https://doi.org/10.1371/journal.pone.0247332.

Okumura, M. & Siew, Y. Y. (2013). An osteological study of trophy heads: unveiling the headhunting practice in Borneo. *International Journal of Osteoarchaeology* 23(6):685–697. https://doi.org/10.1002/oa.1297.

Ortner, D. J. (2008). Differential diagnosis of skeletal injuries. In Kimmerle, E. H. & Baraybar, J. P. (Eds.), *Skeletal Trauma: Identification of Injuries Resulting From Human Rights Abuse and Armed Conflict*, pp. 21–93. Boca Raton, FL: CRC Press. https://doi.org/10.1201/9781420009118.

Outram, A. K. (2002). Bone fracture and within-bone nutrients: an experimentally based method for investigating levels of marrow extraction. In Miracle, P. & Milner, N. (Eds.), *Consuming Passions and Patterns of Consumption*, pp. 51–64. McDonald Institute for Archaeological Research.

Owsley, D. W. & Berryman, H. E. (1975). Ethnographic and archaeological evidence of scalping in the southeastern United States. *Tennessee Archaeologist* 31(1):41–58.

Pérez, V. R. (2012). The politicization of the dead: violence as performance, politics as usual. In Martin, D. L., Harrod, R. P. & Pérez, V. R. (Eds.), *The Bioarchaeology of Violence*, pp. 13–28. Gainesville: University of Florida Press.

Perry, Elizabeth M. (2004). *Bioarchaeology of Labor and Gender in the Prehispanic American Southwest*. Doctoral Dissertation, University of Arizona.

Pollom, T., Harrod, R. P., Herlosky, K., Martin, D. L. & Crittenden, A. (2020). Stories of violent and non-violent injuries among the Hadza of northern Tanzania. Paper presented at the 49th Annual Meeting of the Society for Cross-Cultural Research, Seattle.

Powers, C. H. (2010). *Making Sense of Social Theory: A Practical Introduction*. Washington, DC: Rowman & Littlefield.

Redfern, R. (2006). A bioarchaeological analysis of violence in Iron Age females: a perspective from Dorset, England (fourth century BC to the first century AD). In Davis, O., Sharples, N. M. & Waddington, K. (Eds.), *Changing Perspectives on the First Millennium BC: Proceedings of the Iron Age Research Student Seminar*, pp. 139–160. Oxford: Oxbow.

Redfern, R. (2020). Iron age 'predatory landscapes': a bioarchaeological and funerary exploration of captivity and enslavement in Britain. *Cambridge Archaeological Journal* 30(4):531–554. https://doi.org/10.1017/S0959774320000062.

Redfern, R. & Roberts, C. (2019). Trauma. In Buikstra, J. (Ed.), *Ortner's Identification of Pathological Conditions in Human Skeletal Remains* (3rd ed.), pp. 78–90. New York: Elsevier Inc.

Scheper-Hughes, N. & Lock, M. M. (1987). The mindful body: a prolegomenon to future work in medical anthropology. *Medical Anthropology Quarterly* 1(1):6–41. https://doi.org/10.1525/maq.1987.1.1.02a00020.

Schrader, S. A. & Torres-Rouff, C. (2020). Embodying bioarchaeology: theory and practice. In Cheverko, C. M., Prince-Buitenhuys, J. R. & Hubbe. M. (Eds.), *Theoretical Approaches in Bioarchaeology*, pp. 15–27. Abingdon: Routledge.

Schröder, I. W. (2001). Violent events in the Western Apache past: ethnohistory and ethno-ethnohistory. In Schmidt, B. E. & Schröder, I. W. (Eds.), *Anthropology of Violence and Conflict*, pp. 143–158. Abingdon: Routledge.

Singleton, T. A. (1995). The archaeology of slavery in North America. *Annual Review of Anthropology* 24(1):119–140. https://doi.org/10.1146/annurev.an.24.100195.001003.

Smith, M. (2014). The war to begin all wars? Contextualizing violence in Neolithic Britain. In Knüsel, C. & Smith, M. (2014). *The Routledge Handbook of the Bioarchaeology of Human Conflict*, pp. 109–126. Abingdon: Routledge.

Sofaer, J. R. (2006). *The Body as Material Culture: A Theoretical Osteoarchaeology*. Cambridge: Cambridge University Press.

Sofaer, J. R. (2012). Bioarchaeological approaches to the gendered body. In Bolger, D. R. (Ed.), *A Companion to Gender Prehistory*, pp. 225–243. Chichester: Wiley-Blackwell.

Spradley, M. K. & Jantz, R. L. (2011). Sex estimation in forensic anthropology: skull versus postcranial elements. *Journal of Forensic Sciences* 56(2):289–296.

Standish, K. (2020). Social, cultural and political violence. In Standish, K. (Ed.), *Suicide Through a Peacebuilding Lens*, pp. 163–191. New York: Springer. https://doi.org/10.1007/978-981-13-9737-0_6.

Symes, S. A., L'Abbé, E. N., Chapman, E. N., Wolff, I. & Dirkmatt, D. (2012). Interpreting traumatic injury to bone in medicolegal investigations. In Dirkmatt, D. (Ed.), *A Companion to Forensic Anthropology*, pp. 340–389. John Wiley and Sons.

Tegtmeyer, C. E. & Martin, D. L. (2017). The bioarchaeology of women, children, and other vulnerable groups in times of war. In Martin, D. L. & Tegtmeyer, C. (Eds.), *Bioarchaeology of Women and Children in Times of War: Case Studies from the Americas*, pp. 1–14. New York: Springer International Publishing. https://doi.org/10.1007/978-3-319-48396-2_1.

Toyne, J. M. (2011). Possible cases of scalping from Pre-Hispanic highland Peru. *International Journal of Osteoarchaeology* 21(2):229–242. https://doi.org/10.1002/oa.1127.

Tremblay, L. A. & Reedy, S. (Eds.). (2020). *The Bioarchaeology of Structural Violence: A Theoretical Framework for Industrial Era Inequality*. New York: Springer International Publishing.

Tung, T. A. (2008). Dismembering bodies for display: a bioarchaeological study of trophy heads from the Wari site of Conchopata, Peru. *American Journal of Physical Anthropology* 136(3):294–308. https://doi.org/10.1002/ajpa.20812.

Tung, T. A. & Knudson, K. J. (2008). Social identities and geographical origins of Wari trophy heads from Conchopata, Peru. *Current Anthropology* 49(5):915–925. https://doi.org/10.1086/591318.

Tung, T. A. & Knudson, K. J. (2010). Childhood lost: abductions, sacrifice, and trophy heads of children in the Wari empire of the ancient Andes. *Latin American Antiquity* 21(1):44–66. https://doi.org/10.7183/1045-6635.21.1.44.

Turner, C. G., Turner, I. C. G. & Turner, J. A. (1999). *Man Corn: Cannibalism and Violence in the Prehistoric American Southwest*. Salt Lake City: University of Utah Press.

U.S. Department of Health and Human Services. (2019). *Child Maltreatment 2019*. Administration for Children and Families, Administration on Children, Youth and Families, Children's Bureau. https://www.acf.hhs.gov/sites/default/files/documents/cb/cm2019.pdf.

Walker, P. L. (1989). Cranial injuries as evidence of violence in prehistoric southern California. *American Journal of Anthropology* 80(3):313–323. https://doi.org/10.1002/ajpa.1330800305.

Walker, P. L. (2001). A bioarchaeological perspective on the history of violence. *Annual Review of Anthropology* 30:573–596. https://doi.org/10.1146/annurev.anthro.30.1.573.

Walker, P. L., Sugiyama, L. & Chacon, R. (1998). Diet, dental health, and cultural change among recently contacted South American Indian hunter-horticulturalists. In Lukacs, J. R. (Ed.), *Human Dental Development, Morphology, and Pathology: A tribute to Albert A. Dahlberg*, pp. 355–386. University of Oregon Anthropological Papers (Number 54).

Waters, H. H., Rajkotia, A., Basu, Y., Rehwinkel, S., JA Butchart, A. & World Health Organization. (2004). *The Economic Dimensions of Interpersonal Violence*. http://www.who.int/violence_injury_prevention/publications/violence/economic_dimensions/en/.

Wesp, J. K. (2017). Embodying sex/gender systems in bioarchaeological research. In Agarwal, S. C. & Wesp, J. K. (Eds.), *Exploring Sex and Gender in Bioarchaeology*, pp. 99–126. Albuquerque, NM: University of New Mexico Press.

Whitehead, N. L. (2004). Introduction: Cultures, conflicts, and the poetics of violence practice. In Whitehead, N. L. (Ed.) *Violence*, pp. 3–24. Santa Fe: School of American Research Press.

Wilkinson, R. C. (1997). Violence against women: Raiding and abduction in prehistoric Michigan. In Martin, D. L. & Frayer, D. W. (Eds.), *Troubled Times: Violence and Warfare in the Past*, pp. 21–44. Abingdon: Routledge.

Wilkinson, R. G. & Van Wagenen, K. M. (1993). Violence against women: Prehistoric skeletal evidence from Michigan. *Midcontinental Journal of Archaeology*:190–216. https://www.jstor.org/stable/20708349.

World Health Organization. (2002). *World Report on Violence and Health*. https://www.who.int/violence_injury_prevention/violence/world_report/en/summary_en.pdf.

Wrangham, R. W. & Peterson, D. (1996). *Demonic Males: Apes and the Origins of Human Violence*. Boston: Houghton Mifflin Harcourt.

Zuckerman, M. K. & Crandall, J. (2019). Reconsidering sex and gender in relation to health and disease in bioarchaeology. *Journal of Anthropological Archaeology* 54:161–171. https://doi.org/10.1016/j.jaa.2019.04.001.

28
THE DEVELOPMENTAL ORIGINS OF HEALTH AND DISEASE
Implications for Paleopathology

Rebecca Gowland and Jennifer L. Caldwell

Introduction

Seminal epidemiological research by Barker and colleagues in the 1980s provided evidence linking low birth weight with chronic disease risk in adulthood, including cardiovascular disease (CVD), type 2 diabetes, stroke, and mental health. These results indicated that adverse factors relating to the intrauterine environment were having life-long impacts on morbidity and mortality. Since then, an overwhelming body of evidence has supported these findings, leading to what has become known as the Developmental Origins of Health and Disease (DOHaD) hypothesis. This work characterizes the first 1,000 days of life (from conception) as a particularly sensitive window of developmental plasticity, in which exposure to environmental stimuli can result in adjustments to phenotypic trajectories that increase disease risk (Barker et al., 2002; Gluckman & Hanson, 2006; Barker, 2007).

The plasticity of the human skeleton and phenotypic modifications in response to environmental exposures have long been a central concern for evolutionary anthropologists and bioarchaeologists (Temple, 2019, McPherson, 2021). Research in evolutionary anthropology has focused on plasticity as an adaptive response to social and ecological circumstances to improve biological and reproductive fitness. Within evolutionary anthropology, there is an emphasis on life history trade-offs, referring to the reallocation of energy during periods of stress between the key functions of growth, maintenance (e.g., immune activity), and reproduction (McDade, 2003). Any disruption to homeostasis via disease or malnutrition will result in shifts in energy from one function to another, such as from growth to immune activity (Bogin et al., 2007). Such trade-offs are energetically costly and can result in longer term disease risk; for example, longitudinal studies of growth have demonstrated a relationship between growth disruption and reduced life expectancy, even in those who had experienced catch-up growth (Barker, 2012). DOHaD has strong synergies with life history theory but places a focus on the pathological consequences of plastic responses to adversity (see McKerracher et al., 2020). Both approaches are concerned with the entangled and reactive nature of bodies and their spatial, temporal, and socio-ecological niches.

The emphasis on life history and the life course within paleopathology and bioarchaeology is important because there has long been a tendency to interpret disease in terms of immediate casualties alone. For example, the presence of enamel defects or delayed growth in the skeleton of a young child is often interpreted as direct evidence of weaning-related hazards, with little or no consideration of maternal health. In his seminal paper, "Prisoners of the Proximate", the epidemiologist McMichael (1999) described such a focus as a constraining approach within his own discipline. The integration of DOHaD within paleopathological analysis has heralded a conceptual shift away from proximate factors alone and toward a life course perspective (Gowland, 2015; Agarwal, 2016). Because DOHaD is concerned with intrauterine development, a time when one body is entwined with another, it is also necessary to extend the temporal scale of risk intergenerationally. DOHaD has highlighted the hitherto unexplored potential for direct intergenerational impacts of socio-ecological adversity from parents to grandchildren: a female fetus will produce all the gametes she will have in her lifetime whilst in utero; therefore, stress affecting a pregnant woman could directly impact three generations (Barker, 2012). This has implications for the way in which paleopathologists consider, for example, the intergenerational impact of catastrophic events such as famine in the past.

There are a variety of mechanisms underpinning developmental plasticity in response to adversity, but one garnering much of the attention in recent years is epigenetic change (affecting gene expression rather than gene sequence). What is often overlooked within the DOHaD paradigm are the structural, cultural, and behavioral determinants that perpetuate over generations and their contribution to epigenetic regulation within populations. Environmental cues may trigger epigenetic alterations, which can affect developmental trajectories and have direct intergenerational impacts (Kuzawa, 2005). Normal temporal regulators may become hyper- or hypo-regulated due to these environmental triggers. Epigenetic research reveals how a single genotype can be expressed in phenotypically diverse ways in response to stimuli during development. Adverse environments, including poor diet, exposure to toxins, and stress (trauma), can cause epigenetic changes that alter vulnerabilities to disease in later life and between generations. Subsequently, DOHaD requires paleopathologists and bioarchaeologists to consider the effects of longer term intergenerational adversity as a source of hidden heterogeneity in frailty (McPherson, 2021). DOHaD therefore speaks to well-established debates within bioarchaeology regarding the "osteological paradox" (Wood et al., 1992; DeWitte & Stojanowski, 2015). The inter-weaving of social and biological biographies across generations also requires a theoretical shift in our conceptualization of the life course, and individualized, bounded biologies (Gowland, 2015; Gowland & Newman, 2018). If socio-ecological adversity affecting our grandmother (and mother) has impacts for our own metabolic regulation and disease risk, when does our biography begin and hers end?

Bioarchaeologists are perennially concerned with the genes, environment, and culture triad (Lewontin, 2000); the inter-relationship between these, and how they manifest in the hard tissues of the body. DOHaD likewise emphasizes the centrality of environment and culture in epidemiological research, providing a more integrated paradigm that challenges fundamental disciplinary divides regarding the body and society. Bioarchaeologists have always worked at the interface between culture and biology; therefore, transcending disciplinary divides is comfortable ground. One method to study the socio-ecological effects of our ancestors' past and present health outcomes is by using the model of "Ethnogenetic Layering". This is a non-traditional race model that observes the ancestral, genomic, environmental, cultural, geo-spatial, and behavioral implications of a population. By localizing populations and creating a holistic view of human variation, the explicit details contributing to a population's health outcomes can be observed and effectively treated. The efforts of studying human variation in a localized fashion will advance epigenomic research over time (Jackson, 2008). Contextualized, "local biologies" (referring to the material embedding of bodies geographically, ecologically, temporally and culturally, Lock, 1993) have long been important for the interpretations of past skeletal remains (Appleby, 2019). Such a nuanced approach is also essential for interpreting evidence within a DOHaD framework – there never has been, nor can be, a "one size fits all". This is because history is becoming increasingly important, and a consideration of different temporal scales – evolutionary, developmental, generational, and biographical – are essential to our analysis of disease and what Krieger (2013) has referred to as the emergent "embodied phenotype". The more recent sociological turn within paleopathology and an increasing focus on biographical narratives, means that DOHaD aligns well with existing research approaches and imperatives (Agarwal, 2016). This chapter will explore and summarize some of the key features and applications of DOHaD for paleopathology and bioarchaeology, including theoretical considerations regarding the life course, and the inter-relationship between bodies and societies in the past.

DOHaD: Origins of a Hypothesis

Barker and colleagues' research initially aimed to understand the geographical pattern in CVD within the UK (Barker & Osmond, 1986; Barker et al., 1989). CVD prevalence increased during the 20th century in tandem with increasing national prosperity. Paradoxically, however, the highest rates were amongst individuals living in the most deprived locations. Barker and colleagues' research identified a geographic correlation between the frequency of CVD and areas with high infant mortality six decades previously (Barker & Osmond, 1986; Barker et al., 1989). Other relevant risk factors (e.g., cigarette smoking, or diets high in saturated fats) presented no similar correlation, leading to the novel explanation that factors affecting intrauterine development were pre-disposing people to heart disease in later life (Barker & Osmond, 1986). These findings built on previous research in other countries that had found associations between risk of CVD and childhood poverty (Forsdahl, 1977; Buck & Simpson, 1982).

Since these pioneering studies, the link between low birth weight and coronary heart disease has been established around the world (Gluckman & Hanson, 2006; Heindel & Vandenberg, 2015). Further work by Barker and colleagues' (1989) also highlighted connections between low birth weight and life expectancy, leading to the conclusion that factors affecting intrauterine growth and development, rather than the postnatal environment, were key to life-long health (Barker, 2007). This work has had its detractors; one of the key arguments being that association is not causation, and the range of confounding risk factors that cannot be adequately controlled for in epidemiological studies such as these (Schulz, 2010). Since this early research, however, a wealth of other evidence has demonstrated similar links between intrauterine adversity and chronic disease, including, for example, insulin resistance, obesity, and high blood pressure (Gluckman & Hanson, 2006; Wadhwa et al., 2009). This work then became known as the *Fetal Origins of Adult Disease* hypothesis (Barker, 1995), otherwise referred to as the "Barker hypothesis". Sensitivity to adverse conditions is particularly heightened during embryogenesis, such that under-nutrition or environmental toxins could impact on cell differentiation and influence the epigenome (Heindel & Vandenberg, 2015). These adverse effects do not necessarily manifest in any visible birth defect, but rather create subtle alterations in the function of affected tissues that accumulate in significance over the course of a person's lifetime. The window of developmental sensitivity was subsequently extended into the postnatal period, to recognize infancy and early childhood as a period of continuing developmental plasticity, becoming known as the *Developmental Origins of Health and Disease hypothesis* (Gluckman & Hanson, 2006; Gluckman et al., 2007). The focus of this hypothesis is the first 1,000 days of life; plasticity does occur after this period, but during early development, environmental impacts will have a more profound effect on phenotypic trajectories (McPherson, 2021).

Many DOHaD-related studies focused initially on the impact of maternal nutrition for later life health outcomes. One of the best and most discussed illustrative examples of the impact of nutritional deficits on fetal development is the Dutch Famine, also known as the Dutch Hunger Winter, during World War II. This was a well-documented famine event of clearly delineated, five-month duration, in which food-intake dropped to approximately 400–900 kilocalories for all inhabitants, irrespective of social class. After this period, food intake quickly returned to normal levels, creating an exceptional and distinct period of deprivation (Roseboom et al., 2001, 2006). The availability of detailed records for both the duration of the event and since, has allowed a series of longitudinal studies to assess the repercussions for women who were pregnant, and/or conceived during this period, and their offspring (and grandchildren). These studies demonstrated a range of life-long and intergenerational impacts, which varied depending on the gestational age at which individuals were affected. For example, while birth weight was not affected in those exposed during early gestation, these individuals had a greater likelihood of CVD and obesity in adulthood. By contrast, those who were exposed in late gestation tended to have a low birth weight and were small throughout their lives, but with lower rates of obesity (Roseboom et al., 2006). Those affected in late gestation, however, would also have continued to be impacted by the famine for a short period postnatally, limiting the capacity for catch-up growth in the months after birth. The famine did not necessarily affect linear growth but resulted in disturbed metabolic regulation, resulting in increases in diabetes, cardiovascular disease, hypertension, and schizophrenia (for further details see Ravelli et al., 1999; Roseboom et al., 2001, 2006; Lumey et al., 2011). Further longitudinal studies have provided unequivocal evidence that three generations were *directly* affected by the famine – the expectant mother, her child, and her grandchild; the latter because the ova develop in the fetus during gestation.

As Landecker (2011:177) discusses in relation to the Dutch example, "this is a model in which food enters the body and, in a sense *never leaves it*, because food transforms the organism's being as much as the organism transforms it". It has been argued that one of the reasons for the increase in metabolic disease amongst Dutch famine victims was the mismatch between the intrauterine signaling and the environment into which the child subsequently grew up (Godfrey et al., 2007). Other longitudinal studies of famine events, such as the Great Famine in China from 1959 to 1961, have likewise demonstrated a range of long-term health problems for those who were born during this time, including cognitive issues and stroke (Kim et al., 2017; Li et al., 2020). Such studies should inspire paleopathologists to take a longer term, intergenerational approach to the study of morbidity and mortality in relation to similar catastrophic events in the past, rather than conceptualizing them (as has tended to happen) as a moment in time.

Additional research has explored environmental cues other than nutrition; for example, the impact of exposure to chemical toxins during early life for risk of asthma and immunological problems, psycho-social stress, and social status (Wadhwa et al., 2009; Heindel & Vandenberg, 2015). Factors such as maternal stress have also been shown to be significant for mental as well as physiological well-being in later life (Wadhwa et al., 2009; Hertzman, 2012). Studies have demonstrated that stress during pregnancy can even affect the stress reactivity of offspring after their birth. Differences in maternal care in early infancy have also been shown to have potential life-long consequences, via epigenetic alterations, for the regulation of adult stress reactivity (Weaver et al., 2004). New techniques in paleopathology and bioarchaeology are now allowing us to explore maternal stress in the past via intrauterine isotopic values of carbon and nitrogen in infants, thus opening up new avenues for investigating the mother/infant nexus (e.g., Beaumont et al. 2015).

Much of the original focus of DOHaD was undoubtedly chronic disease risk, and this may be one of the reasons that it was slow to be adopted by bioarchaeologists: much of our work is focused on populations living prior to the epidemiological transition, when infectious disease rather than chronic disease was a far more prevalent threat to mortality. Recent work, however, has shown that early life adversity also has implications for susceptibility to infectious diseases. For example, a series of studies on health in rural Gambia has demonstrated that children born shortly after the "hungry season" suffer from an increased risk of mortality from infectious disease in early adulthood compared to other times of the year. The authors argue that immune function and disease susceptibility is programmed in early life and affected by intrauterine growth retardation (Moore et al., 1999, 2004). Life history trade-offs are an important consideration here: when resources are scarce, growth disruption may occur as they are directed toward supporting the immune response to bolster short-term survival prospects (Temple, 2019, McPherson, 2021). As McDade et al. (2016:7) note "developmental plasticity and ecological sensitivity are defining features of the human immune system". When observing consistent growth delay in non-adults excavated from archaeological cemeteries, paleopathologists could reflect on this as a barometer of immunological stress within the broader populations, with repercussions for adult longevity in the survivors (e.g., Watts, 2015).

The idea that vulnerabilities to chronic disease are programmed into a person's biology prior to birth, via environmentally induced processes, rather than just genetics, represented a profound shift in our understanding of public health, with repercussions for government policies and medical interventions (Müller et al., 2017). In the UK, it shifted the foci of medical policies from adult behaviors/risks, onto mothers, infants, and early childhood, with the instigation of government health initiatives that provided greater social and medical welfare for pregnant women and young children (e.g., the Marmot Review, 2010). Timely and targeted interventions were seen as a cost-effective investment in the overall and longer term health of the population. It has been argued that within a DOHaD paradigm, obesity, diabetes, osteoporosis, cardiovascular morbidity, and neurodegenerative diseases can *all* be considered pediatric diseases: not because they occur in children but because they originate during development (Heindel & Vandenberg, 2015). Early interventions at the time when tissues are forming and biological systems are most sensitive to environmental insults, have the potential to lead to improved lifelong health, although as the sections below illustrate, longer term strategies are needed.

Plastic Fantastic: What is Epigenetic Change

Modifications to the epigenome are a mechanism underpinning developmental plasticity and the alterations in disease risk identified in DOHaD research. Not all DOHaD research presumes an epigenetic origin to phenotypic phenomena; nevertheless, epigenetic processes are frequently conceptualized as a key component. Epigenetics can be broadly defined as "those genetic mechanisms that create phenotypic variations without altering the base-pair nucleotide sequence of the genes" (Gilbert & Epel, 2008:12). Epigenetic factors are those which cause changes in the regulation of gene expression (see, Haig, 2012, for more detail). Epigenetic modifications include DNA methylation, histone modification, and non-coding RNAs. The most heavily researched in terms of maternal exposures is DNA methylation, which refers to the addition of a methyl group to cytosine nucleotides, which then alters gene expression (usually "silencing" it), with subsequent impacts for phenotypic trajectories (Landecker & Panofsky, 2013:338). Epigenetic changes have been identified in response to a range of social and environmental stressors. The analogy of "memory" is often invoked in reference to epigenetic changes: studies often refer to the molecular embedding of social and environmental exposures during the period of development into the "memory" of an organism (e.g., Thayer & Kuzawa, 2011; Meloni, 2014; Kuzawa, 2020).

As the Dutch famine example (discussed above) has demonstrated, the direct effects of a particularly profound episode of adversity can be passed on to three generations, described using the notation F0 (mother) to F1 (daughter) and F2 (grandchild). Any effects beyond this (F3) are classed as transgenerational rather than intergenerational and are much more open to debate (Susser et al., 2012; Heindel & Vandenberg, 2015). Epigenetic information is generally not thought to survive across the germ line, due to post-fertilization re-programming (although see Ryan and Kuzawa, 2020). If the social and environmental circumstances that initiated the epigenetic changes in the F0 generation still exist in F3 then this implies transmission beyond the initial exposure and transgenerationally. However, presumably similar epigenetic markers can be triggered in F3 if the original socio-ecological conditions persist (Susser et al., 2012; Heindel & Vandenberg, 2015). Epigenetic changes have been identified in infants conceived during the hungry season in rural Gambia, and these infants have a greater risk of low birth weight and mortality (Waterland et al., 2010; Dominguez-Salas et al., 2014). Landecker (2011:277) and Landecker and Panofsky (2013) discuss in more detail the potential triggering of an epigenetic response due to sub-optimal nutritional conditions. Research on those affected by the Dutch Famine has also shown that epigenetic effects are strongly influenced by the gestational age of exposure, although further empirical studies are required (Lumey et al., 2011). These early life exposures can invoke phenotypic change which can persist via mitosis throughout an individual's life course, although in some circumstances these may be reversible (Meloni, 2014).

Epigenetics provides a process in which an organism can rapidly alter in response to ecological/social stimuli, without more fundamental genetic changes (Wells, 2010). As Wells (2010:3) states: "Plasticity allows genes to 'stay in the game' through modification of the relationship between genotype and phenotype". While the impact of social and environmental factors for triggering, for example, different patterns of methylation, has been explored intensively, it is important to highlight the nascent status of epigenetic research in terms of broader implications for health and disease in humans (Heijmans & Mill, 2012). Current experiments are mostly focused on rodent species and seek to explore epigenetic responses to different environmental variables (e.g., maternal nutrition, psycho-social stressors) (Hertzman, 2012). The translation of results from rodent species, which have high litter numbers and short life spans, to humans is not straightforward. Further research is expanding to longer lived species, including primates. The majority of epigenetic research has also tended to focus on the triggering of responses rather than potential reversibility (Meloni, 2014).

Bridging the Gap Between the Biological and Social Sciences

Despite some of the limitations, epigenetic research has been regarded as revolutionary; the immutability of DNA has been challenged and the extent of its responsive and reactive nature is now being discovered (Niewöhner & Lock, 2018). Consequently, epigenetic research has been immersed in a considerable amount of hype and excitement (Pickersgill, 2021). Epigenetics explicitly breaks down the barriers between the body and society in understanding human health as never before (Meloni, 2014). The embedding of social factors directly into the epigenome challenges traditionally dichotomized views of the body and society (Niewohner, 2011; Müller et al., 2017). As part of the post-genomic landscape, epigenetics represents a move away from the reductionist turn characterized by genomic research in the 1990s, and instead bridges research in human biology and society (Meloni, 2014; Müller et al., 2017). Even on a biomolecular level, our bodies are malleable and influenced by social environment. It has been argued by some medical anthropologists that there is still a danger that health will be viewed via a "molecular optics", with individuals reduced to their epigenome, potentially contributing to a molecularization of social processes (Lock, 2013). For many though, epigenetics heralds a new and exciting, post-dichotomous, post-genomic era in which human biology has become more fully reconciled with the social (Meloni, 2014; Richardson, 2015; Pickersgill, 2021). Meloni (2014:732) has argued that epigenetics has helped to constitute "a more pluralistic and contingent vision of 'the biological'" (2014:742).

While the epigenetic impact of the Dutch Famine (Heijmans et. al., 2008) is widely accepted, the catastrophic multi-generational impact of the Trans-Atlantic Slave Trade (TAST), enslavement, Jim Crow era, Segregation, and the Prison Industrial Complex seems to be a less acceptable argument for the epigenetic effects of chronic disease and trauma in Legacy African American (LAA) communities. LAAs are the descendants of chattel slavery forcibly brought to the United States for the economic advancement of the country. They are referred to as LAAs because of their ancestry but also to capture the contemporary diversity of African North American populations which includes LAAs and recent, first-, and second-generation African and Caribbean immigrants who significantly contribute to the Black American population (Caldwell & Jackson, 2021).

While LAAs are genetically closely related to the highly diverse ethnic groups in Africa, it is ironic that the population is less well represented in genomic databases, which leads to under-investing in complex disease mapping and epigenetic regulation of disease (Tishkoff et al., 2009; Landry et al., 2018). LAAs are disproportionately affected by chronic disease, major health disparities, and adverse risk factors for disease. To put this into context, 56% of the overall African North American population lives in the Stroke Belt. The Stroke Belt is home to the largest pre-Middle Passage slave port in Charleston, South Carolina, and is called the Stroke Belt due to the high prevalence of stroke and CVD phenotypes that plague populations who live there of all ethnic backgrounds. This flux in CVD and other chronic diseases phenotypes could be the result of intergenerational biological adaptations to social and economic disparities (Sinha et al., 2021). When LAA women were enslaved, they were still responsible for tedious agricultural duties, many breast-fed slave owner's children and their own, and were forced to complete these tasks while experiencing malnourishment and traumatic living conditions. If the Dutch Famine impacted the next generation, the epigenetic damage done during 400 years of enslavement and prejudice experienced by Black mothers is unquantifiable.

Because of their evolutionary history and arrival into the Americas, African Americans contribute greatly to the genomic and thus epigenetic health outcomes exhibited today. Ancestral proportions and degrees of population homogeneity and heterogeneity mirror recent levels of admixture within and across populations. For example, African Americans were born of a large bottle neck migration created by the TAST (Lachance et al., 2018). While great allelic diversity was present in Africa, the TAST forced African Americans to become more genetically homogenous over time. One form of evolutionary effect can be found in the Gullah Geechee, LAA sub-population found in the Lowcountry (<30 miles inland) of South Carolina, North Carolina, Georgia, and Florida coastal areas. Gullah Geechee are an amalgamation of West, West Central, and Windward Coastal Africans. They retained language and customs found in their homelands, and due to their relative isolation in the Lowcountry coast and islands, they usually retain >90% African genomic information with modest gene flow from surrounding populations (Ely et al., 2006). The Gullah Geechee are also a progenitor population for modern African Americans (Caldwell & Jackson, 2021). While geo-spatial restrictions during colonial periods deeply impacted reproductive patterns, the internal Second Middle Passage to the Deep South (1790–1865), and the Great Migrations from the south to northern states (1865–1970s) created genomic re-shuffling that, alongside institutionalized racism, led to clear health disparities between US populations in the past and which are evident today (Baharian et al., 2016).

Decades of research shows that approximately 300,000 Africans were brought to the United States. One-third were women, yielding approximately 70,000 women of childbearing years to "mother" the contemporary LAA populations. This is essential to view through the lens of epigenetic repercussions. During enslavement, African American women carried weighty burdens as field and house workers, "breeders", and objects of sexual and medical exploitation. Pregnancy gave them no reprieve. As medical "subjects" LAAs were characterized as primitive and "animalistic" and were argued to have higher pain thresholds than white people (Booker, 2014); prejudices that continue today. This has led to acute distrust of the medical community and, consequently, discourages genomic testing and research that may improve our understanding of the epigenetic bases of health disparities and assist in ameliorating them.

The repercussions of racial disparities, past and present, are evident. Disparities in environmental, geographical, educational, and socio-economic experiences affect epigenetic mechanisms that alter DNA expression. For example, LAAs infants have a 50% increased risk in being Low Birth Weight and CVD and CVD comorbidities, such as hypertension, obesity, and heart disease, are more common within this population. From the cradle to the grave, and from generation to generation, external and internal stressors have perpetuated health disparities for African Americans (Mohottige et al., 2022).

African Americans today are a young and genetically rich population. Pew Research observed that over 1:3 of the African American population was under 22 years old in 2019, and Millennials constituted an additional 23% of the total population, rendering around 60% of the African American population less than or equal to 38 years old (Tamir, 2022). The diversity in African American sub-populations, many migrations, systemic prejudices, and subsequent intergenerational experiences, contribute to an epigenetic imprint of trauma and resilience. African Americans are thus superb populations to study in order to understand the development and prevalence of human disease, mechanisms that catalyze health disparities, and genetic and environmental factors that contribute to human development, diseases, and mortality.

Hence, the imprinting of social exposures on skeletal biology must be a paradigm that is adopted by paleopathologists, especially since this field operates within the blurred space between the traditional disciplinary divides of science and social theory (Gowland & Thompson, 2021). Research that highlights the impact of environmental cues on phenotype and disease risk fits well within paleopathology's existing remit. For bioarchaeologists and paleopathologists, however, epigenetic research, developmental plasticity, and DOHaD provides a new model for understanding disease etiology and risk, one in which the parameters have expanded to encompass biographical and intergenerational exposures.

Generations of Risk: Back to the Future

One of the key features of DOHaD is that it has altered our perception of timescales of risk and exposure to environmental adversity in early life. Life histories, and in particular the early developmental periods, are taking center stage. For disciplines such as paleopathology and bioarchaeology that have long marginalized the significance of fetal and infant remains, and almost entirely overlooked maternal bodies, this is particularly significant (Han et al. 2017; Gowland & Halcrow, 2020; Halcrow et al., 2020; Hodson, 2021). Infant remains at archaeological sites now take on a new source of significance as windows into overall population health and intergenerational conduits (Gowland, 2018).

DOHaD has also placed a spotlight on maternal health as a key source of vulnerability for the life-long well-being of the developing fetus. Unfortunately, however, within this paradigm, mothers have become conceptualized as a potential source of harm to their fetus, which represents a marked shift away from the previous perception of the maternal body as selfless/nurturing/buffering (Richardson et al., 2014). One consequence of this is that pregnancy within a clinical setting is now regarded as a productive period for medical intervention (Pickersgill et al., 2013). Richardson (2015) argues that DOHaD has essentially produced a deficit model, by presenting ways in which mothers can harm their offspring (Richardson, 2015). There is a danger that pregnant women will be subjected to increasing censure and surveillance from the medical profession because they are viewed as a source of epigenetic triggering that will adversely impact the phenotypic trajectory of their child. The maternal body within DOHaD has been partially re-conceptualized: from protector to "epigenetic vector" (Richardson, 2015:211). Postnatal care is also under scrutiny. For example, well-cited research has revealed that rat pups who were less intensively groomed by their mothers showed epigenetic changes and heightened stress (Weaver et al. 2005). When hastily translated to humans, expectations of maternity become intensified: women must optimize their pre-conception fitness through a regimen of nutrition and exercise, their natal health by adopting a specific lifestyle, and then follow an idealized model of optimum infant care. If she does not then she will pre-dispose her child (and potentially grandchild) to a life of enhanced biological and social disadvantage, including life-long mental health issues. One outcome of DOHaD and cognate research is an increased pressure on pregnant women to be "good reproductive citizens" (Longhurst, 2008), and the privileging of fetal over maternal wellbeing (Richardson, 2015).

Given that DOHaD research has shown that stressors during pregnancy can impact phenotype, it is logical to suppose that interventions during this period, such as nutritional supplementation, will result in more successful birth outcomes and a reduced risk of chronic disease for offspring. Whilst optimal maternal health is clearly desirable, targeting the intra-uterine period, however, has not necessarily proven to be the most effective method of securing the future good health of the developing fetus (Richardson et al., 2014). A growing body of research has demonstrated relatively modest increases in birth weight for the offspring of women provided with nutritional supplements during pregnancy, except perhaps in very marginal environments (Kuzawa, 2005, Chung & Kuzawa, 2014). Birth weight is of course only a very crude indicator of fetal adversity, and very small improvements can result in positive reproductive outcomes (Gluckman & Hanson, 2006). Studies indicate that programs of nutritional intervention may well have a positive outcome on growth and health, but this may happen over intergenerational rather than immediate timeframes (Chung & Kuzawa, 2014). For example, a large-scale randomized nutritional intervention was undertaken in Guatemala between 1969 and 1977, and results showed that the infants of women who were the beneficiaries of nutritional supplements during their own fetal development were significantly larger than those who had received no supplementation (Behrman et al., 2009). This study is significant because it demonstrates the heightened importance of the mother's own birth weight and childhood nutritional experience for her offspring. Sletner et al. (2014), also demonstrated that birth weight of infants was more closely related to the mother's own developmental history than current socio-economic status and living conditions.

The maternal body can, in fact, provide considerable buffering against immediate nutritional deficits through the deployment of glycogen stores, but as Wells (2010) observes, the efficacy of this is dependent upon "maternal somatic capital", which will vary greatly in relation to social, structural, and ecological factors. Wells (2010) and Kuzawa and Thayer (2011) argue that maternal cues to the fetus are constrained by epigenetic "memories", passed via the nutritional experiences of the mother and recent matrilineal ancestors. Within this model, the mother's liabilities are reduced in the face of nutritional deprivation, and conversely, pregnant women have a limited potential to actively improve the wellbeing of their developing fetus through nutritional regimes. This mechanism limits any plastic response to short-term ecological fluctuations, which is prudent from an evolutionary perspective in a long-lived species such as humans, who are exposed to seasonality and other perturbations in resource availability (Wells, 2010).

Research indicates that growth patterns in infancy and childhood, therefore, track the maternal phenotype closely: the mother is essentially a conduit of past generational experiences (Chung & Kuzawa, 2014). Of course, if the infant is born into an environment that is markedly different from ancestral circumstances then the ancestrally derived constraints can potentially result in maladaption. The theoretical model provided by Kuzawa and colleagues is one in which plasticity is not "predictive" of the future as Gluckman and Hanson (2006) have argued, nor reflective of the present, but instead is predicated on past generational experiences (Kuzawa, 2005). Within this model, bodies are backward rather than forward looking and plasticity is constrained rather than facilitated by the "memories" of ancestral experiences (Richardson, 2015). As Han and colleagues note, the fetus "is both materially and metaphorically a product of the past, a marker of the present, and an embodiment of the future" (Han et al. 2017:1). This new body of research also highlights the mechanism by which differing birth outcomes may occur within similar environments: it is because they are contingent upon the diverse life histories of the mothers rather than reflecting current social and ecological settings.

Kuzawa and Thayer (2011) and Thayer et al. (2020) argue that different biological processes are sensitive to different timescales. While nutritional perspectives would more fruitfully consider life history and generational timescales, as outlined above, severe psycho-social stress during pregnancy can have more acute impacts. Kuzawa and Thayer (2011) highlight events such as natural disasters which have had well-documented, detrimental impacts on birth weight and infant mortality, irrespective of nutrition. A well-cited example being the terrorist attack of September 11, 2001 in the US, which resulted in adverse birth outcomes for a significant proportion of female residents with Arabic names (Kuzawa & Sweet, 2009). Some studies of the longer term effects of disasters, including Hurricane Katrina and September 11th, have indicated continuing impacts on reproductive health (Harville et al., 2015). Other studies have likewise highlighted the significance of psycho-social stress, including post-traumatic stress disorder for the developing fetus, although results are sometimes inconclusive (Harville et al., 2010; de Oliveira et al., 2021). Kuzawa and Thayer argue that the biological response to acute stressors is directly transmitted to the fetus and therefore work on a more proximate timescale than nutritional stress. Within DOHaD, therefore, we need to consider the impact of both immediate and ancestral cues and how these might work to both initiate and constrain developmental plasticity (McPherson, 2021). This research provides additional nuance and complexity to our understanding of the effects of intrauterine stress in response to environmental adversity.

As discussed above, current DOHaD-related intervention programs tend to focus on the behaviors, lifestyle, and nutrition of mothers. While the potential of mothers to elicit a developmental response, via intrauterine environment and breastfeeding, is greater than for fathers, it is important for research to also consider paternal influences (Richardson et al., 2014). Sharp et al. (2018) analyzed articles published in the *Journal of Developmental Origins of Health and Disease*, demonstrating that 84% were focused on maternal exposures, while only 4% discussed paternal influences on disease risk. New DOHaD research has started to focus on the importance of patrilineal experiences, with factors such as diet also impacting epigenetically on sperm (Richardson et al., 2014). Recent research is also exploring the impact of epigenetic signaling from the paternal line and is re-evaluating just how complete the epigenetic erasure of the germ-line actually is (Ryan & Kuzawa, 2020). Sharp et al. (2019) and Richardson (2015) also caution against the rushing in of DOHaD findings into public and clinical policy in the absence of a more holistic understanding, which includes paternal factors.

Research shows that routing DOHaD within the context of individualized risks and behaviors will have a minimal impact, compared to wider structural inequities within societies, in which individuals are exposed to adversity over generations. There is now significant evidence that we need to consider health in terms of cumulative, intergenerational biographies. This research creates a new imperative to understand the more insidious effects of deeply entrenched structural inequalities that serve to marginalize the very poorest in society as well as racially marginalized groups. If the social adversity experienced by grandparents continues to impact subsequent generations, it can reinforce the poverty trap and become self-fulfilling. Wells (2010) refers to this as a "metabolic ghetto" stating: "If pregnancy is a niche occupied by the fetus…, then economic marginalization over generations can transform that niche into a physiological ghetto where the phenotypic consequences are long-term and liable to reproduction in future generations" (Wells, 2010:11). The social past literally becomes embodied, and shapes future developmental trajectories (Kuzawa & Sweet, 2009:11).

The Body, Society, and DOHaD in Paleopathology and Bioarchaeology

In paleopathology and bioarchaeology, interpretations of skeletal remains are predicated on the fact that past societies and ecologies become embedded within the chemical and morphological fabric of the hard tissues of the body. It is the role of the paleopathologist to tease these out via a suite of analytical techniques and interpret them in relation to a range of contextual evidence. For bioarchaeologists, embodiment is literal rather than figurative, as the biology of past people yields unique insights into their lives. The plasticity of the human skeleton and the lesions caused by various stressors have long formed an important basis of paleopathological studies. DOHaD provides an extended temporal and life course perspective for our interpretation of skeletal variation and pathology.

One of the implications of DOHaD for paleopathology and bioarchaeology is the new emphasis on mothers and infants. Maternal health and infancy have largely been overlooked in archaeology and very few studies of infants have interpreted their remains with reference to the infant/mother nexus (Gowland, 2018; Gowland & Halcrow, 2020, Riccomi et al., 2021; and Chapter 23, this volume). The varied socio-cultural practices and beliefs surrounding conception and pregnancy have likewise been under-explored. There is a rich ethnographic and sociological evidence that points to a range of culturally specific, spatial, and dietary constraints/taboos that control maternal bodies and by extension affect the developing fetus (e.g., see chapters in Han et al., 2017 and Gowland & Halcrow, 2020). New theoretical developments (including DOHaD), alongside methodological innovations, are now leading to a resurgence of interest.

One such innovation is high-resolution isotopic data from dentine, which can reveal longitudinal dietary changes for the duration of tooth formation. Nitrogen and carbon isotope values can be plotted at intervals of approximately nine months, from just before birth to 15 years of age, depending on the tooth being sampled (Beaumont et al., 2013; Montgomery et al., 2013). Deciduous dentition and the first permanent molar are particularly valuable for comparing pre- and postnatal exposures to adversity. This method also allows, for the first time, a means of making direct comparisons between survivors and non-survivors and has considerable potential for exploring DOHaD within the bioarchaeological record, particularly when integrated with skeletal data (Gowland, 2015; Beaumont et al., 2015, 2018; Kendall et al., 2020).

Incremental stable isotope analysis of deciduous teeth can provide a window into maternal stress during the intrauterine period during which the tooth crowns were developing. Opposing covariance in δ^{15}Nitrogen values and δ^{13}Carbon isotope values potentially indicates physiological stress (Beaumont & Montgomery, 2016). The association between high δ^{15}Nitrogen values and starvation has also been recorded in the clinical literature in studies of hair samples obtained from individuals attending clinics for eating disorders (Mekota & Grupe, 2006). Beaumont et al. (2015) have noted a disparity between maternal δ^{15}Nitrogen values and perinatal offspring. The perinatal values reflect the period of development in utero, whilst maternal values represent pooled data relating to the last five to ten years of the woman's life (depending on the bone sampled). Elevated δ^{15}Nitrogen values in archaeological infants have previously been interpreted exclusively in terms of breastfeeding; instead, Beaumont and colleagues (2015) argue that in some cases, these may reflect the recycling of proteins in the mother in response to environmental adversity. The perinate, therefore, provides high-resolution maternal isotope values, in the absence of the mother herself (Gowland, 2018).

Kendall et al.'s (2020) high-resolution isotope analysis of individuals from a site of putative malaria endemicity (Littleport, Ely, UK) demonstrated a much more erratic pattern of values than the contemporaneous and nearby (but non-malarial) site of Edix Hill. In particular, opposing covariance in δ^{15}Nitrogen and δ^{13}Carbon values in several Littleport individuals indicates maternal malnutrition late in pregnancy. Interestingly, for two of these individuals, a divergence in carbon and nitrogen values continues postnatally alongside skeletal indicators of metabolic stress (Kendall et al., 2020:118). Pregnancy is associated with greater susceptibility to malaria, with one of the associated pathological changes being anemia (Gowland & Western, 2012). Such studies have great potential for exploring reasons underpinning the osteological paradox and hidden heterogeneity in mortality risks.

Preliminary research by Leskovar et al. (2019) indicates that isotope analysis of collagen from ear ossicles also has the potential to provide a signal of maternal health. Formation occurs prior to dental development and therefore provides isotopic information for a hitherto invisible stage of fetal development. This method is still nascent but has enormous potential to improve our understanding of early infant development and maternal stress in the past. The archaeological study of cortisol values from teeth also has the potential to examine aspects of early life adversity (Quade et al., 2021). One application would be to examine cortisol levels in perinatal teeth, with high values potentially related to maternal stress. Comparisons can also be made between cortisol concentrations and other dental indicators of stress. As Kuzawa and Thayer (2011) have noted, acute maternal stress is a risk factor for low birth weight and infant mortality. Should techniques of cortisol analysis become more sensitive, perhaps it would be possible to sample teeth incrementally in a similar way to isotope data to investigate any trends or anomalies in intrauterine values.

A number of studies within paleopathology have provided evidence in support of DOHaD from archaeological contexts, noting correlations between indicators of childhood health stress such as linear enamel hypoplasia (LEH), vertebral neural canal dimensions, cribra orbitalia, growth stunting, and reduced adult longevity (e.g., Armelagos et al., 2009; Watts, 2011, 2013, 2015; Roberts & Steckel, 2018; Temple, 2019; Garland, 2020). Paleopathological analysis of infant remains is often controversial due to the difficulties of differentiating between pathological new bone formation and normal growth (Lewis, 2017; Hodson, 2021). Some studies, however, have provided unequivocal evidence for pathological processes on perinatal remains (e.g., Lewis, 2010; Hodson, 2017). For example, a high proportion of infants from the Roman site of Piddington, Northamptonshire, UK, showed a range of pathological lesions, indicating adverse maternal health that likely reflects a much broader population disease burden (Hodson, 2017). Studies of DOHaD are not limited to the study of infants and young children, and indeed it is the longer terms effects of adversity that are of interest. McPherson (2021) summarizes a series of skeletal indicators that may indicate adversity during the sensitive window of plasticity, and which may be potentially useful for exploring DOHaD.

Both Temple (2014) and Lorentz et al. (2019) demonstrated that the timing and frequency of microscopic dental defects were significant predictors of age-at-death in archaeological samples from Japan and Iran, respectively. Temple (2019) also noted that individuals with dental defects at an earlier age had a higher mortality risk, lending further support to the DOHaD hypothesis. Lawrence et al (2021) analyzed LEH in individuals of known genetic relatedness, finding a correlation that may relate to either genetic or epigenetic factors, suggesting the intergenerational transmission of heterogenous frailty. Brickley et al. (2020) adopted a novel approach for examining vitamin D deficiency in early life. They undertook a histological analysis of inter-globular dentine (diagnostic of vitamin D deficiency), prior to, and after the neonatal line, which forms at birth. They provided an example of a child who died aged three years with evidence of healed rickets at the time of death, and pre-natal evidence of vitamin D deficiency.

The paleopathological evidence, however, does not always straightforwardly map onto DOHaD. For example, Amoroso and Garcia's (2018) study of a 19th–20th-century Portuguese identified skeletal collection, examined the relationship between vertebral neural canal dimensions, indicative of childhood stress, and age-at-death but found no correlation. They argued that cultural or behavioral strategies ameliorated the impact of this developmental response to stress on mortality risk, and also suggest that results align with Gluckman and Hanson's (2006) predictive adaptive response model. It is important, however, to be cognizant of the arguments by Kuzawa (2005) and Wells (2010) against the ability of environmentally induced intrauterine signals to predict postnatal environments.

Holder et al. (2021) integrated a DOHaD and life history theory approach to examine variability in body mass and stature of a sample of Napoleonic soldiers. They found no clear relationship between LEH and final adult stature; however, catch-up growth is a possibility. As discussed in relation to life history theory and the trade-offs between growth, immunity, and reproduction, catch-up growth is energetically costly and growth disruption during childhood can increase morbidity and mortality risks in later life, leading to reduced life expectancy (Barker, 2012; Temple, 2019). LEH may result from acute stressors, whereas reduced stature tends to indicate an extended period of stress (Holder et al., 2021). Studies that focus on permanent teeth, most of which are formed postnatally, are not likely to provide such strong evidence of the DOHaD framework, which is constrained to the first 1,000 days of life. Nevertheless, it is clear that there are sometimes "discrepancies" in terms of what might be expected with regard to early life stressors and adult mortality that requires a nuanced, contextualized analysis, and interpretation.

Bioarchaeological studies utilizing the DOHaD concept have also now started to consider pathology in intergenerational terms. For example, Godde and colleagues (2020) argue that the series of famines that preceded the Black Death in 14th-century England created an environment of chronic stress that contributed, via epigenetic mechanisms, to patterns of mortality observed in a Black Death cemetery assemblage. Yaussy et al. (2016, and see Chapter 4, this volume) also compared stress indicators and mortality amongst famine victims versus an attritional skeletal sample in medieval London and observed an association between early life stressors and mortality. Work by these authors on 14th-century London have highlighted the intergenerational impacts of famine as a source of heterogeneity in frailty.

Well's (2010) "metabolic ghetto" is also evident in intergenerational indicators of stress observed in post-medieval sites in Northern England (Gowland et al., 2018). Severe growth stunting and dental enamel defects on deciduous and permanent teeth can be attributed in this context to low social status and associated health inequality due to a lack of "maternal somatic capital". Early life adversity included chronic, intergenerational under-nutrition, and exposure to environmental pollutants. Life history trade-offs between growth and immunity, compounded by continuing poor living and working conditions for the children, attenuated any likelihood of "catch-up" growth and resulted in a high frequency of adolescent deaths (Gowland et al., 2018).

As discussed above, structural violence in the form of slavery also has long-term, intergenerational consequences that increases disease susceptibility and mortality risks. Continuing structural inequalities today through the racialization of individuals and groups creates adverse social and ecological systems that reproduce and perpetuate vulnerabilities to a wide range of disease risks (Gravlee, 2009). This has been exemplified by the higher rates of mortality experienced by many Black and ethnic minority groups in the UK and US during the COVID-19 pandemic. For many African Americans, living a healthy lifestyle free of complex disease is rare. Racial bias and systemic racism play a pivotal role in the health outcomes for all Americans but access to education and health care, as well as having higher income do not unequivocally lead to better health outcomes for African Americans in comparison to other ethnic minorities. Historical racial beliefs that are infused within modern medical prejudices and practices continue to influence health care dynamics today. CVD and maternal and fetal health are complex health issues with historical relevance to contemporary issues in African American communities. It is important that paleopathological and bioarchaeological research, which seeks to address structural inequalities, avoid narratives of biological disadvantage that creates further stigmatization (Müller et al., 2017) and diminishes the role of individual and collective agency to shield against, and transcend, social adversity. Studying the African Diaspora and LAAs is pivotal in this process and for unveiling biological processes that further our understanding of all human-kind (Clinton & Jackson, 2021).

Conclusions

As always in paleopathology and bioarchaeology, context is everything. Human bodies are constituted within a complex entanglement of molecular, social, ecological, evolutionary, intergenerational, and biographical factors, such that it is no longer adequate to use "interactionist vocabulary" such as biology-culture, nature-nurture (Niewöhner & Lock, 2018).

Current research is increasingly recognizing the constraints of the boundaries we have constructed between disciplines and the ways in which these have shaped a reductionist view of human biology (Meloni, 2014). Sociological, evolutionary, and epigenetic research is also challenging the indivisibility of bodily boundaries and individual biographies in terms of environmental exposures and the accumulation of disease risk across a life course and intergenerationally (Gowland, 2015, 2020). The reactivity and plasticity of the human body in relation to socio-ecological niches has long been considered an important component of human adaptation. For bioarchaeologists, it is crucial to consider the long-term pathological outcomes of early life phenotypic adjustments that are initiated to secure short-term survival advantages.

Paleopathology and bioarchaeology over the last decade have taken a more explicit theoretical turn, embracing sociological understandings of the body and a more integrative approach for interpreting "embodied phenotypes" (Krieger, 2013). Bioarchaeologists have started to utilize detailed, individualized, osteobiographical narratives, and life histories (Agarwal, 2016). A life course approach needs to consider the range of socio-cultural and environmental conditions that could either ameliorate or exacerbate early life adversity in terms of disease risk and mortality in later life. Adopting a life history and life course approach to interpreting socio-ecological entanglements is crucial for our understanding of past disease. DOHaD and epigenetic research expands the temporal framework of our interpretations to encompass intergenerational evidence. For paleopathology and bioarchaeology, embracing the concepts of DOHaD and life histories, also means that the human body is becoming increasingly "particularized" (Niewöhner & Lock, 2018:687). The potential for heterogeneity of individual responses to similar socio-ecological circumstances is governed, in part, by the experiences of our predecessors (Sletner et al., 2014:448). As Krieger (2013:25) writes: "history matters—deeply, at multiple levels and time scales—to claims about disease etiology and causes of health inequities". The integration of DOHaD within paleopathological and bioarchaeological interpretations, and, in particular, the intergenerational dimension, represents a considerable conceptual shift for our interpretations of skeletal growth and disease in the past.

Acknowledgments

Thank you to Tim Thompson, David Bennett-Jones, Anne Grauer, and an anonymous reviewer for their helpful comments on an earlier draft of this chapter.

References

Agarwal, S. C. (2016). Bone morphologies and histories: life course approaches in bioarchaeology. *American Journal of Physical Anthropology* 159(Suppl. 61):S130–149.

Appleby, J. (2019). Osteobiographies: local biologies, embedded bodies, and relational persons. *Bioarchaeology International* 3(1):32–43.

Armelagos, G. J., Goodman, R. H., Harper, K. N. & Blakey, M. L. (2009). Enamel hypoplasia and early mortality: bioarchaeological support for the Barker hypothesis. *Evolutionary Anthropology* 18:261–271.

Amoroso, A. & S J. Garcia. (2018). Can early life growth disruptions predict longevity? Testing the association between vertebral neural canal (VNC) size and age-at-seath. *International Journal of Paleopathology* 22:8–17.

Baharian, S., Barakatt, M., Gignoux, C. R., Shringarpure, S., Errington, J., Blot, W. J., … & Gravel, S. (2016). The great migration and African-American genomic diversity. *PLoS Genetics* 12(5):e1006059.

Barker, D. J. (1995). Fetal origins of coronary heart disease. *British Medical Journal* 311(6998):171–174.

Barker, D. J. & Osmond, C. (1986). Infant mortality, childhood nutrition, and ischaemic heart disease in England and Wales. *The Lancet* 1(8489):1077–1081.

Barker, D. J. P. (2007). The origins of the developmental origins theory. *Journal of Internal Medicine* 261(5):412–417.

Barker, D. J. P. (2012). Developmental origins of chronic disease. *Public Health* 126:185–189.

Barker, D. J. P., Eriksson, J. G. Forsén, T. & Osmond, C. (2002). Fetal origins of adult disease: strength of effects and biological basis. *International Journal of Epidemiology* 31(6):1235–1239.

Barker, D. J., Winter, P. D., Osmond, C., Margetts, B., & Simmonds, S. J. (1989). Weight in infancy and death from ischaemic heart disease. *The Lancet*, 2(8663), 577–580.

Beaumont, J., Atkins, E.-C., Buckberry, J., Haydock, H., Horne, P., Howcroft, R., Mackenzie, K., & Montgomery, J. (2018). Comparing apples and oranges: why infant bone collagen may not reflect dietary intake in the same way as dentine collagen. *American Journal of Physical Anthropology*, 167(3): 524–540.

Beaumont, J., Geber, J., Powers, N., Lee-Thorp, J., Montgomery, J. (2013). Victims and survivors: identifying survivors of the Great Famine in 19th century London using carbon and nitrogen isotope ratios. *American Journal of Physical Anthropology* 150:87–98.

Beaumont, J., & Montgomery, J. (2016). The Great Irish Famine: identifying starvation in the tissues of victims using stable isotope analysis of bone and incremental dentine collagen. *PloS ONE*, 11(8): e0160065.

Beaumont, J., Montgomery, J., Buckberry, J. & Jay. M. (2015). Infant mortality and isotopic complexity: new approaches to stress, maternal health, and weaning. *American Journal of Physical Anthropology* 157(3):441–457.

Behrman, J. R., Calderon, M. C., Preston, S. H., Hoddinott, J., Martorell, R. & Stein, A. D. (2009). Nutritional supplementation in girls influences the growth of their children: prospective study in Guatemala. *American Journal of Clinical Nutrition* 90:1372–1379.

Bogin, B., Inês Varela Silva, M. & Rios, L. (2007). Life history trade-offs in human growth: adaptation or pathology? *American Journal of Human Biology* 19:631–642.

Booker, A. Q. (2014). African Americans' perceptions of pain and pain management: a systematic review. *Journal of Transcultural Nursing* 27(1):73–80.

Brickley, M. B., Kahlon, B. & D'Ortenzio, L. (2020). Using teeth as tools: investigating the mother-infant dyad and Developmental Origins of Health and Disease Hypothesis using vitamin D deficiency. *American Journal of Physical Anthropology* 171(2):342–353.

Buck, C. & Simpson, H. (1982). Infant diarrhoea and subsequent mortality from heart disease and cancer. *Journal of Epidemiology Community Health* 36:27–30.

Chung, G. C. & Kuzawa, C. J. (2014). Intergenerational effects of early life nutrition: maternal leg length predicts offspring placental weight and birth weight among women in rural Luzon, Philippines. *American Journal of Human Biology* 26(5):652–659.

Caldwell, J. & Jackson, F. (2021). Evolutionary perspectives on African North American genetic diversity: origins and prospects for future investigations. *Evolutionary Anthropology* 30(4):242–252.

Clinton, C. K. & Jackson, F. L. (2021). Historical overview, current research, and emerging bioethical guidelines in researching the New York African Burial Ground. *American Journal of Physical Anthropology* 175(2):339–349.

de Oliveira, V., de Ines Lee, H. & Quintana-Domeque, C. (2021). Natural disasters and early human development: Hurricane Catarina and infant health in Brazil. *The Journal of Human Resources*, March. https://doi.org/10.3368/jhr.59.1.0816-8144R1.

DeWitte, S. N. & Stojanowski. C. M. (2015). The osteological paradox 20 years later: past perspectives, future directions. *Journal of Archaeological Research* 23(4):397–450.

Dominguez-Salas, P., Moore, S. E., Baker, M. S., Bergen, A. W., Cox, S. E., Dyer, R. A., ... & Henning, J. (2014). Maternal nutrition at conception modulates DNA methylation of human metastable epialleles. *Nature Communications*. DOI: 10.1038/ncomms4746.

Ely, B., Wilson, J. L., Jackson, F. & Jackson, B. A. (2006). African-American mitochondrial DNAs often match mtDNAs found in multiple African ethnic groups. *BMC Biology* 4(1):1–14.

Forsdahl, A. (1977). Are poor housing conditions in childhood and adolescence an important risk factor for arteriosclerotic heart disease? *British Journal of Preventative Social Medicine* 31:91–95.

Garland, C. J. (2020). Implications of accumulative stress burdens during critical periods of early postnatal life for mortality risk among Guale interred in a colonial era cemetery in Spanish Florida (ca. AD 1605–1680). *American Journal of Physical Anthropology* 172(4):621–637.

Gilbert, S. F. & Epel, D. (2008). *Ecological Developmental Biology.* Sinauer Associates.
Gluckman, P. D. & Hanson, M. A. (2006). *Developmental Origins of Health and Disease.* Cambridge: Cambridge University Press.
Gluckman, Peter D., Hanson, M. A. & Beedle, A. S. (2007). Early life events and their consequences for later disease: a life history and evolutionary perspective. *American Journal of Human Biology* 19(1):1–19.
Godde, K., Pasillas, V. & Sanchez, A. (2020). Survival analysis of the Black Death: social inequality of women and the perils of life and death in Medieval London. *American Journal of Physical Anthropology* 173(1):168–178.
Godfrey, K. M., Lillycrop, K. A., Burdge, G. C., Gluckman, P. D., & Hanson, M. A. (2007). Epigenetic mechanisms and the mismatch concept of the developmental origins of health and disease. *Pediatric Research*, 61(5 Pt 2), 5R–10R.
Gowland, R. L. (2015). Entangled lives: implications of the developmental origins of health and disease hypothesis for bioarchaeology and the life course. *American Journal of Physical Anthropology* 158(4):530–540.
Gowland, R. L. (2018). Infants and mothers: linked lives and embodied life courses. In Crawford, S., Hadley, D. & Shepherd, G. (Eds.), *The Oxford Handbook of the Archaeology of Childhood*, pp. 104–121. Oxford: Oxford University Press.
Gowland, R. L. (2020). Ruptured: reproductive loss, bodily boundaries, time and the life course in archaeology. In Gowland, R. L. & Halcrow, S. (Eds.), *The Mother-Infant Nexus in Anthropology: Small Beginnings, Significant Outcomes*, pp. 257–274. Cham: Springer International Publishing.
Gowland, R. L., Caffell, A. C., Newman, S., Levene, A. & Holst, M. (2018). Broken childhoods: rural and urban non-adult health during the Industrial Revolution in Northern England (Eighteenth-Nineteenth Centuries). *Bioarchaeology International* 2(1):44–62.
Gowland, R. L. & Halcrow, S. (2020). Introduction: the mother-infant nexus in archaeology and anthropology. In Gowland, R. L. & Halcrow, S. (Eds.), *The Mother-Infant Nexus in Anthropology: Small Beginnings, Significant Outcomes*, pp. 1–15. Cham: Springer International Publishing.
Gowland, R. L. & Newman, S. L. (2018). Children of the revolution: childhood health inequalities and the life course during industrialisation of the 18th to 19th Centuries. In Agarwal, S. & Beauchesne, P. (Eds.), *Children and Childhood in Bioarchaeology*, pp. 294–329. Gainsville: University Press of Florida.
Gowland, R. L. & Thompson, T. J. U. (2021). The art of identification: the skeleton and human identity. In Ferguson, R., Littlefield, M. & Purdon, J. (Eds.), *The Art of Identification: Forensics, Surveillance, Identity*, pp. 101–120. Penn State Press.
Gowland, R. L. & Western, A. G. (2012). Morbidity in the marshes: using spatial epidemiology to investigate skeletal evidence for malaria in Anglo-Saxon England (AD410–1050). *American Journal of Physical Anthropology* 147(2):301–311.
Gravlee, C. C. (2009). How race becomes biology: embodiment of social inequality. *American Journal of Physical Anthropology*, 139(1):47–57.
Haig, D. (2012). The epidemiology of epigenetics. *International Journal of Epidemiology* 41:13–16.
Halcrow, S., Warren, R., Kushnick, G. & Nowell, A. (2020). Care of infants in the past: bridging evolutionary anthropological and bioarchaeological approaches. *Evolutionary Human Sciences* 2. https://doi.org/10.1017/ehs.2020.46.
Han, S., Betsinger, T. K. & Scott, A. B. (2017). *The Anthropology of the Fetus: Biology, Culture, and Society.* Berghahn Books.
Harville, E. W., Giarratano, G. Savage, J., Barcelona de Mendoza, V. & Zotkiewicz. T. (2015). Birth outcomes in a disaster recovery environment: new Orleans women after Katrina. *Maternal and Child Health Journal* 19(11):2512–2522.
Harville, E., Xiong, X. & Buekens, P. (2010). Disasters and perinatal health: a systematic review. *Obstetrical & Gynecological Survey* 65(11):713–728.
Heijmans, B. T., Tobi, E. W., Stein, A. D., Putter, H., Blauw, G. J., Susser, E. S., Slagboom, P. E. & Lumey, L. H. (2008). Persistent epigenetic differences associated with prenatal exposure to famine in humans. *Proceedings of the National Academy of Sciences of the USA* 105:17046–17049.
Heijmans, B. T. & Mill, J. (2012). The seven plagues of epigenetic epidemiology. *International Journal of Epidemiology* 41:74–78.
Heindel, J. J. & Vandenberg, L. J. (2015). Developmental Origins of Health and Disease: a paradigm for understanding disease etiology and prevention. *Current Opinion in Pediatrics* 27(2):248.

Hertzman, C. (2012). Putting the concept of biological embedding in historical perspective. *Proceedings of the National Academy of Science* 109 (Suppl. 2):17160–17167.

Hodson, C. M. (2017). Between roundhouse and villa: assessing perinatal and infant burials from Piddington, Northamptonshire. *Britannia* 48:195–219.

Hodson, C. M. (2021). New prospects for investigating early life course experiences and health in archaeological fetal, perinatal and infant individuals. *Childhood in the Past* 14(1):3–12.

Holder, S., Miliauskienė, Z., Jankauskas, R. & Dupras, T. (2021). An integrative approach to studying plasticity in growth disruption and outcomes: a bioarchaeological case study of Napoleonic soldiers. *American Journal of Human Biology* 33(2):e23457.

Jackson, F. L. C. (2008). Ethnogenetic layering (EL): an alternative to the traditional race model in human variation and health disparity studies. *Annals of Human Biology* 35(2):121–144. DOI: 10.1080/03014460801941752.

Kendall, E. J., Millard, A., Beaumont, J. Gowland, R., Gorton, M. & Gledhill, A. (2020). What doesn't kill you: early life health and nutrition in early Anglo-Saxon East Anglia. In Gowland, R. L. & Halcrow, S. (Eds), *The Mother-Infant Nexus in Anthropology*, pp. 103–123. Cham: Springer International Publishing.

Kim, S., Fleisher, B. & Ya Sun, J. (2017). The long-term health effects of fetal malnutrition: evidence from the 1959–1961 China Great Leap Forward Famine. *Health Economics*. https://doi.org/10.1002/hec.3397.

Krieger, N. (2013). History, biology, and health inequities: emergent embodied phenotypes and the illustrative case of the breast cancer estrogen receptor. *American Journal of Public Health* 103(1):22–27.

Kuzawa, C. W. (2005). Fetal origins of developmental plasticity: are fetal cues reliable predictors of future nutritional environments? *American Journal of Human Biology* 17(1):5–21.

Kuzawa, C. W. (2020). Pregnancy as an intergenerational conduit of adversity: how nutritional and psychosocial stressors reflect different historical timescales of maternal experience. *Current Opinion in Behavioral Sciences* 36(December):42–47.

Kuzawa, C. W. & Sweet, E. (2009). Epigenetics and the embodiment of race: developmental origins of US racial disparities in cardiovascular health. *American Journal of Human Biology* 21(1):2–15.

Kuzawa, C. W. & Thayer, Z. M. (2011). Timescales of human adaptation: the role of epigenetic processes. *Epigenomics* 3(2):221–234.

Lachance, J., Berens, A. J., Hansen, M. E., Teng, A. K., Tishkoff, S. A. & Rebbeck, T. R. (2018). Genetic hitchhiking and population bottlenecks contribute to prostate cancer disparities in men of African descent. *Cancer research* 78(9):2432–2443.

Landecker, H. (2011). Food as exposure: nutritional epigenetics and the new metabolism. *Biosocieties* 6:167–194.

Landecker, H. & Panofsky, A. (2013). From social structure to gene regulation, and back: a critical introduction to environmental epigenetics for sociology. *Annual Review of Sociology* 39:333–357.

Landry, L. G., Ali, N., Williams, D. R., Rehm, H. L. & Bonham, V. L. (2018). Lack of diversity in genomic databases is a barrier to translating precision medicine research into practice. *Health Affairs* 37(5):780–785.

Lawrence, J., Stojanowski, C. M., Paul, K. S. Seidel, A. C. & Guatelli-Steinberg, D. (2021). Heterogeneous frailty and the expression of linear enamel hypoplasia in a genealogical population. *American Journal of Physical Anthropology* 176(4):638–651. https://doi.org/10.1002/ajpa.24288.

Leskovar, T., Beaumont, J., Lisić, N. & McGalliard, S. (2019). Auditory ossicles: a potential biomarker for maternal and infant health in utero. *Annals of Human Biology* 46(5):367–377.

Lewis, M. E. (2010). Life and death in a *Civitas* capital: metabolic disease and trauma in the children from late Roman Dorchester, Dorset. *American Journal of Physical Anthropology* 142(3):405–416.

Lewis, M. (2017). *Paleopathology of Children: Identification of Pathological Conditions in the Human Skeletal Remains of Non-Adults*. Academic Press.

Lewontin, R. (2000). *The Triple Helix — Gene, Organism and Environment*. Cambridge, MA: Harvard University Press.

Li, Y., Li, Y., Gurol, M. E., Liu, Y., Yang, P., Shi, J., Zhuang, S., Forman, M. R., Wu, S. & Gao, X. (2020). In utero exposure to the Great Chinese Famine and risk of intracerebral hemorrhage in midlife. *Neurology* 94(19):e1996–e2004. https://doi.org/10.1212/WNL.0000000000009407.

Lock, M. (1993). *Encounters with Aging: Mythologies of Menopause in Japan and North America*. Berkeley, CA: University of California Press.

Lock, M. (2013). The epigenome and nature/nurture reunification: a challenge for anthropology. *Medical Anthropology* 32:291–308.

Longhurst, R. (2008). *Maternities: Gender, Bodies and Space*. London: Routledge

Lorentz, K. O., Lemmers, S. A. M. Chrysostomou, C. Dirks, W., Zaruri, M. R., Foruzanfar, F. & Sajjadi, S. M. S. (2019). Use of dental microstructure to investigate the role of prenatal and early life physiological stress in age at death. *Journal of Archaeological Science* 104(April):85–96.

Lumey, L. H., Stein, A. D. & Susser, E. (2011). Prenatal famine and adult health. *Annual Review of Public Health* 32:237–262.

Marmot, M. (2010). *Fair Society, Healthy Lives. The Marmot Review*. Strategic Review of Health Inequalities in England Post-2010. London.

McDade, T. W. (2003). Life history theory and the immune system steps toward a human ecological immunology. *Yearbook of Physical Anthropology* 46:100–125.

McDade, T. W., Georgiev, A. V. & Kuzawa, C. W. (2016). Trade-Offs between acquired and innate immune defenses in humans. *Evolution, Medicine, and Public Health* 2016(1):1–16.

McKerracher, L., Fried, R., Kim, A. W., Moffat, T., Sloboda, D. M. & Galloway, T. (2020). Synergies between the Developmental Origins of Health and Disease framework and multiple branches of evolutionary anthropology. *Evolutionary Anthropology* 29(5):214–219.

McMichael, A. J. (1999). Prisoners of the proximate: loosening the constraints on epidemiology in an age of change. *American Journal of Epidemiology* 149(10):887–897.

McPherson, C. B. (2021). Examining developmental plasticity in the skeletal system through a sensitive developmental windows framework. *American Journal of Physical Anthropology* 176(2):163–178. https://doi.org/10.1002/ajpa.24338.

Meloni, M. (2014). How biology became social, and what it means for social theory. *The Sociological Review* 62(3):593–614.

Mekota, A. -M. & Grupe, G. (2006). Serial analysis of stable nitrogen and carbon isotopes in hair: monitoring starvation and recovery phases of patients suffering from anorexia nervosa. *Rapid Communications in Mass Spectrometry* 20:1604–1610.

Mohottige, D., Boulware, L. E., Ford, C. L., Jones, C. & Norris, K. C. (2022). Use of race in kidney research and medicine: concepts, principles, and practice. *Clinical Journal of the American Society of Nephrology* 17(2):314–322.

Montgomery, J., Beaumont, J., Jay, M., Keefe, K., Gledhill, A. R., Cook, G. T., Dockrill, S. J. & Melton, N. D. (2013). Strategic and sporadic marine consumption at the onset of the Neolithic: increasing temporal resolution in the isotope evidence. *Antiquity*, 87(338): 1060–1072.

Moore, S. E., Cole, T. J., Collinson, A. C., Postkitt, E. M. E., McGregor, I. A. & Prentice, A. M. (1999). Prenatal or early postnatal events predict infectious death in young adulthood in rural Africa. *International Journal of Epidemiology* 28:1088–1095.

Moore, S. E., Fulford, A.., Streatfield, P., Åke Persson, L. & Prentice, A. M. (2004). Comparative analysis of patterns of survival by season of birth in rural Bangladeshi and Gambian populations. *International Journal of Epidemiology* 33:137–143.

Müller, R., Hanson, C. Hanson, M., Penkler, M., Samaras, G., Chiapperino, L., Dupré, J. & Villa, P. -I. (2017). The biosocial genome? Interdisciplinary perspectives on environmental epigenetics, health and society. *EMBO Reports* 18(10):1677–1682.

Niewohner, J. (2011). Epigenetics: embedded bodies and the molecularisation of biography. *Biosocieties* 6:279–298.

Niewöhner, J. & Lock, M. (2018). Situating local biologies: anthropological perspectives on environment/human entanglements. *BioSocieties* 13(4):681–697.

Pickersgill, M. (2021). Negotiating novelty: constructing the novel within scientific accounts of epigenetics. *Sociology* 55(3):600–618.

Pickersgill, M., Niewöhner, J., Müller, R., Martin, P. & Cunningham-Burley, S. (2013). Mapping the new molecular landscape: social dimensions of epigenetics. *New Genetics and Society* 32:429–447.

Quade, L., Chazot, P. L. & Gowland, R. (2021). Desperately seeking stress: a pilot study of cortisol in archaeological tooth structures. *American Journal of Physical Anthropology* 174(3):532–541.

Ravelli, A. C. J., van der Meulen, J. H. P., Osmond, C., Barker, D. J. P. & Bleker, O. P. (1999). Obesity at the age of 50 years in men and women exposed to famine prenatally. *American Journal of Clinical Nutrition* 70:811–816.

Riccomi, G., Felici, C. & Giuffra, V. (2021). Maternal–fetal death in Medieval Pieve Di Pava (central Italy, 10th–12th Century AD). *International Journal of Osteoarchaeology* 31(5):701–715. https://doi.org/10.1002/oa.2983.

Richardson, S. S. (2015). Maternal bodies in the postgenomic order: gender and the explanatory landscape of epigenetics. In Richardson, S. & Stevens, H. (Eds.), *Postgenomics: Perspectives on Biology after the Genome*, pp. 210–231. Duke University Press.

Richardson, S. S., Daniels, C. R., Gillman, M. W., Golden, J., Kukla, R., Kuzawa, C. & Rich-Edwards, J. (2014). Society: don't blame the mothers. *Nature* 512(7513):131–132. DOI: 10.1038/512131a.

Roberts, C. & Steckel, R. (2018). The developmental origins of health and disease: early life health conditions and adult age at death in Europe. In Steckel, R., Larsen, C., Roberts, C. & Baten, J. (Eds.), *The Backbone of Europe: Health, Diet, Work and Violence over Two Millennia*, pp. 325–351. Cambridge: Cambridge University Press.

Roseboom, T. J., van der Meulen, J. H. P. & Ravelli, A. C. J. (2001). Effects of prenatal exposure to the Dutch famine on adult disease in later life: an overview. *Molecular and Cellular Endocrinology* 185:93–98.

Roseboom, T., de Rooij, S. & Painter, R. (2006). The Dutch famine and its long-term consequences for adult health. *Early Human Development* 82(8):485–491.

Ryan, C. P. & Kuzawa, C. J. (2020). Germline epigenetic inheritance: challenges and opportunities for linking human paternal experience with offspring biology and health. *Evolutionary Anthropology* 29(4):180–200.

Schulz, L. C. (2010). The Dutch Hunger Winter and the developmental origins of health and disease. *Proceedings of the National Academy of Sciences of the United States of America* 107(39):16757–16758.

Sinha, A., Gupta, D. K., Yancy, C. W., Shah, S. J., Rasmussen-Torvik, L. J., McNally, E. M., ... & Khan, S. S. (2021). Risk-based approach for the prediction and prevention of heart failure. *Circulation: Heart Failure* 14(2):e007761.

Sharp, G. C., Lawlor, D. A. & Richardson, S. S. (2018). It's the mother!: how assumptions about the causal primacy of maternal effects influence research on the developmental origins of health and disease. *Social Science Medicine* 213:20–27.

Sharp, G. C., Schellhas, L., Richardson, S. S. & Lawlor, D. A. (2019). Time to cut the cord: recognizing and addressing the imbalance of DOHaD research towards the study of maternal pregnancy exposures. *Journal of Developmental Origins of Health and Disease* 10(5):509–512. DOI: 10.1017/S204017441900007.

Sletner, L., Jenum, A. K., Mørkrid, K., Vangen, S., Holme, I. M., Birkeland, K. I. & Nakstad, B. (2014). Maternal life course socio-economic position and offspring body composition at birth in a multi-ethnic population. *Paediatric and Perinatal Epidemiology*, 28(5): 445–454.

Susser, E., Kirkbride, J. B., Heijmans, B. T., Kresovich, J. K., Lumey, L. H. & Stein, A. D. (2012). Maternal prenatal nutrition and health in grandchildren and subsequent generations. *Annual Review of Anthropology* 41:577–610. https://doi.org/10.1146/annurev-anthro-081309-145645.

Tamir, C. (2022, January 31). Key findings about Black America. *Pew Research Center*. Retrieved May 31, 2022, from https://www.pewresearch.org/fact-tank/2021/03/25/key-findings-about-black-america/.

Temple, D. H. (2014). Plasticity and constraint in response to early-life stressors among late/final Jomon period foragers from Japan: evidence for life history trade-offs from incremental microstructures of enamel. *American Journal of Physical Anthropology* 155(4):537–545.

Temple, D. H. (2019). Bioarchaeological evidence for adaptive plasticity and constraint: exploring life-history trade-offs in the human past. *Evolutionary Anthropology* 28(1):34–46.

Thayer, Z. M. & Kuzawa, C. W. (2011). Biological memories of past environments: epigenetic pathways to health disparities. *Epigenetics: Official Journal of the DNA Methylation Society* 6(7):798–803.

Thayer, Z. M., Rutherford, J. & Kuzawa, C. W. (2020). The maternal nutritional buffering model: an evolutionary framework for pregnancy nutritional intervention. *Evolution, Medicine, and Public Health* 2020(1):14–27.

Tishkoff, S. A., Reed, F. A., Friedlaender, F. R., Ehret, C., Ranciaro, A., Froment, A., ... & Williams, S. M. (2009). The genetic structure and history of Africans and African Americans. *Science* 324(5930):1035–1044.

Wadhwa, P. D., Buss, C., Entringer, S. & Swanson, J. M. (2009). Developmental Origins of Health and Disease: brief history of the approach and current focus on epigenetic mechanisms. *Seminars in Reproductive Medicine* 27:358. NIH Public Access.

Waterland, R. A., Kellermajer, R., Laritsky, E., Rayoo-Solon, P., Harris, R. A., Travisino, M., ... & Prentiss, A. (2010). Season of conception in rural Gambia affects DNA methylation at putative metastable epialleles. *PLoS Genetics* 6(12):e1001252.

Watts, R. (2011). Non-specific indicators of stress and their relationship to age-at-death in medieval York: using stature and vertebral canal neural size to examine the effects of stress occurring during different stages of development. *International Journal of Osteoarchaeology* 21:568–576.

Watts, R. (2013). Childhood development and adult longevity in an archaeological population from Barton-upon-Humber, Lincolnshire, England. *International Journal of Paleopathology* 3:95–104.

Watts, R. (2015). The long-term impact of developmental stress: evidence from later medieval and post-medieval London (AD1117–1853). *American Journal of Physical Anthropology* 158(4):569–580.

Weaver, I. C., Cervoni, N., Champagne, F. A., D'Alessio, A. C., Sharma, S., Seckl, J. R., Dymov, S., Szyf, M. & Meaneyet, M. J. (2004). Epigenetic programming by maternal behaviour. *Nature Neuroscience* 7:847–854.

Weaver, I. C., Champagne, F. A., Brown, S. E., Dymov, S., Sharma, S., Meaney, M. J. & Szyf, M. (2005). Reversal of maternal programming of stress responses in adult offspring through methyl supplementation: altering epigenetic marking later in life. *Journal of Neuroscience* 25(47):11045–11054.

Wells, J. C. K. (2010). Maternal capital and the metabolic ghetto: an evolutionary perspective on the transgenerational basis of health inequalities. *American Journal of Human Biology* 22(1):1–17.

Wood, J. W., Milner, G. R., Harpending, H. C. & Weiss, K. M. (1992). The osteological paradox: problems of inferring prehistoric health from skeletal samples. *Current Anthropology* 33:343–370.

Yaussy, S. L., DeWitte, S. N. & Redfern, R. C. (2016). Frailty and famine: patterns of mortality and physiological stress among victims of famine in Medieval London. *American Journal of Physical Anthropology* 160(2):272–283.

29
DISEASE IN THE FOSSIL RECORD

Florian Witzmann and Patrick Asbach

Introduction

Paleopathology in paleontology is the study of injury and disease that can be recognized in fossils, i.e., organismal remains that are by definition older than 10,000 years or pre-Holocene in age (Rothschild & Martin, 2006). Compared to archaeological human paleopathology and zooarchaeology, paleontological paleopathology is by far the smallest and most "exotic" field within paleopathology, with probably only less than a dozen scientists worldwide working permanently on this subject. Strictly speaking, paleontological paleopathology studies all fossil organisms, including protozoans, plants, invertebrates and vertebrates, including prehistoric humans (Moodie, 1923). Although the studies of all these different organismal groups are important for our understanding of the evolutionary history of life and diseases on earth, the present contribution will focus on the paleopathology of fossil non-human vertebrates (in the following referred to as "paleontological paleopathology" for simplicity) because its results and their implications can best be compared to those in human and archaeozoological paleopathology.

Paleontological paleopathology is an ideal complement and extension to human and archaeozoological paleopathology because it significantly expands the timespan from thousands up to hundreds of millions of years and considers diverse groups of vertebrates throughout their evolutionary history. Many diseases of modern humans are significantly older than the origin of humans themselves. Therefore, the origin of most human diseases and the evolution of pathophysiologic response and repair mechanisms (e.g., bone healing after fracture) must be seen in the context of the distant evolutionary past among our remote ancestors and relatives. The study of fossils can provide this deep-time perspective on the origin and evolution of diseases. Furthermore, greater knowledge of the origin and distribution of diseases among animals (including fossil taxa) is important for our understanding of zoonotic diseases (Thomas, 2012).

Similar to the other fields of paleopathology, paleontological paleopathology takes a highly interdisciplinary approach. Although it lacks the inclusion of social science and humanities disciplines, which characterize human paleopathology, paleontological paleopathology overlaps broadly with paleobiology (including paleoecology) and geology and seeks to understand the mode of life and physiology of extinct organisms and their interactions with each other and the environment. It requires the expertise of paleontologists, physicians and veterinarians, biologists and geologists, but increasingly also of material scientists and geochemists due to modern methods of examination and analytics.

Paleontological paleopathology primarily deals with fossil (or "petrified") skeletal hard components of the body, like bones and teeth. However, fossil bones and teeth are not simply "rocks". While they usually have a more complex taphonomic history than bones and teeth recovered archaeologically and are permineralized to varying degrees, the structure remains largely unchanged and allows for microstructural and histological analyses. The pathological alterations found in fossil bones include injury, joint disease, toxic-metabolic diseases (e.g., gout), infection, neoplastic disease ("cancer") or congenital malformations. In rare cases, trackways, remains of eggshells, the impression of skin and even preserved pathogens may be recovered and provide valuable insight into pathological conditions suffered by ancient organisms.

Modern paleontological paleopathology is basically hypothesis- and problem-driven and seeks to explore specific paleobiological and medical questions. Such questions may include: Have diseases always been concomitants of organismal life? How did healing evolve in vertebrate evolution? How did the prevalence of certain diseases change through time, and can they be compared to those in extant humans? Can we correlate pathologies in earth history with certain environmental factors? Can we identify time-periods in which organisms were exposed to natural pollutants before the anthropogenic influence on the environment started? This chapter attempts to show how paleontological paleopathology can contribute to the understanding of the origin and history of present-day diseases, where its common roots with archaeological paleopathology lie, and some current scientific approaches and research topics.

Short History of Paleontological Paleopathology

Although it is centered on archaeological and mummified human remains today, paleopathology, both as a scientific discipline and in name, has its roots in paleontological paleopathology. The first published paleopathological work was authored by Johann Friedrich Esper (1732–1781) who described a fractured cave bear femur (Esper, 1774). Other early paleopathological studies dealt with Pleistocene non-human mammals (e.g., Goldfuss, 1810; von Walther, 1825), although the early paleopathological publications often included Pleistocene human *and* non-human mammalian remains together (e.g., Schmerling, 1835). Even by the 20th century, Sir Marc Armand Ruffer (1859–1917) considered both archaeological human and fossil animal remains in his famous *Studies in the Paleopathology of Egypt* (Ruffer, 1921). These exemplars show that human and non-human paleopathology was not strictly separated, as it is today.

Subsequent to the earliest studies dealing with Pleistocene mammals, several publications of pathological lesions in Mesozoic reptiles, in particular dinosaurs, were published in the later course of the 19th century, starting with the work on Jurassic dinosaurs by Eudes-Deslongchamps (1838). As more discoveries of fossil reptiles and mammals were made, the number of paleopathological descriptions increased considerably in the second half of the 19th and the beginning of the 20th century, many of which were descriptions of isolated cases – often incidentally mentioned within morphological descriptions and often incorrectly diagnosed without emphasis on the etiology. In 1893, Robert W. Shufeldt published a study on pathological bones of Pliocene birds and formally introduced the name "palaeopathology": "Palaeopathology […] is a term here proposed under which may be described all diseased or pathological conditions found fossilized in the remains of extinct or fossil animals" (Shufeldt, 1893:679, footnote).

At the beginning of the 20th century, pathological lesions in fossil vertebrates aroused the interest of paleobiology, a new discipline within paleontology that aimed to reconstruct the mode of life of extinct animals and their adaptations to their environments. Othenio Abel (1875–1946), one of the founding fathers of paleobiology (Kutschera, 2007), described and discussed a number of skeletal injuries in fossil vertebrates (Abel, 1912). He was more interested in the paleobiological and behavioral context of these injuries like inter- and intraspecific fights than in medical questions. In spite of the paleobiological approaches, paleontological paleopathology at the beginning of the 20th century was dominated by Roy Lee Moodie (1880–1934), a paleontologist who can rightly be designated the founder of paleontological paleopathology as a discipline (Rega, 2012). Moodie published a great number of paleopathological studies between 1904 and 1931 on nearly all aspects of paleopathology, culminating in his major work *Paleopathology: An Introduction to the Study of Ancient Evidences of Disease* (Moodie, 1923). Moodie's methodological approach was innovative and involved X-rays and histological thin sections of pathological fossil bone, although many of his diagnoses and conclusions must be treated with caution today (see Waldron, 2015).

After Moodie's untimely death in 1934, the interest of scientists in paleopathology of fossil organisms decreased markedly, and in the following decades, paleontological paleopathology appeared to wane. However, most notable in this time-period is the publication of a general compendium on fossil animal paleopathology by the Hungarian paleontologist András Tasnádi-Kubacska (1902–1977), which summarized the state of knowledge in the middle of the 20th century (Tasnádi-Kubacska, 1960).

Starting in the 1980s and 1990s, a new generation of paleontologists and medical scientists developed an interest in paleontological paleopathology. This took place along with the rise of new non-invasive techniques like X-ray-computed tomography (e.g., micro-CT) and neutron- and synchrotron scanning to study the internal structure of fossil bones and teeth. Since then, paleontological paleopathology has turned into a problem-driven field of research that focuses increasingly on the etiology of diseases by the formulation of testable hypotheses. It seeks to quantify data and answer-specific paleobiological and epidemiological questions in correlation with environmental and evolutionary factors (e.g., Hanna, 2002; Rothschild et al., 2003; Rothschild & Martin, 2006; Wolff, 2008, 2009; Rega, 2012; Tanke & Rothschild, 2014; Foth et al., 2015; Pardo-Pérez et al., 2019; Hamm et al., 2020; Witzmann et al., 2021).

Diagnosis in Paleontological Paleopathology and the Extant Phylogenetic Bracket

The diagnostic pathway in paleontological paleopathology corresponds directly to that in human paleopathology. It encompasses hypotheses-testing of pathological conditions by differential diagnosis and the comparison of fossil bone lesions with those in modern humans and other animals (Buikstra et al., 2017; Mays, 2018). However, diagnosis is complicated by the fact that we have to deal with phylogenetically very disparate groups of vertebrates from fossil fishes, amphibians and reptiles, including birds to non-human mammals. Thus, the paleopathologist working with fossils has to decide which is the appropriate morphological and physiological extant analog for comparison (see below).

As pointed out by Ortner (1991) and Hanna (2002), it is essential to provide an accurate, careful description of each paleopathological bone alteration (preferably in a standardized manner) before providing a differential diagnosis (see Chapters 2 and 3, this volume). This enhances the comparability of data derived from different authors, and furthermore, diagnoses may change in the future with increasing knowledge about manifestation of disease in fossil vertebrates. If ever possible, a multimodal approach encompassing macroscopic, radiological and histological investigation is most desirable (Barbosa et al., 2016; Hedrick et al., 2016; Ekhtiari et al., 2020). When interpreting bone alterations, we must apply the uniformitarian principle (Shufeldt, 1893; Rega, 2012; Buikstra et al., 2017), i.e., we must assume that diseases in the past proceeded in the same way as they do today, although environmental conditions and the nature of pathogens, for example, might have changed over time. Considering the fact that only very few skeletal lesions are truly pathognomonic (Rega, 2012; Hamm et al., 2020), even a careful, objective differential diagnosis may leave two or more plausible candidate diseases. Therefore, authors often use a classification of bone pathologies that is based on a broader etiology (e.g., traumatic; infectious; developmental; idiopathic) to avoid any over-interpretation of the data (e.g., Hanna, 2002; Bell & Coria, 2013). A new approach combining the extant phylogenetic bracket (EPB) and epidemiological methods with radiologic imaging was recently used by Hamm et al. (2020) to diagnose skeletal alterations in a specimen of *Tyrannosaurus rex*. In the EPB, a completely extinct taxon (e.g., a species, genus or family) is bracketed in the phylogenetic tree by two taxa with living representatives. The presence of a certain disease in both bracket taxa indicates that a homolog of this disease must have been present also in the extinct taxon. For example, skeletal lesions in dinosaurs are usually bracketed between their closest extant archosaurian relatives, i.e., crocodilians and birds (Wolff, 2009; Rega, 2012; Foth et al., 2015). In the study by Hamm et al. (2020), the differential diagnosis based on outer morphology and CT revealed that neoplasia and infection were the most likely diagnoses, and therefore, an epidemiological likelihood estimation by phylogenetic disease bracketing was conducted. It showed that infectious diseases are considerably more common in reptiles, including birds, than are neoplastic diseases, suggesting that the bony lesions in *Tyrannosaurus* probably represent infection. However, it should be kept in mind that even with extant bracketing taxa, there is often restricted possibility for direct comparison. For example, although being the closest extant relatives of dinosaurs, the bone structure of most extant birds differs from that of non-avian dinosaurs in the lack of cyclical bone growth and adaptations for active flight (Rega, 2012).

The question regarding which group(s) of extant animals should be considered the adequate model(s) for diagnosis of ancient diseases is still a matter of debate in paleontological paleopathology. Basically, two competing conceptual frameworks for diagnosis exist: (1) the trans-phylogenetic and (2) the phylogenetic approach. Both are based upon comparison to extant groups and follow common principles of pathologic diagnosis. However, the proponents of the trans-phylogenetic approach regard manifestation of disease in the skeleton of vertebrates as not (or only to a minor extent) determined by phylogeny (Rothschild & Martin, 2006; Rothschild, 2017) and argue that the same fundamental physiological and cellular mechanisms are shared by most vertebrates (Beatty & Rothschild, 2009). Consequently, skeletal pathologies in human medicine can be used as reference for the diagnosis of paleopathologies in mammalian and non-mammalian fossils. In contrast, the supporters of the phylogenetic approach recognize fundamental differences in immunology, disease physiology, anatomy and behavior between the different vertebrate groups and criticize the direct reference to human pathology (Wolff, 2009). Rather, they apply the method of the EPB as a framework for diagnosis. Two examples in extinct reptiles shall illustrate these two competing conceptual frameworks.

The first example is osteomyelitis in dinosaurs, which has often been compared with osteomyelitis in humans as an extant model (e.g., Gross et al., 1993; Hanna, 2002). It has been shown, however, that the immune response to infection in extant reptiles (including birds) includes the immobilization of infectious particles in a local fibriscess, which prevents the hematogenous spread of the infection; this stands in contrast to mammals, in which liquid pus is produced and hematogenous transmission occurs (Montali, 1988; Huchzermeyer & Cooper, 2000). Thus, the EPB suggests that dinosaurs had an immune response more similar to extant reptiles than to mammals, and many of the observed pathomorphological features

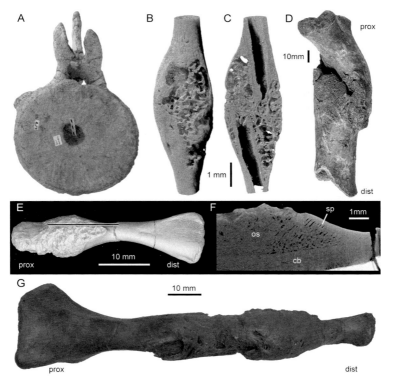

Figure 29.1 (a) caudal vertebra (SNMB 1695-R) of an indeterminate sauropod dinosaur from the Middle-Late Jurassic of Niger, anterior view with erosive lesion on the articular surface of the vertebral body (© Achim Ritter); (b) and (c) CT-scans of a fractured tibia of a frog (*Rana* sp.; MB.Am.1352) from the late Pleistocene/early Holocene of Pisede, Germany, with callus formation in external view (b) and longitudinal section (c) (© Mario Thiele); (d) fractured femur of a juvenile cave bear (*Ursus spelaeus*; MB.Ma.3852) with callus formation from the late Pleistocene of Letmathe, Germany (© Carola Radke); (e) and (f) femur of the stem-turtle *Proganochelys rosinae* (SMNS 91680) from the Middle Triassic of Germany with osteosarcoma as revealed by external view (e) and internal structure (f) (© Yara Haridy). The black line in (e) indicates the location of the section shown in (f); (g) fibula of *Tyrannosaurus rex* (FMNH PR 2081) from the Late Cretaceous of South Dakota, USA with rugose surface indicating osteomyelitis (modified from Hamm et al. 2020, © The authors, under CC BY 4.0, https://creativecommons.org/licenses/by/4.0/). Abbreviations: cb, cortical bone; dist, distal; FMNH, Field Museum of Natural History, Chicago, USA; MB, Museum für Naturkunde Berlin, Germany; os, osteosarcoma; prox, proximal; SMNS, Staatliches Museum für Naturkunde Stuttgart, Germany; SNMB, Staatliches Naturhistorisches Museum Braunschweig, Germany; sp, spicular outgrowth

of affected dinosaur bones correspond to this interpretation (Foth et al., 2015; Romo-de-Vivar-Martínez et al., 2017; Hamm et al., 2020). However, to complicate this matter, Vittore and Henderson (2013) and Hunt et al. (2019) identified a Brodie abscess, which is a type of hematogenous osteomyelitis, in two dinosaurs. This suggests that spread of the infection via the blood stream might have been more common in dinosaurs than initially thought. Nevertheless, this would still conform to modern reptiles as extant analogs for dinosaur osteomyelitis because although hematogenous osteomyelitis does not occur in non-avian reptiles, it indeed occurs in birds, albeit it is less common than in mammals (Hunt et al., 2019).

The second example is Schmorl's nodes, i.e., the herniation of intervertebral disc material in the vertebral body causing deep erosive lesions. While Schmorl's nodes are well known in human paleopathology (Weiss, 2005), they are extraordinarily rare in the non-human fossil record and have been demonstrated only in a few Pleistocene mammals (Barbosa et al., 2019, and references therein). Similar erosive lesions have also been detected on the articular surfaces of vertebral bodies of a marine reptile (Hopley, 2001) and two dinosaurs (Witzmann et al., 2016; Barbosa et al., 2018) (see Figure 29.1a). However, because extant reptiles, inclusive of birds, do not have intervertebral discs, but rather synovial joints between their vertebral bodies, the EPB indicates that these lesions can be interpreted as subchondral cysts rather than Schmorl's nodes (Witzmann et al., 2016).

In conclusion, the reference to human medicine in diagnosis of pathological lesions in fossil non-mammalian vertebrates is certainly valuable when cautiously used, especially considering the large body of evidence on human diseases, highly developed diagnostic techniques, and the fact that the largest part of the osteopathological literature deals with humans (Hunt et al., 2019; Ekhtiari et al., 2020). Furthermore, bone dynamics (e.g., Haversian remodeling and growth rate) is similar in humans (and other mammals) and in archosaurs, like birds and many dinosaurs (Rega, 2012). However, the EPB should be applied more regularly in diagnosis of pathological lesions in non-mammalian fossils, especially when significant differences in morphology and physiology (e.g., immune response and bone dynamics) between humans and the taxon under study are apparent.

Examination Methods

As in human and archaeozoological paleopathology, macroscopic investigation of the morphology of pathologic bone is still the basis for paleopathological analysis (see Chapter 2, this volume). To investigate the internal bone structure, histological sections of pathologic fossil bone are extremely valuable tools toward understanding pathological alterations (e.g., Barbosa et al., 2016; Hedrick et al., 2016; Ekhtiari et al., 2020), but since it is an invasive method, it is often restricted by curatorial policies. Therefore, most studies of the internal structure are performed by non-invasive cross-sectional imaging techniques like X-ray-computed tomography or micro-CT (e.g., Anné et al., 2015), neutron tomography (e.g., Cisneros et al., 2010), and synchrotron X-ray phase contrast tomography (e.g., Witzmann et al., 2011, and see Chapter 6, this volume).

In recent years, an increasing number of geochemical analyses of fossil pathological bone, in comparison to adjacent healthy areas, have been performed to demonstrate differences in tissue temperature (Straight et al., 2009), in distribution of certain trace elements (Anné et al., 2014), or to assess how crystallinity and structure of pathological bone tissue differ from that of "normal" fossil and extant bones (Surmik et al., 2017). The application of biomechanics in paleopathology has also proven to be fruitful, although it has so far been rarely performed. Bishop et al. (2015) applied Finite Element Analysis (FEA) to study the partially healed fracture in the limb of an Early Carboniferous stem-tetrapod to reconstruct the loading scenario under which the fracture occurred. In contrast to archaeological paleopathology, microbiological or biochemical clues are preserved only in exceptional cases in paleontology, and they are restricted to the geologically youngest fossils. For example, 17,000-year-old DNA fragments of tuberculosis pathogens have reportedly been isolated from skeletal elements of Pleistocene bison (Rothschild et al., 2001).

Paleoepidemiological Studies of Fossil Populations

Although descriptions of individual cases are important because they might deal with a rare disease or a rare fossil taxon, modern paleontological paleopathology increasingly seeks to analyze the types and frequencies of pathologies in fossil populations or larger taxonomic groups. Discrete fossil assemblages or bonebeds may represent catastrophic mass death assemblages, natural trap caves or tar pits, and include a large number (or a population) of individuals of one or more particular species. However, admittedly, such "populations" do not represent true populations in an epidemiological sense. Only if all preserved individuals of a fossil assemblage died in a catastrophic event at the same time, would they represent a former true population. In most cases, however, the preserved populations are time averaged, i.e., they include individuals of several consecutive populations that accumulated over a time span of hundreds or thousands of years. For example, the fossils found in the famous La Brea Tar Pits in California have accumulated over a period of at least 35,000 years (Shaw & Ware, 2018). A further limiting factor in fossil populations is that they often contain incomplete or disarticulated specimens, or sometimes only bone fragments, rather than complete skeletons.

Examples of population studies in paleontological paleopathology are Bell and Coria (2013) who documented bone alterations of the theropod dinosaur *Mapusaurus* from a Late Cretaceous monospecific bonebed. They found that the majority of skeletal pathologies in this predator are injury-related, supporting an active and probably aggressive mode of life. Schlüter and Kohring (2002) demonstrated a correlation between the presence of hyperostotic bones in cichlid fishes from a Pliocene/Pleistocene lake in Tanzania with an unusually high content of fluorine in the water, while Duckler and Van Valkenburgh (1998) used the prevalence of Harris lines (areas of hypercalcification in long bones created when growth is forced to cease due to disease or the presence of a severe stressor and then resumes) in limb bones as an indicator of environmental stress in populations of large mammals from the La Brea Tar Pit locality prior to the end-Pleistocene extinctions. Pardo-Pérez et al. (2019) quantitatively investigated the correlation between individual age, adult body size and environmental stress with the type and frequency of skeletal pathologies in different ichthyosaur genera from the Early Jurassic Posidonia Shale in southwestern Germany. They found that adult ichthyosaurs show only slightly more skeletal injuries than juveniles but were more susceptible to age-related skeletal alterations like articular disease and ankyloses. Interestingly, a minor mass extinction event in the Posidonienschiefer Formation, which affected ichthyosaur diversity and body size, did not have an impact on the prevalence of their osseous pathologies.

Research in Paleontological Paleopathology

In the following, a selection of current research topics in paleontological paleopathology is provided, which potentially link fossil with human paleopathological and medical research, since they focus on diseases that affect ancient and modern humans.

Traumatic Injuries

Injury-related pathologies, like bite wounds or bone fractures, are the most common types of pathologies in fossil vertebrates (Figure 29.1b–d). They are of special interest for two reasons. First, each traumatic lesion is related in some way to the behavior or mode of life of an animal and may have been caused by interspecies predator-prey relationships or intraspecies aggression, such as hierarchical and territorial conflict and competition for mates and carcasses. Injuries are thus of great importance for the paleobiologist in order to reconstruct behavior of fossil animals and their interactions within a given ecosystem (Abel, 1912; Tanke & Currie, 1998; Brown et al., 2017). Second, fossil bone injuries in the state of healing are unique in providing direct evidence of the origin and evolution of healing and regeneration of skeletal tissues.

Evolution of Skeletal Healing

The first known mineralized skeletal elements in vertebrates are dermal plates consisting of acellular bone (aspidin) and an outer layer of dentin that formed the exoskeleton of Paleozoic jawless fishes, the so called heterostracans (Keating et al, 2018). Johanson et al. (2013) provided evidence that wound repair in these dermal plates occurred by reactive dentinous tissue that sealed the bony lesion, before bone repair by formation of reactive bone tissue had evolved. In the first jaw-bearing vertebrates, the placoderm fishes, the earliest known cellular bone healing has been described combined with dentin healing (Capasso et al., 1996). Because cellular bone is evolutionary derived from aspidin (Keating et al. 2018), Herbst et al., (2019) concluded that bone healing, as observed today in all extant vertebrates, evolved once in their earliest common ancestor. Furthermore, secondary formation of dentin as a repair mechanism in teeth of humans and other tetrapods appears to have its roots in the wound repair by dentin in heterostracans (Johanson et al., 2013; Herbst et al., 2019).

A further point of interest in the evolution of bone healing, in particular fracture repair, is that the formation of repair tissue (callus) differs between extant ectothermic and endothermic vertebrates, leading to a proportionally smaller callus size, larger amount of cartilage, and a higher degree of vascularization and remodeling in endotherms (Pritchard & Ruzicka, 1950). Thus, the morphology, microstructure and histology of a fossil fracture callus are illuminative for the metabolism of an extinct animal. Straight et al. (2009) conducted a multi-approach analysis of fracture callus of neural spines in hadrosaurid dinosaurs, which indicates that hadrosaurids were more similar to birds than to non-avian reptiles in the formation of dense Haversian bone and in the faster rate of remodeling. A systematic survey of the inner and outer structure of fracture callus in fossil vertebrates would certainly be an important future study.

Evolution of Regenerative Capacities

Salamanders are the only group of modern tetrapods that can fully regenerate their limbs and other organs throughout their life after amputation. On the basis of comparison with the unique pattern of salamander limb regeneration abnormalities, Fröbisch et al. (2015) showed that Permo-Carboniferous stem-amphibians (temnospondyls) and stem-amniotes (microsaurs) had the capacity for salamander-like, complete limb regeneration. This indicates that the striking regenerative capabilities of modern salamanders are not evolutionary derived as previously thought but rather represent an ancient character of tetrapods that was subsequently lost at the base of amniote evolution and retained only in salamanders. This new deep-time perspective on the evolution of regenerative capacities in tetrapods has implications for modern regenerative medicine, as well, since it might indicate that the capability of limb regeneration is still present – albeit concealed – in amniotes, including humans.

Neoplastic Disease

To understand the relatively high prevalence of neoplasms (or tumors) in modern human populations (see Chapter 15, this volume), it is certainly instructive to look at the deep-time perspective of neoplastic disease, given its extremely low prevalence in wild animals and in the fossil record (Capasso, 2005; Tu, 2010; Hamm et al., 2020). In Paleozoic vertebrates, findings of neoplastic diseases are exceptional with only two undisputed cases, an osteoma in an Early Carboniferous ray-finned fish (Moodie, 1927) and an odontoma in an early Permian mammalian ancestor, a gorgonopsian (Whitney et al., 2017). In Mesozoic vertebrates, diagnoses of neoplasms are still extremely rare, although their numbers have increased. Three cases of neoplasm are known in the Triassic, consisting of an osteoma and a parostotic osteosarcoma – the first known malignant tumor – in two Early Triassic amphibians (Gubin et al., 2001; Novikov et al., 2020), and a further malignant form, an osteosarcoma, in a Middle Triassic stem-turtle (Haridy et al., 2019a) (Figure 29.1e,f).

Apart from osteomas in Late Cretaceous mosasaurs (Moodie, 1923; Rothschild & Martin, 2006), documentations of Jurassic and Cretaceous occurrences of neoplasms are restricted to dinosaurs. An epidemiologic study revealed a predisposition of the Late Cretaceous hadrosaurs for neoplastic disease, showing 2–3% benign tumors (hemangiomas), whereas only one case of malignant cancer was found (Rothschild et al., 2003). Neoplasms in other dinosaurs were extremely rare, encompassing mostly benign forms like ameloblastoma (Dumbravă et al., 2016), osteoma and hemangioma (Rothschild & Martin, 2006; Barbosa et al., 2016), and osteoblastic tumor (Gonzalez et al., 2017), whereas only two cases of malignant forms of cancer have been reported (Rothschild & Martin, 2006; Ekhtiari et al., 2020).

The prevalence of neoplasms in the Cenozoic remained very low, with benign neoplasms documented in a Paleocene crocodilians (Sawyer & Erickson, 1998) and in a Miocene sea turtle (Rothschild et al., 2012). Among mammals, osteoma has been diagnosed in a Pliocene balaenopterid whale (Hampe et al., 2014), and in wholly mammoths, an odontoma (van Essen, 2004) and a probably malignant tumor of the mandible (Lister & Bahn, 2009) have been reported. Prehistoric and historic populations of humans also show a markedly low prevalence of neoplastic disease, with a significant increase appearing after the 13th century and with the industrial revolution, and this has been associated with several aspects of human civilization like environmental pollution, diet and increasing individual age (Capasso, 2005; Tu, 2010; and see Chapter 15, this volume).

Summarized, the fossil record suggests that the prevalence of neoplasms is generally low but has increased through geological time, and that benign tumors may be older and much more common than malignant forms in the history of vertebrates. However, the fossil record also attests that unregulated neoplastic cell growth is not a modern phenomenon; rather, it is deeply rooted in the origin of vertebrate evolution hundreds of million years ago.

Infection

Nonspecific Bone Infection – Osteomyelitis

Bone infection has rarely been documented in the fossil record, but it has a long geological history. The earliest known bone infections were described in the Early Carboniferous stem-tetrapod *Crassigyrinus* (Herbst et al., 2019) and in a Late Carboniferous ray-finned fish (Rothschild & Martin, 2006), and further Paleozoic reports encompass post-traumatic osteomyelitis in an early Permian captorhinid reptile (Reisz et al., 2011) and in two non-mammalian synapsids from the early and Middle Permian, respectively (Moodie, 1923; Shelton et al., 2017). Most cases of fossil osteomyelitis, both post-traumatic and non-traumatic, have been described in different groups of dinosaurs (e.g., Hunt et al., 2019; Hamm et al., 2020, and references therein) (Figure 29.1g), and other reptiles like lepidosaurs (Schulp et al., 2006; Romo-de-Vivar-Martínez et al., 2017) and in turtles (Rothschild et al., 2012). Rare cases of osteomyelitis have been reported in Pleistocene mammals like cave bears (Tasnádi-Kubacska, 1960), macropods (Rothschild & Martin, 2006), and proboscideans (Lister & Bahn, 2009; Barbosa et al., 2016).

Tuberculosis and Treponemal Infection

In the last years, paleontological paleopathology has been able to contribute to our understanding of the evolutionary history of infectious diseases that plagued humans for thousands of years – tuberculosis and treponemal disease (see Chapters 16 and 17, this volume). Rothschild et al. (2001) reported the presence of ancient DNA of the human-type tubercle bacteria (i.e., *Mycobacterium tuberculosis* rather than the bovine form *Mycobacterium bovis*) in skeletal remains of more than 17,000-year-old bison from Wyoming. This is inconsistent with the classic view that *M. tuberculosis* evolved from *M. bovis* during domestication of cattle in the Neolithic. Rather, it supports the alternative hypothesis that the human form *M. tuberculosis* existed before *M. bovis* (Brosch et al., 2002). Rothschild & Turnbull (1987) diagnosed treponemal infection – most probably yaws – in a late Pleistocene short faced bear, *Arctodus simus* from Indiana, US, based on skeletal lesions and direct immunofluorescent analysis. This find supports the view that treponemal infection like yaws and/or syphilis have been present in the New World for thousands of years.

Metabolic Disease

Bone alterations similar to Paget's Disease of Bone (PDB) indicating increased bone turnover rates have been diagnosed in only two fossil specimens, a dorsal vertebra of a Late Jurassic dinosaur (Witzmann et al., 2011) and in two tail vertebrae of a basal amniote from the early Permian (Haridy et al., 2019b) (Figure 29.2a,b). This suggests that PDB-like disturbances of bone metabolism are of considerable antiquity, and that the susceptibility for this kind of disease evolved at the base of the evolution of amniotes. Providing that a viral component was present, as presumed for extant PDB, this would be the earliest indirect evidence of the existence of a virus in the fossil record. Also, in human paleopathology, diagnoses of PDB are rare, whereas this disease is quite common among elderly people in modern humans (Waldron, 2009). The apparently low prevalence of PDB in paleontological and archaeological remains, however, might be due to the fact that PDB is recognized mainly by radiological investigation, and the more frequent application of CT-scans might change this picture in

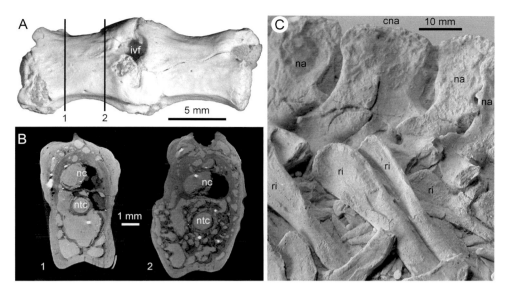

Figure 29.2 (a) and (b) fused caudal vertebrae of an early amniote (varanopid; MB.R.5931) from the early Permian of Oklahoma, USA showing Paget's disease of bone-like alterations; the locations of transverse sections illustrated in (b) are shown in 1 and 2; (a), right lateral view, (b) cross sections as revealed by micro-CT (modified from Haridy et al. 2019b, © The authors, under CC BY 4.0, https://creativecommons.org/licenses/by/4.0/); (c) two conjoined neural arches of the early amphibian *Glanochthon lellbachae* (SMNS 91279) from the early Permian of Germany in left lateral view (© Florian Witzmann). Abbreviations: cna, conjoined neural arches; ivf, intervertebral foramen; MB, Museum für Naturkunde Berlin, Germany; na, neural arch; nc, neural canal; ntc, notochordal canal; ri, rib; SMNS, Staatliches Museum für Naturkunde Stuttgart, Germany.

the future (see Waldron, 2009). A further metabolic disease, rickets, appears to be a very old disease in humans (see Chapter 19, this volume), known from mid-Holocene human remains (Waldron, 2009). This corresponds with deformed bones (osteomalacia) and teeth attributed to rickets that were described in juvenile cave bears from the Alps and were correlated with diet poor in vitamins and calcium in this environment (Tasnádi-Kubacska, 1960). Moodie (1923) diagnosed osteomalacia in the hind limb of an Eocene hyaenodontid carnivore, which is the oldest case known.

Developmental Anomalies

Witzmann et al. (2021) surveyed the occurrence of developmental (or congenital) anomalies throughout the fossil record of vertebrates, from the Silurian to the Pleistocene. The authors showed that such malformations were part of the common history of all groups of vertebrates for more than 400 million years. Teeth (e.g., supernumerary and malformed teeth) and vertebral column (e.g., failure of formation and segmentation of vertebrae; Figure 29.2c) are the most commonly affected anatomical regions, and the mechanisms causing these malformations apparently remained the same through geological time. An interesting aspect of developmental anomalies is their possible correlation with environmental factors. For example, van der Geer and Galis (2017) asserted that the appearance of cervical ribs connected with an anomalous number of cervical vertebrae in shrinking populations of the woolly rhinoceros and mammoth from the North Sea might be the result of stress and possible inbreeding close to the end-Pleistocene extinction.

Last, paleontological paleopathology might help to answer to what extent deviation from the norm can be regarded as "disease". Types of discontinuous variation like polydactyly or congenital block vertebrae, which might usually be regarded as pathological, became taxon-specific and adaptive under altered environmental conditions in certain fossil vertebrates, so that the determination of what is "healthy" and what is "disease" is neither absolute nor evident across deep time (Witzmann et al., 2021).

Outlook and Future Directions

We expect that one problem in paleopathological investigation, the rare opportunity to produce thin sections of fossil pathological bone, will be overcome by the further development and improvement of non-invasive imaging techniques enabling virtual histological studies. High-resolution micro-CT already has the potential to image the internal structure of fossil bone, including bone cell lacunae and different tissue types (e.g., Haridy et al., 2019b), and phase-contrast synchrotron imaging enables the three-dimensional paleohistological reconstruction of fossil bone on a sub-micron scale (Sanchez et al., 2016).

We also think that the already existing trend away from single case descriptions to more comprehensive population studies with increasingly larger data sets will continue. In this respect, it would be interesting to focus on the different environmental factors acting on population health, for example, in smaller or larger mass extinctions or faunal crises (e.g., caused by climatic changes).

We predict that the significance of paleopathology for paleobiological studies, including works on behavior, paleophysiology, feeding, locomotion and other biomechanical aspects in extinct animals, will increase and be methodologically refined. For example, in an innovative population study, Brown et al. (2017) recently calculated the frequencies of traumatic injuries in the skeletons of the sabre-tooth cat and dire wolf from the La Brea Tar Pits, which can be attributed to hazards of predation. Statistical analysis of the anatomical regions in which most of the injuries are concentrated showed significant differences between the two predators, reflecting alternative hunting behaviors of the ambush (sabertooth cat) and the pursuit predator (dire wolf).

As outlined above, considering the EPB is important for the diagnosis of a disease, especially in non-mammalian fossil vertebrates. However, because the veterinary literature on bone pathologies in extant fishes, amphibians, and reptiles is scarce, paleontological paleopathologists should seek to carry out first-hand investigations in osteological museum collections of the skeletal impact of disease in these potential bracketing taxa.

Finally, we would advocate moving "back to the roots", to a more holistic concept of paleopathology in the way advocated by Robert W. Shufeldt and Roy Lee Moodie. These early pioneers envisioned paleopathology as a discipline that encompasses pathologies in organismal remains from both archaeology and paleontology and from humans and other animals. In our opinion, the separation between the different areas is artificial because both aim to unravel the origin and evolutionary history of disease and use similar approaches and methodologies. Increased collaboration would shift from a rather limited focus to a broader context and would create large synergistic effects. This would certainly increase our understanding of how modern human and non-human diseases are rooted in the deep past and better prepare us for the emergence of new diseases.

Acknowledgments

We are indebted to Anne L. Grauer for the kind invitation to contribute to this volume. The thorough reviews of Anne L. Grauer and an anonymous reviewer substantially improved the manuscript. Yara Haridy, Carola Radke, Achim Ritter and Mario Thiele are thanked for providing pictures of fossil specimens.

References

Abel, O. (1912). *Grundzüge der Palaeobiologie der Wirbeltiere*. Stuttgart: E. Schweizerbart'sche Verlagsbuchhandlung.

Anné, J., Edwards, N. P., Wogelius, R. A., Tumarkin-Deratzian, A. R., Sellers, W. I., van Veelen, A., ... & Manning, P. L. (2014). Synchrotron imaging reveals bone healing and remodelling strategies in extinct and extant vertebrates. *Journal of the Royal Society Interface* 11(96):20140277.

Anné, J., Garwood, R. J., Lowe, T., Withers, P. J. & Manning, P. L. (2015). Interpreting pathologies in extant and extinct archosaurs using micro-CT. *PeerJ* 3:e1130.

Barbosa, F. H., da Costa, P. V. L. G., Bergqvist, L. P. & Rothschild, B. M. (2016). Multiple neoplasms in a single sauropod dinosaur from the Upper Cretaceous of Brazil. *Cretaceous Research* 62:13–17.

Barbosa, F. H., da Costa Ribeiro, I., da Costa, P. V. L. G. & Bergqvist, L. P. (2018). Vertebral lesions in a titanosaurian dinosaur from the Lower-Upper Cretaceous of Brazil. *Géobios* 51(5):385–389.

Barbosa, F. H., da Silva Marinho, T., Iori, F. V. & Paschoa, L. S. (2019). A case of infection in an Aeolosaurini (Sauropoda) dinosaur from the Upper Cretaceous of São Paulo, southeastern Brazil, and the impact on its life. *Cretaceous Research* 96:1–5.

Beatty, B. L. & Rothschild, B. M. (2009). Paleopathologies are features of an organism and its interaction with the environment and should not be treated like organisms unto themselves: commentary. *Historical Biology* 21(3–4):229–233.

Bell, P. R. & Coria, R. A. (2013). Palaeopathological survey of a population of *Mapusaurus* (Theropoda: Carcharodontosauridae) from the Late Cretaceous Huincul Formation, Argentina. *PloS One* 8(5):e63409.

Bishop, P. J., Walmsley, C. W., Phillips, M. J., Quayle, M. R., Boisvert, C. A. & McHenry, C. R. (2015). Oldest pathology in a tetrapod bone illuminates the origin of terrestrial vertebrates. *PLoS One* 10(5):e0125723.

Brosch, R., Gordon, S. V., Marmiesse, M., Brodin, P., Buchrieser, C., Eiglmeier, K., ... & Cole, S. T. (2002). A new evolutionary scenario for the *Mycobacterium tuberculosis* complex. *Proceedings of the National Academy of Sciences* 99(6):3684–3689.

Brown, C., Balisi, M., Shaw, C. A. & Van Valkenburgh, B. (2017). Skeletal trauma reflects hunting behaviour in extinct sabre-tooth cats and dire wolves. *Nature Ecology & Evolution* 1(5):1–7.

Buikstra, J. E., Cook, D. C. & Bolhofner, K. L. (2017). Introduction: scientific rigor in paleopathology. *International Journal of Paleopathology* 19:80–87.

Capasso, L. L. (2005). Antiquity of cancer. *International Journal of Cancer* 113(1):2–13.

Capasso, L. L., Bacchia, F., Rabottini, N., Rothschild, B. M. & Mariani-Costantini, R. (1996). Fossil evidence of intraspecific aggressive behaviour of Devonian giant fishes (Arthrodira, Dinichthyidae). *Journal of Paleopathology* 8:153–160.

Cisneros, J. C., Cabral, U. G., De Beer, F., Damiani, R. & Fortier, D. C. (2010). Spondarthritis in the Triassic. *PLoS One* 5(10):e13425.

Duckler, G. L. & Van Valkenburgh, B. (1998). Exploring the health of late Pleistocene mammals: the use of Harris lines. *Journal of Vertebrate Paleontology* 18(1):180–188.

Dumbravă, M. D., Rothschild, B. M., Weishampel, D. B., Csiki-Sava, Z., Andrei, R. A., Acheson, K. A. & Codrea, V. A. (2016). A dinosaurian facial deformity and the first occurrence of ameloblastoma in the fossil record. *Scientific Reports* 6:29271.

Ekhtiari, S., Chiba, K., Popovic, S., Crowther, R., Wohl, G., Kin On Wong, A., ... & Evans, D. C. (2020). First case of osteosarcoma in a dinosaur: a multimodal diagnosis. *The Lancet Oncology* 21(8):1021–1022.

Esper, J. F. (1774). *Ausführliche Nachricht von neuentdeckten Zoolithen unbekannter vierfüsiger Thiere, und denen sie enthaltenden, so wie verschiedenen andern denkwürdigen Grüften der Obergebürgischen Lande des Marggrafthums Bayreuth*. Nürnberg: Georg Wolfgang Knorr.

Eudes-Deslongchamps, J. A. (1838). Mémoire sur le *Poekilopleuron bucklandii*, grand saurien fossile, intermédiaire entre les crocodiles et les lézards. *Mémoire de la Société Linnéenne de Normandie* 6:37–146.

Foth, C., Evers, S. W., Pabst, B., Mateus, O., Flisch, A., Patthey, M. & Rauhut, O. W. M. (2015). New insights into the lifestyle of *Allosaurus* (Dinosauria: Theropoda) based on another specimen with multiple pathologies. *PeerJ* 3. https://peerj.com/articles/940/.

Fröbisch, N. B., Bickelmann, C., Olori, J. C. & Witzmann, F. (2015). Deep-time evolution of regeneration and preaxial polarity in tetrapod limb development. *Nature* 527(7577):231–234.

Goldfuss, G. A. (1810). *Die Umgebungen von Muggendorf. Ein Taschenbuch für Freunde der Natur und Alterthumskunde. Fränkische Schweiz.* Erlangen: Verlag Johann Jakob Palm.

Gonzalez, R., Gallina, P. A. & Cerda, I. A. (2017). Multiple paleopathologies in the dinosaur *Bonitasaura salgadoi* (Sauropoda: Titanosauria) from the Upper Cretaceous of Patagonia, Argentina. *Cretaceous Research* 79:159–170.

Gross, J. D., Rich, T. H. & Vickers-Rich, P. (1993). Chronic osteomyelitis in a hypsilophodontid dinosaur in Early Cretaceous, Polar Australia. *Research and Exploration* 9:286–286.

Gubin, I., Petrovichev, N. N., Solov'ev, I., Kochergina, N. V., Luk'ianchenko, A. B. & Markov, S. M. (2001). Cranial bone neoplasm in Early Triassic amphibia. *Voprosy onkologii* 47(4):449–455.

Hamm, C. A., Hampe, O., Schwarz, D., Witzmann, F., Makovicky, P. J., Brochu, C. A., Reiter, R. & Asbach, P. (2020). A comprehensive diagnostic approach combining phylogenetic disease bracketing and CT imaging reveals osteomyelitis in a *Tyrannosaurus rex*. *Scientific Reports* 10:18897.

Hampe, O., Witzmann, F. & Asbach, P. (2014). A benign bone-forming tumour (osteoma) on the skull of a fossil balaenopterid whale from the Pliocene of Chile. *Alcheringa* 38(2):266–272.

Hanna, R. R. (2002). Multiple injury and infection in a sub-adult theropod dinosaur *Allosaurus fragilis* with comparisons to allosaur pathology in the Cleveland-Lloyd Dinosaur Quarry collection. *Journal of Vertebrate Paleontology* 22:76–90.

Haridy, Y., Witzmann, F., Asbach, P., Schoch, R. R., Fröbisch, N. & Rothschild, B. M. (2019a). Triassic cancer—osteosarcoma in a 240-million-year-old stem-turtle. *JAMA Oncology* 5(3):425–426.

Haridy, Y., Witzmann, F., Asbach, P. & Reisz, R. R. (2019b). Permian metabolic bone disease revealed by microCT: Paget's disease-like pathology in vertebrae of an early amniote. *Plos One* 14(8):e0219662.

Hedrick, B. P., Gao, C., Tumarkin-Deratzian, A. R., Shen, C., Holloway, J. L., Zhang, F., Hankenson, K. D., Liu, S., Anné, J. & Dodson, P. (2016). An Injured *Psittacosaurus* (Dinosauria: Ceratopsia) From the Yixian Formation (Liaoning, China): implications for *Psittacosaurus* Biology. *Anatomical Record* 299:897–906.

Herbst, E. C., Doube, M., Smithson, T. R., Clack, J. A. & Hutchinson, J. R. (2019). Bony lesions in early tetrapods and the evolution of mineralized tissue repair. *Paleobiology* 45(4):676–697.

Hopley, P. J. (2001). Plesiosaur spinal pathology: the first fossil occurrence of Schmorl's nodes. *Journal of Vertebrate Paleontology* 21(2):253–260.

Huchzermeyer, F. W. & Cooper, J. E. (2000). Fibriscess, not abscess, resulting from a localised inflammatory response to infection in reptiles and birds. *Veterinary Record* 147(18):515–516.

Hunt, T. C., Peterson, J. E., Frederickson, J. A., Cohen, J. E. & Berry, J. L. (2019). First documented pathologies in *Tenontosaurus tilletti* with comments on infection in non-avian dinosaurs. *Scientific Reports* 9(1):1–8.

Johanson, Z., Smith, M., Kearsley, A., Pilecki, P., Mark-Kurik, E. & Howard, C. (2013). Origins of bone repair in the armour of fossil fish: response to a deep wound by cells depositing dentine instead of dermal bone. *Biology Letters* 9(5):20130144.

Keating, J. N., Marquart, C. L., Marone, F. & Donoghue, P. C. (2018). The nature of aspidin and the evolutionary origin of bone. *Nature Ecology & Evolution* 2(9):1501–1506.

Kutschera, U. (2007). Palaeobiology: the origin and evolution of a scientific discipline. *Trends in Ecology & Evolution* 22(4):172–173.

Lister, A. & Bahn, P. (2009). *Mammuts: Riesen der Eiszeit* (2nd ed.). Eschbach: Jan Thorbecke Verlag.

Mays, S. (2018). How should we diagnose disease in palaeopathology? Some epistemological considerations. *International Journal of Paleopathology* 20:12–19.

Montali, R. (1988). Comparative pathology of inflammation in the higher vertebrates (reptiles, birds and mammals). *Journal of Comparative Pathology* 99:1–26.

Moodie, R. L. (1923). *Paleopathology. An Introduction to the Study of Ancient Evidences of Diseases.* Urbana: University of Illinois Press.

Moodie, R. L. (1927). Tumors in the lower Carboniferous. *Science* 66:540.

Novikov, I. V., Haiduk, P. A., Gribanov, A. V., Ivanov, A. N., Novikov, A. V. & Starodubtseva, I. A. (2020). The earliest case of neoplastic bonelesion in tetrapods. *Paleontological Journal* 54(1):68–72.

Ortner, D. J. (1991). Theoretical and methodological issues in paleopathology. In Ortner, D. & Aufderheide, A. (Eds.), *Human Paleopathology: Current Syntheses and Future Options*, pp. 5–11. Smithsonian Institution Press.

Pardo-Pérez, J. M., Kear, B. & Maxwell, E. E. (2019). Palaeoepidemiology in extinct vertebrate populations: factors influencing skeletal health in Jurassic marine reptiles. *Royal Society Open Science* 6(7):190264.

Pritchard, J. J. & Ruzicka, A. J. (1950). Comparison of fracture repair in the frog, lizard and rat. *Journal of Anatomy* 84:236–261.

Rega, E. A. (2012). Disease in dinosaurs. In Brett-Surman, M. K., Holtz Jr., T. R. & Farlow, J. O. (Eds.), *The Complete Dinosaur* (2nd ed.), pp. 667–711. Bloomington: University of Indiana Press.

Reisz, R. R., Scott, D. M., Pynn, B. R. & Modesto, S. P. (2011). Osteomyelitis in a Paleozoic reptile: ancient evidence for bacterial infection and its evolutionary significance. *Naturwissenschaften* 98(6):551–555.

Romo-de-Vivar-Martínez, P. R., Martinelli, A. G., Paes Neto, V. D. & Soares, M. B. (2017). Evidence of osteomyelitis in the dentary of the late Triassic rhynchocephalian *Clevosaurus brasiliensis* (Lepidosauria: Rhynchocephalia) from southern Brazil and behavioural implications. *Historical Biology* 29(3):320–327.

Rothschild, B. M. (2017). Transcending human spondylarthritis: implications of the ecologic record from the Permian to the present. *Rheumatology Research* 2(2):45–50.

Rothschild, B. M., Martin, L. D., Lev, G., Bercovier, H., Bar-Gal, G. K., Greenblatt, C., Donoghue, H., Spigelman, M. & Brittain, D. (2001). *Mycobacterium tuberculosis* complex DNA from an extinct bison dated 17,000 years before the present. *Clinical Infectious Diseases* 33(3):305–311.

Rothschild, B. M. & Martin, L. R. (2006). Skeletal impact of disease. *New Mexico Museum of Natural History Science Bulletin* 33:1–226.

Rothschild, B. M., Schultze, H.-P. & Pellegrini, R. (2012). Osseous and other hard tissue pathologies in turtles and abnormalities of mineral deposition. In Brinkman, D. B., Holroyd, P. A. & Gardner, J. D. (Eds.), *Morphology and Evolution of Turtles*, pp. 501–534. Springer.

Rothschild, B. M., Tanke, D. H., Helbling, M. & Martin, L. D. (2003). Epidemiologic study of tumors in dinosaurs. *Naturwissenschaften* 90:495–500.

Rothschild, B. M. & Turnbull, W. (1987). Treponemal infection in a Pleistocene bear. *Nature* 329(6134):61–62.

Ruffer, M. A. (1921). *Studies in the Paleopathology of Egypt*. Edited by R. L. Moodie. Chicago: University of Chicago Press.

Sanchez, S., Tafforeau, P., Clack, J. A. & Ahlberg, P. E. (2016). Life history of the stem tetrapod *Acanthostega* revealed by synchrotron microtomography. *Nature* 537(7620):408–411.

Sawyer, G. T. & Erickson, B. R. (1998). *Paleopathology of the Paleocene Crocodile* Leidyosuchus. St. Paul, Minnesota: Science Museum of Minnesota.

Schlüter, T. & Kohring, R. (2002). Palaeopathological fish bones from phosphorites of the Lake Manyara area, Northern Tanzania—fossil evidence of a physiological response to survival in an extreme biocenosis. *Environmental Geochemistry and Health* 24(2):131–140.

Schmerling, M. (1835). Description des ossements fossiles à l'état pathologique provenant des cavernes de la province de Liège. *Bulletin des la Société Géologique de France* 7:51–61.

Schulp, A. S., Walenkamp, G. H. I. M., Hofman, P. A., Stuip, Y. & Rothschild, B. M. (2006). Chronic bone infection in the jaw of *Mosasaurus hoffmanni* (Squamata). *Oryctos* 6:41–52.

Shaw, C. A. & Ware, C. S. (2018). *Smilodon* paleopathology: a summary of research at Rancho La Brea. In Werdelin, L., Mcdonald, H. G. & Shaw, C. A. (Eds.), Smilodon: *The Iconic Sabertooth*, pp. 196–206. Johns Hopkins University Press.

Shelton, C. D., Chinsamy, A. & Rothschild, B. M. (2017). Osteomyelitis in a 265-million-year-old titanosuchid (Dinocephalia, Therapsida). *Historical Biology* 2017. https://doi.org/10.1080/08912963.2017.1419348.

Shufeldt, R. W. (1893). Notes on palaeopathology. *Popular Science Monthly* 42:679–684.

Straight, W. H., Davis, G. L., Skinner, C. W., Haims, A., McLennan, B. L. & Tanke, D. H. (2009). Bone lesions in hadrosaurs: computed tomographic imaging as a guide for paleohistologic and stable-isotopic analysis. *Journal of Vertebrate Paleontology* 29(2):315–325.

Surmik, D., Rothschild, B. M., Dulski, M. & Janiszewska, K. (2017). Two types of bone necrosis in the Middle Triassic *Pistosaurus longaevus* bones: the results of integrated studies. *Royal Society Open Science* 4(7):170204.

Tanke, D. H. & Currie, P. J. (1998). Head-biting behavior in theropod dinosaurs: paleopathological evidence. *Gaia* 15:167–184.

Tanke, D. H. & Rothschild, B. M. (2014). Paleopathology in Late Cretaceous Hadrosauridae from Alberta, Canada. In Eberth, D. A. & Evans, D. C. (Eds.), *Hadrosaurs*, pp. 540–571. Indiana University Press.

Tasnádi-Kubacska, A. (1960). *Az Ősállatok Pathologiája*. Budapest: Medicina Könyvkiadó.

Thomas, R. (2012). Nonhuman paleopathology. In Buikstra, J. E. & Roberts, C. A. (Eds.), *The Global History of Paleopathology: Pioneers and Prospects*, pp. 652–664. Oxford University Press.

Tu, S.-M. (2010). *Origin of Cancers: Clinical Perspectives and Implications of a Stem-Cell Theory of Cancer*. New York: Springer.

van der Geer, A. A. & Galis, F. (2017). High incidence of cervical ribs indicates vulnerable condition in Late Pleistocene woolly rhinoceroses. *PeerJ* 5:e3684.

van Essen, H. (2004). A supernumerary tooth and an odontoma attributable to *Mammuthus primigenius* (Blumenbach, 1799) (Mammalia, Proboscidea) from The Netherlands, and various related finds. *Acta Zoologica Cracoviensia* 47:81–121.

Vittore, C. P. & Henderson, M. D. (2013). Brodie abscess involving a tyrannosaur phalanx: imaging and implications. In Molnar, R., Currie, P. J. & Koppelhus, E. B. (Eds.), *Tyrannosaurid Paleobiology*, pp. 223–237. Indiana University Press.

Waldron, T. (2009). *Palaeopathology*. Cambridge, UK: Cambridge University Press.

Waldron, T. (2015). Roy Lee Moodie (1880–1934) and the beginnings of palaeopathology. *Journal of Medical Biography* 23(1):8–13.

Walther, F. von. (1825). Ueber das Alterthum der Knochenkrankheiten. *Journal der Chirurgie und Augenheilkunde* 8:1–16.

Weiss, E. (2005). Schmorl's nodes: a preliminary investigation. *Paleopathological Newsletter* 132:6–10.

Whitney, M. R., Mose, L. & Sidor, C. A. (2017). Odontoma in a 255-million-year-old mammalian forebear. *JAMA Oncology* 3(7):998–1000.

Witzmann, F., Claeson, K. M., Hampe, O., Wieder, F., Hilger, A., Manke, I., Niederhagen, M., Rothschild, B. M. & Asbach, P. (2011). Paget disease of bone in a Jurassic dinosaur. *Current Biology* 21:R647–R648.

Witzmann, F., Hampe, O., Rothschild, B. M., Joger, U., Kosma, R., Schwarz, D. & Asbach, P. (2016). Subchondral cysts at synovial vertebral joints as analogies of Schmorl's nodes in a sauropod dinosaur from Niger. *Journal of Vertebrate Paleontology* 36:e1080719.

Witzmann, F., Haridy, Y., Hilger, A., Manke, I. & Asbach, P. (2021). Rarity of congenital malformation and deformity in the fossil record of vertebrates – a non-human perspective. *International Journal of Paleopathology* 33:30–42.

Wolff, E. D. S. (2008). The discovery of two novel archosaur diseases with implications for future paleopathological exploration. *Historical Biology* 20:185–189.

Wolff, E. D. S. (2009). Reply: the limitations of homology in vertebrate paleopathology. *Historical Biology* 21:235–238.

30
ZOOARCHAEOLOGY AND THE PALEOPATHOLOGICAL RECORD

László Bartosiewicz and Khashaiar Mansouri

Introduction

Animal disease in the past has been a typically interdisciplinary subject. Historians have recovered ancient veterinary literature in many parts of Europe and Asia. The earliest texts, related to curing horses, are known from the third millennium BCE, found among the ruins of the former Hittine capital Boğazköy/Ḫattuša on the Anatolian plateau (McMiken, 1990: 75). Similarities of their language to Sanskrit led to the assumption that they were recorded by Indo-Europeans (Hrozný, 1931). Additional tablets referring to horses were unearthed at Boğazköy (Kammenhuder, 1961; Tāj'bakhsh, 2003). In India, Salihotra became known as the "veterinarian" of horses around 2350 BCE, recommending medicinal plants to cure various diseases (Froehner, 1922). Urlugaledinna was named as "expert in healing animals" in Mesopotamia, where rabies control and veterinary fees were codified by around the early second millennium BCE (Jones, 2010). The earliest texts on animal health in China are sporadic references to the treatment of horses dated to the Qin (255–206 BCE) and Han (206 BCE–AD 220) periods. In the 6th century AD, the medical book on the *Essential Arts to Assist the People* also contained veterinary recipes (Buell et al., 2018).

In Europe, *Historia Animalium* by Aristotle (384–322 BCE) is the earliest work dealing with animal disease. During the late antiquity, the health of animals became more widely discussed. Pelagonius, "Chiron" and Vegetius were among the most influential authors on this topic. Veterinary medicine in Iran was first documented from the Sassanid Period (AD 212–652). Livestock were treated with drugs and surgical operations. General practice was the same in human and veterinary medicine (Tāj'bakhsh, 2016: 43–46). Written in the mid-4th century AD, *Ars Veterinaria* by Pelagonius was influenced by Apsyrtus, a likely veterinarian from Greece who served in the court of Constantine I (AD 306–337), emperor of Rome. Although *Mulomedicina Chironis* mostly deals with equids, discussion of diseases of other livestock also appear in two of its ten volumes. These two works inspired *Mulomedicina* by Vegetius around the turn of the 4th–5th centuries AD (Mezzabotta, 2000: 63).

A direct, empirical way of studying ancient animal disease is the analysis of excavated osseous remains. An advantage of this method is that it offers information on prehistoric animal health pre-dating the written record. Even in historical times, the study of bone finds has the potential to reveal conditions not mentioned in documentary sources.

Although rooted in paleontology, zooarchaeology focuses on animal remains from archaeological contexts. The study of animal-human relations amounts to "an indirect psycho, philosophic and natural historic analysis of man himself" (Murthy & Padmanabha, 1990). As human and animal health have become inseparable, animal disease offers a special perspective on past societies, sometimes holding a mirror to our present conditions. In order to understand the changing roles played by animal paleopathology in archaeological inquiry, basic concepts are essential to discuss: archaeozoology, zooarchaeology, and paleopathology. Within the field of *archaeozoology*, traditional analyses of animal remains aim to identify and document human impacts on animals. This is an inductive approach. The accumulation of zoological information (e.g., morphotypes, bone measurements), for instance, focuses on understanding aspects of animal domestication (Bartosiewicz, 2001). In *zooarchaeology*, however, interpreting faunal remains is deductive and framed within larger archaeological hypotheses that incorporate socio-cultural aspects of human/animal interactions, at times referred to as social zooarchaeology (Russell, 2011). The subtle difference in nomenclature reflects developments in the discipline. Terminology also varies when pathology is added to the analyses. Shufeldt (1893: 679, footnote (1)) first defined paleopathology as the study of "all diseased or pathological conditions found fossilized in the remains of extinct or fossil animals", but later, the term (and the field, itself) focused on human diseases. However, choosing a label for the study of ancient animal disease proved difficult. Thomas (2012) highlights many recommended terms (Brothwell, 1995; Dieguez et al., 1996; Thomas & Hammon, 1999; Bartosiewicz, 2002; Brothwell, 2008a). Conventionally, zooarchaeologists use the term "animal paleopathology" for the sake of simplicity.

History

Fossils were popular items in 15th–16th-century-curio cabinets but were not always recognized as past living organisms; they were seen as *ludi naturae*, games of nature. The intellectual movement that grew out of Renaissance humanism in 17th–18th century Europe offered a systematic and rational approach to phenomena in nature. The anatomical collection in the "King's Cabinet" of Louis XV in Paris, for example, became the subject of the third volume of *Natural History* by Georges-Louis Leclerc, Comte de Buffon (1749). It was Swedish botanist Carl Linnaeus, however, who sought to coherently classify all known organisms and conditions (Linnaeus, 1735) and ventured further to divide human disease into 11 classes and 325 genera based on symptoms (Linnaeus, 1763).

The earliest known documentation of a case in animal paleopathology is the mandibula of a "war elephant" published by Count Luigi Ferdinando de Marsigli (1726), found near the Roman fort of Tibiscum in Romania during his survey of Roman ruins along the Danube. The buccal side of this mandible appears to be deformed by *actinomycosis*. Although the proboscid bone was later identified by Tasnádi Kubacska (1960) to have belonged to a mammoth (*Mammuthus primigenius* Blumenbach, 1799), Marsigli's illustration shows the lesion itself in remarkable detail.

As discussed below, the history of animal paleopathology can be divided into four general periods paralleling the development of zooarchaeology as outlined by Robison in 1987.

The Formative Period

The first known paleopathological diagnosis was "a callus by which nature healed a fracture" on a cave bear (*Ursus spelaeus* Rosenmüller, 1794) femur published by Johann Friedrich Esper

(1774). During the following century, paleopathological research was mostly carried out on Quaternary animals, such as mammoths, ancient deer and other game. The "formative period" of zooarchaeology commenced in the last quarter of the 18th century between 1774 and 1870, when Steenstrup concluded that shell mounds on the Danish coast were deposited by prehistoric humans (Forchammer et al., 1851–1856), and Rütimeyer (1861) analysed the remains of domestic animals recovered from prehistoric pile dwellings in Switzerland. When emphasis shifted onto trauma in human paleopathology between 1870 and 1900 (Ubelaker, 1982), zooarchaeology also focused attention on animal hunting injuries (Babington, 1863; Nilsson, 1868; Steenstrup, 1870, 1880). Shufeldt (1893) actually coined the term paleopathology while researching hunting injuries on bird bones found in association with lithic blades. Cordier (1990) published a historical inventory of perimortem injuries in both humans and animals, with survivors noted by the presence of healed wounds. For example, bone remodeling was recorded around a flint arrowhead wedged into the atlas of a Neolithic aurochs (*Bos primigenius* Bojanus, 1827) from Hungary (Bökönyi, 1974: 104, Fig. 4).

Zooarchaeological research decelerated in the first half of the 20th century, while close cooperation between human paleopathology and archaeology persisted. Between 1918 and the 1960s, an evolutionary perspective on human disease developed (Grauer, 2018). Moodie (1923) wrote the first comprehensive work on the paleopathology of plants, animals and humans. The first paleopathological synthesis dealing exclusively with animals was published by Tasnádi Kubacska (1960). However, due to its distinctly paleontological scope, his book had no visible impact in zooarchaeology.

The Systematization Period

In the 1950s, radiocarbon dating stimulated a second scientific revolution in archaeology (Kristiansen, 2014). A new generation of archaeozoologists – paleontologists, veterinarians and zoologists – started regularly studying archaeological animal remains. However, since they published in flagship journals in zoology and animal science (e.g., Nobis 1954; Zalkin 1960), their work fell outside the purview of most archaeologists. Many of these works were written in languages other than English, which also isolated them from international communication concerning animal paleopathology. It appears that language divided the development of archaeology more strongly than the East-West dichotomy perpetuated by Cold War propaganda (Bartosiewicz, 2001).

The 1950s thru the 1970s brought standardization of key methods into zooarchaeology, such as withers height estimations (Vitt, 1952; Boessneck, 1956), caprine identification (Boessneck et al., 1964), dental ageing (Payne, 1973) and bone measurement (von den Driesch 1976). The potential of studying animal disease was yet to be recognized. The classic volume by Cornwall (1956) *Bones for the Archaeologist* does not mention pathological lesions within the methodological discussions of animal bones, although the importance of paleopathology is mentioned among the possible interpretations of human remains (Cornwall, 1956: 244). The handbook *Science in Archaeology* (Brothwell & Higgs, 1963) devoted ten pages to human paleopathology (Goldstein, 1963), while the paleopathology of other mammals is summarized in only four (Brothwell, 1963). Consequently, no paleopathological protocols were developed in zooarchaeology during the systematization period and inconsistent and inadequate recording remained a problem (Thomas & Hammon, 1999).

Beginning in 1964, an increase occurs in reporting animal paleopathology, as animal bone assemblages formed the core of dissertation topics assigned to veterinary students at the *Institut für Paläoanatomie, Domestikationsforschung und Geschichte der Tiermedizin* in München (Germany).

These authors had the skills and supervision to reliably diagnose sporadically occurring pathological conditions and their work incorporated technical medical disease paradigms that had already been synthesized into human paleopathology during the 1930s (Grauer, 2018).

The Integration Period

With the emergence of "processual" or New Archaeology in the mid-1960s, the application of scientific methods to archaeological data became central to interdisciplinary discourse. In this intellectual environment, zooarchaeology contributed to the formulation of testable archaeological hypotheses. However, some new practitioners – trained primarily in archaeology – did not possess the biological training indispensable to paleopathological research. Traditional archaeozoologists could be characterized as lonesome specialists accumulating data. Few countries in Europe employed more than one or two such experts. The establishment of the International Council for Archaeozoology (ICAZ) in 1971 marked a historic step forward, as it intensified the international exchange of methods and ideas between archaeozoologists who had worked in isolation in a then politically divided Europe (Bartosiewicz, 2020).

Although sporadic paleopathological data had accumulated in mainstream archaeozoology, major syntheses were first undertaken in the 1970s (Haimovici & Haimovici, 1971; von den Driesch, 1975; Wäsle, 1976; Siegel, 1976; Van Wijngaarden-Bakker & Krauwer, 1979). A review of animal paleopathology in North America followed (Shaffer & Baker, 1997). Information reached critical threshold by the end of this period, when the first ever specialized book entitled *Animal Diseases in Archaeology* was published by Baker and Brothwell (1980) and they unequivocally stated that "Archaeology in the future must be seen more and more as an ecological science" (Baker & Brothwell, 1980: 1). Although ancient human disease had already been studied within ecological contexts as early as the 1930s, the approach within zooarchaeology only took root when modern environmentalism, heralded by the publication of *Silent Spring* (Carson 1962), resonated with scientific thought in archaeology. When viewed as a reaction to the environment, disease was seen as "a very useful source of information in archaeology" (Hillson, 1986: 283). However, even at the turn of the millennium, integration between animal paleopathology and other forms of archaeological evidence remained inadequate (Thomas & Hammon, 1999).

The Diversification Period

From the viewpoint of zooarchaeology, the 1980s ended with an adverse research trend. An emphasis on culture history began to prevail within archaeology, represented by the post-processual movement, a diverse school of thought largely united by the rejection of the "false objectivity" of science and scientific methods (Shanks & Tilley, 1987). This archaeological approach created a noticeable lull in interest in zooarchaeology, especially marked among works published in Great Britain (Bartosiewicz, 2019: 30, Figure 2).

Recovery took decades, aided by a third scientific revolution in archaeology (Kristiansen, 2014). This included advances in cutting-edge natural sciences (applications of mass spectrometry, DNA analyses etc.), as well as the increasing specialization and global spread of zooarchaeology. At last, efforts were made to draft protocols for the systematic recording of paleopathological phenomena in animals, some using contemporary clinical reference materials (Bartosiewicz et al., 1997; Dobney & Ervynck, 1998; Vann & Thomas, 2006; Bendrey, 2007). Specialist studies began to be devoted to pathological changes on bird (Brothwell, 1993; Gál, 2008, 2013), as well as fish bones (Wheeler & Jones 1989; von den Driesch,

1994; Harland & Van Neer, 2018). Sophisticated imaging techniques, already promoted in taphonomic studies (e.g., Shipman, 1981) and human paleopathology (e.g., Bell, 1990), drew attention within the study of animal disease (O'Connor, 2005; Brothwell, 2008b).

In 1999, the specialist Animal Palaeopathology Working Group of the increasingly diversifying ICAZ was established (Thomas & Hammon, 1999). Since then, this working group has regularly organized triennial conferences and published their proceedings (Davies et al., 2005; Miklíková & Thomas, 2008; Bartosiewicz & Gál, 2018).

Materials and Methods

Prior to evaluating critical aspects of our research materials, a few concepts are worth reviewing. The term *lesion* refers to a structural change in a body part caused by disease or trauma. Paleopathology deals with skeletal lesions accumulated during life or inflicted perimortem, at the time of death. Taphonomy, on the other hand, is the study of postmortem changes that affect a body until its archaeological recovery. Since animals were typically dismembered for consumption and are rarely recovered anatomically complete, the basic observational unit in zooarchaeology is a *specimen*, "a bone or tooth, or fragment thereof" (Grayson, 1984).

A perpetual problem in paleopathology is the limited way in which bone can respond to disease. Due to the narrow range of morphological responses, it can be difficult if not impossible to determine the etiology, or causes, of disease. This general difficulty is further compounded by the unique nature of most zooarchaeological assemblages, which tend to consist of an admixture of fragmented and commingled bones from various species.

Skeletal Integrity – Taphonomy and Sampling

Most zooarchaeological assemblages, generated through butchery and meat consumption, were prone to scavenging, multiple re-deposition and other destructive forces. While human burials often contain relatively complete individuals, finding articulated animal skeletons is rare. When articulated animal remains come to light, they often belong to companion animals (e.g., mounts or putative pets) and are more commonly encountered in structured "ritual" deposits or proper burials alongside humans. On the other hand, commingled and fragmented human remains pose taphonomic histories different from those of animals (Outram et al., 2005). In zooarchaeology, this leads to lesions being typically noted on isolated single bones; hence, lacking key associated information on age, sex and skeletal changes to other areas of the animal's body (Bartosiewicz, 2008a). This taphonomic loss of information has unfortunately contributed to and preserved the tradition of pathological cases being reported as "curious examples" devoid of biological context (Thomas, 2012).

Another recurring problem in animal paleopathology has been the lack of quantitative information on the occurrence of animal disease in the past (Upex & Dobney, 2012). The concept of prevalence – the proportion of a population affected by a particular condition – is an essential component in our understanding of human disease in the past, but remains impossible to reliably apply in animal paleopathology. The size and demographic structure of ancient animal populations (the denominator of this value) are unknown. Pathological finds (the numerator) are unlikely to be representative, as archaeological data, in general, are non-random in nature. Moreover, the effects of sampling are critical in appraising animal paleopathology.

In the case of commonly occurring lesions found on bones of livestock, broad-based quantification may facilitate a quasi-epidemiological approach to animal disease. Synthetic studies of large assemblages of refuse bone may reveal patterning in the relative frequency of various conditions. For example, in caprines, including sheep (*Ovis aries* L., 1758) and goats (*Capra hircus* L., 1758), parodontal disease is marked by the dissolution of alveolar margins, swelling and eventual *in vivo* tooth loss and fistulation (see Figure 30.1). In a study by Bartosiewicz (2008b), cases of the lesion were compared between 36 sites in Europe and Southwest Asia, representing a total of over half million identifiable specimens. The results reflect the remarkably low incidence of this modern clinically common pathological condition (Table 30.1), even if the resulting percentages of diseased fragments are derived from bones that were archaeologically recovered as food refuse. What does stand as reasonably reflective of the disease in the past is that a significantly greater proportion of parodontal disease was noted among the fewer caprine remains published from Europe than in Southwest Asia ($\chi^2=9.677$, d.f.=1, p=0.002). The reason for this difference is difficult to determine since the etiology of this disease is multicausal. It can be linked to differences in the natural environment and human-controlled access to quality graze, as well as the fact that sheep mandibles from Europe come from older individuals, possibly resulting from increased emphasis on sustainable wool production, especially in later archaeological periods.

Utilizing an epidemiological approach in animal paleopathology has led to a number of other insights into the health of animal populations in the past. For instance, mapping the anatomical patterns of potentially work-related lesions on disarticulated cattle (*Bos taurus* L., 1758) bones from Europe and Southwest Asia delineated a diachronic trend of increasing morbidity, commensurate with intensifying draught exploitation between the Neolithic and Middle Ages (Bartosiewicz, 2006). On the other hand, an increase in distal limb lesions in cattle at medieval/post-medieval Dudley Castle, England (Thomas, 2008) was attributable to a demographic trend in the cattle population, as beasts were simply slaughtered at an increasingly old age. This is a warning that similarly to the aforementioned example of parodontal

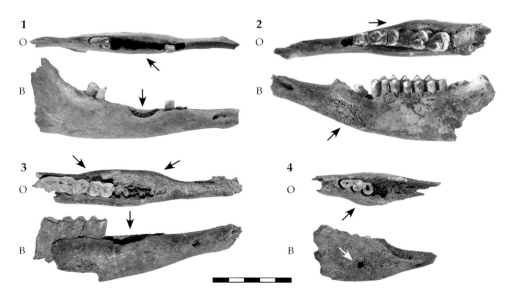

Figure 30.1 Parodontal disease in sheep. 1: Neolithic Endrőd 23B, Hungary; 2: Neolithic Tell Karanovo, Bulgaria; 3: Chalcolithic Horum Höyük, Anatolia/Turkey; 4: Chalcolithic Polyanitsa, Bulgaria. Occlusal (O) and buccal (B) aspects. Arrows mark various lesions. Scale: 50 mm.

Table 30.1 Frequencies of parodontal disease among caprines in 36 zooarchaeological assemblages from Europe and Southwest Asia* Incidence is significantly (p=0.000) higher in assemblages from Europe

NISP (Number of identifiable specimens)	Europe	Southwest Asia
Number of assemblages	28	8
Total NISP	283,473	327,184
Caprine NISP	74,553	124,003
Caprine %	26.3	37.9
Caprine parodontal disease NISP	36	14
Parodontal disease among caprines %	0.048	0.011

*Numbers are pooled by region (Bartosiewicz 2008b).

disease in sheep, the age structure of animals may interfere with interpretations of exploitation. Age is not a disease in itself, but is a predisposing factor that must always be considered.

Large-scale analyses of isolated fragments, born out of taphonomic necessity, help to circumvent some problems inherent to the absence of complete skeletons. These analyses are no substitute, however, for a detailed qualitative study of intact animal burials. Thanks to the latter, the paleopathology of horse (*Equus caballus* L., 1758) and dog (*Canis familiaris* L., 1758) and even domestic hen (*Gallus domesticus* L., 1758) tend to be better understood than that of ordinary livestock (e.g., Bartosiewicz & Bartosiewicz, 2002; Baron, 2018).

Taxonomic Diversity

Animal paleopathology is not focused on a single species. Diverse human lifeways are reflected in the anatomical patterns of disease appearing on the skeleton (Berger & Trinkaus, 1995). In zooarchaeology, at least a dozen mammalian species are a subject to regular study, each with their own skeletal features and various ways of life conducive to different diseases. Even general conditions – such as injuries or congenital defects – vary between taxa depending on body size and specific skeletal morphology. Different body regions are affected by disease in different ways in various animals. After death, taphonomic loss (fragmentation, excavation techniques) also affects the bones of various animal species differently.

The distribution of 1257 lesions by taxa and body region is summarized for domesticates in Figure 30.2 (in this graph, "Caprine" stands for the sum of all sheep and/or goat remains). These cases represent various archaeological periods in Europe and Southwest Asia, but articulated skeletons were excluded. Lesions in the "head" also include dental pathologies, "trunk" refers to vertebrae and bones of the rib cage, "limb" to the pectoral and pelvic girdles, and the stylo- and zygopodium. "Foot" bones are carpals/tarsals, metapodia and phalanges. Wild animals display fewer pathological lesions, which in part is an artifact of their underrepresentation in most studied assemblages. Distribution by body region, thus, cannot be meaningfully discussed for rarely occurring game animals.

Although there is a seven-fold difference between the total number of pathological specimens in horse and cattle in Figure 30.2, the ratio of lesions on the head was significantly increased by horn deformations and dental disorders in cattle. Without considering lesions on the head and on limb bones (the latter being rather rarely recorded in horses), the distribution of lesions between cattle and horse was homogeneous within the trunk and feet (χ^2=3.87; d.f.=2, p=0.144), a phenomenon partly attributable to the comparable body sizes of these large ungulates.

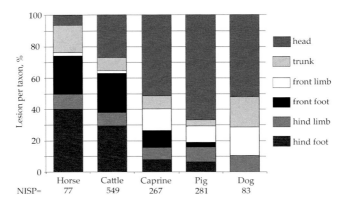

Figure 30.2 The distribution of pathological lesions by body region in domestic animals.

The numerical representation of lesions in all caprines (all identifiable remains of sheep and goat) and pig (*Sus domesticus* Erxleben, 1777) is more balanced, with both groups approaching 300 pathological specimens. The comparison of all body regions showed a significant difference between these two major taxa (χ^2=23.911, d.f.=5, p=0.000). The distribution, however, was homogeneous when the head and front feet were not considered (χ^2=4.149, d.f.=3, p=0.246). Among pathological phenomena on the head, crowded teeth – a symptom of domestication in pigs – are rare in caprines. On the other hand, the fused 3rd–4th metacarpal bones of sheep or goat are more often impacted by disease than the smaller, more differentiated metapodia in pig.

The small group of osteological lesions on dispersed dog remains shows a remarkable absence of all foot bones. These elements being the smallest among the bones summarized here are prone to taphonomic loss, and they are less likely to be found. Metacarpal lesions have been observed during the more careful excavation of articulated dog skeletons (e.g., Bathurst & Barta, 2004; Bartosiewicz, 2013). The consistent recovery of small dog phalanges usually requires water-sieving.

Biomolecular Methods

Biomolecular tests provide important information about ancient diseases that are difficult or impossible to obtain using traditional, morphology-based paleopathological methods (Prendergast et al., 2017). Importantly, these analyses help diagnosis directly even in the absence of osteological symptoms, for example in the case of acute infections. By the 1990s, the identification of tuberculosis, one of the diseases best investigated in ancient humans, entered a new phase facilitated by ancient mycobacterial DNA (aDNA) and the analysis of lipid biomarkers recovered from the 8th century AD cemetery of Bélmegyer–Csömöki-domb, Hungary (Molnár et al., 2015). By isolating and identifying microbes and analyzing their aDNA extracted from affected bones, it is possible to determine the evolutionary history of the disease. This is best illustrated by how various *Mycobacterium* species adapted to particular host species (see Chapters 8 and 17, this volume).

Defining and Grouping Animal Disease in Archaeology

Defining and classifying animal disease in archaeology is challenging. Inconsistencies in nomenclature (derived from both veterinary medicine and human paleopathology) originate from the heterogeneous evolution of animal paleopathology under the influence of other disciplines. The recognition and classification of disease is made even more difficult by the fine line between lesions indicating "disease" and those within the boundaries of normal variation. This latter variation is hard to define in domesticates, as the boundary between "pathological" and "normal" can be blurred (O'Connor, 2000) by variability. Some hereditary conditions became selected for by breeders, sometimes leading to "the production of slobbering brutes with severe endocrine pathology. Only our daft species would keep some of these varieties alive, and regard them acceptable as breeds" (Brothwell, 2016: 166). However, a more consequential methodological problem persists in animal paleopathology. Many lesions on archaeological specimens have no known parallels in modern veterinary medicine, as today's animals are either slaughtered (on both economic and humane grounds) or treated before skeletal manifestations of disease can develop. This limits the availability of reference skeletons with known clinical diagnoses. For want of such materials, many researchers resort to using illustrations from handbooks (e.g., Baker & Brothwell 1980; Bartosiewicz, 2013) as visual thesauri in diagnosing specimens, even though such works were never intended to serve as systematic and comprehensive identification manuals.

Comparing present-day cases of pathological lesions of known etiology with archaeological specimens is essential to creating reliable and explicit paleopathological protocols (Baker, 1978). Visually observed similarities between modern lesions and those found on archaeological bone is an insufficient criterion for diagnosis. Circumspect differential diagnoses are necessary as, in spite of some commonalities; food-producing livestock, beasts of burden, companion animals and game have differing disease spectra (Upex & Dobney, 2012; Lawler, 2017). O'Connor (2000) has long emphasized the importance of detailed documentation (textual and pictorial), rather than ad hoc diagnosis, since the latter may be inadvertently biased by hypothetical interpretations. This common practice was prevalent in human paleopathology prior to the 1970s (Buikstra & Cook, 1980). Some works in animal paleopathology are still rife with simplistic, monocausal interpretations, especially regarding evidence for working animals, an important archaeological topic. Observations must be presented alongside alternative hypotheses. Differential diagnoses must include a proper range of possible diseases, as well as their multicausal origins.

At least since the time of Hippocrates, classifying disease has posed a challenge in medicine (Bálint et al., 2006). Buffon (1749) listed human skeletal anomalies in six categories. Miller et al. (1996) set up seven groups, based on recognizable, although often non-specific, symptoms encountered in human paleopathology. Given the variety of animal species and diverse forms of exploitation, this scheme is difficult to apply in zooarchaeology. Diagnoses based on isolated symptoms on disarticulated fragments are even more problematic to integrate within a coherent system. For purely practical purposes, an empirical grouping in animal paleopathology was proposed by von den Driesch (1972), which included:

(1) Traumatic lesions: With the exception of extremely complex cases, healed trauma is relatively easy to identify. Causes are rarely evident. This category is direct and empirical.
(2) Lesions caused by overworking: Osteological responses of animal work coincide with those of age. Animals kept under harsh conditions also tend to "age" faster. Distinguishing between these two factors is difficult using isolated bones. This category is by definition etiological and deductive.
(3) Dental anomalies: Teeth preserve well, are easily identifiable, allow age at death and in some species sex of the individual to be estimated, permitting more accurate diagnoses than the analysis of lesions on skeletal bone. This category is taxonomic-anatomical.

These three gross categories conveniently cover the majority (over 90%) of recognizable lesions in animal paleopathology (Bartosiewicz, 2021) and their simplicity provides a practical advantage. However, the groups of lesions represent three very different, intersecting paradigms of animal morbidity. Baker (1978) pointed out that grouping diseases in animal paleopathology can be based on either the type of pathology (such as 1: trauma – empirical) or etiology (2: overworking – deductive). Defining a third group on the basis of dental anatomy adds yet another dimension to diagnosis.

The limitations of this grouping include the overlap between the three categories and the fact that several rare but important forms of disease are not explicitly included. Elusive metabolic and endocrinological conditions, many hereditary in nature, are not addressed. Infections and neoplasms are likewise missing. It is understood, however, that they need to be added to the list as they occur. Subsequent classifications of pathological lesions into eight and nine categories, respectively (Baker & Brothwell 1980; Bartosiewicz, 2013), reflect this necessity.

Human Agency

By its exclusive focus on animal remains from archaeological contexts, animal paleopathology in zooarchaeology is inseparable from the study of human agency, distinguishing it from applications in paleontology. Interactions between animal and human populations have been argued to lead to natural selection among animals and social adaptation by humans (Norris, 1979). This simplistic dichotomy, however, represents merely theoretical end points of a continuum. Animal-human interactions intensified as a consequence of the domestication of animals. Humans have, often inadvertently, manipulated animal heredity mimicking genetic drift that eventually made domesticates different from their wild ancestors. Although wild animal morbidity is difficult to study due to its underrepresentation in archaeological assemblages, Moodie (1923: 235) points out that, "No constitutional diseases of the bison are known, nor should we expect to meet any". These diseases in the wild include malfunctions and lesions whose etiology is significantly influenced by heritability. Moodie's point is reflected in European, Asian and African archaeological assemblages: the relatively few healed skeletal lesions in game tend to appear on the bones of large and strong individuals of aurochs (*B. primigenius* Bojanus, 1827), wild boar (*Sus scrofa* L., 1758) or brown bear (*Ursus arctos* L., 1758) and the like. Such animals were less threatened by either animal or human predation, but ultimately succumbed to hunters. The range of diseases is far broader in domesticates sheltered from natural selection by humans.

Care and Neglect

Human agency in fostering, as well as handling animal disease has recently taken center stage in research illustrating how ancient people and animals coexisted in their shared natural environments and immediate living spaces. While examples of animal abuse or simply neglect may be suspected in the presence of serious lesions, possible therapeutic intervention to heal animal bone fractures has also been explored. Udrescu and Van Neer (2005) examined healed fractures in small domestic ungulates (pig, caprines) and dog, although they also reported healed metacarpal fractures among the finds of roe deer and klipspringer antelope (*Oreotragus oreotragus* Zimmermann, 1783). Even in the absence of archaeological evidence for direct therapeutic intervention, one may hypothesize that in domestic animals, recovery was aided by humans. Rare examples of natural recovery in wild ungulates exist, although chances are better in smaller species: the live weights of roe deer (15–25 kg) and klipspringer antelope (8–18 kg) may be an advantage in retaining some mobility after injury.

Without veterinary care, limb fracture recovery is hampered by body mass in large ungulates. Small Iron Age horses in Europe weighed at least 250–360 kg and the weight of coeval cattle probably ranged between 180 and 300 kg. Even if these values look modest by modern standards, they are an order of magnitude greater than those for small ungulates. In addition to size, the age of the individual is important in the prognosis: physiological fracture healing is easier in young individuals whose weights are, logically, also smaller.

Due to their strategic and status value, treating horses appears to have the longest documented tradition in veterinary history (von den Driesch & Peters, 2002; Xu 2021). Thanks to the special efforts devoted to curing horses, in spite of their large live weight, chances of fracture healing are known to be good in the distal limb segment of modern horses (Schatzman, 1998). Most paleopathological cases in horse and cattle indeed appear in the foot region, while healed injury in proximal limb segments is rare. An exceptional case appears in a femur diaphysis fracture in Roman period cattle reported by Van Neer & Udrescu (2015). In the absence of parallels to this healed trauma in modern veterinary collections, the authors cite a present-day example in giant eland antelope (*Taurotragus derbianus* Gray, 1847; live weight: 300–900 kg) comparable to cattle in size. This distant parallel, however, is very telling: the femur originated from a zoo specimen that recovered under close veterinary supervision.

Compound fractures in the metacarpal bones of two Iron Age horses (Celtic Manching, Germany: von den Driesch, 1989; 4th–7th century BCE Sindos, Greece: Antikas, 2008) healed at an obtuse angle (*dislocatio ad axim*), accompanied by the physiological dissolution of bone mineral content. These animals may have been spared due to their symbolic or emotional value but show no signs of treatment. Another healed fracture of a horse metacarpus (Late Roman Mühlberg, Germany: Teichert, 1988) healed with a well-developed callus on the palmar side, although the animal may have been well attended. Lastly, a simple metacarpal fracture in another Iron Age horse (Stična, Slovenia: Bökönyi, 1994) healed with only minor dislocation and shortening (Figure 30.3). This example raises the possibility that the horse received expert care, including suspension (slinging) of the beast for weeks as recommended by the 4th-century Greek veterinary surgeon Apsyrtos (Zellwecker, 1981). Several historical images of horse slinging, summarized by Schatzman (1998), include a

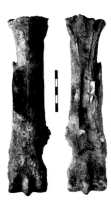

Figure 30.3 Healed fracture of a horse left third metacarpal showing slight dislocation and shortening (Early Iron Age Stična, Slovenia). Anterior (left) and palmar aspects. Scale: 50 mm

mid-15th-century illumination by Johan Alvarez de Salamiellas showing not only the suspension of the animal, but also the splinting of its lower front leg.

Front limbs support, on average, two-thirds of the live weight in ungulates, while hind legs provide primary dynamic force in locomotion (Bartosiewicz, 2006). Therefore, the prognosis of spontaneous fracture healing seems better in metatarsal than the weight-bearing metacarpal bones. A broken cattle metatarsus with only a slight dislocation along its longitudinal axis, and another with minor overriding of the healed fracture ends (Middle Ages, Haithabu, Germany: Johansson, 1982) match an example of a healed metatarsus of an Iron Age horse (Skedemosse, Sweden: Boessneck et al., 1968). Although the possibility of treatment can never be ruled out in domesticates, the broken metatarsus of a wild guanaco (*Lama guanicoe* Müller, 1776) from Argentina also healed with only a slight deviation from the bone's long axis (Bartosiewicz, 2013; the live weight of guanacos ranges between 100 and 120 kg, falling between the weights of small and large domestic bovids). This example indicates that we need to be careful when asserting that treatment was provided to an animal.

Zoonoses

In Europe, Asia and Africa, the conduit for human infection by wildlife was significantly amplified by the onset of domestication (Pearce-Duvet, 2006). The combined effect of increasing human population density supported by emerging agriculture, in correlation with close and regular contact between people and their animals, led to a much richer pool of dangerous pathogens. Eighty percent of infections in humans are shared with other vertebrates and two-thirds of zoonoses have their origins in domesticates (Schwabe, 1984). Risks of infection were multiplied by the intensification of both human and animal contact within early farming communities (Fournié et al., 2017). The earliest biomolecular evidence of tuberculosis in humans was found in a 25-year-old woman and a 12-month-old infant from the Pre-Pottery Neolithic B settlement of Atlit-Yam, Israel, dating from 9250 to 8160 years ago. These cases were confirmed by both aDNA and lipid biomarker analysis (Hershkovitz et al., 2008).

In Figure 30.4, the numbers of diseases shared bilaterally between humans and their domesticates (McNeill, 1976) are plotted against the estimated time of domestication (Zeder, 2008). While humans share the greatest numbers of diseases with dogs, the four domestic artiodactyl species (sheep, goat, cattle and pig) of the so-called "Neolithic package" form a

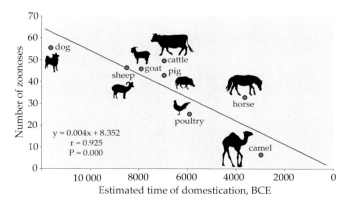

Figure 30.4 The number of bilateral zoonoses shared by humans and various animals as a function of the time since domestication

cluster associated with more zoonoses than expected on the basis of their chronological positions (above the trend line). Horse, domesticated later, shows the same tendency. Within this complex scenario, parasites also played a role in the evolution and spread of new pathogens. Recent analyses of the Neolithic sediment sequence from Els Trocs cave in Spain show a major increase in the abundance and diversity of parasites, as pastoral resources were increasingly exploited through time (Tejedor-Rodríguez et al., 2021).

The presence of tuberculosis and brucellosis in humans and animals serves as an example of dangerous contacts noted in zooarchaeological findings. Microbes causing tuberculosis (*Mycobacterium* spp.) and spontaneous abortion (linked to brucellosis) have the potential to affect the skeletons of both humans and animals. Symptoms of these two diseases are not always easily distinguishable morphologically in animals and possibilities of their molecular identification depend on chemical preservation (Bendrey et al., 2007; Bendrey, 2008).

Tuberculosis is caused by 11 known species of *Mycobacteria*, collectively called the *Mycobacterium tuberculosis complex* (MTC). At first, evidence of Late Pre-Pottery Neolithic B period tuberculosis in humans in the Levant supported the hypothesis that shortly after domestication, coexistence between early domesticates and humans contributed to the emergence of this zoonotic disease (Horwitz & Smith, 2000), aided by aerosols or by eating contaminated milk and meat particularly of *Mycobacterium bovis*. aDNA evidence of tuberculosis has been confirmed in humans from Late Neolithic Hungary (Masson et al., 2013; Pósa et al., 2015, and see Chapters 8 and 17, this volume). Morphological identification of a tuberculous lesion on a cow metatarsus from a contemporaneous tell settlement at Herpály in Hungary (Bartosiewicz, 2013: 101, Figure 81) has also been reported. However, biomolecular analyses indicate that *M. tuberculosis* in humans did not originate from *M. bovis* (Smith et al., 2009). *M. tuberculosis* has evolved over thousands of years, and variables such as transmission dynamics, host tolerance and human population patterns may have shaped the evolution of mycobacterial genomes (Saelens et al., 2019). *M. tuberculosis* appears to be one of the most ancient pathogens among the MTC. There is a possibility that *M. bovis* evolved as it spread to members of the Bovidae family and that it can thrive in taxonomically disparate animals displaying a most extensive host range (Mostowy et al., 2005; Buzic & Giuffra, 2020).

Although zoonoses have always been common, some diseases might have been mitigated or prevented if humans treated animals better (Benatar, 2007: 1545). Future work in animal paleopathology should consider power relations and practices of care, as well as domination and exploitation that shape animal-human relations (Fredengren, 2021: 13). Importantly, diets, animal husbandry and interactions developed within colonial and settler cultures have influenced the evolution of zoonotic diseases as much, if not more than practices of indigenous human groups. The racist trope that cultural practices such as the development of "wet markets" or that the consumption of "bushmeat" is filthy and creates an "unhealthy" intimacy with and between animals perpetuates a dangerous ignorance regarding the effects of colonial practices on zoonotic diseases (Rosenberg, 2020: 652; Bartosiewicz, 2021: 64). Hence, beyond simply focusing on animals and microbiota, understanding animal disease requires exploring past and present human-human relationships.

Concluding Remarks

Human health and animal health are integral aspects of human history. Their co-evolution, an exciting area of academic inquiry, is unimaginable without understanding animal disease in archaeology. However, the brief summary of research presented here supports the view of Thomas (2012) that animal paleopathology saw a relatively protracted methodological development compared to zooarchaeology as a whole, or compared to work in human paleopathology. Although zooarchaeological advances are intertwined with achievements in paleopathology, unique aspects of archaeological animal bone assemblages (taphonomic loss, taxonomic diversity) make them very different from the analysis of human bone and limit the possibilities of direct intellectual cross-fertilization between these two related fields. Regardless, Upex and Dobney (2012) emphasize the need for large syntheses and more detailed analyses. A delicate balance between the quality and quantity of information, however, is difficult to strike. Rare pathological finds require differential diagnosis and epidemiological interpretation, while synthetic analyses of large series of bones usually become possible only at the expense of individual diagnostic detail. This paradox in animal paleopathology illustrates a greater general dilemma; the horizontal expansion of scientific applications in archaeology is hard to reconcile with in-depth, vertical specialization. The limited understanding of complex biological processes behind pathological phenomena in archaeology, along with the introduction of highly sophisticated laboratory techniques, has hindered the accessibility of animal paleopathology to archaeologists and the broader public. The only solution is to intensify substantive cooperation between highly specialized experts, a welcome trend in many areas of archaeological research.

References

Antikas, T. G. (2008). They didn't shoot horses: fracture management in a horse of the 5th century BCE from Sindos, Central Macedonia, Greece. *Veterinarija ir Zootechnika* 43(64):21–27. https://vetzoo.lsmuni.lt/data/vols/2008/42/pdf/antikas.pdf.

Babington, C. C. (1863). On a skull of Bos primigenius associated with flint implements. *Proceedings of the Cambridge Antiquarian Commission* II:285–288.

Baker, J. R. (1978). The differential diagnosis of bone disease. In. Brothwell, D. R., Thomas, K. D. & Clutton-Brock, J. (Eds.), *Research Problems in Zooarchaeology*, pp. 107–112. Occasional Publication No. 3. London: Institute of Archaeology.

Baker, J. R, & Brothwell, D. (1980). *Animal Diseases in Archaeology*. Academic Press.

Bálint, G. P., Buchanan, W. W. & Dequeker, J. (2006). A brief history of medical taxonomy and diagnosis. *Clinical Rheumatology* 25:132–135. DOI 10.1007/s 10067-004-1051-z.

Baron, H. (2018). *Quasi liber et pictura. Die Tierknochenfunde aus dem Gräberfeld an der Wiener Csokorgasse – eine anthrozoologische Studie zu den awarischen Bestattungssitten*. Monographien des Römisch-Germanischen Zentralmuseums Band 143. Verlag Schnell und Steiner.

Bartosiewicz, L. (2001). Archaeozoology or zooarchaeology?: a problem from the last century. *Archaeologia Polona* 39:75–86.

Bartosiewicz, L. (2002). Pathological lesions on prehistoric animal remains from south-west Asia. In Buitenhuis, H., Choyke, A. M., Mashkour, M. & Al-Shiyab, A. H. (Eds.), *Archaeozoology of the Near East V. Proceedings of the Fifth International Symposium on the Archaeozoology of Southwestern Asia and Adjacent Areas*, pp. 320–336. ARC Publications 62.

Bartosiewicz, L. (2006). Mettre le chariot devant le boeuf. Anomalies ostéologiques liées à l'utilisation des boeuf pour la traction. In Pétrequin, P., Arbogast, R.-M., Pétrequin, A.-M., Van Willigen, S. & Bailly, M. (Eds.), *Premiers Chariots, Premiers Araires. La Diffusion De La Traction Animale En Europe Pendant Les IVe et IIIe Millénaires Avant Notre Ère*, pp. 259–267. CRA Monographies 29. CNRS Editions.

Bartosiewicz, L. (2008a). Taphonomy and palaeopathology in archaeozoology. *Geobios* 41(1):69–77. http://math.unife.it/interfacolta/lm.preistoria/insegnamenti/archeozoologia-1/materiale-didattico/a-a-2013-2014/presentazioni-8-13-14-gennaio/13-gennaio/bartosiewicz-2008_geobios.pdf.

Bartosiewicz, L. (2008b). Environmental stress in early domestic sheep. In Miklíková, Z. & Thomas, R. (Eds.), *Current Research in Animal Palaeopathology*, pp. 3–13. British Archaeological Reports, IS S1844. Archaeopress.

Bartosiewicz, L. (2013). *Shuffling Nags, Lame ducks. The Archaeology of Animal Disease*. Oxford: Oxbow.

Bartosiewicz, L. (2019). Animal palaeopathology: between archaeology and veterinary science. In Peters, J. (Ed.), *Animals: Cultural Identifiers in Ancient Societies?*, pp. 27–36. Verlag Marie Leidorf GmbH.

Bartosiewicz, L. (2020). International council for archaeozoology (ICAZ). In Smith, C. (Ed.), *Encyclopedia of Global Archaeology*, pp. 1–3. Springer Nature Switzerland AG. DOI: https://doi.org/10.1007/978-1-4419-0465-2_2112.

Bartosiewicz, L. (2021). What is a rare disease in animal paleopathology? *International Journal of Paleopathology* 33:13–24. https://doi.org/10.1016/j.ijpp.2021.02.001.

Bartosiewicz, L. (2021). Herding cats. *Current Swedish Archaeology* 29:56–71. https://doi.org/10.37718/CSA.2021.07.

Bartosiewicz, L. & Bartosiewicz, G. (2002). "Bamboo spine" in a migration period horse from Hungary. *Journal of Archaeological Science* 29.8:819–830.

Bartosiewicz, L. & Gál, E. (2018). Introduction: care, neglect and the "osteological paradox". In Bartosiewicz, L. & Gál, E. (Eds.), *Care or Neglect? Evidence of Animal Disease in Archaeology*, pp. 1–3. Oxford: Oxbow.

Bartosiewicz, L., Van Neer, W. & Lentacker, A. (1997). *Draught Cattle: Their Osteological Identification and History*. Annalen, Zoologische Wetenschappen Vol. 281. Koninklijk Museum voor Midden-Afrika.

Bathurst, R. R. & Barta, J. L. (2004). Molecular evidence of tuberculosis induced hypertrophic osteopathy in a 16th-century Iroquoian dog. *Journal of Archaeological Science* 31:917–925. https://doi.org/10.1016/j.jas.2003.12.006.

Bell, L. S. (1990). Palaeopathology and diagenesis: an SEM evaluation of structural changes using backscattered electron imaging. *Journal of Archaeological Science* 17:85–102. https://doi.org/10.1016/0305-4403(90)90016-X.

Benatar, D. (2007). The chickens come home to roost. *American Journal of Public Health* 97(9):1545–1546. doi:10.2105/AJPH.2006.090431. PMC 1963309. PMID 17666704.

Bendrey, R. (2007). Ossification of the interosseous ligaments between the metapodials in horses: a new recording methodology and preliminary study. *International Journal of Osteoarchaeology* 17:207–213. https://doi.org/10.1002/oa.875.

Bendrey, R. (2008). A possible case of tuberculosis or brucellosis in an Iron Age horse skeleton from Viables farm, Basingstoke, England. In Miklíková, Z. & Thomas, R. (Eds.), *Current Research in Animal Palaeopathology*, pp. 19–26. British Archaeological Reports, IS S1844. Archaeopress.

Bendrey, R., Taylor, G. M., Bouwman, A. S. & Cassidy, J. P. (2007). Suspected bacterial disease in two archaeological horse skeletons from southern England: paleopathological and biomolecular studies. *Journal of Archaeological Science* 35:1–10. https://doi.org/10.1016/j.jas.2007.11.002.

Berger, T. D. & Trinkaus, E. (1995). Patterns of trauma among the Neandertals. *Journal of Archaeological Science* 22:841–852. https://doi.org/10.1016/0305-4403(95)90013-6.

Boessneck, J. (1956). Ein Beitrag zur Errechnung der Widerristhöhe nach Metapodienmaßen bei Rindern. *Zeitschrift für Tierzüchtung und Züchtungsbiologie* 68/1:75–90.

Boessneck, J., Müller, H-H. & Teichert, M. (1964). Osteologische unterscheidungsmerkmale zwischen Schaf (*Ovis aries* Linné) und Ziege (*Capra hircus* Linné). *Kühn Archiv* 78:1–129.

Boessneck, J., von den Driesch-Karpf, A. & Gejvall, N.-G. (1968). *Die Tierknochenfunde von Säugetieren und vom Menschen. The Archaeology of Skedemosse III*. Stockholm: Royal Academy of Letters, History and Antiquities.

Bökönyi, S. (1974). *History of Domestic Mammals in Central and Eastern Europe*. Akadémiai Kiadó.

Bökönyi, S. (1994). Analiza zivalskih kosti (Die Tierknochenfunde). In Gabrovec, S. (Ed.), *Stična I. Naselbinska izkopovanja*. Siedlungsausgrabungen, pp. 190–213. Catalogi et Monographiae 28.

Brothwell, D. R. (1963). The palaeopathology of pleistocene and more recent mammals. In Brothwell, D. R. & Higgs, E. S. (Eds.), *Science in Archaeology: A Survey of Progress and Research*, pp. 275–278. Thames and Hudson.

Brothwell, D. (1993). Avian osteopathology and its evaluation. *Archaeofauna* 2:33–43.

Brothwell, D. (1995). The special animal pathology. In Cunliffe, B. (Ed.), *Danebury: An Iron Age Hillfort in Hampshire. Volume 6. A Hillfort Community in Perspective*, pp. 207–233. Council for British Archaeology, Research Report.

Brothwell, D. (2008a). Problems of differential diagnosis in Pleistocene mammal pathology. *Veterinarija ir Zootechnika* 44(66):88–90. https://vetzoo.lsmuni.lt/data/vols/2008/44/en/brothwell.pdf.

Brothwell, D. R. (2008b). Chapter 5: Paleoradiology in the service of zoopaleopathology. In Chhem, R. K. & Brothwell, D. R. (Eds.), *Paleoradiology Imaging Mummies and Fossils*, pp. 119–145. Springer-Verlag.

Brothwell, D. (2016). *A Faith in Archaeological Science: Reflections on a Life*. Archaeopress.

Brothwell, D. & Higgs, E. S. (Eds.) (1963). *Science in Archaeology: A Survey of Progress and Research*. Thames and Hudson.

Buell, P. D., May, T. & Ramey, D. (2018). Chinese horse medicine: texts and illustrations. In Lo, V. & Barrett, P. (Eds.), *Imagining Chinese Medicine*, pp. 315–326. Sir Henry Wellcome Asian Series, 18. Brill.

Buffon, Comte de. (1749). *Histoire Naturelle, Générale et Particulière, Avec la Description du Cabinet du Roi*. Tome Troisième. L'Imprimerie Royale.

Buikstra, J. E. & Cook, D. C. (1980). Palaeopathology: an American account. *Annual Review of Anthropology* 9:433–470. https://www.annualreviews.org/doi/pdf/10.1146/annurev.an.09.100180.002245.

Buzic, I. & Giuffra, V. (2020). The paleopathological evidence on the origins of human tuberculosis: a review. *Journal of Preventive Medicine and Hygiene* 61(Suppl 1): E3–E8. DOI:10.15167/2421-4248/jpmh2020.61.1s1.1379.

Carson, R. (1962). *Silent Spring*. Houghton Mifflin Harcourt.

Cordier, G. (1990). Blessures préhistoriques animales et humaines avec armes ou projectiles conservés. *Bulletin de la Société Préhistorique Française* 87(10):462–482. https://www.persee.fr/doc/bspf_0249-7638_1990_hos_87_10_9929.

Cornwall, I. W. (1956). *Bones for the Archaeologist*. Macmillan.

Davies, J., Fabiš, M., Mainland, I., Richards, M. & Thomas, R. (2005). *Diet and Health in Past Animal Populations. Current Research and Future Directions*. Oxford: Oxbow.

Dieguez, C., Isidro, A. & Malgosa, A. (1996). An introduction to zoo-paleopathology and an update on fossil phyto-paleopathology from Spain. *Journal of Paleopathology* 8(3):133–142.

Dobney, K. M. & Ervynck, A. (1998), A protocol for recording enamel hypoplasia on archaeological pig teeth. *International Journal of Osteoarchaeology* 8:263–273. https://doi.org/10.1002/(SICI)1099-1212(199807/08)8:4<263::AID-OA427>3.0.CO;2-P.

Driesch, A. von den. (1972). *Osteoarchäologische Untersuchungen auf der Iberischen Halbinsel*. Studien über frühe Tierknochenfunde von der Iberischen Halbinsel 3. München: Uni-Druck.

Driesch, A. von den. (1975). Die Bewertung pathologisch-anatomischer Veränderungen an vor- und frühgeschichlichen Tierknochen. In. Clason, A.T (Ed.), *Archaeozoological Studies*, pp. 413–425. Elsevier.

Driesch, A. von den. (1976). *Das Vermessen von Tierknochen aus vor- und frühgeschichtlichen Siedlungen*. Dissertation. Institut für Paläoanatomie, Domestikationsforschung und Geschichte der Tiermedizin der Universität München.

Driesch, A. von den. (1989). La paléopathologie animale. Analyse d'ossements animaux pathologiques pré- et protohistoriques. *Revue de Médecine Vétérinaire* 140(8–9):645–652.

Driesch, A. von den. (1994). Hyperostosis in fish. In Van Neer, W. (Ed.), *Fish Exploitation in the Past*, pp. 37–45. Annalen, Zoologische Wetenschappen Vol. 274. Koninklijk Museum voor Midden-Afrika.

Driesch, A. von den & Peters, J. (2002). *Geschichte der Tiermedizin. 5000 Jahre Tierheilkunde*. Schattauer, F. K. Verlag.

Esper, J.F. (1774). *Déscription des Zoolithes Nouvellement Découvertes d'Animaux Quadrupedes Inconnus et des Cavernes Qui les Renferment Quand Même Que de Plusieurs Autres Grottes Remarquables Qui se Trouvent dans le Margraviat de Baireuth au delà des Monts*. Georg Wolfgang Knorr.

Fredengren, C. (2021). Beyond entanglement. *Current Swedish Archaeology* 28:11–33.

Forchhammer, G., Steenstrup, J. C. H. R. & Worsaae, J. (1851–1856). *Undersøgelser i Geologisk-Antikvarisk Retning* [Studies in geological-antiquarian direction]. Kongliga Hofbogtrykker Bianco Luno.

Fournié, G., Pfeiffer, D. U. & Bendrey, R. (2017). Early animal farming and zoonotic disease dynamics: modelling brucellosis transmission in Neolithic goat populations. *Royal Society Open Science* 4:160943. http://dx.doi.org/10.1098/rsos.160943.

Froehner, R. (1922). Salihotra. *Veterinärhistorische Mitteilungen* 2(1):1–2.

Gál, E. (2008). Broken-winged: Fossil and subfossil pathological bird bones from recent excavations. In Miklíková, Z. & Thomas, R. (Eds.), *Current Research in Animal Palaeopathology*, pp. 80–86. British Archaeological Reports, IS S1844. Archaeopress.

Gál, E. (2013). Pathological changes in bird bones. In Bartosiewicz, L. (Ed.), *Shuffling Nags, Lame Ducks: The Archaeology of Animal disease*, pp. 217–238. Oxford: Oxbow.

Goldstein, M. S. (1963). The palaeopathology of human skeletal remains. In Brothwell, D. R. & Higgs, E. S. (Eds.), *Science in Archaeology: A Survey of Progress and Research*, pp. 480–489. Thames and Hudson.

Grauer, A.L. (2018). A century of paleopathology. *American Journal Physical of Anthropology* 165:904–914. DOI: 10.1002/ajpa.23366.

Grayson, D. K. (1984). *Quantitative Zooarchaeology: Topics in the Analysis of Archaeological Faunas.* Academic Press.

Haimovici, A. & Haimovici, S. (1971). Sur la presence de parodontopathies marginales sur des restes subfossiles de mammifères de stations pre- et protohistoriques du territoire de la Roumanie. *Bulletin de l'Groupe International des Rècherches Stomatologiques* 14:259–271.

Harland, J. & Van Neer, W. (2018). Weird fish: defining a role for fish palaeopathology. In Bartosiewicz, L. & Gál, E. (Eds.), *Care or Neglect? Evidence of Animal Disease in Archaeology,* pp. 256–275. Oxbow.

Hershkovitz, I., Donoghue, H. D., Minnikin, D. E., Besra, G. S., Lee, O.Y-C., Gernaey, A. M., … & Spigelman, M. (2008). Detection and molecular characterization of 9000-year-old *Mycobacterium tuberculosis* from a Neolithic settlement in the Eastern Mediterranean. *PLoS One* 3:e3426. http://dx.doi.org/10.1371/journal.pone.0003426.

Hillson, S. W. (1986). *Teeth.* Cambridge University Press.

Horwitz, L. K. & Smith, P. (2000). The contribution of animal domestication to the spread of zoonoses: a case study from the southern levant. *Ibex, Journal of Mountain Ecology* 5/*Anthropozoologica* 31:77–84. https://sciencepress.mnhn.fr/sites/default/files/articles/pdf/az2000n2a9.pdf.

Hrozny, B. (1931). L' entraînement des chevaux chez les anciens Indo Europiens. *Archiv Orientální* 3:431–461.

Johansson, F. (1982). *Untersuchungen an Skelettresten von Rindern aus Haithabu (Ausgrabung 1966–1969).* Berichte über die Ausgrabungen in Haithabu 17. Karl Wachholtz Verlag.

Jones, B. V. (2010). *Global Veterinary Medicine Timeline.* London: Knowledge. Royal College of Veterinary Surgeons. https://knowledge.rcvs.org.uk/heritage-and-history/.

Kammenhuber, A. (1961). *Hippologie Hethitica.* Harrassowitz.

Lawler, D. F. (2017). Differential diagnosis in archaeology. *International Journal of Paleopathology* 19:119–123. https://doi.org/10.1016/j.ijpp.2016.05.001.

Linnaeus, C. (1735). *Systema Naturæ, Sive Regna Tria Naturæ Systematice Proposita per Classes, Ordines, Genera, & Species.* Lugduni Batavorum.

Linnaeus, C. (1763). *Genera Morborum, in Auditorum Usum.* C. E. Steinert.

Marsigli, L. F. (1726). *Danubius Pannonico- Mysicus, Observationibus Geographicis, Astronomicis, Hydrographicis, Historicis, Physicis Perlustratus et in Sex Tomos Digestus. Tomus Secundus. De Antiquitates Romanae Militares ad Utramque Ripam Danubii.* P. Grosse, R. Chr. Alberts, P. de Hondt, Herm. Uytwert and Franç.

Masson, M., Molnár, E., Donoghue, H. D., Besra, G. S., Minnikin, D. E., Wu, H. H. T., Lee, O.Y-C., Bull, I. D. & Pálfi, G. (2013). Osteological and biomolecular evidence of a 7000-year-old case of hypertrophic pulmonary osteopathy secondary to tuberculosis from neolithic Hungary. *PLoS One* 8(10):e78252. http://dx.doi.org/10.1371/journal.pone.0078252.

McMiken, D. F. (1990). Ancient origins of horsemanship. *Equine Veterinary Journal* 22(2):73–78.

McNeil, W. H. (1976). *Plagues and People.* Doubleday/Anchor.

Mezzabotta, M. R. (2000). Aspects of multiculturalism in the *Mulomedicina* of Vegetius. *Akorterion* 45:52–64.

Miklíková, Z. & Thomas, R. (2008). *Current Research in Animal Palaeopathology.* British Archaeological Reports, IS 1844. Archaeopress.

Miller, E., Ragsdale, B. D. & Ortner, D. J. (1996). Accuracy in dry bone diagnosis: a comment on palaeopathological methods. *International Journal of Osteoarchaeology* 6:221–229. https://doi.org/10.1002/(SICI)1099-1212(199606)6:3<221::AID-OA267>3.0.CO;2-2.

Molnár, E., Donoghue, H. D., Lee, O. Y.-C., Wu, H. H. T., Besra, G. S., Minnikin, D. E., Bull, Ian D., Llewellyn, G., Williams, C. M., Spekker, O., & Pálfi, G. (2015). Morphological and biomolecular evidence for tuberculosis in 8th century AD skeletons from Bélmegyer-Csömöki domb, Hungary. *Tuberculosis* 95 (Supplement 1):S35–S41. https://doi.org/10.1016/j.tube.2015.02.032.

Moodie, R. L. (1923). *Palaeopathology: An Introduction to the Study of Ancient Evidences of Disease.* The University of Illinois Press.

Mostowy, S., Inwald, J., Gordon, S., Martin, C., Warren, R., Kremer, K., Cousins, D. & Behr, M. A. (2005). Revisiting the evolution of *Mycobacterium bovis. Journal of Bacteriology* 187(18):6386–6395. DOI: 10.1128/JB.187.18.6386-6395.2005.

Murthy, K. & Padmanabha, K. (1990). *A Dictionary of Archaeo-Zoology.* Ajanta Publications.

Nobis, G. (1954). Zur Kenntnis der ur- und frühgeschichtlichen Rinder Nord- und Mitteldeutschlands. *Zeitschrift für Tierzüchtung un Züchtungsbiologie* 63:155–194.

Norris, J. (1979). Plagues and Peoples by William H. McNeill. Review. *Bulletin of the History of Medicine* 53(1):145–147. https://www.jstor.org/stable/44451303.

O'Connor, T. P. (2000). *The Archaeology of Animal Bones*. Sutton Publishing Ltd.

O'Connor, T. P. (2005). Digitising and image-processing radiographs to enhance interpretation in avian palaeopathology. In Grupe, G. & Peters, J. (Eds.), *Feathers, Grit and Symbolism. Birds and Humans in the Ancient Old and New Worlds*, pp. 69–82. Marie Leidorf Verlag Gmbh.

Outram, A. K., Knüsel, C. J. Knight, S. & Harding, A. F. (2005). Understanding complex fragmented assemblages of human and animal remains: a fully integrated approach. *Journal of Archaeological Science* 32(12):1699–1710. https://doi.org/10.1016/j.jas.2005.05.008.

Payne, S. (1973). Kill-off patterns in sheep and goats: the mandibles from Aşvan Kale. *Anatolian Studies* 23:281–303.

Pearce-Duvet, J. M. C. (2006). The origin of human pathogens: evaluating the role of agriculture and domestic animals in the evolution of human disease. *Biology Review* 81:369–382. DOI: 10.1017/S1464793106007020.

Prendergast, M.E., Buckley, M., Crowther, A., Frantz, L., Eager, H., Lebrasseur, O., ... & Boivin, N. L. (2017). Reconstructing Asian faunal introductions to eastern Africa from multi-proxy biomolecular and archaeological datasets. *PLoS One* 12(12):e0190336. https://doi.org/10.1371/journal.pone.0182565.

Pósa, A., Maixner, F., Mende, B. G., Köhler, K., Osztás, A., Sola, C., Dutour, O., Masson, M., Molnár, E., Pálfi G. & Zink A. (2015). Tuberculosis in Late Neolithic-Early Copper Age human skeletal remains from Hungary. *Tuberculosis* 95:518–522. https://doi.org/10.1016/j.tube.2015.02.011.

Robison, N. D. (1987). Zooarchaeology: its history and development. In Bogan, A. E. & Robison, N. D. (Eds.), *The Zooarchaeology of Eastern North America: History, Method and Theory, and Bibliography*, pp. 1–26. Miscellaneous Paper No. 12. Tennessee Anthropological Association.

Rosenberg, G. N. (2020). On the scene of zoonotic intimacies. Jungle, market, pork plant. *Transgender Studies Quarterly* 7(4):646–656. DOI 10.1215/23289252-8665341.

Russell, N. (2011) *Social Zooarchaeology: Humans and Animals in Prehistory*. Cambridge University Press.

Rütimeyer, L. (1861). *Die Fauna der Pfahlbauten der Schweiz. Untersuchungen über die Geschichte der wilden und der Haus-Säugetiere von Mittel-Europa*. Allgemeine Schweizerische Gesellschaft für die gesammten Naturwissenschaften/Société Helvétique des Sciences Naturelles 19.

Saelens, J. W., Viswanathan, G. & Tobin, D. M. (2019). Mycobacterial evolution intersects with host tolerance. *Frontiers in Immunology* 10:528. https://doi.org/10.3389/fimmu.2019.00528.

Schatzman, U. (1998). Suspension (slinging) of horses: history, technique and indications. *Equine Veterinary Education* 10(4):219–223. https://doi.org/10.1111/j.2042-3292.1998.tb00880.x.

Schwabe, C. W. (1984). *Veterinary Medicine and Human Health* (3rd ed). Williams & Wilkins.

Shaffer, B. S. & Baker, B. W. (1997). Historic and prehistoric animal pathologies from North America. *Anthropozoologica* 25/26:255–261. https://sciencepress.mnhn.fr/sites/default/files/articles/pdf/az1998n25-26a31.pdf.

Shanks, M. & Tilley, C. (1987). *Social Theory and Archaeology*. University of New Mexico Press.

Shipman, P. (1981). *Life History of a Fossil: An Introduction to Taphonomy and Paleoecology*. Harvard University Press.

Shufeldt, R. W. (1893). Notes on paleopathology. *Popular Science Monthly* 42:679–684.

Siegel, J. (1976). Animal palaeopathology: possibilities and problems. *Journal of Archaeological Science* 3:349–384. DOI: 10.1016/0305-4403(76)90070-4.

Smith, N., Hewinson, R., Kremer, K., Brosch, R. & Gordon, S. V. (2009). Myths and misconceptions: the origin and evolution of *Mycobacterium tuberculosis*. *Nature Reviews Microbiology* 7:537–544. https://doi.org/10.1038/nrmicro2165.

Steenstrup, J. C. H. R. (1870). Vidnesbyrd om samtigheden mellem Kæmpe-Oxen (*Bos primigenius* Boj.) og landets ældre Fyrreskove og om Flintskjaerver invoxne i Dyreknogler, som Minder om Stenalderna Forfølgerser af de vilde Dyr [Evidence of the contemporaneity between the giant ox (*Bos primigenius* Boj.) and the country's ancient pine forests and of flint shards embedded in animal bones, reminiscent of the Stone Age pursuers of the wild animals]. *Oversigt over det Kongelige Danske videnskabernes selskabs forhandlinger og dets Medlemmers Arbejder i Aaret* 1870:105–114.

Steenstrup, J. C. H. R. (1880). Nogle i året 1879 til Universitetsmuseet indkomm bidrag til landets forhistoriske fauna [Some contribution to the country's prehistoric fauna brought to the University Museum during the year 1879]. Foredragsreferat. *Oversikt over det Kongelige Danske videnskabernes selskabs forhandlinger og dets Medlemmers Arbejder i Aaret* 1880:132–146.

Tasnádi Kubacska, A. (1960). *Az ősállatok pathológiája*. Medicina Könyvkiadó. German translation: *Paläopathologie. Pathologie der vorzeitlichen Tiere*. Veb Gustav Fischer Verlag, 1962.

Tāj'bakhsh, H. (2003). *History of Medicine and Veterinary Medicine in Iran*. Vol. 1. Lyon: Fondation Mérieux.

Tāj'bakhsh, H. (2016). Veterinary medicine in Iran. In Selin, H. (Ed.), *Encyclopaedia of the History of Science, Technology, and Medicine in Non-Western Cultures*, pp. 4346–4351. Springer. https://doi.org/10.1007/978-94-007-7747-7_8913.

Teichert, M. (1988). Gebissanomalien und pathologish-anatomische Veränderungen an Tierknochen aus der germanischen Siedlung bei Mühlberg, Kreis Gotha. *Archiv für Experimentelle Veterinärmedizin* 42:294–301.

Tejedor-Rodríguez, C., Moreno-García, M., Tornero, C., Hoffmann, A., García-Martínez de Lagrán, Í., ... & Rojo-Guerra, M. (2021). Investigating neolithic caprine husbandry in the Central Pyrenees: insights from a multiproxy study at Els Trocs cave (Bisaurri, Spain). *PLoS ONE* 16(1):e0244139. https://doi.org/10.1371/journal.pone.0244139.

Thomas, R. (2008). Diachronic trends in lower limb pathologies in later medieval and post-medieval cattle from Britain. In Grupe, G., McGlynn, G. & Peters, J. (Eds.), *Limping Together Through the Ages. Joint Afflictions and Bone Infections*, pp. 187–201. Verlag Marie Leidorf Gmbh.

Thomas, R. (2012). Nonhuman paleopathology. In Buikstra, J. E. & Roberts, C. A. (Eds.), *The Global History of Paleopathology. Pioneers and Prospects*, pp. 652–664. Oxford University Press.

Thomas, R. & Hammon, A. (1999). Veterinary palaeopathology working group. *Newsletter of the Osteoarchaeology Research Group* 20:2–3.

Ubelaker, D.H. (1982). The development of American paleopathology. In F. Spencer (Ed.), *A History of American Physical Anthropology 1930–1980*. Academic Press, 337–356.

Udrescu, M. & Van Neer, W. (2005). Looking for human therapeutic intervention in the healing of fractures of domestic animals. In Davies, J., Fabiš, M., Mainland, I., Richards, M. & R. Thomas (Eds.), *Diet and Health in Past Animal Populations. Current Research and Future Directions*. pp. 24–33. Oxbow.

Upex, B. & Dobney, K. (2012). More than just mad cows: exploring human-animal relationships through animal paleopathology. In Grauer, A. L. (Ed.), *A Companion to Paleopathology*, pp. 191–213. Wiley-Blackwell Publishing Ltd. DOI: 10.1002/9781444345940.ch11.

Van Neer, W. & Udrescu, M. (2015). Healed mid-shaft fracture of an early Roman bovine femur. *International Journal of Paleopathology* 8:24–28. DOI: 10.1016/j.ijpp.2014.09.003.

Van Wijngaarden-Bakker, L. & Krauwer, M. (1979). Animal palaeopathology: some examples from the Netherlands. *Helinium* XIX:37–53.

Vann, S. & Thomas, R. (2006). Humans, other animals and disease: a comparative approach towards the development of a standardised recording protocol for animal palaeopathology. *Internet Archaeology* 20. https://intarch.ac.uk/journal/issue20/5.

Vitt, V. O. [Витт, В. О.] (1952). Лошади Пазырыкских курганов. *Советская археология*, 16: 163–205.

Wäsle R. (1976). *Gebissanomalien und pathologisch-anatomische Veränderungen an Knochenfunden aus archäologischen Ausgrabungen*. Dissertation. Institut für Paläoanatomie, Domestikationsforschung und Geschichte der Tiermedizin der Universität München.

Wheeler, A. & Jones, A. K. G. (1989). *Fishes*. Cambridge Manuals in Archaeology. Cambridge University Press.

Xu, Z. (2021). Imperial horse policy and the publication of equine veterinary medicine books in Ming China: a case study on Yuanheng Liaomaji. In Bartosiewicz, L. & Choyke, A. M. (Eds.), *Medieval Animals on the Move. Between Body and Mind*, pp. 41–65. Palgrave–MacMillan.

Zalkin, V. I. [Цалкцн, В. И.] (1960). Изменчивость метаподий и ее значение для изучения крупного рогатого скота древности. *Бюллетенб Московского Общества Испытателеуй Природы, Отдел биологии отдебиый оттиск* LXV: 109–126.

Zeder, M. A. (2008). Domestication and early agriculture in the Mediterranean Basin: origins, diffusion, and impact. *Proceedings of the National Academy of Sciences* 105(33):11597–11604. https://doi.org/10.1073/pnas.0801317105.

Zellwecker, L. (1981). *Die Kapitel über Erkrankungen an den Extremitäten im Corpus Hippiatricorum Graecorum. Übersetzung und Besprechung*. Dissertation. Institut für Paläoanatomie, Domestikationsforschung und Geschichte der Tiermedizin der Universität München.

31
PLAGUES AND PANDEMICS

Sharon N. DeWitte, Ziyu R. Wang and Saige Kelmelis

Introduction

Several devastating disease epidemics and pandemics in recent years have captured the attention of people around the world, generated fear and anxiety, and directly affected the biological and mental health and livelihoods of many people. These include the Ebola epidemic of 2014–2016 and the ongoing (at the time of writing) Covid-19 pandemic. These recent examples are caused by novel pathogens, but epidemics and pandemics are not new phenomena. Infectious diseases have affected humans and been shaped by our behavior, demography, and social, political, and economic conditions for much of our recent history, and indeed have been major threats since the Neolithic Revolution established conditions that promoted their spread and maintenance.

Epidemiological Transitions and Emerging Diseases

Over the last ~10,000 years, there have been important, sweeping changes in "disease-scapes", the predominant diseases that cause mortality in human populations, as described by epidemiological transition theory (Omran, 1971; Gage, 2005; McKeown, 2009; Harper & Armelagos, 2010). This model, originally described by A.R. Omran (1971), provides a general framework for understanding transitioning mortality rates observed in high-income nations – primarily in the northern western hemisphere – from acute infectious diseases to mortality largely caused by chronic, non-infectious, degenerative diseases over time in three transitional stages associated with changes in subsistence strategies, settlement patterns, and demography (Harper & Armelagos, 2010).

Although the epidemiological transition model is often viewed as broadly applicable to studies of trends in mortality and morbidity, the universality of this model has been widely criticized (Santosa et al., 2014). Omran's proposed transitions are largely informed by historical events in the US and Western Europe, and, as such, may not reflect patterns in the vast majority of global populations (Mackenbach, 1994). One of the model's underlying assumptions is a step-wise structure and continuous progression, which has been strongly criticized based on examinations of geographic development of those later stages in light of emerging and re-emerging diseases and the effects of historical context on those transitions

(Frenk et al., 1991; Smallman-Raynor & Phillips, 1999). There are several other challenges to Omran's model, many of which point to its oversimplification of global and historical trends in mortality transitions, lack of consensus on the role of medicine and public health in prevention methods and interventions, disregard for the nuanced relationship between social inequalities and co-existing diseases (syndemics), and so on (Caldwell, 2001; Caselli, Meslé, & Vallin, 2002; Pearson, 2003; McKeown, 2009; Santosa et al., 2014). While there are several important conceptual drawbacks to the epidemiological transition model, it does provide a general framework for understanding the fundamental relationships between human behavior and biology and emerging and re-emerging pathogens.

The optimism of medical and public health experts in the mid-20th century that we would eventually conquer infectious diseases through the use of antibiotics and vaccines (see, e.g., Burnet, 1962) was undermined by increasing recognition by the 1990s of emerging infectious diseases and the re-emergence of those that had previously been on the decline (Morse, 1995). There are several factors that contribute to the emergence and re-emergence of diseases including those related to host behavior (i.e., urban-rural migration, the increasing scale and speed of long-distance mobility and trade, war and conflict, encroachment on previously uncultivated natural environments, and human-induced climate change), as well as the evolution of the pathogen in response to human action (i.e., antimicrobial-resistant (AMR) strains of diseases) (Weiss & McMichael, 2004). Some diseases have re-emerged as a result of the overuse or misuse of antibiotics or because of the syndemic effects of multiple conditions, such as co-infection with HIV and tuberculosis or syphilis.

Our futures will undoubtedly be marked by repeated disease outbreaks, caused both by currently existing and novel pathogens. Whether we will, on a global scale, improve strategies to prepare for and respond adequately to those threats remains to be seen. Regardless, one way to build capacities for disease preparedness is to better understand how disease pandemics have affected us in the past: how human biology, demography, social, economic, and environmental conditions affect the emergence and epidemiology of diseases; how those diseases affect our bodies, well-being, and populations; and what is at least theoretically possible for us to do in order to prevent deaths from infectious diseases in the future.

Syndemics

The concept of the syndemic, developed within medical anthropology but applied more broadly, is crucial for understanding and responding to epidemic disease. A syndemic refers to the interrelated complex of health and (importantly) social crises or "synergies of co-occurring epidemics" faced by vulnerable populations (Singer, 1994, 1996; Mendenhall & Singer, 2020). Key to this concept is that the interaction of two (or more) diseases/conditions occurring at the same time and place has health consequences greater than simply the sum of their individual effects. Infectious diseases, and the burdens they cause, are not solely responses to biological stimuli (Singer & Clair, 2003). Rather, the existence and persistence of infectious diseases in our populations and their effects are all deeply intertwined with human sociocultural systems. The disproportionate incidence and prevalence of diseases among certain populations are strongly influenced by social factors like poverty, stigma and ostracization, racism, sexism, and structural violence, and, ultimately, these directly contribute to the excess burden on these communities irrespective of the causative agent of the pathogen (Singer & Clair, 2003; Bentley, 2020). Therefore, it is imperative that researchers interested in epidemics examine pathogens within the complex "bio-social" contexts in which they occur (Singer & Claire, 2003).

Paleopathological Contributions to Understanding Epidemics and Pandemics

What can we uniquely learn from studying diseases in the (sometimes distant) past that is worth diverting time, energy, and resources away from efforts to understand and control diseases that affect people today? Public health and emerging disease experts are mainly devoted to understanding and mitigating current or impending global health crises, as well as developing and distributing effective medical treatments for those whose lives are at stake now. However, there are important questions about the interrelationships between humans and pathogens that require deeper understanding of the biocultural factors that have contributed to the emergence and re-emergence of diseases in the distant past, and can potentially inform us about future epidemics (DeWitte, 2016). Paleopathology and bioarchaeology provide perspectives on time periods for which there is neither surviving documentary nor oral history to provide insights on past epidemics. They also serve to humanize our reconstructions of the past and to populate them with those who are typically absent from documentary sources, i.e., individuals who were socially, politically, and economically marginalized or otherwise deemed to be inconsequential. Paleopathological and bioarchaeological data can also improve our understanding of syndemics in the past. Disease processes themselves can leave physical or molecular traces on and in our skeletons, and further, as posited by ecosocial theory (Krieger, 2005), skeletal data represent an embodiment of the social, economic, and other larger, structural contexts that affect our exposure to causative pathogens, the severity of our symptoms, and our risks of dying from those diseases. Lastly, paleopathological and paleogenomic evidence combined provide unparallel insights on the evolution and phylogeographies of pandemic pathogens.

Which Plagues and Pandemics are Visible Paleopathologically?

To date, most paleoepidemiological studies have leveraged diagnostic skeletal pathological lesions that resulted from chronic infections, such as tuberculosis, leprosy, and treponemal infections. It is also possible to identify the victims of epidemic disease outbreaks based on mortuary contexts, e.g., atypical burial patterns, or associated documentary evidence (DeWitte, 2016). For example, in addition to plague burials detailed below (see list of sites in Kacki, 2019), archaeological evidence indicates that a cemetery with inconsistent burial positions and mass burials from the Mixtec site of Teposcolula Yucundaa, Mexico is associated with a historically documented disease (*cocoliztli*) outbreak in 1544–1550 (Warinner et al., 2012), possibly caused by *Salmonella enterica* (Vågene et al., 2018). It is also possible to use medical records associated with documented skeletal collections to identify people who suffered from specific diseases, such as the 1918 influenza pandemic (Wissler, 2019). Further, ancient biomolecule analyses (e.g., of DNA or proteins) are increasingly yielding insights on the phylogeography and evolutionary history of several diseases (e.g., Blevins et al., 2020), though their destructive nature and expense currently precludes using them to screen for diseases not already suspected to be present based on other lines of evidence. Ultimately, given the low specificity and/or sensitivity of many skeletal pathologies and the fact that not all individuals who died during past epidemics have been or will be excavated or are otherwise unavailable for study (e.g., in deference to the wishes of descendant communities), most past epidemics are, and will likely remain, inaccessible to paleopathologists.

The Black Death and the Second Pandemic of Plague

One of the most devastating disease pandemics in human history, and the one that comes immediately to the minds of many people when they hear the word "plague", was the mid-14th-century pandemic of bubonic plague, now commonly referred to as the Black Death. Recent molecular evidence indicates that the pathogenic strain that caused the Black Death emerged in Central or East Asia (Spyrou et al., 2019) perhaps in the 12th or 13th century (Spyrou et al., 2018; Green, 2020) and spread from there across Afro-Eurasia. Currently, the bulk of historical evidence regarding the spread and effects of the Black Death comes from European sources (though the Eurocentric nature of historic plague scholarship is changing), from which scholars have estimated that the pandemic killed between 30% and 60% of affected populations between 1346 and 1353 (Green, 2014). Following the Black Death, there were repeated outbreaks of plague in Afro-Eurasia for centuries during what is now called the Second Pandemic of Plague (the First Pandemic of Plague began in the 6th century CE and lasted for about 200 years, and the Third Pandemic of Plague began in the 19th century and ended by the mid-20th century (Ziegler, 2014)).

Molecular evidence has confirmed that the Second Pandemic was caused by *Yersinia pestis*, the bubonic plague bacterium that continues to cause plague around the world today (Schuenemann et al., 2011; Bos et al., 2016, 2011). Between 2010 and 2015, there were over 3000 reported cases of plague worldwide and nearly 600 deaths from the disease (WHO, 2017). Modern cases of plague are commonly reported in the media, often in a sensationalized manner with speculations about whether the Black Deaths is "back" (Mathers, 2020), reflecting general ignorance of the fact that the disease is continuously maintained in wild animal populations.

Plague is a zoonotic infection and is most often transmitted to humans from animals (typically wild rodents) via the bite of an ectoparasite (e.g., a flea or louse) feeding on the original animal host, though *Y. pestis* can also be transmitted from animals via the consumption of contaminated meat (Perry & Fetherston, 1997; Ziegler, 2014). Infection with *Y. pestis* can produce several different clinical forms of disease that vary in their symptoms and case-fatality rates: bubonic, septicemic, pneumonic, gastrointestinal, and pharyngeal plague. Contemporary reports during the Black Death note symptoms consistent with both bubonic and pneumonic plague (e.g., respiratory distress, coughing up of blood or sputum, rapid progression to death) (Horrox, 2004), though it has not yet been established which clinical form predominated during the Second Pandemic. Much of the literature reproduces the unexamined assumption that rats and fleas were the primary or sole culprits during the Black Death; however, many animals are natural reservoirs of plague and many ectoparasites can transmit the disease to humans, including the human louse (Houhamdi et al., 2006), and there is, as of yet, no conclusive evidence regarding the animal reservoir(s) and insect vector(s) that were involved in the Second Pandemic.

No form of plague has been reported to affect the skeleton, and thus plague does not leave diagnostic skeletal lesions that can be identified in the archaeological record. However, pathological conditions of varying etiologies have been examined in documented historical plague burials, not to identify victims of the disease, but rather to assess the characteristics of those who succumbed to it. Specifically, several studies have tested the assumption that past plague epidemics killed indiscriminately with respect to health or frailty (and by extension that associated burials will more closely reflect health conditions in the living populations than is true of attritional assemblages). To date, these studies have yielded contradictory findings. Waldron (2001) found similar frequencies of degenerative conditions, dental disease, trauma, and skeletal evidence of infections between the East Smithfield Black Death cemetery and a post-epidemic cemetery from London, contrary to what would be expected if the epidemic killed indiscriminately and thus produced a skeletal sample with a relatively low proportion of skeletal pathologies. Using a hazards-model based approach (see Chapter 4, this volume for more information on mathematical modeling) to address heterogeneous frailty and selective mortality, DeWitte and colleagues examined patterns of skeletal stress markers (linear enamel hypoplasia – LEH, dental calculus, short adult stature, cribra orbitalia, and periosteal new bone formation) in East Smithfield in comparison to attritional assemblages. Their results showed that the risk of death during the Black Death was higher for people with these skeletal indicators of stress (all of which were found to be associated with elevated risks of death under ordinary circumstances and thus reflective of underlying frailty) compared to peers without them (DeWitte & Wood, 2008; DeWitte, 2010; DeWitte & Hughes-Morey, 2012; Yaussy & DeWitte, 2019), suggesting that the Black Death was selective with respect to frailty. DeWitte and Kowaleski (2017) produced similar findings applying this same approach to burials from the Cistercian Abbey of St. Mary Graces London that are associated with an outbreak subsequent to the Black Death (possibly the *pestis secunda* of 1361). Godde et al. (2020) also examined selectivity in the East Smithfield Black Death cemetery using survival and hazards analysis and found that cribra orbitalia, short femora, and LEH were associated with elevated risks of death during the Black Death, providing further evidence of the selective nature of Black Death mortality.

In contrast, Kacki (2017) found that frequencies of LEH, cribra orbitalia, endocranial lesions, and periosteal reactions were lower in plague burials compared to non-plague burials from France (*c.* 14th–16th centuries). These results might indicate better health among plague victims (prior to death during the epidemic) compared to people who died under normal conditions of mortality, and thus that plague in these outbreaks was not selective with respect to pre-existing health. It should be noted that there was variation in methodological and analytical approaches among these studies. In contrast to the frequentist approach used by Kacki, DeWitte and colleagues and Godde and colleagues use hazards analysis and age-structured data (and both groups used Bayesian approaches to age estimation, which are designed to address the limitation of age mimicry inherent to the more conventional methods). The differences in approaches among these studies raise the question of whether the inconsistencies in their findings are an artifact of those approaches or reflect true differences in plague mortality patterns by location or time period.

Burials associated with the Second Pandemic have also been the focus of ancient DNA and immunoassay studies, initially aimed at verifying the cause of the Black Death and other outbreaks (Raoult et al., 2000; Haensch et al., 2010; Kacki et al., 2011), but more recently examining genomic variation with a goal of assessing the phylogeography and evolution of *Y. pestis* (Bos et al., 2016, 2011; Spyrou et al., 2019). Microbial detection array analysis of a tooth from East Smithfield, London (Devault et al., 2014) revealed evidence of dozens of pathogenic, environmental, and microbiomic taxa, demonstrating the feasibility of this approach for addressing questions of broader anthropological and evolutionary consequence, e.g., the hypothesis that co-infection with multiple pathogens, and resulting within-host competition (i.e., a syndemic), contributed to high levels of mortality during the Black Death.

Tuberculosis

Tuberculosis, an ancient mycobacterial disease (see Chapter 17, this volume), is considered a global epidemic by the World Health Organization (WHO). In 2019, tuberculosis was attributed to an estimated 1.4 million deaths (including 208,000 who were co-infected with

HIV) and infected another 10 million (WHO, 2020). This is in grim contrast to the optimism expressed by Smith and others nearly 30 years ago that tuberculosis had been vanquished in the industrialized world (Smith, 1988), based on decreases in incidence rates since the turn of the 19th century and the discovery of streptomycin in 1944 by Albert Schatz and Selman Waksman (Sherman, 2017). Yet, in the 1980s, the US reported the re-emergence of tuberculosis (Singer, 1994; CDC, 2012; Poteat et al., 2016), which occurred because of syndemic interactions with the HIV epidemic, rising poverty, and immigration; insufficient control measures; and improper use and application of therapeutic treatments for individuals with co-morbidities, thus contributing to the growing threat of multi-drug-resistant and extreme multi-drug-resistant forms (MDR and XMDR) (Wood et al., 2007; Harries et al., 2010; Khan et al., 2010; Swaminathan et al., 2010; Kwan & Ernst, 2011; Zumla et al., 2012; Poteat et al., 2016; Hargreaves et al., 2020). The modern associations among tuberculosis, poverty, and individuals who suffer from HIV/TB co-infection are unfortunately stigmatized, which promotes additional health problems, mortality risk, and contributes to the re-emergence of the disease.

In humans, tuberculosis is the result of infection by members of the *Mycobacterium tuberculosis* complex (MTBC) (Roberts & Buikstra, 2003; Taylor et al., 2005), which are transmitted through airborne infected droplets (i.e., coughing, sneezing, speaking, singing, spitting) into the lungs (respiratory route), or through the gastrointestinal route via consumption of infected foods (i.e., milk or dairy products). A primary infection of the lungs can further disseminate into other adjacent tissues, including the associated skeletal elements (i.e., ribs, vertebrae, and joint surfaces) where it can produce distinctive bony lesions (Ortner, 2003; Roberts & Buikstra, 2003; Wiley & Allen, 2019). There is a rich literature on paleopathological criteria for identification and diagnosis of tuberculosis in archaeological remains and paleoepidemiological reconstruction from cemetery samples (Ortner, 2003; Roberts & Buikstra, 2003; Stone et al., 2009; Dangvard Pedersen et al., 2019a, 2019b; Kelmelis & Dangvard Pedersen, 2019). Modern tuberculosis and its skeletal effects have been well explored, and it is assumed that lesions produced by ancient TB are unlikely to be significantly different from those in clinical case studies (Kelley & El-Najjar, 1980; Kelley & Micozzi, 1984; Santos & Roberts, 2006 Redman et al., 2009; Dangvard Pedersen et al., 2019b). It is not yet known whether paleopathological indicators differ across MTBC species. Further, tuberculosis tends to have low skeletal involvement possibly as a result of competing co-morbidities (i.e., only severely affected individuals who survive long enough to develop lesions will be counted) and resulting lesions may appear similar to those caused by other maladies, including other mycobacteria (Roberts & Buikstra, 2003; Stone et al., 2009). New paleoepidemiological methods using sensitivity and specificity measures estimated from modern, diagnosed TB cases have promising potential to provide more accurate estimates of tuberculosis in cemetery samples without necessarily over or undercounting cases based on incomplete data (Milner & Boldsen, 2017; Dangvard Pedersen et al., 2019a, 2019b; Kelmelis & Dangvard Pedersen, 2019).

Bioarchaeological research on tuberculosis is invaluable for reconstructing the co-evolutionary history of humans and tuberculosis and clarifying the socio-ecological factors influencing disease dynamics prior to contemporary medical treatment. Such work has illustrated the importance of living conditions, diet, population growth, and urban intensification in the skeletal prevalence of tuberculosis in Afro-Eurasia and the Americas (see Roberts & Buikstra, 2003 and references therein). For instance, Stone and colleagues (2009) describe several early examples of tuberculosis in Afro-Eurasia, but note that there was not a significant number of populations in much of Europe with definitive evidence of tuberculosis until the medieval period; similarly, higher prevalence of tuberculosis in the Americas is associated with population growth and poor living conditions (they do, however, note that the absence of these data in other regions may be an artifact of sampling bias). These conditions, which are ultimately created by human action, permit the persistence of tuberculosis in human populations and contribute to the re-emergence and worsening of the current tuberculosis epidemic.

Considerable progress has been made in biomolecular research in conjunction with paleopathology in assessing the antiquity, lesion-formation processes, and evolutionary history of human mycobacteria (Mays et al., 2001; Mays et al., 2002; Mays & Taylor, 2003; Roberts & Buikstra, 2003; Stone et al., 2009; Stone, 2017). Current genomic data indicate that ancient lineages of MTBC originated in Africa approximately 70,000 years ago and dispersed globally with migrations of anatomically modern humans (Gutierrez et al., 2005; Hershberg et al., 2008; Comas et al., 2013). Researchers have suggested that repeated waves of migration into Europe and Asia promoted the spread and diversification of the bacteria that had, until the advent of agriculture and increased population sizes and density, been sustained in mobile hunter-gathering groups via its long latency period (Comas et al., 2013; Harper & Armelagos, 2013). To date, the earliest known case of TB was recorded from an Iron Age male (c. 2200 BP) whose remains showed signs of Pott's disease (skeletal lesions and vertebral collapse resulting from severe pulmonary infection) and was positively identified with molecular evidence of *M. tuberculosis* (Taylor et al., 2005).

Paleopathological study of tuberculosis provides a unique opportunity to examine host-pathogen co-evolution while providing valuable context for disease susceptibility within and between populations. A collection of studies on the influence of medieval urbanization on tuberculosis and leprosy prevalence in Denmark have revealed that, in addition to host factors like age, sex, and dwelling environment, disease prevalence may have been strongly affected by human economic behaviors and disease-stigma (Kelmelis & Dangvard Pedersen, 2019a; Kelmelis et al., 2020). Using paleoepidemiological methods developed by Dangvard Pedersen and colleagues (2019b), maximum likelihood estimates showed that tuberculosis was far more prevalent among medieval populations – regardless of whether they were urban or rural residents – compared to leprosy, which may have been strongly selected against as individuals with visible signs of sickness were secluded in leprosaria. Interestingly, these studies indicated that rural populations, on average, scored higher for tuberculosis, which could indicate a number of things. First, it could indicate that rural populations became more exposed to pathogens by increased contact with urban populations through widening economic markets. Conversely, urban populations may have also been significantly affected by the disease but either (a) died of other complications before lesions could manifest (thereby, more significantly affecting immune compromised people), and/or (b) urban survivors were more immunologically robust. Regardless, these findings indicate that the rise in tuberculosis was correlated with increased urban poverty, contact with domestic animals, diet change, and migration.

These observations coincide with the historical literature from England and other regions, where tuberculosis is believed to have risen in prevalence steadily until the Industrial period when it reached epidemic heights. As part of a larger disease ecology, tuberculosis likely would have competed with other pathogens. In fact, archaeological evidence from the Roman period to the 13th century shows that some individuals infected with leprosy (*Mycobacterium leprae*) also carried *M. tuberculosis*, linking the eventual decline of leprosy to the prevalence and co-infection of tuberculosis (Donoghue et al., 2005). Nevertheless, by the 19th century, tuberculosis became a leading cause of death in industrialized nations, facilitated by rapid population growth and migration to urban centers where, in addition to opportunities, rural-migrants, immigrants, and minorities were subjected to congested, unsanitary living and working conditions.

Tuberculosis is once again a leading cause of death globally. Given the relative ease of global travel and that over 50% of the world population lives in cities, we have created conditions in which tuberculosis can infect and, worse, co-infect communities that are more likely to have compromised immune systems – the poor, disenfranchised, and minority groups. The dangers of TB co-infection cannot be understated. The clinical failure to identify the underlying risks of latent and active TB co-infection has dire consequences for patients who are already suffering from socially stigmatizing and physically debilitating diseases (Sendrasoa et al., 2015; Mangum et al., 2018). In 2018, the United Nations along with the WHO and the Russian Federation developed global strategies to end the tuberculosis epidemic. The goals of the WHO are to end the TB epidemic by 2030 – a mere ten years from the writing of this document (WHO, 2020). Despite the policies, guidelines, and plans in place by global and national health agencies, the rise in HIV-associated tuberculosis has yet to be quelled, and the effects of this epidemic are most harshly felt in sub-Saharan Africa, where early diagnosis and treatment of TB/HIV is sorely needed (Harries et al., 2010). It is perhaps useful to know that paleopathology can continue to contribute to our longitudinal understanding of tuberculosis as it will most assuredly continue to affect people.

Syphilis

Syphilis is a highly infectious disease caused by *Treponema pallidum* subsp. *pallidum* (TPA). It is usually acquired through sexual contact or congenitally from infected mother to offspring. Syphilis has become endemic in many low-income counties with antibiotic treatments. Recently, in concurrence with emergence of a macrolide-resistant TPA cluster, incidences of syphilis have resurged in several high-income counties in North America, Western Europe, and Australia (Beale et al., 2019). The disease disproportionately impacts many already vulnerable populations, particularly in high-risk groups, such as men who have sex with men (MSM). Now, syphilis poses a global health threat with 6 million new cases reported each year (Kojima & Klausner, 2018).

The origin and subsequent spread of syphilis epidemics is an enigma. Because its transmission is linked with direct sexual contacts, syphilis has been closely intertwined with negative social and moral attitudes toward infected individuals for their perceived promiscuity. Over the past centuries, discussions of its evolutionary history have been structured on several assumptions. First, researchers generally believed that the "first" syphilis epidemic occurred in Europe in 1495 during a time of many socially transformative events, particularly with the beginning of frequent global interconnections through advances in maritime technology. Thus, views on the origin of syphilis (see Chapter 16, this volume) are generally divided by a temporal point with Columbus' transatlantic travel: the Columbian hypothesis and the pre-Columbian hypothesis (includes Hudson's "unified" hypothesis proposed in 1964). Second, our understanding of syphilis is largely framed within the four-disease model of treponematoses: syphilis, yaws (*T. pallidum* subsp. *pertenue*; TPE), endemic syphilis (also known as bejel; *T. pallidum* subsp. *endemicum*; TEN), and pinta (*Treponema carateum*, which has an unknown phylogenetic placement and thus is not a focus here). All treponematoses are multi-staged infections. Lastly, researchers have exclusively associated syphilis with the most virulent *T. pallidum* variant that can cross the blood-brain barrier and cause severe damage to vital organs, invade the cardiovascular system and the central nervous system (CNS), and transmit through vertical transmission (Turner & Hollander, 1957).

These assumptions, however, have been criticized for lacking scientific basis. Conventionally, scholars suggest reports of the 1495 syphilis epidemic unequivocally documented a disease that was distinct and easily recognizable. Yet, close examination of historical documents and scientific knowledge of syphilis suggest otherwise (Tampa et al., 2014). A malady, called the "great pox" (*grande verole*), was reportedly widely spread among the mercenary army assembled by Charles VIII of France. Descriptions of this disease shared many similarities with modern clinical signs of syphilis, as well as other skin diseases that were present during this time (Peterman, 2009). Given the virulence and un-treatability of this highly visible and detrimental disease, people associated the "great pox" with divine punishment for immoral behavior and conveniently blamed the plague on those viewed as morally and politically inferior (i.e., "the French disease" by the Italians, the "Jew disease" by the Christian church, the "Turkish disease" by the Persians) (Hayton, 2005). It was only during the early 19th century that "syphilis" was adapted from a poetic source broadly connecting with venereal diseases (as derived from the goddess of Venus) (Krumbhaar, 1927).

Meanwhile, early western physicians documented diseases, known by many local names, with signs and symptoms that closely resemble those of "syphilis" across colonized regions around the world (Hudson, 1946). Conversely to acquired syphilis, these diseases were often documented in children and, thus, were purposely disassociated from sexual sin (Mitjà et al., 2013). This practice continued even after identifying the spirochaete bacterium, *T. pallidum*, as the causative agent of syphilis and other treponematoses in 1905 (Castellani, 1905). In efforts to consolidate the "array of thousand" local names, the WHO and United Nations Children's Fund (UNICEF) proposed the existing four-disease model of human treponematoses in the 1950s (Hackett, 1955, 1963). Without a way to accurately differentiate the causative agents of each treponematosis, the WHO's handbook specified that the organism that caused syphilis was "identical in almost all respects" to other agents of endemic form. Recommendations for distinction were solely based on careful assessments of narrow differences in symptoms, epidemiological characteristics, ecological boundaries, and the transmission routes thought to be disease-specific by general consensus, despite overlapping disease signs (Turner & Hollander, 1957; Giacani & Lukehart, 2014).

Advancements in molecular technology have offered new tools to study treponematoses. Our ability to generate genomic data provides evidence relevant to challenging many long-held beliefs regarding the pathogen's basic biology and evolutionary relationships. Early molecular studies of limited *T. pallidum* strains revealed closely related genetic relations among TPA, TPE, and TEN (< 0.2% genomic differences) but with several genetically distinct regions (e.g., *arp* and several genes in the *tpr* family) for subspecies-level differentiations supporting the four-model view (Centurion-Lara et al., 1998, 2006, 2013; Harper et al., 2008). Follow-up studies, however, have shown inconsistencies. For example, genetic signatures of TPA are found in other subspecies (Centurion-Lara et al., 2013). With expanded sampling and genome-wide data, researchers additionally found a high degree of intra-subspecies genetic heterogeneity within each lineage than initially believed and between subspecies (Pinto et al., 2016; Beale et al., 2019). Further, molecular clock estimation of 39 modern *T. pallidum* genomes using Bayesian statistical procedures calculated the emergence of the modern TPA cluster to be between the 17th and 18th centuries (Arora et al., 2016), thereby raising questions about whether the 1495 syphilis epidemic in Europe was truly caused by the TPA subspecies alone.

By accurately and confidently identifying the responsible agent in clinically diagnosed cases, molecular tools offer a means to generate data to reexamine many long-held dogmas. Clinicians have long been puzzled regarding whether the four-disease model of treponematoses correlates with the pathogen's true biological and genetic variants (e.g., Grin, 1952). Patient reports further raise questions about the common divide between the sexual versus non-sexual mode of transmission in treponematoses. For example, non-sexual transmission of syphilis can occur through exposure to body fluids from contagious patients (i.e., dentists and wet nurses) (Lydston, 1886). Further, increased rate of miscarriages seen in women with bejel, together with neurological and cardiovascular complications documented in yaws patients, suggest TPE and TEN subspecies may not truly lack the ability to cross the blood and brain barrier (Wilson & Mathis, 1930; Grin, 1952; Edington, 1954; Román & Román, 1986; Tabbara et al., 1989). Recent genetic studies confirmed genetically characterized TPE and TEN from patients' samples taken from genital primary lesions (Grange et al., 2013; Mikalová et al., 2017). These studies imply possible cases of sexual transmission of yaws and bejel. Additionally, animal model studies demonstrate that not all TPA strains are capable of crossing placental barriers as was expected from typical syphilis manifestations (Wicher et al., 2000). Collectively, there is growing evidence that challenges the established view of the diagnostic condition of each disease form, as each pathogen variant is biologically capable of crossing the transmission and epidemiological boundaries rigidly defined in the four-disease model. This legacy classification system may merely reflect the discomfort over sexuality imposed by the Christian church and implicitly promotes an Eurocentric colonial view of human sociocultural conditions and moral values (Engelstein, 1986). This raises the question of the relevance of using the current four-disease model and its associated diagnostic criteria when interpreting treponematoses in antiquity.

Paleopathological analyses have emphasized methods to distinguish syphilis from other treponematoses in skeletal records. Inferring the presence of treponematoses, not a specific infection form, is possible with large mortuary assemblages that permit systematic scoring and analysis of lesion types and their distribution throughout the skeleton. Nevertheless, skeletal evidence lacks the precision (sensitivity and specificity) needed to confidently link archeological cases with the etiological agents to evaluate the evolutionary dynamics of *T. pallidum*. Yet, in paleopathological studies, the etiological pathogen variants are assumed from clinical assigned disease forms and used interchangeably in discussions regarding the evolutionary dynamics of *T. pallidum* pathogen. This interferes with studying *T. pallidum's* evolutionary history and necessitates that researchers first gain comprehensive knowledge of the social and medical history of all human treponematosis, not just of syphilis. Only then can we critically examine evidence, free of bias, of the underlying causes for the emergence and spread of syphilis.

Given the lack of known sensitivity and specificity of treponemal lesions in bone, researchers have turned to paleogenomics studies of targeted-capture of *T. pallidum* genomes in human remains. Currently, four paleogenomic studies reported successful reconstructions of nine near-complete ancient *T. pallidum* draft genomes from skeletons dated to the late 15th to mid-19th centuries (Schuenemann et al. 2018; Barquera et al., 2020; Giffin et al., 2020; Majander et al., 2020). Although with small sample sizes and challenges of ancient DNA studies, these studies have been promising in providing novel insights and highlight the limitations of relying on skeletal lesions alone to identify specific forms of treponemal infection in archaeological collections. For example, Schuenemann and colleges identified a TPE genome, instead of a TPA, from an infant from colonial Mexico City (A.D. 1681–1861). This evidence pointed to a possible congenital transmission of a variant in the TPE linage. Genomes of the TPE linage were identified in several adult individuals (>25 years old) in Mexico and in Europe, who would otherwise have been diagnosed with syphilis using a classic paleopathology approach. The recovered pathogen genomes revealed a wide range of genetic diversity in the treponemes that likely circulated in Europe between AD 1464 and 1727 than found contemporaneously in Mexico. Existing studies have assumed that either a sexually transmitted or non-sexually transmitted form of treponemal infection existed in a past community, but the possibility of multiple disease forms or pathogen subspecies co-existing in the same community was rarely considered. The new paleogenomic evidence calls for critical evaluation of our currently established perception on treponemal infections in antiquity. This presents a research opportunity to develop theoretical framework and methodological approaches that consider the variability of pathogens, their syndemic impacts in past communities, and changing prevalence of a pathogen variant/linage through time. By combining evidence from genetic, skeletal, and modern disease clinical data, it is important to advance disease identification and studies of past epidemics from a focus on the individual to the population level in mortuary assemblages and evaluate effects of disease on demographic patterns.

Finally, our current ability to confidently draw inferences is still limited by few available genomes and with a restrictive set of single-nucleotide polymorphisms (SNPs). Nevertheless, there is a clear branching pattern indicating the divergence between TPA and non-TPA (TPE and TEN) clades likely occurred deeper in time than previously thought (Schuenemann et al., 2018; Barquera et al., 2020; Giffin et al., 2020; Majander et al., 2020). This branching pattern may signal independent evolutionary trajectories for the TPA and the non-TPA lineages through adaptation to different environmental niches in different geographic regions. Yet, if both TPA and TPE lineages have had a long history of co-existing in the same populations in both AfroEurasia and, possibly, the lands now referred to as the Americas, it is unclear what selective factors caused this branching pattern. For now, the divergent hypotheses favor pre-existing TPA lineage in Europe before Columbus' travels (Majander et al, 2020) while others support a radiation of the TPE lineage linked with Western African slave trade (Majander et al. 2020; Giffin et al., 2020; Barquera et al. 2020). Regardless, a recent global spreading event at the end of the 15th century would fall short of explaining the large number of North American skeletal evidence with lesions consistent with treponemal infection well before European colonization (Baker et al, 2020). As it stands, the origin and spread of syphilis (treponematoses) epidemics are still highly debated. While the ancient *T. pallidum* genome evidence has proven to provide important value, they still lack considerable temporal and geographic representations from archaeological contexts around the world. More importantly, the interpretation of genomic evidence needs to be contextualized with other lines of evidence, such as historical records and bioarchaeological evaluation of skeletal remains in order to construct a complete picture of the pathogen's evolutionary history.

Relevance of Pandemic Paleopathology to Current Concerns

We have outlined in this chapter some of the cautionary tales provided by historical emerging disease epidemics and the application of paleopathology to understanding the origins, spread, and lasting impacts of past diseases on once-living populations. Many of these diseases continue to affect contemporary populations and are, to the surprise of many, not long-gone plagues of antiquity. These old foes are, unfortunately, not without their new tricks as it has become apparent that many are re-emerging despite medical advancements in vaccination and treatment. Yet, they are not the only challenge that we will continue to face, as the past 100 years have observed a number of new emerging diseases, including HIV, Ebola, Zika, SARS, MERS, and, now, Covid-19. These pathogens, like those that are re-emerging, have the ability to become major global health threats because their spread, prevalence, and divergence is facilitated by modern means of transportation, population growth and density, as well as other human behaviors like the anti-vaccination movement.

We arrive again at the question of why should the study of past epidemics matter? It is perhaps obvious, given our own research foci, that we are convinced of the utility and relevance of bioarchaeological perspectives on disease. However, like other bioarchaeologists, our interests are not driven solely by curiosity about life in the past; rather, we are also motivated to do work that can benefit living people. Crucially, we can draw parallels with conditions that still exist today and that we can (at least theoretically) address in order to lessen the negative impacts of disease on people in the future. A case can be made that studies on previous pandemics have the potential to provide important lessons about systems resilience, planning and prevention, and best practices in the wake of an emerging or re-emerging disease.

We also want to promote another potential benefit of paleopathological studies of past epidemics and pandemics: teaching. Researchers have the luxury of writing scholarship that is often primarily aimed at an audience who is already, in some capacity, familiar with the literature and the underlying premises of how epidemics happen and who thus need little convincing of the relevance of bioarchaeological research. However, many of the authors in this volume – as well as those who will inevitably read it – are educators, and we engage with other audiences, be they students, community members, or family and friends, about the importance of understanding epidemics. This is an invaluable skill, and we have seen first-hand the impact this information can have on people, many of whom are not anthropologists, but some of whom might have the power to enact change using this knowledge. The authors of this chapter have taught courses and given talks on ancient diseases and epidemics, and we are constantly amazed by the feedback from our students and the public – ranging from overwhelmingly positive to shock and appall. Many have told us they feel enlightened by what they learned and feel strongly that if this information was more readily accessible to others that we might be more adequately prepared to deal with pandemics. Ultimately, what the public can take from classes and talks that focus on disease in the past is an arsenal of information that they will apply to their lives and, hopefully, convey to others who might not readily engage with the literature discussed here.

References

Arora, N., Schuenemann, V. J., Jäger, G., Peltzer, A., Seitz, A., Herbig, A. … & Bagheri, H. C. (2016). Origin of modern syphilis and emergence of a pandemic Treponema pallidum cluster. *Nature Microbiology* 2:16245. https://doi.org/10.1038/nmicrobiol.2016.245

Barquera, R., Lamnidis, T. C., Lankapalli, A. K., Kocher, A., Hernández-Zaragoza, D. I., Nelson, E. A., … & Krause, J. (2020). Origin and health status of first-generation Africans from early colonial Mexico. *Current Biology* 30(11): P2078–2091.E11 https://doi.org/10.1016/j.cub.2020.04.002

Beale, M. A., Marks, M., Sahi, S. K., Tantalo, L. C., Nori, A. V., French, P., … & Thomson, N. R. (2019). Genomic epidemiology of syphilis reveals independent emergence of macrolide resistance across multiple circulating lineages. *Nature Communications* 10(1):1–9.

Bentley, G. R. (2020). Don't blame the BAME: ethnic and structural inequalities in susceptibilities to COVID -19. *American Journal of Human Biology* 32(5):e23478. https://doi.org/10.1002/ajhb.23478

Blevins, K. E., Crane, A. E., Lum, C., Furuta, K., Fox, K. & Stone, A. C. (2020). Evolutionary history of *Mycobacterium leprae* in the Pacific Islands. *Philosophical Transactions of the Royal Society B: Biological Sciences* 375(1812):20190582. https://doi.org/10.1098/rstb.2019.0582

Bos, Herbig, A., Sahl, J., Waglechner, N., Fourment, M., Forrest, S. A., … & Poinar, H. N. (2016). Eighteenth century *Yersinia pestis* genomes reveal the long-term persistence of an historical plague focus. *ELife* 5:e12994. https://doi.org/10.7554/eLife.12994

Bos, K., Schuenemann, V., Golding, G., Burbano, H., Waglechner, N., Coombes, B., … Krause, J. (2011). A draft genome of *Yersinia pestis* from victims of the Black Death. *Nature* 478:506–510.

Burnet, M. (1962). *Natural History of Infectious Disease* (3rd edition). Cambridge: Cambridge University Press.

Caldwell, J. C. (2001). Population health in transition. *Bulletin of the World Health Organization* 79(2):159–160.

Caselli, G., Meslé, F. & Vallin, J. (2002). Epidemiologic transition theory exceptions. *Genus*, 9–51. https://www.demogr.mpg.de/Papers/workshops/020619_paper40.pdf

Castellani, A. (1905). Further observations of parangi (yaws). *British Medical Journal* 2(2342):1330–1331. https://doi.org/10.1136/bmj.2.2342.1330-a

CDC, (2012). CDC Grand Rounds: the TB/HIV Syndemic. Last accessed January 3, 2021 at: https://www.cdc.gov/mmwr/preview/mmwrhtml/mm6126a3.htm

Centurion-Lara, A., Castro, C., Castillo, R., Shaffer, J. M., Van Voorhis, W. C. & Lukehart, S. A. (1998). The flanking region sequences of the 15-kDa lipoprotein gene differentiate pathogenic treponemes. *Journal of Infectious Diseases* 177(4):1036–1040.

Centurion-Lara, A., Molini, B. J., Godornes, C., Sun, E., Hevner, K., Van Voorhis, W. C. & Lukehart, S. A. (2006). Molecular differentiation of *Treponema pallidum* subspecies. *Journal of Clinical Microbiology* 44(9):3377–3380. https://doi.org/10.1128/JCM.00784-06

Centurion-Lara, A., Giacani, L., Godornes, C., Molini, B. J., Brinck Reid, T. & Lukehart, S. A. (2013). Fine analysis of genetic diversity of the *tpr* gene family among treponemal species, subspecies and strains. *PLoS Neglected Tropical Diseases* 7(5):e2222.

Comas, I., Coscolla, M., Luo, T., Borrell, S., Holt, K. E., Kato-Maeda, M., ... & Gagneux, S. (2013). Out-of-Africa migration and Neolithic co-expansion of mycobacterium tuberculosis with modern humans. *Nature Genetics* 45(10):1176–1182. https://doi.org/10.1038/ng.2744

Dangvard Pedersen, D., Milner, G. R., Kolmos, H. J. & Boldsen, J. L. (2019a). Tuberculosis in medieval and early modern Denmark: a paleoepidemiological perspective. *International Journal of Paleopathology* 27:101–108. https://doi.org/10.1016/j.ijpp.2018.11.003

Dangvard Pedersen, D., Milner, G. R., Kolmos, H. J. & Boldsen, J. L. (2019b). The association between skeletal lesions and tuberculosis diagnosis using a probabilistic approach. *International Journal of Paleopathology* 27:88–100. https://doi.org/10.1016/j.ijpp.2019.01.001

Devault, A. M., McLoughlin, K., Jaing, C., Gardner, S., Porter, T. M., Enk, J. M., ... & Poinar, H. N. (2014). Ancient pathogen DNA in archaeological samples detected with a microbial detection array. *Scientific Reports* 4:4245. https://doi.org/10.1038/srep04245

DeWitte, S. N. (2010). Age patterns of mortality during the black death in London, A.D. 1349–1350. *Journal of Archaeological Science* 37(12):3394–3400. https://doi.org/10.1016/j.jas.2010.08.006

DeWitte, S. N. (2016). Archaeological evidence of epidemics can inform future epidemics. *Annual Review of Anthropology* 45(1):63–77. https://doi.org/10.1146/annurev-anthro-102215-095929

DeWitte, S. N. & Hughes-Morey, G. (2012). Stature and frailty during the black death: the effect of stature on risks of epidemic mortality in London, A.D. 1348–1350. *Journal of Archaeological Science* 39(5):1412–1419.

DeWitte, S. N. & Kowaleski, M. (2017). Black death bodies. *Fragments: Interdisciplinary Approaches to the Study of Ancient and Medieval Pasts* 6:1–37.

DeWitte, S. N. & Wood, J. W. (2008). Selectivity of black death mortality with respect to preexisting health. *Proceedings of the National Academy of Sciences of the United States of America* 105(5):1436–1441. https://doi.org/10.1073/pnas.0705460105

Donoghue, H. D., Marcsik, A., Matheson, C., Vernon, K., Nuorala, E., Molto, J. E., ... & Spigelman, M. (2005). Co–infection of *Mycobacterium tuberculosis* and *Mycobacterium leprae* in human archaeological samples: a possible explanation for the historical decline of leprosy. *Proceedings of the Royal Society B: Biological Sciences* 272(1561):389–394. https://doi.org/10.1098/rspb.2004.2966

Edington, G. M. (1954). Cardiovascular disease as a cause of death in the Gold Coast African. *Transactions of the Royal Society of Tropical Medicine and Hygiene* 48(5):419–425.

Engelstein, L. (1986). Syphilis, historical and actual: cultural geography of a disease. *Reviews of Infectious Diseases* 8(6):1036–1048.

Frenk, J., Bobadilla, J. L., Stern, C., Frejka, T. & Lozano, R. (1991). Elements for a theory of the health transition. *Health Transition Review* 1(1):21–38.

Gage, T. B. (2005). Are modern environments really bad for us?: revisiting the demographic and epidemiologic transitions. *American Journal of Physical Anthropology* 128(S41):96–117. https://doi.org/10.1002/ajpa.20353

Giacani, L. & Lukehart, S. A. (2014). The endemic treponematoses. *Clinical Microbiology Reviews* 27(1):89–115. https://doi.org/10.1128/CMR.00070-13

Giffin, K., Lankapalli, A. K., Sabin, S., Spyrou, M. A., Posth, C., Kozakaitė, J., ... & Bos, K. I. (2020). A treponemal genome from an historic plague victim supports a recent emergence of yaws and its presence in 15th century Europe. *Scientific Reports* 10(1):9499 https://doi.org/10.1038/s41598-020-66012-x

Godde, K., Pasillas, V. & Sanchez, A. (2020). Survival analysis of the black death: social inequality of women and the perils of life and death in medieval London. *American Journal of Physical Anthropology* 173(1):168–178. https://doi.org/10.1002/ajpa.24081

Grange, P. A., Allix-Beguec, C., Chanal, J., Benhaddou, N., Gerhardt, P., Morini, J. P., … & Dupin, N. (2013). Molecular subtyping of *Treponema pallidum* in Paris, France. *Sexually Transmitted Diseases* 40(8):641–644. https://doi.org/10.1097/OLQ.0000000000000006

Green, M. H. (2014). Editor's introduction to "pandemic disease in the medieval world: rethinking the black death." *The Medieval Globe* 1:9–26.

Green, M. H. (2020). The four black deaths. *The American Historical Review* 125(5):1601–1631. https://doi.org/10.1093/ahr/rhaa511

Grin, E. I. (1952). Endemic syphilis in Bosnia: clinical and epidemiological observations on a successful mass-treatment campaign. *Bulletin of the World Health Organization* 7(1):1–74.

Gutierrez, M. C., Brisse, S., Brosch, R., Fabre, M., Omaïs, B., Marmiesse, M., … & Vincent, V. (2005). Ancient origin and gene mosaicism of the progenitor of *Mycobacterium tuberculosis*. *PLOS Pathogens* 1(1):e5. https://doi.org/10.1371/journal.ppat.0010005

Hackett, C. J. (1955). *An International Nomenclature of Yaws Lesions*. Geneva: World Health Organization.

Hackett, C. J. (1963). On the origin of the human treponematoses (pinta, yaws, endemic syphilis and venereal syphilis). *Bulletin World Health Organization* 29:7–41.

Haensch, S., Bianucci, R., Signoli, M., Rajerison, M., Schultz, M., Kacki, S., … & Bramanti, B. (2010). Distinct clones of *Yersinia pestis* caused the black death. *PLoS Pathog* 6(10):e1001134. https://doi.org/10.1371/journal.ppat.1001134

Hargreaves, S., Himmels, J., Nellums, L. B., Biswas, G., Gabrielli, A. F., Gebreselassie, N., … & Maher, D. (2020). Identifying research questions for HIV, tuberculosis, tuberculosis-HIV, malaria, and neglected tropical diseases through the world health organization guideline development process: a retrospective analysis, 2008–2018. *Public Health* 187:19–23. https://doi.org/10.1016/j.puhe.2020.03.028

Harper, K. & Armelagos, G. (2010). The changing disease-scape in the third epidemiological transition. *International Journal of Environmental Research and Public Health* 7(2):675–697. https://doi.org/10.3390/ijerph7020675

Harper, K. N. & Armelagos, G. J. (2013). Genomics, the origins of agriculture, and our changing microbe-scape: time to revisit some old tales and tell some new ones: genomics, agriculture, and human microbes. *American Journal of Physical Anthropology* 152:135–152. https://doi.org/10.1002/ajpa.22396

Harper, K. N., Ocampo, P. S., Steiner, B. M., George, R. W., Silverman, M. S., Bolotin, S., … & Armelagos, G. J. (2008). On the origin of the treponematoses: a phylogenetic approach. *PLoS Neglected Tropical Diseases* 2(1):e148. https://doi.org/10.1371/journal.pntd.0000148

Harries, A. D., Zachariah, R., Corbett, E. L., Lawn, S. D., Santos-Filho, E. T., Chimzizi, R., … & De Cock, K. M. (2010). The HIV-associated tuberculosis epidemic—When will we act? *The Lancet* 375(9729):1906–1919. https://doi.org/10.1016/S0140-6736(10)60409-6

Hayton, D. (2005). Joseph Grünpeck's astrological explanation of the French Disease. In Siena, K. (Ed.), *Sins of the Flesh: Responding to Sexual Disease in Early Modern Europe, Essays and Studies, Vol 7*, pp. 81–104. Centre for Reformation and Renaissance Studies.

Hershberg, R., Lipatov, M., Small, P. M., Sheffer, H., Niemann, S., Homolka, S., … & Gagneux, S. (2008). High functional diversity in *Mycobacterium tuberculosis* driven by genetic drift and human demography. *PLoS Biology* 6(12):e311. https://doi.org/10.1371/journal.pbio.0060311

Houhamdi, L., Lepidi, H., Drancourt, M. & Raoult, D. (2006). Experimental model to evaluate the human body louse as a vector of plague. *Journal of Infectious Diseases* 194(11):1589–1596. https://doi.org/10.1086/508995

Hudson, E. H. (1946). Treponematosis. In Christian, H. A. (Ed.), *Treponematosis*. New York: Oxford University Press.

Kacki. (2019). Black death: cultures in crisis. In *Encyclopedia of Global Archaeology*, pp. 1–12. Cham: Springer International Publishing. https://doi.org/10.1007/978-3-319-51726-1_2858-1

Kacki, Rahalison, L., Rajerison, M., Ferroglio, E. & Bianucci, R. (2011). Black death in the rural cemetery of Saint-Laurent-de-la-Cabrerisse Aude-Languedoc, southern France, 14th century: immunological evidence. *Journal of Archaeological Science* 38(3):581–587. https://doi.org/10.1016/j.jas.2010.10.012

Kacki, S. (2017). Investigation of the relationship between health status and plague mortality in past populations: contribution to palaeoepidemiology. *Bulletins et Memoires de La Societe d'Anthropologie de Paris* 29(3–4):202–212. Scopus. https://doi.org/10.1007/s13219-017-0189-6

Kelley, M. A. & El-Najjar, M. Y. (1980). Natural variation and differential diagnosis of skeletal changes in tuberculosis. *American Journal of Physical Anthropology* 52(2):153–167. https://doi.org/10.1002/ajpa.1330520202 PMID:7369337

Kelley, M. A. & Micozzi, M. S. (1984). Rib lesions in chronic pulmonary tuberculosis. *American Journal of Physical Anthropology* 65(4):381–386. https://doi.org/10.1002/ajpa.1330650407 PMID:6395694

Kelmelis, K.S., Kristensen, V. R. L., Alexandersen, M. & Dangvard Pedersen, D. (2020). Markets and mycobacteria – a comprehensive analysis of the influence of urbanization on leprosy and tuberculosis prevalence in Denmark (AD 1200–1536). In Betsinger, T. K. & DeWitte, S. N. (Eds.), *The Bioarchaeology of Urbanization: The Biological, Demographic, and Social Consequences of Living in Cities* (pp. 147–182). Cham: Springer International Publishing. https://doi.org/10.1007/978-3-030-53417-2_7

Kelmelis, K. S. & Dangvard Pedersen, D. (2019). Impact of urbanization on tuberculosis and leprosy prevalence in medieval Denmark. *Anthropologischer Anzeiger*. https://doi.org/10.1127/anthranz/2019/0962

Khan, F. A., Minion, J., Pai, M., Royce, S., Burman, W., Harries, A. D. & Menzies, D. (2010). Treatment of active tuberculosis in HIV-coinfected patients: a systematic review and meta-analysis. *Clinical Infectious Diseases* 50(9):1288–1299. https://doi.org/10.1086/651686

Kojima, N. & Klausner, J. D. (2018). An update on the global epidemiology of syphilis. *Current Epidemiology Reports* 5(1):24–38. https://doi.org/10.1007/s40471-018-0138-z

Krieger, N. (2005). Embodiment: a conceptual glossary for epidemiology. *Journal of Epidemiology & Community Health* 59(5):350–355. https://doi.org/10.1136/jech.2004.024562

Krumbhaar, E. B. (1927). The lure of medical history. *Science* 66(1696):1–4. https://doi.org/10.1126/science.66.1696.1

Kwan, C. K. & Ernst, J. D. (2011). HIV and tuberculosis: a deadly human syndemic. *Clinical Microbiology Reviews* 24(2):351–376. https://doi.org/10.1128/CMR.00042-10

Lydston, F. (1886). Syphilis in its relations to dental and oral surgery. *Journal of the American Medical Association* 1886VI(24):652–657. https://doi.org/10.1001/jama.1886.04250060036002

Majander, K., Pfrengle, S., Neukamm, J., Kocher, A., Plessis, L., du, Pla-Díaz, M., … & Schuenemann, V. J. (2020). Ancient bacterial genomes reveal a formerly unknown diversity of *Treponema pallidum* strains in early modern Europe. *BioRxiv* 2020.06.09.142547. https://doi.org/10.1101/2020.06.09.142547

Mangum, L., Kilpatrick, D., Stryjewska, B. & Sampath, R. (2018). Tuberculosis and leprosy coinfection: a perspective on diagnosis and treatment. *Open Forum Infectious Diseases* 5(7):ofy133. https://doi.org/10.1093/ofid/ofy133

Mathers, M. (2020, July 14). Teenager dies of black death in Mongolia amid fears of new outbreak. Last accessed January 20 2021 *The Independent* website: https://www.independent.co.uk/news/world/asia/black-death-mongolia-china-teen-dead-new-outbreak-a9617731.html

Mays, S., Fysh, E. & Taylor, G. M. (2002). Investigation of the link between visceral surface rib lesions and tuberculosis in a medieval skeletal series from England using ancient DNA. *American Journal of Physical Anthropology* 119(1):27–36. https://doi.org/10.1002/ajpa.10099

Mays, S., Taylor, G. M., Legge, A. J., Young, D. B. & Turner-Walker, G. (2001). Paleopathological and biomolecular study of tuberculosis in a medieval skeletal collection from England. *American Journal of Physical Anthropology* 114(4):298–311. https://doi.org/10.1002/ajpa.1042

Mays, Simon, & Taylor, G. M. (2003). A first prehistoric case of tuberculosis from Britain. *International Journal of Osteoarchaeology* 13(4):189–196. https://doi.org/10.1002/oa.671 e

McKeown, R. E. (2009). The epidemiologic transition: changing patterns of mortality and population dynamics. *American Journal of Lifestyle Medicine* 3(1 Suppl):19S–26S. https://doi.org/10.1177/1559827609335350

Mikalová, L., Strouhal, M., Oppelt, J., Grange, P. A., Janier, M., Benhaddou, N., … & Šmajs, D. (2017). Human *Treponema pallidum* 11q/j isolate belongs to subsp. *endemicum* but contains two loci with a sequence in TP0548 and TP0488 similar to subsp. *pertenue* and subsp. *pallidum*, respectively. *PLoS Neglected Tropical Diseases* 11(3):1–14. https://doi.org/10.1371/journal.pntd.0005434

Milner, G. R. & Boldsen, J. L. (2017). Life not death: epidemiology from skeletons. *International Journal of Paleopathology* 17:26–39. https://doi.org/10.1016/j.ijpp.2017.03.007

Mitjà, O., Asiedu, K. & Mabey, D. (2013). Yaws. *The Lancet* 381(9868):763–773. https://doi.org/10.1016/S0140-6736(12)62130-8

Morse, S. S. (1995). Factors in the emergence of infectious diseases. *Emerging Infectious Diseases* 1(1):7–15. (8903148).

Omran, A. R. (1971). The epidemiologic transition. A theory of the epidemiology of population change. *The Milbank Memorial Fund Quarterly* 49(4):509–538.

Ortner, D. J. (2003). *Identification of Pathological Conditions in Human Skeletal Remains*. San Diego, CA: Academic Press.

Pearson, T. A. (2003). Education and income: double-edged swords in the epidemiologic transition of cardiovascular disease. *Ethnicity & Disease* 13(2 Suppl 2):S158–163.

Perry, R. D. & Fetherston, J. D. (1997). Yersinia pestis—etiologic agent of plague. *Clinical Microbiology Review* 10(1):35–66.

Peterman, T. A. (2009). Sex, sin, and science: a history of syphilis in America. *Emerging Infectious Diseases* 15(6):999. https://doi.org/10.3201/eid1506.090308

Pinto, M., Borges, V., Antelo, M., Pinheiro, M., Nunes, A., Azevedo, J., … &Vieira, L. (2016). Genome-scale analysis of the non-cultivable *Treponema pallidum* reveals extensive within-patient genetic variation. *Nature Microbiology* 2(1):1–11.

Poteat, T., Scheim, A., Xavier, J., Reisner, S. & Baral, S. (2016). Global epidemiology of HIV infection and related syndemics affecting transgender people: *JAIDS Journal of Acquired Immune Deficiency Syndromes* 72:S210–S219. https://doi.org/10.1097/QAI.0000000000001087

Raoult, D., Aboudharam, G., Crubezy, E., Larrouy, G., Ludes, B. & Drancourt, M. (2000). Molecular identification by "suicide PCR" of *Yersinia pestis* as the agent of medieval black death. *Procedings of the National Academy of Sciences* 97(23):12800–12803.

Redman, J. E., Shaw, M. J., Mallet, A. I., Santos, A. L., Roberts, C. A., Gernaey, A. M. & Minnikin, D. E. (2009). Mycocerosic acid biomarkers for the diagnosis of tuberculosis in the Coimbra Skeletal Collection. *Tuberculosis (Edinb)* 89(4):267–277. https://doi.org/10.1016/j.tube.2009.04.001

Roberts, C. A. & Buikstra, J. E. (2003). *The Bioarchaeology of Tuberculosis: A Global View on a Reemerging Disease*. Gainesville: University Press of Florida.

Román, G. C. & Román, L. N. (1986). Occurrence of congenital, cardiovascular, visceral, neurologic, and neuro-ophthalmologic complications in late yaws: a theme for future research. *Reviews of Infectious Diseases* 8(5):760–770.

Santos, A. L. & Roberts, C. A. (2006). Anatomy of a serial killer: differential diagnosis of tuberculosis based on rib lesions of adult individuals from the Coimbra identified skeletal collection, Portugal. *American Journal of Physical Anthropology* 130(1):38–49. https://doi.org/10.1002/ajpa.20160

Santosa, A., Wall, S., Fottrell, E., Högberg, U. & Byass, P. (2014). The development and experience of epidemiological transition theory over four decades: a systematic review. *Global Health Action* 7(1):23574. https://doi.org/10.3402/gha.v7.23574

Schuenemann, Bos, K., Dewitte, S., Schmedes, S., Jamieson, J., Mittnik, A., … Poinar, H. N. (2011). Targeted enrichment of ancient pathogens yielding the pPCP1 plasmid of *Yersinia pestis* from victims of the black death. *Proceedings of the National Academy of Sciences of the United States of America* 108:E746–E752. https://doi.org/10.1073/pnas.1105107108

Schuenemann, V. J., Kumar Lankapalli, A., Barquera, R., Nelson, E. A., Iraiz Hernandez, D., Acuna Alonzo, V., … Krause, J. (2018). Historic *Treponema pallidum* genomes from Colonial Mexico retrieved from archaeological remains. *PLoS Neglected Tropical Diseases* 12(6):e0006447. https://doi.org/10.1371/journal.pntd.0006447

Sendrasoa, F. A., Ranaivo, I. M., Raharolahy, O., Andrianarison, M., Ramarozatovo, L. S. & Rapelanoro Rabenja, F. (2015). Pulmonary tuberculosis and lepromatous leprosy coinfection. *Case Reports in Dermatological Medicine* 2015:898410. https://doi.org/10.1155/2015/898410

Sherman, I. (2017). *The Power of Plagues* (Second). Washington, DC: ASM Press.

Singer, M. (1994). AIDS and the health crisis of the U.S. urban poor; the perspective of critical medical anthropology. *Social Science & Medicine* 1982 39(7):931–948. https://doi.org/10.1016/0277-9536(94)90205-4

Singer, Merrill. (1996). A dose of drugs, a touch of violence, a case of AIDS: conceptualizing the SAVA syndemic. *Free Inquiry in Creative Sociology* 24:99–110.

Singer, Merill & Clair, S. (2003). Syndemics and public health: reconceptualizing disease in bio-social context. *Medical Anthropology Quarterly* 17(4): 423–441. https://doi.org/10.1525/maq.2003.17.4.423

Smallman-Raynor, M., & Phillips, D. (1999). Late stages of epidemiological transition: health status in the developed world. *Health & Place* 5(3):209–222. https://doi.org/10.1016/S1353-8292(99)00010-6

Smith, E. R. (1988). *The Retreat of Tuberculosis, 1850–1950*. London: Croom Helm.

Spyrou, M. A., Keller, M., Tukhbatova, R. I., Scheib, C. L., Nelson, E. A., Andrades Valtueña, A., … & Krause, J. (2019). Phylogeography of the second plague pandemic revealed through analysis of historical *Yersinia pestis* genomes. *Nature Communications* 10(1):4470. https://doi.org/10.1038/s41467-019-12154-0

Spyrou, M. A., Tukhbatova, R. I., Wang, C.-C., Valtueña, A. A., Lankapalli, A. K., Kondrashin, V. V., ... & Krause, J. (2018). Analysis of 3800-year-old *Yersinia pestis* genomes suggests Bronze Age origin for bubonic plague. *Nature Communications* 9(1): 2234. https://doi.org/10.1038/s41467-018-04550-9

Stone, A. C., Wilbur, A. K., Buikstra, J. E. & Roberts, C. A. (2009). Tuberculosis and leprosy in perspective. *American Journal of Physical Anthropology* 140(S49):66–94. https://doi.org/10.1002/ajpa.21185

Swaminathan, S., Padmapriyadarsini, C. & Narendran, G. (2010). HIV-associated tuberculosis: clinical update. *Clinical Infectious Diseases* 50(10):1377–1386. https://doi.org/10.1086/652147

Tabbara, K. F., Al Kaff, A. S. & Fadel, T. (1989). Ocular manifestations of endemic syphilis (bejel). *Ophthalmology* 96(7):1087–1091.

Tampa, M., Sarbu, I., Matei, C., Benea, V. & Georgescu, S. R. (2014). Brief history of syphilis. *Journal of Medicine and Life* 7(1):4–10.

Taylor, G. M., Young, D. B. & Mays, S. A. (2005). Genotypic analysis of the earliest known prehistoric case of tuberculosis in Britain. *Journal of Clinical Microbiology* 43(5):2236–2240. https://doi.org/10.1128/JCM.43.5.2236-2240.2005

Turner, T. B. & Hollander, D. H. (1957). Biology of the treponematoses based on studies carried out at the International Treponematosis Laboratory Center of the Johns Hopkins University under the auspices of the world health organization. *Monograph Series World Health Organization* (35):3–266.

Vågene, Å. J., Herbig, A., Campana, M. G., Robles García, N. M., Warinner, C., Sabin, S., ... & Krause, J. (2018). *Salmonella enterica* genomes from victims of a major sixteenth-century epidemic in Mexico. *Nature Ecology & Evolution* 2(3):520–528. https://doi.org/10.1038/s41559-017-0446-6

Waldron, H. A. (2001). Are plague pits of particular use to palaeoepidemiologists? *International Journal of Epidemiology* 30(1):104–108. (11171868).

Warinner, C., García, N. R., Spores, R. & Tuross, N. (2012). Disease, demography, and diet in early colonial New Spain: investigation of a sixteenth-century Mixtec cemetery at Teposcolula Yucundaa. *Latin American Antiquity* 23(4):467–489.

Weiss, R. A. & McMichael, A. J. (2004). Social and environmental risk factors in the emergence of infectious diseases. *Nature Medicine* 10(12 Suppl):S70–76. https://doi.org/10.1038/nm1150

WHO, (2020). Tuberculosis (TB). Last accessed December 23 2020 at: https://www.who.int/news-room/fact-sheets/detail/tuberculosis

Wicher, K., Wicher, V., Abbruscato, F. & Baughn, R. E. (2000). *Treponema pallidum* subsp. *pertenue* displays pathogenic properties different from those of *T. pallidum* subsp. *pallidum*. *Infection and Immunity* 68(6). https://doi.org/10.1128/IAI.68.6.3219-3225.2000

Wiley, A. & Allen, J. (2019). *Medical Anthropology: A Biocultural Approach* (3rd). New York: Oxford University Press.

Wilson, P. W. & Mathis, M. S. (1930). Epidemiology and pathology of yaws: a report based on a study of one thousand four hundred and twenty-three consecutive cases in Haiti. *Journal of the American Medical Association* 94(17):1289–1292.

Wissler, A. (2019). The impact of frailty in the Spanish influenza pandemic of 1918. *American Journal of Physical Anthropology* 168(S68):273.

Wood, R., Middelkoop, K., Myer, L., Grant, A. D., Whitelaw, A., Lawn, S. D., ...& Bekker, L.-G. (2007). Undiagnosed tuberculosis in a community with high HIV prevalence. *American Journal of Respiratory and Critical Care Medicine* 175(1):87–93. https://doi.org/10.1164/rccm.200606-759OC

Yaussy, S. L. & DeWitte, S. N. (2019). Calculus and survivorship in medieval London: the association between dental disease and a demographic measure of general health. *American Journal of Physical Anthropology.* 168(3):552–565. https://doi.org/10.1002/ajpa.23772

Ziegler, M. (2014). The black death and the future of the plague. *The Medieval Globe* 1:259–284.

Zumla, A., Atun, R., Maeurer, M., Kim, P. S., Jean-Philippe, P., Hafner, R. & Schito, M. (2012). Eliminating tuberculosis and tuberculosis–HIV co-disease in the 21st century: key perspectives, controversies, unresolved issues, and needs. *The Journal of Infectious Diseases* 205(suppl2):S141–S146. https://doi.org/10.1093/infdis/jir880

32
PUBLIC PERCEPTIONS OF PALEOPATHOLOGY AND THE FUTURE OF OUTREACH

Kristina Killgrove and Jane E. Buikstra

Introduction

The previous chapters in this volume have been directed primarily towards researchers and students of paleopathology, as various authors have explored current methods for identifying diseases in the past, the present state of knowledge concerning a range of conditions identified in past peoples, and commonly addressed theoretical issues. In this contribution, we extend our gaze outwards and ask how paleopathology is perceived by non-specialists, including collaborating scholars and members of the public, in order to better understand what themes and ideas are being consumed through various media. To address this question, we consider three sources: first, we evaluate the top eight articles published in the *International Journal of Paleopathology* (*IJPP*) across the dimensions of citations, downloads, and social media presence; second, we explore how our field is marketed to the public through press releases from the news aggregator *Science Daily*; and third, we employ a frame analysis of popular paleopathology news articles in *Forbes* to glean information on key topics of interest to the general public. Finally, we reiterate our longstanding support of anthropologists engaged in public outreach and highlight some of the current work being done by our colleagues to communicate the core tenets of both our broader research field and the specialty of paleopathology. As we have seen with the ongoing COVID-19 pandemic, effective communication with non-specialist audiences is of the utmost importance in producing beneficial public health outcomes. We therefore aim in this chapter to better understand what intrigues non-specialists about paleopathology, with the hope that the themes we draw out of our analysis can be used to better communicate information about health in the past and in the present.

Perceptions of Paleopathology

Analysis of non-specialists' understanding of paleopathology is a relatively new line of research. While US anthropology as a broader field engaged in a post-modern turn in the 1990s, bringing in ideas like public accessibility of practitioner-generated knowledge (e.g., Borofsky & De Lauri, 2019; Borofsky, 2000), the concept of communicating information about ancient diseases to multiple audiences is much more recent. With a rise in user-generated web content and social media starting around 2005, academic archaeologists began dipping toes into the Web 2.0 waters, producing research websites, specialty blogs, and social media profiles in addition to retrospective and summary research articles on the value of this new form of public outreach (McDavid, 2004; Joyce & Tringham, 2007; De Koning, 2013; Meyers Emery & Killgrove, 2015; Morgan & Winters, 2015; Perry & Beale, 2015).

The first journal article to reflect broadly on the state of media engagement with the practice of paleopathology specifically, however, was Stojanowski and Duncan's (2015) paper in the *American Journal of Human Biology*. Their wide-ranging article included quantitative information on academic journal publication rankings and a qualitative investigation into articles published through the news aggregator *Science Daily*. At the time, they concluded that "'old bones' continue to capture the public imagination, but perhaps in ways not completely in line with professional interests" and suggested that "it is better for professional bioarchaeologists to help capture and shape public imagination about what we do" (2015:57–58). Since their article was published, Kristina Killgrove spent four and a half years (2015–2020) writing news articles for *Forbes* as a professional bioarchaeologist. We therefore sought both to replicate the methods that Stojanowski and Duncan used to reflect on media engagement with paleopathology since 2015 and to apply methods drawn from communications research to Killgrove's robust textual data set as a case study in discerning how various publics understand our work.

Academic Perceptions: International Journal of Paleopathology (IJPP)

In the past decade, publication of paleopathology-related articles has accelerated, with papers coming out frequently in the *International Journal of Osteoarchaeology*, *Bioarchaeology International*, and the *American Journal of Biological Anthropology*. The flagship journal of the Paleopathology Association, the *International Journal of Paleopathology* (*IJPP*), first published in 2011, is unique in its publication of large numbers of review articles, case studies, and differential diagnoses of past health concerns (Mays, 2021). Because the *IJPP* includes articles reflecting all "four pillars" of paleopathology – human and nonhuman skeletal pathology, desiccated soft tissue pathology, and paleoparasitology (Buikstra, 2011; Mays, 2021) – an analysis of its content is an ideal starting point for evaluating how paleopathology is perceived by specialists, non-specialists, and the public.

We gathered the most frequently cited (three years), downloaded (90 days), and visible articles in social media (three years) published in the *IJPP* and report them in Table 32.1, assuming that high article citations reflect research interest by practitioners, that downloaded articles represent more general interest to non-specialist researchers and academic audiences, and that social media visibility is a proxy for public interest. We classified each article into one or more broad topical categories, including: case studies, differential diagnoses, evolutionary focus, interdisciplinary work, methodological, and response or review papers.

When the most popular or engaging articles published in the *IJPP* are split into broad topical categories, interesting patterns emerge. Methodological subject matter is of disproportionate interest to practitioners, for example, as five of the most frequently cited articles can be categorized as methods articles, whereas only one of the most downloaded and none of the popular social media articles focus on methods. Articles that focus on case studies are of interest to all audiences, but they are disproportionately represented among those that got the most social media attention, with seven of the top eight articles falling into this category. This finding suggests that a specific individual's or their community's health status may be the most intriguing aspect of paleopathology to the general public, while methods are more often cited by practitioners moving the discipline of paleopathology forward with their research.

Table 32.1 Most engaging peer-reviewed articles in the *International Journal of Paleopathology* (as of 27 December 2021) and their category codes

	Most cited (prev. three years)		Most downloaded (prev. 90 days)		Most social media attention (prev. three years)	
1	New world origin of canine distemper: Interdisciplinary insights (Uhl et al., 2019)	E I	New world origin of canine distemper: Interdisciplinary insights (Uhl et al., 2019)	E I	On engagement with anthropology: Response to Bhattacharya et al. (Halcrow et al., 2018)	Resp CS-I
2	Multi-proxy stable isotope analyses of dentine microsections reveal diachronic changes in life history adaptations, mobility, and tuberculosis-induced wasting in prehistoric Liguria (Goude et al., 2020)	I M CS-R	The pathology of vitamin D deficiency in domesticated animals: An evolutionary and comparative overview (Uhl, 2018)	E Rev	Advances in regional paleopathology of the Southern Coast of the Central Andes (Tomasto-Cagigao, 2020)	CS-R
3	Identification of working reindeer using paleopathology and entheseal changes (Salmi et al., 2020)	M	Towards a definition of Ancient Rare Diseases (ARD): Presenting a complex case of probable Legg-Calvé-Perthes Disease from the North Caucasian Bronze Age (2200–1650 cal BCE) (Fuchs et al., 2021)	DD CS-I	Sensationalism and speaking to the public: Scientific rigour and interdisciplinary collaborations in paleopathology (Snoddy et al., 2020)	Resp
4	The association between skeletal lesions and tuberculosis diagnosis using a probabilistic approach (Pedersen et al., 2019a)	M DD	Survival after trepanation – Early cranial surgery from Late Iron Age Switzerland (Moghaddam et al., 2015)	CS-I CS-R	A bioarchaeological and biocultural investigation of Chinese footbinding at the Xuecun archaeological site, Henan Province, China (Lee, 2019)	CS-R
5	Multiple myeloma in paleopathology: A critical review (Riccomi et al., 2019)	DD Rev	Fancy shoes and painful feet: Hallux valgus and fracture risk in medieval Cambridge, England (Dittmar et al., 2021)	CS-C	Skeletal evidence for violent trauma from the bronze age Qijia culture (2,300–1,500 BCE), Gansu Province, China (Dittmar et al., 2019)	CS-C

(*Continued*)

| | Most cited
(prev. three years) | | Most downloaded
(prev. 90 days) | | Most social media attention
(prev. three years) | |
|---|---|---|---|---|---|---|
| 6 | Tuberculosis in medieval and early modern Denmark: A paleoepidemiological perspective (Pedersen et al., 2019b) | E M | How rare is rare? A literature survey of the last 45 years of paleopathological research on ancient rare diseases (Gresky et al., 2021) | Rev | Osseous mass in a maxillary sinus of an adult male from the 16th–17th-century Spain: Differential diagnosis (González-Garrido et al., 2020) | DD CS-I |
| 7 | Environmental correlates of growth patterns in Neolithic Liguria (Dori et al., 2020) | CS-R | Neoplasm or not? General principles of morphologic analysis of dry bone specimens (Ragsdale et al., 2018) | DD M | Evidence of congenital block vertebra in Pleistocene Cave Bear (*Ursus spelaeus*) from Cueva de Guantes (Fuentes-Sánchez et al., 2019) | DD CS-I |
| 8 | Spatial paleopathology: A geographic approach to the etiology of cribrotic lesions in the prehistoric Andes (Scaffidi, 2020) | M CS-R | Periodontal disease in sheep and cattle: Understanding dental health in past animal populations (Holmes et al., 2021) | CS-R E | Gastrointestinal infection in Italy during the Roman Imperial and Longobard periods: A paleoparasitological analysis of sediment from skeletal remains and sewer drains (Ledger et al., 2021) | CS-R |

*Category codes: CS (case study) -I/-C/-R (individual, community, regional); DD (differential diagnosis); E (evolutionary); I (interdisciplinary); M (methods); Resp (response); Rev (review)

Also significant is the social media popularity of two brief communication articles cautioning researchers from other fields not to sensationalize archaeological discoveries and urging interdisciplinary rigor. The *IJPP* article with the most social media engagement is a critical response to a non-specialist analysis of an Andean fetal mummy (Halcrow et al., 2018), while the *IJPP* article with the third-highest social media engagement highlights how non-specialist journals often publish studies with poor paleopathological methods and no interdisciplinary communication (Snoddy et al., 2020).

This small sample of peer-reviewed publications in the *IJPP* points us towards general trends in popularity of topics among practitioners, the broader scientific research community, and the general public. To focus more specifically on the non-specialist understanding of paleopathology, we turn to a summary of media communication through press releases.

Public Relations Perceptions: Science Daily

Much of the news coverage of paleopathology research that reaches the general public initially comes through press releases. Written by a media professional at a scholar's institution or by the media wing of a journal or its publisher, a press release in paleopathology is typically a summary of a published, peer-reviewed research article or an explanation of an individual or group research program. While press releases are ostensibly accurate encapsulations of a specialty topic for the general public, they can often exaggerate the implications of the findings or show bias towards the contributions of certain scholars (Killgrove, 2019a; Snoddy et al., 2020).

Public Perceptions of Paleopathology and the Future of Outreach

In their 2015 article, Stojanowski and Duncan reviewed 27 bioarchaeological articles featured by the press release aggregator *Science Daily* for the years 2011–2013. They found that mummies and King Richard III dominated the *Science Daily* press releases in that time period, with additional stories falling into their qualitative categories of disease, curiosities, superlatives (e.g., "the first…"), Vikings, and diet. Only about one-third of their sample involved paleopathology specifically, however.

We present in Table 32.2 summary information for the 13 paleopathology-related press releases from *Science Daily* for the year 2021. Of the institutional media offices that created these posts, Cambridge University led with four postings, or one-third of the total. Other institutions, such as the Max Planck Institute, the University of Warwick, and the University of Otago, have one each. These press releases summarize papers published in top tier journals – one each in *Nature*, *Science*, and *Proceedings of the National Academy of Sciences* – and represent research that institutions wished to promote. As above, we classified each article into one or more broad categories, including: DNA, pathogen/human evolution, virus/bacterium/plague, case study, care/empathy/violence, methods, and interdisciplinary. Table 32.2 presents the titles of the *Science Daily* pieces alongside those of the original articles.

Table 32.2 Paleopathology press releases in *Science Daily* from January–December 2021 (Accessed 28 December 2021 from the Anthropology & Archaeology section)

Science Daily title (source)	Research article (journal)	Categories
Ten millennia of hepatitis B virus evolution described (Max Planck Institute)	Ten millennia of hepatitis B virus evolution (Kocher et al. 2021, *Science*)	DNA Pathogen/Human Evolution and Dispersal Virus
Transatlantic slave trade introduced novel pathogenic viruses in the Americas (*eLife*)	Ancient viral genomes reveal introduction of human pathogenic viruses into Mexico during the transatlantic slave trade (Guzmán-Solís et al. 2021, *eLife*)	DNA Empathy Pathogen/Human Evolution and Dispersal Virus
First evidence that medieval plague victims were buried individually with "considerable care" (University of Cambridge)	Beyond plague pits: Using genetics to identify responses to plague in Medieval Cambridgeshire (Cessford et al. 2021, *European Journal of Archaeology*)	Bacterium Care Case Study – Community DNA Empathy Plague
Vitamin D deficiency for the first time visible after cremation (Vrije Universiteit Brussel)	Interglobular dentine attributed to vitamin D deficiency visible in cremated human teeth (Veselka & Snoeck, 2021, *Scientific Reports*)	Experimental Methods Superlative
Scientists dig deep to understand the effects of population pressure on violence levels (Okayama University)	Population pressure and prehistoric violence in the Yayoi period of Japan (Nakagawa et al. 2021, *Journal of Archaeological Science*)	Case Study – Region Evolutionary Violence

(*Continued*)

Science Daily title (source)	Research article (journal)	Categories
Tooth cavities provide unique ecological insight into living primates and fossil humans (University of Otago)	Dental caries in wild primates: Interproximal cavities on anterior teeth (Towle et al. 2022, *American Journal of Primatology*) Dental caries in South African fossil hominins (Towle et al. 2021, *South African Journal of Science*)	Empathy Evolutionary Human and Nonhuman
Justinianic plague was nothing like flu and may have struck England before it reached Constantinople, new study suggests (University of Cambridge)	Viewpoint: New approaches to the "Plague of Justinian" (Sarris, 2021, *Past & Present*)	Bacterium DNA Plague Dispersal
Fashion for pointy shoes unleashed plague of bunions in medieval Britain (University of Cambridge)	Fancy shoes and painful feet: Hallux valgus and fracture risk in Medieval Cambridge, England (Dittmar et al. 2021, *International Journal of Paleopathology*)	Case Study – Community Empathy Interdisciplinary
Early migrations of Siberians to America tracked using bacterial population structures (University of Warwick)	*Helicobacter pylori*'s historical journey through Siberia and the Americas (Moodley et al. 2021, *PNAS*)	Bacteria DNA Pathogen/Human Evolution and Dispersal
Ancient gut microbiomes may offer clues to modern disease (Joslin Diabetes Center)	Reconstruction of ancient microbial genomes from the human gut (Wibowo et al. 2021, *Nature*)	Coprolites DNA Interdisciplinary Microbiomes
Cancer rates in medieval Britain around ten times higher than previously thought (University of Cambridge)	The prevalence of cancer in Britain before industrialization (Mitchell et al. 2021, *Cancer*)	Cancer Case Study – Community Interdisciplinary
Nits on ancient mummies shed light on South American ancestry (University of Reading)	Ancient human genomes and environmental DNA from the cement attaching 2,000-year-old head lice nits (Pedersen et al. 2022, *Molecular Biology & Evolution*)	DNA Interdisciplinary Lice Methods Mummies Pathogen/Human Dispersal
Ancient feces shows people in present-day Austria drank beer and ate blue cheese up to 2,700 years ago (*Cell* Press)	Hallstatt miners consumed blue cheese and beer during the Iron Age and retained a non-Westernized gut microbiome until the Baroque period (Maixner et al. 2021, *Current Biology*)	Case Study – Community Coprolites Diet DNA Fungi Microbiome Proteomic Analysis

This small sample shows that 2021 was a year when DNA (n=9) and plague (n=3) dominated *Science Daily* press releases. Neither is surprising, given the remarkable advances made in the direct recovery and amplification of aDNA and phylogenetic models based on molecular databases of increasing size and resolution (see Chapter 8). Additionally, plague was a subject of popular interest well before COVID-19 (see Chapter 31), but its heightened visibility during a global pandemic is to be expected. Prior to 2020, for example, part of the allure of the Black Death was as an exotic and morbid event – something that could only happen in the distant past. The continuing coronavirus pandemic, however, may have stimulated public interest in learning more about past plagues, and interdisciplinary scholarship on the Black Death provides rich and personal historical accounts that could be providing a mirror for our own experiences as we struggle to cope with illness, death, quarantine, and isolation.

Press release aggregators such as *Science Daily*, however, largely reflect work produced by scholars at research-intensive universities with dedicated PR departments interested in communicating the work their faculty accomplish. These releases become intertwined in the science news cycle, where they sometimes yield an accurate and interesting summary of a new research study, but where they are more often republished uncritically, passing along sensationalized and exaggerated information to a non-specialist public. In order to fully understand what the general public is learning about paleopathology, we move to a detailed, text-based analysis of popular science articles.

General Public Perceptions: Killgrove Forbes Column

In his 1996 Distinguished Lecture in Archaeology at the American Anthropological Association's annual meeting, Jeremy Sabloff remarked that "While archaeologists may think they are talking clearly to the public, what the latter often hears, I believe, is 'blah, blah, blah, *tomb*, blah, blah blah, *sacrifice*, blah, blah, blah, *arrowhead*'" (1998:869). Here we attempt to identify what directly piques the public's interest and how the information is presented to them through frame analysis, a technique from communication studies that "can offer insight into the choices and interpretations journalists make when framing a story, which can ultimately define the nature of the debate and suggest to audience members how an issue can be interpreted" (Touri & Koteyko, 2015:602). Using article hit counts and journalistic research methods on a single-authored online science news column, we identify both the vocabulary and journalistic frames that have particularly intrigued the public in recent years.

Frame analysis in culture studies dates back at least to 1974, when sociologist Erving Goffman wrote the book *Frame Analysis: An Essay on the Organization of Experience*. Based on his understanding of anthropologist Gregory Bateson's concept of psychological framing, Goffman worked to understand how conceptual frames – which are often linguistically mediated – help people perceive themselves and their society and construct meaning from their world. A frame analysis of a newsworthy topic can be accomplished inductively, deductively, or using a combination of the two (e.g., Touri & Koteyko, 2015; VanGorp & Vercruysse, 2012). For inductive analysis, keywords and concordances among these words in the examined set of media are statistically identified to pull out instances of unusually high usage of particular language. These terms are therefore assumed to indicate journalistic emphasis and, when paired with data on article popularity, can suggest ideas or meanings that piqued the public's interest. Deductive frame analysis skips this step and uses already defined frames to understand how the information is presented. In combining these methods, communications researchers such as Touri and Koteyko (2015) have employed inductive analysis to generate basic frames and then deductive analysis to understand news issues. Frame analyses generated in this manner include inductively generated statistics followed by a matrix of deductively generated news frames.

One archaeologically relevant example of frame analysis comes from a 2005 article by communication researchers Cynthia-Lou Coleman and Erin Dysart on the news media's framing of Kennewick Man/The Ancient One. They performed a close reading of 155 articles published over an eight-year period to identify frames and assess the extent of the scientific-cultural dichotomy of the news coverage. In their analysis, Coleman and Dysart discovered frames often highlighted "conflicts using war and battle metaphors, religion versus science or rationality, the legal and moral rights of stakeholders within the rationality of the court system, the political rights and motives of stakeholders, and the persuasive nature of progress" (2005:13). Further, in investigating the statistical use of specific words, Coleman and Dysart found that, for example, "the term *significance* is used to refer to the scientific perspective but is rarely used in framing Indian accounts" (2005:15). The framing of the news coverage they analyzed "has resulted in a disservice to publics," they concluded, particularly because the Kennewick Man news frames "channel stereotypes of cowboy-and-Indian skirmishes of the past, thus confusing contemporary arguments, such as repatriation, with vestigial visions of a conquered people" (2005:22).

For our frame analysis, we focus on a *Forbes* Science column that was written by bioarchaeologist Kristina Killgrove from May 2015 through January 2020. During this period, Killgrove wrote 325 articles; of those, 108 were focused on paleopathology, or about one-third of all articles (see Killgrove, 2021 and Table 32.3). At the time of publication, all *Forbes* articles were widely accessible and free to read (albeit with ads). Using a multiscalar approach – deductive analysis of frames based on inductive analysis of keywords – we identified patterns in word frequencies, concordances with popularity, and journalistic news frames that signal how the general public both consumes and understands paleopathology news.

Inductive Frame Analysis

In just over four years' time, the 79 paleopathology-focused *Forbes* articles for which we have popularity data received about 2.6 million hits from individuals interested in these news stories. Although no hit numbers were available for the additional 29 articles, we can extrapolate from the available data to estimate that the total number of hits on all 108 articles was likely closer to 3.5 million. It is worth further exploring where the information on paleopathology came from and what the general themes were that these millions of readers viewed.

Table 32.3 includes a title, source, hit count, and topic(s) for each of the 108 articles. Most of the news items came from information published in the *International Journal of Paleopathology* (n=17) and the *International Journal of Osteoarchaeology* (n=17), for a total of 31.5% of all the news articles. Additional journals with more than one newsworthy paleopathology article included *PLOS* (6), *Antiquity* (4), *American Journal of Physical/Biological Anthropology* (4) and its conference (4), *Journal of Archaeological Science: Reports* (3), *Latin American Antiquity* (3), *Archaeometry* (2), and *Nature Communications* (2). All told, 57% of paleopathology news articles came from information published in these academic journals.

In coding topics for this step, we used essentially the same categories as above (see Table 32.2). Each news article was coded as *individual* when focused on one person and *community* when focused on multiple individuals; the number of individual case studies in these *Forbes* pieces (59 or 55%) slightly outweighed the community studies (49 or 45%). Each article was also coded for one or more themes, as follows: (1) specific disease or named condition (57%);

Table 32.3 Characteristics of paleopathology articles in *Forbes* (2015–2020)

Forbes title	Source	Hits	Individual (I)/Community (C)/Case Study (C)	Empathy/Sympathy (Vulnerable)	Macabre/Curiosity	Methods	Superlative (S)/Unique (U)	DNA	Violence/War	Virus, Bacteria	Pathogen Evolution and Disease Dispersal	Specific Disease or Condition	Coprolites/Microbiome/Paleoparasitology
Healthy Vampires Emerge From Graves in Medieval Polish Cemetery	AAPA conf	292,749	C		X								
Alexander The Great's Father Found in Tomb with Foreign Princess	IJOA	212,697	I				U		X				
Archaeologists Find Bound Bodies of Enslaved Africans in Portuguese Trash Dump	IJOA	170,177	C	X					X				
Here's How Corsets Deformed the Skeletons of Victorian Women	NEXUS	154,292	I	X	X								
Archaeologists Discover a New Profession in an Ancient Egyptian Woman's Teeth	Edited volume	142,552	I				U						
Skeleton of Medieval Giantess Unearthed from Polish Cemetery	Edited volume	136,983	I		X		U					X	
How Castration and Opera Changed the Skeleton of 19th-Century Singer Pacchierotti	Nature Scientific Reports	117,447	I	X	X		U					X	
Castration Affected Skeleton of Famous Opera Singer Farinelli Archaeologists Say	IJPP/J of Anatomy	109,532	I	X	X		U					X	
Archaeologists Discover Amazon Warrior in Ancient Armenian Grave	IJOA	106,301	I		X		U		X				

(Continued)

Forbes title	Source	Hits	Individual (I)/Community (C)/Case Study (C)	Empathy/Sympathy/(Vulnerable)	Macabre/Curiosity	Methods	Superlative (S)/Unique (U)	DNA	Violence/War	Virus, Bacteria, Pathogen Evolution and Disease Dispersal	Specific Disease or Condition	Coprolites/Microbiome/Paleoparasitology
This Ancient Greek's Breastbone Shows He Was Executed with Terrifying Precision	Access Archaeology	80,765	I		X				X			
Archaeological Skeletons from London Prove Some Romans Were Lead Poisoned	Archaeometry	70,199	C								X	
DNA Analysis from Colonial Delaware Skeletons Reveals Beginning of American Slave Trade	AJPA	58,303	C					X				
Industrial Revolution Caused Rise in Cancer, Obesity, and Arthritis, Archaeologists Suggest	Press release – MOLA	50,599	C								X	
Mystery Of Morbid Aztec Skull Masks Solved by Archaeologists	Current Anthropology	49,509	C		X	X			X			
Bronze Arrowhead Embedded in Spine Shows Elite Iron Age Warrior Survived Battle	IJOA	41,751	I		X				X			
Skeletons of Napoleon's Soldiers Discovered in Mass Grave Show Signs of Starvation	Master's theses	41,418	C						X		X	
What Does an Ancient Skull from Tennessee Tell Archaeologists about the Evolution of Syphilis?	IJPP	39,260	I							X	X	
Ancient Mesoamerican Recipe for Cooking Human Flesh Decoded by Archaeologists	Archaeometry	38,443	C		X	X						
Evil Twin Ovarian Tumor Found in Skeleton from 16th-Century Peru	IJPP	36,499	I		X						X	

Forbes title	Source	Hits	Individual (I)/Community (C) Case Study	Empathy/Sympathy (Vulnerable)	Macabre/Curiosity	Methods	Superlative (S)/Unique (U)	DNA	Violence/War	Virus, Bacteria Pathogen Evolution and Disease Dispersal	Specific Disease or Condition	Coprolites/Microbiome/Paleoparasitology
Mass Grave from War of 1812 Gives Archaeologists First Evidence of Buckshot Injuries	JAS:R	35,623	C			X			X			
Archaeologists Discover Elite 6th Century AD Cavalryman with Unique Foot Prosthesis	IJPP	35,019	I	X			U				X	
This Bone is the Only Skeletal Evidence for Crucifixion in the Ancient World	Various	31,885	I				S		X		X	
Man Bound to Tree Has Right Hand Cut Off in 14th-Century Blood Feud	IJPP	28,604	I						X		X	
Mass Grave from 30 Years' War Reveals Brutal Cavalry Attack	PLOS	27,747	C						X			
Heel Bone from Italy is Only Second Example of Crucifixion Ever Found	Archaeol & Anthropol Sciences	26,311	I				S		X		X	
Babies in Ancient Ecuador Were Buried with Human Skull Helmets	Latin AmAntiq	25,750	C	X	X							
Mass Grave Reveals Ottoman Soldiers Fought to the Death in 16th-Century Romania	IJOA	24,003	C		X				X			
This Skeleton is the Oldest Known Ancient Olympic Athlete	Various	22,692	I				S				X	
Revolutionary War Hero's Skeleton Suggests He Was Intersex	Documentary	22,305	I	X	X		U		X		X	
Prehistoric Native American Woman Shot with Four Arrows Died While Pregnant	AAPA conf	20,821	I	X					X		X	

(Continued)

Forbes title	Source	Hits	Individual (I)/Community (C)/Case Study (C)	Empathy/Sympathy (Vulnerable)	Macabre/Curiosity	Methods	Superlative (S)/Unique (U)	DNA	Violence/War	Virus, Bacteria	Pathogen Evolution and Disease Dispersal	Specific Disease or Condition	Coprolites/Microbiome/Paleoparasitology
Gruesome Evidence of Political Torture Found on Precolumbian Skulls	Latin AmAntiq	20,648	C		X				X				
Archaeologists Discover How Women's Bodies Were Dissected in Victorian England	Bioarch Int'l	19,758	C	X	X								
Mass Sacrifice of Children and Llamas in Ancient Peru Reflects Trauma Over Climate Change	PLOS	16,631	C		X				X				
This Woman from Medieval Iceland Lived with a Disfiguring Facial Anomaly	IJPP	16,321	I	X	X							X	
Brutal Brawls and Cranial Surgery Discovered on Ancient Skeletons from Lake Titicaca	IJOA	16,143	C						X			X	
Pot Polish on Bones from Franklin's 1845 Arctic Expedition is Evidence of Cannibalism	IJOA	14,387	C		X				X				
How a Pregnant Woman's Love of Dogs Led to Death by Parasite in Ancient Greece	IJOA	14,343	I	X								X	X
Intestinal Worm Discovered in Ancient Roman Coffin	Korean J of Parasitology	13,654	I									X	X
Bones of Saint Nicholas Reveal What Santa Claus Really Looked Like	Various	12,413	I				U		X				
Skeletons of Two Possible Eunuchs Discovered in Ancient Egypt	AAPA conf	11,589	I	X	X							X	

Forbes title	Source	Hits	Individual (I)/Community (C) Case Study (C)	Empathy/Sympathy (Vulnerable)	Macabre/Curiosity	Methods	Superlative (S)/Unique (U)	DNA	Violence/War	Virus, Bacteria Pathogen Evolution and Disease Dispersal	Specific Disease or Condition	Coprolites/Microbiome/Paleoparasitology
Did Toxic Rum Kill These 19th-Century British Soldiers?	Conf proceedings	11,250	C						X		X	
Bones of Indigenous Victim Reveal Brutality of European Colonization of Gran Canaria	IJOA	10,514	I	X					X			
Roman Forum Yields Stash of Teeth Extracted by Ancient Dentist	Int'l J of Anthropology	10,426	C				U				X	
Inside the Last Meals of Ancient Victims of Sacrifice and Murder	Various	10,391	C	X	X				X			
Infant Burials and Decapitated Men in Ancient Teotihuacan Neighborhood Reveal Diverse Origins	PLOS	10,227	C	X	X			X	X			
Archaeologists Find Case of Dwarfism in 3rd Millennium BC China	IJPP	8,819	I		X						X	
Brawny Bones Reveal Medieval Hungarian Warriors Were Accomplished Archers	Acta Bio. Szegediensis	7,946	C						X		X	
World's Oldest Cold Case: A 430,000-Year-Old Murder Victim Found in Pit of Bones	PLOS	7,620	I		X		S		X			
Plague Genome Sequenced from 6th-Century Woman's Teeth	Molecular Bio & Evolution	7,587	I					X		X	X	
Mysteries of the Black Death, Shroud of Turin, and Origins of Early Americans Solved with DNA	Various	6,969	C					X		X	X	

(Continued)

Forbes title	Source	Hits	Individual (I)/Community (C)/Case Study (C)	Empathy/Sympathy (Vulnerable)	Macabre/Curiosity	Methods	Superlative (S)/Unique (U)	DNA	Violence/War	Virus, Bacteria	Pathogen Evolution and Disease Dispersal	Specific Disease or Condition	Coprolites/Microbiome/Paleoparasitology
In Ancient Peru, Archaeologists Find Rare Spinal Condition and Possible Inbreeding	AAPA conf	6,852	C		X							X	
Christian Cemetery from Viking Age Iceland Reveals Strenuous Lives and Early Deaths	IJOA	6,600	C						X			X	
Earliest Case of Leprosy in Britain Reveals Scandinavian Origins of the Disease	AAPA conf	6,517	I				S			X		X	
DNA Confirms Headless Roman-Era Gladiator Not from Britain – and Maybe Not a Gladiator	Nature Comms.	6,188	I		X			X	X				
London Crossrail Dig Hits Beheaded Romans	Press release	6,048	C		X				X				
How Grave Robbers and Medical Students Helped Dehumanize 19th-Century Blacks and The Poor	Various	5,631	C	X									
This Defender of a Byzantine Fort Was Decapitated by the Ottomans	Byzantina Symmeikta	5,345	I		X				X				
Skeletons of Jewish Victims of Inquisition Discovered in Ancient Portuguese Trash Heap	JAA	5,062	C	X					X				
To Drug Test Shakespeare's Bones Or Not to Drug Test Them? That is the Question	Media	4,856	I				U					X	
Ancient Pompeians Had Good Dental Health but Were Not Necessarily Vegetarians	Media	4,479	C									X	

Forbes title	Source	Hits	Individual (I)/Community (C)/Case Study (C)	Empathy/Sympathy (Vulnerable)	Macabre/Curiosity	Methods	Superlative (S)/Unique (U)	DNA	Violence/War	Virus, Bacteria	Pathogen Evolution and Disease Dispersal	Specific Disease or Condition	Coprolites/Microbiome/Paleoparasitology
Ancient Roman Man Tiptoed Through Life from a Hip Fracture	IJPP	4,293	I	X								X	
Cannibalism Is Much Older Than Drew Barrymore's Santa Clarita Diet	Various	4,236	I		X				X				
Skinned, Carved and Boiled Skull Cup Reveals Cannibalism in Neolithic Spain	AJPA	4,004	I		X				X				
Earliest Case of Scurvy in Ancient Egypt Detected by Archaeologists	IJPP	3,894	I				S			X		X	
Young Woman with Disabilities Found in Artifact-Packed Bronze Age Burial	IJPP	3,740	I	X								X	
A Case of Death in Childbirth in Neolithic China	IJOA	3,653	I	X								X	
Rotten Roman Baby Teeth Blamed on Honey, Porridge	IJOA	3,383	I	X								X	
Kids' Skulls Reveal Traumatic Death in Ancient France	IJOA	3,254	C	X					X				
Twisted Knee Might Identify Alexander the Great's Father but Some Are Skeptical	PNAS	3,243	I				U		X				
Why Was This Medieval Sicilian Stabbed in the Back and Buried Face-Down?	IJOA	2,987	I		X				X				
Children in Manhattan Got Scurvy and Rickets, 19th-Century Skeletons Reveal	PhD diss	2,487	C	X						X		X	

(Continued)

Forbes title	Source	Hits	Individual (I)/Community (C)/Case Study	Empathy/Sympathy (Vulnerable)	Macabre/Curiosity	Methods	Superlative (S)/Unique (U)	DNA	Violence/War	Virus, Bacteria	Pathogen Evolution and Disease Dispersal	Specific Disease or Condition	Coprolites/Microbiome/Paleoparasitology
Teenager in Ancient Panamanian Ritual Burial Had Bone Cancer	IJPP	2,405	I		X							X	
Archaeologists Find Medieval Foot Fungus in Portuguese Cemetery	IJPP	2,162	I							X		X	
What Does Ancient Human Sacrifice Look Like?	Various	2,156	C		X				X				
Heart Disease Found in 16th-Century Greenland Mummies	Various	2,145	C									X	
Archaeologists Uncover the Skeleton of a Medieval Christian Pilgrim with Leprosy	PLOS Neglected Tropical Diseases	1,962	I									X	
Paleopoop from Neolithic Çatalhöyük Reveals Parasitic Infections	Antiquity	1,579	C										X
DNA Evidence of Malaria Found in Imperial-Era Skeletons in Southern Italy	Current Biology	1,553	C					X		X		X	
Ancient Skeleton Yields Earliest Diagnosis of Legg-Calvé-Perthes Disease in China	IJPP	1,146	I									X	
Aborted Fetus and Pill Bottle in 19th-Century New York Outhouse Reveal History of Family Planning	Historical Archaeology	N/A	I	X	X							X	
Ancient Baby Teeth Tell Archaeologists That Life in This South American Desert Was Stressful	AJPA	N/A	C		X							X	

Public Perceptions of Paleopathology and the Future of Outreach

Forbes title	Source	Hits	Individual (I)/Community (C)/Case Study (C)	Empathy/Sympathy (Vulnerable)	Macabre/Curiosity	Methods	Superlative (S)/Unique (U)	DNA	Violence/War	Virus, Bacteria	Pathogen Evolution and Disease Dispersal	Specific Disease or Condition	Coprolites/Microbiome/Paleoparasitology
Ancient Italian Skeletons Had Hemp in Their Teeth, Archaeologists Discover	AJPA	N/A	C									X	
Ancient Roman Poop Shows Rich and Poor Were Infected by Different Parasites	JAS:R	N/A	C									X	X
Archaeologists Find Ancient Knife Hand Prosthesis on Medieval Warrior	JAS	N/A	I		X							X	
Archaeologists Find Deformed Dog Buried Near Ancient Child in the Philippines	IJOA	N/A	I	X								X	
Archaeologists Find Intestinal Worms in Burials from the Time of Hippocrates	JAS:R	N/A	C									X	X
Archaeologists Study Medieval Mass Graves in Latvia for Evidence of Plague and Famine	PLOS	N/A	C									X	
Archaeologists Test Feces from Roman Latrine, Find Roundworm and Dysentery	IJPP	N/A	C			X						X	X
Basketball-Sized Jaw Tumor Found on Skeleton Of 17th-Century Woman in West Virginia	IJOA	N/A	I		X							X	
Castrated Egyptian Mummy Is an Archaeological Mystery	Press release	N/A	I		X							X	
How the Black Death Caused Medieval Women to Shrink	AJHB	N/A	C			X						X	
Human Sacrifices at Massive Pyramid Along Great Wall Change Archaeologists' View of Early China	Antiquity	N/A	C		X					X			

(Continued)

Forbes title	Source	Hits	Individual (I)/Community (C)/Case Study (C)	Empathy/Sympathy (Vulnerable)	Macabre/Curiosity	Methods	Superlative (S)/Unique (U)	DNA	Violence/War	Virus, Bacteria, Pathogen Evolution and Disease Dispersal	Specific Disease or Condition	Coprolites/Microbiome/Paleoparasitology
International Experts Refute Alien Mummy Analysis, Question Ethics and Legality	IJPP	N/A	I		X	X		X				
Painted Bones Spark 4,500-Year-Old Burial Mystery in Ukraine	Baltic–Pontic Studies	N/A	I		X						X	
Skeleton Found at Late Roman Fortress in Egypt Reveals Violent Death	IJOA	N/A	I							X		
Skeleton of Famed Astronomer Tycho Brahe Finally Reveals Cause of Death	PLOS	N/A	I				U				X	
Skeleton Reveals 19th-Century Peoria Woman Had Chronic UTIs	IJPP	N/A	I			X					X	
Skeletons from Killing Fields Remind Visitors That Violence Is Not Easily Erased	PhD Diss	N/A	C							X		
Skeletons from Napoleonic Battlefield Shed Light on Soldiers' Health	IJPP	N/A	C			X					X	
Skeletons of Executed Immigrants Found in Neolithic Mass Grave in Germany, Archaeologists Report	Nature Comms.	N/A	C							X		
Skeletons of Pregnant Egyptian Woman and Fetus Found by Archaeologists Suggest Death in Childbirth	Press release	N/A	I	X							X	
Smashed Skulls on Spikes Show Violence in Ancient Scandinavia	Antiquity	N/A	C		X					X		

Forbes title	Source	Hits	Individual (I)/Community (C)/Case Study (C)	Empathy/Sympathy/(Vulnerable)	Macabre/Curiosity	Methods	Superlative (S)/Unique (U)	DNA	Violence/War	Virus, Bacteria, Pathogen Evolution and Disease Dispersal	Specific Disease or Condition	Coprolites/Microbiome/Paleoparasitology
Suicide, Sacrifice, and Mutilations in Precolumbian Cemetery Questioned by Archaeologists	Latin AmAntiq	N/A	C			X			X			
This Napoleonic Soldier Survived for Two Months with Horrific Facial Wound Following 1812 Battle	IJOA	N/A	I	X	X				X			
This Pregnant Medieval Woman with Head Wound "Gave Birth" in Her Grave	World Neurosurgery	N/A	I		X				X		X	
Tiny Mummified Girl Not an Alien, May Be Result of Fatal Birth Defects	Genome Research	N/A	I		X						X	
Two Dozen People Massacred at Ancient Swedish Fort, Archaeologists Report	Antiquity	N/A	C						X			
What Causes Lion Face Syndrome of the Skull?	Various	N/A	I								X	

(X = present)
★ Full text of all articles can be found in Killgrove (2021)

(2) violence [including structural] or war (44%); macabre or curiosity (41%); vulnerable people/empathy and sympathy (26%); superlative or unique individual (18%); focus on or presentation of methods (8%); DNA analysis (7%); coprolites, microbiome, or paleoparasites (6%); and pathogen evolution or disease dispersal (2%). If we look at the top ten articles by popularity, however, the percentages change. In these most-read *Forbes* pieces, which represent 58% of all hits, 80% are individual case studies, 70% can be coded as macabre or curiosities, 60% coded as superlative or unique, 40% of the articles provide discussion of vulnerable individuals, 40% focus on violence or war, and 30% focus on a specific condition the individual(s) had. Both of these topical analyses, however, suggest that high-popularity news items are those that pique the public's curiosity about human differences and interest in transgressive deaths.

To explore further, we ran a Pearson correlation on individual words/phrases in the articles and their hit counts to see which words were positively correlated with the interest of the general public in the news article. Table 32.4 provides this correlation, separated into grammatical categories of noun, adjective, verb, and adverb. None of the Pearson statistics rises above a moderate positive correlation, but the correlative words that appear most frequently are interesting to note. For example, among the nouns, the word *life* appears in 52 documents and *people* in 55, while *burials* and *graves* appear in 33 and 19 news pieces, respectively. This suggests that popular paleopathology news articles are focused both on people's lived experiences and on their deaths. The category of adjective shows a Pearson correlation greater than 0.5 between hit count and use of the words *degenerative* and *strange*, while other adjectives that commonly appeared in popular articles include *pathological*, *longstanding*, and *intriguing*. These would seem to parallel the macabre/curiosity theme noted above. Action verbs such as *excavate* and *investigate* are moderately positively correlated with popularity of these *Forbes* articles, while basic demonstrative verbs *show* and *give* occur most frequently. Finally, the adverb *why* turns up in 18 articles and shows a moderate positive correlation with frequency, perhaps speaking to the themes of curiosity about and explanation of ancient disease.

Table 32.4 Pearson correlation of word frequency with popularity of *Forbes* articles

	Word	Number of articles appeared in	Pearson correlation with hit count
NOUNS	Scholar(s)	6	0.573
	Friend(s)	3	0.520
	Tuberculosis	6	0.402
	Perception	4	0.384
	Grave(s)	19	0.363
	Sense	4	0.343
	Correlation	4	0.332
	People	55	0.327
	Burial(s)	33	0.326
	Fear	3	0.323
	Ribs	15	0.307
	Life	52	0.306
	Trait(s)	3	0.303
	Student(s)	4	0.302

	Word	Number of articles appeared in	Pearson correlation with hit count
ADJECTIVES	Degenerative	5	0.582
	Strange	4	0.539
	Pathological	11	0.385
	Disabled	4	0.368
	Longstanding	7	0.349
	Intriguing	8	0.336
	Alone	3	0.333
	Professional	4	0.327
	Lunar	3	0.306
	Respiratory	4	0.305
	Enslaved	3	0.301
VERBS	Excavate	5	0.461
	Admit	3	0.437
	Investigate	6	0.401
	Show	35	0.388
	Regard	3	0.385
	Call	7	0.356
	Born	10	0.340
	Give	35	0.324
	Wear	9	0.305
ADVERBS	Why	18	0.454
	Necessarily	5	0.405
	Certain	8	0.394
	Slightly	5	0.356
	Suddenly	4	0.319

The themes that arise from an inductive analysis of news article topics and correlative words, then, suggest that the general public is most interested in reading and sharing paleopathology news items that focus on past people's lives and deaths, but particularly on those individuals who are deemed different, strange, or intriguing today or in the past.

Deductive Frame Analysis

A challenge raised by both Stojanowski & Duncan (2015:54) and the various scholars writing in the edited volume *Bioarchaeologists Speak Out* (Buikstra, 2019a) is for practitioners to contribute to larger societal discussions about topics that echo through time, such as warfare and violence, through outreach. Quantitative analysis of the *Forbes* pieces demonstrates that there is public interest in the topic of violence from a bioarchaeological perspective, so it is an ideal candidate for an issue frame analysis (cf. Touri & Koteyko, 2015). Loosely following the methodology of VanGorp and Vercruysse (2012), key terms and phrases were extracted from the text using an open coding method in addition to linguistic elements suggesting a cognitive framework for the reader for each of the 47 paleopathology-focused *Forbes* pieces that dealt with violence. These frames were collapsed into broader logical categories and correlated with values and morals in a frame matrix (Table 32.5).

Table 32.5 Frame matrix for *Forbes* articles related to violence

Frame	Cultural/moral values	Common words and phrases	Conclusions…
1 Identification of an individual or group	Individualism Authority Self-reliance Loyalty	PEOPLE: archers, assailant, diplomat, foreigners, king, ruler, soldier, troops, warrior LOCATIONS: battle, mass grave, combat, public, shipwreck ACTIONS: amputate, assassinate, beat, boil, cannibalize, conquer, cook, escape, explore, feud, fight, hack, imprison, inflict, penetrate, plunder, punish, raid, scrape, slash, smash, starve, strip, succumb, suffer DESCRIPTIONS: ambiguous, bound, brutal, chaotic, chained, conclusive, debilitating, difficult, frightening, furious, gruesome, haphazard, hastily, horrific, painful, political, shocking, surprising, tossed in, tragic, twisted ITEMS/RESULTS: buckshot, flesh removal, fracture, guns, injury, knife marks, musket, pot polish, trauma, weapon, wound	• Famous people are more interesting than unnamed folks of the past • Osteobiography of individuals is compelling • Historically important individuals within paleopathology are likely to have been warriors or soldiers
2a Broad, socially sanctioned violence (e.g., war, slavery)	Authority Betrayal Inequality Oppression	PEOPLE: archers, casualties, children/infants, criminals, ethnic group, elites, foreigners/immigrants, gladiator, grave robber, heretics, hostage, Inca, Jews, labor force, raiders, rebels, regime, soldiers, victim, warrior LOCATIONS: battle, burial, fort, jail, mass grave, pyramid, temple, trash dump ACTIONS: abandon, autopsy, colonize, conquer, cut, defend, discipline, dissect, execute, kill, massacre, raid, remove, sacrifice, slit, stab, torture, toss, transition DESCRIPTIONS: angry, beheaded/decapitated, bloody, broken, brutal, carved up, charred, conclusive, contaminated, cracked, defleshed, dehumanized, demanding, different, difficult, disarticulated, discarded, diverse, economic, elaborate, enigmatic, extracted, fatal, genetic, ghoulish, gouged-out, gruesome, hard work, historical, improper, Indigenous, largest, marginalized, massive, medical, mistreated, mixed-heritage, modified, naked, nefarious, non-lethal, peaceful, poisoned, political, puncture, race, rotting, significant, split, systematic, terrifying, tied, unique, unstable, unusual, urban	• General empathy with the oppressed • Understanding of the role of violence in sociopolitical systems

Frame	Cultural/moral values	Common words and phrases	Conclusions…
		ITEMS/RESULTS: activity, ancestry, armor, blunt force trauma, child abuse, class differences, climate change, collapse, cut marks, DNA, genocide, hierarchy, injury, Inquisition, isotopes, power, pressure, ritual, rum, slavery, stress, surgery, sword, trauma, trepanation, weaponry	
2b Specific, public violence or torture (e.g., crucifixion)	Individualism Authority Degradation Oppression	PEOPLE: attacker, bog body, cadaver, defender, prisoner, soldier, victim LOCATIONS: battle, fort, ruins, spikes/stakes ACTIONS: beat, colonize, execute, penetrate, torture DESCRIPTIONS: amputated, bound, brutal, condemned, contorted, cracked, decapitated, dismembered, displayed, dropped, drugged, extraordinary, face-down, forced, healed, historical, humiliated, important, Indigenous, medical, murdered, naked, oldest, painful, pierced, preserved, public, rare, shallow, sharp, shattered, significant, slow, smashed, split, stabbed, unburied, unusual ITEMS/RESULTS: alcohol, armor, artery cut, blood loss, blunt force trauma, coca, cold case, crimes, fracture, injury, last meal, organ failure, punishment, swords, trauma, trophy head, vultures	• Specific empathy with the victim • Lack of understanding of oppressor's need to enact violence
3 Improper burial	Degradation Oppression Inequality	PEOPLE: criminals, ethnic group, fetus, foreigners, grave robber, heretics, Jews, victims LOCATIONS: burial, jail, mass grave, ruins, trash pit ACTIONS: autopsy, dehumanize, dissect, dump, excise, execute, hack, inflict, mistreat, punish, sacrifice, shoot, stab, torture DESCRIPTIONS: angry, bound, contorted, discarded, disturbing, enslaved, face-down, forced, gruesome, humiliating, improper, left to rot, marginalized, medical, outside, painful, pierced, pregnant, public, rare, shallow, shocking, slow, unusual ITEMS/RESULTS: arrowhead, climate change, crime, fertility, musket, trauma	• Dead bodies are different than other refuse • People deserve respect and dignity, even in death

(Continued)

Frame	Cultural/moral values	Common words and phrases	Conclusions...
4 Human nature is violent, but often as a last resort	Action Authority Care/Harm Practicality	PEOPLE: cadaver, victim, warrior LOCATIONS: battle, shipwreck ACTIONS: butcher, boil, cannibalize, chop, cook, cut, drop, eat, explore, grill, murder, prove, remove, scrape, smash, train, work DESCRIPTIONS: cold case, gruesome, horrific, injured, modified, oldest, shattered, tragic ITEMS/RESULTS: blood, blunt force trauma, brain, famine, knife marks, pot polish, recipe, skull cup, trophy head	• Violence has been with us since we evolved • But violence is often framed as a last resort, to preserve oneself or one's community
5 Transgression of "natural" order	Individualism Subversion Degradation	PEOPLE: hero, martyr, warrior, woman LOCATIONS: civilization, mass grave, pyramid ACTIONS: collapse, decapitate, sacrifice DESCRIPTIONS: elaborate, intersex, massive ITEMS/RESULTS: biology, DNA, gender, ritual, political power, social hierarchy	• Violence against the vulnerable (especially women and children) is frowned upon • Individuals who subvert the "natural order" of things are fascinating
6 Administering care in the past	Care Community Loyalty Fairness	PEOPLE: assailant, children, community, elite, fetus, Inca, military, nomad, soldier, warrior, community LOCATIONS: battle, fort, hospital, mass grave ACTIONS: abuse, combat, discipline, pierce, punish, reconstruct, succumb DESCRIPTIONS: amputated, brutal, decapitated/headless, disappeared, fertility, healed, historical, horrific, important, judicial, killed, massive, non-lethal, outside, pain, political, pregnant, scattered, severe, shot, unburied ITEMS/RESULTS: arrowhead, blunt force trauma, copper, fracture, knife, medical care, pressure, prosthesis, stress, surgery, survival, trauma, trepanation, trophy head, wound	• Families and social groups took care of their injured members
7 Past experts were wrong	Fairness Authority	WORDS: historical, mortuary ritual, mutilation, sacrifice, suicide, trauma	• Science is self-correcting

Because the *Forbes* column was written by an American for an English-speaking audience, we sought out literature from social psychology and American culture studies on values and moral framing, assuming the author would be communicating – intentionally or not – within this milieu. Haidt's (2012) moral foundations theory includes care (harm), fairness (cheating), loyalty (betrayal), authority (subversion), purity (degradation), and liberty (oppression) as the most important categories of moral intuition, while Kohls' (1984) "values Americans live by" include equality, individualism, self-reliance, competition, optimism, action, informality, directness/honesty, practicality/efficiency, and materialism. We therefore assessed the 47 violence-focused articles, subjectively coding them with the above values and morals, and pulled out relevant keywords in order to create seven frames (Table 32.5), which we discuss here in order of popularity:

1. Identification of an individual or group. By far, the most popular *Forbes* articles by hit count included new information on historical individuals such as Philip II, Napoleon's soldiers, or the Franklin Expedition. This result correlates with a general American interest in crime scene investigation (CSI), forensic anthropology, and corpses (Foltyn, 2008; Meyers Emery and Killgrove, 2015; Penfold-Mounce, 2016; Buikstra, 2019b). The cultural values influencing this frame include authority and loyalty to political or military figures, as well as themes of individualism and self-reliance. We can surmise from this frame that the *Forbes* readership felt that celebrities were more interesting than average people of the past, that osteobiography of these individuals was compelling, and that historically important individuals within paleopathology were likely to have been warriors or soldiers.

2a. Broad, socially sanctioned violence. The second most popular frame was that of socially sanctioned violence, which we split here into a collective category (e.g., war, slavery) and a more individual one (e.g., crucifixion, sacrifice). From the word list, it is evident that the actors relevant to this framing included groups engaging in the violence, such as *archers* and *raiders*, and those subject to violence, such as *hostages* and *children*. Descriptive words used in these articles, such as *ghoulish* and *genocide*, are evocative of the scale of violence being reported. Values displayed in this framing include authority (noted in frame 1 above), but also betrayal, inequality, and oppression. Although this frame elicits empathy with oppressed groups, it does not reflect values noted by researchers in social psychology and American culture studies, which include care, fairness, and equality.

2b. Specific, public violence or torture. The noted popularity of articles referencing socially sanctioned violence may be correlated with the uniqueness of the deaths – crucifixion, trophy heads, and sacrifices – which can pique morbid curiosity. Descriptive words reporting the violent events ranged from neutral (*amputated*, *unburied*, *rare*) to evocative and potentially triggering (*forced*, *naked*, *humiliated*). The values in this frame are similar to 2a but with an important addition: degradation, which is antithetical to the American value of purity and also opposed to the concepts of fairness and care. With this addition, readers' empathy towards the victim is evoked, as both reader and victim fail to understand the motivations of the oppressor.

3. Improper burial. Articles on mass graves are popular with readers, as are pieces indicating mistreatment at death (e.g., being bound or buried face-down). Words such as *unusual* and *shocking* were employed to signal that, even within the context of a particular culture, various types of burial were anomalous. Three actions in opposition to common American values are evident: degradation, oppression, and inequality. Readers are encouraged to conclude that all individuals deserve dignity during life and in death, and that human remains should not be treated as refuse.

4. Human nature is violent, but often as a last resort. Several articles framed violence as integral to human nature, but most often elicited in dire circumstances or as a last resort. These news items included terms such as *pot polish* when focused on the topic of

cannibalism and *skull cup* and *trophy head* to communicate the violence inherent in war. By considering violence a part of human nature, this frame appeals to the values of action and practicality, while violence as a last resort displays a struggle between the value of care and its opposite, harm.

5. <u>Transgression of "natural" order</u>. Some articles fit into a transgressive frame, focusing on rebellion, exemplified by articles on an Amazon warrior woman and an intersex Revolutionary War hero (see Killgrove, 2021 for full text). These articles signal the value of individualism, but also subversion of what many readers would consider to be "natural" categories like sex/gender. This frame further suggests to the reader that violence against vulnerable bodies, especially women and children, is not acceptable.

6. <u>Administering care in the past</u>. With the rise of the bioarchaeology of care approach in recent years (e.g., Tilley, 2015; and see Chapter 25 this volume), a growing number of publications have identified skeletal evidence of care in past populations. The articles within this frame elicit values of fairness and loyalty, in addition to care and community, which lead the reader to conclude that social groups in the past acted similarly to those in the present.

7. <u>Past experts were wrong</u>. Only one paleopathology article fit this frame, but this was a theme in non-paleopathological news items in the *Forbes* column. While American school children are generally taught that science is self-correcting, the reality of published academic science is much more complicated (Peterson & Panofsky, 2021), and the public's understanding of the scientific process is often poorly informed (Kennedy & Hefferon, 2019). This frame demonstrates to the reader that values of fairness and authority are relevant within science.

Deductive issue frame analysis has provided clues to seven broad themes that Killgrove used to help *Forbes* readers understand the topic of violence in the past. Values of individualism and authority run through many of the top posts on the paleopathology of violence, to contribute to how past individuals' lives are framed. Adding in the anti-values of degradation and oppression, readers were pointed to different or strange deaths in the past, echoing results from the inductive analysis. The moral dichotomy between the value of a human life and the harm in taking one was communicated to readers, along with challenges to readers' cultural assumptions versus scientific realities.

The sample of Killgrove's *Forbes* articles in this analysis – 108 full-text news items over a 4.5-year span – is far larger than that found in other popular news sources or press release outlets such as *Science Daily*. While this sample represents the interest of over 3 million readers of paleopathology news, there are a couple of major caveats. First, using a single-author site is not without bias. Killgrove writes, as we all do, through a personal lens. Her writing, including her linguistic predilections and her values as, for example, an American, a woman, a mother, and a bioarchaeologist, all influence her perspective. A similar critique has been raised about Margaret Mead's *Redbook* column, which totaled 108 pieces and 3 million readers over 16 years (Shankman, 2018). Nevertheless, in her *Forbes* column, Killgrove intentionally directed attention away from the traditional research university press bias, and focused on work and expert commentary from early career researchers, BIPOC scholars, geographically diverse scholars, and from a wide range of institutions (Killgrove, 2019b). The second important point to address is that the hit count of an article is influenced by external factors such as date and time of release, promotion by *Forbes* itself, appearance on social media, and search engine optimization (SEO). Low hit counts can also be linked to churnalism – when a larger and more popular news outlet summarizes a published story and promotes it to their own audience. In these instances, people are more likely to share the churned article than the original piece, thus obscuring its popularity rather than reflecting lack of interest (see Killgrove, 2019a).

While the above analysis may help us better understand what the general public finds interesting about paleopathology and the way that that information is framed, it does not address impact, which is a point raised by Stojanowski & Duncan (2015) and addressed directly by all authors in *Bioarchaeologists Speak Out* (Buikstra, 2019a). Hit count or article popularity is a weak proxy for impact; it shows that we have been able to capture the public's imagination about ancient bodies but not what the public *does* with that knowledge. If we want bioarchaeology in general or paleopathology in particular to "directly engage policy debates on topics such as violence, gender, health policy, and matters of the body" (Stojanowski & Duncan, 2015:58), we need to address this goal specifically. Moving forward, anthropologists interested in conveying their research on ancient violence to the general public, for example, can learn from this popularity-mediated issue frame analysis that the values of individualism, liberty, and authority are useful ways to present their work for maximum interest.

Incorporating interdisciplinary methods and theory into public outreach is therefore an ideal place to start, particularly in understanding how ideology frames a discussion, a topic popular as far back as the 1980s, when archaeologist Mark Leone reframed patterns of thought and meaning as the "givens of life held unawares" (1982:742). As an example, a recent paper by Sarah E. Jackson and colleagues (2020) used computational meta-analytical techniques to survey the text of nearly 600 published archaeology journal articles for language that practitioners used to discuss "bone." Their multi-method analysis revealed that bone was discussed in regular and patterned ways, often as an extension of the body in general, but additionally as fragmentation, parts, and objects. More importantly, they were able "to uncover indications of scholarly assumptions and beliefs about bone, not all of which are overtly acknowledged or expressed" (2020: sect. 7.1, para. 2). There is a new opportunity, they argue, to investigate textual datasets at varying scales using machine learning techniques in order to engage more fully and reflexively with the narratives that make up our field of research.

What additional tools might communications researchers, journalists, museum interpreters, assessment and evaluation researchers, and policy experts have that would help us better market our discipline and, more importantly, understand its impact on the contemporary world? We argue that any analysis of public perception of our field should be done in an interdisciplinary and systematic way if we wish to understand what topics are newsworthy and how we can better educate the public on the importance of paleopathology. Tapping into this rich vein of research and methodology is a necessary next step, as it will help bioarchaeologists translate our conclusions about the past into impactful public policy in the present.

Current and Future Outreach

Over half a century ago, John Fritz and Fred Plog wrote that "unless archaeologists find ways to make their research increasingly relevant to the modern world, the modern world will find itself increasingly capable of getting along without archaeologists" (1970:412). Archaeology is, of course, still here, and outreach practitioners have ably pivoted in the last decade to the "fragmented future" of Web 2.0 (DiNucci, 1999), highlighting user-generated content on blogs and social media accounts communicating news.

Today, though, podcasts have grown immensely in popularity, with more than 40% of Americans over the age of 12 having listened to at least one podcast episode in the past month (Shearer and Liedke, 2021). With a low barrier to entry – a microphone and recording device are the main tools needed – podcasting has given many anthropologists their own channel of communication. One excellent example is bioarchaeologist Michael Rivera's *The Arch & Anth Podcast* (https://archandanth.com/), which ran for 150 episodes from May 2019 to July 2020. Rivera interviewed anthropologists from around the world working in all subfields, for a fantastic snapshot of the diversity of research and researchers in the field. His podcast reached up to 10,000 listeners per month in over 100 countries (Rivera, 2020). Another example is *The Dirt* (https://thedirtpod.com/), an ongoing podcast started in July 2018 and hosted by zooarchaeologist Anna Goldfield and archaeologist Amber Zambelli. Their episodes cover a wide range of topics, such as "mythbusting," the archaeology of childbirth, human remains trafficking, and disability and queerness in archaeology. A newly created podcast called *Digging to the Other Side* (https://anchor.fm/diggingtotheotherside) was developed in 2022 by "Asian-hyphenated archaeologists" to communicate how they approach and are approached by the field of archaeology. Wenner-Gren's *SAPIENS* outlet has its own podcast as well (https://www.sapiens.org/podcast/). The current Season 4 – "Our Past is the Future" – is hosted by Ora Marek-Martinez and Yoli Ngandali, who are exploring how Black and Indigenous people are helping change archaeology research. And the long-running *Sausage of Science* podcast (https://www.humbio.org/podcasts/) sponsored by the Human Biology Association is hosted by Cara Ocobok and Chris Lynn, focusing on the work of graduate students and early career researchers. As a final example, when the COVID-19 pandemic shut down her opportunities to engage in classroom outreach, bioarchaeologist Myeashea Alexander, the "Rockstar Anthropologist," created a YouTube series called *Science & …*, where she talks to STEM researchers about their interests and work outside of academia (https://therockstaranthropologist.com/announcing-science-and-a-new-series/).

As public outreach in anthropology continues to move away from the more traditional and unidirectional outlets of print, online news, and public talks and moves towards diverse, community-based, and interactive engagement, we are hopeful that paleopathology will lift up new voices and new forms of outreach. It remains difficult, however, for people within academia to get outreach to "count," even as anthropologists in general admit that engagement benefits everyone (Mennear, 2017; Killgrove, 2019a; Tommy and Hawks, 2021). Rewarding these anthropologists, particularly those early in their career, for trying something new is critical for the ongoing evolution of outreach.

Twenty years ago, Charlotte Roberts wrote that "we must also promote our [paleopathology] studies through the media, whatever we think of that opportunity, because it is through informing the public of our work that we can show its value" (2002:15–16). In spite of our disciplinary hand-wringing on communicating the value of our work over the past several decades, we have shown in this chapter that paleopathology outreach is increasing over time, and we remain optimistic that 21st-century practitioners will continue to blaze a clear path forward.

Acknowledgments

Thanks are owed to Patrick Reynolds for his assistance parsing text and hit counts of the *Forbes* articles, as well as to all the anthropologists who graciously allowed KK to cover their research over the years.

References

Borofsky, R. (2000). Commentary: public anthropology. Where to? What next? *Anthropology News* 41(5):9–10. DOI: 10.1111/an.2000.41.5.9.

Borofsky, R. & De Lauri, A. (2019). Public anthropology in changing times. *Public Anthropologist* 1(1):3–19. DOI: 10.1163/25891715-00101002.

Buikstra, J. E. (2019a). *Bioarchaeologists Speak Out: Deep Time Perspectives on Contemporary Issues*. Springer. DOI: 10.1007/978-3-319-93012-1.

Buikstra, J. E. (2019b). Knowing your audience: reactions to the human body, dead and undead. In Buikstra, J. E. (Ed.), *Bioarchaeologists Speak Out: Deep Time Perspectives on Contemporary Issues*. pp. 19–57. Springer. DOI: 10.1007/978-3-319-93012-1_2.

Buikstra, J. E. (2011). Welcome to the *International Journal of Paleopathology*. *International Journal of Paleopathology* 1(1):1–3. DOI: 10.1016/j.ijpp.2011.03.001.

Cessford, C., Scheib, C. L., Guellil, M., Keller, M., Alexander, C., Inskip, S. A. & Robb, J. E. (2021). Beyond plague pits: using genetics to identify responses to plague in Medieval Cambridgeshire. *European Journal of Archaeology* 24(4):496–518. DOI: 10.1017/eaa.2021.19.

Coleman, C. L. & Dysart, E. V. (2005). Framing of Kennewick Man against the backdrop of a scientific and cultural controversy. *Science Communication* 27(1):3–26. DOI: 10.1177/1075547005278609.

De Koning, M. (2013). Hello world! Challenges for blogging as anthropological outreach. *The Journal of the Royal Anthropological Institute* 19(2):394–397.

DiNucci, D. (1999). Fragmented future. *Print* 53(4):32, 221–222.

Dittmar, J. M., Berger, E., Zhan, X., Mao, R., Wang, H. & Yeh, H. Y. (2019). Skeletal evidence for violent trauma from the Bronze Age Qijia culture (2,300–1,500 BCE), Gansu Province, China. *International Journal of Paleopathology* 27:66–79. DOI: 10.1016/j.ijpp.2019.08.002.

Dittmar, J. M., Mitchell, P. D., Cessford, C., Inskip, S. A. & Robb, J. E. (2021). Fancy shoes and painful feet: hallux valgus and fracture risk in medieval Cambridge, England. *International Journal of Paleopathology* 35:90–100. DOI: 10.1016/j.ijpp.2021.04.012.

Dori, I., Varalli, A., Seghi, F., Moggi-Cecchi, J. & Sparacello, V. S. (2020). Environmental correlates of growth patterns in Neolithic Liguria (northwestern Italy). *International Journal of Paleopathology* 28:112–122. DOI: 10.1016/j.ijpp.2019.12.002.

Foltyn, J. L. (2008). Dead famous and dead sexy: popular culture, forensics, and the rise of the corpse. *Mortality* 13(2):153–173. DOI: 10.1080/13576270801954468.

Fritz, J. M. & Plog, F. T. (1970). The nature of archaeological explanation. *American Antiquity* 35(4):405–412. DOI: 10.2307/278113.

Fuchs, K., Atabiev, B. C., Witzmann, F. & Gresky, J. (2021). Towards a definition of Ancient Rare Diseases (ARD): presenting a complex case of probable Legg-Calvé-Perthes Disease from the North Caucasian Bronze Age (2200-1650 cal BCE). *International Journal of Paleopathology* 32:61–73. DOI: 10.1016/j.ijpp.2020.11.004.

Fuentes-Sánchez, D., Mateos, A., Aldea, J. & Rodríguez, J. (2019). Evidence of congenital block vertebra in Pleistocene Cave Bear (*Ursus spelaeus*) from Cueva de Guantes (Palencia, Spain). *International Journal of Paleopathology* 24:165–170. DOI: 10.1016/j.ijpp.2018.10.010.

Goffman, E. (1974). *Frame Analysis: An Essay on the Organization of Experience*. Harvard University Press.

González-Garrido, L., González, C. V., Ramos, R. C. & Wasterlain, S. N. (2020). Osseous mass in a maxillary sinus of an adult male from the 16th–17th-century Spain: differential diagnosis. *International Journal of Paleopathology* 31:38–45. DOI: 10.1016/j.ijpp.2020.08.003.

Goude, G., Dori, I., Sparacello, V. S., Starnini, E. & Varalli, A. (2020). Multi-proxy stable isotope analyses of dentine microsections reveal diachronic changes in life history adaptations, mobility, and tuberculosis-induced wasting in prehistoric Liguria (Finale Ligure, Italy, northwestern Mediterranean). *International Journal of Paleopathology* 28:99–111. DOI: 10.1016/j.ijpp.2019.12.007.

Gresky, J., Dorn, J., Teßmann, B. & Petiti, E. (2021). How rare is rare? A literature survey of the last 45 years of paleopathological research on ancient rare diseases. *International Journal of Paleopathology* 33:94–102. DOI: 10.1016/j.ijpp.2021.03.003.

Guzmán-Solís, A. A., Villa-Islas, V., Bravo-López, M. J., Sandoval-Velasco, M., Wesp, J. K., Gómez-Valdés, J. A., ... & Arcos, M. C. Á. (2021). Ancient viral genomes reveal introduction of human pathogenic viruses into Mexico during the transatlantic slave trade. *Elife* 10:e68612. DOI: 10.7554/eLife.68612.

Halcrow, S. E., Killgrove, K., Robbins Schug, G. R., Knapp, M., Huffer, D., Arriaza, B., Jungers, W. & Gunter, J. (2018). On engagement with anthropology: a critical evaluation of skeletal and developmental abnormalities in the Atacama preterm baby and issues of forensic and bioarchaeological research ethics. Response to Bhattacharya et al. "Whole-genome sequencing of Atacama skeleton shows novel mutations linked with dysplasia" in *Genome Research* 28(2018):423–431. *International Journal of Paleopathology* 22:97–100. DOI: 10.1016/j.ijpp.2018.06.007.

Haidt, J. (2012). *The Righteous Mind: Why Good People are Divided by Politics and Religion*. Vintage.

Holmes, M., Thomas, R. & Hamerow, H. (2021). Periodontal disease in sheep and cattle: understanding dental health in past animal populations. *International Journal of Paleopathology* 33:43–54. DOI: 10.1016/j.ijpp.2021.02.002.

Jackson, S. E., Richissin, C. E., McCabe, E. E. & Lee, J. J. (2020). Data-informed tools for archaeological reflexivity: examining the substance of bone through a meta-analysis of academic texts. *Internet Archaeology* 55. DOI: 10.11141/ia.55.12.

Joyce, R. A. & Tringham, R. E. (2007). Feminist adventures in hypertext. *Journal of Archaeological Method & Theory* 14:328–358. DOI: 10.1007/s10816-007-9036-2.

Kennedy, B. & Hefferon, M. 2019. What Americans know about science. *Pew Research Center*. Last accessed 17 February 2022 at: https://www.pewresearch.org/science/wp-content/uploads/sites/16/2019/03/PS_2019.03.28_science-knowledge_FINAL.pdf.

Killgrove, K. (2019a). Bioarchaeology and the media: anthropology scicomm in a post-truth landscape. In Buikstra, J. E. (Ed.), *Bioarchaeologists Speak Out*, pp. 305–324. Springer.

Killgrove, K. (2019b). Gender ratio in bioarchaeology media coverage. Blog post last accessed 14 January 2022 at: http://www.poweredbyosteons.org/2019/03/gender-ratio-in-bioarchaeology-media.html.

Killgrove, K. (2021). Forbes palaeopathology blog posts, 2015–2020. Access to text files can be found at: https://github.com/killgrove/KKpalaeopatharticles. Last accessed 28 February 2022.

Kocher, A., Papac, L., Barquera, R., Key, F. M., Spyrou, M. A., Hübler, R., ... & Moiseyev, V. (2021). Ten millennia of hepatitis B virus evolution. *Science* 374(6564):182–188. DOI: 10.1126/science.abi5658.

Kohls, L. Robert. (1984). *The Values Americans Live By*. Meridian House International.

Ledger, M. L., Micarelli, I., Ward, D., Prowse, T. L., Carroll, M., Killgrove, K., Rice, C., Franconi, T., Tafuri, M.A., Manzi, G. & Mitchell, P. D. (2021). Gastrointestinal infection in Italy during the Roman Imperial and Longobard periods: a paleoparasitological analysis of sediment from skeletal remains and sewer drains. *International Journal of Paleopathology* 33:61–71. DOI: 10.1016/j.ijpp.2021.03.001.

Lee, C. (2019). A bioarchaeological and biocultural investigation of Chinese footbinding at the Xuecun archaeological site, Henan Province, China. *International Journal of Paleopathology* 25:9–19. DOI: 10.1016/j.ijpp.2019.03.001.

Leone, M. P. (1982). Some opinions about recovering mind. *American Antiquity* 47(4):742–760. DOI: 10.2307/280280.

Maixner, F., Sarhan, M. S., Huang, K. D., Tett, A., Schoenafinger, A., Zingale, S., ... & Kowarik, K. (2021). Hallstatt miners consumed blue cheese and beer during the Iron Age and retained a non-Westernized gut microbiome until the Baroque period. *Current Biology* 31(23):5149–5162. DOI: 10.1016/j.cub.2021.09.031.

Mays, S. A. (2021). A content analysis by bibliometry of the first ten years of the *International Journal of Paleopathology*. *International Journal of Paleopathology* 34:217–222. DOI: 10.1016/j.ijpp.2021.07.007.

McDavid, C. (2004). Towards a more democratic archaeology? The Internet and public archaeological practice. In Merriman, N. (Ed.), *Public Archaeology*, pp. 173–202. Routledge. DOI: 10.4324/9780203646052.

Mennear, D. J. (2017). Highlighting the importance of the past: public engagement and bioarchaeology of care research. In Tilley, L. and Schrenk, A. A. (Eds.), *New Developments in the Bioarchaeology of Care*, pp. 343–364. Springer. DOI: 10.1007/978-3-319-39901-0_18.

Meyers Emery, K. & Killgrove, K. (2015). Bones, bodies, and blogs: outreach and engagement in bioarchaeology. *Internet Archaeology* 39. DOI: 10.11141/ia.39.5.

Mitchell, P. D., Dittmar, J. M., Mulder, B., Inskip, S., Littlewood, A., Cessford, C. & Robb, J. E. (2021). The prevalence of cancer in Britain before industrialization. *Cancer* 127(17):3054–3059. DOI: 10.1002/cncr.33615.

Moghaddam, N., Mailler-Burch, S., Kara, L., Kanz, F., Jackowski, C. & Lösch, S. (2015). Survival after trepanation—early cranial surgery from Late Iron Age Switzerland. *International Journal of Paleopathology* 11:56–65. DOI: 10.1016/j.ijpp.2015.08.002.

Moodley, Y., Brunelli, A., Ghirotto, S., Klyubin, A., Maady, A. S., Tyne, W., ... & Achtman, M. (2021). *Helicobacter pylori*'s historical journey through Siberia and the Americas. *Proceedings of the National Academy of Sciences* 118(25). DOI: 10.1073/pnas.2015523118.

Morgan, C. & Winters, J. (2015). Introduction: critical blogging in archaeology. *Internet Archaeology* 39. DOI: 10.11141/ia.39.11.

Nakagawa, T., Tamura, K., Yamaguchi, Y., Matsumoto, N., Matsugi, T. & Nakao, H. (2021). Population pressure and prehistoric violence in the Yayoi period of Japan. *Journal of Archaeological Science* 132:105420. DOI: 10.1016/j.jas.2021.105420.

Pedersen, D. D., Milner, G. R., Kolmos, H. J. & Boldsen, J. L. (2019a). The association between skeletal lesions and tuberculosis diagnosis using a probabilistic approach. *International Journal of Paleopathology* 27:88–100. DOI: 10.1016/j.ijpp.2019.01.001.

Pedersen, D. D., Milner, G. R., Kolmos, H. J. & Boldsen, J. L. (2019b). Tuberculosis in medieval and early modern Denmark: a paleoepidemiological perspective. *International Journal of Paleopathology* 27:101–108. DOI: 10.1016/j.ijpp.2018.11.003.

Pedersen, M. W., Antunes, C., De Cahsan, B., Moreno-Mayar, J. V., Sikora, M., Vinner, L., … & Perotti, M. A. (2022). Ancient human genomes and environmental DNA from the cement attaching 2,000-year-old head lice nits. *Molecular Biology and Evolution* 39(2):msab351. DOI: 10.1093/molbev/msab351.

Penfold-Mounce, R. (2016). Corpses, popular culture and forensic science: public obsession with death. *Mortality* 21(1):19–35. DOI: 10.1080/13576275.2015.1026887.

Perry, S. & Beale, N. (2015). The social web and archaeology's restructuring: impact, exploitation, disciplinary change. *Open Archaeology* 1(1). DOI: 10.1515/opar-2015–0009.

Peterson, D. & Panofsky, A. (2021). Self-correction in science: the diagnostic and integrative motives for replication. *Social Studies of Science* 51(4):583–605. DOI: 10.1177/03063127211005551.

Ragsdale, B. D., Campbell, R. A. & Kirkpatrick, C. L. (2018). Neoplasm or not? General principles of morphologic analysis of dry bone specimens. *International Journal of Paleopathology* 21:27–40. DOI: 10.1016/j.ijpp.2017.02.002.

Riccomi, G., Fornaciari, G. & Giuffra, V. (2019). Multiple myeloma in paleopathology: a critical review. *International Journal of Paleopathology* 24:201–212. DOI: 10.1016/j.ijpp.2018.12.001.

Rivera, M. B. (2020). The Arch and Anth Podcast: education, outreach and representation. *American Journal of Physical Anthropology* 171(S69):235. DOI: 10.1002/ajpa.24023.

Roberts, C.A. (2002) Palaeopathology and archaeology: the current state of play. In Arnott, R. (Ed.), *The Archaeology of Medicine*, pp. 1–20. BAR International Series 1046. Oxford: Archaeopress.

Sabloff, J. A. (1998). Distinguished lecture in archeology: communication and the future of American archaeology. *American Anthropologist* 100(4):869–875.

Salmi, A. K., Niinimäki, S. & Pudas, T. (2020). Identification of working reindeer using palaeopathology and entheseal changes. *International Journal of Paleopathology* 30:57–67. DOI: 10.1016/j.ijpp.2020.02.001.

Sarris, P. (2021). New approaches to the 'Plague of Justinian'. *Past & Present* 254(1):315–346. DOI: 10.1093/pastj/gtab024.

Scaffidi, B. K. (2020). Spatial paleopathology: a geographic approach to the etiology of cribrotic lesions in the prehistoric Andes. *International Journal of Paleopathology* 29:102–116. DOI: 10.1016/j.ijpp.2019.07.002.

Shankman, P. (2018). The public anthropology of Margaret Mead: Redbook, women's issues, and the 1960s. *Current Anthropology* 59(1):55–73. DOI: 10.1086/695987.

Shearer, E. and Liedke, J. (2021). Audio and podcasting fact sheet. *Pew Research Center*. Last accessed 28 February 2022 at: https://www.pewresearch.org/journalism/fact-sheet/audio-and-podcasting/.

Snoddy, A. M. E., Beaumont, J., Buckley, H. R., Colombo, A., Halcrow, S. E., Kinaston, R. L. & Vlok, M. (2020). Sensationalism and speaking to the public: scientific rigour and interdisciplinary collaborations in palaeopathology. *International Journal of Paleopathology* 28:88–91. DOI: 10.1016/j.ijpp.2020.01.003.

Stojanowski, C. M. & Duncan, W. N. (2015). Engaging bodies in the public imagination: bioarchaeology as social science, science, and humanities. *American Journal of Human Biology* 27(1):51–60. DOI: 10.1002/ajhb.22522.

Tilley, L. (2015). *Theory and Practice in the Bioarchaeology of Care*. New York: Springer.

Tomasto-Cagigao, E. (2020). Advances in regional paleopathology of the southern coast of the central Andes. *International Journal of Paleopathology* 29:141–149. DOI: 10.1016/j.ijpp.2019.11.003.

Tommy, K. & Hawks, J. (2021). Strategizing public-facing work within an academic career. *American Journal of Human Biology* 34(S1):e23699. DOI: 10.1002/ajhb.23699.

Towle, I., Irish, J. D., Groote, I. D., Fernée, C. & Loch, C. (2021). Dental caries in South African fossil hominins. *South African Journal of Science* 117(3–4):1–8. DOI: 10.17159/sajs.2021/8705.

Towle, I., Irish, J. D., Sabbi, K. H. & Loch, C. (2022). Dental caries in wild primates: interproximal cavities on anterior teeth. *American Journal of Primatology* 84(1):e23349. DOI: 10.1002/ajp.23349.

Touri, M. & Koteyko, N. (2015). Using corpus linguistic software in the extraction of news frames: towards a dynamic process of frame analysis in journalistic texts. *International Journal of Social Research Methodology* 18(6):601–616. DOI: 10.1080/13645579.2014.929878.

Uhl, E. W. (2018). The pathology of vitamin D deficiency in domesticated animals: an evolutionary and comparative overview. *International Journal of Paleopathology* 23:100–109. DOI: 10.1016/j.ijpp.2018.03.001.

Uhl, E. W., Kelderhouse, C., Buikstra, J., Blick, J. P., Bolon, B. & Hogan, R. J. (2019). New world origin of canine distemper: interdisciplinary insights. *International Journal of Paleopathology* 24:266–278. DOI: 10.1016/j.ijpp.2018.12.007.

Van Gorp, B. & Vercruysse, T. (2012). Frames and counter-frames giving meaning to dementia: a framing analysis of media content. *Social Science & Medicine* 74(8):1274–1281. DOI: 10.1016/j.socscimed.2011.12.045.

Veselka, B. & Snoeck, C. (2021). Interglobular dentine attributed to vitamin D deficiency visible in cremated human teeth. *Scientific Reports* 11(1):1–9. DOI: 10.1038/s41598-021-00380-w.

Wibowo, M. C., Yang, Z., Borry, M., Hübner, A., Huang, K. D., Tierney, B. T., … & Kostic, A. D. (2021). Reconstruction of ancient microbial genomes from the human gut. *Nature* 594(7862):234–239. DOI: 10.1038/s41586-021-03532-0.

33
BIG PICTURES IN 21ST-CENTURY PALEOPATHOLOGY
Interdisciplinarity and Transdisciplinarity

Jane E. Buikstra, Elizabeth W. Uhl and Amanda Wissler

The development of advanced imaging technologies and methods for recovering and analyzing ancient pathogen DNA provide remarkable opportunities for studies at a global scale. Here we consider recent advancement in evolutionary paleopathology, which develops from evolutionary medicine and has clear transdisciplinary applications. ONE Paleopathology historically aligns most closely with ONE Medicine and ONE Health movements, which link human medical science with veterinary medicine. A ONE Paleopathology approach encourages us to address questions of global significance, past, present, and future.

Introduction

Paleopathology has been interdisciplinary from its very inception, uniting those who excavated and studied the past with those whose special biological knowledge provided significant insights concerning diseased fossils, archaeological bone, and mummified remains. Other professionals from the biomedical and social sciences added their expertise as the field matured. Within the 21st century, we have opportunities to further advance our discipline by engaging in transdisciplinary studies that bring knowledge from deep time to contemporary issues. Similarly, combining recent biomedical methodological advances in genomics and pathophysiology with theoretical "big pictures" drawn from evolutionary insights and comprehensive ONE Health (OH) approaches will also serve to advance paleopathology.

Transdisciplinarity and Paleopathology

Transdisciplinarity emerged in reaction to the strict boundaries between academic disciplines that discouraged collaboration and knowledge sharing. The term is used to describe research approaches that transcend individual disciplines, drawing on methods, theories, and knowledge from many fields, often to solve real-world problems. Transdisciplinarity emphasizes creativity, collaboration, and community-engagement, encouraging the integration of non-academics into research and the production of knowledge (Rigolot, 2020). Transdisciplinary studies speak to issues relevant to the biomedical sciences today and therefore to an audience of non-specialist researchers and the public. As noted in the previous chapter, four of the 14 paleopathology papers identified in *Science Daily* posts included subject-matter we would consider transdisciplinary, including risk factors for cancer and bone fractures. Adding the temporal dimension to interpretations of the human biome and the propagation of violence also has significance well beyond our profession.

The transdisciplinary nature of paleopathology extends to our understanding of bone architecture and physiology. For instance, archaeological skeletons have been studied to assess whether abnormal bone loss (osteopenia) and bone loss leading to increased risk of fractures (osteoporosis) are very recent phenomena attributable to contemporary lifestyles or whether today's patterns extend into deep time (Brickley et al., 2020). Bioarchaeological and historical evidence for 19th-century London, for example, identifies patterns of age-related bone loss and osteoporosis similar to that of today (Brickley, 2002). By contrast, Medieval (11th–16th centuries) remains from North Yorkshire, United Kingdom, present patterns of age-related bone loss that are distinctly different from more recent historical and contemporary models (Agarwal et al., 2004).

Similarly, in a comprehensive review of the oft-cited normative perspective that uncritically accepts age and sex as the primary or perhaps exclusive risk factors for osteoporosis and osteopenia, Agarwal (2021) underscores variability across the globe in societies of different scales, past and present. She emphasizes the multifactorial nature of bone loss and that features "such as genetics, ethnicity, nutrition, physical activity, parity, and lactation" are key influences on bone maintenance (Agarwal, 2021:5). Informed by bioarchaeological data from Nubian groups and Medieval rural and urban people from the United Kingdom, Agarwal abundantly illustrates the significance of using the past as a natural laboratory for studying bone quality and loss with compelling implications for health today. These and other comparative studies help inform our contemporary perspective on osteopenia, osteoporosis, and other metabolic disorders affecting bone, and the variables instrumental in predicting and potentially ameliorating these conditions in modern populations.

Another example of transdisciplinary work in paleopathology centers on today's growing recognition of the presence and effects of cardiovascular disease. Like osteoporosis, atherosclerosis is not a condition found solely in modern populations. Expanding upon Ruffer's 1911 studies of blood vessels in ancient Egyptian mummies, the Horus Research Group (Thompson et al., 2013) has investigated atherosclerosis in a global sample of mummies using C-T scanning technology. They concluded that this condition was common in ancient peoples, including pre-industrial hunter-gatherers. Extending this line of research, Nerlich, Galassi, and Bianucci (2021) infer that genetic predispositions and chronic infections were more significant risk factors for atherosclerosis in the past than those commonly cited today, which include diabetes, hypertension, and other metabolic disorders. This knowledge suggests that, as in the case of bone loss cited above, the definition of "normative" risk factors for atherosclerosis must be reevaluated and that modern medicine will benefit from mummy science and paleopathology.

Paleopathological methods have also been used in conjunction with techniques drawn from immunology and microbiology to create a broader understanding of epidemics. Research into influenza not only provides perspectives on the evolution of the pathogen, but also the keys to developing tools for the prevention and treatment of influenza today. The 1918–1919 "Spanish flu" killed an estimated 40–50 million people. Using 20th-century frozen remains and archival samples, researchers have isolated ancient DNA (aDNA) of the deadly influenza virus. Results indicate that this influenza strain is intermediate between birds and mammals, having been transmitted to mammals only shortly before 1918. Hence, human manipulation of the environment, which can force otherwise widespread species closer together, or direct human actions, such as the creation of markets selling live animals or farming practices that geographically concentrate domesticated species, can serve as the catalyst for viral change from a relatively benign strain to one that is deadly. Such pioneering paleopathological research led to complete sequencing of these viral pathogens and facilitated the development of antiviral drugs and vaccines (Reid et al., 1999; Drancourt & Raoult, 2005). It also led to reconstitution of the 1918 influenza virus, which has increased concerns about the dangers of engineering pathogens (Tumpey et al., 2005; Lipsitch, 2018).

Paleopathology, in addition to other academic disciplines, can also be explored through the lenses of current events and popular culture, creating a transdisciplinary perspective on the field that is embedded in modern times. For instance, epidemics have been a subject of popular interest well before COVID-19 (see Chapter 32, this volume), but their heightened visibility during a pandemic era is clear. Scholarship on the Black Death is rich with personal historical accounts, artwork depicting suffering and death, and mass burials where the seemingly unending carts of victims were interred. These stories evoke interest due to their macabre, sometimes morbid nature. Prior to 2020, part of the allure of the Black Death and plague was that it was viewed as an exotic event – something that could only happen in the distant past. The continuing coronavirus pandemic, however, has stimulated public interest in comparing plague in the past to today's COVID pandemic. As we struggle to cope with illness, death, quarantine, and isolation, we seek to find people whose experiences mirror our own. Exploring the past helps us contextualize the shock of this moment within broader history. That the plague was deadly, eliminating as much as 60% of Europe population over four years (1347–1351), but did not eliminate our species also inspires hope. Discussions of plague in the popular media also addressed our ongoing fears and uncertainty about the future. In the spring of 2020, Jenny Nicholson's [@JennyENicholson] June 11 Twitter thread went viral, commenting on the assertion that "We're gonna have to retire the expression 'avoid it like the plague' because it turns out people do not do that" (https://twitter.com/jennyenicholson/status/1271267475963838467?lang=en). In July of 2020, a news report of two cases of bubonic plague in Mongolia was picked up by news outlets around the world and spread across Twitter like wildfire. Many people were unaware that plague in any form still existed. Occasional reports of plague continue today in the US and elsewhere. According to the World Health Organization, there were over 3,000 cases of plague between 2010 and 2015. This recent public awareness of epidemics, public health initiatives, and syndemics provides a new platform up on which we can move the field of paleopathology in new directions.

One of these directions may be how our knowledge of how disease has behaved in the past can be used to inform public health initiatives in the present. Paleopathologists understand that pandemics must be conceptualized as long-term processes, whose impact is framed by prior conditions, both social and medical, with outcomes that can vary significantly depending upon political, economic, and environmental factors. Decades of paleopathological and historical studies of plague and other pandemics can be leveraged to engage with our current health crisis (DeWitte, 2016, 2019; DeWitte & Wissler, 2021; Buikstra, 2022). From past experiences, we have learned that public health measures that ensure effective responses and health care delivery can figure heavily in dampening the impact of a pandemic. These measures can be instrumental to the trajectory of a pandemic, and alongside biomedical advances, such as vaccine development, shape the course and evolution of the pathogen. We have also learned that morbidity and mortality directly depend upon individuals mounting effective immune responses, which are greatly influenced by life history stressors that begin in the womb and continue through the life course. Hence, proactive initiatives to reduce global poverty and encourage trust in responsible leadership and science would also be significant steps in protecting humankind from pandemics that will doubtless threaten our future.

BIG PICTURE Challenges of the 21st Century

Issues of Scale in Research: Evolutionary Paleopathology and ONE Paleopathology

The field of paleopathology is inherently interdisciplinary since it incorporates the expertise of medical practitioners, historians and biological, social, and biomedical scientists. Published contributions, regardless of the perspective of the author, range from case reports to general research articles. While the significance of research articles goes unquestioned, the role played by case studies has garnered attention. The *IJPP*, for example, has from its inception (Buikstra, 2011:1) deliberately invited case reports of special significance. Recently, Mays (2021:220) has identified two important aspects of case studies: (1) value in contributing to medico-historical debates; and (2) illustrating rigorous differential diagnoses. Stojanowski and Duncan (2015:57) highlight the significance of case studies in advancing the "anthropological veto" or as referenced above, questioning the normative (risk factors for osteoporosis, atherosclerosis). Individual case studies, such as those of Ötzi (Zink & Maixner, 2019), often anchor broader discussions of the time period ("if you lived in Ötzi's time, then…) or the results of methods (in fact, studies of the microbiome have…). The promise for case studies to decrease fear of and prejudice against "the other" has also been highlighted by Boutin and Callahan (2019) in their work that draws readers' attention toward humanistic aspects of life in the past rather than evaluating individuals as samples, mere bones, or worse, defined simply by their condition or disease.

At the other end of the scale, paleopathologists have contributed significantly to large issues, such as the effects of the rise of agriculture on health (Cohen & Armelagos, 1984) and the exploration of change through time and urban-rural differences tackled by big data projects such as the Western Hemisphere (Steckel & Rose, 1997) and Western Europe (Steckel et al., 2019) Projects. The products of these expansive efforts also excite public interest, perhaps best translated through blogs such as the important Killgrove *Forbes* postings (see Chapter 33, this volume).

Here we propose two broad, theoretical approaches with salience in the 21st century. Both have developed from interdisciplinary efforts uniting biomedical science with social science. Evolutionary anthropology and evolutionary medicine (EM) are not novel approaches, but to explicitly formulate an Evolutionary Paleopathology links them to the transdisciplinarity discussed in the previous section.

Evolutionary Paleopathology

Whether one approaches the topic of health and disease from a life history viewpoint, as do Gowland and Caldwell in Chapter 28 in this volume, or from an explicit evolutionary perspective (Plomp et al 2022a), it is clear that the perceived division between proximate and ultimate causes for disease has become blurred. Nuanced appreciation of developmental plasticity, knowledge of epigenetic factors, intergenerational influences upon health are all features that influence the course of disease, whether embodied in an individual or abstracted to focus upon the condition itself. As Gowland and Caldwell emphasize in their discussion of the DoHaD hypothesis, "history is becoming increasingly important, and a consideration of different temporal scales – evolutionary, developmental, generational and biographical – are essential to our analysis of disease and what Krieger (2013) has referred to an the emergent 'embodied phenotype'".

For paleopathology, this means that our appreciation of health in the past must be informed by context, at varying temporal scales. As with DoHaD (Developmental Origins of Health and Disease), EM provides another important point of departure for an explicit evolutionary focus in paleopathology. As the editors of *Palaeopathology and Evolutionary Medicine: An Integrated Approach* (Plomp et al., 2022a) emphasize in their introductory chapter (Plomp et al., 2022b:2), "a major goal of EM should be to integrate ultimate explanations to create a broader, synergistic framework that seeks to improve health and well-being in contemporary populations". Thus, the goals of an evolutionary paleopathology should be transdisciplinary, as discussed above.

Plomp et al. (2022a) organize their interdisciplinary treatment of evolutionary paleopathology around six key categories originally proposed for the study of EM (Williams & Nesse, 1991): (1) co-evolution of host and pathogen; (2) constraints on selection; (3) mismatch with current industrialized societies; (4) physiological defenses; (5) reproduction at the expense of health; and (6) trade-offs. Ranging widely across the globe, their chapters include impressive examples wherein evolutionary perspectives usefully inform clinical practice. Predictive models for clinicians advising about prospective sport or other activity regimes, as well as in rehabilitation, can develop from knowledge of variations in spine morphology that predispose a person to painful lower back conditions. Cancer, often considered a modern disease, has a long history noted in paleopathology (see Chapter 15, this volume) that can be evolutionarily linked to the complex trade-offs between an organism's need for cellular growth and genetic suppressors to limit it (Casás-Selves & DeGregori, 2011; Somarelli et al., 2019). The recognized effects of environmental conditions, alongside organismal senescence, on tumor proliferation and suppression can be tested and more fully understood through a paleopathological lens. Similarly, long-term trajectories in the oral microbiome and human health are recorded in dental calculus, as histories of parasitic infections explore the beneficial nature of certain bacteria. Knowledge of the way people with leprosy and other disfiguring conditions were stigmatized (or not) in the past forces us to question "essentialized" universal reactions to such alterities (Buikstra, 2022). Thus, it is crucial to think about current health and interventions in a manner that employs evolutionary principles.

ONE Medicine, ONE Health and ONE Paleopathology

ONE Medicine

The ONE Health (OH) movement, popular today, was preceded by ONE Medicine (OM), both with deep roots within the development of medical professions within the US. OM was first articulated by Dr. Carl F. Schmidt, MD (1893–1988), who notably advanced the field of pharmacology and had international experience in China, where he taught at the Peking Union Medical College (1922–1924). Based at the University of Pennsylvania for most of his professional life, he wrote of "One Medicine for More than One World" (1962) in an editorial in *Circulation Research*, a journal of the American Heart Association, alluding to space travel and the cardiovascular challenges faced during rocket acceleration. Two earlier physicians at the University of Pennsylvania are also cited for concepts essential to the OM concept. Linking the study of animal diseases with a physician's responsibility for health writ large, Benjamin Rush (1745–1843) presented a lecture entitled, "The Duty and Advantages of Studying the Diseases of Domestic Animals and the Remedies Proper to Remove Them" on Nov. 2, 1807. During his brief tenure (1884–1888) at the University of Pennsylvania, (Sir) William Osler (1849–1919) argued successfully for the geographical proximity of the University of Pennsylvania veterinary and (human) medical schools.

Calvin W. Schwabe (1927–2006) is the person most commonly cited for the development of the OM initiative. Schwabe (DVM 1954) specialized in tropical public health, parasitology, and epidemiology, having spent the first ten years of his career (1956–1966) at the American University School of Medicine in Beruit, Lebanon. His developed interest in hydatid disease led to his joining the faculty of the Medical School at the University of California – Davis where he founded the Department of Epidemiology. He explicitly developed the OM concept in the third edition (1984) of his popular text, *Veterinary Medicine and Human Health*, first published in 1964, with a second edition in 1969.

OM first morphed into OH in a briefing booklet for the 2003 World Parks Congress held in Durban, South Africa, "As socioeconomic progress demands sustained improvements in health for humans, their domestic animals, and the environment, our institutions recognize the need to move towards a "one health" perspective- an approach that we hope will be the foundation of our discussions in Durban" (pg. 3). Since that time, OH has outpaced OM in popularity, as witnessed by Cassidy's (2018) discussion of the OH movement. The integration of the medical sciences in a fully ecological perspective appears most well developed in the veterinary sciences and organizations focused upon preserving endangered species or studying natural history.

Animal Paleopathology

Just as the OM and OH approaches had strong grounding in veterinary medicine and attendant environmental contexts, a unified ONE Paleopathology must appreciate the broad perspective that the study of nonhuman animals and the veterinary sciences contribute to the study of ancient global health. As Bartosiewicz and Mansouri emphasize in Chapter 31, this volume, the study of animal disease is an interdisciplinary counterpart of human paleopathology. Even so, the two fields have converged and departed from one another, reflecting the distinctive histories of veterinary medicine and the clinical practice of medicine directed toward humans. Within the 20th century, veterinary training institutions and medical schools have specialized, with the former being much more contextually oriented, reflecting the global diversity of species that require treatment. The human species is indeed global, but its disease susceptibilities, both historical and modern, are often similar to those of animals, as manifestations of disease in humans and animals are embedded and entangled within shared evolutionary and environmental contexts. However the focus of clinical human medicine on treating the individual patient, has often obscured these critical contexts, which has resulted in public health being a separate, often less emphasized specialty. In contrast, veterinary medicine has incorporated consideration of these broader contexts in its foundation, especially in the treatment of large animals.

A more extended history of animal paleopathology appears in Chapter 31, this volume, which includes discussions of similar and dissimilar trends in studies of animal disease and that of our species. Post-dating Moodie's (1923) integrated perspective, the fields had separated, as witnessed by texts produced for the study of human diseases (Ortner & Putschar, 1981) and those of other animals (Baker & Brothwell, 1980). These two volumes have very different orientations, as revealed in their contrastive tables of contents. The second and third chapters of Baker and Brothwell (1980) focus upon interpreting mortality tables and the natural history of disease. By contrast, Ortner and Putchar (1981) engage with methods of analysis and bone biology at the outset. An ecological approach thus contrasts with a clinical emphasis.

As emphasized by zooarchaeologist Thomas (2012), the study of animal disease in the past faces special challenges not frequently encountered by those who study humans. The archaeological record of faunal remains, for example, includes relatively few complete burials, most instead being fragmented and dispersed. An ability to use clinical studies in direct analogy is limited by the fact that animals of economic significance are normally slaughtered at a young age, when diseases have not followed a full life course. For humans, the issue is not length of life in clinical examples, but the efficacy of modern medical treatments, not the least being antibiotics and vaccinations, which attenuate the impact of infectious conditions. Both necropsies and autopsies focus upon soft tissues and the cause and manner of death rather than the extent of disease in osseous tissues. As we argue below, a global ONE Paleopathology problem-oriented perspective driven by the ecological, contextual focus of veterinary science, coupled with advances in genomics, may override concerns about fragmented and incompletely preserved remains, along with the failure of many infectious diseases to manifest pathognomonically in bone.

ONE Paleopathology

In light of the great strides taken within paleopathology over the past century, we suggest that now is the time for paleopathogists to speak to even broader, global issues by conceptualizing and emphasizing a "ONE Paleopathology" approach to the study of ancient disease. Through the integration of an evolutionary perspective with OM/OH perspectives, we generate a more complete, more impactful narrative of the past, with implications for contemporary veterinary and human biomedical sciences. This initiative requires combining the study of ancient remains of all forms, faunal and human, and subscribing to expansive global and environmental inquiry that characterizes much of veterinary science. This approach differs significantly from the relatively decontextualized diagnostic strategies of human biomedicine. A ONE Paleopathology approach also unites molecular methods with problem-oriented paleopathology to identify instances wherein significant evolutionary changes occurred and fully incorporates these findings within human/animal/environmental contexts. Genomic studies, for example, are highly visible today and have truly revolutionized our knowledge of ancient infectious diseases, but without archaeological and historical contextualization, their significance may be limited and their remarkable potential incompletely realized. We offer here three examples, two ongoing and reported, and the other with potential to illustrate the power of a ONE Paleopathology approach.

TUBERCULOSIS

The spirit of ONE Paleopathology is not foreign to the study of ancient mycobacterial disease (see Chapter 18, this volume, for detailed discussion of these diseases). For example, by initiating a long-term field program in the Andes specifically focused upon addressing the presence and evolution of ancient tuberculosis through the analysis of mummified tissues, Buikstra (1995) collaboratively combined bioarchaeological problem-solving with paleopathological approaches and biomedical research (Salo et al., 1994; Bos et al., 2014) to uncover the remarkable and unexpected introduction of the *Mycobacterium tuberculosis* complex (MTBC) into the western hemisphere by pinnipeds. This investigation has led to further bioarchaeological inquiries and focused molecular studies in Mexico (Blevins, 2020), which have stimulated nuanced models for repeated introductions of MTBC in the South-central coastal Andes. The research has also succeeded in defining pathological tissues most likely to yield aDNA, a critical contribution given that destructive sampling of tuberculosis lesions remains the method of genomic choice. Hence, it has become clear through the adoption of a ONE Paleopathology perspective that the presence of tuberculosis in the Americas involves a complex interplay of environmental conditions, mammalian and pathogen biology and evolution, and human culture. Our understanding of the real impact of tuberculosis is greatly limited by simply focusing on finding the oldest example of the disease in human remains or mapping the genome of the pathogen. Through an integrated ONE Paleopathology approach, broader hemispheric questions about the introduction and evolution of infectious disease can be explored.

CANINE DISTEMPER

Another example of a ONE Paleopathology approach is found in the Uhl et al. (2019) evolutionary study of morbilliviruses, a closely related cluster of viruses that cause canine distemper (CDV), human measles (HMV), and rinderpest (RPV) in cattle. By engaging faunal paleopathology, historical sources, molecular analyses and morbilliviral pathogenesis, and epidemiology, this interdisciplinary effort argued convincingly for a South American origin of CDV developing out of the measles epidemics that ravaged Andean populations during the Colonial Period (1500–1700 CE). Specifically, epidemiological studies showing the morbillivirus' ability to jump to new host species were used to confirm that the HMV epidemics, along with human's close association with canine populations at that time, provided conditions that facilitated the transmission and adaptation of the pathogen to dogs. This transmission fits the historically documented emergence and global dissemination of CDV. Molecular, genetic, and codon usage analysis was used to document CDV's close relationship to HMV and to provide evidence that it had only recently evolved from HMV to become a canine pathogen. This study illustrates how considering evidence from multiple disciplines and deeply contextualizing multiple forms of data can fill in the "missing pieces" and provide an essential context for studying disease.

GLANDERS AND MELIOIDOSIS

Another important advantage of the cross-disciplinary and the holistic ONE Paleopathology approach is that diseases without distinctive bone lesions can be investigated. Many of these diseases have had major historical impacts and are still problematic today, including, for example, those caused by *Burkholderia mallei* (glanders) and *Burkholderia pseudomallei* (melioidosis). Glanders is primarily a disease of equids and their human handlers (Dvorak and Spickler, 2008; Van Zandt et al., 2013). It was transmitted to humans before mechanization, when horses were used extensively for transportation and were often crowded into urban environments (Bierer, 1939; Wilkinson, 1981; Uhl & Thomas, 2022). Although glanders has been historically documented since the time of Aristotle, was well-noted during wars, and was used as a biological weapon – most recently in Afghanistan – it has not been well-documented in paleopathological studies because it is not characterized by distinctive bone lesions (Wilkinson, 1981; Sharrer, 1995; Dance, 2009; Uhl & Thomas, 2022).

Melioidosis is caused by *B. pseudomallei* and is primarily documented as a human pathogen. Its clinical presentation can vary (Wiersinga et al., 2006). Like *B. mallei*, it can infect multiple tissues including bone and does not induce unique lesions. Thus, it is difficult to diagnosis from pathological findings alone. Even today, when encountered outside its endemic regions of tropical and subtropical Southeast Asia, northern Australia, and the Indian subcontinent, melioidosis may not be readily diagnosed and thus can lead to severe infections and death (Gassiep et al., 2020). Hence, the disease still poses a significant health risk to human populations, and vaccine research is currently being promoted. Interestingly, recent deaths due to melioidosis in the US have been traced to rocks from endemic regions introduced into aromatherapy products: "Better Homes & Gardens Lavender & Chamomile Essential Oil Infused Aromatherapy Room Spray with Gemstones" (https://www.cdc.gov/meliodosis/outbreak/2021/index.html).

Epidemiological and genomic research informs ONE Paleopathological studies centering on these diseases, as they direct investigations into how *Burkholderia* pathogens emerged and the factors facilitating their spread. These studies indicate that the facultative pathogen *B. pseudomallei* (melioidosis) initially arose in Australia, with the SE Asian strain emerging approximately 16,000–225,000 years ago (Pearson et al., 2009; Gassiep et al., 2020). Genomic analysis shows that *B. mallei* (glanders) arose when a single clone of the free-living *B. pseudomallei* entered an animal host and underwent genome reduction to evolve into an obligate intracellular pathogen (Losada et al., 2010). Genetic and epidemiological studies also indicate that the virulence traits of *Burkholderia* pathogens initially evolved as adaptations to the rhizosphere environment (French et al., 2020). Since the rhizosphere is heavily impacted by farming, irrigation, and the introduction of animals and non-native vegetation, human activities potentially played a role in the emergence of these pathogens (French et al., 2020).

Such phylogenomic and epidemiological evidence and phylogeographic reconstructions tell us where and when evolutionary change took place but needs rigorous contextualization through historical, archaeological, and aDNA data. Ongoing research using the ONE Paleopathology approach will provide this perspective by overcoming limitations inherent in the narrow foci of individual specialties. For the genus *Burkholderia*, important holistic questions to address include:

- What factors facilitated the emergence of *B. pseudomallei* (opportunistic pathogen; melioidosis), which originated in Australia/Asia 16,000–225,000 years ago? Were they instigated by climate change? Effects of glaciation? Flooding? Human activities?
- How did *B. pseudomallei* spread from Asia to Europe, Africa, and the Americas: Through migrations? Along trade routes? By the movement of armies and/or enslaved groups?
- What conditions allowed glanders emerge from the single transfer of *B. pseudomallei* to a mammalian host (horse? human?) and what facilitated its spread throughout the world?

We would also like to know how human activities influenced the rise of *B. pseudomallei* and *B. mallei* and be able to better document the historical and health impacts of glanders and melioidosis on humans and animals. In these explorations, the following questions arise:

- Can paleopathological evidence of the presence of these diseases be directly or indirectly inferred from skeletal remains, or will aDNA analysis be the primary means of detecting the pathogens in the absence of definitive bone lesions?
- Why did the pathogens originate in Australia/Asia? Did the presence of moist environments, flooding, the development of rice farming, and/or disruption of soil rhizosphere serve as accommodating niches?
- Why are horses a common mammalian host and how did close associations with humans affect the evolution and transmission of the pathogen? Glanders was described very early in Greece – how did it get there and how did it spread through the Mediterranean/Europe and to Africa and the Americas?
- How were the host/pathogen relationships of *Burkholderia* impacted by war, trade, migration, animal husbandry, environmental climate (wet conditions, flooding from storms?), and subsistence farming practices? Did rice farmers in the southern US suffer more frequently from melidosis/glanders?

Posing these questions illustrates the power of a global ONE Paleopathology approach to address broad questions of infectious disease origins and spread. In the case of tuberculosis, problem-oriented archaeological studies anchor startling genomic results. For CDV, historical records directed the paleopathological, epidemiological, and codon usage studies, while for glanders, the results of genetic analyses guide us where to initiate historical and paleopathological investigations. Importantly, in addition to documenting the evolution and impact of pathogens in the past, interdisciplinary investigations provide critical insights into future threats. For example, nonpathogenic, soil-dwelling *Burkholderia sp.* shares the same virulence traits as the pathogenic forms. Isolating the conditions that allowed *B. pseudomallei* and *B. mallei* to emerge as pathogens is essential to our understanding and prediction of future change. It clearly elevates the study of these pathogens (and many others) beyond mere historical interest (French et al., 2020).

Concluding Statement

A truly transdisciplinary paleopathology will be a vital force that not only builds upon traditional strengths but is also looking for partnerships with emerging fields such as sustainability, indigenous studies, and decolonizing programs. These will facilitate answering questions significant in the profession, but also relate importantly to contemporary social, economic, and cultural issues. Paleopathology cannot and should not address these issues alone, but neither should they be addressed in the absence of the long-term perspective of global history that paleopathology affords. A special challenge for the field, with an appended opportunity, is to direct our discipline toward 21st-century ethical concerns, including decolonization and public engagement. Ultimately, this inclusive effort will enrich our studies, as it will our lives.

References

Agarwal, S. C. (2021). What is normal bone health? A bioarchaeological perspective on meaningful measures and interpretations of bone strength, loss, and aging. *American Journal of Human Biology* 33(5):e23647. https://doi.org/10.1002/ajhb.23647.

Agarwal, S. C., Dumitriv, M. & Tomlinson, G. A. (2004). Medieval trabecular bone architecture: the influence of age, sex, and lifestyle. *American Journal of Physical Anthropology* 124:33–44.

Baker, J. R. & Brothwell, D. (1980). *Animal Diseases in Archaeology.* Academic Press.

Bierer, B. W. (1939). *History of Animal Plagues of North America*, Reproduced ed. Washington, DC: United States Department of Agriculture.

Blevins, K.E. (2020). *Evolution and Disease Ecology of the Mycobacterium tuberculosis Complex in the Americas Prior to European Contact: Inter-continental and Intra-site Perspectives.* Doctoral Dissertation. Arizona State University. Tempe: Arizona State University.

Bos, K. I., Harkins, K. M., Herbig, A., Coscolla, M., Weber, N., Comas, I., … & Krause, J. (2014). Pre-columbian mycobacterial genomes reveal seals as a source of New World human tuberculosis. *Nature* 514:494–497.

Boutin, A. T. & Callahan, M. P. (2019). Increasing empathy and reducing prejudice: an argument for fictive osteobiographical narrative. *Bioarchaeology International* 3(1):78–87. https://doi.org/10.5744/bi.2019.1001.

Brickley, M. (2002). An investigation of historical and archaeological evidence for age-related bone loss and osteoporosis. *International Journal of Osteoarchaeology* 12:364–371.

Brickley, M. B. Ives, R. & Mays, S. (2020). *The Bioarchaeology of Metabolic Bone Disease*, (2nd ed.). Academic Press. DOI -10.1016/B978-0-08–101020-4.00018-5.

Buikstra, J. E. (1995). Tombs for the living … or for the dead: the osmore ancestors. In Dillehay, T. (Ed.), *Tombs for the Ancestors*, pp. 229–280. Washington, DC: Dumbarton Oaks Research Library and Collection.

Buikstra, J. E., (2011). Editorial. *International Journal of Paleopathology* 1:1–3.
Buikstra, J. E. (2022). Afterword. In Plomp, K., Roberts, C. A., Elton, S. & Bentley, G. R. (Eds.), *Palaeopathology and Evolutionary Medicine: An Integrated Approach*, pp. 354–355. Oxford: Oxford University Press.
Casás-Selves, M. & DeGregori, J. (2011). How cancer shapes evolution and how evolution shapes cancer. *Evolution: Education Outreach* 4:624–634. https://doi.org/10.1007/s12052-011-0373-y.
Cassidy, A. (2018). Humans, other animals and 'one health' in the early twenty-first century. In Woods, A., Bresalier, M., Cassidy, A & Dentinger, R. M. (Eds.), *Animals and the Shaping of Modern Medicine: One Health and Its Histories*, pp. 193–236. Cham, Switzerland, Palgrame Macmillan, Springer Nature. https://doi.org/10.1007/978-3-319-64337-3_6.
Cohen, M. N. & Armelagos G. J. (1984). *Paleopathology at the Origins of Agriculture*. Orlando, FL: University Press of Florida.
Dance, D. A. B. (2009). Melioidosis and glanders as possible biological weapons. In Fong, I. W. & Alibek, K. (Eds.), *Bioterrorism and Infectious Agents: A New Dilemma for the 21st Century*, pp. 99–145. Cham, Switzerland: Springer Nature. DOI: 10.1007/978-1-4419-1266-4_4.
DeWitte, S. N. (2016). Archaeological evidence of epidemics can inform future epidemics. *Annual Review of Anthropology* 45:63–77.
DeWitte, S. N. (2019). Misperceptions about the bioarchaeology of plague. In Buikstra, J. E. (Ed.), *Bioarchaeologists Speak Out*, pp. 109–131. Cham, Switzerland: Springer Nature.
DeWitte, S. N. & Wissler, A. (2021). Demographic and evolutionary consequences of pandemic diseases. *Bioarchaeology International* 6(Special Issue):15–39.
Drancourt, M. & Raoult, D. (2005). Palaeomicrobiology: current issues and perspectives. *Nature Reviews: Microbiology* 3:3–35.
Dvorak, G. D. & Spickler, A. R. (2008). Glanders. *Journal of the American Veterinary Medical Association* 233:570–577.
French, C. T., Bulterys, P. L., Woodward, C. L., Tatters, A. O., Ng, K. R. & Miller, J. F. (2020). Virulence from the rhizosphere: ecology and evolution of Burkholderia pseudomallei-complex species. *Current Opinion in Microbiology* 54:18–32.
Gassiep, I., Armstrong, M. & Norton, R. (2020). Human melioidosis. *Clinical Microbiology Reviews* 33(2):e00006–19. doi: 10.1128/CMR.00006–19.
Krieger, N. (2013). History, biology, and health inequities: emergent embodied phenotypes and the illustrative case of the breast cancer estrogen receptor. *American Journal of Public Health* 103(1):22–27.
Lipsitch, M. (2018). Why do exceptionally dangerous gain-of-function experiments in influenza? *Influenza Virus: Methods and Protocols, Methods in Molecular Biology* 1836:589–608. Springer Science+Business Media, LLC, part of Springer Nature. https://doi.org/10.1007/978-1-4939-8678-1_29.
Losada, L., Ronning, C. M., DeShazer, D., Woods, D., Fedorova, N., Kim, H. S., ... & Nierman, W. C. (2010). Continuing evolution of *Burkholderia mallei* through genome reduction and large-scale rearrangements. *Genome Biology and Evolution* 2:102–116.
Mays, S. (2021). A content analysis by bibliometry of the first ten years of the *International Journal of Paleopathology*. *International Journal of Paleopathology* 34:217–222.
Moodie, R. L. (1923). *Palaeopathology: An Introduction to the Study of Ancient evidences of Disease*. The University of Illinois Press.
Nerlich, A. G., Galassi, F. M. & Bianucci, R. (2021). The burden of arteriosclerotic cardiovascular disease in ancient populations. In Hoon, D. & Bianucci, R. (Eds.), *The Handbook of Mummy Studies* pp. 147–162. Springer Nature.
Ortner. D. J. & Putschar, W. G. J. (1981). *Identification of Pathological Conditions in Human Skeletal Remains*. Washington, DC: Smithsonian Institution Press.
Pearson, T., Giffard, P., Beckstrom-Sternberg, S., Auerbach, R., ... Keim, P. (2009). Phylogeographic reconstruction of a bacterial species with high levels of lateral gene transfer. *BMC Biology* 7:78. 10.1186/1741-7007-7-78.
Plomp, K., Roberts, C. A., Elton, S. & Bentley, G. R. (2022a). *Palaeopathology and Evolutionary Medicine: An Integrated Approach*. Oxford: Oxford University Press.
Plomp, K., Roberts, C. A., Elton, S. & Bentley, G. R. (2022b). What's it all about? A legacy for the next generation of scholars in evolutionary medicine and palaeopathology. In Plomp, K., Roberts, C. A., Elton, S. & Bentley, G. R. (Eds.), *Palaepathology and Evolutionary Medicine: An Integrated Approach*, pp. 1–16. Oxford: Oxford University Press.

Reid, A. H., Fanning, T. G., Hultin, J. V. & Taubenberger, J. (1999). Origin and evolution of the 1918 "Spanish" influenza virus hemagglutinin gene. *Proceedings of the National Academy of Sciences* 96:1651–1656.

Rigolot, C. (2020). Transdisciplinarity as a discipline and a way of being: complementarities and creative tensions. *Humanities and Social Sciences Communications* 7(1):1–5.

Ruffer, M. A. (1911). On arterial lesions found in Egyptian mummies (1580BC-525 AD). *The Journal of Pathology and Bacteriology* 15:453–462.

Salo, W. L, Aufderheide, A. A, Buikstra, J. E. & Holcomb, T. A. (1994). Identification of *Mycobacterium tuberculosis* DNA in a Pre-Columbian Peruvian mummy. *Proceedings of the National Academy of Sciences* 91:2091–2094.

Somarelli, J. A., Gardner, H., Cannataro, V., Gunady, E., Boddy, A., … & Townsend, J. (2019). Molecular biology and the evolution of cancer: from discovery to action. *Molecular Biology Evolution* 37(2):320–326. DOI: 10.1093/molbev/msz242.

Schmidt, C. F. (1962). Editorial: one medicine for more than one world. *Circulation Research* 11:901–903.

Sharrer, G. T. (1995). The great glanders epizootic, 1861–1866: a Civil War legacy. *Agricultural History* 69:79–97.

Steckel, R. H., Larsen, C. S., Roberts, C. A., & Baten, J. (2019). *The Backbone of Europe: Health, Diet, Work and Violence Over Two Millennia*. Cambridge: Cambridge University Press.

Steckel, R. H. & Rose, J. C. (1997). *The Backbone of History: Health and Nutrition in the Western Hemisphere*. Cambridge: Cambridge University Press.

Stojanowski, C. M., & Duncan, W. N. (2015). Engaging bodies in the public imagination: bioarchaeology as social science, science, and humanities. *American Journal of Human Biology* 27(1):51–60.

Thomas, R. (2012). Nonhuman paleopathology. In Buikstra, J. E. & Roberts, C. A. (Eds.), *The Global History of Paleopathology: Pioneers and Prospects*, pp. 652–664. Oxford University Press.

Thompson, R. C., Allam, H., Lombardi, G. P., … & Thomas, G. (2013). Atherosclerosis across 4000 years of human history: the Horus study of four ancient populations. *Lancet* 381:1211–1222.

Tumpey, T. M., Basler, C. F., Aguilar, P. V., Zeng, H., Solórzano, A., Swayne, D. E., … & García-Sastre, A. (2005). Characterization of the reconstructed 1918 Spanish influenza pandemic virus. *Science* 310:77–80.

Uhl, E. W., Kelderhouse, C., Buikstra, J. E., Blick, J. P., Bolon, B. & Hogan, R. J. (2019). New World origin of canine distemper: interdisciplinary insights. *International Journal of Paleopathology* 24:266–278.

Uhl, E. W. & Thomas, R. (2022). Uncovering tales of transmission. In Plomp, K. A., Roberts, C. A., Bentley, G. & Elton, S. (Eds.), *Palaeopathology and Evolutionary Medicine*. Oxford: Oxford University Press. DOI: 10.1093/oso/9780198849711.003.0017.

Van Zandt, K. E., Greer, M. T. & Gelhaus, H. C. (2013). Glanders: an overview of infection in humans. *Orphanet Journal of Rare Diseases* 8:131.

Wiersinga, W. J., van der Poll, T., White, N. J., Day, N. P. & Peacock, S. J. (2006). Melioidosis: insights into the pathogenicity of *Burkholderia pseudomallei*. *Nature Reviews. Microbiology* 4:272–282.

Wilkinson, L. (1981). Glanders: medicine and veterinary medicine in common pursuit of a contagious disease. *Medical History* 25:363–384.

Williams, G. C. & Nesse, R. M. (1991). The dawn of Darwinian medicine. *The Quarterly Review of Biology* 66(1):1–22.

Zink, A. R. & Maixner, F. 2019. The current situation of the Tyrolean Iceman. *Gerontology* 65(1):1–8. https://doi.org/10.1159/000501878.

INDEX

Note: **Bold** page numbers refer to tables; *italic* page numbers refer to figures.

Aboriginal Australians 202
abscess *28,* **327**, 330, 331, 332, 333, 546; *see also* dental abscess
achondroplastic dwarfism 198, 217; *see also* development (developmental) conditions
actinomycosis 558
activity patterns **55**, 197, 198, 220, 511; *see also* stress indicators
adaptation 2, 4, 122, 146, 193, 264, 324, 343, 399, 449, 505, 526, 534, 543, 544, 566, **595,** 632, 633
adenocarcinoma 218
aDNA *see* DNA
adolescence, adolescent 30, 71, 124, 125, 194, 196, 298, 316, 317, 329, 330, 345, 405, 406, 417–427, 471, 533
adult(s): dental disease 368, 372; developmental conditions *253*, 260, 261; developmental origins of disease 522–524, 532, 533; differential diagnosis 48, **54**, **55**; disability and care **467**, **468**, 470, 472, 473; fossil record 547; genetic analyses 148; histopathology 69, 70, 71, 73, 75, 76, **91**, 96; infectious diseases 329, *330*, 331, 333, 334; isotopic analyses 121; macroscopic analyses **25**, 27, 30; marginalization 487, 491; metabolic and endocrine diseases 340, 341, 346, 352; mummified remains 217; mycobacterial infection 307, 310, 312, 316, 317; osteobiographies 194, 196, 197, 198; parasitology 165, **168**; plagues and pandemics 580, 585; perceptions of **596**; stress 402, 406, 407; structural violence 420, 421, 422, 423, 426, 506, 509, 511, 512, 513, 514; traumatic injuries 234, 235, 238, 243; treponemal infection 273, **277**, 285, 298, 300
adulthood 70, 71, 120–121, 124, 263, 284, 330, 360, 512, 520, 523, 524
Africa, African(s) 2, **54**, 167, 169, 202, 256, 280, 297, 298, 299, 300, 307, 309, 315, 509, 526, 527, 568, 582, 583, 586, **598**, **601**, 630, 633
African American 5, 203, 365, 372, 441, 448, 485, 526–527, 533; descendant communities 384, 391; Grave and Repatriation Protection Act (AAGPRA) 383, 489; Legacy 526, 527; *see also* New York African American Burial Ground
African sleeping sickness 167
Aggregatibacter actinomycetemcomitans 365
age-at-death 76, 121, 215, 407, 513, 532, 565; distribution 69, 73, *330;* estimation 68, 76, 94, 95–96, 284, 387
aging, effect on bone 96, 339, 352, 422, 444
agency, human 7, 122, 349, 388, 418, 420, 421, 422, 435–451, 461, 462, **466**, 490, 504, 533, 566
aggression 8, 400, 507, 548
agriculture 122, 568; effects of 65, 66, 197, 353, 582, 628; isotopes 122; impact on dentition 362, 363, 371
AIDS *see* HIV
Alaska 31
Alexander the Great 185, **601**, **607**
allostasis 398–399, 407, 408
ameloblastoma 28, 549
amelogenesis 293
American *see* United States
American Anthropological Association (AAA) 599

637

American Association of Biological (Physical) Anthropologists (AABA, AAPA) 10, 381; Code of Ethics 383; Statement on Race 439
Amish 72
amphibians 280, 543, 548, 549, 552
amputation 331, 346, 347, **464**, 472, 486, 548; *see also* trauma
anatomical collections 4, 5, 9, 28, 45, **46**, 202, 204, 389, 391, 444, 448, 486, 488, 506, 558
Anatolia *see* Turkey
ancient DNA (aDNA) *see* DNA
Ancient One, The 202, 257, 383, 600
anemia 65, 343–344, 401, 513, 531; chronic 124, 146, 147, 401–402; diagnosis of 30, 45, **54**, 69, 122, 181; effects on bone 343, **344, 348,** 349–350, 352; etiology of 171, 172, 338, 343, 349, 401, 402; hemolytic 348, 402; iron-deficiency (acquired) 343, 348; megaloblastic 402; and red blood cells (RBC) 344, 349; sickle cell 147, 402; thalassemia 148, 343, 402; *see also* cribra orbitalia; porotic hyperostosis
Anglo-Saxon 182, 198, 310
animal(s) 3, 6, 8, 9, 71, 86, 487; abuse and neglect 566; as food 122, 307, 561; cancer (neoplasm) 280, 282, 549; congenital defects 252; dental pathologies 562, **563,** 565, 566, **596;** domestic 169, 313, 563, **564,** 582, **595;** human interaction 158, 167, 199, 306, 314, 324, 325, 558, 568, 579, 626; lesions in 95, 258, 565; paleopathology 1, 124, 146, 169, 213, 252, 313, 541, 542, 543, 544, 552, 558–562, 570, 630–634; and trauma 548, 565, 567; and tuberculosis 306, 313, 314, 315, 569; wild 563; *see also* archaeozoology; fauna; zooarchaeology; zoonoses
ankylosis 24, 240, 253, 328
anthrax 84
anthropophagy 504, 514
antibiotics **54**, 283, 284, 286, 307, 329, *330*, 332, 577, 583, 631; resistance 307, 335, 577
apatite dissolution 87
archaeoparasitology *see* parasitology
archaeozoology 558, 560; *see also* zooarchaeology
Archaic Period, USA 470, 471, 472
archive 44, 59, 107, 141, 159, 160, 219, 296
archosaurs 546
Argentina 371, 568
armadillos 167, 307, 313
Arroyo Hondo, New Mexico 194
arsenic 86, 293, 294
arteries 114, 217, 333, 403
arteriosclerosis 84
arthritis: osteoarthritis 23, 34, **35, 55,** 65, 75, 110, *111,* 112, 124, 196, 198, 204, 253, 255, **275, 276,** 328, 329, 469, 473, 486, 513, **602;** rheumatoid **55**, 196, 218, **275,** 328; septic 334; *see also* joint disease
Ascaris sp. 145, 163, 167, **168**, 216
Asia 2, 149, 162, 166, 169, 171, 192, 197, 216, 256, 297, 307, 309, 364, 471, 488, 489, 557, 562, **563**, 568, 579, 582, 632, 633
Athens 198, 240
atherosclerosis 85, 114, 214, 217, 626, 628
Aufderheide, Arthur 212
aurochs 559, 566
Australian Aboriginal 202
Australopithecus sediba 280
autolysis 210
autopsy 181, 201, 202, 211, 212, 213, 284, 339, 486–487, **614**, **615**

Bacillus anthracis 84
bacteria, bacterial 6, 83, 84, 86, 87, 148, 166, 186, 187, 240, 279, 306, 308, 315, 316, 317, 324, 365, 400, 550, 582, 598, **601–611**; DNA 143–144, 145, 148–150, 214–215; oral 363, 364; pyogenic 326, 335; *see also specific bacteria taxa*
bacteriology 329
Barker Hypothesis 522
Bartonella quintana 166
bears (cave) 550, 551
bejel *see* treponemal infection
bias: in disease identification 20, 31, 36, **50, 51,** 272, 585; and ethical concerns 310, 393; racial 533; skeletal samples and sampling 64, 66, 67, 121, 140, 252, 283, 286, 297, 315, 364, 448, 582; social 2, 10, 241, 293, 435, 437, 441, 446, 447, 450, 451, 491, 565; systemic 45, 310, 382, 389, 596, 618
bibliometric survey 20–24, 29, 193
bioarchaeology 9, 47, 118, 147, 192, 193, 211, 219, 292, 300, 309, 312, 368, 371, 382, 387, 388, 397, 418, 419, 435, 442, 459, 462, 483, 510, 511, 619; of care model 197, 201, 311, 460, 461, 464, 459, 460, 461, 465–474, 618; and case studies 195, 203; and ethics 383–385, 387, 391, 393, 419; life history, life course approach 520, 521, 522, 524, 530–534; population approach 195, 578; social 7, 121, 220, 241, 442, 482, 486, 504, 505, 506, 528
biocultural approach 193, 220, 241, 419, 505
bioethics *see* ethics
biological approach **26**, 45, **46**
biomechanics 88, 95, 255, 261, 366, 406, 546, 552; of trauma 231–233, 236, 242
biomolecules, biomolecular: methods 162–163; and *Mycobacteria* 309, 310, 313–317, 568, 569; stable isotopes 6, 76, 128, 325, 526, 578, 582; and tumors and neoplasms 272, 278–279; and zooarchaeology 564; *see also* DNA

Index

BIPOC (Black, Indigenous, People of Color) 202, 203, 387, 393, 618
Biraben, Jean 183
birds 280, 542, 543, 544, 545, 546, 548, 559, 560, 626
birth 31, 71, 72, 194, 215, 251, 263, 307, 316, 406, 424, 425, 436, 443, 450, 484, 503, 520, 522, 523, 524, 528, 529, 531, 532, **611**; *see also* childbirth (birthing)
birth weight 407, 484, 520, 522, 523, 525, 527, 528, 529, 531
bison 547
Black, women 201, 440, 448, 490
Black Death 70, 73, 74, 143, 148, 149, 533, 579–580, 599, **605**, **609**, 627; *see also* plague
Black feminist theory 448, 490
Black, Indigenous, and People of Color *see* BIPOC
Boas, Franz 386
body modification 201, 234, 242, 443; *see also* trauma
bog bodies *see* mummified remains
bone: composition of 88, 108, 112, 124, 511; cortical (dense; compact) 27, 30, 83, 87, 88, **89**, **91**, 92, 94, 96, 328, 331, 332, **344**, 345, *348*, 349, 350, 402, 406, 445, *545*; effects of aging on 96, 339, 352, 422, 444; formation **26**, 27, 29, 30; growth 424, 445, 544; lamellar 30, 88, **90**, **91**, 92, 96, 238, 402; loss 47, 236, 338, 339, 345, 352, 353, 365, 626; mineralization and demineralization 27, 30, **55**, 86, 92, 122, 127, 338, 341, **342**, 346, *348*, 350, *351*; remodeling 27, **28**, 29, 30, 32, 48, **54**, **55**, **89**, **91**, 92, 96, 231, 234, 238, *239*, 326, **342**, 349, 368, 365, 412, 546, 548, 559; repair 56, 88, 92, 238, 273, 326, 328, 360, 541, 548; trabecular (spongy; cancellous) 26, 27, *28*, **88**, **89**, **90**, 92, 112, 255, 331, **344**, 346, 350, 402; woven 30, 47, 48, 88, **90**, **91**, 92, 238
bone cells *see* osteoblasts; osteoclasts; osteocytes
brachydactyly 251, 254, 256, 259, 262
Brazil 5, 163, 166, 197, 214, 217, 296, 307, 363, 367, **468**
Britain *see* United Kingdom
British Columbia 256
Brodie's abscess 331, 333, 546
Bronze Age 113, 148, 149, 169, 240, 260, **468**, **595**, **607**
Brucella melitensis 144, 326
brucellosis 25, 122, 326, 328, 569
bubonic plague *see* plague; *Yersinia pestis*
burial(s) 2, 28, 87, 148, 149, 161, **169**, 198, 202, 281, 317, 386, 446, *467*, 473, 487, **607**, **608**, **610**; practices, treatment 70, 71, 86, 184, 203, 252, 259, 261, 162, 263, 364, 310, 360, 369, *403*, 441, 442, 446, 448, *467*, 487, 488, 508, 509, 514, 578; perceptions of **612**, **614**, **615**, **617**
Burkholderia 632, 633, 634

calcaneus 256, 259
calculus *see* dentition, calculus
California, US 241, 364, 506, 547, 630
callus 238, *239*, *545*, 548, 558, 567
Canada 199, 309, 426
Canary Islands 299
cancer: aDNA 147, 151, 278–279; breast 57, 186; carcinoma 27, 110, 218, 220, **274**, **275**, **276**; evolution of 281–282; histology 278; metastatic **25**, **26**, 27, 29; metastatic carcinoma 27, 110, 275; past prevalence 280, 281, 282–286, 549; sarcoma (osteosarcoma) 97, 112, **274**, **276**, 278, 280, 281, 545, 549; *see also* neoplasm; tumors
Cancer Research in Ancient Bodies (CRAB) 281
canaliculi 88, 89
canine distemper 595, 632
cannibalism *see* anthropophagy
caprine(s) 559, 562, **563**; *see also* goats; sheep
captive, captive-taking 450, 503, 504, 509
carbon 119, 121, 124, 315, 316, 484, 524, 531; carbon 13 ($\delta^{13}C$) 119, 121, 122, 124, 125, 126, 315, 316, 317, 371
Carboniferous 547, 548, 549, 550
care *see* bioarchaeology of care; Index of Care
caregivers 48, 460, 462, **466**, 471, 474, 475, 512
carcinoma 27, 110, 218, 220, **274**, **275**, **276**; *see also* tumor and cancer
caries *see* dental, caries
caries sicca 294, 295
carpal bones 253
Caribbean 299, 300, 526
cartilage 92, 211, 238, 240, **274**, 334, 548
Cartagena, Colombia 299
case studies 8, 21, 22, 23, **25**, 51, 141–150, 192, 200–204, 215, 219, 241, 264, 286, 388, 447; best practices 193–196; and biohistorical approach 199–200; and developmental conditions 254–255; and disability and impairment 198–199, **467–469**, 471; history of 192–193; in paleopathology 23–25, 388, 504, 505, 506, 511, 594, 600, 612, 628; and personhood 199; and stigma 198; and trauma and violence 196–197; *see also* osteobiography
case control studies 64
castration, *castrati* 445, **601**
catabolism 124, 125, 317
catacombs 86, 260, 386
cattle 170, 364, 507, 550, 562, 563, 567, 568, **596**, 632
cell, bone 96, 552; *see also* osteoblasts; osteoclasts; osteocytes

cemetery (cemeteries) 5, 252, 259, 264, 283, 285, 310, 311, 312, 317, 488, 491, 511, 513, 524
Cenozoic 549
chagas disease 167, 214, 216, 217, 472
charcot joint 347
cherubism 217, 220
chi-square analyses 22, 23, 75
child abuse *see* trauma
childbirth (birthing) 202, 424, 425, 428, 449, 450, 451, 487, **607**, **610**, 620
child sacrifice 421, 602
children, childhood 8, 42, 71, 73, 119, 120, 121, 124, 125, 197, 217, 311, 312, 317, 447, 450, 522, 524, 528, 602, **618**; cancer (neoplasm) 217, **274**, **275**, **277**, 320; care 417, 424, 426, **428**, 471, **616**; dental disease and conditions 293, 360, 369, 372; developmental conditions 263; disability/impairment 462, 471; growth 30, 48, **54**, **90**, 330, 529; infectious disease 72, 317, 329, *330*, 331, 332, 333, 334, 335, 584; metabolic disorders **55**, 197, 312, 341, 344, 345, 403, **607**; stress 372, 399, 402, 418, 485, 486, 524, 526, 532, 533; trauma (fractures) 231, 234, 235, 236, 242, 243, 420–421, 484; violence 417, 418–420, 421–423, 426, 484, 489, 491, 509–512, 513, **614**, **616**, **617**; *see also* infant; juveniles; subadult
Chile 165, 170, 172, 214, 216, 309, 316, 370, 472
China 166, 169, 180, 309, 315, 371, 503, 523, 557, **595**, **605**, **607**, **608**, **609**, 629
cholera 84, 144, 182
chronic conditions: dental 365, 367, 403; and development 120, 522, 524, 526, 528; and growth 520; and impairment and care **468**, **469**, 472, 487; infectious diseases **55**, 122, 125, 128, 167, 215, 217, 218, 311, **332**, 333, 400, **468**, 472, 486, 578, 626; metabolic disorders 124, 128, 146, 338, 352, 401, 402, **403**; in paleopathological literature 610; and parasites 170; and stress 201, 399, 400, 533; trauma (fractures) 261, 486; and violence 443, 444, 460, 484, 486, 513
church registers 184
climate change 8, 128, 296, 360, 474, 515, 577, **604**, **615**, 633
cleft palate 251, 253, 262
cloaca 331, 332, 333
Clonorchis sinensis **168**, 169, 216
Cobb, William Montague Human Skeletal Collection 5, 390, 391, 488
Cockburn, Aidan 211, 212, 324
Cocoliztli 578
coevolution 76, 365
collagen 89, 90, 91, 92, 121, 122, 124, 125, 127, 211, 232, 316, 339, 402, 531
colonial, colonization 2, 4, 9, 200, 209, 365, 385, *403*, 485, **602**, 632; effects and consequences of 9, 371, 387, 393, 409, 426, 463, 489, 509, 527, 569, 585
Columbian 299; hypothesis 299, 300, 583
commingled 48, 198, 259, 352, 361, 362, 369, 561
communication 6, 48, 59, 140, 213, 296, 372, 391, 559, 593, 594, 596, 599, 600, 619, 620; *see also* publications
community 66, 106, 137, 138, 141, 142, 148, 159, 161, 170, 203, 308, 335, 340, 344, 345, 364, 368, 371, 372, 384, 418, 421, 438, 442, 444, 509, 596, 597, 598, 600, **601–611**, **616**; of care 194, 197, 220, 261, 311, 457, 459, 461, 462, 466, **468**, 469, 487, 488; descendent 9, 138, 390, 391, 392; of engagement 9, 202, 382, 620, 625; health 196, 201, 316, 317, 347, 350, 353, 364, 401, 421, 444, 447, 585, 586, 594
co-morbidity 239, 463, **465**, 470, 527
comparative approach 32, 45, **46**
compassion 201, 459, 461
computerized tomography (CT) *see* imaging techniques
congenital abnormalities 8, 21, **22**, 24, 49, 211, 214, 236, **250**, 251, 254, 255, 258, 261, 293, 294, 298, 369, 407, 417, **437**, 460, 464, 473, 542, 551, 552, 563, 583, 585, **596**; *see also* developmental disorder
contaminated, contamination 324, 328, 329, 333; in DNA analyses 137, 138, 139, 140, 142, 144, 149, 279; food 170; in parasitology 163, 171
coprolites 139, 145, 158, 159, *160*, 163, 164, 165, **168**, **169**, 171, 172, 210, 472, **598**, **601–611**, 612
coronary artery disease *see* atherosclerosis
COVID–19 307, 313, 533, 576, 586, 593, 599, 620, 627; *see also* SARS CoV–2
cows *see* cattle
cranium 65, 197, 234, 256, 261, 362, 369, 402, 486, 510, 514
Charles Creighton 182–183
cremation 127, 369, **597**
Cretaceous 547, 549
cribra orbitalia 65, 69, 73, **74**, 76, 348, 401, 402, 532, 580; interpretation of 109, 122, 172, 348, 407; and isotope analysis 125; *see also* anemia
cross-cultural 363, 419, 425, 436, 464, 508
cross-tabulation analyses 75
crucifixion **603**, 615, 617
Cunningham debate *see* diagnosis of disease
Cyprus 65, 198
cysts 55, 110, *111*, 112, 166, **168**, **169**, 170, 217, 252, 273, 366, 546
cytopathic effect 326

Danish 73, 74, 112, 259, 310, 316, 559
data 20–21, 59; analysis and interpretation 10, 32–33, 65, 68, 69–76, 118, 122, 123, 125, 126, 127, 213, 220, 231, 371, 389, 390, 436,

438, 443, 449, 465, 487–488, 505, 511, 544; clinical 6, 114, 198, 215, 282, 511, 586; collection, recording 1, 24, 26, 30, 31, 49, 65, 68, 86, 139, 142, 233, 372, 435, 448; genomic 8, 137, 138, 139, 146–147, 148–151, 296–298, 300, 584; population-level 32–33, 139, 256, 257, 280, 283, 580, 628; standardization 5, 194, 219, 242; types of 32–33, 36, 46, 50–52, 106, 113, 120, 121, 123, 128, 136, 140, 164, 170, 172, 212, 241, 279, 307, 325, 408, 435, 447, 482, 485, 508, 619; *see also* database(s)

database(s) 114, 123, 145, 162, 183, 186, 188, 315, 504, 526, 599; bibliometric 20, *21*; Cancer Research in Ancient Bodies (CRAB) 28; European Nucleotide Archive 296; IMPACT 219; National Center for Biotechnology Information 296; Wellcome Osteological Database, Museum of London 312

death 28, 32, 53, 68, 72, 144, 195, 197, 198, 201, 202, 261, 271, 272, 326, 332, 338, 349, 388, 419, 442, 474; cause of 2, 30, **46**, **55**, 70, 185, 187, 199, 200, 201, 218, 253, 262, 307, 311, 421, 424, 443, 450, 470, 483, 456, 502, 508, 514, 582, 583, 603, **606**, **607**, **610**, 617, 631, 632; registers 182, 184; risk of 64, 66, 67, 69, 70, 71, 72, 73, **74**, 361, 450; time of 239, 314, **342**, 532, 561; treatment after 311, 390, 425, 426, **466**, **468**, 482, 489, 503, 507, 563, **615**, 617

decalcification 84, 93, 94

decolonization 1, 5, 10, 203, 381, 383, 385–387, 391, 426, 634

decomposition 82, 84, 86, 87, 210, 386, 508

deductive (reasoning, analysis) 558, 565, 566, 599, 600, 613–619

deer 559, 566, 567

degenerative diseases conditions 460, 472, 524, 576; *see also* specific diseases

degenerative joint disease *see* joint disease

demography 48, 74, 197, 200, 212, 231, 232, 233, 240, 262, 273, 283, 284, 285, 292, 295, 296, 301, 324, 344, 360, 421, 443, 448, 449, 450, 470, 471, 485, 510, 562, 576, 577, 586

Denmark 70, **74**, 169, 170, 259, 310, 582, **596**

dental enamel hypoplasia *see* enamel hypoplasia

dentin, dentine 96, 119, 121, 124, 125, 126, 138, 316, **342**, 360, 363, 366, 367, 408, 531, 532, 548, **595**, **597**

dentition, dental: abfraction 366, *367*, 368; ablation 368, 369; abrasion 293, 366, *367*; abscess **35**, 326, 366, 371; agenesis 263, 370; attrition 366; ante-mortem tooth loss 361, 368–369; calculus 75, 127, 139, 143, 144, 312, 314, 361, 362, 363–365, 371, 372, 373, 580, 629; caries **35**, **54**, 65, 73, 294, 362–363, 365, 366, 368, 369, 370, 371, 372, 485, 486, **598**; defects (anomalies) 251, 486, 513, 532, 565; disease 6, 21, 22, 24, 108, 196, 202, 360–373, 579; and subsistence strategies 363, 37; transposition 263, 264, 370; trauma **22,** 484; and treponemal diseases 293, 294, 299; wear 366, 368, 369, 371; *see also* enamel hypoplasia

dermal plates 548

descendant, descendant community 126–127, 138, 140, 141, 142, 147, 202, 203, 204, 381, 382, 384, 385, 388, 389, 390–391, 392, 489, 578

desiccation 86, 93, 165, 213, 278

destructive analyses 31, 52, 82, 92, 95, 105, 118, 126, 138, 141, *143*, 212, 260, 279, 280, 295, 313, 314, 326, 333, 361, 423, 489, 561, 578, 631

developmental conditions: anomalies 250–264, 273, 361, 417, 458, 513, 544, 551–552; of enamel 403–405; *see also* specific conditions/disorders

Developmental Origins of Health and Disease (DOHaD) hypothesis 120, 399, 418, 490, 520–534

diabetes mellitus 339, 484, 523, 524, 626; Type 2 338, 346–347, 520

diagenesis 87, 92

diagnosis 10, 19, 20, 24, 25, 27, 30, 32, 82, 83, 86, 95, 96–97, 186, 254, 325, 352, 460, 463, 632; accuracy and rigor of 4, 6, 23, 27; and aDNA 278–279, 564; and anemia 343–350; Cunningham debate 186–187; and diabetes 346; and historical texts 184, 186; of historical figures, individuals 185; macroscopy 272; microscopy and histology 82, 83, 95, 96–97, 278; modern biological 188, 487; and mycobacterial diseases 310–311, 314, 581, 583, **595**; and paleontology 543–546; and parasites 162, 167, **168**; retrospective 180, 185, 186, 187, 188, 466; and rickets 350, and radiography 105, 110, 112, 114, 214, 273–278, social 180, 487; and treponemal disease 293–296; and zooarchaeology 565, 566; *see also* differential diagnosis

diet 4, 6, 8, **57**, **58,** 196, 220, 260, 422, 569; and care **464**, 471, 472; and dental disease 360, 362, 363, 364, 365, 366, 367, 368, 370, 371, 372, 404, 409, 531; and development 521, 522, 530, 531; and isotopic analysis 119, 120–121, 123, 124, 127, 423, 514; and metabolic diseases 339, 340, 341, 343, 346, 347, 349, 351, 352, 402, 551; and mycobacterial diseases 308, 314, 316, 317, 581, 582; and neoplasms 283, 284, 549; and parasitology 158, 159, 160, 163, 170, 171, 172; *see also* food; nutrition; subsistence strategies

differential diagnosis 6, 23, 43–59, 188, 404, 447, 543, 544, 570; and histology 96–97; and infectious disease 333, 334, 335, 351; and macroscopy 25–27; and neoplastic disease 273, 278; and pseudopathology 29; and treponemal disease 293–296

differential mortality *see* mortality
diffuse idiopathic skeletal hypertrophy (DISH) 197
dinosaurs 280, 542, 544, 545, 546, 548, 549, 550
diphtheria 182, 183
disability 196, 198–199, 200, 233, 241, 308, 311, 418, 422, 423, 426, 444, 457–475, 483, 487, 491, 508, 620; theory of 7, 8; *see also* impairment
disarticulated remains 253, 421, 547, 562, 565, **614**
discrimination 147, 214, 307, 383, 439, 490
disease *see specific diseases*
disease categories 56
disenfranchisement, social 5, 482, 488, 583
dislocation *see* trauma
dissection 83, 181, 185, 201, 202, 211, 212, 238, 260, 386, 444, 445, 448, 449, 486–487
DNA (aDNA), analysis 6, 7, 56, 76, 136–151, 181, 295, 388, 423, 472, 509, 524, 525, 527, 560, 564, 568, 580, **597**, **598**, 599, **601–611**, **615**, **616**, 625, 626, 633; archive 141; anemias 146; *Ascaris lumbricoides* 145, 163; bacterial (bacteria) 143–144, 214; *Bordetella pertussis* 214; *Borrelia recurrentis* 144; *Brucella melitensis* 144; contamination/decontamination 142; *Enterobius vermicularis* 163; *Escherichia coli* 214; ethics 140–141, 142, 145–147; extraction 138; eukaryotic 145–146; *Gardnerella vaginalis* 144; and genetic disorders 217–218, 264; *Helicobacter pylori* 144; and hepatitis 215–216; history in paleopathology 137; laboratory methods 138–139; and microbiome 144–145; *Mycobacteria sp.* 26, 142, 144, 150, 214, 309, 313–314, 315, 335, 365, 547, 550, 569, 631; *Mycolicibacterium* 142; methylation 524; in parasitology 159, 160, 162, 166, 167, 216–217; PCR 137; *Plasmodium spp.* 145, 167; *Salmonella enterica* 144, 578; sampling 138, *143;* sequencing 140; single nucleotide polymorphisms (SNPs) 139; *Staphylococcus spp.* 144; *Tannerella forsythia* 365; *Teania spp.* 145; terms used 136; *Treponema spp.* 144, 214, 293, 297, 298, 585; *Trichuris trichiura* 163; *Trypanosoma cruzi* 167, 216; tumors and neoplasms 147, 278–279; *Yesinia pestis* 141, 148–149, 335; *Variola ssp.* 215; viral (virus) 145, 215
documents (historical) 182, 183, 283, 317, 332, 485, 506, 584; *see also* church, registers; death, registers
dogs 163, 167, 170, 199, 563, 564, 566, 568, **604**, **609**, 632
domestic abuse *see* violence
domestication, domesticated 371, 550, 558, 564, 566, 568, 569, **595**, 626
Down's syndrome 251, 263, 264
draught (draft) animals 562

dual process model (DPM) **25**
dwarfism 23, 198, 217, 253, 255, 261, **276**, 462, 605
dysentery 171, 182, **609**
dysplasia 252, 253, 255, 260

Ebola 576, 586
ectoparasites 160, 165–166, 181, 579
Echinococcus **169**, 170
Echinostomiasis 169
ecological, ecology 4, 47, 65, 118, 120, 128, 137, 145, 151, 159, 164, 187, 195, 220, 295, 313, 396, 389, 399, 404, 520, 522, 524, 525, 529, 533, 560, 582, 584, **598**, 630, 631; determinism 122
economy 66, 371, 418, 512
Egyptian, Egypt 4, 106, 181, 216, 217, 258, 261, 263, 281, 283, 284, 308, 309, 339, 346, 368, 542, **601**, **604**, **607**, **609**, **610**; mummified remains (mummification) 3, 84, 85, 93, 105, 108, 112, 114, 137, 166, 167, 169, 213, 214, 626
electron microscopy *see* imaging techniques
embalming 112, 213
embodiment 368, 373, 392, 486, 529, 530, 578; theory 369, 372, 436, 445–446, 451, 483, 484, 490
empathy 203, 425, **597**, **598**, **601–611**, 612, **614**, **615**, 617
enamel hypoplasia (linear enamel hypoplasia 'LEH') 2, 29, **34**, 65, 73, 74, 76, 125, 202, 293, 299, 369–370, 403–404, *405,* 423, 485, 532, 580
endocranium 309, 310, **340**, 403, 580
endocrine system 88; diseases 7, **276**, 277, 338–353, 402, 565
endosteum **26**, 27, 88, **89**, 91, 92, 109, **275**, 333, 512
England *see* United Kingdom
Enlightenment Period/Era 385, 386, 387–388
enslaved, enslavement 9, 203, 241, 298–300, 372, 384, 420, 426, 484, 487, 489, 503, 504, 509, 526, 527, 533, 586, 597, **601**, **602**, **613**, **614**, **615**, **617**, 633
Enterobius vermicularis 161, 162, 163, **168**, 171, 216
entheseal change 255, **595**
enthesopathy 233
environment, environmental: conditions 2, 3, 10, 31, 47, 58, 65, 67, 69, 76, 86, 88, 164, 210, 220, 232, 250, 260, 283, 284, 308, 386, 388, 389, 390, 393, 419, 445, 459, 485, 490, 549, 630, 631, 633; and bioarchaeology of care **465**, 474, 482, 483, 485; change 4, 8, 9, 324, 485, 577, 626; and childhood 418, 422, 425; and dentition 360, 363, 364, 370, 372; and disease 3, 114, 123, 146, 147, 542, 543, 544, 551, 552, 560, 627, 629, 632, 633; and DNA analysis 139, 142, 144, 149, 217;

and epigenetics 521, 522, 523, 524, 525, 527, 533, 534; genetic 256; maternal 251, 252, 520, 530, 531, 532; and metabolic/endocrine diseases 341, 343, 345, 351, 353; mismatch 282, 529; and mycobacterial infection 306, 307, 312, 313, 314, 316, 582; and parasitology 165, **168**; and stress 398, 406, 409, 547; and treponemal infection 292, 295, 300, 586; and violence 54, 505, 507, 510

Enzyme-Linked Immunosorbent Assay (ELISA) 162, 163, 166

epidemic(s) 7, 8, 69, 70, 74, 166, 182, 183, 297, 299, 325, 406, 576, 577, 578, 579, 580, 581, 582, 583, 584, 586, 626, 627, 632

epidemiology, epidemiological 163, 164, 166, 171, 172, 183, 188, 193, 197, 198, 216, 307, 339, 393, 482, 485, 490, 520, 521, 522, 584, 585, 632, 633, 634; approach/models 64–76, 161, 408, 543, 544, 561, 562, 570; transition 524, 576–577

epigenetics 279, 521, 523, 524–525, 526, 527, 528, 529, 530, 532, 533, 534, 628

equifinality 126, 352

error, observer 32–35, 36, 45, 48–49

Escherichia coli (E. coli) 214, 329

Esper, Johann Friedrich 1, 542, 558

estrogen **54**, 365, 437

ethics, ethical 10, 118, 187, 202, 204, 212, 311, 420, 461–463, 474, 634, **610**; and aDNA 140, 142, 146; codes of 383, 490; and issues involving human remains 52, 126–127, 203, 310, 381–393, 463

ethnic groups, ethnicity **58**, 240, 241, 296, 301, 444, 510, 512, 513, 514, 526, 533, 614, 615, 626

Eudes-Deslongchamps, E. 542

eugenics 382, 384, 386, 387

eukaryote 143, 144, 145–146, 163, 166

Europe, European 2, 3, 4, 8, 170, 256, 298, 300, 315, 386, 605; colonization/contact 66, 170, 171, 202, 292, 299, 314, 439, 514, 586; samples/populations 69, 285, 297, 313, **468**, 566, 579

European Nucleotide Archive 296

evolution, evolutionary 150, 219, 383, 385, 397, 407, 443, 449, 450, 451, 461, 463, 552, 526, 529, 533, 534, 577; anthropology 520; biology 425; of *Burkholderia* 632–634; of cancer 271, 272, 281–282, 286, 549; of canine distemper 632; of disease/pathogens 1, 4, 6, 8, 47, 56, 114, 123, 136, 137, 139, 140, 151, 210, 218, 219, 220, 262, 329, 343, 347, 372, 373, 541, 543, 552, 559, 579, 586; of healing 542, 548–549; and life history model 407, 408, 409; and *Mycobacterium* 313, 314–315, 564, 569, 583, 631; of parasites 159, 162, 163, 167, 569; publications 594, 595, **597**, 598, **601–611**, 612, 620; pyogenic bacteria 335; of treponemal diseases 292, 299, 300, 550, 584, 585; of violence 503; viral 215, 216, 626; of *Yersia pestis* 149, 580; paleopathology 625, 628–634; zoonoses 569

exostosis 110, 281, 368

fauna 9, 87, 138, 552, 558, 630, 631, 632

feces, paleofeces 137, 138, 145, 158, 159, 163, 166, 167, **168**, **169**, 598, **609**

fecundity 164, 167, 282

feet 112, 233, 252, 254, 259, 262, 275, 308, 444, 563, 564, **595**, **598**

female(s) 7, **25**, **54**, **57**, **168**, 447, 508, 521, 529; and agency 441–442; analysis of 25, 194, 196, 198, 200, 214, 217, 472, 487; and cancer 283; and dental disease 363, 365, 366, 368, 371, 372; and infectious disease 333, 338; and leprosy 314, 316; lesions in **54**, 253, 261; and the obstetrical dilemma 449–451; and osteoporosis 345; parasites **168**; patients **57**, 469; and plague 298; and race 440, 441; scholar 392; and sex and gender determination 436–438, 446; stress 485; and trauma/fractures 241, 242, 346, 441, 442, 506, 507, 509, 513, 514; and violence 241, 243, 444, 488, 509–512; *see also* women

feminism, feminist: approaches 7, 9, 201, 241, 442, 482, 488, 490; archaeology 38; Black 448, 490

femur 25, 73; cancer in 280, 281; cave bear 542, *545*, 558; fracture of 236, 567; infectious disease in 111, 329, *330*, *332*, 333, 336; length **74**, **75**

Fenlanders 426

fetal: bone 92, 401, 449, 528; development 120, 125, 345, 399, 443, 523, 528, 531; hemoglobin production 148; maternal nexus 418, 423, 424, 425, 528, 533; mummy 596; Origins of Adult Disease 522

Finite Element Analysis 546

First African Baptist Church 372

fish 280, 343, 543, 547, 548, 552, 560; and infection 550; and parasites 167, 169, 170, 171, 172; neoplasm in 549

fishing 122

fleas 165, 166, 579

flu *see* influenza

fluke 161, 167, **168**, 169

fluctuating asymmetry 33, 407

fluorine 547

fluorosis 281, 401

folate (folic acid) 252, 260, 338

food 54, 118, 170, 341, 422, 523, 562, 565; and care **464**; contamination 167, 169, 170, 307, 513, 581; and dental disease 360, 361, 363, 364, 365, 366, 367, 368, 370, 371, 372; insecurity/famine 31, 340, 406, 523; and

isotopes 118, 119, 121, 122, 126; and parasites 170, 171; preference 423; and scavenging/gathering 163, 507; *see also* diet
foodborne 145, 167, 169
foot binding 242, 444, **595**
Forbes 593, 594, 599–611
forensic 95, 105, 237, 242, 252, 372, 388, 392, 462, 484, 485, 502, 512; anthropology 195, 242, 383, 384, 387, 503, 505, 617; taphonomy 47
fossils, fossil record 1, 8, 85, 541; developmental disorders in 551–552; diagnosis of disease 543–546, 552; examination methods 546–547; history of study 542–543, 558; infection in 550; metabolic disease in 550–551; neoplasms in 550–551; paleoepidemiological studies of 547; in publications **598;** and teeth 113; traumatic injuries and healing 548–549
Fournier's (mulberry) molars 294
fractionation 118, 119, 121, 126, 127; *see also* kinetic isotope effects
fractures: accidental 242; in animals 567, 568; and biomechanical force 232, 233, 234; complications 239, 328; depression 198; in the fossil record 547, 558; healing of 198, 233, 234, 238–239, 541, 548, 567; interpretation of 242, 492; mechanisms of 236–237; recording 233; and osteoporosis 232, 345; pathological 232, 236, **274, 275, 277**, 403; patterns of 240, 242, 234, 441, 511; stress 236; types of 233, 234, **235**, 240; and violence 443, 485, 508; *see also* trauma
fragments: bone 234, 547, 562, 563, 565; DNA 137, 139, 162, 214, 547; osteon 96
frailty 128, 579; heterogeneity in 66–67, 69, 72, 74, 124, 370, 485, 491, 521, 532, 573, 580, 627; index 408
frame analysis: deductive 613–619; inductive 600–613
France 83, 84, 169, 183, 194, 450, **467**, 580, 584, **607**
Franklin Expedition 213, 617

gastrointestinal 144, 145, 308, 309, 400, **464**, 472, 579, 581, **596**; *see also* intestines
gender: definition of 436; and diseases 7, 57, 201, 365, 368, 469, 507; binary/nonbinary 8, 438, 491; and race 419, 424, 425, 438, 439–441, 512; and identity 241, 423, 435–451; perception of **616,** 618, 619; and social practices (roles) 166, 201, 242, 363, 365, 368, 370, 422, 503, 515; theory 442–443, 483, 490; and violence/trauma 241, 423, 443–445, 485, 506, 507, 510–512
genes, genetic, genome 66, 136–151, 232, 325, 521, 524; analyses 6, 8, 52, 136, 139, 217, 256, 259, 260, 262, 364, 372, 439, 440, **597;** and cancer 147, 218, **277**, 278–280, 282, 629; differential diagnosis 55, 58; disorders (heritable) 146–147, 217, 250, 251, 252, 255, 256, 258, 260–262, 263, 369, 370, 402, 407, 626; drift 260, 566; flow 260, 262, 527; and infectious disease 141–146, 148–150, 214–216, 292, 296–298, 300, 313–315, 584–585, 632, 633, 634; and metabolic diseases 343, 345, 347, 402; and mummified remains 211, 214–218; mutations 58, 137, 217, 218, 250, 251, 272, 297, 402; of parasites 162, 163, 216; and race 8, 383, 439, 440; and relatedness 149, 252, 256, 259, 262, 508, 532; *see also* epigenetics
general adaptation syndrome 2, 399
germ theory 84, 183
Germany 84, 148, 170, 213, 264, 281, 309, 385, *545, 547, 551*, 559, 567, 568, **610**
Gerszten, Enrique 211
Giardia ssp. 166
gigantism 146, 198, **276**, 470
glanders 632–634
Global Burden of Disease 470
Global History of Health Project 69
goats 563, 564, *568; see also* caprines
Gompertz (Gompertz-Makeham) mortality model 70–73
Gorlin syndrome 273, **277**
granuloma, granulomatous 326, **327**, 328
grave(s) 47, 612; goods (accompaniments) 5, 123, 194, 196, 198, 261, 421, 441, **468**, 487; mass or clusters 184, 252, 423, **602, 614, 616**, 617; perceptions of **601, 602, 603, 606, 609, 610, 611**, 612, **614, 615, 616**; robbing 5, 382, 284, 386, **614, 615**
Great Britain *see* United Kingdom
Greece 65, 181, 198, 240, 339, 557, 567, **604**, 633
Greek 83, 271, 567, **602**
growth 30, **54, 55, 90**, 95, 121, 329, 334, 443, 445, 490, 513, 522, 528, 529, 534, 596; disorders 250; disruption (arrest) 73, 109, 121, 125, 170, 299, 316, 369, 404, 405–407, 408, 422, 423, 424, 485, 520, 523, 524, 532, 533; in fossil taxa 544, 546, 547; hormone 400; and metabolic disease 339, 341, 342, 344, 345, 347, 350, *351*, 353; plate 48, 255, 330, 331, 340; of populations 197, 311, 324, 581, 582, 586; of tumors 272, 273, **276**, 280, 281, 282; *see also* development, disorders
gunshot wounds/trauma 27, 238

habitation sites and structures 161, 164, 165, 171
Hamann-Todd Human Osteological Collection 4, 389, 391, 488
hands 114, 197, 218, 256, 309, 311, 441, **603, 609**
Hansen's disease *see* leprosy
Harris lines 109, 407, 409, 484, 547
Haversian canal/bone 83, 88, **90, 91**, 92, 95, 96, 546, 548

Index

hazard model(s) 68, 69–72
healing/ healed 30, 32, 54, 55, 197, 384, 422, 512; evolution of 541, 542, 548–549; of fractures and trauma 90, 109, 110, 124, 198, 233, 235, 237, 238, 239, **468**, 506, 509, 512, 513, 514, 547, 558, 559, 565, 566, 567, 568; infectious disease 295, 328, 333, 334; metabolic disease 55, 197, 341, 342, 351, 491, 532
health: animal 557, 558, 562, 569, 630, 632, 634; belief about 82; of bone 345, 346, 444; and care 461, **464**, **468**, 470, 471, 475; definitions of 64, 458; disparity in 352, 382, 392, 399, 439, 483, 485, 534; of enslaved 299, 484; gut 397; infant/child 418, 420, 422, maternal 252, 340, 345, 407, 408, 423–425; measures of 43, 64, 65, 67–76, 119, 122, 124, 127, 128, 136, 143, 163, 172, 192, 194, 200, 201, 203, 210, 214, 220, 260, 261, 306, 315, 343, 349, 352, 361, 418; and microbiome 144; and mobility 123; and personhood 199; outcomes 352, 353, 439, 440, 490, 507; and pandemics 307, 586–587; public 335, 338, 343, 577, 578, 593, 627, 630; respiratory 312; and violence 418–420, 421–423, 484, 512, **610**
heirloom parasites 159, 162
Helicobacter pylori 144, **598**
helminths 145, 167–172, 342
hemangioma 281, 549
hepatitis 145, 215, 326, 328, **597**
hidden heterogeneity 66–67, 73, 285, 485, 491, 521, 531; *see also* frailty
hierarchical log-linear analyses 68, 75–76
Hippocrates 82, 339, 565, **609**
histology, histological 19; and disease diagnosis 48, 52, 84, 86, 96–97, 251, 260, 309, 372, 402, 404, 532, 542, 543, 544, 552; in mummied remains 86, 212, 214, 215; and tumors and neoplasms 272, 278–279, 281
histomorphology 83, 92, 96, 97, 507
histopathology 85; methods and techniques 24, 84, 85, 92–94, 361, 546
historical documents; and diagnosis 151, 182–183, 185, 200, 283, 293, 298–300, 301, 311, 317, 332, 471, 506, 578, 579, 583, 584, 632; types of 148, 182, 184, 199, 200, 450, 485; *see also* anatomical collections
history: of aDNA 137; of biological anthropology and bioarchaeology 381–382, 387–388; of endocrinology 339; of disease identification and diagnosis; gender and identity 435, 438; of infants and children 417–418; of microscopy 82–84; of mummy studies 212; of neoplasm 271; of paleoepidemiology 65–66; of paleoparasitology 158; of paleontology 542–543; of paleopathology 1–5, 84–86, 192–193; of stress 398–399; of zooarchaeology 557–561

HIV/AIDS 297, 307, 308, 446, 447, 577, 581, 583, 586
Holocene 197, 363, 541, *545*, 551
holistic 9, 19, 193, 211, 231, 255, 325, 389, 417, 426, 427, 521, 530, 552, 632, 633
Homo erectus 281, 460
Homo naledi 280, 368
Homo neanderthalensis see Neanderthals
Homo sapiens 279, 293, 324
homeostasis 210, 398–399, 418, 520
Hooton, Earnest 4, 65, 193
hormones 88, 273, **276;** and endocrine and metabolic disease 338, 341, 344, 345, 401; and growth 405; sex **54**, 437, 443; stress 399, 400, 407
horses 90, 199, 557, 563, 567, 568, 569, 632, 633
horseback riding 199
hospitals 27, 150, 182, 332, 341, 487, **616**; leprosy 150, 310; tuberculosis 311
Hounsfield Units (HU) 106, 108
Hrdlička, Aleš 2, 4, 385, 386
human papillomavirus (HPV) 216
human-pathogen coevolution 76, 365
humerus 25, 73, *111*, 112, 260, 329, **330**, *334*, **344**
Hungary 214, 281, 309, 314, 599, **562**, *564*, 565
hunting 552, 559; and gathering/foraging 65, 66, 122
Hutchinson's teeth 251, 294
hydatid disease **169**, 170, 630
hydrocephaly 253, 273, **276**, 277
hypercalcification 547; *see also* Harris lines
hyperparathyroidism 97, 338, 344–345

Iceland 170, 197, **604**, **606**
Iceman, The *see* Ötzi
Ichthyosaur 547
iconographic, iconography 194, 196, 261, 420
identity 8, 127, 195, 389, 393, 417, 418, 425, 440, 447, 451, 492; children 418, 419, 420; community/group 371, 420, 421, 507; gender 423, 436–439, 443, 448, 510; individual 387–388, 466; social 138, 369, 422, 465, 468, 483, 490, 503, 512
imaging, techniques: 3D visualizations 105, 106, 108, 138, 273, 278, 361; computerized tomography (CT) 20, 23, 24, 32, 85, 105, 106, 107–109, *110*, 112, 113, 213, 255, 345, 372, *545*, 550; cone beam (CBCT) 112–113, 361; confocal laser scanning microscopy (CLSM) 85, 161; magnetic resonance imaging (MRI) 113, 114, 213, 219; radiography (X-ray) 19, 20, 27, 53, 105, 106–109, 211, 213, 219, 233, 260, 273, 278, 285, 345; scanning electron microscope (SEM) 85, 94–95, 361; terahertz imaging 114, 213
immobilization 239, 345, **464**, 545
immigration *see* migration

immune system 483; competence/strength 3, 308, 311; compromised 307, 308, 484, 582, 583; function 120, 312, 397, 520, 524; response 54, 55, 66, 147, 238, 277, 282, 326, 327, 328, 338, 343, 365, 400, 401, 545, 546, 627
immunocompetence 76, 401
immunocompromised 582, 583
immunofluorescence assay (IFA) 162
immunology, immunological 121, 144, 159, 162, 166, 212, 214, 216, 292, 422, 523, 524, 544, 582, 626; response 54, 55, 66, 147, 238, 277, 282, 326, 338, 343, 365, 400, 401, 524, 545, 546, 627
impairment 7, 194, 196, 197, 198–199, 200, 233, 239, 240, 241, 308, 309, 351, 457, 459, 467, 468, 469, 473
Inca 172, 371, 487, 614, 616
Index of Care 194, 200, 201, 465, 466, 468, 470, 471
India 5, 58, 166, 201, 465, 466, 468, 470, 471
Indigenous Peoples 126, 127, 202, 371, 426, 489, 605, 614, 615, 620
inductive reasoning 558, 599, 600, 613, 618
industrialization 144, 343, 423, 486, 581, 629; and health 66, 486, 582, 598
inequality *see* social, inequality
infant 8, 30, 47, 48, 120, 121, 197, 198, 263, 298, 300, 329, *330*, 331, 340, 352, 403, 417–427, 468, 485, 487, 522, 524, 525, 527, 528, 529, 520, 531, 532, 569, 585, 605, 614
infant mortality 421, 522, 529, 531
infanticide 263, 264, 420
infection: acute 128, 148, 240, 564, 576; angiitic pattern of 326, 327, 328; bacterial 144, 317; chronic 365, 578, 626; in the fossil record 550; pyogenic 334, 326, 328, 333, 334, 335; infectious disease 4, 7, 324–335; and dental disease 362, 372; detection of 26, 84, 110, 183; diagnosis of 43, 55, 56, 58, 273, 324–326, 486, 631; and DNA analysis 141–146, 314–315, 631; epidemiology 70, 164, 299, 576, 577; evolutionary history of 123, 313, 550, 583, 634; in the fossil record 544; and the life course 408, 524; osteomyelitis 329–333; periostitis 334–335; pyogenic bacteria 335; septic arthritis 334; specific vs. Nonspecific 326–328, 329; spondylodiscitis 333–334; and stress 400; terminology 182, 328; and tissue damage 328; transmission pathways 84, 123, 128, 183, 197, 283, 317; and vitamin D deficiency 352; *see specific pathogens and diseases*
inflammation, inflammatory 2, 47, 88, 124, 218; and dental disease 365, 366; and infectious disease 328, 349; and metabolic disease 350, 352, 403; and stress 397, 407, 409, 484;

influenza 182, 326, 626; 1918 "Spanish Flu" 145, 578, 626, 627
injury *see* trauma
interdiscipline, interdisciplinary 64, 150, 158, 159, 161, 172, 188, 211, 242, 292, 300, 469, 490, 491, 541, 557, 560, 594, 595, 596, 597, 598, 599, 619, 625, 628, 629, 630, 632, 634
International Academy of Pathology 211
International Council for Archaeozoology (ICAZ) 560, 561
International Journal of Osteoarchaeology (IJO) 21, 44, 594, 600
International Journal of Paleopathology (IJPP) 44, 49, 158, 194, 593, 594, 595–596, 598, 600, 601, 602, 603, 604, 605, 607, 608, 609, 610, 628
interpersonal violence 8, 123, 196–197, 234, 243, 441, 442, 468, 485, 503, 505, 506, 508, 509, 510, 511, 513; *see also* trauma
intersectionality 127, 200, 241, 440, 441, 444, 445, 451, 490, 491, 506, 507
intervertebral disks 236, 328, 333, 546
intestines 85, 144, 145, 162, 163, 166, 169, 170, 210, 472, 604, 609; *see also* gastrointestinal
Inuit 165
invertebrates 167, 541
involucrum 331, 332
Irish Famine 124, 423
Iron Age 170, 194, 196, 198, 364, 511, 567, 568, 582, 595, 598, 602
iron 127, 338; *see also* anemia, iron deficiency
isotopes *see* stable isotopes
Israel 148, 163
Istanbul Terminological Protocol 52, 53, 295
Italy 5, 167, 184, 196, 198, 215, 217, 218, 309, 315, 316, 347, 369, 445–446, 569, 603, 608

Jamaica 300
Japan 3, 71, 216, 315, 364, 365, 405, 532, 597
joint disease 3, 23, 346, 542; degenerative joint disease 65, 197, 368, 484; rheumatoid arthritis 55, 196, 218, 275, 328
Jones, Frederic Wood 1
Jurassic 542, 545, 547, 549, 550
juvenile 71, 162, 165, 196, 472, 545, 547, 551

Kaplan-Meier survival analysis 68–69
kappa statistic 33, 34
Kennewick Man *see* Ancient One, The
Kenya 280, 506
King Richard III 199, 597
Kingella kingae 326, 327, 329, 335
kinetic isotope effects 118; *see also* fractionation
Kolmogorov-Smirnov Test 21
Korea 158, 169, 171, 215, 217, 604

La Brea Tar Pits, California 547, 552
La Plata, New Mexico 241, 441, 442, 485

lamellar bone *see* bone
Lateral-Flow Immunoassays (LFIA) 162
Latin 250, 298
Latin America 192, 216
Latin American Antiquity 600, **603**, **604**, **611**
Latrines 144, 145, 161, 163, 164, 165, 166, 167, 169, 170, 171, 180, **609**
Latvia 149, 163, **609**
Legacy African Americans 526, 527, 533
Leishmania sp. 166, 216
leishmaniasis 166
leprosarium (leprosaria) 310, 311, 312, 313, 316, 471
leprosy: and care 426, 470, 471; and disability 198; evolution of 313, 314–316; detection and diagnosis 6, 55, 57, 150, 182, 293, 310–312, 313–314, 326, 365, 463; lapromatous 308; paleoepidemiology of 84, 182, 307, 578, 582; in past populations 69, 123, 198, 299, 308–309, 316; pathogenesis 307, 308, 328, 400; perceptions of **606**, **608**; and poverty 306–307; and respiratory disease 312; stigma of 488, 629; treatment of 293; and Vitamin D deficiency 312–313; and zoonoses 313; *see also* Mycobacterial diseases; *Mycobacterium spp.*
Leri-Weill dyschondrosteosis 255, 259
lice 165, 166
life course 7, **54**, 194, 196, 200, 201, 232, 243, 255, 348, 351, 365, 399, 401, 417, 420, 421, 423, 426, **468**, 510, 520, 521, 522, 525, **598**, 627, 631
Life course theory/model 194, 195, 197, 199, 200, 204, 241, 371, 373, 407, 408, 409, 422, 472, 473, 490, 491, 521, 530, 534
life expectancy 283, 520, 522, 532
life history 151, 196, 282, 363, 369, 399, 407, 408, 409, 484, 490, 520, 524, 529, 532, 533, 534, **595**, 627, 628
life tables 69
lifespan 70–71, 282, 284, 399, 407, 408, 409, 417, 422
ligaments 114, 234, 236, 240, 333
linear enamel hypoplasia *see* enamel hypoplasia
Lithuania 215, 217, 298
livestock 122, 311, 324, 557, 561, 563, 565
logistic regression 74–75
London 70, 73, 76, 148, 200, 259, 285, 312, 424, 462, 485, 486, 491, 506, 533, 580, **602**, **606**, 626
longevity 218, 250, 284, 361, 524, 532
Lycopodium spores 163, 164
lytic **25**, 27–30, 32, 273, **275**, 310

macropods 550
macroscopy, macroscopic 2, 19; bibliometric study of 20–27; description and images 31–32, 36, 53, *111*, 300, 363 and diagnosis 20–27, 112, 233, 252, 255, 260, 272–273, 278, 279, 309, 325, 341, 342, 349, 361, 365, 402, 404; in mummified remains 86, 87, 88, 112; observer error 32–35; in paleopathology 20–25, 544, 546; in pseudopathology 27–29; reliance on 105, 109, 110; and stress indicators 29–31; and theory 36
Madeira 299
Madelung's deformity 255, 259
magnetic resonance imaging (MRI) *see* imaging techniques
maize 122, 371; agriculture 122
malaria 24, **58**, 72, 125, 128, 145, 146, 147, 167, 181, 299, 402, 531, **608**
male(s): castration 445, **601**; cancer 283, 384; care 467; dental disease 365, 366, 368, 371; developmental anomalies 259, disease 54, 196; enslaved; 372; and estrogen 365; fractures/trauma 346, 441, 442, 506, 509, 511; intersectionality 166, 200; and leprosy 309, 316; and race 439, 447; social violence 507, 513; spondylodiscitis 333; testosterone 436, 437, 445; *see also* men
malignant 28, 109, 147, 271, 272, 273, **275**, **276**, **277**, 278, 280, 281, 282, 286, 549; *see also* cancer *and specific types*
malnutrition 67, 124, 126, 183, 316, 484, 531; and health risks 122, 422, 520; *see also* nutrition
mammals 95, 148, 166, 280, 281, 282, 542, 543, 544, 545, 546, 547, 549, 550, 552, 559, 563, 626, 631, 633
mammoth 549, 552, 558, 559
mandible 110, 217, 234, 280, **330**, **340**, 402, 403, 513, 549, 558, 562
Mantel-Cox log-rank test 69
Marfan syndrome 251, 260
Maria of Aragon 214, 215, 216
marginalization, social; and autopsy and dissection 486–487; definition of 482–483; and dental disease 365, 372; and ethics 391, 382, 384, 395, 386, 387, 390, 391, 392, 393, 488–490; and intersectionality 490–492; and metabolic disease 40, multiple lines of data 487–488; and structural violence/inequality 200, 409, 419, 424, 426, 448, 484–486, 490, 503, 530; and trauma/fractures 231, 241, 421; perceptions of **614**, **615**
marine economies 122
marrow 48, **54**, **89**, 114, 216, **274**, **275**, 343, **344**, *348*, 349, 350, 401, 402; hypertrophy 401, 402
mass graves 184, 423, **602**, **603**, **609**, **610**, **614**, **615**, **616**, 617
mass spectrometry 364, 560
massacre 420, 421, 504, 508–509, **611**, **614**
maternal health 252, 340, 345, 407, 408, 521, 528, 530, 531, 532

Maya(n) civilization 128, 195, 197
measles 145, 182, 326, 632
medieval (period): archaeological sites 169; Black Death **609;** bone lesions 285, 312; Britain 182, **598;** Brussels 171; cancer **598;** Croatia 370; Cyprus 198; Czech Republic 196, 199; Denmark, Danish 73, 74, 259, 310, 316, 582, **596;** dental pathology 371; developmental anomalies 258, 259, 260; disability 198; early 73, 125, 148, 196, 199, 370; England, English 125, 200, 308, 345, 364, 471, **595**, **598**; Europe 7, 150, 166, 285, 309, 314, 315; feet 608; frame of mind 183; Germany 148, 170; gigantism 470, **601;** Hungarian archers **605;** Iceland 170, **604;** Italian 364, **607;** Kazakhstan 199; late 309, 316, 333, 471; latrines 166; leprosy, leprosarium 150, 198, 308, 312, 314, 315, 316, 426, 470, 471, 533, 582, **608;** London 76, 424, 533; mortality risks 75, 364; Nubian 626; osteomyelitis 333; osteoporosis 345; parasite 169, 170; plague **597;** Poland 198, 470, **601;** Portugal 608; prosthesis **609;** protozoa 171; rickets 312; Riga, Latvia 163, **609;** Romania 371; texts 186; tuberculosis 285, 312, 581, 582, **596;** United Kingdom 626
Mediterranean 148, 166, 198, 299, 633
melioidosis 632–633
men: disease rates **54**, **57;** injuries 421; infectious disease 446, 583; and perceptions **605;** and socioeconomic status 485
Mesoamerica 309, 420, 421, **602**
Mesopotamia 180, 181, 557
Mesozoic 542, 549
mercury 86, 181, 185, 293, 294
MERS 586
metabolic disease 7, 21, 22, 24, 56, 92, 119, 121, 127, 128, 210, 236, 273, 334, 338–353, 399, **464**, 483, 530, 542, 626; in animals 566; co-morbidity, co-occurrence 351–352, 486; disruption/dysfunction 120, 401, 402, 421, 484, 531; in fossil record 550–551; "ghetto" 530, 533; rate/regulation 282, 400, 521, 523; syndrome 346–347; vitamin A deficiency 252; vitamin B_9 (folate, folic acid) deficiency 402; vitamin B_{12} deficiency 172, 338, 402; vitamin C deficiency 338, 339–441, 402, *403*; vitamin D deficiency 24, 30, 194, 312–313, 338, 341–343, 345, 351, 352, 353, 402, 532, **595**, **597**; *see also* anemia; diabetes; hyperparathyroidism; osteomalacia; osteoporosis; rickets; scurvy
metacarpals, metacarpal bones **330**, 564, 566, 567, 568
metagenomics next generation sequencing (mNGS) 162, 163

metatarsals, metatarsal bones 236, 257, 280, **330**, 346, 568
metastatic carcinoma *see* cancer
metastasize 27, 97, 147, 272, 273, **274**, **275**, **276**, **277**, 279, 284
Methanobrevibacter oralis 366
metopic trait 73
Mexico 162, 196, 298, 299, 365, 370, 421, 471, 578, 585, **597**, 631
miasma theory 183
microbiome 137, 144–145, 163, 164, 598, **601**–**611**, 612; oral 144, 145, 314, 360, 362, 364, 365, 629; gastrointestinal 144, 145, 365, **598**
micronutrient deficiencies 128, 421
microscopic, microscopy: and dental conditions 31, 342, 361, 364, 404, 532; and developmental conditions 255; and diagnosis 26, 27, 31, 36, 52, 96–97, 113, 165; and DNA 162–163; history of 82–85, 212, and metabolic diseases 24, 344, 345; methods 92–94; in mummy studies 86, 93; and neoplasms 278; in parasitology 160, 161–162, 165, 166, 167, 169; in publications 20, 21, 22, 23, 24; scanning electron 94–95; and taphonomy 86, 87; *see also* histology
microscopic focal destruction (MFD) 87
middle ear infection 109, 312
Middle East 162, 166, 170
migration 119, 120, 123, 128, 194, 315–317, **595**
mineralization: defective 27, 30, **55**, 86, 96, 122, 341, **342**, 346, **348**, 350, *351*; *see also* bone mineralization
mineralogy 52
miscarriage 585
mobility: cellular **277**, 545; geographic 123, 171, 172, 203, **577;** migrant 120, 123; physical 194, 198, 239, 240, 309, 345, **464**, **468**, 470, 567; social 509; *see also* migration; paleomobility
modification *see* body modification
molecular *see* biomolecular
molecular paleoparasitological hybridization (MPH) 162
Møller-Christensen 3
Moodie, Roy L. 3, 85, 106, 543, 551, 552, 559, 566, 630
moral(s) 126, 466, 583, 585, 600, **614**–**615**, 616, 617, 618
morbidity 64, *72*, 76, 120, 231, 271, 272, 338, 351, 398, 399, 408, 424, 425, 451, 570, 520, 523, 524, 532, 562, 566, 576, 627
morbilliviruses 632
morphology, morphological 7, 20, 23, 27, 30, 31, **54**, 86, 92, 108, *109*, 110, 123, 126, 137, 161, 162, **168**, 210, 211, 212, 216, 217, 218, 219, 237, 238, 242, 250, 251, 252, 253, 254, 255, 260, 263, 264, 273, **274**, 278, **348**, 350, 269, 370, 401, 402, 438, 440, 449, **468**, 470, 510,

511, 514, 530, 548, 561, 563, 564, 542, 543, 544, 546, 561, 563, 564, 569, **596**, 629; *see also* histomorphology; pathomophological
mortality: Developmental Origins of Health and Disease 120, 399, 520, 522, 523, 524, 525, 527, 529, 531, 532, 533, 534, 627; of infants and children 421, 423, 425, 471; and infectious disease 215, 324, 332, 338, 400, 576; and isotopic studies 121, 122, 128; maternal 443, 449, 450, 451; and metabolic and endocrine diseases 351; models of 65, 69–71, 72–74, 406, 485, 576, 577, 580; and neoplasm 271, 272, 284, 285; patterns of 64, 67, 580: risks of 64, 76, 398, 399, 404, 406, 407, 484, 532, 581; selective 66, 67, 75, 406, 580; and violence 418, 420, 422, 424
Morton, Samuel 384, 488
mortuary 4, 58, 194, 198, 370, 426, 441, 474, 485, 487, 488, 504, 506, 507, 508, 509, 515, 578, 585, 586; practices 197, 198, 199, 212, 213, 214, 263, 426, **466, 467, 468**, 487, **616;** *see also* burial
most recent common ancestor (MRCA) 140, 150, 297
MOVE 383, 384, 489
MRI (magnetic resonance imaging) 113, 114, 213, 219
multidimensional analysis 268
multidiscipline (multidisciplinary) 1, 10, 118, 170, 172, 260, 272, 279, 325, 482, 502
multi-state models 68, **72**, 73, 74; assumptions of 72; Usher 72, 73, 74
multiple myeloma, plasmacytoma **57**, **58**, 272, **275**, 281, 285, 286, 472, **595**
multivariate analyses 259
mummified remains: access to 2, 218; aDNA 137, 214, 313; alien **610**, **611**; animal 105, 112, 213, 263; autopsies 211–212; bioarchaeology of care **468**, **469**, 471, 472; Brazilian 166; cherubism 217; Christian Nubian 166; diseases in 2, 3, 10, 84, 85, 145, 147, 167, 472, 180, 210, 213, 215, 216, 217, 218, 325, **469,** 472, 626; Egyptian 1, 3, 4, 84, 85, 93, 106, 112, 137, 166, 167, 169, 217, 263, **609**, 626; Greenland 108, **608**; histology 84, 85, 86, 97, 212; and imaging techniques 105, 106, 108, 112, 113, 114, 212, 213, 214, 219, 260, **468**, 626; Joseon Korean 169, 215, 217; Lithuanian 215; microscopy 6, 84, 92, 168; molecular studies 159, 169, 212; parasitology 158–159, *160*, 166, **168**, **169**, 216, 217; Peruvian 106, 169, 213, 216, 217; Siberian 215; tissue preservation 86, 93, 138, 180, 210, 463
Muramoto, Osamu 187, 188
musculo-skeletal stress markers 277, 484, 511
Mycenae 128

Mycobacterial diseases: clinical and statistical approaches 310–311; DNA analyses 140, 142, 150, 214, 313–314, 564; evolution of 314–315, 569, 582, 631; and isotopic studies 315–317; and respiratory disease 312; and vitamin D deficiency 312; zoonotic transmission 313; *see also* leprosy; tuberculosis
Mycobacterium ssp: *bovis* 306, 550, 569; *leprae* 140, 149–150, 306, **327**, 328, 335, 365, 582; *lepromatosis* 306, **327**; *pinnipedii* 144, 306; *tuberculosis* 84, 214, 306, **327**, 328, 335, 550, 582, 631; *see also* leprosy; tuberculosis
Mycobacterium Tuberculosis Complex (MTBC) 306, 313, 314, 315, 569, 581, 582, 631
myositis ossificans 110, 233, 240, 281

Napoleon 166, 532, **602**, **610**, **611**, 617
nasopharyngeal cancer 281
Native American Graves Protection and Repatriation Act (NAGPRA) 4, 383, 489
National Institute of Standards and Technology (NIST) 242
Native American 2, 4, 257, **603**; and health experiences 66
natural selection 282, 364, 566
Neanderthals 146, 253, 281, 368, **468**
Neolithic Era 149, 170, 171, 197, 257, 324, 343, 365, 368, 369, **486**, **471**, 550, 559, 562, 568, 569, **596**, **607**, **608**, **610**; revolution 353, 576
neoplasm: in the fossil record 280, 283, 549; past prevalence of 280, 281, 282–286, 549; *see also* cancer; tumors
nerves 88, 114, 210, 240, 261, 272, 308, **327**, 328, 346, 347, 367
neural tube 252
neurofibromatosis 214, 272, 273, **277**, 281
"New archaeology" 4, 560
New York African Burial Ground 9, 383, 391, 487
New York City 9, 197, 201, 372, 470
New World 216, 257, 550
New Zealand 200, 202, 311, 426, 470
Next Generation Sequencing (NGS) 137, 145, 162, 163, 279, 314, 315, 325
nitrogen 15 ($\delta^{15}N$) 119, 121, 124, 125, 126, 127, 315, 316, 317, 371, 484, 524, 531
nomenclature in paleopathology 49
non-human primates 95, 280, 313, 404
non-specific infection 97, 306, 326, **327**, 335
non-specific stress 3, 21, 22, 196, 299, 399
nonstationarity 385
Norman conquest 340
normative perspective 628
North America 2, 3, 8, 122, 127, 158, 166, 170, 171, 172, 216, 217, 296, 297, 300, 341, 421, 489, 526, 560, 583, 586
Norway 84, 314
Nova Scotia 170

Nubia 166, 368, 626
nutrition, nutritional 120, 121, 511, 514, 528, 529: deficiency 7, 31, 54, 58, 67, 120, 122, 124, 125, 126, 404, 406, 407, 513, 520 (*see also* metabolic disease); and dentition 372; and gender **57**; and growth and development 258, 406, 407; infants and children 120, 121, 196, 345, 417, 420, 422, 423, 522; and infectious disease 183, 197; maternal 252, 344, 522, 523, 525, 528, 529, 530, 531; and metabolic diseases 338, 343, 349, 352; and status/social inequity 58, 201, 393, 443, 484, 485, 490; and tuberculosis 316; variation 67; of vitamins (*see* vitamin deficiency); *see also* diet; food; malnutrition; metabolic disease

observer error *see* error, observer
obstetrical dilemma 449–450
odds ratios 68; interpretation of 75; limitations of 75
Odense 74
Odontoma 549
oncogenes 218, 279, 282, 283
oncology *see* cancer; neoplasm; paleo-oncology; tumors
One Health 9, 313, 625, 629–630
One Medicine 625, 629
One Paleopathology 9, 618, 625, 628, 629, 630, 631, 632, 633, 634
oppression 7, 9, 385, 418, 426, 439, 461, **614**, **615**, 617, 618
oral: bacteria 214; cavity 144, 361, 362, 364, 365; conditions 339; disease pathogen 312; diseases 365, 366, 372; environment 363; health **54**, 309, 361, 365, 369, 372, 513; history 299, 576; infections 314; medications 346; microbiome 144, 145, 314, 360, 362, 364, 365, 629; mucosa 114, **327**, 328; pathologies 361; pH 363; surgery 112; traditions 301; *see also* dentition
Organization of Scientific Area Committees for Forensic Science (OSAC) 242
os acromiale 252, 260
os intermetatarseum 256
os odontoideum 254, 255
osteitis deformans *see* Paget's disease
osteoarthritis *see* joint disease
osteobiography *see* case studies
osteoblasts **54**, **55**, 88, **89**, **90**, 92, 273, **274**, **275**, 279, 339, 401, 405, 549
osteoblastoma 275, 281
osteochondroma 110, 281
osteoclastogenic 407
osteoclasts 88, **90**, 92, 273, **274**, **275**, 279, 339, 402, 405, 549
osteocytes 88, **89**, 90
osteogenesis imperfecta 236, 251, 252, *253*

osteoid **55**, 88, **90**, 92, 281, 341, **342**, 402
Osteological Paradox 53, 66–67, 68, 69, 73, 285, 311, 332, 370, 426, 491, 521, 531
osteomalacia 27, 338, 341, **342**, 551; *see also* scurvy
osteoma 276, 280, 281, 549
osteomyelitis 25, 56, *111*, 112, 124, 309, 326, **327**, 328, 329, 330, 331, 332, 333, 334, 335, 400, 468, 545; in animals 550; in the fossil record 280, 545, 546, 550
osteopenia 124, 236, **274**, **275**, 309, 626
osteoporosis 24, 55, 109, 110, 236, 232, 273, 309, 338, 339, 345–346, 352, 524, 626, 628
osteosarcoma 97, 112, **274**, **276**, 278, 280, 281, 545, 549
Ötzi 217, 218, 628
oxygen (δ^{18}O) 87, 118, 119, 121, 124, 147, 315, 316, 317, 343, 349, 350, 401

Pacific Islands 150, 197, 309, 315, 339, 347
Paget's disease (of bone) 92, 97, 217, 550, *551*
paleobiology 325, 541, 542, 543, 548, 552
paleodemography 284
paleodiet *see* diet
paleoecology 541
paleoepidemiology: and fossil record 547; general approach 195, 215, 393, 578; and heterogenous frailty 66–67; history of 65–66; methods 68–69, 75, 76, 163, 581, 582; and public perceptions **596**; *see also* epidemiology
paleogenetics, paleogenomics *see* gene (genetic, genome)
paleohistology 85, 552
paleohistopathology *see* histopathology
paleoimaging techniques *see* imaging
paleomobility 120; *see also* mobility
paleo-oncology 272–273, 278, 279, 280, 282, 283, 285, 286, 287; *see also* cancer; neoplasm; tumor
paleoparasitology 52, 122, 158–172, 325
Paleopathology Association 4, 10, 31, 211, 324, 492, 594
paleo-proteomic 76, 278, 279, 325, 329
paleoradiology *see* imaging techniques
palynology 159, 161, 167
pandemic 8, 128, 145, 148, 297, 307, 382, 512, 533, 576–580, 586–587, 493, 599, 620, 627
parametric models 69, 70, 71
parasites (parasitism) 401, 402, 404, 569; DNA 216–217, 279; ectoparasites 165–166; helminths 167–172; *Plasmodium* **58**, 145; protozoa 166–167
parasitology *see* paleoparasitology
pathogen 1, 2, 3, 4, 6, 7, 9, 56, 58, 76, 84, 120, 123, 136, 137, 138, 139, 140, 141, 142, 143, 144, 145, 146, 147, 148, 150, 151, 166, 169, 183, 214, 215, 240, 279, 282, 286, 292, 295,

296, 300, 308, 312, 313, 314, 315, 324, 325, 326, 328, 329, 333, 334, 335, 362, 542, 544, 547, 568, 569, 576, 577, 578, 579, 580, 582, 584, 585, 586, 597, 598, 601–611, 612, 625, 626, 627, 629, 631, 632, 633, 634
pathogenesis, pathogenicity 123, 165, 297, 307, 309, 327, 361, 366, 400, 402, 417, 632
pathogen load 76
pathognomonic 53, **57**, 97, 125, 254, 264, 273, 293, 294, 295, 296, 368, 403, 544, 631
pathomorphological 545; *see also* morphology
PCR (polymerase chain reaction) 137, 162
peak bone mass (PBM) 338, 345, 353
Pecos Pueblo 2, 4, 193
Pediculosis capitis see lice
Pediculus humanus capitis 165
Penn Museum 384
Perikymata 369, 404, *405*
periodontal disease 76, 145, 362, 363, 365, 368, 371, 372, 409, 463; apical lesions 366, 372; in caprines 562, **562**, **596**; etiology 365; sex differences 363, 365, 366
periodontitis *see* periodontal disease
perimortem 47, 148, 196, 197, 201, 202, **237**, 239, 421, 504, 509, 511, 559, 561
periosteal new bone reaction (PNB, PNBR) 2, 31, 97, 109, *111*, 112, *351*; active and inactive 30; and anemia **344**, 350; in children 30; and neoplasms **274**, 275; and nonspecific infection 329, 334–335; in plague burials 580; and scurvy **340**, 350; as stress indicators 29
periosteal reaction *see* periosteal new bone reaction
periosteum 48, 83, 88, **89**, 328, 329, 331, 332, 334, 339, 401, 403, 512
periostitis **25**, 85, 124, 328, 334–335
periostosis 47, 400–401, 407, 409
Permian 549, 550, *551*
personhood 196, 199, 241, 406, 417, 421, 426, **468**, 470, 483
Peru 4, 144, 217, *257*, *258*, 260, 261, 281, 339, *403*, **468**, 472, 485, 487, 513, 514, **602**, **604**, **606**; Chiribaya 166, 214, 314; mummified remains 85, 106, 169, 213, 214, 216, 217, 311, **468**; tuberculosis 214, 311, 314
Philip II 617
phocomelia 251
Phthirus pubis 165
Phylogeny 136, 279, 297; in fossil record 543–546; of *M. leprae* 159; of T lymphotropic virus 216; of *T. pallidum* 583; of *Variola* 215; of *Y. pestis* 146
phylogeography 578, 580, 633
pigs (*Sus*) 170, 564, 566, 568
pinta *see* treponemal infection
pituitary gigantism 146
Plasmodium vivax 125

plague 6, 7, 128, 148–149, 166, 182, 183, 184, 186, 298, 382, 400, 526, 578–580, 584, 587, 627; perceptions of **597**, **598**, 599, **605**, **609**; *see also Yersinia pestis*
plants 171, 313, 363, 364, 371, 541, 557, 559
Pleistocene 262, 280, 362, 363, 542, *545*, 546, 547, 550, 551, 552, **596**
Pliocene 542, 547, 549
Poland 198, 309, 470
polydactyly *257*, 261, 552
polymerase chain reaction (PCR) 137, 162
poorhouse 487, 491
porotic hyperostosis 26, 29, 65, 73, 74, 76, 348; and Black Death **74**; etiology 122, 172, 348, 401; interpretations of 197, 402; *see also* anemia
positionality 382, 389–390, 392, 488, 489
positivism 4, 122
post-deposition 27, 28, 29, 211; breaks/fractures 27, 344, 348
post medieval 309, 312, 364, 424, 533, 562
post-mortem 47, 86, 144, 210, 212, **237**, 239, 273, 278, 361, 368, 382, 390, 392, 448, 486, 504, 508, 561
post-processual archaeology 122, 560
Pott's disease 85, 110, 125, 309, 311, 333, 582; *see also* tuberculosis
poverty 125, 166, 170, 306, 419, 420, 423, 424, 445, 490, 491, 522, 530, 577, 581, 582, 627
Pre-Columbian 172, 259, 286, 421, 470, 472, **604**, **611**; hypothesis 292, 299, 583
pre-Hispanic 365, **403**
pre-industrial 187, 285
pregnancy 54, 72, 125, 202, 251, 252, 263, 264, 344, 422, 423, 424, 427, 443, 450, 451, 521, 523, 524, 527, 528, 529, 530, 531, **603**, **604**, **610**, **611**, **615**, **616**
preservation: of bone 85, 87, 127, 243, 292, 309, 348, 508, 569; of dentition 362; DNA 138, 142, 144, 314; intrinsic factors 86; and neoplasms 272, 279, 280, 284, 285, 286; of parasites 159, 164–165, **168–169**; of tissues 85, 86, 93, 210, 211, 217, 219, 254, 463
prevalence, of diseases 24, 31, 464, 527, 542, 586; calculations 24, 31, 33, 34, 67, 68, 75, 309, 470, 561; cardiovascular 522, 526; Chagas disease 217; dental 31, 54, 363, 369, 404; and nutritional stress 125; Pagets disease 550; parasites 164, 165, 170, 171; and social factors 577, 582, 527; and stress 485; tuberulosis 54, 581, 582; and violence and fractures 240, 511
privilege 1, 4–5, 10, 126–127, 389–390, 391, 461, 463, 488–489, 492
probabilistic statistical approaches 310, **595**
processual archaeology 121, 122, 352, 560
proliferation (of bone) 30, 73, 165, **276**, **277**, 350

proteomic 6, 364, 373, **598**
protozoa 162, 166–167, 171, 216, 293, 324, 541
pseudopathology: identification of 27–29; *see also* taphonomy
public health 335, 338, 343, 483, 524, 577, 578, 593, 627, 630
public policy 389, 390, 619
publication(s), analysis of 20–25, 44, 593–620
Pueblo cultures 2, 4, 193, 194, 196, 201, 442, 485, 514
Pulex irritans 165, 216

quantitative 32, 95, 128, 163, 164, 167, 172, 192, 233, 345, 561, 594, 613; research 4, 24, 36, 254, 547
queer, queerness, queering 438; theory 7, 241, 436, 446–447

rabies 557
race, racial 439–441, 450, 483; definitions of 8, 439; and ethics 383; and inequality 8, 9, 383, 424, 425, 444, 445, 490; and intersectionality 436, 441, 451, 507; perceptions of **614**; and structural violence 419, 512; theory 9, 241, 438, 521; typology 385, 386, 441
racism 9, 383; scientific 384–387, 382
radiodense 106, 110, **111**, 112
radiography *see* imaging techniques
radiolucent 106, 107, 110, *111*, 112, **274**
radiopaque 106, 107, 108, 112, **237**
Ramses V 215
random amplified polymorphic (RAPD) 162
rare disease 220, 283, 286, 473, 547, **595**, **596**
reburial 59, 200, 203, 390; *see also* repatriation
recidivism *see* trauma
recrystallization 87
red blood cells (RBC); and anemia 147, 343, 344, 348, 349, 401
reflexivity 10, 435, 446
re-emerging infection 9, 159, 164, 576–577, 578, 581, 582, 586–587
regeneration 548, 549
regression analyses 96, 406; logistic 68, 74–75
relative risk 67, 68, **72**
religion 184, 197, 301, 391, 421, 445, 470, 512, 600
Renaissance 171, 212, 339, 558
repatriation 4, 5, 383, 489, 600
reptiles 280, **464**, 542, 543–546, 548, 550, 552
resorption 30, **54**, 88, **90**, 92, 96, 338, 345, 349
respiratory disease 128; and Vitamin D deficiency 312–313
retrospective diagnosis 180, 184–185, 186–188, 331, 349, 466, 594
rheumatic disease 273
rheumatoid arthritis *see* joint disease
ribs 27, 96, 252, 253, 257, 259, 261, 274, 309, 330, 334, 402, 403, 446, 486, 551, 581, 612

rickets 341–343; diagnosis of **55**, 350, 491; effects on skeleton 30, **342**, *351*; in past populations 194, 312, 339, 345, 350, 352, 532, 551; pathophysiology of 228, 486; perceptions of **607**; and skin pigmentation 352
rigor 5, 6, 36, 43, 44, 48, 59, 159, 160, 162, 172, 184, 193, 194, 300, 596
rinderpest 632
RNA 145, 215
rodents 167, 508, 525, 579
Roman Era 71, 165, 167, 170, 171, 198, 299, 317, 341, 346, 351, 368, 532, 558, 567, 582, **596**, **604**, **605**, **606**, **607**, **609**, **610**
Romania 371, 558, **603**
Rome 128, 557
roundworm 145, 161, **168**, 170, **609**
Rovisco Pais Hospital-Colony, Tocha, Portugal 311
Ruffer, Sir Marc Armand 1, 3, 85, 169, 210, 215, 325, 542, 626
rural 69, 200, 285, 300, 310, 311, 371, 524, 525, 577, 582, 626, 628

sacral cleft 258
sacrifice, human and animal 418, 420, 421, 487, 504, 599, **604**, **605**, **608**, **609**, **611**, **614**, **615**, **616**, **617**
sampling: bias 64, 66, 67, 121, 140, 252, 283, 286, 297, 315, 364, 448, 582; bone 27, 96, 119, 123, 127, 138, 139, 140, 142, **143**, 144, 159, 212, 214, 293, 297, 300, 313, 314, 315, 361, 561–563, 631; teeth 121, 124, 127, 142, 313, 361
Salmonella enterica 144, 578
SARS-CoV-2 307, 317, 586
sarcomas *see* cancer
Sardinia 163
Schistosoma ssp. 85, **168**, 169
schistosomiasis 85, 169, 216, 220
scalping 504, 514
scanning electron microscopy (SEM) 20, 94–95; and histology 24, 85, 361; *see also* imaging techniques
scapula **26**, 252, **330**, 403
Schufeldt, Robert Wilson 542, 552, 558, 559
Schmorl's nodes 236, 546
Science Daily 593, 594, 596–599, 618, 625
scurvy 339–441; diagnostic criteria 45, 97, 402; effects on skeleton *340*, *403*; in past populations 29, 197, 351, 486; pathophysiology 30, **54**, **55**, 338, 343, 349, 350; perceptions of **607**
sedentism 65, 197, 296, 401
selective mortality 66, 67, 72–75, 285, 406, 580
Selye, Hans 2, 20, 398
sensitivity estimates 33, 52, 68, 295, 310, 524, 578, 581, 585

sequestrum 332, 333
sex: bias 252; and bone properties 232; determination/estimation 76, 273, 387, 423; and cancer 282, 284; definition of 7, 436–439, 510–511; and dental disease 363, 365, 369, 371, 565; and disease presence **57**, 70, 75, 76, 121, 252, 626; and DNA 423; and frailty 67; hormones **54**, 400, 437; and infectious disease 308, 329, 582; and lesion severity **54**; problems with 363; perceptions of 618, 626; and race 440–441; techniques 448–449; theory 442–443; and trauma/injury/violence 240, 241, 445, 504, 506, 507, 509, 511; *see also* gender; female; male
sex hormones **54**, 400, 437
sexism 419, 447, 448, 577
Shakespeare, William 185, **606**
sheep 363, 562, 563, 564, 568, **596**; *see also* caprines
Siberia 169, 170, 214, 215, 257, 511, **598**
sickle cell anemia (disease) *see* anemia
single nucleotide polymorphism (SNP) 137, 139, 217, 218, 297, 586
sinusitis 312
skeletonization 2, 45, **50**, 87, 92, 93, 114, 161, 180, 278
smallpox 6, 85, 145, 182, 215, 299, 300, 326
Smith, Grafton Elliot 1, 210
Snow, Clyde 195
Smithsonian Institution 5, 199, 310, 365
social: inequality 121, 122, 201, 241; diagnosis 180, 181, 184, 186–188, 487; environment 3, 526; media 141, 381, 384, 593, 594, **595–596**, 618, 619; science 33, 36, 200, 525, 541, 625, 628; stigma 198; theory 6–8, 127, 194, 195, 200, 204, 231, 388, 408, 418, 451, 504, 505, 527; *see also* status, social
South Africa(n) **54**, 280, **598**, 630
South America(n) 2, 24, **58**, 122, 158, 162, 207, 216, 217, 259, 297, 309, 371, 513, **598**, **608**, 632
souvenir parasites 159
Spain 170, 298, 316, 569, **596**, **607**
Spanish flu *see* influenza
specificity 52, 68, 97, 279, 295, 310, 326, **327**, 578, 581, 585
spermatozoa 83
spondylodiscitis **327**, 328, 329, 333
spina bifida 252, 260
Sri Lanka 72, 293
stable isotope analysis 6, 86, 118, 119, 120, 260, 317, 360, 370, 371, 373, 403, 441, 470, 472, 531, 532, **615**; calcium 127; carbon 119, 121, 122, 124, 125, 126, 127, 315, 316, 317, 371, 484, 524, 531; and descendant communities 126, 127; and diet 119, 120, 121, 122, 123, 124, 125, 126, 127, 128, 196, 316, 340, 370, 371, 423, 472, 514, 531; and disease-mediating factors 120–123, 128; ethics of 126, 127; limitations of 121, 124, 126, 127; and mobility 119, 120, 123, 128, 194, 316, 317, **595**; and mycobacterial diseases (TB and leprosy) 125, 128, 315, 316, 317, **595**; nitrogen 119, 121, 124, 125, 126, 127, 315, 316, 317, 371, 484, 524, 531; oxygen 118, 119, 121, 124, 315, 316, 317; and tissue sampling 119, 127, 360; strontium 119, 315, 316, 317; sulphur 119, 121, 127, 315, 316
stakeholders 52, 138, 140, 141, 142, *143*, 147, 202, 203, 204, 600
Standards for Data Collection from Human Skeletal Remains 448
Stannington Children's Sanatorium 311
Staphylococcus sp. 84, 144, 240, **327**, 329, 335, 401
stature 255, 364, 406, 437, 439, 442, 462, 484, 485, 513, 532, 580
status (social): in death 261, 488, 507; and health 192, 195, 196, 199, 200, 299, 352, **464**, 469, 515, 594; nutritional **54**, **57**, 345, 349; and risk of mortality 71; social 4, **58**, 66, 71, 75, 194, 197, 220, 262, 360, 363, 389, 423, 440, 463, 470, 485, 487, 488, 491, 506, 509, 510, 511, 512, 523, 533, 567; socioeconomic **58**, **67**, 241, 352, 422, 423, 425, 444, 463, 485, 506, 507, 510, 512, 529
sterility 72
stigma *see* social, stigma
Streptococcus spp. **56**, **327**, 329, 362, 401
streptomycin 581
stress, stress indicators 23, 24, 27, 36, 126, 217, 316, 352, 397, 439, 440, 44; biocultural 418; biomechanics of 95, 232, 235, 236, 252, 260; chronic 201, 443, 444, 484, 533; environmental 547; and growth disruption 405–407, 424; infant and children 125, 369, 370, 372, 422, 424, 485, 532; and infection 400–401; and linear enamel hypoplasia 367, 403–405, 423, 532, 580; and macroscopy 29–31; mechanisms of 399–400; maternal 523, 524, 531; modeling of 407–409; nutritional 124, 125, 258, 372, 393, 401–403, 484, 485, 529; and periosteal new bone formation 29–30; physiological 67, 69, 120, 121, 124, 340, 350, 400, 424, 472; psychological 2, 200, 368, 484, 523, 529, 531; perceptions of **615**, **616**; theoretical models of 2–3, 20, 397, 398–399, 520, 521, 527–530
striae of Retzius 96, 404
strontium ($^{87}Sr/^{86}Sr$) 119, 315, 316, 317
structural apathy 392, 393
structural violence *see* violence
subadult 69, 71, 243, 254, 255, 263, 422, 423, 513
subchondral cysts 546
subperiosteal: abscess 330, 331, 332; deposits 27, 29, 30, 32, 274; hematomas 331, 403; hemorrhage 403

subsistence strategies 3, 31, 158, 172, 197, 423, 515, 576; agriculture 65, 66, 633; and dental disease 363, 369, 370; and stable isotope analysis 120, 121–123
Sudanese Nubia *see* Nubia
sulphur (δ34S) 119, 121, 127, 315, 316
surgery 5, 112, 181, 284, **464**, 472, **595**, **604**, **615**, **616**; *see also* trauma
survival analysis, Kaplan-Meier 68–69
survivorship 64, 69, 124, 363, 370, 400, 426
Swartkrans Cave 280
Sweden 85, 314, 316, 368, **468**, 508, 568
sympathy **601–611**, 612
syndemics 7, 490, 577, 578, 627
syphilis *see* treponemenal infection

Taiwan 72, 234
Tannerella forsythia 145, 365
tapeworms 145, 161, 167, 169–172
taphonomy (taphonomic) 5, 6, 34, 199, 202, 231, 262, 273, 489, 508; and differential diagnosis 47–48; and DNA 279; identification of 5, 27, 28, 29, 278, 283, *348*, 502; and imaging 112, 113; and microscopy and histology 86, 87, 92, 95, 278; and mummified remains 211, 213, 219; and paleoparasitology 158, 161, 162, 164–165, 167, 171; and zooarchaeology 561–563, 564, 570
taphognomonic 47
Tasnádi-Kubacska, A. 543, 558, 559
targeted-capture 585
Tarone-Ware test 69
teeth *see* dentition
tarsals, tarsal bones 253, **330**; coalition 256, 259, 260, 262
tendons 86, 114, 236, 240, 316
teratomas 273, **276**, 281
Terminologia anatomica 49
terminology 5, 19, 31, 32, 36, 48, 49, 59, 119, 194, 251, 328, 558
Terry, Robert J. Collection 4, 310, 389, 441, 448, 488, 506
testosterone 309, 400, 436, 437, 445
Thailand 363
thalassememia *see* anemia
Tirup 73
tobacco 251, 283, 284, 361, 364
Tollund Man 112
tool marks 181, **237**
tooth *see* dentition
torture 420, 504, **604**, **614**, **615**, 617
trace elements 360, 546
trauma: accidental 240–241, 242, 328, 485, 505, 506, 507; antemortem 202, **237**, 504; biomechanics of 232, 233; blunt force 236, **237**, 242, 331, 509, 513, **615**, **616**; body modification 201, 234, 242, 443; and care 460, 464, **468**, 469; case studies of 196–197, 198, 200, 201, 202, 468; classification of 47, 56, 234–236, 444, 544, 565, 566; complications/consequences of 56, 88, 110, 199, 239–240, 280, 309, 328, 331, 334, 349, 401, 469, 470, 521, 579; diagnosis 213, 253, 254, 256, 273, 502, 512; dislocations 234; in the fossil record 548, 550, 552; healing 238–239, 567; high-velocity projectile 236, 238; interpretation(s) of 65, 67, 95, 97, 196, 200, 220, 232, 240–242, 261, 401, 404, 417, 421, 436, 445, 483, 502, 506, 509, 511; perimortem 37, 128, 201, 202, 237, **504**, 509; recidivism 200, 507; recording of 233, 512; sharp force 47, 238, 511; and structural violence 418, 441, 442, 484–485, 502–515, 526–527; and weapons 196, 197, 199, 240, 505, 509, **614**, **615**; *see also* fractures
trabecular bone 27, *28*, 88, **89**, 92, 255, 331, 346
trans-Atlantic African slave trade 299, 526
transdisciplinary 9, 313, 462, 469, 625–628, 629, 634
treatment: of animals 557, 567, 568, 630; antibiotic 583; arsenic 293, 294; of bodies 425, 484, 504, 512; burial 261, 262, 264; of data 139, 161; of dental pathology 113; of ectoparasites 181; of HIV 583; of influenza 626; of leprosy 307, 309, 311, 426; medical 2, **46**, **51**, **54**, **57**, **58**, 114, 181, 182, 188, 234, 299, 386, 426, 464, **468**, 470, 471, 472, 578, 581, 583, 586, 631; mercury 185, 293, 294; mortuary 197, 198, 263, **466**, **468**, 617; of osteomyelitis 332, 333; of syphilis 181, 300; of treponemal disease 293, 294, 300; of tuberculosis 306, 307, 309, 311, 312, 583; of Type 2 Diabetes (T2D) 346
trematode 167, **168**
trepanation, trephination 254, 273, **464**, **468**, 472, **595**, **615**
Treponema spp. 144, 214, 293, 297, 298, 585
treponemal infection 292–301; caries sicca 294, 295; Columbian hypothesis 299, 300, 583; differential diagnosis 293–296, 584, 585; epidemic 583–585; evolution of **55**, **56**, 295, 297, 298, 550, 584, 586; evolutionary hypothesis 292; Fournier's (mulberry) molars 294; in historical documents 298–300; Hutchinson's teeth 251, 294; Moon molars 294; pathogenesis 294; pinta 292, 293, 296, 485, 583; Pre-Columbian hypothesis 292, 583; saber shins 294, 295; syphilis, congenital 293, 298; syphilis, endemic (bejel) 292, 294, 295, 298, 329, 485, 583, 585; syphilis, venereal 9, 55, 124, 181, 185, 214, 292, 299, 583; tertiary syphilis 214; trans-Atlantic African slave trade 299–300; treatment, remedies 293, 300; Unitarian hypothesis 292,

299; venereal 185, 214, 292, 299, 583; yaws 292, 293, 294, 295, 298, 299, 300, 328, 485, 550, 583, 585
Teposcolula Yucundaa, Mexico 578
Triassic 280, 283, *545*, 549
Trichuris trichiura 163, **168**
trophy heads, trophy taking 508, 513, 514, **615**, **616**, 617, 618
Trypanosoma spp: *brucei* 167; *cruzi* 167, 216, 217
typhus 166
tuberculosis: DNA analyses 6, 142, 143, 144, 214, 220, 314, 335, 365, 547, 564, 568; epidemiology 69, 310, 311, 578, 580–583; imaging and microscopy 84, 214; and isotopic analyses 122, 123, 125, 128, 315–317; methods of diagnosis **25**, 26, **28**, 29, **54**, **56**, 200, 201, 308, 326, 463; and ONE Paleopathology 631–632, 634; in past populations 285, 308–310, 484, 485, 486; pathogenesis 252, 294, 306, 307–308, **327**, 400; perception of and publications **595**, **596**, **612**; reemergence 577; synergistic approach 312–313; zoonotic evolution (origins) of 313, 314–315, 550, 569; *see also Mycobacteria spp.*; mycobacterial diseases
tumors 88, 92, 110, 112, 271–287, 334; benign 271, 280, 281, 282, 283, 345; definitions 271–277; DNA analyses of 278–279; in fossil record 280, 549; genes 282, 400, 629; in mummified remains 211; in publications **602**, **609**; types of **274–277** *see also* cancer; neoplasm
Turkey (Anatolia) 65, 260, 557, *562*
Turner syndrome 251
Turtles 280, *545*, 549, 550
Tyrannosaurus rex 544, *545*
Tyrolean Iceman *see* Ötzi

ultraviolet light, radiation (UVA/UVB) 138, 212, 341, 343, 352
Umm an-Nar period Tell Abraq, U.A.E 194
Ungulates 563, 566, 567, 568
unconscious bias 393
uniformitarian principle 544
Unitarian hypothesis 292, 299
United Kingdom (UK) and Britain 4, 5, 8, **59**, 182, 183, 286, 286, 316, **351**, 450, 585, 491, 511, 522, 524, 531, 532, 533, 560, **598**, **606**
United Nations' Sustainable Development Goals 306
United States (US) 4, 193, 199, 202, 211, 218, 263, 295, 296, 297, 309, 426, 439, 484, 486, 487, 490, 518, 527
urban 69, 170, 197, 285, 300, 309, 310, 311, 312, 341, 371, 485, 577, 581, 582, **614**, 626, 628, 632
urbanization 474; consequences of 66, 171, 197, 285, 310, 343, 360, 362, 486, 582

vaccines, vaccination 84, 183, 283, 284, 286, 306, 577, 586, 627, 631, 632
variation (human) 8, 69, 387, 438, 521
Variola major, Variola minor 6, 215, 326
vascular impressions 47
venereal syphilis *see* Treponematosis
vertebrae 27, *28*, 29, 89, 144, 252, 257, 402, 563; cervical 255, 551; fractures 255, 551; and infection 328, 333, 581, 582; lumbar 113, 240; metabolic disease 344, 550; neoplasm **274**, **275**, **277**, 280; neural canal 33, 406, 423, 532; segmentation errors 251, 253, 258, 259, 551, 552, **596**; thoracic **25**
vertebrates 280, 281, 282, 283, 397, 399, 541, 542, 543, 544, 546, 548, 549, 551, 552, 568
veterinarian 542, 557, 559, 630
veterinary medicine 557, 564, 565, 625, 630
Viborg 74
Vibrio cholerae 84, 144
Vietnam 197, 203
Vilnius, Lithuania 298
violence: anthropophagy (cannibalism) 504, 514; definitions of 503–504, 418–420, 443–444, 483, 512; enslavement 9, 203, 298–300, 372, 384, 484, 487, 489, 509, 526, 527, 601, 613, 615, 633; gendered 241, 423, 443–445, 485, 506, 507, 510–512; and infants and children 417–427, 512; institutionalized 419, 427, 513; intergroup 505, 508–510; intragroup 510; interpersonal 8, 123, 196, 197, 234, 243, 441, 442, 468, 485, 503, 505, 506, 508, 509, 510, 511, 513; massacres 420, 421, 504, 508–509, 611, 614; scalping 504, 514; social 1, 10, 381, 502–551; structural 8, 10, 201, 202, 204, 242, 243, 384, 390, 392–393, 417–427, 436, 441, 443–444, 445, 446, 448, 451, 482, 483, 484–486, 488, 490, 512, 533, 577; *see also* trauma; trophy taking; warfare
virulence **55**, 149, 297, 325, 584, 633, 634
virus(es) *see specific taxa*
visual analysis *see* macroscopy, macroscopic
vitamin(s) 7, 69; A 252; B_9 402; B_{12} 172, 338, 402; C 339, 402; D 24, 30, 194, 312, 341, 343, 345
VITAMIN disease classification 56, 273
Volkmann's canals 88

war 166, 197, 185, 339, 385, 387, 420, 421, 507, 523, 558, 559, 577, 600, **601–611**, 612, **614**, 617, 618, 632, 633
warfare 196, 238, 360, 419, 420, 468, 503, 504, 506, 507, 508, 511, 613
warrior 196, 199, 438, 511, 514, **601**, **602**, **605**, **609**, **614**, **616**, 617, 618
weaning, weanling 198, 316, 340, 372, 404, 406, 409, 425, 485, 521; diarrhea 404

weapons 196, 297, 299, 240, 505, 509, **614, 615**, 632
Wellcome Osteological Research Database (WORD) 312
Wells, Calvin 193
Wharram Percy, England 27, *28*, 345
whipworms 161, 170
whooping cough 182
women: agency/roles 122, 438; and care **468, 469**, 470, 472, 473; of color 201, 411, 448, 451, 490, 527; and dental disease 363, 366; and disability 198, 201; disease rates **54, 57**; enslaved 384, 526; and gender 438, 440; and leprosy 198; and marginalization 486, 487, 490, 491; and metabolic diseases 344, 346; mummified remains of 218; perceptions of **601, 603, 604, 605, 607, 609, 610, 611, 616**, 618; post menopausal 236, 237; and pregnancy/maternity 202, 251, 263, 344, 443, 449, 450, 487, 521, 523, 524, 527, 528, 529, 531, 585; and structural/social violence 419, 420, 426, 427, 509, 510–512; and trauma/fractures 201, 202, 421, 442, 470; and treponemal diseases 300; and tuberculosis 568; *see also* females
World Health Organization (WHO) 307, 344, 425, 459, 503, 580, 627
woven bone *see* bone

X-rays *see* imaging techniques

yaws *see* treponemal infection
yellow fever 299
Yersinia pestis 141, 143, 148–150, 166, 335, 579, 580
Yersinia pseudotuberculosis 148

Zika virus 586
zooarchaeology 95, 170, 199, 242, 260, 340, 541, 557–570, 620, 630; and disease 564–566; history 558–561; human interactions 566–568; issues 561–562, 630–631; scope of 558; *see also* archaeozoology
zoonoses 313, 324, 568–569